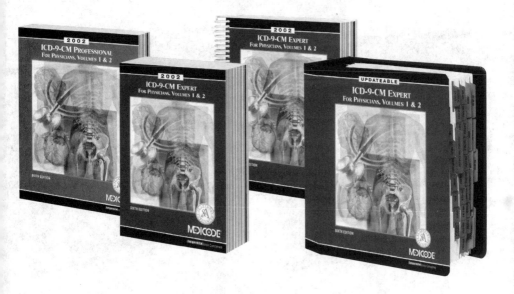

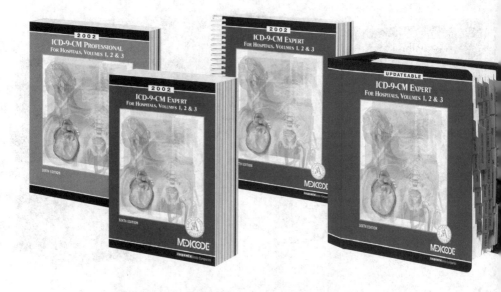

ST. ANTHONY PUBLISHING/MEDICODE 2002 PUBLICATIONS

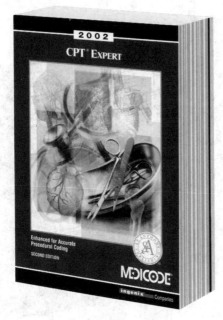

Your Enhanced Handbook to CPT®

CPT® Expert

CPT Expert is designed to help maximize reimbursement and save your office time and money. You get each CPT code with comprehensive coding tips, illustrations and definitions. A fantastic tool that helps experienced coders take procedural coding to a new level.

- **NEW — Special Reports Via E-mail.** Keep up to date with quarterly CPT changes.
- **NEW — Complete Description.** Includes all CPT codes and full official descriptions.
- **NEW — Deleted Codes.** 2002 deleted codes with strikeouts will help you finish claims from last year.
- **NEW — Appendix of Codes Most Frequently Miscoded.** Know which codes to watch out for, and learn why they can be miscoded.

8 1/2 x 11 Spiral bound
ISBN No. 1-56329-830-9   Item No. 4509 **$79.95**

6 x 9 Soft bound
ISBN No. 1-56329-831-7   Item No. 4507 **$69.95**

Available: December 2001

Publisher's Note: *CPT Expert is not a replacement for AMA's CPT 2002 Standard or Professional Code Book.*

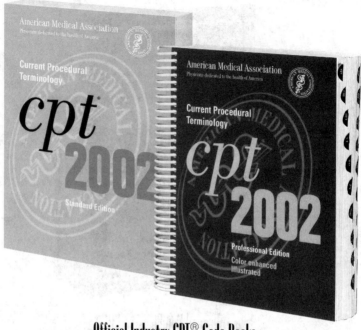

Official Industry CPT® Code Books

American Medical Association's (AMA) CPT®

Many of the changes you've anticipated from CPT-5 project will be seen in CPT 2002, including revamped Category I procedural and service codes and terms, new Category II "Performance Measure" codes, and new Category III "Emerging Technology" codes. New icons refer to the AMA's *CPT Changes* 2000, 2001, and 2002 books. Don't code without this book, which unveils the work of the CPT-5 project! All St. Anthony Publishing/ Medicode CPT 2002 buyers who provide an e-mail address will receive e-mail special reports that provide code updates and changes.

CPT 2002 Standard

The AMA's economical, perfect bound classic. Features self-stick tabs and an extensive index.

ISBN No. 1-57947-220-6   Item No. 4368 **$49.95**

Available: December 2001

CPT 2002 Professional

Color coded and spiral bound for ease of use, this product includes illustrations, preinstalled thumbtabs, and references to *CPT Assistant* along with the features of the *CPT 2002 Standard*.

ISBN No. 1-57947-221-4   Item No. 4372 **$74.95**

Available: December 2001

*CPT is a trademark of the American Medical Association

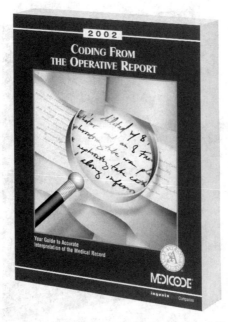

Accurate Coding Using Actual Operative Reports and Notes!

Coding From The Operative Report

This manual provides instruction on gathering the proper information from physician's documentation. Beginning with a discussion of operative reports and their importance to the coding process, this book gives you information you need to successfully and accurately code, from different situations based on specialty, and the CPT chapter in which the service falls.

- **Real Operative Reports and Operative Notes.** This manual reveals the complexities of accurate procedural coding and provides the solutions.
- **Organized by CPT Chapter.** Gives you an overview of each CPT category and its specialty.
- **Definitions, Key Points, Tips and Glossaries.** Helps you interpret cryptic shortcuts, abbreviations and nomenclature used by physicians.
- **Checklists, Guidelines, and Special Situations.** Foolproof guidance through the entire operative report interpretation, abstracting and coding process. Includes scenarios for CPT, ICD-9-CM, HCPCS, DRG and more.

ISBN: 1-56337-396-X

Item No. 4268 **$99.95**

Available: October 2001

Educators: Call for multi-copy discounts

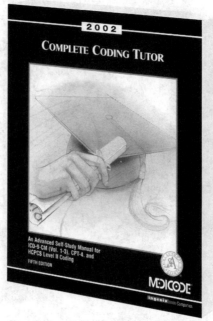

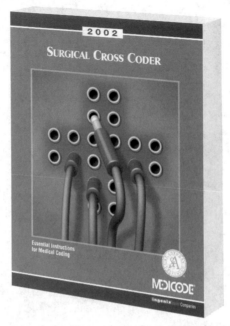

Simplify Your Coding Process with This Surgical Code Link Tool

Surgical Cross Coder

You face a myriad of codes and coding systems. How do you connect? This comprehensive illustrated coding guide links more than 4,000 CPT surgical codes to their corresponding diagnostic, procedural and supply codes. Based on sound clinical assumptions and with the input of extensive data and clinical expertise, *Surgical Cross Coder* is a one-source cross-coding book that simplifies the coding of surgical procedures.

- **Organized by CPT Surgical Codes.** Provides a one-step source for coders who need information on a variety of code sets based on surgical procedures.

- **Complete Code Descriptions.** Prevent miscoding and time-consuming corrective action.

- **Comprehensive Appendices.** Includes notes on exempt and excluded codes, modifiers, as well as recommendations for inpatient and outpatient diagnostic coding.

- **Notations.** Serve as a reminder to coders to seek out the causes of the infection, their manifestations and underlying diseases.

ISBN: 1-56337-400-5

Available: December 2001

Item No. 3237 **$149.95**

5 CEUs from AAPC

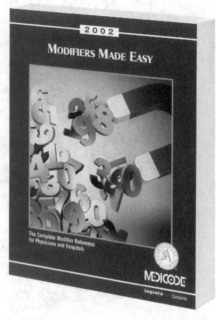

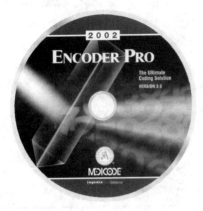

Publication Order and Fax Form

FOBA3

Customer No. _____   Purchase Order No. _____
(Attach copy of Purchase Order)

Contact Name _____

Company_____ Title_____

Address _____
(no P.O. Boxes, please)

City_____ State_____ Zip_____

Phone (_____)_____ Fax (_____)_____
(in case we have questions about your order)

IMPORTANT: EMAIL REQUIRED FOR ORDER CONFIRMATION AND SELECT PRODUCT DELIVERY.

Email _____

❑ YES, I WANT TO RECEIVE PRODUCT UPDATES AND INFORMATION
❑ YES, I WANT TO RECEIVE INGENIX NEW PRODUCT ANNOUNCEMENTS AND SPECIAL OFFERS

Item #	Qty	Item Description	Price	Total
4025	1	(Sample) book	$89.95	$89.95

Shipping and Handling	
No. of Items	**Fee**
1	9.95
2-4	11.95
5-7	14.95
8-10	19.95
11+	Call

Sub Total _____

OH and VA residents please add applicable sales tax _____

Shipping & handling (see chart) _____
(11 plus units, foreign and Canadian orders, please call for shipping costs)

Total enclosed _____

Payment Options:

◯ Bill Me. (St. Anthony, Medicode, CHIPS & St. Anthony Consulting are doing business as Ingenix).

◯ Check enclosed. (Make payable to St. Anthony Publishing) Check #_____

◯ Charge my: ◯ MasterCard   ◯ VISA   ◯ AMEX   ◯ Discover

Card # | | | | | | | | | | | | | | | | | | | | | Exp. Date: | | | |
                                                                    MM   YR

Signature _____

---

 ❹ Easy Ways to Order

100% Money Back Guarantee

❶ **Mail** this form with payment and/or purchase order to:
PO Box 27116
Salt Lake City, UT 84127-0116

❷ **Call toll-free (800) 765-6588** and mention Source Code: FOBA

❸ **FAX** this order form with credit card information and purchase order to (801) 982-4033

❹ **Visit our website at** www.IngenixOnLine.com

If our merchandise ever fails to meet your expectations, please contact our Customer Service Department at (800) 765-6588 for an immediate response. We will resolve any concern without hesitation.

Coders'
Desk
Reference

ACRONYMS, SYNDROMES, PROCEDURAL EPONYMS

SURGICAL CPT® EXPLANATIONS AND CODING TIPS

MEDICAL TERMS, ABBREVIATIONS, ANATOMY CHARTS

Notice

Coders' Desk Reference was conceived to be an accurate and authoritative source of information about coding and reimbursement issues. Every effort has been made to verify accuracy and information is believed reliable at the time of publication. Absolute accuracy cannot be guaranteed, however. This publication is made available with the understanding that the publisher is not engaged in rendering legal or other services requiring a professional license. Please address correspondence regarding this product to:

Bonnie Schreck
Coders' Desk Reference, Product Manager
2525 Lake Park Blvd
Salt Lake City, UT 84120

American Medical Association Notice

Acknowledgments

The following staff contributed to the development and/or production of this book:

Bonnie G. Schreck, CCS, CPC, CPC-H, CCS-P	*Product Manager*
Elizabeth Boudrie	*Publisher; Vice President, Essential Regulatory Group*
Lynn Speirs	*Senior Director, Publishing Services Group*
Sheri Poe Bernard, CPC	*Product Director, Essential Regulatory Group*
Christine B. Fraizer, MA, CPC	*Project Editor*
Charlene Neeshan, LPN, CCS, CCS-P, CPC, CPC-H	*Clinical/Technical Editor*
Kerrie Hornsby	*Desktop Publishing Manager*

AAPC Continuing Education Units

This publication has prior approval by the American Academy of Professional Coders for five continuing education units. Granting of prior approval in no way constitutes endorsement by AAPC of the publication content nor the publisher. Please contact the AAPC for the appropriate form to apply for these CEUs. (800) 626-2633

Copyright

Contents

Introduction

Coding is a complicated business. It's not enough to have current copies of ICD-9-CM, CPT®, and HCPCS Level II books. Medical coders also need dictionaries and specialty texts if they are to accurately translate physicians' operative reports or patient charts into reimbursement codes.

That's why Ingenix originally developed *Coders' Desk Reference* — to provide a one-stop resource with answers to a wide variety of coding questions. We polled the medical reimbursement community and our own technical staff to determine the issues causing bottlenecks in a coder's workload.

We found that experienced coders are frustrated by limited definitions accompanying many CPT® and ICD-9-CM codes. Beginning coders need guidelines on the use of ICD-9-CM, CPT®, and HCPCS codes and basic information about medical and reimbursement issues. Everyone requires up-to-date information about the anticipated changes in diagnostic and procedural coding.

Coders' Desk Reference (CDR), Seventh Edition, answers the questions of both experienced and novice medical coders. Coders, physicians, dentists, registered nurses, physician assistants, and physical therapists contributed to the technical information contained in *CDR*. The result is a compendium of answers to a wide variety of coding questions and an introduction to new systems in coding structures.

Since the first release of *CDR* in 1995, coders' corrections, suggestions, and tips have been incorporated into every printing, making this book as informative and useful as possible. Changes reflecting the dynamic world of coding are ongoing, and Ingenix encourages input for inclusion in future editions of the book.

Format

CDR is divided into convenient sections for easy use, with each section organized in alphabetic or numeric order. Simply access the section by thumbing through the convenient tabbing system to find the specific item of interest by referencing the headings at the top of the page. For quick identification, the range of numbers or words within a page are shown at the top of each page, just as in a traditional dictionary.

Using ICD•9•CM

Diagnostic coding not only serves the needs of coders and payers, it assures the accurate collection of data regarding morbidity. This easy-to-understand chapter outlines the history, logic, and use of the ICD-9-CM diagnostic codes, including the index and other aspects.

Getting Ready for ICD•10

Diagnostic and procedural coding systems are at the crossroads. Current methods are inadequate, and replacements are under development. This chapter briefly explains what's going on and what to expect.

Using CPT® Codes

For the new coder, and even for the veteran, this chapter provides an overview of the CPT® book: what it is and how best to use this coding system for identifying procedures.

CPT® Modifiers

Modifiers augment CPT® codes to the satisfaction of private and government payers. Ingenix Publishing coding experts interpret CPT® modifiers and identify their advantage in reimbursement.

Using HCPCS Codes

HCPCS Level II (national) codes identify available medical goods, pharmaceuticals and some services in claims filed for Medicare and some private payers.

Acronyms, Abbreviations, and Symbols

The medical profession has its own shorthand for documentation. Here, acronyms, abbreviations and symbols commonly seen on operative reports or medical charts are listed for easy reference.

Prefixes and Suffixes

The uniquely efficient language of medicine is based on prefixes and suffixes attached to root words to modify the meaning. Medical prefixes and suffixes evolved from the Greek and Latin used by pioneering physicians.

Surgical Terms

Operative reports contain words and phrases that not only communicate the importance and urgency of surgery, but they communicate the techniques as well. CDR's glossary of surgical terms includes the terms most commonly used in operative reports to describe techniques and tools.

Procedural Eponyms

What is the Marshall-Marchetti procedure? What is the Binet test? Eponyms honor the developer of a procedure or test, but do little to clarify what the procedure is. Editors have researched the procedural eponyms found in the index of the CPT® book and provide simplified explanations of what the procedures are, along with some biographical data about the physician or scientist for whom the procedure is named.

Syndromes

Syndromes are defined as the aggregate of signs and symptoms of any disease process. *CDR* lists more than 1,000 syndromes. Editors have researched, defined, and cross-referenced these syndromes and presents them alphabetically. Related or similar syndromes are listed in parentheses and the ICD-9-CM code of each syndrome is listed with the entry.

Mental Health Terms

This glossary provides definitions for the mental health and substance abuse terms. It is organized alphabetically and explains terms, concepts, and diagnoses used in the profession. Terms are cross-coded to diagnostic codes.

Anatomical Charts

Illustrations are included by body system with additional plates showing the planes of the body and Rule of Nines for burns.

Anesthesia Crosswalk

This quick reference provides a quick crosswalk to acceptable CPT® anesthesia codes used with each surgical CPT® code. It is organized numerically by CPT® surgical code.

CPT® Code Lay Descriptions

The CPT® book lay descriptions are written by Ingenix Publishing for people with medical training and may not offer the details office personnel need to choose a code based on the contents of an operative report or patient's chart. Ordered numerically, each CPT® code is followed by a detailed description of the procedure that code represents.

Coders' Desk Reference was developed to help providers comply with the emerging standards by which medical services are coded, reported, and paid. Remember that *Coders' Desk Reference* is a post-treatment medical reference and, as such, it is inappropriate to use this manual to select medical treatment.

The *International Classification of Diseases, Ninth Revision, Clinical Modification* (ICD-9-CM) ranks as the single source for diagnostic coding in this country. As a medical coding reference, it works "hand-in-glove" with the *Physicians' Current Procedural Terminology* (CPT), its correlative physician and outpatient procedural coding manual used everywhere in the United States.

The origins of ICD-9 lie in methodology developed to compile and analyze morbidity and mortality data. ICD-9-CM codes translate written terminology or descriptions into universal numeric and alphanumeric codes that can be processed electronically.

The role of ICD-9-CM codes for health care reimbursement is relatively simple: Diagnostic codes serve to establish medical necessity for the resultant procedures, treatments, and medical supplies. Coded medical data from recent decades verifies that associations between disorders and their treatments are generally appropriate. Treatments and procedures once cultivated following years of clinical experience can now be developed by consulting statistically driven treatment protocols.

While ICD-9-CM is still useful for statistical purposes, this more recent role has arisen as a means to precisely convey a patient's clinical picture to third-party payers. This role is firmly established, since government payers, as well as most commercial insurers, require ICD-9-CM diagnostic codes before payment can be made on a claim.

Despite the strengths of ICD-9-CM, the current structure is decidedly flawed. It's not always precise and there are concerns about ambiguity. But rather than refining the current structure, the United States is moving to an advanced system, *International Classification of Diseases, Tenth Revision* (ICD-10), developed by the World Health Organization (WHO), same as ICD-9. Similar to ICD-9 is the clinical modification of ICD-10 for use in the United States.

Coders' Guide

This chapter offers coders a guide to many areas of diagnostic coding. A comprehensive glossary comprises the body of the chapter and should be consulted as needed. However, a primer of ICD-9-CM coding conventions and methods follows.

Among the most important aspects of diagnostic coding is its role as a means to convey a patient's health status. An ICD-9-CM code usually represents a patient's condition, and in many instances is contained in the medical record for the life of the patient. This significant fact warrants absolute accuracy in the designation of diagnostic codes.

The sole source of any diagnosis is the treating physician. Medical coders should exercise extreme care that an ICD-9-CM diagnostic code specifically represents the physician's documented decision. The physician and the coding staff must work closely to develop a process that guarantees coding accuracy. In some offices the treating physician actually assigns ICD-9-CM codes. In others, coding staff derives codes from the physician's documentation of the encounter. Whatever system is employed, clear communication is absolutely essential.

Contents

Volume 1 of ICD-9-CM is a tabular listing of disease and injury and is divided into 17 sections, generally along anatomic, or body, sites. Two supplementary classifications contain alphanumeric codes to report factors influencing health status and other contact with health services (V codes) and causes of injury and poisoning (E codes). Appendixes to Volume 1 provide additional information and references.

Volume 2 is an alphabetic index of codes contained in Volume 1 and is important in locating proper diagnoses. An index to external causes of injury (E codes) is included. Three tables are included to assist in the selection of proper codes for hypertension, neoplasms, and drugs and chemicals.

A third volume of ICD-9-CM contains codes developed for coding inpatient facility procedures and is not ordinarily consulted for physician or outpatient services. Volume 3 contains both a tabular listing, arranged along anatomic lines, and an alphabetic index. Volume 3 coding issues are outside the framework of this reference manual.

Glossary of ICD-9-CM Coding Terms

Consult the following glossary as needed to solve ICD-9-CM coding problems.

Adverse Effect — An adverse effect occurs when a drug was correctly prescribed and administered but the patient has an adverse reaction to it in spite of correct use. Terms commonly associated with an adverse effect include adverse reaction, side effect, and idiosyncratic reaction. Adverse effects occur due to individual differences among patients, including genetic factors, disease state, age, and sex.

To code an adverse effect, first identify the effect as tachycardia, hallucinations, vomiting, respiratory failure, and gastritis. The effect is sequenced first. Next, identify the drug or medicinal substance that caused the adverse effect and select the E-code in the Table of Drugs and Chemicals from the column titled Therapeutic Use. Sequence the E-code second.

Adverse effect always means that the drug was correctly prescribed and administered so it can never be used with a poisoning code indicating that an error in prescription or administration was made. Only a code from the Therapeutic Use column can be selected as the second code because all other external causes identified in the table also imply an error was made. See Poisoning for definition and examples.

Assigning Codes — The six-step process for assigning diagnostic codes can be summarized as follows:

1. Determine the main terms that describe the patient's condition or symptoms.

2. Look up the main term in Volume 2 where the condition is alphabetized as a noun or adjective.

3. If indicated, follow cross-references such as see, see also, and see category to find the correct code.

4. Review subterms and modifying words. Refer to any indented terms under the main term to further clarify the code selection.

5. Verify the code as listed in Volume 2, the alphabetic index, by checking it against Volume 1, the tabular listing.

6. Review all instructions and notes in Volume 1 such as includes, excludes, code first underlying disease or use additional code to assure that the correct code has been selected.

Brackets ([ ]) — Brackets enclose synonyms, alternative wordings, or explanatory phrases. The brackets may be square [ ] or italicized [ ].

460 Acute nasopharyngitis [common cold]

Category — In ICD-9-CM, a category refers to the three-digit form of each code, such as 384 other disorders of tympanic membrane. Category codes can be further broken down into subcategories (fourth digits) 384.2 perforation of tympanic membrane, and subcategories can be broken down into subclassifications (fifth digits) 384.21 central perforation of tympanic membrane.

Code Also — This instructional note dictates the use of two diagnostic codes. List the etiology (cause) first, followed by the manifestation that is being treated. The two codes combined represent the primary diagnosis.

Code First Underlying Disease — Code first underlying disease identifies diagnoses that are not primary and are incomplete when used alone. In such cases the code, its title, and instructions are italicized. This type of instructional note appears only in Volume 1. A code with this instructional note should be recorded second, with the underlying cause recorded first. Italicized brackets identify this situation in Volume 2.

Coding Symptoms — ICD-9-CM has no codes and offers no provisions to rule-out any given diagnosis. Do not attempt to code diagnoses documented as "probable," "suspected," "questionable," or "rule-out." Although rule-out statements remain common in physician documentation, insurers generally do not pay for probable or rule-out diagnoses; they do, however, reimburse for symptoms. Volume 1, Category 16 (780–799) contains codes for signs, symptoms, and ill-defined conditions. Use these codes for generalized complaints and symptoms. They may also be appropriate to identify provisional diagnoses, transient signs, and additional problems.

Coexisting Conditions — Some patients present with coexisting conditions that affect the management of care. These conditions should be reported as supplemental information. The HCFA-1500 form accommodates up to three supporting diagnostic codes to establish clear medical necessity. The following situations require multiple diagnostic codes to identify medical necessity of each service performed: multiple injuries; multiple diseases; surgical and postoperative complications; injury and trauma, late effects. Codes that contain the instructional notes, Code Also or Code first underlying disease, require additional codes.

Colon — A colon (:) is used in Volume 1 of ICD-9-CM to identify a term that is incomplete without one or more of the descriptors following it. Do not assign the code unless one or more of the descriptors is present in the physician's diagnostic statement.

Conventions — Each space, type face, indentation, and punctuation mark determines how to interpret ICD-9-CM codes. These "conventions" were developed to match correct codes to the diagnoses encountered. Conventions include format, typeface, punctuation, symbols, and notes.

Cross-references — In Volume 2 several types of cross-references are encountered:

See — This cross-reference indicates that you should see the condition listed instead of the term you've found in order to assign the correct diagnostic code.

See also — See also indicates that additional information is available. This cross-reference may provide a more specific code or an additional code.

See category — See category directs you to an additional three-digit category, not just a single code. Again, you cannot assign an appropriate code unless you follow this instruction.

Drugs and Chemicals, Table of — This table identifies drugs and other chemical substances associated with poisonings and adverse effects. The table lists the substance alphabetically. Each substance up to six codes is identified. The first code identified is the poisoning classification (960–989). Next, up to five E-codes are listed. These are listed under the following headings: accident, therapeutic use, suicide attempt, assault, undetermined. The codes listed under these headings identify the external cause.

Correct code assignment is dependent on a thorough understanding of the definitions for a poisoning and an adverse effect. A poisoning is defined as occurring whenever an error is made in drug prescription or administration. A poisoning can be accidental, intentional (suicide attempt or assault), or undetermined. Terms normally associated with a poisoning include poisoning, overdose, wrong substance given or taken, intoxication. See Poisoning for additional information and coding examples. See Adverse Effect for additional information and coding examples.

E Codes — The second set of supplemental codes in Volume 1 is the Supplementary Classification of External Causes of Injury and Poisoning (E800–E999), also known as E codes. The E codes are never listed as the primary diagnosis; they are adjunctive. You may even need to use more than one E code to describe fully the circumstances of an accident. Use them to establish medical necessity, identify causes of injury and poisoning, and to identify drugs. The index for the E codes is found in Volume 2, following the Table of Drugs and Chemicals.

EXCLUDES — "Excludes" indicates terms that are not ordinarily coded under the referenced term. The word "Excludes" is surrounded by a box for easy identification and the corresponding note is italicized. This note does not prevent you from using the excluded code in addition to the code from which it was excluded when both conditions are present.

Italics — Italicized type in either volume of ICD-9-CM alerts the user to a code that cannot be reported as a primary diagnosis. Italicized type is also used for exclusion notes.

Late Effects — A late effect is a residual condition occurring after the acute phase of an illness or injury has passed. The original illness or injury is healed, but a chronic or long-term condition remains. Watch for key phrases in documentation, such as "due to old injury" to justify a late effect code. There is no time limit between the acute phase and the late effect.

The current, or residual, problem is always coded first followed by the late effect code, which serves to identify the underlying cause.

268.1   Rickets, late effect

A late effect code can technically be used as a principal diagnosis to specify the cause of the late effect when no residual effects are specified. Keep in mind, however, that ICD-9-CM codes are never assigned for diagnoses or conditions that are no longer detectable.

Multiple Injuries — To code multiple injuries, list the conditions treated by the physician in order of importance with the major problem listed first. As a rule of thumb, when medical and surgical problems are being managed, list the surgical problem first. If in doubt as to which problem should be listed, first consult with the physician.

NEC (not elsewhere classifiable) — This nonspecific diagnosis indicates the main term is broad or not well defined. Use an NEC code only when more information is unavailable. This term is used only in Volume 2.

NOS (not otherwise specified) — This nonspecific diagnosis is the equivalent of NEC (*see* NEC) and is used only in Volume 1.

Notes — Notes are found in Volumes 1 and 2 and have no fixed length. They give general coding instructions. Notes in Volume 1 are indented and printed in plain type, while those in Volume 2 are boxed and italicized. The placement of these notes is as important as their content. Notes at the beginning of a section apply to all categories within the section. Those at the beginning of a subsection apply to all categories within the subsection. Likewise, notes preceding three-digit categories apply to all fourth-digit and fifth-digit codes within that category.

Notes, Instructional — To assign diagnostic codes at the highest level of specificity, coders must follow four additional kinds of notes:

INCLUDES (appear immediately under three-digit code titles and provide further definition or give an example of the category contents); **EXCLUDES** (indicates terms not to be coded under the referenced term); Code first underlying disease (identifies a code deemed not primary and, therefore, incomplete when used alone). Use additional code (identifies Volume 1 categories where additional coding provides a more complete picture). For additional information on instructional notes, see individual listing.

Primary Diagnosis — The primary diagnosis reflects the current, most significant reason for the services or procedures provided. When coding pre-existing conditions, make certain the diagnostic code assigned identifies the current reason for medical management.

You may code for a chronic disease as often as you treat the patient for that condition, but if the patient presents and you treat a condition other than the chronic problem, code only the new condition. Also, never code a diagnosis that is no longer detectable. If the disease or condition has been successfully treated and no longer exists, it is not billable and should not be coded. Signs and symptoms should be coded when a definitive diagnosis is not provided.

Sequence of Codes — Diagnostic codes are sequenced, or listed, according to the diagnosis that reflects the reason for the current medical encounter (primary code). Additional codes sometimes further describe the primary code, but may also report underlying conditions, coexisting conditions, additional injuries, or numerous other conditions.

Supplemental Classifications — Volume 1 contains two supplemental code classifications: V codes and E codes. V codes can be used as primary diagnoses when reporting services not related to current medical problems or conditions such as periodic or routine medical exams. E codes are never used as primary diagnoses, providing supplemental information only on the causes of injury and poisoning. See the individual listings for more information.

Tables, Drugs and Chemicals — The Table of Drugs and Chemicals contains an extensive list of drugs, industrial solvents, corrosives, gases, noxious plants, pesticides, and other toxic agents set in a six-column format. *See* the following glossary headings for more information: Adverse Effect; Drugs and Chemical, Table of; Poisoning.

Tables, Hypertension — The complications, etiology (cause), and clinical manifestations of hypertension are listed alphabetically under the bold heading Hypertension, hypertensive. The table includes categories 401 through 405 plus additional codes, such as hypertension, that may complicate pregnancy, childbirth, or puerperium. Read the diagnostic statement carefully, watching for the words "due to" and "with." The term "due to" identifies hypertension caused by another condition. The term "with" identifies hypertension in conjunction with another condition. These terms are critical for accurate coding. Also note that categories 402 through 405 require fifth digits.

The Neoplasm table lists neoplasms alphabetically by location under the behavioral rubrics of Malignant, Benign, Uncertain Behavior, or Unspecified. The Malignant heading is further divided into Primary, Secondary, and Ca in situ. See Neoplasm for more specific information.

Tips for Coding — Follow the steps of assigning diagnostic codes. Reference the main terms first in the index (Volume 2) then verify the code in Volume 1. Pay careful attention to the following ICD-9-CM coding guidelines:

- Assign each medical service and surgical procedure a corresponding diagnostic code.

- Select an ICD-9-CM code to describe the diagnosis, symptom, complaint, condition, or problem, indicating why the service was performed.

- Code the primary diagnosis first, followed by the secondary, then tertiary, and so on. Code all coexisting conditions that pertain to the treatment of the patient during the visit or procedure.

- Read the code categories and subcategories carefully. Use fourth and fifth digits when they are available.

- Code what you know. Use symptom codes when a definitive diagnosis is not determined. Do not code "rule-out" statements as if they exist.

- Code a chronic diagnosis only as often as it is applicable to the patient's treatment.

- Code the diagnosis appropriate to the procedure for surgical procedures. If the postoperative diagnosis differs from the preoperative diagnosis use the postoperative diagnosis.

- For postoperative care, use a V code, followed by the postoperative diagnosis.

- List commonly used codes on your charge ticket, including the numerical designator and an accurate ICD-9-CM written description. Allow ample room for write-ins.

- Revise your billing forms periodically to ensure they contain only accurate and complete codes.

Undetermined — Undetermined codes apply when the cause of the poisoning or injury is unknown. See Drugs and Chemicals, Table of Poisoning for more information.

Unspecified Codes — Unspecified codes and general terms do not clarify the medical necessity issue; therefore, be as specific as possible in describing the patient's condition, illness, or disease. For those instances when a specific diagnosis is not yet determined clinically, "unspecified" codes are available. An unspecified diagnosis may be the only information available at the patient's first visit. When specific clinical information is determined, however, and the diagnosis is documented in the patient's chart, assign more definitive codes. A patient's diagnosis may change several times through the course of treatment as more specific information is available.

Use Additional Code — Use additional code placed in Volume 1 in those categories where an additional code is available to provide further information and to give a more complete picture of the diagnosis or procedure. The additional code should identify other aspects of the disease, including manifestation, cause, associated condition, and nature of the condition itself.

358.2 Toxic myoneural disorders
Use additional E code to identify toxic agent

V Codes — V codes (V01–V82) describe circumstances that influence a patient's health status and identify reasons for medical encounters resulting from circumstances other than a disease or injury classified in the main part of ICD-9-CM.

V codes are generally used in three instances:

- When a physician identifies a circumstance or problem in a person who is not currently sick but has nonetheless come in contact with health services (e.g., to act as an organ donor or to receive a prophylactic vaccination)

- When an ill or injured patient requires specific treatment (such as chemotherapy for malignancy or removal of pins or rods in postoperative orthopedic care)

- When a problem or circumstance that influences the patient's health is not itself a current illness but may affect future medical treatment

The main terms used with V codes reflect the nature of the medical service provided such as:

Admission	Observation
Aftercare	Problem (with)
Attention (to)	Screening
Examination	Status
History (of)	Supervision (of)

Volume 1, Appendixes — These appendixes provide further information about areas of Volume 1 and should be consulted as needed.

Appendix A	Morphology of Neoplasms
Appendix B	Glossary of Mental Disorders
Appendix C	Classification of Drugs by American Hospital Formulary Service List Number and Their ICD-9-CM Equivalents
Appendix D	Classification of Industrial Accidents According to Agency
Appendix E	List of Three-Digit Categories

See also listings for Morphology of Neoplasms, Mental Disorders, Industrial Accidents, and Three-Digit Categories.

Volume 3 — This volume is used primarily by hospitals. It is the basis for Diagnosis Related Groups (DRGs), a coding system for inpatient care that links diagnoses with appropriate procedures and treatments.

The major divisions of Volume 3 are:

- Numerical List and Alphabetic Index to Procedures

- Numerical List by Anatomical Site

- Miscellaneous Diagnostic and Therapeutic Procedures

Getting Ready for ICD-10

Introduction

The diagnosis and treatment of diseases are not stagnant, so neither are the structures used to report and record the information. Continual strides in our understanding of medicine and the inherent affect on clinical applications require coding systems that keep the same pace. The two prominent coding systems used in the United States for reporting clinical information, however, have not kept up, as acknowledged by those relying on the codes for both statistical and reimbursement issues.

International Classification of Diseases

The World Health Organization (WHO) originally developed ICD in the as a statistical tool for the international exchange of mortality data. In other words, ICD-9 was and still is used to code and classify mortality data from death certificates. In 1955, almost 30 years after WHO published the original ICD, the United States looked into the international system as a way to classify operations and treatments.

Acceptance was slow in the United States. An eighth edition published by WHO in 1965 did not provide the depth of clinical data many believed necessary for America's emerging health care system. A subsequent clinical modification produced two widely accepted publications in 1968: the *Eighth Revision International Classification of Diseases Adapted for Use in the United States* (ICDA-8) and the Hospital Adaptation of ICDA (H-ICDA).

In 1975 WHO published the ICD version still used in its clinical modification by health care providers and payers in the United States. *The International Classification of Diseases, Ninth Edition, Clinical Modification* (ICD-9-CM) has been the structural basis of diagnostic coding — inpatient and outpatient — since the National Center for Health Statistics (NCHS) in 1978 modified ICD-9 for hospital indexing and retrieving case data for clinical studies. The NCHS and the newly created Council on Clinical Classifications developed a companion procedural classification. This classification, published as Volume 3 of ICD-9-CM, revised a portion of WHO's International Classification of Procedure Modification (ICPM). In 1978, the 3-volume set was published in the United States for use one year later.

There were no changes in the direction to ICD-9-CM until the October 1983 implementation of Diagnosis Related Groups (DRGs), which gave ICD-9-CM a new significance. After almost 30 years since ICD's arrival in the United States, the classification system proved indispensable to hospitals interested in payment schedules for health care services.

ICD-10 and its Clinical Modification

The evolution of ICD took another step in 1994 when WHO published ICD-10. This is a major revision as indicated by the full title of the tenth edition: *International Statistical Classification of Diseases and Related Health Problems*. The new name not only clarifies the classification's content and purpose but shows how the scope of the classification has moved beyond the classification of disease and injuries to the coding of ambulatory care conditions and risk factors frequently encountered in primary care.

NCHS developed a clinical modification of ICD-10 for the United States, with an emphasis on problems that had been identified in the current ICD-9-CM. ICD-10-CM is planned as the replacement for ICD-9-CM, Volumes 1 and 2. There is not yet an anticipated implementation date for the ICD-10-CM. The date a new system takes affect is based on the process for adoption of standards under the Health Insurance Portability and Accountability Act of 1996 (HIPAA). There will be a two-year implementation window once the final notice has been published in the *Federal Register*.

As agreed upon by the NCHS and WHO, all modifications to the ICD-10 must conform to WHO conventions for the ICD. Except in rare instances, no modifications have been made to existing three-digit categories and four-digit codes, with the exception of title changes that did not change the meaning of the category or code.

The Center for Health Policy Studies (CHPS) was awarded the NCHS contract to analyze ICD-10 and to develop the appropriate clinical modifications. ICD-10-CM was developed following an evaluation by a Technical Advisory Panel and additional consultation with physician groups, clinical coders, and others to assure clinical accuracy and utility. The current draft of ICD-10-CM contains a significant increase in codes over ICD-10 and ICD-9-CM. Notable improvements in the content and format include:

- Adding information relevant to ambulatory and managed care encounters

- Expanding injury codes
- Creating combination diagnosis/symptom codes to reduce the number of codes needed to fully describe a condition
- Adding a sixth character
- Incorporating common 4th and 5th digit subclassifications
- Laterality (e.g., left, right, bilateral)
- Granularity, a term that describes greater specificity in code assignment

Procedural Coding

Parallel procedural coding systems have been in place in United States medical reimbursement circles for decades. Volume 3 of ICD-9-CM contains the procedural codes to use with the diagnostic codes found in Volume 1. The American Medical Association's *Physicians Current Procedural Terminology* (CPT), first published in 1966 and now in its fourth edition, covers outpatient (office) services, and inpatient (hospital) procedures and services performed specifically by the physician. HCPCS (Healthcare Common Procedural Coding System) is used to report services not found in the CPT book (CPT is Level I), and HCPCS Level III codes were created for local use.

Two options are available to replace the present procedural coding systems:

- The *International Classification of Diseases, Tenth edition, Procedural Coding System* (ICD-10-PCS): Several years ago the Centers for Medicare and Medicaid Services (CMS), formerly the Health Care Financing Administration (HCFA), contracted with 3M to design an alphanumeric procedure coding system that could be implemented at the same time as ICD-10-CM. The 3M procedural coding product is a numeric key of "smart codes." The 7-character code structure in ICD-10-PCS is sequenced to specify the type of procedure being performed (e.g., imaging, laboratory), while the other characters specify additional information such as approach and specific organ.

- *Current Procedural Terminology, Fourth Edition* — The AMA holds the copyright to CPT, and it is both the coding system required for Medicare and Medicaid reimbursement and the system of choice among most physicians. AMA's CPT-5 project is an attempt to enhance the coding system for use beyond the millenium.

Glossary

Many of the terms found in ICD-10-CM are similar to those you are familiar with from ICD-9-CM. In some cases, the meanings may be slightly altered and, thus, affect the coding application. There are also new terms to learn. Following is a list of terms that may be found in the proposed systems of diagnostic and procedural coding.

Abbreviations — The abbreviations NEC and NOS are found in the Tabular List of ICD-10-CM.

The term NEC means "not elsewhere classified" or "not elsewhere classifiable." At the three-character level, NEC means that documentation lacks the necessary information for coding to a more specific category.

In the Tabular List, the phrase "not elsewhere classified" is applied to residual categories that do not appear in sequence with (i.e., immediately following) the pertinent specific categories.

Administrative Simplification — Under the Administrative Simplification provisions of the Health Insurance Portability and Accountability Act of 1996 (HIPAA), the Secretary of Health and Human Services (HHS) must adopt standards to simplify electronic transmission for all health plans, health care clearinghouses, and health care providers who choose to conduct transactions electronically. Standards include those for code sets, defined as "any set of codes used for encoding data elements, such as tables of terms, medical concepts, medical diagnosis codes, or medical procedural codes." Code sets for medical data are required for administrative and financial health care transaction standards for diagnoses, procedures, and drugs.

Alphanumeric Codes — All codes in ICD-10 are alphanumeric, i.e., one letter followed by two numbers at the three-character level as opposed to three numeric characters in the main classification of ICD-9-CM. Of the 26 available letters, all but the letter U is used. Some three-character categories have been left vacant for future expansion and revision.

Axis of Classification — ICD-10-CM is an arrangement of similar entities, diseases, and other conventions on the basis of specific criteria. Diseases can be arranged in a variety of ways: according to etiology, anatomy, or severity. The particular criteria chosen is called the axis of classification. Anatomy is the primary axis of classification of ICD-10-CM.

Blocks — After the appropriate includes and excludes notes, each chapter ICD-10-CM starts with a list of subchapters or "blocks" of three-character categories. These blocks provide an overview of the structure of the chapter.

Cross References — In the Alphabetic Index, cross references point to all the possible information for a term or its synonyms.

Deactivated Codes — To meet data-gathering goals desired by the federal government for coding in the United States, some codes that are valid in ICD-10 have been deactivated for ICD-10-CM. These codes fall into several categories: procedure codes, death codes, and codes considered to be highly unspecific.

Granularity — A term used in coding application to describe greater specificity in code assignment.

International Classification of Diseases, Ninth Revision (ICD-9) — The system of diagnostic coding lists codes published by WHO and is required documentation on all physician-submitted Medicare B claims, as well as a reimbursement and reporting tool for many private payers. The United States uses a clinically modified version.

The International Classification of Diseases, Tenth Revision, Procedural Coding System (ICD-10-PCS) — The procedural coding product is a numeric key of "smart codes." The 7-character code structure in ICD-10-PCS is sequenced to specify the type of procedure being performed (e.g., imaging, laboratory), while the other characters specify additional information such as approach and specific organ. There are no multiple meanings among the code schemes, and a specific definition is supplied to each term in the system. There is no diagnostic information. There is no numeric listing of codes. Rather, there are 16 sections filled with tables that determine code selection.

Laterality — In the past, there have been proposals to add laterality codes (i.e., right, left, or bilateral) to diagnostic coding classifications. ICD-10-CM does not add laterality in all cases, though the modification enhances particularly the Neoplasm and Injury chapters. For example, with the reporting of laterality, providers will need to document where the injury occurred.

Manifestation — As applied to medicine, a manifestation is the display or disclosure of characteristic signs or symptoms of an illness.

Modifiers — Two types of descriptors — called modifiers — are found in the Alphabetic Index:

  Essential — The modifiers affect code selection for a given diagnosis due to the axis of classification.

  Non-essential — The modifiers may be present or absent for the diagnosis to be codes. Either way, the code stays the same.

Morbidity — Term describes the disease rate or number of cases of a particular disease — in a given age range, gender, occupation, or other relevant population-based grouping.

Mortality — Term describes the death rate reflected by the population in a given region, age range, or other relevant statistical grouping.

Notes — The tenth revision contains notes that describe the general content of the succeeding categories and provide instructions for using the codes. These include:

  Code First — A "code first" note tells you that two codes are necessary to describe the condition.

  Excludes — An "excludes" note prevents a code from being applied incorrectly.

  Use — A "use" note gives specific instructions for using an additional code to completely describe a condition.

Punctuation — The ICD-10-CM Tabular list employs certain punctuation that must be clearly understood to use the classification correctly. These include:

  Braces — Braces enclose a series of terms, each of which is modified by the word(s) following the brace.

  Brackets — These enclose synonyms, alternative wordings, or explanatory phrases.

  Colon — The colon is applied rather than a comma for a term that has more than one essential modifier.

  Comma — Words following a comma are essential modifiers.

  Parentheses — Supplementary words that are present or absent in the statement of a disease or procedure, but do not affect the code, are enclosed in parentheses.

  Point Dash — It instructs you to turn to the category or subcategory referenced to review the subdivisions available for coding.

Residual Category — This is a place for classifying a specified form of a condition that does not have its own specific subdivision.

Rubric — In ICD-10-CM rubric — a grouping of similar conditions — denotes either a three-character category or a four-character subcategory.

Tabular List (Volume 1) — The Tabular List is comprised of 21 chapters vs. the 17 main chapters and two supplemental classifications (V and E codes) for ICD-9-CM. As in ICD-9-CM, many of the chapters classify diseases of an organ system. Others are devoted to specific types of conditions grouped according to etiology or nature, e.g., neoplasms, referred to in ICD-10 as "special group" chapters. Three chapters do not fall into either of these categories: Symptoms, Signs and Abnormal Clinical and Laboratory Findings, Not Elsewhere Classified; External Causes of Morbidity and Mortality; and Factors Influencing Health Status and Contact with Health Services.

Volumes — Similar to ICD-9-CM, the tenth edition is separated into three volumes:

- Volume 1 contains the listing of alphanumeric codes. The same hierarchical organization of ICD-9 applies to ICD-10: All codes with the same first three digits have common traits. Each digit beyond three adds more specificity. In ICD-10, valid codes can contain anywhere from three to five digits. In ICD-10-CM, valid codes may contain a sixth digit.

- If Volume 2 remains the title of the instructional manual after clinical modification in the United States, coders will need to remember that Volume 2 in ICD-10-CM refers to instructions, and not the index, which is what Volume 2 provides in ICD-9-CM.

- Volume 3 provides the index to the codes in the Tabular List. As in the ICD-9-CM index, terms in the ICD-10 index are found alphabetically, by diagnosis.

Using CPT®

The numeric and alphanumeric codes of ICD-9-CM constitute the diagnostic component of the reimbursement language. The codes of the *Physicians Current Procedural Terminology* (CPT®) book constitute procedural and medical service components. The CPT® book is in its fourth edition.

The CPT® coding system was selected as one of the National Code Sets mandatory for use by October 1, 2002 to facilitate electronic transactions, including health claims, enrollments, eligibility, payment / remittance and referral authorization. The current CPT-5 Project was developed by the American Medical Association, holder of the CPT® code copyright, in response to the Health Insurance Portability and Accountability Act of 1996 (HIPAA). In addition, exclusive of HIPAA demands, CPT® codes will be divided into three categories to enhance the use of the CPT® system by practicing physicians, managed care and other payer organizations, and researchers. Category I codes refer to the accustomed five-digit numerical system. Category II codes are a set of optional tracking codes, developed principally for performance measurement. The CPT® 2002 book includes a section of Category III codes, which are temporary tracking codes to identify new and emerging technologies.

History of CPT®

The CPT® book creates is a standardized system of five-digit codes and descriptive terms used to report medical services and procedures performed by physicians. The system was developed and is updated and published annually by the AMA. CPT® codes communicate to payers, and in some instances other providers and even patients, the procedures and services performed during a medical encounter.

The AMA published the first edition of the CPT® book in 1966 as a companion piece to its *Current Medical Terminology* (CMT), a manual of preferred medical nomenclature, then in its third edition. The first edition of CPT® (5 x 7-inches, 163 pages) contained a listing of four-digit codes and brief descriptions to report a full range of medical procedures and services. Each code was cross-referenced to then-available diagnostic codes: the *Standard Nomenclature of Diseases and Operations* (SNDO) and the *International Classification of Diseases, Adapted* (ICDA).

Editors of the first edition cited a variety of sources in developing the work, including the Social Security Administration, the Blue Shield Manual of Statistical Requirements, and the Relative Value Studies of the California Medical Society. The four-digit codes do not approximate those of today's CPT®. The task of modifying them to the present format was reserved for the editors of the second edition, published in 1970.

The 1970 edition of the CPT® book marks the genesis of the coding manual familiar to today's medical office workers. Many of the 1970 edition's five-digit codes and expanded descriptions in this work remain unchanged. The number of coded procedures far exceeds those available to users of the first edition and guidelines to the various sections appear for the first time. The second edition was developed with assistance from a handful of members of medical professional societies, a practice that would evolve into the 75-member CPT® Advisory Panel listed in CPT® 1997.

The third edition of the CPT® book published in 1973 and offered new features, such as alphabetic modifiers and starred procedures marked by an asterisk. Deleted codes (but not new codes) could be found in an appendix. This edition also saw the medical codes moved to the front of the code listings, a benchmark that would stand for almost 20 years until the introduction of the Evaluation and Management (E/M) codes in 1992.

The fourth edition of the CPT® book was originally published in 1977, and this current edition is sometimes referred to as CPT®-4. This edition began the custom of significant yearly revisions, usually concentrated on a limited number of sections. Since then, medical office coders across the country have made an annual ritual of anticipating the code changes and the related effects on coding and billing habits for their practices.

The CPT® Book Conventions

The CPT® book is self-referencing. Its introductory material provides information about its rules, format, and guidelines. The introduction to the CPT® book should be carefully studied at least once by medical coders and reviewed annually for changes. Classes and correspondence courses teach medical coding and several good introductory coding books convey the CPT® book fundamentals. Additionally, the AMA and private consultants sponsor coding seminars to discuss changes and methods to implement these changes into regular coding practice.

The heart of this chapter is a glossary of the CPT® book terminology. Consult these listings as needed to solve procedural coding problems. However, a brief primer to conventions, rules, and anomalies is presented below.

The six major sections of the CPT® book are:

- Evaluation and Management (E/M)

- Anesthesiology

- Surgery

- Radiology (including nuclear medicine and diagnostic ultrasound)

- Pathology and Laboratory

- Medicine

A common misconception about the CPT® book is that its organization serves to arrange procedural codes according to the major medical specialties that can report them. This is simply not the case. Any qualified physician can render any service or procedure listed by code. A physician's advanced medical training dictates the types of services and procedures customarily performed. Many physicians, particularly those in primary care, can in the course of a day perform work coded from all six sections.

The CPT® book is, however, primarily a reference for physicians' work; only a very small code set can be reported by non-physicians (e.g., chiropractic, physician assistants, nurse practitioners). The rest of the codes report the physicians' work or, in some instances, the work of others under close physician supervision. Payers almost universally assume a physician performs the work coded. Since that is no the case, non-physician work and coding must be clearly negotiated in advance with all involved payers.

Although required by almost all third-party payers, the mere existence of a procedure does not in any way guarantee payment when the work is performed. Insurance plans vary widely in reimbursement.

Format
The printed format is designed to save a great deal of space while still making a great deal of sense. A key to interpreting this space-saving scheme involves the use of the semicolon (;).

A main code is typically a single-sentence description, constructed so that pertinent adjunct information follows the semicolon. The following indented codes appear only as brief adjunct information. An important coding axiom is that an indented code always includes the common portion of the preceding main code description as it appears up to and including the semicolon.

25500   Closed treatment of radial shaft fracture; without manipulation

25505   with manipulation

The complete description of code 25505 is: Closed treatment of radial shaft fracture; with manipulation. Although 25505 appears under 25500, it stands alone to describe a treatment requiring manipulation.

Symbols and Appendix B
Symbols alert users to changes or other attributes of a code. The symbols appear in the left margin, just in front of the code number, as shown here:

- A closed black circle designates a new code.

- A black triangle indicates a code description has been changed or altered.

- A star (appearing more as an asterisk) indicates a minor surgical procedure not subject to global fee policies. See also Starred Procedures.

These symbols may have a bearing on assignment of codes for a practice.

Modifiers
Code modifiers were introduced to the CPT® book 25 years ago to flag a service that is altered in some way from the stated description. The basic definition of the coded service remains intact. Modifiers more precisely convey the nature of the service or procedure. Modifiers are two-digit codes and those commonly used in a practice become second nature. They may or may not affect the level of reimbursement.

Modifiers can indicate:

- A service or procedure represents only a professional or a technical component

- A service or procedure was performed by more than one physician

- Only part of a service was performed

- An adjunct service was performed

- A bilateral service was performed

- A service or procedure was provided more than once

- Unusual events occurred

- A procedure or service was altered in some way

Consult Appendix A of the CPT® book for a listing with full descriptions of modifiers. Additionally, individual sections of the CPT® book will contain special instructions for the use of modifiers to codes in that particular section. See the Modifiers chapter of this book for further discussion.

CPT® only © 2001 American Medical Association

Glossary of Terms

Use the following glossary of terms to troubleshoot and solve CPT® code related claims problems. Other chapters of this book will be useful for modifier-related and E/M problems. And, as stated earlier, the CPT® book introduction and introductory material at the section heads can help coders sort out problem areas.

Add-on Codes — Procedure performed in addition to the primary procedure and designated with a **+**. Add-on codes are never reported as stand-alone services. They are reported secondarily in addition to the primary procedure.

Alphabetical Reference Index — The coding process begins with a careful examination of the medical record to determine primary and secondary procedures as well as any modifying or extenuating circumstances. The alphabetical index is the starting point of all CPT® coding. Do not select codes solely on the basis of information in the index — it is only a reference to the full listing of codes. The alphabetic index is not a substitute for the main text. You must refer to the main text to ensure appropriate code selection.

Anesthesia 00100–01999, 99100–99140 — The Anesthesia section of includes codes to report "general, regional, supplementation of local anesthesia, or other supportive services. See the anesthesia chapter in this book for code-to-code crosswalks.

Appendixes — Six appendixes appear toward the back of the CPT® book. Appendix A is a listing of modifiers and their descriptions. Appendix B is a listing of additions, deletions, and revisions that were accomplished to compile the current edition. Appendix C pertains to changes in short descriptions as they appear in the data file. Appendix D is a series of clinical examples for E/M codes. Appendix E is a summary of add-on codes. Appendix F is a summary of CPT® codes exempt from Modifier '-51.'

Bilateral Procedure — Modifier 50 is used in those instances where a bilateral code for the same operative session is unavailable. The second (or bilateral) procedure is identified by the primary procedure code along with the modifier. An anatomical counterpart must exist for the procedure. See the Modifier chapter of this book for more information.

Category Codes — The CPT-5 Project places CPT® codes into three categories to enhance the use of the CPT® by practicing physicians, managed care and other payer organizations, and researchers. The existing CPT® codes are considered Category I. Category I CPT® codes describe a procedure or service identified with a five-digit CPT® code and descriptor nomenclature. CPT® Category II codes are optional tracking codes intended to facilitate data collection by coding certain services and test results that contribute to positive health outcomes and quality patient care. CPT® Category III codes are tracking codes to identify new and emerging technologies. Category II CPT® codes facilitate data collection for new services and procedures to substantiate usage and clinical efficacy.

Consultations — This term defines times when a treating physician asks the advice or opinion of another physician. A consulting physician has a wide degree of latitude in providing services, but does not assume care or provide treatment plans. The E/M code range 99241–99275 reports consultation services and the E/M chapter of this book can be consulted for more information.

Code Changes — To keep up with the dynamic nature of medicine, the AMA revises and publishes the CPT® book on an annual basis. Appendix B consists of a summary of additions, deletions, and revisions to the current edition. Of these three types of changes, only the descriptions of new codes appear in Appendix B, so you must compare the new edition to the previous one to identify how the code descriptions have been revised. These changes are indicated as follows:

● New codes — New codes are identified by a blackened circle.

11981   Insertion, non-biodegradable drug delivery implant

▲ Revised codes — Revised codes are identified by a blackened triangle.

20550*   Injection; tendon sheath, ligament, ganglion cyst

● Deleted codes — Deleted codes are identified by parentheses.

     (Code 88170 has been deleted. To report, see 10021)

Code Ranges — Whenever more than one code applies to a given entry in the index, a code range is listed. If only two sequential codes or several non-sequential codes apply, they are separated by a comma. For example:

Antepartum Care

Cesarean Section   59510

     Previous   59610, 59618

If a range of codes applies, a hyphen is used. For example:

Aneurysm Repair

Aorta

     Abdominal Aorta 35081–35103

Correct Coding Initiative — Centers for Medicare and Medicaid Services (CMS) correct coding initiative

Using CPT®

(CCI) provides edits that determine the appropriateness of CPT® code combinations in billing for Medicare claims. The edits are designed to detect "fragmentation," or separate coding of the component parts of a procedure.

Cross-references — Two types of references appear in CPT® to direct coders to additional material:

• See — this directs the user to refer to the term listed after the word "see."

• See also — this directs the user to look under another main term if the procedure is not listed under the first main entry.

Evaluation and Management (E/M) 99201–99499 — The E/M system is a relative value approach to assessing the medical services provided. The series of codes provides a means to classify and report the extent of a physician's involvement for a full range of common physician/patient encounters.

E/M codes describe the intensity of a medical encounter as measured by the risks and complexities associated with the diagnosis and medical decision making. The more detailed the components and the more complex the diagnosis and treatment plan, the more valuable the E/M service.

The simplest, most basic treatment constitutes what many refer to as level 1 in treatment. Higher levels are assigned consequential to the complexity of services and diagnoses. See the E/M chapter in this book for more information about this series of codes.

Global Surgery Package — This denotes a normal surgical procedure with no complications that includes all of the elements needed to perform the procedure. Fragmentation, or "unbundling," refers to providers who may intentionally or accidentally charge separately for procedures included in the global package for that given surgical procedure.

Guidelines — Guidelines appear at the beginning of each of the six major sections of CPT®. The guidelines define items that are necessary to interpret and report the procedures and services contained in that section.

Home Infusion and Home Visit — Two series of codes were added to the CPT® 2002 book, of which both report the provision of services at the patient's home. Home infusion codes include health care professional home visit and all the necessary supplies, excluding drugs, required to deliver the therapy in a 24-hour period. Home visit health services consist of part-time or intermittent skilled nursing, physical, occupational, and speech therapy, and certain related services, including social work and home health aide services, all furnished in a patient's home, including assisted living residences, group homes, custodial care facilities, nontraditional private homes, and schools.

Incidental Procedures — An incidental procedure is generally minor and considered an integral part of the primary procedure. Incidental procedures are not separately reimbursable and are included in the primary charge.

Indented Code Description — Indented code descriptions include all words up to the semicolon of the main description preceding it. See also Format.

Main Terms, Listing in Index — Procedures are listed in the CPT® book index by:

• Procedure or service (endoscopy or splint)

• Organ or other anatomic site (tibia or colon)

• Condition (abscess or entropion)

• Key synonyms

• Key eponyms (disease or procedure named after a person, e.g., Moh's technique)

• Abbreviations such as MRI for magnetic resonance imaging

Medicine Services 90281–99569 — The CPT® book's Medicine section is found at the end of the book. Among the many diagnostic and therapeutic services included under medicine are immunizations, injections, specialty specific codes, and special services.

The guidelines begin with instructions on billing multiple procedures. Coders are instructed to report each procedure separately. Note that the word "procedures" may include medical and/or evaluation and management services.

Modifying Terms — A main term may be followed by a series of up to three indented terms that modify the main term. Subterms affect the selection of appropriate codes.

Modifiers, CPT® — CPT® modifiers show that a service was altered from the stated description without actually changing the basic definition of the service. The CPT® Modifiers chapter of this book explains how modifiers are used and which modifiers affect reimbursement. For example, Modifier -27: Multiple Outpatient Hospital E/M Encounters on the Same Date. This modifier identifies hospital resources used in relation to separate and distinct E/M encounters performed by the same physician in multiple outpatient settings on the same date.

Note: This modifier should not be appended to designated "add-on" codes.

Outpatient Services — This term usually refers to physician office, clinical, and hospital outpatient department settings. The E/M code range 99201–99215 reports services in these settings. See the E/M chapter of this book for more information.

Parenthetical — Information specific to a given code may be included as a parenthetical phrase following the code. These constitute directions to the coder and should be followed. Read all the rules, guidelines, and general information in each section and subsection.

Pathology and Laboratory 80048–89399 — The Pathology and Laboratory section of the CPT® book is divided into fourteen subsections. Many procedures are performed by various methods and coders must know the methodology used. In many instances, identification of method is the key to appropriate coding.

Pathology and Laboratory services are provided by pathologists or technologists under supervision of a physician. If the pathologist must review a test result and/or render an opinion, the appropriate code should be selected and a modifier -26 attached to indicate that only a professional component was provided.

Radiology 70010–79999 — Reporting radiological procedures involves two components: the technical and the professional. The technical component is that part of the procedure specific to the equipment, including the services of a technician. The professional component is specific to the physician's evaluation of the images. CPT® coding and nomenclature in the radiology section is under constant review in an effort to reflect current standards of service for this broad specialty.

Separate Procedures — Separate procedures are still defined in the CPT® book as services that are "commonly carried out as an integral part of a total service, and as such do not warrant a separate identification." These services are noted in the CPT® book with the parenthetical phrase (separate procedure) at the end of the description. When this phrase appears before the semicolon, all indented descriptions that follow are covered by it.

To reduce fragmented billing, review pertinent surgical codes that include the notation (separate procedure), and apply these guidelines:

- Code separate procedures only when the procedure is performed alone rather than in conjunction with related procedures.

- When a procedure that is ordinarily a component of a larger procedure is performed alone for a specific purpose, you can list it by itself or as a multiple procedure with modifier -51 attached. In other words, it is unrelated to the other procedure performed in a multiple setting. The operative report and associated ICD-9-CM code must be very clear and specific to substantiate a separate procedure in conjunction with another major surgical procedure.

Starred Procedures — Some surgical services are characterized by indefinite pre- and postoperative services. Because of these indefinite parameters, the usual package concept for surgical services cannot be applied. Such procedures are identified by a star (*) following the procedure code.

When a star (*) follows a surgical procedure code, the service listed includes only the surgical procedure, no associated pre- and postoperative services. This is the guideline as stated in the CPT® book. Medicare national policy for starred procedures may differ from this. Contact your Medicare carrier for this listing.

Surgery 10021–69990 — The Surgery section of CPT® includes three types of procedures: package, diagnostic, and starred services. To select CPT® surgical codes that accurately reflect the service performed, read surgical code descriptions carefully and remember that modifiers may have a significant impact on reimbursement. See the lay description chapter of CDR for general explanations of procedures.

Surgical Package Procedures — The CPT® book defines a surgical package in terms of a normal, uncomplicated performance of specific surgical services, with the assumption that on average, all surgical procedures of a given type are similar with respect to skill level, duration, and length of normal follow-up care. The majority of CPT® surgical codes are package services; they include related minor procedures and normal follow-up. Reimbursement for package procedures includes the actual surgical service, local infiltration, metacarpal and digital block or local anesthesia (when used), and an allowance for normal postoperative care. Pre-operative care provided after the decision for surgery has been made is also normally included. See also Unbundling and Separate Procedures.

Unbundling — Unbundling a code is similar to coding an incidental procedure but usually involves less subtle fragmenting of a bill. Never divide the components of a procedure when one code covers all the components. Examples of minor procedures always included in the primary surgical package include the following:

- Local infiltration of medication

- Closure of surgically created wounds, minor debridement, and wound culture

- Exploration of operative area

- Lysis of moderate amounts of adhesion and fulguration of bleeding points

- Application of dressings

- Application of splints with musculoskeletal procedures

Unlisted Procedure or Service — Codes have been designated to report services or procedures that are not found in the CPT® book. These codes usually end in the number 99. When an unlisted procedure code is used, a manual review by the payer is necessary. Documentation, such as operative notes and a cover letter, should be submitted with the claim. The provider should establish the fee for an unlisted procedure. It may help the payer if the provider relates the service's value to a procedure of similar value and worth.

Using CPT® Modifiers

Modifiers, introduced in the third edition of the CPT® book, allow coders to indicate that a service was altered in some way from the stated CPT® description without actually changing the basic definition of the service. This 1973 addition to CPT® adds a useful variable to coding that is easy to use. Proper use of modifiers may or may not have an impact on reimbursement. Modifiers can indicate the following:

- A service or procedure represents only a professional or technical component.

- A service or procedure was performed by more than one physician.

- Only part of a service was performed.

- An adjunctive service was performed.

- A bilateral procedure was performed.

- A service or procedure was provided more than once.

- Unusual events occurred.

- A procedure or service was altered in some way.

Physical Status Modifiers
New to CPT® 2002 are the physical status modifiers that, consistent with guidelines of the American Society of Anesthesiologists, ranks the patient's physical status as well as differentiates complexity levels of the anesthesia services provided.

-21 Prolonged Evaluation and Management Services
Modifier -21 is used to report services performed that take more time or are greater than the highest level E/M code in a category.

- Modifier -21 may be reported with CPT® codes, 99205, 99215, 99223, 99233, 99245, 99255, 99263, 99303, 99313, 99323, 99333, 99343.

- Modifier -21 is used to report physician face-to-face or floor/unit service(s); do not report with non-physician service(s).

Note: an additional value for this modifier has not been established. Payers will determine a percentage increase based upon individual contracts, medical necessity, and documentation.

-22 Unusual Procedural Services
Modifier -22 is not appropriate for CPT® codes with the term "simple" as part of the code description.

Rather, modifier -22 is used to indicate that a procedure was complicated, complex, difficult, or took significantly more time than usually required by the provider to complete the procedure. (Note: Do not use modifier -22 to report procedures complicated by altered surgical sites, such as scarring or trauma. Procedures complicated by altered surgical sites are reported using modifier -60.) Documentation should be provided with the billing and kept in the medical record when this modifier issued. When a modifier -22 is used, an operative report should always be attached to the claim.

The fee for modifier -22 should be the usual and customary amount for the procedure plus an additional 20 to 30 percent for the unusual circumstances. If modifier -22 is appended to a code that is not the primary code, and a modifier -51 has been appended, modifier -22 should be paid in full in addition to the cut contract rate paid for the code.

Modifier -22 often produces an automatic review or audit by payers. If the operative report attached to the claim does not indicate appropriate use of the modifier, the 20 to 30 percent increase in payment will be denied. The difficulty here is that the physician is not always the one who dictates operative reports, and the person who does the dictation may not realize the impact insufficient documentation has on reimbursement. Periodic orientations for all involved in the coding process are a good idea from both a legal and reimbursement perspective.

Because modifier -22 is often used when complications are encountered during surgical procedures, medical necessity is substantiated by additional diagnostic codes that identify the complication. These diagnostic codes should reflect the operative condition and the complication(s) encountered during the surgery.

-23 Unusual Anesthesia
This modifier is used by anesthesiologists to indicate that this procedure is normally performed under local or regional block but due to unusual circumstances, general anesthesia is needed. This modifier is not appropriate for use with codes that include the term "without anesthesia" in the descriptor, or for procedures normally performed under general anesthesia.

Using CPT® Modifiers

-24 Unrelated Evaluation and Management Service by the Same Physician During a Postoperative Period

This modifier reports that an unrelated E/M service was provided by the surgeon within the global period. Use of this modifier needs to be correlated to a diagnosis code that is unrelated to the surgical diagnosis code.

-25 Significant, Separately Identifiable Evaluation and Management Service by the Same Physician on the Same Day of the Procedure or Other Service

This modifier indicates that on a day a procedure or service identified by a CPT® code performed, the patient's condition required a significant, separately identifiable E/M code beyond the usual level of service required for the procedure. In addition, the modifier denotes that the patient's condition required services that were above and beyond the usual preoperative and postoperative care associated with the actual procedure performed.

This modifier is not appropriate with an E/M code that has a minimum level of service. Assign the proper E/M code and amount as appropriate for service rendered. Most payers will allow payment for significant E/M services on the day of a procedure. Performance of a procedure includes an evaluation of the patient as it relates to that procedure or service code. When the patient's condition causes the evaluation to exceed that usual level of service, the appropriate E/M code is listed and appended with modifier -25 or with the five-digit modifier 09925.

Paper documentation does not need to accompany the claim, but the medical record must clearly show the medical necessity for billing E/M code in addition to the procedure/service code.

Note: Modifier -25 has been approved for ambulatory surgery center (ASC) hospital outpatient use.

-26 Professional Component

Modifier -26 identifies the physician's component of a two-component service. Do not use this modifier with procedures that are either 100 percent technical or 100 percent professional. It is only used on procedures having both components, such as x-rays or pathology codes; and it results in payment being made for only the professional component of the service. Using modifier -26 also alerts payers to expect a separate claim from the facility for the technical component.

-27 Multiple Outpatient Hospital E/M Encounters on the Same Date

Modifier -27, new to CPT® 2001, gives physicians the means for reporting the use of hospital resources when providing E/M services in multiple outpatient settings on the same date. (Note: Modifier -27 has been approved for ASC hospital outpatient use.)

-32 Mandated Services

Modifier -32 identifies services that are mandated by Medicare, a peer review organization, a state, local, or government agency, and private payers. Reimbursement may be made at 100 percent of the allowable amount for the service or procedure (such as confirmatory consultations and related diagnostic services). Deductibles or co-payments may also be waived by the payer. Keep in mind, however, that not all payers cover services when they are mandated, and often expect the government agency to pay for the service (e.g., an examination to determine abuse or confirm rape).

-47 Anesthesia By Surgeon

Modifier -47 identifies that the surgeon administered regional or general anesthesia. The most common use of this modifier is for a Bier block, which is not identified with its own code. The claim should identify the time spent administering the block. The charge for anesthesia by a surgeon is usually based on time increments instead of a percentage of the total charge for the surgical service. Reimbursement policies for these situations vary dramatically. The predominant attitude of most payers is that a physician should perform the role of the operating surgeon or the anesthesiologist, but not both. Contact frequently billed payers for specific instructions.

-50 Bilateral Procedure

Modifier -50 identifies an identical procedure performed bilaterally during a single operative session. Depending upon payer rules, you will either have to (1) list the procedure twice and append modifier -50 to the second procedure, or (2) only list the code once with the bilateral modifier appended. Or, in either example, you can use the separate five digit modifier 09950.

Do not use modifier -50 when a procedure code description specifically states that the procedure is bilateral, such as code 58700 Salpingectomy, complete or partial, unilateral or bilateral (separate procedure). Also, modifier -50 should not be used on procedures where the organ is considered to be midline, such as the bladder, uterus, esophagus, and nasal septum.

Note: Medicare and many national payers are moving toward the single line entry to identify a bilateral situation. However, careful monitoring will ensure correct reimbursement for both sides. Some payers allow 100 percent for each side if a separate incision is involved. Payers that do not allow 100 percent for the second side usually allow from 50 to 75 percent. Because of the varying allowances, monitor your reimbursement to determine the percentage allowed for the second side.

Note: Modifier -50 has been approved for ASC Hospital Outpatient use.

-51 Multiple Procedures

Modifier -51 designates multiple procedures that are rendered at the same operative session or on the same day. CPT® states that modifier -51 should be used when a combination of surgical services, medical services, or surgical and medical services are provided. Modifier -51 is not used with E/M services. It is applicable when multiple related procedures are performed and there is no single inclusive code available. List the primary procedure first on the HCFA-1500 claim form, then attach modifier -51, or the five digit modifier code 09951, to each secondary procedure code.

The following guidelines make good billing and coding practice for modifier -51:

- List the procedure code with the highest value first when billing Medicare and commercial payers.

- List additional procedures by descending value.

- Clearly state in your operative reports which procedures were accomplished through separate incisions and which were done through the same incision.

- Do not combine charges when coding multiple, unrelated procedures. List each procedure separately on the claim form and indicate each charge.

- If a comprehensive procedure has a single CPT® code, report that code rather than "unbundling" or listing the individual components.

Note: This modifier should not be appended to designated "add-on" codes.

-52 Reduced Services

Modifier -52 and the five-digit modifier code 09952 identify situations where the physician elects to reduce or eliminate a portion of a service or procedure. Cover letters or operative reports are not necessary when modifier -52 is used since these claims are not usually sent to medical review. Cover letters and operative reports may even impede claims processing. However, physicians may find it helpful to provide the payer with an explanation of the reduced fee compared to the usual fee. The reduction in charge reflects the reduction or elimination of a portion of the service.

Note: For hospital outpatient reporting of a previously scheduled procedure or service that is reduced or cancelled due to extenuating circumstances or those

that threaten the well-being of the patient prior to or after administration of anesthesia, see modifiers -73 and -74. These modifiers are new to CPT®1999.

Note: Modifier -52 has been approved for ASC Hospital Outpatient use.

-53 Discontinued Procedure

Modifier -53 is used to denote a surgical l or diagnostic procedure terminated by the physician because of concerns about the procedure's impact on the patient's well-being. Add modifier -53 to the code for the discontinued procedure or use the five-digit modifier code 09953. This code can only be used if the procedure was discontinued after anesthesia was administered and/or the patient was prepped in the operating suite.

Note: This modifier reports the elective cancellation of a procedure prior to the patient's anesthesia induction and/or surgical preparation in the operating suite. For outpatient hospital/ambulatory surgery center (ASC) reporting of a previously scheduled procedure or service that is reduced or cancelled due to extenuating circumstances or those that threaten the well being of the patient prior to or after anesthesia, see modifiers -73 and -74. These modifiers are new to 1999.

-54 Surgical Care Only

Modifier -54 is used when one physician performs a surgical procedure and another provides preoperative and/or postoperative management. The surgeon who performs the procedure reports modifier -54. Both physicians need to determine what percentage of the overall fee each will bill for their individual services (for example, 70 percent for the surgery and 30 percent for the postoperative care). Do not bill more than 100 percent for the service provided. HCFA identifies the percentage assigned the intraoperative column in the Medicare Reimbursement Table.

-55 Postoperative Management Only

Modifier -55 is used when one physician provides postoperative management after another physician has performed the surgical procedure. The physician providing preoperative management bills the surgical procedure code at the percentage agreed upon (see modifier -54) with modifier -55 attached. HCFA identifies the percentage assigned the postoperative column in the Medicare Reimbursement Table.

-56 Preoperative Management Only

Modifier -56 identifies the physician providing preoperative care during the preoperative care during the preoperative time clause established by the payer but not performed in the actual surgery. Use this modifier only with codes from the Surgery and Medicine sections of the CPT® book. It does not appear in guidelines of the E/M codes. CMS identifies

Using CPT ® Modifiers

the percentage assigned the intraoperative column in the Medicare Reimbursement Table.

-57 Decision for Surgery

Modifier -57 identifies an E/M service that resulted in the initial decision to perform surgery. Even though modifier -57 is included in the guidelines for E/M, Surgery, and Medicine services, it should only be reported with E/M codes. Because the CPT® book does not designate whether the surgery decided upon is major or minor, diagnostic or therapeutic, use modifier -57 to identify when the decision for any surgery is made.

The prevailing industry standard, is to use modifier -25 for minor non-starred procedures and modifier -57 on major procedures. CMS identifies minor as having 10 follow-up days and major as having 90 follow-up days assigned. Providers are more likely to use modifier -25 to identify that a significant, separately reportable E/M service was provided on the same day a minor procedure was performed.

-58 Staged or Related Procedure or Service by the Same Physician during the Postoperative Period

When reporting modifier -58, the physician may need to indicate that the procedure or service was one of the following: 1) planned prospectively at the time of the original procedure, or staged; 2) more extensive than the original procedure; or 3) for therapy following a diagnostic surgical procedure. Do not use this modifier to report the treatment of a problem that requires a return to the operating room (see modifier -78). Modifier -58 is included in the guidelines for E/M, Surgery, Radiology, and Medicine services.

Note the following about modifier -58:

- The existence of CPT® modifier -58 does not negate the global fee concept; therefore, services that are included in CPT® as multiple sessions are otherwise defined as including multiple services or events may not be billed with this modifier.

- Modifier -58 should not alter the amount charged or paid for subsequent unrelated or staged procedures that are performed during the postoperative period of a previous procedure.

-59 Distinct Procedural Service

Sometimes, a physician is required to report modifier -59 to indicate that a procedure or service is distinct from other services performed on the same day. Modifier -59 is used to identify procedures that are not normally reported together, but are appropriate under the circumstances. According to the CPT® book, "This may represent a different session or patient encounter, different procedure or surgery, different site or organ system, separate incision/excision, separate lesion, or separate injury

(or area of injury in extensive injuries) not ordinarily encountered or performed on the same day by the same physician.

Note: Modifier -59 has been approved for ASC Hospital Outpatient use.

-62 Two Surgeons:

Modifier -62 indicates that the skills of two or more surgeons (sometimes with different skills) are required to manage a specific surgical procedure. Multiple-surgeon procedures may be related or unrelated. When the procedures are unrelated, identify the separate services performed by each surgeon. List multiple related procedures as though one physician performed all procedures and add modifier -62. The surgeons should agree on charges, procedure codes, and reimbursement percentage splits prior to submission. Because of many variables, it is imperative you coordinate the physicians' billing, and submit complete and detailed documentation.

Note: If a co-surgeon assists in performing additional procedures during the same surgical session, those are reported using separate procedure codes with the modifier -80 or -81, as appropriate.

-66 Surgical Team

Modifier -66 identifies complex procedures that require concomitant services. Several physicians, from the same or different specialties, other highly skilled and specially trained personnel, and different types of complex equipment may be used in the surgery. Team surgery is usually confined to organ transplants and re-transplants. Identify these circumstances for team surgery by listing all procedures as though performed by one physician and add modifier -66 to each procedure code used. The surgeons should agree on charges, procedure codes, and reimbursement splits prior to claims submission. Because of many variables, carefully coordinate the physicians' billing and submit complete and detailed documentation. Also, include a cover letter explaining the reimbursement distribution for each member of the team. The total of charges for all procedures performed may be increased up to 50 percent for team surgery. The reimbursement is divided among the surgeons, contingent upon actual fees, complexity of procedures, and medical review.

-73 Discontinued Out-Patient Hospital/Ambulatory Surgery Center (ASC) Procedure Prior to the Administration of Anesthesia

Modifier -73 identifies those situations when a physician may cancel a surgical or diagnostic procedure subsequent to the patient's surgical prep (including sedation — when provided — and being taken to the room where the procedure is to be performed) but prior to the administration of anesthesia (local, regional block(s) or general). The physician may cancel a surgical or diagnostic procedure due to extenuating circumstances or those that threaten the well being of the patient. Under these circumstances, the intended service that is prepared for but cancelled can be reported by its usual procedure number and the addition of the modifier -73 or by use of the separate five digit modifier code 09973.

Note: The elective cancellation of a service prior to the administration of anesthesia and/or surgical preparation of the patient should not be reported. For physician reporting of a discontinued procedure, see modifier -53.

Note: Modifier -73 has been approved for ASC Hospital Outpatient use.

-74 Discontinued Outpatient Hospital/Ambulatory Surgery Center (ASC) Procedure after Administration of Anesthesia

Modifier -74 identifies those situations when a physician may terminate a surgical or diagnostic procedure after the administration of anesthesia (local, regional block(s) or general) after the procedure was started (incision made, intubation started, scope inserted, etc.) due to extenuating circumstances or those that threaten the well-being of the patient. Under these circumstances, the procedure started but terminated can be reported by its usual procedure number and the addition of the modifier -74 or by use of the five-digit modifier code 09974.

Note: The elective cancellation of a service prior to the administration of anesthesia and/or surgical prep of the patient should not be reported. For physicians reporting a discontinued procedure, see modifier -53.

Note: Modifier -74 has been approved for ASC Hospital Outpatient use.

-76 Repeat Procedure By Same Physician

Modifier -76 indicates that the exact procedure had to be repeated by the same physician. Use this modifier to identify a procedure or service that was repeated subsequent to the original procedure or service. This distinguishes the procedure or service from either a duplicate service or billing error. Payers may require additional documentation to establish medical necessity. Modifier -76 is easily misused, so note the following applications of other modifiers:

- A staged or related procedure or service by the same physician during the postoperative period is reported with modifier -58.

- A return to the operating room for a related procedure or service during the postoperative period is reported with modifier -78.

- An unrelated procedure or service by the same physician during the postoperative period is reported with modifier -79.

Note: Modifier -76 has been approved for ASC Hospital Outpatient use.

-77 Repeat Procedure by Another Physician

Modifier -77 indicates that a service or procedure performed by one physician was repeated by another physician. This modifier is usually used during the postoperative period of the procedure or service. The second physician adds the modifier to the procedure or service code used by the first physician.

It is appropriate to use modifier -22 when the procedure is unusually complicated, or modifier -52 when only a portion of the procedure or service is repeated. The ICD-9-CM diagnostic codes must substantiate the medical necessity of repeating the procedure. Because payers often require additional documentation to establish medical necessity, it is advisable to submit the operative report with a cover letter.

Note: Modifier -77 has been approved for ASC Hospital Outpatient use.

-78 Return to the Operating Room for a Related Procedure during the Postoperative Period

Modifier -78 is used to report related procedures performed in the operating room within the assigned postoperative period of a surgical procedure.

-79 Unrelated Procedure or Service by the Same Physician During the Postoperative Period

Modifier -79 was added to notify payers that the procedure was performed during a postoperative period of another procedure but is not related to that surgery. The diagnostic codes must document the medical necessity of the service, so the ICD-9-CM codes are usually different for this service from those reported with the initial procedure. Do not use modifier -79 to report staged or related procedures or services performed by the same physician during the assigned postoperative period of a procedure.

-80 Assistant Surgeon

Modifier -80 identifies surgical assistant services and is applied to the surgical procedure code(s). Assisting physicians usually charge 16 to 30 percent of their normal fee for performing the surgery alone. Be aware that payers may use the surgeon's contract rate to figure the assistant's percentage, and usually will not pay a resident for an assistant surgeon fee.

Using CPT ® Modifiers

-81 Minimum Assistant Surgeon

Modifier -81 identifies minimal surgical assistant service when assistance is required for a short time. Minimal assistant surgeons usually charge from 10 to 15 percent for their services. Be aware that not all payers will allow this modifier to be used for that purpose. Always bill for non-physician assistants at surgery as instructed by the payer.

-82 Assistant Surgeon (when qualified resident surgeon not available)

Modifier -82 identifies situations when a qualified resident is unavailable to assist in surgery and another physician must be brought in to assist. Assisting physicians usually charge 16 to 30 percent of their normal fee for performing the surgery alone. Be aware that modifier -80 is used more frequently than modifier -82 by surgeon assistants. Bill according to the payer rules for assistant surgery modifiers.

-90 Reference (Outside) Laboratory

Modifier -90 identifies laboratory procedures performed by a party other than the treating or reporting physician. HMOs and private payers will often allow a fee for a blood draw (arterial and/or venous) and a fee for transport to an outside facility. Use codes 99000-99001 to report this type of service — not modifier -90.

-91 Repeat Clinical Diagnostic Laboratory Test

Modifier -91 identifies tests repeated on the same day for the same patient to obtain multiple results. Do not use this modifier, however, for tests rerun to confirm initial results or due to testing problems.

-99 Multiple Modifiers

Modifier -99 identifies circumstances when two or more modifiers are necessary to delineate a service. Attach modifier -99 to the procedure code and list all appropriate modifiers as subsequent line items.

Using E/M Codes

The medical community relies on E/M codes for patient care and reimbursement, yet the codes cause more of an uproar than any other code set. E/M codes are difficult to understand. Coders and physicians have grappled over the complex guidelines defining the use of E/M codes since introduced to the CPT® book in 1992. In 1997, E/M documentation guidelines were revised by the American Medical Association (AMA), which holds the copyright to the CPT® book, and the Centers for Medicare and Medicaid Services (CMS), formerly the Health Care Financing Administration (HCFA). Their attempt to simplify E/M coding, however, did not come to fruition by the anticipated effective due to widespread physician dissatisfaction regarding the revisions. Until formal adoption, Medicare carriers are to use either the 1995 or 1997 guidelines, depending upon which set is more advantageous to the physician.

The jointly developed E/M framework is available from the AMA (by mail or the AMA website).

Categories and Subcategories of Service

Office or Other Outpatient Services
New Patient   99201-99205

Established Patient   99211-99215

Hospital Observation Services
Observation Care Discharge Services   99217

Initial Observation Care   99218-99220

Hospital Inpatient Services
Initial Hospital Care   99221-99223

Subsequent Hospital Care   99231-99233

Observation or Inpatient Care
Services (Including Admission
and Discharge Services)   99234-99236

Hospital Discharge Services   99238-99239

Consultations
Office Consultations   99241-99245

Initial Inpatient Consultations   99251-99255

Follow-up Inpatient Consultations   99261-99263

Confirmatory Consultations   99271-99275

Emergency Department Services
New or Established Patient   99281-99285

Other Emergency Services   99288

Patient Transport
99289-99290

Critical Care Services
99291-99292

Neonatal Intensive Care
99295-99298

Nursing Facility Services
Comprehensive Nursing Facility
Assessments   99301-99303

Subsequent Nursing Facility Care   99311-99313

Nursing Facility Discharge Services   99315-99316

Domiciliary, Rest Home or Custodial Care Services
New Patient   99321-99323

Established Patient   99331-99333

Home Services
New Patient   99341-99345

Established Patient   99347-99350

Prolonged Services
With Direct Patient Contact   99354-99357

Without Direct Patient Contact   99358-99359

Standby Services   99360

Case Management Services
Team Conferences   99361-99362

Telephone Calls   99371-99373

Care Plan Oversight Services
99374-99380

Preventive Medicine Services
New Patient   99381-99387

Established Patient   99391-99397

Individual Counseling   99401-99404

Group Counseling   99411-99412

Other   99420-99429

Newborn Care
99431-99440

Special E/M Services
99450-99456

Other E/M Services
99499

Glossary of Coding Terms

Care Plan Oversight Services — These codes report the services of a physician providing ongoing review and revision of a patient's care plan involving complex or multidisciplinary care modalities. Only one physician may report this code per patient per 30-day period and only if more than 30 minutes is spent during the 30 days. Also, low intensity and infrequent supervision services are not reported separately.

Case Management Services — These codes report the care a physician coordinates with an interdisciplinary team of physicians or health professionals/agencies without a patient encounter. Documentation must spell out the services each team member renders to the care plan.

Chief Complaint — The chief complaint is a concise statement describing the symptom, problem, condition, diagnosis or other factor for the patient encounter. The chief complaint is often written in the patient's words. The medical record should clearly reflect the chief complaint.

Components — Three key components — history, examination, and medical decision making — appear in the descriptors for office and other outpatient services, hospital observation services, hospital inpatient services, consultations, emergency department services, nursing facility services, domiciliary care services, and home services. Refer to CPT 2001 for E/M services and instructions for selecting a level of service.

The descriptors for the levels of E/M services recognize a total of seven components, including the three key components, used in defining the levels of E/M services. These components are as follows:

- History
- Examination
- Medical decision making
- Counseling
- Coordination of care
- Nature of presenting problem, and
- Time

Concurrent Care — Concurrent care describes similar services provided to the same patient on the same day by more than one physician. No special reporting is required for concurrent care. The diagnosis codes and physician specialties should mesh.

Consultations — The CPT book provides four subcategories of consultations: (1) Office or Other Outpatient Consultations, (2) Initial Inpatient Consultations, (3) Follow-up Inpatient Consultations, and (4) Confirmatory Consultations. If counseling dominates the encounter, time determines the correct code in three of the four subcategories. Confirmatory consultations have no times established.

The general rules and requirements of a consultation are as listed below:

- Most requests for consultation come from an attending physician or other appropriate source, and the necessity for this service must be documented in the patient's record. Include the name of the requesting physician on the HCFA-1500 form or electronic billing. Confirmatory consultations may be requested by the patient and/or family or may result from the second (or third) opinion required by the patient's insurance company.

- The consultant may initiate diagnostic and/or therapeutic services, such as writing orders or prescriptions and initiating treatment plans.

- The opinion rendered and services ordered or performed must be documented in the patient's medical record and a report of this information communicated to the requesting entity.

- Report separately any identifiable procedure or service performed on, or subsequent to, the date of the initial consultation.

- When the consultant assumes responsibility for the management of any or all of the patient's care subsequent to the initial consultation, consult codes are no longer appropriate. Depending on the location, identify the correct subsequent or established patient codes.

Contributory Components — Counseling, coordination of care, and the nature of the presenting problem are not major considerations in most encounters and, thus, provide contributory information to the code selection process. The exception arises when counseling or coordination of care dominates the encounter (more than 50 percent of the time spent). In these cases, time determines the proper code. Documentation of the exact amount of time spent substantiates the selected code. For office encounters, count only the time spent face-to-face with the patient and/or family; for hospital or other inpatient encounters, count the time spent in the patient's unit or on the patient's floor, but be sure the time spent and counted is directed at caring only for one patient. The time assigned to each code is an average and varies by physician.

Coordination of Care — This is one of the contributory factors in determining E/M service levels. Care coordinated with other providers or agencies without a patient encounter on that day is reported using the case management codes.

When coordination of care dominates (more than 50 percent) the physician/patient and/or family visit time is considered the key or controlling factor to qualify for a particular level of E/M services.

Counseling — A discussion between the physician and the patient and/or family concerning one or more of the following areas as designated by the American Medical Association:

- Diagnostic results, impression, and/or recommended diagnostic studies
- Prognosis
- Risks and benefits of management (treatment) options
- Instructions for management (treatment) and/or follow-up
- Importance of compliance with chosen management (treatment) options
- Risk factor reduction
- Patient and family education

When counseling dominates (more than 50 percent) the physician/patient and/or family encounter, time is considered the key or controlling factor to qualify for a particular level of E/M services.

Critical Care Services — Critical care is not specific to a location such as an ICU or CCU. Critical care is determined by the patient's critically ill or critically injured condition requiring this type of physician care. Routine visits to a stabilized patient in an ICU are not necessarily critical care. General guidelines for critical care are as follows:

- Critical care codes include evaluation and management of the critically ill or injured patient, requiring constant attendance of the physician.
- AMA and CMS have assigned procedures that should not be reported separately.
- Care provided to a patient who is not critically ill or critically injured but happens to be in a critical care unit should be identified using subsequent hospital care codes or inpatient consultation codes as appropriate.
- Although critical care typically requires interpretation of multiple physiologic parameters and/or application of advanced technology, critical care may be provided in life-threatening situations when these elements are not present.
- Critical care codes identify the total duration of time spent by a physician on a given date, even if the time is not continuous. Code 99291 reports the first hour of critical care and is used only once per date. Code 99292 reports each additional 30 minutes of critical care per date.
- Critical care of less than 15 minutes beyond the first hour or less than 15 minutes beyond the final 30 minutes should not be reported.
- Refer to the CPT® book for examples of correct reporting of critical care services.

Documentation — The Basics

The following basic principles of documentation apply to all types of medical and surgical services in all settings:

1. The medical record should be complete and legible.

2. The documentation of each patient encounter should include or provide reference to the reason for the encounter and, as appropriate,

   - Relevant history, examination findings and prior diagnostic test results
   - Assessment, clinical impression or diagnosis
   - Plan for care

3. Date and legible identity of the observer must be in the medical record.

4. If not specifically documented, the rationale for ordering diagnostic and other ancillary services should be easily inferred.

5. Past and present diagnoses should be accessible to the treating and/or consulting physician.

6. Appropriate health risk factors should be identified.

7. The patient's progress, response to and changes in treatment, and revision of diagnosis should be documented.

8. The CPT® and ICD-9-CM codes reported on the health insurance claim form or billing statement should be supported by the documentation in the medical record.

Domiciliary, Rest Home, or Custodial Care Services — These codes report care given to patients residing in a long-term care facility that provides room and board, as well as other personal assistance services that do not include a medical component.

Emergency Department Services — Emergency Department (ED) service codes do not differentiate between new and established patients and are used by hospital based and non-hospital based physicians.

Time is not a descriptive component for the emergency department levels of E/M services since services are on a variable basis and usually involve multiple encounters with several patients over extended periods of time.

Associated with ED services is 99288 Physician direction of emergency medical systems (EMS) emergency care, advanced life support. The physician must be located in the ED or critical care department, be in two-say voice communication with the ambulance or rescue personnel outside the hospital, and direct the performance of necessary medical procedures.

Established Patient — This patient has received professional services within the past three years from

Using E/M Codes

the physician, or another physician of the same specialty who belongs to the same group practice.

Examination Component Guidelines — History, physical examination, and medical decision making are considered key to selecting the correct level of E/M codes. Four levels characterize the examination component, as follows:

- Problem Focused — A limited exam of the affected body area or organ system.

- Expanded Problem Focused Examination — A limited exam of the affected body area or organ system(s) and other symptomatic or related organ system(s).

- Detailed — An extended exam of the affected body area(s) and other symptomatic or related body system(s).

- Comprehensive — a general multi-system exam or a complete exam of a single organ system. The comprehensive exam performed as part of the preventive medicine evaluation and management service is multi-system, but its extent is based on age and risk factors identified.

Examinations — CPT® recognizes the following body areas:

- ENT (Ears, Nose, Mouth and Throat)
- Eyes
- Cardiovascular
- Respiratory
- Gastrointestinal
- Genitourinary
- Musculoskeletal
- Skin
- Neurological
- Psychiatric
- Hematologic/Lymphatic/Immunologic

History Component Guidelines — History, examination, and medical decision making are considered key to selecting the correct level of E/M codes. Four levels characterize the history component, as follows:

- Problem Focused: Chief complaint; brief history of present illness or problem.

- Expanded Problem Focused: Chief complaint; brief history or present illness; problem-pertinent system review.

- Detailed: Chief complaint; extended history of present illness; problem-pertinent system review extended to include a review of a limited number of additional systems; pertinent past, family, and/or social history directly related to the patient's problems.

- Comprehensive: Chief complaint; extended history of present illness; review of systems related to present illness/problems and a review of all additional body systems; detailed past, family, and social history.

Each category is comprised of two to four of the following elements:

Chief complaint (CC);
History of present illness (HPI);
Review of systems (ROS); and
Past, family, and/or social history (PFSH).

The guidelines supplement the information found in CPT® and are summarized as follows (for the full test, refer to CPT® 2001):

- The chief complaint, review of systems, and the past, family, and/or social history may be included as separate elements of the history. Or, this information may be included in the description of the history of the present illness.

- The comprehensive history obtained as part of the preventive medicine evaluation and management service is not problem-oriented and does not involve a chief complaint or present illness. It does, however, include a comprehensive system review and comprehensive or interval past, family, and social history as well as a comprehensive assessment/history of pertinent risk factors.

- A review of systems and/or past, family, and/or social history obtained during an earlier encounter does not need to be re-recorded if there is evidence that the physician reviewed and updated the previous information. This may occur when a physician updates his or her own record, or in an institutional setting or group practice where many physicians use a common record. The review and update may be documented by describing any new review of systems and/or past, family, and/or social history information. Or, the documentation may note no change in the information since the date and location of the earlier review of systems and/or past, family and/or social history.

- The review of systems and/or past, family, and/or social history may be recorded by ancillary staff or on a form completed by the patient. To document that the physician reviewed the information, there must be a notation supplementing or confirming the information recorded by others.

- If the physician cannot obtain a history from the patient or other source, the record should describe the patient's condition or other circumstance that precludes obtaining a history.

- The medical record should clearly reflect the chief complaint.

- To qualify for a brief history of the present illness, the medical record should describe one to three elements of the present illness.

- To qualify for an extended history of the present illness, the medical record should describe four or more elements of the present illness or associated comorbidities.

- To qualify for a problem pertinent review of systems, the patient's positive responses and pertinent negatives for the system related to the problem should be documented.

- To qualify for an expanded review of systems, the patient's positive responses and pertinent negative responses for two or more two systems should be documented.

History of Present Illness (HPI) — The HPI describes the patient's history of present illness from the first sign and/or symptom to the present condition. The description of the developing illness includes location, quality, severity, timing, context, modifying factors, and associated signs and symptoms significantly related to the present problem.

Brief and extended HPIs are distinguished by the amount of detail needed to accurately characterize the clinical problem(s).

- A brief HPI consists of one to three elements of the HPI.

- An extended HPI consists of at least four elements of the HPI.

Home Services — These are services and care provided at the patient's home. Home services to new patients (99341-99345) and those for established patients (99347-99350) include typical times the physician may spend with the patient and/or family.

Hospital Discharge Services — These codes vary depending upon the patient's hospital status. Code 99217 is reported when a patient is discharged from "observation status" on a day other than the initial date of "observation status." Services include final exam of the patient, discussion of the hospital stay, instructions for continuing care, and preparation of the discharge records. Use 99234-99236 to report services to a patient designated as "observation status" or "inpatient status" and discharged on the same date. Codes 99238-99239 apply to all services provided to a patient on the date of discharge when other than the initial date of inpatient status. Use 99238 for 30 minutes or fewer minutes, and 99239 for more than 30 minutes. Use Subsequent Hospital Care codes (99231-99233) for reporting concurrent care provided on discharge day by another physician.

Hospital Inpatient Services — These codes (99221-99239) report admission to a hospital setting, follow-up care provided in a hospital setting, and hospital discharge day management. For inpatient care, the time component includes not only face-to-face time with the patient but also the physician's time spent in the patient's unit or on the patient's floor. This time may include family counseling or discussing the patient's condition with the family; establishing and reviewing the patient's record; documenting within the chart; and communicating with other healthcare professionals such as other physicians, nursing staff, respiratory therapists, and so on.

Hospital Observation Services — These codes (99217-99220, 99234-99236) report E/M services provided to patients designated or admitted as observation status in a hospital. It is not necessary that the patient be located in an observation area designated by the hospital to use these codes; however, whenever a patient is placed in a separately designated observation area of the hospital or emergency department, these codes should be used.

- Observation Care Discharge Services: Use 99217 only if discharge from observation status occurs on a date other than the initial date of observation status. The code includes final examination of the patient, discussion of the hospital stay, instructions for continuing care, and preparation of discharge records.

- Observation or Inpatient Care Services (99234-99236) are used to report observation or inpatient hospital care services provided to patients admitted and discharged on the same date of service.

Level of E/M Services — The level of E/M service is dependent on two or three key components - history, physical exam, medical decision making. The other levels include components considered contributory to the level of E/M service. They are as follows:

- Counseling

- Coordination of Care

- Nature of Presenting Problem

- Time

Medical Decision Making — This term is one of three key components necessary in determining the correct level of E/M services, as it describes the complexity of establishing a diagnosis and/or selecting a management options, as measured by:

- The number of possible diagnoses and/or the number of management options that must be considered;

- The amount and/or complexity of medical records, diagnostic tests, and/or other information that must be obtained, reviewed and analyzed; and

- The risk of significant complications, morbidity and/or mortality, as well as comorbidities, associated with the patient's presenting problem(s), the diagnostic procedure(s) and/or the possible management options.

CPT® lists four types of medical decision making, as described here:

- Straightforward: Minimal risk of complications and/or morbidity or mortality; minimal or no complexity of the data to be reviewed; and a minimal number of diagnoses or management options.
- Low Complexity: Low risk, limited complexity of the data to be reviewed, and a limited number of diagnoses or management options.
- Moderate Complexity: Moderate risk, moderate complexity of the data to be reviewed, and multiple diagnoses.
- High Complexity: High risk, extensive complexity of data to be reviewed, and an extensive number of diagnoses.

The medical decision making component guidelines are summarized as follows:

- An assessment, clinical impression, or diagnosis should be documented for each encounter. This information may be explicitly stated or implied in documented decisions regarding management plans and/or further evaluation.
- The initiation of or changes in treatment should be documented. Treatment includes a wide range of management options including patient instruction, nursing instructions, therapies, and medications.
- If referrals are made, consultations requested, or advice sought, the record should indicate who receives the advice, who requests the advice, and where the referral or consultation is made.
- If a diagnostic service (test or procedure) is ordered, planned, scheduled, or performed at the time of the E/M encounter, the type of service, e.g., lab or x-ray, should be documented.
- The review of lab, radiology and/or other diagnostic tests should be documented. The review may be documented by initialing and dating the report containing the test results.
- A decision to obtain old records or decisions to obtain additional history from the family, caretaker, or other source to supplement that obtained from the patient should be documented.
- Relevant findings from the review of old records, and/or the receipt of additional history from the family, caretaker, or other sources should be documented. If there is no relevant information beyond that already obtained, that fact should be documented.
- The results of discussion of laboratory, radiology or other diagnostic test with the physician who performed or interpreted the study should be documented.

- Comorbidities, underlying disease, or other factors that increase the complexity of medical decision making by increasing the risk of complications, morbidity, and/or mortality should be documented.
- The direct visualization and independent interpretation of an image, tracing, or specimen previously or subsequently interpreted by another physician should be documented.
- If a surgical or invasive diagnostic procedure is prescribed, planned, or scheduled at the time of the E/M encounter, the type of procedure (e.g., laparoscopy) should be documented.
- If a surgical or invasive diagnostic procedure is performed at the time of the E/M encounter, the specific procedure should be documented.
- The referral for or decision to perform a surgical or invasive diagnostic procedure on an urgent basis should be documented or implied.
- If the physician elects to report the level of service based on counseling and/or coordination of care, the total length of time of the encounter (face-to-face floor time, as appropriate) should be documented and the record should describe the counseling and/or activities to coordinate care.

Neonatal Intensive Care — Codes 99295-99298 report services provided by a physician directing the care of a neonate or infant in a neonatal intensive care unit (NICU). Initial NICU care does not include services provided prior to admission to the NICU. Code 99295 is the only code among the four NICU codes that pertains to the date of admission. Codes 99296-99298 encompass intensive care provided on dates subsequent to the admission date. A new code to CPT® '99 - 99298 - applies to low birth weight neonates who are no longer critically ill though require NICU services, and who may require infrequent therapy as indicated by codes 99296-99297.

New Patient — This patient has not received any professional services within the past three years from the physician, or another physician of the same specialty who belongs to the same group practice.

Nursing Facility Services — These E/M services have been grouped into three subcategories: Comprehensive Nursing Facility Assessments (99301-99303), Subsequent Nursing Facility Care (99311-99313), and Nursing Facility Discharge Services (99315-99316). The two former subcategories include services provided to patients in psychiatric residential treatment centers. The facilities must provide a "24 hour therapeutically planned and professionally staffed group living and learning environment." Report other services, such as medical psychotherapy, separately when provided in addition to E/M services. The discharge service subcategory reports the time spent by a physician for the final nursing facility discharge of a patient, such as the final exam and a discussion of the nursing facility stay.

Office or Other Patient Services — Use these codes (99201-99215) to report the services for most patients' encounters. Multiple office or outpatient visits provided on the same calendar date are billable if medically necessary. Support the claim with documentation.

Past, Family and/or Social History (PFSH) — The PFSH provides information relevant to the patient's past illnesses and treatments, the patient's family, and an age appropriate review of the patient's past and current activities.

Past History — A review of the patient's past experiences with illnesses, injuries, and treatments that includes significant information as designated by the AMA:

- Allergies
- Tobacco/alcohol/drug abuse
- Operations
- Injuries/trauma
- Pregnancy history
- Growth and development history
- Immunization history
- Behavioral/functional history
- Other relevant past history

Family History — A review of medical events in the patient's family that includes significant information as designated by the AMA:

- Cardiovascular disease: stroke, myocardial infarction or other cardiovascular illness
- Cancer
- Alcohol/tobacco/drug abuse
- Domestic violence, child abuse
- Lipid disorders
- Hereditary disorders
- Other relevant family history

Social History — An age appropriate review of past and current activities that includes significant information as designated by the AMA:

Status of immediate and extended family

- Marital status
- Employment status
- Occupational history
- Education
- Housing/source of drinking water
- Financial status

- Other relevant social factors

Other relevant social factors consist of a review of three areas:

- Past history (the patient's past experiences with illnesses, operations, injuries and treatments)
- Family history (a review of medical events in the patient's family, including diseases which may be hereditary or place the patient at risk)
- Social history (an age appropriate review of past and current activities)

A pertinent PFSH is a review of the history area(s) directly related to the problem(s) identified in the HPI.

- At least one specific item from any of the three history areas must be documented for a pertinent PFSH.

A complete PFSH is of a review of two or all three of the PFSH history areas, depending on the category of the E/M service. A review of three history areas is required for services that by their nature include a comprehensive assessment or reassessment of the patient. A review of two of the three history areas is sufficient for other services.

Patient Transport — Patient transport codes report the physician's direct face-to-face contact with a critically ill patient during transport between facilities.

Place of Service — The E/M code section is divided into subsections by type and place of service. Keep the following in mind when coding each service setting:

- A patient is considered an outpatient at a health care facility until formal inpatient admission occurs.
- Consultation codes are linked to location.
- Admission to a hospital or nursing facility includes evaluation and management services provided elsewhere (e.g., office or emergency department) by the admitting physician on the same day.

Presenting Problem (Nature of) — A disease, condition, illness, injury, symptom, sign, finding, complaint, or other reason for an encounter, with or without the physician establishing a diagnosis at the time of the encounter. E/M codes recognize five types of presenting problems, defined as follows:

- Minimal: A problem that may not require the presence of the physician, but service is provided under the physician's supervision.
- Self-Limited Or Minor: A problem that runs a definite and prescribed course, is transient in nature, and is not likely to permanently alter the patient's health status OR has a good prognosis with management/compliance.

- Low Severity: A problem where the risk of morbidity without treatment is low; there is little to risk of mortality without treatment; full recovery without functional impairment is expected.

- Moderate Severity: A problem where the risk of morbidity without treatment is moderate; there is moderate risk of mortality without treatment; uncertain prognosis OR increased probability or prolonged functional impairment.

- High Severity: A problem where the risk of morbidity without treatment is high to extreme; there is a moderate to high risk of mortality without treatment OR high probability of severe, prolonged functional impairment.

Prolonged Services — This section of E/M codes includes three service categories, as described here:

- Prolonged Physician Service With Direct Face-To-Face Patient Contact: These codes report services involving direct patient contact beyond the usual service, with separate codes for office or outpatient encounters (99354 and 99355) and for inpatient encounters (99356 and 99357). Prolonged physician services are reportable in addition to other physician services, including any level of E/M service. The codes report the total duration of face-to-face time spent by the physician on a given date, even if the time is not continuous.

- Prolonged Physician Service Without Face-To-Face Direct Patient Contact: These prolonged physician services without direct patient contact may include review of extensive records and tests, and communication (other than telephone calls, 99371-99373) with other professionals and/or the patient and family. These are beyond the usual services and include both inpatient and outpatient settings. Report these services in addition to other services provided, including any level of E/M service. Use 99358 to report the first hour and 99359 for each additional 30-minute period. All aspects of time reporting are the same as explained above for direct patient contact services.

- Physician Standby Services: Code 99360 identifies when a physician is requested by another physician to be on standby, and the standby physician has no direct patient contact. The standby physician may not provide services to other patients or be proctoring another physician for the time to be reportable. Also, if the standby physician ultimately provides services subject to a surgical package, the standby is not separately reportable. This code reports cumulative standby time by date or service. Less than 30 minutes is not reportable, and a full 30 minutes must be spent for each unit of service reported. For example, "25

minutes" is not reportable, and "50 minutes" is reported as one unit (99360 x 1).

Review of Systems — The physician asks a series of questions to identify the signs of and/or symptoms the patient is experiencing or has experienced. The ROS is divided into three types, as follows:

- Problem Pertinent: Questions directly relating to the present illness

- Extended: Questions relating to the present illness and a limited

- Complete: Questions relating to the present illness and all additional body systems

For purposes of ROS, the following systems are recognized

- Constitutional symptoms (e.g., fever, weight loss)

- Eyes

- Ears, Nose, Throat, Mouth

- Cardiovascular

- Respiratory

- Gastrointestinal

- Genitourinary

- Musculoskeletal

- Integumentary (skin and/or breast)

- Neurological

- Psychiatric

- Endocrine

- Hematologic/Lymphatic

- Allergic/Immunologic

A problem pertinent ROS inquires about the system directly related to the problem(s) identified in the HPI.

- The patient's positive responses and pertinent negatives for the system related to the problem should be documented.

An extended ROS inquires about the system directly related to the problem(s) identified in the HPI and a limited number of additional systems.

- The patient's positive responses and pertinent negatives for two or more systems should be documented.

A complete ROS inquires about the system(s) directly related to the problem(s) identified in the HPI plus all additional body systems.

- At least 10 organ systems must be reviewed. These systems with positive or pertinent negative responses must be individually documented. For the remaining systems, a notation indicating all other systems are negative is permissible. In the absence of such a notation, at least 10 systems must be individually documented.

Service components — The seven components used in defining levels of E/M are as follows:

- History
- Examination
- Medical Decision Making
- Counseling
- Coordination of Care
- Nature of Presenting Problem
- Time

The three components of history, examination, and medical decision making are key to selecting the correct level of E/M codes. In most cases, all three components must be addressed in the documentation. However, in established, subsequent, and follow-up categories, only two of the three must be met or exceeded for a given code.

The key components (history, exam, decision making) must meet or exceed the stated requirements to qualify for a particular level of E/M service for the following new or initial patient categories and subcategories:

- Office, new patient; hospital observation services
- Initial hospital care
- Office consultations
- Initial inpatient consultations
- Confirmatory consultations; emergency department services
- Comprehensive nursing facility assessments
- Domiciliary care, new patient; and home, new patient

Two of the three key components (history, exam, decision making) must meet or exceed the stated requirements to qualify for a particular level of E/M service for the following established or follow-up patient categories and subcategories:

- Office, established patient
- Subsequent hospital care
- Follow-up inpatient consultations
- Subsequent nursing facility care
- Domiciliary care
- Established patient; and home, established patient

Service Levels — E/M services within subcategories are arranged in levels, each with the same basic format:

- A unique code
- Place and/or type of service

- What is included in the service
- The nature of the presenting problem
- Time spent

Special Evaluation and Management Services — This series of codes reports physician evaluations to establish baseline information for insurance certification and/or work related or medical disability.

Standby Services — *See* under "Prolonged Services: Physician Standby Services."

Subsequent Nursing Facility Care — *See* under "Nursing Facility Services."

Time — Adding time in CPT® 1992 was done to assist physicians in selecting the most appropriate level of E/M services. The time frames are based on data on the amount of time and work associated with typical E/M services as obtained from surveys of practicing physicians. Subsequently, specific times expressed in the visit code descriptors are averages and represent a range of time that may be higher or lower depending on actual clinical circumstances.

Time, however, is not a descriptive component for the emergency department levels of E/M services since these services are typically provided on a variable intensity basis, often involving multiple encounters with several patients over an extended period of time. It is often difficult for physicians to provide accurate estimates of the time spent face-to-face with the patient.

Diagnosis or Management Options

The number of possible diagnoses and/or the number of management options a physician must consider is on the number and types of problems addressed during the encounter, the complexity of establishing a diagnosis and the management decisions that are made by the physician.

Generally, decision making with respect to a diagnosed problem is easier than that for an identified but undiagnosed problem. The number and type of diagnostic tests employed may be an indicator of the number of possible diagnoses. Problems that are improving or resolving are less complex than those that are worsening or failing to change as expected. The need to seek advice from others is another indicator of complexity of diagnostic or management problems. Document the information, as noted in the following:

- For each encounter, an assessment, clinical impression, or diagnosis should be documented. It may be explicitly stated or implied in documented decisions regarding management plans and/or further evaluation.

- For a presenting problem with an established diagnosis the record should reflect whether the problem is: a) improved, well controlled, resolving or resolved, or b) not adequately controlled, worsening, or failing to change as expected.

- For a presenting problem without an established diagnosis the assessment or clinical impression may be stated in the form of differential diagnoses or as a "possible," "probable," or "rule out" diagnosis.

- The initiation of, or changes in, treatment should be documented. Treatment includes a wide range of management options including patient instruction, nursing instructions, therapies, and medications.

- If referrals are made, consultations requested or advice sought, the record should indicate to whom or where the referral or consultation is made or from whom the advice is sought.

Amount and/or Complexity of Data to Review

The amount and complexity of data to be reviewed is based on the types of diagnostic testing ordered or reviewed. A decision to obtain and review old medical records and/or obtain history from sources other than the patient increases the amount of complexity of data to be reviewed.

Discussion of contradictory or unexpected test results with the physician who performed or interpreted the test is an indication of the complexity of data being reviewed. On occasion the physician who ordered a test may personally review the image, tracing or specimen to supplement information from the physician who prepared the test report or interpretation; this is another indication of the complexity of data being reviewed.

For additional information, review the section "Medical Decision Making."

Assessing Risk

The risk of significant complications, morbidity, and/or mortality is based on the risks associated with the presenting problem(s), the diagnostic procedure(s), and the possible management options.

- Comorbidities/underlying disease or other factors that increase the complexity of medical decision making by increasing the risk of complications, morbidity, and/or mortality should be documented.

- If a surgical or invasive diagnostic procedure is ordered, planned or scheduled at the time of the E/M encounter, the type of procedure, e.g., laparoscopy, should be documented.

- If a surgical or invasive diagnostic procedure is performed at the time of the E/M encounter, the specific procedure should be documented. The referral for or decision to perform a surgical or invasive diagnostic procedure on an urgent basis should be documented or implied.

The accompanying table may be used to help determine whether the risk of significant complications, morbidity, and/or mortality is minimal, low, moderate, or high. Since risk is complex and not readily quantifiable, the table includes common clinical examples rather than absolute measures of risk. Keep in mind the following:

- The assessment of risk of the presenting problem(s) is based on the risk related to the disease process anticipated between the present encounter and the next one.

- The assessment of risk of selecting diagnostic procedures and management options is based on the risk during and immediately following any procedures or treatment.

- The highest level of risk in any one category (presenting problem(s), diagnostic procedure(s), or management options) determines the overall risk.

Table of Risk

Level of Risk	Presenting Problem	Diagnostic Procedure(s) Ordered	Management Options Selected
Minimal	• One self-limited or minor problem, e.g., cold, insect bite, tinea corporis	• Laboratory tests requiring venipuncture • Chest x-rays • EKG/EE.G. • Urinalysis • Ultrasound, e.g., echocardiography • KOH prep	• Rest • Gargles • Elastic bandages • Superficial dressings
Low	• Two or more self-limited or minor problems • One stable chronic illness, e.g., well controlled hypertension, non-insulin dependent diabetes, cataract, BPH • Acute uncomplicated illness or injury, e.g., cystitis, allergic rhinitis, simple sprain	• Physiologic tests not under stress, e.g., pulmonary function tests • Non-cardiovascular imaging studies with contrast, e.g., barium enema • Superficial needle biopsies • Clinical laboratory tests requiring arterial puncture • Skin biopsies	• Over-the-counter drugs • Minor surgery with no identified risk factors • Physical therapy • Occupational therapy • IV fluids without additives
Moderate	• One or more chronic illnesses with mild exacerbation, progression, or side effects of treatment • Two or more stable chronic illnesses • Undiagnosed new problem with uncertain prognosis, e.g., lump in breast • Acute illness with systemic symptoms, e.g., pyelonephritis, pneumonitis, colitis • Acute complicated injury, e.g., head injury with brief loss of consciousness	• Physiologic tests under stress, e.g., cardiac stress test, fetal contraction stress test • Diagnostic endoscopies with no identified risk factors • Deep needle or incisional biopsy • Cardiovascular imaging studies with contrast and no identified risk factors, e.g., arteriogram, cardiac catheterization • Obtain fluid from body cavity, e.g. lumbar puncture, thoracentesis, culdocentesis • Minor surgery with identified risk factors	• Elective major surgery (open, percutaneous or endoscopic) with no identified risk factors • Prescription drug management • Therapeutic nuclear medicine • IV fluids with additives • Closed treatment of fracture or dislocation without manipulation
High	• One or more chronic illnesses with severe exacerbation, progression, or side effects of treatment • Acute or chronic illnesses or injuries that pose a threat to life or bodily function, e.g., multiple trauma, acute MI, pulmonary embolus, severe respiratory distress, progressive severe rheumatoid arthritis, psychiatric illness with potential threat to self or others, peritonitis, acute renal failure • An abrupt change in neurologic status, e.g., seizure, TIA, weakness, sensory loss	• Cardiovascular imaging studies with contrast with identified risk factors • Cardiac electrophysiological tests • Diagnostic Endoscopies with identified risk factors • Discography	• Elective major surgery (open, percutaneous or endoscopic) with identified risk factors • Emergency major surgery (open, percutaneous or endoscopic) • Parenteral controlled substances • Drug therapy requiring intensive monitoring for toxicity • Decision not to resuscitate or to de-escalate care because of poor prognosis

Using E/M Codes

Using HCPCS Codes

Codes in the HCPCS Level II National Code set are one component of the three-level coding system that is collectively known as HCPCS. This chapter is primarily dedicated to these Level II codes. However, the following discussion addresses the formal structure of this larger medical coding system while sorting through the popular terminology and taking a brief look at how electronic technology will change the way we code.

HCPCS is an acronym that stands for the Healthcare Common Procedural Coding System (pronounced 'hick-picks').

Level I — CPT

The first level of the three-tier HCPCS system is the American Medical Association's CPT (*Current Procedural Terminology*). This code set reports a broad spectrum of medical procedures and services. The previous three chapters of CDR can be consulted for details about its uses.

Level II — HCPCS/National Codes

The codes are alphanumeric and each starts with a single letter followed by four numerals. The letters (A through V) serve to divide the types of services or supplies, while the numerals denote the specific service or supply. These HCPCS codes are commonly known by their alphabet categories (i.e., J codes, L codes, etc.). The codes are maintained and updated annually by the Centers for Medicare and Medicaid Services, or CMS (formerly the Health Care Financing Administration, or HCFA).

Level III — Local Codes

Individual state and regional Medicare carriers assign and maintain the third tier of procedure related codes, the so-called local codes, or sometimes 'carrier codes.' As with Level II codes, these are alphanumeric and always begin with W, X, Y, or Z. Local codes are slated for replacement by October 2002.

System Goals

This system has grown to become a uniform method for health care providers and medical suppliers to report professional services, procedures, and supplies.

CMS integrated the system in 1983 to accomplish the following:

1. Meet the operational needs of Medicare/ Medicaid

2. Coordinate government programs by uniform application of CMS's policies

3. Allow providers and suppliers to communicate their services in a consistent manner

4. Ensure the validity of profiles and fee schedules through standardized coding

5. Enhance medical education and research by providing a vehicle for local, regional, and national utilization comparisons

Standardizing Codes

The Administrative Simplification rule of the Health Insurance Portability and Accountability Act (HIPAA) will change the way we code. Among the impacts of the legislation is the move to standardized code sets for the electronic data interchange (EDI) of health care claims. Standard coding guidelines may include eliminating the redundancy among some code sets, and will certainly affect code sets in use by most health plans, health care clearinghouses, and health care providers. The codes sets include ICD-9-CM, HCPCS Levels I, II, and III, Current Dental Terminology (CDT), and the National Drug Codes (NDC).

Level II Conventions

Level II codes are organized first according to the type of service or procedure provided. This is accomplished through the use of an alphabetic prefix to the code (A through V). This initial sorting serves to divide HCPCS into the main categories for which it is best known. For example, dental and oral and maxillofacial surgical services and supplies appear under the rubric D codes.

All Medicare payers and almost all Medicaid authorities now require the use of HCPCS codes to reimburse a claim. Additionally, many private payers also demand HCPCS Level II codes to report reimbursable services. Most HCPCS references show keyed information to indicate whether Medicare coverage is available or even probable. While not strictly a part of HCPCS coding convention, these references to Medicare policy and legislation can be valuable to determine reimbursable services and supplies. These references generally have no bearing on claims submitted to private payers. Again, the methods to reference coverage issues will vary among publishers and whether the medium is print or electronic.

Another convention of HCPCS Level II coding involves the guidelines that accompany the code subsections. These guidelines should be followed. Users of this product may be alerted to additional information in an appendix, general definitions, or the use of eponyms within a series of listings. Within the code descriptions themselves, instructions sometimes cross-reference to specific CPT codes, or to the CPT book generally. But the most significant instructions involve the use of Level II modifiers.

....

Modifiers

Modifiers are used in all three code levels to generally identify circumstances that alter or enhance the description of a service or supply. Three levels of HCPCS modifiers have been developed. The Level I modifiers of CPT are discussed in detail in a previous chapter. The Level III carrier modifiers are best referenced through the local carrier's newsletters and correspondence.

The HCPCS Level II modifiers are ordinarily two alphanumeric digits (AA through ZZ), although a handful of single-letter modifiers are also used. These modifiers are recognized by carriers nationally and, as with the codes themselves, are updated annually by HCFA.

Many Level II modifiers can accompany a Level I CPT code for Medicare-related claims submitted via the HCFA-1500 form. For example, modifier -QB designates that a physician provided a service in a rural health shortage area and can be applied to an applicable CPT code.

Ambulance Origin and Destination Modifiers

Single-digit modifiers for ambulance transport are used in combination in reporting services to HCFA. The first digit indicates the transport's place of origin, and the destination is indicated by the second digit.

-D Diagnostic or therapeutic site other than 'P' or 'H' when these codes are used as origin codes

-E Residential, domiciliary, custodial facility (other than an 1819 facility)

-G Hospital-based dialysis facility (hospital or hospital-related)

-H Hospital

-I Site of transfer (e.g., airport or helicopter pad) between types of ambulance vehicles

-J Non hospital-based dialysis facility

-N Skilled nursing facility (SNF) (1819 facility)

-P Physician's office (includes HMO non-hospital facility, clinic, etc.)

-R Residence

-S Scene of accident or acute event

-X (Destination code only) intermediate stop at physician's office on the way to the hospital (includes HMO non-hospital facility, clinic, etc.)

PET Scan Modifiers

Use the following single digit alpha characters, in combination as two-character modifiers to indicate the results of a current PET scan and a previous test.

-N Negative

-E Equivocal

-P Positive, but not suggestive of extensive ischemia

-S Positive and suggestive of extensive ischemia (>20 percent of the left ventricle)

Reimbursement Terms

An increasingly complex reimbursement climate means new terminology develops every year. The following glossary includes terms not only used when coding, it includes terms used by major insurers and the federal government.

AAPA — American Academy of Physician Assistants.

AAPC — American Academy of Professional Coders.

AAPCC — Adjusted average per capita cost. The best estimate of the amount of money it costs to care for Medicare recipients in a given area.

AAPPO — American Association of Preferred Provider Organizations.

Abstractor — Selects and extracts data from the medical record entered into computer files. The data and coded diagnoses track morbidity and mortality, infectious disease, and index disease. Information may be gathered to track data for departments such as quality assurance and utilization review within the facility.

Accrual — The amount of money set aside to cover the benefit plan's expenses. Estimated using a combination of data including the claims system and plan's prior history.

ACLS — Advanced Cardiac Life Support. A certification often required of professionals who serve seriously injured or ill patients.

ACR — Adjusted community rate. A calculation of what premium the plan charges to provide Medicare-covered benefits for greater frequency of use by participants.

ACS contract — See ASO

Activities of daily living — Activities often used to determine eligibility for long-term care. They include bathing, dressing, using a toilet, transferring in and out of bed or chair, continence, eating, and walking.

Actuarial assumptions — Characteristics used in calculating the risks and costs of a plan. Assumptions include age, sex, and occupation of enrollees; location; utilization rates; and service costs.

Adjudication — The judging of a claim.

Admission — Registration of a patient for services in a healthcare facility.

ADS — Alternative delivery system. Any method of providing healthcare benefits that differs from traditional indemnity methods.

Adverse selection — The risk of enrolling members who are sicker than assumed and who will utilize more expensive services more frequently.

Age restriction — Limitation of benefits when a patient reaches a certain age.

Age/sex rating — Structuring capitation payments based on a members' ages and genders.

Aggregate amount — The maximum for which a member is insured for any single event.

AHA — American Hospital Association.

AHIMA — American Health Information Management Association.

Al-Anon, Alateen — Alcoholic support groups.

ALOS — Average length of stay. A benchmark average used for analysis of utilization.

AMA — American Medical Association.

Ambulatory Surgery — Surgical procedure in which the patient is admitted, treated, and released on the same day.

AMCRA — American Managed Care Review Association.

AMLOS — Arithmetic mean length of stay — Average numbers of days within a given DRG stay in the hospital.

ANA — American Nursing Association.

AOA — American Osteopathic Association.

APA — American Psychiatric Association.

AP-DRG — All Patient Diagnostic Related Group. 3M HIS made revisions and adjustments to the DRG system, now referred to as the All Patient DRGs (AP-DRGs). Early features of AP-DRGs included MDC 24, specifically devoted to the human immunodeficiency virus (HIV), and restructuring of the MDC governing newborns.

APG — Ambulatory patient group. A reimbursement methodology developed for the Centers for Medicare and Medicaid Services.

Appeal — A request for reconsideration of a negative claim decision.

Appropriateness of care — Term often used to denote proper setting of medical care that best meets the patient's diagnosis.

APR — Average payment rate. The amount of money the Centers for Medicare and Medicaid Services could pay a Health Maintenance Organization for service to Medicare recipients under a risk contract.

ART — Accredited Record Technician. *See* RHIT.

AS — Associate of Science.

ASN — Associate of Science, Nursing.

ASO — Administrative service only. A contract stipulation between a self-funded plan and an insurance company in which the insurance company assumes no risk and provides administrative services only.

Assignment — An arrangement in which the provider submits the claim on behalf of the patient and is reimbursed directly by the patient's plan. By doing so, the provider agrees to accept what the plan pays.

Assignment of benefits — Payment of benefits directly to the provider of the services rather than to the member who received the benefits.

At risk — A contract between Medicare and a payer or a payer and a provider in which the payer (in the case of Medicare) and the provider (in the case of the payer contracts) gets paid a set amount for care of a patient base. If costs exceed the amount the payer or provider were paid, the patients still receive care during the term of the contract.

Attained age — The age of the member as of the last birthday.

Auditor — A professional who evaluates a provider's utilization, quality of care, or level of reimbursement.

AWP — 1) Average wholesale price. A pharmaceutical price based on common data that is included in a pharmacy provider contract. 2) Any willing provider. Statutes requiring a provider network to accept any provider who meets the network's usual selection criteria.

Backlog — The queue of claims that have not been adjudicated.

Balance billing — When providers charge the patient the amount not paid by the insurance carrier above the agreed deductible.

Basic coverage — Insurance providing coverage for hospital care.

Basic health services — Benefits all federally qualified HMOs must offer.

Board certification — A certification in a particular specialty based on the physician's expertise and experience.

Boarder — An individual who receives lodging — a parent, caregiver, or other family member — who is not a patient but may wish or need to be near the patient.

Boarder baby — 1) A newborn who remains in the nursery following discharge because the mother is still hospitalized; 2) A premature infant who no longer needs intensive care but who remains for observation.

Book of business — A payer's list of clients and contracts.

BSN — Bachelor of Science, Nursing

Bundled — 1) The gathering of several types of health insurance policies under a single payer; 2) The inclusive grouping of codes related to a procedure when submitting a claim.

Business coalition — Employers who form a cooperative to purchase health care less expensively.

Cafeteria plan — A benefit by an employer where various services of many payers are offered to members as separate elements in the health care plan.

Cap — Contract maximum.

Capitation — A system in which a set amount of money is received or paid out based on membership rather than on a number of services rendered.

Care unit — A specific department or facility within a hospital or long-term care facility designed and staffed for the treatment of a particular type of patient.

Carrier — Insurance company responsible for processing claims.

Carve-out — 1) Term often used when referring to the integrated plan method of providing coverage to Medicare-eligible employees;

2) Medical benefits for a specific type of care that are not provided by the carrier of the members' insurance (e.g., Mental/Nervous provided by company A while company B carries the medical plan).

Case management — The ongoing review of cases by professionals to assure the most appropriate utilization of services.

Case manager — A medical professional (usually a nurse or social worker) who reviews cases every few days to determine necessity of care and to advise provider on payer's utilization restrictions. Certifies ongoing care.

Case-mix index — Sum of all DRG relative weights, divided by number of Medicare cases.

Catastrophic case management — Also called large case management. A method of review of ongoing cases in which the patient sustains catastrophic or extremely costly medical problems.

Catchment area — The geographical area from which a healthcare organization draws its members.

CC — Complication or comorbidity affecting payment.

CCU — Coronary Care Unit. A facility dedicated to patients suffering from heart attack, stroke, or other serious cardiopulmonary problems.

CDC — Center for Disease Control.

Census — The number and demographics of patients or members.

Certification — Approval by a payer's case manager to continue care for a given number of days or visits.

Cherry picking — Practice of enrolling only healthy individuals and excluding those with existing problems.

Chief complaint — The presenting problem.

Churning — 1) A performance-based reimbursement system emphasizing provider productivity; 2) When a provider sees a patient more than medically necessary with the intent of generating more revenue.

CLA — Certified Laboratory Assistant.

Claim — Statement of medical services rendered requesting payment from insurance company or government entity.

Claim lag — 1) The time between the incurred date of the claim and its submission; 2) The time between the incurred date of the claim and its payment.

Claim manual — The administrative guidelines used by claims processors to adjudicate claims according to company policy and procedure.

Claims manager — Payer's manager who oversees employee who processes routine claims.

Claims reviewer —Payer employee who reviews claims like an auditor, looking at coding, prior authority, contract violations, etc.

CLIA — Clinical Laboratory Improvement Amendments. Requirements set in 1988 CLIA to impose varying levels of federal regulation on clinical procedures, and few laboratories, including those in physician offices, are exempt. Adopted by Medicare and Medicaid, CLIA regulations redefine laboratory testing in regard to laboratory certification and accreditation, proficiency testing, quality assurance, personnel standards, and program administration.

Closed claim — A claim for which all apparent benefits have been paid.

Closed panel — An arrangement in which a managed care organization contracts providers on an exclusive basis, restricting the providers from seeing patients enrolled in other payers' plans.

Closed treatment — A fracture site that is not surgically opened. There are three methods of closed treatment of fractures: without manipulation, with manipulation, and with or without traction.

CMA — Certified Medical Assistant.

CMI — Case mix index. Sum of all DRG relative weights, divided by the number of Medicare cases.

CMP — Competitive medical plan. A federal designation allowing plans to obtain eligibility to receive a Medicare risk contract without having to qualify as an HMO.

CMS — Centers for Medicare and Medicaid Services, formerly HCFA. The federal agency that administers the public health programs.

CMT — Certified Medical Transcriptionist

COA — Certificate of authority. A state license to operate as an HMO.

COB — Coordination of benefits. An agreement that prevents double payment for services when the member is covered by two or more sources. The

agreement dictates which organization is primarily and secondarily responsible for payment.

COBRA — Consolidated Omnibus Reconciliation Act. Legislation that in part requires employers to offer terminated employees the opportunity to continue buying coverage as part of the employer's group.

Coder — Professional who translates documented, written diagnoses and procedures into numeric and alphanumeric codes.

Coding conventions — Each space, type face, indentation, and punctuation mark determining how ICD-9-CM codes are interpreted. These "conventions" were developed to help match correct codes to the diagnoses that are encountered.

Coinsurance — A limitation of the amount payable by the payer to the provider or member for care in traditional plans or in parts of managed care plans. For example, most traditional plans only pay 80 percent of care costs.

Commercial carriers — For-profit insurance companies issuing health coverage.

Common working file — All beneficiary entitlement information (Part A, Part B, Medicare Secondary Payer, and Health Maintenance Organization), deductible status, and all Part A and Part B claims history are maintained in CWF.

Community rating — Methodology of state and federal governments that requires qualified HMOs to request the same amount of money for each member in a plan.

Comorbidity — Preexisting condition that causes an increase in length of stay by at least one day in around 75 percent of cases. Used in DRG reimbursement.

Comparative performance reports — CPRs. CPRs annually compare a physician's services and procedures to those of physicians in the same specialty and geographic area.

Complex repair — The repair of wounds requiring reconstructive surgery, complicated wound closure, debridement, skin grafting, or intricate, unusual, and time-consuming techniques to obtain the maximum functional and cosmetic result. Complex repairs include the creation of a defect, (e.g., extending excisions), necessary preparations for repairs, and moderate debridement of complicated lacerations, avulsions, and other wounds.

Complication — From an insurer's point of view, this is a condition that arises during a hospital stay prolonging patients' stays by at least one day in 75 percent of the cases.

Component code — In CCI, the code following the comprehensive code that cannot be charge Medicare when the comprehensive code is charged.

Component coding — Standardizes the reporting of interventional radiological services. Component coding allows a physician, regardless of specialty, to specifically identify and report those aspects of the service he or she provided, whether the procedural component, the radiological component, or both.

Comprehensive codes — The code behind which component codes fall. *See also* CCI.

Consultation — Advice or an opinion rendered by a medical professional at the request of the primary care provider.

Continuity of coverage — Transfer of benefits from one plan to another without a lapse of coverage.

Conversion — Shifting of a member under a group contract to an individual contract.

Conversion factors — National multipliers that convert the geographically adjusted relative value units into Medicare Fee Schedule dollar amounts and applies to all services paid under the MFS.

Coordinated care — *See* managed care.

Copayment — A portion of the medical expense the member must pay out of pocket. In managed care plans, the member pays the copayment while checking in for his or her appointment.

Correct Coding Initiative — CCI Provides edits that determine the appropriateness of CPT code combinations in Medicare billing. Updated quarterly.

Corridor deductible — A fixed out-of-pocket amount that the member must pay before benefits are available. Also called simply "deductible."

COT — Certified Ophthalmic Technician.

COTA — Certified Occupational Therapy Assistant.

Counseling — A discussion with a patient and/or family concerning one or more of the following areas: diagnostic results, impressions, and/or recommended diagnostic studies; prognosis; risks and benefits of management (treatment) options; instructions for management (treatment) and/or follow-up; importance of compliance with chosen management (treatment) options; risk factor reduction; patient and family education.

Coverage issues manual — CIM. The CIM is a CMS publication containing national coverage decisions and presenting specific medical items, services, treatment procedures, or technologies paid for under the Medicare program. The CIM is used by Part A Intermediaries, Part B Carriers, and Peer Review Organizations (PROs).

Covered charges — Charges for medical care and supplies that the insurance plan will pay.

Covered person — Any person entitled to benefits under the policy, whether a member or dependent.

CPR — Computerized patient record — A computer application that allows all or most elements of a patient's medical record to be stored in a computerized database.

CPT® — *Physicians' Current Procedural Terminology, Fourth Edition.* The American Medical Association's list of five-digit codes used to report medical services. A standard reference for billing.

CPT® code — A descriptor of a procedure with a five-digit identifying code number. CPT codes are developed, maintained, and copyrighted by the American Medical Association.

CPT® modifiers — Additional codes to indicate that a service was altered in some way from the stated CPT code description without actually changing the basic definition of the service. Modifiers can indicate a service or procedure has both a professional and a technical component, a service or procedure was performed by more than one physician, only part of a service was performed, an adjunctive service was performed, a bilateral procedure was performed, a service or procedure was provided more than once, unusual events occurred, a procedure or service was altered in some way. A complete listing of modifiers is located in an appendix of the CPT book.

Credentialing — Reviewing the medical degrees, licensure, malpractice and any disciplinary record of medical providers for panel and quality assurance purposes.

Critical care — The care of critically ill patients in a variety of medical emergencies that requires the constant attendance of the physician (e.g., cardiac arrest, shock, bleeding, respiratory failure, postoperative complications, critically ill neonate).

CRNA — Certified Registered Nurse Anesthetist

Crosswalk — The cross-referencing of CPT codes with ICD-9-CM, anesthesia, dental, or HCPCS codes.

CRT — 1) Cathode ray tube. An old term for the computer used by coders. Refers specifically to the monitor; 2) Certified Respiratory Therapist.

CSO — Clinical service organization — Health care organization developed by academic medical centers to integrate medical school, faculty practice plan, and hospital.

CST — Certified Surgical Technologist.

Cutback — Reduction of the amount or type of insurance for a member who attains a specified age or condition (e.g., age 65, retirement).

Daily benefit — A specified maximum benefit payable for room and board charges at a hospital.

Database — The electronic store of utilization information used by payers to pay claims, negotiate contracts, and track utilization and cost of services.

Date of Service — *see* Service date

DAW — Dispense as written. The notation from a physician to a pharmacist requesting that the brand-name medication be given in lieu of a generic medication.

Days per thousand — A standard unit of measurement of utilization determined by calculating the number of hospital days used in a year for each thousand covered lives.

DC — Doctor of Chiropractic medicine.

Decapitation — Inadequate capitation.

Deductible — Member's medical services that must be paid out of pocket before the payer begins to pay.

Diagnosis — Determination of condition, disease, or syndrome and its implications.

Diagnostic — Services provided to determine the nature of the member's complaints.

Direct claim payment — A method where members deal directly with the payer rather than submitting claims through the employer.

Direct contract model — A plan that contracts directly with individual private practice physicians rather than through an intermediary.

Discharge plan — A plan submitted by a provider to the case manager as part of the treatment plan that details follow-up care after discharge.

Discharge status — Circumstance of patient at discharge. Examples include "expired,""transferred" to another facility, "left against medical advice."

Discharge transfer — Discharge of a patient from one facility to another.

Disposition of patient — A term used for data and quality assurance purposes that is accompanied by a description of the patient's status and destination at discharge (for example, "discharged to home").

DME — Durable medical equipment. Permanent equipment meant for medical treatment.

DO — Doctor of Osteopathy.

DOS — Date of service. The date on which care was provided.

DPM — Doctor of Podiatric Medicine.

DRG — Diagnosis Related Groups. The method CMS uses to pay hospitals for Medicare recipients based on a statistical system of classifying any inpatient stay into one of 25 groups. It is a classification scheme whose patient types are defined by patients diagnoses or procedures and in some cases, by the patient's age or discharge status. Each DRG is intended to be medically meaningful and would ordinarily require an approximately equal resource consumption as measured by length of stay and cost.

Drug formulary — *See Formulary.*

DSM-IV — Diagnostic and Statistical Manual of Mental Disorders, Fourth edition. The manual used by mental health workers as the diagnostic coding system for substance abuse and mental health patients.

Dual option — The offering of an HMO and traditional plan by one carrier.

DUR — Drug utilization review. A review to assure prescribed medications medically necessary and appropriate.

DVM — Doctor of Veterinary Medicine.

E codes — ICD-9-CM codes describing circumstances of an injury or illness. Their use establish medical necessity, identify causes of injury and poisoning, and identify medications. Their use can also be pivotal in reimbursements from payers such as medical insurance plans, car insurers, home insurers or workers compensation programs. Also known as the Supplementary Classification of External Causes of Injury and Poisoning (E800—E999) The index for the E codes is found in Volume 2, following the Table of Drugs and Chemicals.

EAP — Employee assistance program. Short-term counseling offered to members to quickly resolve transient emotional problems and to identify on-going mental or substance abuse problems for subsequent referral. Often limited to a handful of visits.

EdD — Doctor of Education.

EDI — Electronic data interchange. The transference of claims, certifications, quality assurance reviews, and utilization data via computer.

EHO — Emerging healthcare organizations — Hospitals and other providers that are emerging or affiliating.

Elective admission — An admission made at the discretion of the patient and facility based on available resources.

ELOS — Estimated length of stay. The average number of days of hospitalization required for a given illness or procedure. Base on prior histories of patients who have been hospitalized for the same illness or procedure.

E/M — Evaluation and management services. Contacts with the patient for assessment, counseling, and other services provided to a patient and reported through CPT-4 codes.

E/M service components — The key components in determining the correct level of E/M codes are history, examination, and medical decision making.

Emergency admission — An admission in which the patient requires immediate medical or psychiatric attention because of life-threatening, severe, and potentially disabling conditions.

Emergency department — An organized hospital-based facility for the provision of unscheduled episodic services to patients who present for immediate medical attention. The facility must be available 24 hours a day.

Emergency outpatient — A patient admitted for diagnosis and treatment of a condition requiring immediate attention but who will not stay at that facility or be transferred to another.

EMT — Emergency medical technician.

EMT-P — Paramedic.

Encoder — A computer application that helps assign a DRG.

Encounter — Contact with a patient.

Enrollee — A person who subscribes to a specific health plan.

Enrollment — The number of lives covered by the plan.

EOB — Explanation of benefits. A statement mailed to member (and sometimes provider) explaining claim adjudication and payment.

Episode of care — One or more health care services received during a period of relatively continuous care by a hospital or health care provider.

EPO — Exclusive provider organization. Similar to an HMO but the member must remain within the provider network to receive benefits. EPOs are regulated under insurance statutes rather than HMO legislation.

ERISA — Employee Retirement Income Security Act. An act with several provisions protecting both payer and member, including requiring that payers send the member an EOB when a claim is denied.

Established patient — An individual who has received professional services from the physician, or another physician of the same specialty who belongs to the same group practice, within the past three years.

Exclusions — Also called exceptions. Services excluded from a plan's coverage by the employer or payer because of risk or cost.

Experience rating — The designation of a group's previous claims history to help determine premium rates.

Extramural birth — An infant born outside of a sterile environment.

Facility — A building house a place of patient care, including inpatient and outpatient, acute or long term.

Facility of payment — A contractual relationship that permits the payer to pay someone other than the member or provider.

Fact-oriented V codes — Do not describe a problem or a service; they simply state a fact. These generally do not serve as an outpatient primary or inpatient principal diagnosis.

FAR — Federal Acquisition Regulations. Regulations of the federal government's acquisition of services.

FDA — Food and Drug Administration.

Federal Register — A government publication listing all changes in regulations and federally-mandated standards, including HCPCS and ICD-9-CM.

Federally qualified HMO — An HMO that meets CMS guidelines for Medicare reimbursement.

Fee schedule — The maximum fees a plan will pay for services, primarily listed by CPT codes.

FEHBARS —Federal Employee Health Benefits Acquisition Regulations. Federal regulations for acquisition of health services used by government agencies and subcontractors.

FEHBP — Federal Employee Health Benefits Program. Provides health plans to federal workers.

FFS — Fee for service. Situation in which payer pays full charges for medical services.

Formulary — A listing of drugs providers may prescribe as dictated by the plan or Medicare. Prescription of a medication not included in the formulary usually is not reimbursed.

FPP — Faculty practice plan. A form of group practice developed around a teaching program or medical school.

Fragmentation — *See* unbundling.

Fraternal insurance — A cooperative plan provided to members of an association or fraternal group.

FTE — Full time employee. The accounting equivalent of one full time employee that includes wages, benefits, and other costs.

Gatekeeper — A practice in which a member's care must be provided by a primary care physician, unless the physician refers the member to a specialist or approves the care provided by a specialist.

GHAA — Group Health Association of America — An HMO trade organization.

Global surgery package — A code denoting a normal surgical procedure with no complications that includes all of the elements needed to perform the procedure.

GMLOS — Geometric mean length of stay. A component that figures in the reimbursement calculation for a DRG.

Government mandates — Services mandated by state or federal law. In government claims, the correct use of ICD-9-CM codes is required by law. In 1988, Congress passed the Medicare Catastrophic Coverage Act. Although the act itself was later repealed, the mandate requiring ICD-9-CM codes on all physician-submitted Part B claims was upheld. Medicare's rules changed again in 1996, when it began to reject any claim that did not assign the most specific ICD-9-CM code available.

Grace period — The period after a member has terminated employment for which he or she is still covered.

Group model — An HMO that contracts with a group of providers.

Group practice — A group of providers that shares facilities, resources, and staff, and who may represent a single unit in a managed care network.

Grouper — Computer application that assigns DRGs.

Guidelines — Information appearing at the beginning of each of the six major sections of the CPT book. They also may appear at the beginning of subsections and code ranges. The information contained in the guidelines provides definitions, explanations of terms, and factors relevant to the section.

HCFA — Health Care Financing Administration, *see* CMS.

HCFA-1500 — A standard claim form.

HCPCS — Healthcare Common Procedural Coding System. Codes used by Medicare and other payers to describe procedures and supplies.

HCPCS modifiers — Modifiers should, or in some cases must, be used to identify circumstances that alter or enhance the description of a service or supply. Level II/HCPCS modifiers are two alphabetic digits (AA–ZZ). They are recognized by carriers nationally and are updated annually by CMS. Level III /Local modifiers are assigned by individual Medicare carriers and are distributed to physicians and suppliers through carrier newsletters. The carrier may change, add, or delete these local modifiers as needed.

HHS — Health and Human Services. The cabinet department that oversees CMS, Medicare, and other entities.

HIAA — Health Insurance Association of America. A trade organization for payers.

Hierarchy — The rank or order of codes. Numerical hierarchy plays a key role in ICD-9-CM coding because each digit beyond three adds more detail.

HMO — Health maintenance organization. A health plan that uses primary care physicians as gatekeepers. Emphasis is on preventive care.

Hold harmless — The contractual clause stating that if either party is held liable for malpractice, the other party is absolved.

Home health — Palliative and therapeutic care and assistance in the activities of daily life to home bound Medicare and private plan members.

Hospice — A service program, either inpatient or outpatient, that offers palliative support, counseling, and daily resources to the terminally ill and their family members.

Hospital admission plan — Used to facilitate admission to the hospital and to assure prompt payment to the hospital.

IBNR — Incurred but not reported. The amount of money the payer's plan accrues to forestall unknown medical expenses.

ICD-9-CM — International Classification of Diseases, Ninth edition, Clinically Modified for use in reimbursement and statistical reporting in the United States. Classification is primarily numeric.

ICD-10 — *International Classification of Diseases, Tenth Revision.* Classification of diseases by alphanumeric code, used by the World Health Organization but not yet adopted in the United States.

ICD-10-CM — Clinical modification of ICD-10 developed for use in the United States.

ICF — Intermediate care facility. A step-down facility for patients leaving the hospital but who cannot be discharged to home because of continuing medical needs.

ID card — The wallet card carried by the member providing name, member number, group number, effective dates, deductibles, and other information.

Immediate maternity — Coverage provided for pregnancies that began prior to the date the member became insured.

In plan — Services chosen from a network provider.

Incontestable clause — A provision in a policy that prohibits the plan from disputing coverage for certain conditions after a specified period of time.

Inpatient hospitalization — A period in which a patient is housed in a single hospital usually without interruption.

Inpatient reimbursement — The payment to an hospital for the costs incurred to treat a patient.

Intermediate repair — Repair performed for wounds and lacerations where one or more of the deeper layers of subcutaneous tissue and non-muscle fascia are repaired in addition to the skin and subcutaneous tissue. Single-layer closure can also be coded as an intermediate repair if the wound is heavily contaminated and requires extensive cleaning or removal of particulate matter.

Internal skeletal fixation — Repair involves wires, pins, screws, and/or plates placed through or within the fractured area to stabilize and immobilize the injury.

IPA — Individual practice association. An organization made up of providers who along with the rest of a group contract with payers at a discounted fee-for-service or capitated rate.

IPO — Individual practice organization. *See* IPA.

IS — Information services. The administrators of the computer systems used by payers and providers.

JCAHO — Joint Commission for the Accreditation of Health Organizations. The primary accrediting body for hospitals, out-patient facilities, and other facilities. This non-profit organization audits these facilities and was previously known as the Joint Commission for the Accreditation of Hospitals.

JD — Doctor of Jurisprudence.

Key Components — The three components of history, examination, and medical decision making are considered the keys to selecting the correct level of E/M codes. In most cases, all three components must be addressed in the documentation. However, in established, subsequent, and follow-up categories, only two of the three must be met or exceeded for a given code.

Lag study — A report used by plan managers to determine how long claims are pending and how much is paid out each month.

Lapse — A terminated policy.

Late effect — A residual condition occurring after the acute phase of an illness or injury has terminated. The original illness or injury is healed, but a chronic or long-term condition remains.

LCSW — Licensed Clinical Social Worker.

Limiting charge — The maximum amount a nonparticipating physician can charge for services to a Medicare patient.

Limits — The ceiling for benefits payable under a plan.

Line of business — Different health plans offered by a larger insurer or insurance broker as a product line.

Lives — The unit of measurement used by plans to determine the number of people covered. Calculated by multiplying the number of members by 2.5.

Local medical review policy — A policy that is carrier specific and used in the absence of a national coverage policy and is used to make local Medicare medical coverage decisions when needed. Developing local Medicare policy includes creating a draft policy based on review of medical literature, understanding local practice, soliciting comments from the medical community and Carrier Advisory Committee, responding to and incorporating into final local policy comments received, and notifying providers of the policy effective date.

Long-term care facility — A nursing home or, more specifically, a facility offering extended, non-acute care to a resident patient whose illness does not require acute care.

Loss ratio — The ratio between the cost to deliver medical care and the amount of money taken in by the plan.

LPN — Licensed Practical Nurse.

LVN — Licensed Vocational Nurse/Licensed Visiting Nurse.

MA — Master of Arts degree/Medical Assistant.

MAC — Maximum allowable charge. The maximum a pharmacy vendor can charge for something.

Malingering — The feigning of illness, either as the result of intentional deceit or as the result of mental illness.

Managed healthcare — 1) The concept of managing cases while in progress to assure care is the most appropriate, efficient, and effective; 2) A system of health care meant to manage overall cost; 3) A method of health care where contracted physicians participate in the management of health care costs.

Mandated benefits — Services mandated by state or federal law such as in child abuse or rape, not necessarily covered by insurers.

Maximum allowable charge — Amount set by insurer as highest amount to be charge for particular medical service.

MCE — Medical care evaluation. A part of the quality assurance program that reviews process of medical care.

MCO — Managed care organization. A generic term for EPA, IPO, HMO, and others.

MD — Medical Doctor.

MDC — Major diagnostic category — Classification of diagnoses typically grouped by body system. Used in DRG reimbursement.

ME — Medical Examiner.

MEd — Master of Education.

Medicaid — Federal-state health insurance for qualified low-income people.

Medical consultation — Advice or an opinion rendered by a physician at the request of the primary care provider.

Medical loss ratio — *See* loss ratio.

Medical meaningfulness — Patients in the same DRG can be expected to evoke a set of clinical responses which result in a similar pattern of resource use.

Medicare — A national program that provides medical care to the elderly, people with disabilities, and those who have End Stage Renal Disease (ESRD).

Medicare Carriers Manual — MCM. The manual CMS provides to Medicare carriers. It contains instructions for processing and payment of Medicare claims, preparing reimbursement forms, billing procedures, and Medicare regulations. As processes and regulations change, CMS issues revisions to the manual.

Medicare Fee Schedule — MFS. A fee schedule designed to slow the rise in cost for services and standardizes payment to physicians regardless of specialty or location. Payments vary through geographic adjustments. Different payment for the same service performed by physicians of different specialties is eliminated. The MFS is based on the Resource Based Relative Value Scale (RBRVS). A national total relative value unit (RVU) is given for each procedure (HCPCS Level I [CPT], Level II codes) by a physician. Each total RVU has three components: physician work, practice expense, and malpractice insurance.

Medicare Part A — Coverage includes hospital, nursing home, hospice, home health, and other inpatient care. Claims are submitted to intermediaries for reimbursement. Ten regional offices provide the Centers for Medicare and Medicaid Services (CMS) with a decentralized administration and delivery of Medicare programs. Each regional office manages private insurance companies that contract with the government to process and make payment for Medicare services.

Medicare Part B — Coverage provides payment for physician and outpatient services. Physicians submit their claims to carriers for reimbursement. Regional offices provide the Centers for Medicare and Medicaid Services (CMS) with a decentralized administration and delivery of Medicare programs. Each regional office manages private insurance companies that contract with the government to process and make payment for Medicare services.

Medicare Secondary Payer — MSP. Medicare becomes secondary when patients are 65 or older and have group health benefits through their own employer or their spouse's. Also covered under the MSP program are patients of any age who have End-Stage Renal Disease (ESRD), are covered by an employer group plan, and are in the first 18 months of treatment. Variables apply to this program.

Medicare supplement — Private insurance coverage that pays costs of services not covered by Medicare.

Medigap policy — A health insurance or other health benefit plan offered by a private company to those entitled to Medicare benefits. The policy provides payment for Medicare charges not payable because of deductibles, coinsurance amounts, or other Medicare imposed limitations.

Member — A subscriber of a health plan.

Member months — Total of months each member was covered.

Member services — A payer department that works as a patient advocate to solve problems. The department also works with the patient to take claims appeals to a final committee after all other processes have been exhausted.

Mental health/Substance abuse — A payer term for services rendered to members for emotional problems or chemical dependency.

Mental/Nervous — *See* Mental health/Substance abuse.

MeSH — Medical Staff-Hospital Organization. Organization that bonds hospital and attending medical staff as a network.

MET — Multiple employer trust. A group of employers which joins together to purchase health insurance on a self-funded approach. This approach lowers cost by preventing an adverse selection by broadening the membership pool.

MEWA — Multiple Employer Welfare Association. *See* MET.

MHA — Master of Health Administration.

Minor procedures — Procedures considered by many payers to be part of the package for a primary surgical service.

MIS — Management information system. Hardware and software that facilitates claims management.

Mixed model — An HMO that includes both an open panel and closed panel option.

MLP — Midlevel practitioners. Professionals such as nurse practitioners, nurse midwives, physical therapists, physician assistants, and others who provide medical care but do so with physician input.

MLT — Medical Laboratory Technician.

Modality — 1) A form of imaging. These include x-ray, fluoroscopy, ultrasound, nuclear medicine, duplex Doppler, CT, and MRI; 2) Any physical agent applied to produce therapeutic changes to biologic tissue; includes but is not limited to thermal, acoustic, light, mechanical, or electric energy.

Modifier — A descriptive code attached to a CPT code as a suffix.

Morbidity rate — Actuarial term describing predicted medical expense rate.

MPH — Master of Public Health.

MSA — Medical savings account.

MSN — Master of Science in Nursing.

MSW — Master of Social Work.

MT — Medical Technologist.

Multiple birth — Two or more infants delivered with no complications.

Multiple employer group — A group of employers who contract together to subscribe to a plan, broadening the risk pool and saving money. Different from a multiple employer trust.

NA — Nurse Assistant.

NAHMOR — National Association of HMO Regulators.

NAIC — National Association of Insurance Commissioners. An organization of state insurance regulators.

National coverage policy — Policy outlining Medicare coverage decisions that apply to all states and regions. National coverage policy indicates whether and under what circumstances items/services are covered. These policies are published in CMS regulations in the *Federal Register*, contained in CMS rulings, or issued as program memorandums, manual issuances to Coverage Issues Manual or the Medicare Carriers Manual.

NBICU — Newborn Intensive Care Unit. A special care unit for premature and seriously ill infants.

NCHS — National Center for Health Statistics

NCQA — National Committee on Quality Assurance. The organization that accredits payers' quality assurance programs.

ND — Doctor of Naturopathy.

NEC — Not elsewhere classifiable. Indicates that the main term in ICD-9-CM is broad or ill-defined. Use an NEC code only when you lack the information necessary to code to a more specific category. This term is used only in Volume 2.

Neonatal period — The period of an infant's life from birth to the age of 27 days, 23 hours, and 59 minutes.

Network model — A plan that contracts with multiple groups of providers, or networks, to provide care.

New patient — Patient who is receiving care from the provider for the first time within three years.

Newborn admission — An infant born in the facility.

Normal delivery — A baby delivered without complication.

NOS — Not otherwise specified. The equivalent of NEC, indicating that the main term in ICD-9-CM is broad or ill-defined. Use an NOS code only when you lack the information necessary to code to more specific category. NOS is used only in Volume 1.

NP — Nurse practitioner.

OB — Obstetrician.

Observation patient — A patient who needs to be monitored and assessed for inpatient admission or referral to another site for care.

Occupational therapy — Therapy meant to help a member who is recovering from a serious illness or injury retain activities of daily life.

OL — Outlier threshold. A component that figures in the reimbursement calculation for a DRG.

Open enrollment period — A period of usually one month annually during which members can revise their medical coverage.

Open panel — An arrangement in which a managed care organization that contracts providers on an exclusive basis is still seeking providers.

OPL — Other party liability. In COBs, the decision that the other plan is the primary plan.

Orthotics — Braces and other appliances worn to alleviate a medical condition.

OTR — Occupational Therapist Registered.

Out of plan— Choosing a provider who is not a member of the preferred provider network.

Out of service area — Medical care received out of the geographic area that may or may not be covered, depending on plan.

Outliers — Medical cases that statistically fall outside of established parameters of length of stay or cost.

Outpatient — A patient who receives care without being admitted for inpatient or resident care.

Outpatient visit — A patient's visit to a recognized outpatient facility or service.

Overutilization — Services rendered by providers more frequently than desired by payers.

PA — 1) Physician's Assistant. 2) Physician Association.

Paneled — A provider contracted with an HMO.

Par provider — Shorthand for a provider who is participating in the plan.

Partial disability — Inability to perform part of one's job.

Partial hospitalization — A situation in which the patient only stays part of each day over a long period. Cardiac, rehabilitation, and chronic pain patients, for example, could use this service.

Partial payment — A payment to the provider or member in which it is expected that other payments will be made before the claim is closed.

PAS norms — Professional acuity study. Based on a professional activity study performed regularly by the Commission Professional and Hospital Activities and broken out by average length of stay (ALOS) by region.

PBM — Prescription benefit managers — HMO staff who monitor amount and use of drugs prescribed.

PCP — Primary care physician. The physician who makes initial diagnosis and referral and retains control over the patient and utilization of services both in and outside the plan.

Pediatric patient — A patient usually under the age of 14 years.

Peer review — Evaluation of physician's performance by his or her peers.

PEPM — Per employee per month.

PEPP — Payment error prevention program. Program to help reduce Medicare PPS inpatient hospital payment errors.

Per diem reimbursement — Reimbursement to an institution based on a set rate per day rather than on a charge by charge basis.

Percutaneous skeletal fixation — Describes fracture treatment that is neither open nor closed. Fixation, such as pins, is placed across the fracture site, usually under x-ray imaging.

Perinatal death — Refers to both stillborn births and neonatal deaths.

PharmD — Doctor of Pharmacy.

PhD — Doctor of Philosophy.

PHO — Physician-hospital organization. *See* MeSH

Physician Assistant — A medical professional who receives additional training and can assess, treat, and prescribe medications under a physician's review. *See also* PA.

PIN — Physician identification number.

Plan manager — Payer employee managing all of the contracts and contract negotiations for one or more specific plans.

PMPM — Per member per month.

PMPY — Per member per year.

Pooling — Health payers' practice of combining risk.

POS — Point of service. A plan in which members do not have to choose services (HMO vs. traditional) until they need them. Benefits may differ by choice and members may be financially motivated to choose managed care plans.

Posting date —The date a charge is posted to a patient account by the provider. The posting date is frequently not the same as the actual date of service, but usually within five days of the actual date of service. Some providers list the posting date and the actual date of service for a charge.

PPA — Preferred provider arrangement. Similar to a PPO.

PPO — Preferred provider organization. A plan contracting with providers to provide services on a discounted basis. Members must stay within the plan or pay a greater copay.

PPS — Prospective payment system. A payment system, such as DRGs, that pays on historical data of case mix and regional differences.

Pre-existing condition — A condition that existed prior to the effective date of the plan. There is often a short-term or permanent limitation to reimbursement for care of this condition.

Precertification — Preadmission certification. The approval of a procedure or hospital stay before the act by a payer employee, who considers the diagnosis, the planned treatment, and expected length of stay.

Premature delivery — An infant delivered with weight and time of gestation qualifying it as premature.

Presenting problem — A disease, condition, illness, injury, symptom, sign, finding, complaint, or other reason for the patient encounter.

Primary care — First contact and continuing care, including diagnosis and treatment. *See* PCP.

Primary diagnosis — The code reflecting the current, most significant reason for the services or procedures provided. If the disease or condition has been successfully treated and no longer exists, it is not billable and should not be coded.

Principal diagnosis — The condition established after study to be chiefly responsible for occasioning the admission of the patient to the hospital of care.

Principal procedure — The procedure performed for definitive treatment rather than one performed for diagnostic or exploratory purposes, or was necessary to take care of a complication. If there appears to be two procedures that are principal, then the one most related to the principal diagnosis should be selected as the principal procedure.

PRO — Peer review organization. An organization that reviews costs charges in Medicare reimbursement.

Problem-oriented V codes — ICD-9-CM codes that identify circumstances that could affect the patient in the future but are neither a current illness or injury.

Use these codes to describe an existing circumstance or problem that may influence future medical care.

Professional association plans — A plan provided by a professional association that affords self-employed professionals (e.g., physicians, CPAs, lawyers) less expensive coverage.

Provider — A business entity that furnishes health care to a consumer.

PT — Physical Therapy. Physical Therapist.

PTA — Physical Therapy Assistant.

PTMPY — Per thousand members per year.

QA — Quality assurance. Monitoring and maintenance of established standards of quality for patient care.

QM — Quality management. Monitoring and maintenance of established standards of quality using techniques proposed by Crosby, Demming, and Juran. *See* TQM.

RBRVS — Resource-based relative value study. A relative value scale originally developed by Harvard for use in Medicare. The scale assigns value to procedures based on the related resources rather than based on historical data.

Reasonable and customary — The prevailing fees for services in a given geographical area.

Referral — In managed care, the primary care physician's act of sending a member to specialist within or outside the panel.

Regional Medical Center — A descriptive term for a hospital that provides comprehensive services to a large regional area but that may not be a tertiary care facility. Largely used in the west, where facilities may serve hundreds of square miles.

Rehabilitation — Physical and mental restoration of disabled members.

Reimbursement — Payment of actual charges incurred as a result of accident or illness.

Reinsurance — Insurance purchased by a payer to protect itself from extremely high losses.

Relative weight — Assigned weight intended to reflect relative resource consumption associated with each DRG.

Review committee — A multidisciplinary committee that considers denied cases being appealed, catastrophic cases, or fee-for-service cases.

RHIA — Registered Health Information Administrator. Formerly known as RRA (Registered Record Administrator). An accreditation for health information administrators.

RHIT — Registered Health Information Technologist. Formerly known as ART (Accredited Records Technician). An accreditation for health information practitioners.

Risk contract — *See* At risk.

Risk factor reduction — The reduction of risk in the pool of members.

Risk manager — The person charged with keeping financial risk low, including malpractice cases.

Risk pool — The pool of people who will be in the insured group, their medical and mental histories, other factors such as age, and their predicted health.

RN — Register nurse.

RPh — Registered Pharmacist.

RPT — Registered Physical Therapist.

RRA — Registered Records Administrator. *See* RHIA.

RRT — Registered Respiratory Therapist.

Rush charge — A charge for expeditious test results.

RVS — Relative value study. A guide that shows the relationship between the time, resources, competency, experience, severity, and other factors necessary to perform procedures.

RVU — Relative value unit. A value assigned a procedure based on difficulty and time consumed used for computing relative value study.

Sanction — Imposition of penalties or exclusion of a provider for infractions such as using services inappropriately, using procedures that are harmful to the patient, and using technique that is inferior in quality. Fraud will also earn a sanction for the provider.

Schedule — The listing of amounts payable for specific procedures.

Second opinion — Another professional's opinion to help determine the necessity of a medical procedure. This is often required by plans before a surgical procedure.

Secondary insurer — In a COB arrangement, the insurer that reimburses for benefits pending after payment by the primary insurer.

Self-insured or self-funded plan — A plan where the risk is assumed by the employer rather than an insurer.

Self-pay patients — Patients who pay for medical care out-of-pocket.

Separate procedures — Services that are commonly carried out as an integral part of a total service, and as such do not warrant a separate identification. These services are noted in the CPT book with the parenthetical phrase (*separate procedure*) at the end of the description. When this phrase appears before the semicolon, all indented descriptions that follow are covered by it.

Service date — The date a charge is incurred for a service.

Service-oriented V codes — ICD-9-CM codes that identify or define examinations, aftercare, ancillary services, or therapy. Use these V codes to describe the patient who is not currently ill but seeks medical services for some specific purpose such as follow-up visits. You can also use this type of V code as a primary diagnosis for outpatient services when the patient has no symptoms that can be coded and screening services are provided.

Service plan — 1) A plan that has contracts with providers but is not a managed care plan; 2) Another name for Blue Cross/Blue Shield plans.

Shadow pricing — Setting rates just below a competitor's rates. This procedure, maximizes profits but raises medical costs.

Short stay patients — In-patients admitted for 48 hours or less, or outpatients who stay 24 hours or less.

Sick baby — An infant with medical complications not resulting from premature birth.

Simple repair — Is performed when the wound is superficial, e.g., involving partial or full thickness damage to the skin and/or subcutaneous tissues. There is no significant involvement of deeper structures and only simple, primary suturing is required.

Skeletal traction — The application of a force to a limb segment through a wire, pin, screw, or clamp attached to bone.

Skin traction — The application of a force to a limb using felt or strapping applied directly to skin only.

Small subscriber group aggregate — An aggregate of professional associations, small business, or other entities formed to be considered a single, large subscriber group.

SNF — Skilled nursing facility. A facility that cares for long-term patients with acute medical needs.

Specimen — Tissue submitted for individual and separate attention, requiring individual examination and pathologic diagnosis.

SSN — Social security number.

Staff model — An HMO that employs its own providers.

Standard anesthesia formula — Reimbursement formula that consists of basic value (units) + time units + modifying units (e.g., physical status and qualifying circumstances) + other allowed unit/charges. An abbreviation is B + T + M (basic + time + modifying circumstances). The formula may also include O (other) for other allowed unit charges.

Starred procedure — Identified surgical procedures in the CPT book.

Stat charge — A charge for expeditious test results.

State insurance commission — The state group that approves insurance certificates for each state and regulate the industry based on statutes.

Steering — The act of providing financial incentives to members to use the managed care provider panel.

Stop loss — A form of reinsurance that protects health insurance above a certain limit and minimizes risks for providers.

Subrogation — Recovery of monies or benefits from a third party who is liable for the payment.

Subsidiary "In Addition To" codes — Services not included as part of the primary procedure. Key phrases are used throughout the CPT book to indicate that a code is to be used "in addition" to the primary code. Phrases that help identify subsidiary codes include, but are not limited to: each additional, list in addition to, and done at time of other major procedure.

Substantial co-morbidity — A pre-existing condition that will, because of its presence with a specific principle diagnosis, cause an increase in the length of stay by at least one day in approximately 75 percent of the cases.

Substantial complication — A condition that arises during the hospital stay that prolongs the length of stay by at least one day in approximately 75 percent of the cases.

Subtraction — The removal of an overlying structure in order to better visualize the structure in question. This is done in a series by imposing one x-ray on top of another.

Supplemental health services — Benefits HMOs offer in addition to base services.

Surgical package — A normal, uncomplicated performance of specific surgical services, with the assumption that on average, all surgical procedures of a given type are similar with respect to skill-level, duration, and length of normal follow-up care.

Swing beds — Hospital beds designated to serve varying needs, depending on census. This is usually done to convert acute care beds to long-term care to meet a rural community's needs.

TCC — Transitional care center. Used in lieu of extended care facility or prior to discharge to an extended care facility.

Technical component — a part of a radiology service that includes the provision of the equipment, supplies, technical personnel, and costs attendant to the performance of the procedure other than the professional services.

TEFRA — Tax Equity and Fiscal Responsibility Act. An act that protects the rights of full-time employees to remain on the company's plan to age 69.

Tertiary care facility — A hospital providing specialty care to patients referred from other hospitals because of the severity of their injuries or illnesses.

Therapeutic — An act meant to alleviate a medical or mental condition.

Therapeutic procedures — A manner of effecting change through the application of clinical skills and/or services that attempt to improve function.

Therapeutic services — Are performed for treatment of a specific diagnosis. These services include performance of the procedure, various incidental elements, and normal, related follow-up care.

Third party payer — Payer responsible for claims paid by a health plan or member for claims incurred for which the health plan or member should not have primary liability.

Three-digit diagnostic codes — Are used only when no fourth or fifth digit is available. There are only about 100 codes at the highest level of specificity in the three-digit form. Many payers, including Medicare, do not accept three-digit codes when higher levels of specificity exist.

Time limit — Set number of days in which a claim can be filed.

TPA — Third party administrator. A firm that performs administrative functions for a self-funded plan but assumes no risk.

TPL — The third party payer liable for the cost of an illness or injury, such as auto or homeowner insurer.

TQM — Total quality management. The concept that quality is an organic part of a plan's service and a provider's care and can be quantified and constantly improved.

Transfer — Movement of a patient from one treatment service or location to another.

Treatment plan — The plan of care submitted by the provider to the case manager when seeking certification for a member.

Triage — 1) Medical screening of patients to determine priority of treatment based on severity of illness or injury and resources at hand; 2) Charge levied by health care facilities for emergency and other patients.

Triple option — The offering of an HMO, indemnity plan, and PPO by one insurance firm.

UB-92 — The common claim form used by facilities to bill for services.

UCR — Usual, customary, and reasonable. The prevailing fees for services in a given geographical area.

Unbundling — Breaking a single service into its multiple components to increase total billing charges.

Underwriting — Evaluating and determining the financial risk a member or member group will have on an insurer.

Unlisted procedures — Procedural descriptions in each section of the CPT book used when the overall procedure and outcome of the surgery is not adequately described by an existing CPT code. Use unlisted procedures as a last resort in finding an appropriate CPT code.

Unspecified — A term in ICD-9-CM that indicates more information is necessary to code the term to further specificity. In these cases, the fourth digit of the code is always 9. Fourth digits 0 through 7 identify more specific information of the main term or condition. The fourth-digit number 8 is reserved for identifying other information.

Upcoding — Provider billing for a procedure that reimburses more than the procedure actually performed.

UPIN — Unique physician identification number.

URAC — Utilization Review Accreditation Commission. The accrediting body of case management.

Urgent admission — An admission in which the patient requires immediate attention for treatment of a physical or psychiatric problem.

USP — United States Pharmacopeia.

USPHS — United States Public Health Service.

Utilization review — Review of the utilization of medical services based on the diagnosis, site, ALOS, and other factors in each case.

Utilization review nurse — A nurse who evaluates cases for appropriateness of care and length of service and can plan discharge and services needed after discharge in home health appointments.

V codes — ICD-9-CM codes also known as The Supplementary Classification of Factors Influencing Health Status and Contact with Health Services

(V01—V82), V codes describe circumstances that influence a patient's health status and identify reasons for medical encounters resulting from circumstances other than a disease or injury already classified in the main part of ICD-9-CM.

Volume — 1) The number of services performed; 2) the number of patients; 3) The number of patients in a DRG during a specific time.

Weighting — The practice of assigning more worth to a fee based on the number of times it is charged, "weighting" the RBRVS fees for an area.

Well-baby care — Medical services, immunizations, and regular provider visits considered routine for an infant.

Withhold — Percentage of payment to providers held by HMO until cost of referral or services has been determined. If the provider goes over the amount determined appropriate, that amount is kept by the HMO.

Workers Compensation — Laws requiring employers to furnish care to employees injured on the job.

Wraparound plan — Insurance or health plan coverage for copays and deductibles not covered under a member's base plan.

Abbreviations, Acronyms, & Symbols

The acronyms, abbreviations, and symbols used by health care providers speed communications. The following list includes the most often seen acronyms, abbreviations, and symbols. In some cases, abbreviations have more than one meaning. Multiple interpretations are separated by a slash (/). Abbreviations of Latin phrases are punctuated.

<	less than
>	greater than
@	at
A	assessment/blood type
a (ante)	before
a fib	atrial fibrillation
a flutter	atrial flutter
A2	aortic second sound
a.a.	of each
AA	Alcoholics Anonymous
AAHP	American Association of Health Plans
AAL	anterior axillary line
AAMT	American Association for Medical Transcription
AAPCC	adjusted average per capita cost
AAPPO	American Association of Preferred Provider Organizations
AAROM	active assistive range of motion
ab	abortion
AB	blood type
abd	abdomen
ABE	acute bacterial endocarditis
ABG	arterial blood gas
abn.	abnormal
ABO	referring to ABO incompatibility
abs. fev.	without fever
a.c.	before eating
ACD	absolute cardiac dullness
ACE	angiotensin converting enzyme/adrenal cortical extract
ACL	anterior cruciate ligament
ACLS	advanced cardiac life support
ACP	acid phosphatase
ACR	adjusted community rating
acq.	acquired
ACSW	Academy of Certified Social Workers
ACTH	adrenocorticotropic hormone
ACVD	acute cardiovascular disease
ad lib	as desired, at pleasure
ad part. dolent.	to the aching parts
a.d.	right ear/to, up to
ad. us. ext.	for external use
ADA	American Dental Association, or Americans with Disabilities Act
ADH	antidiuretic hormone
ad. hib.	to be administered
ADL	activities of daily living
ad. lib.	as desired
adm	admission, admit
ADM	alcohol, drug or mental disorder
ADP	adenosine diphosphate
ADS	alternative delivery system
adst. feb.	when fever is present
AE	above the elbow
AF	atrial fibrillation
AFB	acid fast bacilli
A/G	albumin-globulin ratio
ag. feb.	when the fever increases
AGA	appropriate (average) for gestational age
AgNO3	silver nitrate
AHA	American Hospital Association
AHC	alternative health care
AHIMA	American Health Information Management Association
AHP	accountable health plan

AI	aortic insufficiency	APC	Ambulatory Payment Classification
AICD	automatic implant cardioverter defibrilator	APM	arterial pressure monitoring
AID	artificial insemination donor/acute infectious disease	approx	approximately
		appy.	Appendectomy
AIDS	acquired immunodeficiency syndrome	APT	admissions per thousand
		aq.	water (aqua)
AIH	artificial insemination by husband	ARC	AIDS-related complex
AK	above the knee	ARD	Acute respiratory disease
AKA	above knee amputation	ARDS	adult respiratory distress syndrome
ALA	aminolevulinic acid	ARF	acute respiratory/renal failure
alb. (albus)	white	AROM	active range of motion/artificial rupture of membranes
alk. phos.	alkaline phosphatase		
ALL	acute lymphocytic leukemia	art.	artery, arterial
ALOS	average length of stay	AS	aortic stenosis/ arteriosclerosis
ALP	alkaline phosphatase	a.s.	left ear
ALS	advanced life support	ASAP	as soon as possible
ALT	alanine aminotransferase	ASC	ambulatory surgery center
alt. dieb.	every other day	ASCVD	arteriosclerotic cardiovascular disease
alt. hor.	every other hour		
alt. noc.	every other night	ASCX12N	American Standard Committee standard for claims and reimbursement
a.m.	morning		
ama	against medical advice		
AMA	American Medical Association	ASD	atrial septal defect
amb	ambulate	ASHD	arteriosclerotic heart disease
AMCRA	American Managed Care and Review Association	ASO	administrative services only
		ASR	age/sex rate
AMGA	American Medical Group Association	Asst	assistance (min= minimal; mod= moderate)
AMI	acute myocardial infarction	AST	aspartate aminotransferase
AML	acute myelogenous leukemia	ATP	adenosine triphosphate
AMML	acute myelomonocytic leukemia	a.u.	each ear, both ears
AMP	adenosine monophosphate/ampule	AUR	ambulatory utilization review
ANA	American Nursing Association, or antinuclear antibodies	A-V	arteriveneous
		AV	atrioventricular
ANS	autonomic nervous system	AVF	arteriovenous fistula
ANSI	American National Standards Institute	AWP	average wholesale price
		ax	auxiliary
ANSI/HISB	ANSI Health Information Standards Board	AZT	azidothymidine
		Ba	barium
ant	anterior	bal.	bath
AOD	arterial occlusive disease	B&B	bowel and bladder
AODM	adult onset diabetes mellitus	BB	blow bottles
A&P	auscultation and percussion	BBA	Balanced Budget Act of 1997
A-P	anterior posterior	BBB	bundle branch block
Ap	apical	BCC	basal cell carcinoma
AP	antepartum/anterior-posterior	BCP	birth control pill

BE	barium enema/below the elbow	caps.(capsula)	capsule
BI	biopsy	CAT	computerized axial tomography
bib.	drink	cath	catheterize
BICROS	bilateral routing of signals	CBC	complete blood count
b.i.d.	two times a day	CBR	complete bed rest
b.i.n.	twice a night	cc	chief complaint
b.i.s.	twice	CCPD	continuous cycling peritoneal dialysis
BK	below the knee		
BKA	below knee amputation	CCU	coronary care unit
BLS	basic life support	CDC	Centers for Disease Control
BM	bowel movement	CDH	congenital dislocation of hip
BMR	basal metabolic rate	CE	cardiac enlargement
BMT	bone marrow transplant	CEA	carcinoembryonic antigen
BO	body order	CF	cystic fibrosis
BOW	bag of water	CH,Chol	cholesterol
BP	blood pressure	CHAMPUS	Civilian Health and Medical Program of the Uniformed Services
BPD	bronchopulmonary displasia		
BPH	benign prostatic hypertrophy	CHD	congenital heart disease/congestive heart disease
Br	breastfeeding		
BrC	breast care	CHF	congestive heart failure
BRM	biological response modifier	chgd	changed
BRP	bathroom privileges/bathroom, private	chr.	chronic
		CI	confidence interval/chloride
BS	bachelor of surgery/breath sounds/bowel sounds	CIS	carcinoma in situ
		cl liqs	clear liquids
BSA	body surface area	CLC	creative living center
BSC	bedside commode	CLD	chronic lung disease/chronic liver disease
BSD	bedside drainage		
BUN	blood urea nitrogen	CLL	chronic lymphatic leukemia
BUR	back-up rate (ventilator)	c/m	counts per minute
BUS	Bartholin urethra skenes	c.m.	tomorrow morning
bx	biopsy	cm	centimeter
C&S	culture and sensitivity	cm2	square centimeters
C	centigrade/complements/cervical vertebrae	CMC	carpometacarpal
		CMG	cystometrogram
c	with	CMHC	community mental health center
C-collar	cervical collar	CML	chronic myelogenous leukemia
CA	cancer	CMP	competitive medical plan
Ca	calcium/cancer	CMRI	cardiac magnetic resonance imaging
CABG	coronary artery bypass graft		
CAC	Certified Alcoholism Counselor	CMS	circulation motion sensation
CAD	coronary artery disease	CMV	cytomegalovirus
Cap	Capitation	cn	cranial nerves
CAPD	continuous ambulatory peritoneal dialysis	c.n.	tomorrow night
		CNM	certified nurse midwife

CNP	continuous negative airway pressure	CTZ	chemoreceptor trigger zone
		cu	cubic
CNS	central nervous system	CV	cardiovascular
co	cardiac output	CVA	cerebral vascular accident/cerebrovascular accident/costovertebral angle
c/o	complaints of		
CO2	carbon dioxide		
COA	certificate of authority	CVD	cardiovascular disease, cerebrovascular disease
COB	coordination of benefits		
COBRA	Consolidated Omnibus Budget Reconciliation Act	CVI	chronic venous insufficiency
		CVL	central venous line
COC	certificate of coverage	CVMS	clean voided midstream urine
COLD	chronic obstructive lung disease	CVP	central venous pressure
CON	certificate of need	CVU	cerebrovascular unit
conc.	concentration	CW	closed ward
cont.	continue	CXR	chest x-ray
COPD	chronic obstructive pulmonary disease	CXy	chest x-ray
		cysto	cystoscopy
CP	cerebral palsy	D	day/diopter
CPAP	continuous positive airway pressure	DAW	dispense as written
		D&C	dilation and curettage
CPHA	Commission on Professional and Hospital Activities	D/C	discharge/discontinue
		dc	discontinue
CPB	cardiopulmonary bypass	DC	dual choice
CPD	cephalopelvic disproportion	DCid	discharged/discontinued
CPK	creatine phosphokinase	DCA	deferred compensation administrator
CPM	continuous passive motion		
CPR	cardiopulmonary resuscitation, or computer-based patient record	DCI	duplicate coverage inquiry
		DCR	dacrocytstorhinostomy
CPT	chest physical therapy	DD	down drain
CPT	Physicians' Current Procedural Terminology	DDST	Denver Developmental Screening Test
		DE	dose equivalent
CQI	Continuous Quality Improvement	decem	ten
CR	carrier replacement	decub.	decubitus ulcer/lying down
CR	creatine	def.	deficient, deficiency
CRC	community rating by class	del	delivery
CRF	chronic renal failure	dep.	dependent
CRH	corticotropic releasing hormone	det.	let it be given
crit.	hematocrit		
CROS	contralateral routing of signals	DEXA	dual energy x-ray absorptiometry
CRP	C-reactive protein	dexter, dextra	the right
C/S	cesarean section	DHEA	dehydroepiandrosterone
CS	central service	DHHS	Department of Health and Human Services
CSF	cerebrospinal fluid		
CT	computerized tomography/corneal thickness/ carpal tunnel syndrome	DHT	dihydrotestosterone
		DIC	disseminated intravascular coagulopathy
CTLSO	cervical-thoracic-lumbar-sacral-orthosis		

DIF	direct immunofluorescence	ead.	the same
dim.	divide in half	EAP	employee assistance program
disp	disposition	EBL	estimated blood loss
DJD	degenerative joint disease	EBV	Epstein-Barr virus
DKA	diabetic ketoacidosis	ECCE	extracapsular cataract extraction
DM	diabetes mellitus	ECF	extended care facility, extracellular fluid
DMD	Duchenne muscular dystrophy		
DME	durable medical equipment	ECG	electrocardiogram
DNA	deoxyribonucleic acid	ECHO	enterocytopathogenic human orphan virus/echocardiogram
DNP	do not publish		
DNR	do not resuscitate	ECMO	extracorporeal membrane oxygenation
DNS	do not show	ECT	electro-convulsive therapy/emission computerized tomography
DO	Doctor of Osteopathy		
DOA	dead on arrival		
DOB	date of birth	ectopic	ectopic pregnancy (OB)
doc.	doctor	ED	emergency department/effective dose
DOE	dyspnea on exertion		
DOH	Department of Health	EDC	estimated date of confinement/ expected date of confinement
DOS	date of service	EDI	electronic data interchange
DPR	drug price review	EEG	electroencephalogram
DPT	days per thousand	EENT	eye, ear, nose, and throat
DPT	diphtheria - pertussis - tetanus	EGA	estimated gestational age
D/R	dayroom	EGD	esophagus, stomach and duodenum
DR	delivery room		
dr.	dram	EKG	electrocardiogram
Dr	doctor	E/M	evaluation and management
DRG	diagnosis related group	EMG	electromyogram
Dsg	dressing	e.m.p.	as directed
DSM-IV	Diagnostic and Statistical Manual of the American Psychiatric Association's Task Force on Terminology, Fourth Edition	en	an enema, a clyster
		en bloc	in total
		eng.	engorged
DSS	dioctyl sulfosoccinate	ENG	electronystagmogram
DTs	delirium tremens	ENT	ear, nose, and throat
DTRs	deep tendon reflexes	EO	elbow orthosis
DUE	drug use evaluation	EOB	explanation of benefits
duo	two	EOG	electrooculography
duodecim.	twelve	EOI	evidence of insurability
dur. dolor.	while pain lasts	EOM	end of month
DUR	drug utilization review	EOM	extraocular motion
DVT	deep vein thrombosis	EOMB	explanation of Medicare benefits
D/W	dextrose in water	EOMI	extraocular motion intact
dx	diagnosis	EOP	external occipital protuberance
DX	diagnosis code	EOY	end of year
dz	disease	Epis.	episiotomy
		EPO	epoetin alfa

EPO	exclusive provider organization	fluro	fluoroscopy
EPS	electrophysiologic stimulation	FM	face mask
EPSDT	early periodic screening, diagnosis and treatment	f.m.	make a mixture
		FME	full-mouth extraction
ER	emergency room	FMG	fine mesh gauze
ERC	endoscopic retrograde cholangiography	FNP	family nurse practitioner
		FOD	free of disease
ERCP	endoscopic retrograde cholangiopancreatography	fort.	strong (fortis)
ERG	electroretinogram	FP	family planning/family practitioner
ERISA	Employee Retirement Income Security Act of 1974	FR	family relationship
		FRAT	free radical assay test
ESR	erythrocyte sedimentation rate	FSA	flexible spending account
ESRD	end stage renal disease	FSE	fetal scalp electrode
EST	electroshock therapy	FSH	follicle stimulating hormone
ESWL	extracorporeal shockwave lithotripsy	FTND	full term normal delivery
		FTSG	full thickness skin graft
et	and	FTT	failure to thrive
ET	endotracheal	F/U	follow-up
ETG	episode treatment group	FUO	fever of unknown origin
ETOH	alcohol	FVC	forced vital capacity
EVR	evoked visual response	fx	fracture
Ex	examination	fxBB	fracture, both bones
exc	excise	G	gram
ext.	extremity	GA	gastric analysis
extr.	extract	gav.	gavage
F (on OB)	firm	GB	gallbladder
F	Fahrenheit/female	GDM	gestational diabetes mellitus
FAS	fetal alcohol syndrome	GFR	glomerular filtration rate
FB (fb)	fingerbreadth	GH	growth hormone
FB	foreign body	GHAA	Group Health Association of America
FBR	foreign body removal		
FBS	fasting blood sugar	GI	gastrointestinal
FDP	fibrin degradation products	GIFT	gamete intrafallopian transfer
Fe	female/iron	GLC	gas liquid chromatography
FEV	forced expiratory volume	Gly. supp.	glycerin suppository
FFP	fresh frozen plasma	GMP	guanosine monophosphate
FFS	fee for service equivalency	GNID	gram-negative intracellular diplocci
FFS	fee for service reimbursement	GnRH	gonadotropin-releasing hormone
FH	family history	GP	general practitioner
FHR	fetal heart rate	gr.	grain
FHT	fetal heart tone	grav	number of pregnancies
FI	firm one finger down from umbilicus	GS	general surgeon
		GSR	galvanic skin response
fl	fluid	gsw	gunshot wound
FLK	funny looking kid	gt./gtt.	drop/drops

GU	genitourinary		HHA	home health agency
Gu	guiac		HHS	Department of Health and Human Services
GxT	graded exercise test			
gyn	gynecology		HIAA	Health Insurance Association of America
H	hertel measurement			
h (hora)	hour		HIAA	hydroxyindolacetic acid
H2O	water		Hib	Hemophilus influenzae vaccine
H2O2	hydrogen peroxide		HIPAA	Health Insurance Portability and Accountability Act of 1996
HA	headache/hearing aide		HIPC	health insurance purchasing cooperative
HAA	hepatitis antigen B			
HAAb	hepatitis antibody A		HIV	human immunodeficiency virus
HaAg	hepatitis antigen A		HLV	herpes-like virus
HAI	hemaglutination test		HMD	hyaline membrane disease
HAV	hepatitis A virus		HMO	health maintenance organization
HB	headbox/hepatitis B		HMS	hepatosplenomegaly
HBsAb	hepatitis surface antibody B		HNAD	hypersmolar nonacidotic diabetes
HBcAg	hepatitis antigen B		H.O.	house officer
HBD	hydroxybutyril dehydrogenase		HOB	head of bed
Hbg	hemoglobin		hor. decub.	at bedtime
HBO	hyperbaric oxygen		HORF	high output renal failure
HbO2	oxyhemoglobin		H&P	history and physical
HBP	high blood pressure		HPs	hot packs
HBsAg	hepatitis antigen B		HPF	high power field
HBV	hepatitis B vaccine		HPG	human pituitary gonadotropin
HCFA	Health Care Financing Administration. *See* CMS		HPI	history of present illness
			HPL	human placental lactogen
HCFA-1500	a universal billing form developed by HCFA		HPV	human papilloma virus
			HR	Harrington rod/heart rate/hour
HCG	human chorionic gonadotropin		hrt.	heart
HCl	hydrochloric acid		HRT	hormone replacement therapy
HCPCS	Healthcare Common Procedural Coding System		HS	heelstick/hour of sleep
			h.s.	at bedtime
HCPP	health care prepayment plan		HSA	health service agreement
Hct	hematocrit		HSBG	heelstick blood gas
Hctz	hydrochlorothiazide		HSG	hysterosalpingogram
HCVD	hypertensive cardiovascular disease		HSP	health service plan
HD	hip disarticulation		HSV	herpes simplex virus
h.d.	at bedtime		ht.	height
HDL	high-density lipoproteins		HTLV/III	human T-cell lymphotropic virus /three
HEDIS	Health Plan Employer Data and Information Set			
			HTN	hypertension
HEENT	head, eyes, ears, nose, and throat		HVA	homovanillic acid
HGH	human growth hormone		Hx	history
Hg/Hgb	hemoglobin		hypo	hypodermic injection
HH	hard of hearing		IA	intra-arterial

Abbreviations & Acronyms

IAB	intra-aortic balloon	I& O	intake and output
IABC	intra-aortic balloon counterpulsation	IOL	intraocular lens
		IOP	intraocular pressure
IABP	intra-aortic balloon pump	IP	intraperitoneal/interphalangeal
IBNR	incurred but not reported	IPA	individual practice association
IBS	irritable bowel syndrome	IPD	intermittent peritoneal dialysis
IBW	ideal body weight	IPPB	intermittent positive pressure breathing
IC	infant care		
ICAT	indirect Coombís test	IQ	intelligence quotient
ICCE	intracapsular cataract extraction	IRDS	idiopathic respiratory distress syndrome
ICD-9-CM	International Classification of Diseases, Ninth Revision, Clinical Modification	ISC	infant servo-control
		ISG	immune serum globulin
ICD-10	International Classification of Diseases, Tenth Revision	ISN	integrated service network
		IT	intrathecal administration
ICD-10-PCS	International Classification of Diseases, Tenth Revision, Procedural Coding System	ITP	idiopathic thrombocytopenia purpura
		IU	international units
ICF	intermediate care facility	IUD	intrauterine device
ICH	intracranial/cerebral hemorrhage	IV	intravenous
ICP	intracranial pressure	IVC	inferior vena cava, intravenous cholangiogram
ICS	intercostal space		
ICSH	interstitial cell stimulating hormone	IVF	in vitro fertilization
		IVH	intraventricular hemorrhage
ICU	intensive care unit	IVP	intravenous pyelogram
ID	infective dose	JCAHO	Joint Commission on Accreditation of Healthcare Organizations
I& D	incision and drainage		
Id31	radioactive iodine	JODM	juvenile onset diabetes mellitus
IDDM	insulin dependent diabetis mellitus	JVD	jugular venous distention
IDH	isocitric dehydrogenase	JVP	jugular venous pressure
IDM	infant of diabetic mother	K	potassium
Ig	immunoglobulin, gamma	Kcal	kilocalorie
IH	infectious hepatitis	KCL	potassium chloride
II	icteric index	kg	kilogram
IM	internal medicine/intramuscular/infectious mononucleosis	KJ	knee jerk
		KO	keep open/knee orthosis
IMC	intermediate care	KUB	kidneys, ureters, bladder
IME	independent medical evaluation	KVO	keep vein open
IMO	integrated multiple option	L	left/lumbar vertebrae
IMV	intermittent mandatory ventilation	L&A	light and accommodation
inc.	incision	LA	left atrium
indep	independent	LAD	left anterior descending
INF	inferior, infusion	lap.	laparotomy, laparoscopy
INH	inhalation solution	LAP	leucine aminopeptidase
INJ	injection	LAT	lateral
instill	instillation	LAV	lymphadenopathy associated virus

LAVH	laparascopic assisted vaginal hysterectomy	LS fusion	lumbar sacral fusion
LB	legbag	LSA	left sacrum anterior position
LBB	left bundle branch	LSB	left sternal border
LBBB	left bundle branch block	LSO	lumbar sacral orthosis
LBP	lower back pain	LT	left
LCP	licensed clinical psychologist	LTC	long term care
LCSW	licensed clinical social worker	lul	left upper lobe
LD	lethal dose	luq	left upper quadrant
LDH	lactate dehydrogenase	LV	left ventricle
LDL	low-density lipoproteins	L&W	living and well
LE	lower extremity/lupus erythematosis	lymphs	lymphocytes
		lytes	electrolytes
LEEP	loop electrocautery excision procedure	M	manifest refraction/male
		M1	mitral first sound
LGA	large for gestational age	M2	mitral second sound
LH	luteinizing hormone	MA1	volume respirator
LHF	left heart failure	MAC	maximum allowable cost
LHR	leukocyte histamine release	MAD	monoamine oxidase (inhibitor)
Li	lithium	man. prim.	first thing in the morning
lido	lidocaine	MAP	mean arterial pressure
liq.	solution (liquor)	MASER	microwave amplification by stimulated emission of radiation
LKS	liver, kidneys, spleen		
LLETZ	large loop excision of transformation zone of cervix of uterus	MAST	military antishock trousers
		MBC	minimum bactericidal concentration/maximum breathing capacity
LLL	left lower lobe		
LLQ	left lower quadrant	MBD	minimal brain dysfunction
LMD	local medical doctor	mcg	microgram
LML	left medio lateral position	MCH	mean corpuscular hemoglobin
LMN	lower motor neuron	MCHC	mean corpuscular hemoglobin concentration
LMP	last menstrual period		
LMS	left mentum anterior position (chin)	MCL	midclavicular line
		MCP	metacarpophalangeal
LMT	left mentum transverse position	MCR	modified community rating
LOA	leave of absence	MCT	mediastinal chest tube
LOC	level of consciousness/loss of consciousness	MCV	mean corpuscular volume
		MD	medical doctor
LOM	limitation of motion	MD	muscular dystrophy/myocardial disease/manic depression
LOP	left occiput posterior position		
LOS	length of stay	MDC	major diagnostic category
LOT	left occiput transverse position	MDD	manic-depressive disorder
LP	lumbar puncture	Mec	meconium
LPC	licensed professional counselor	MED	minimal effective dose
LPM	liters per minute	med/surg	Medical, surgical
LR	lactated Ringer's/log roll	Medigap	Medicare supplemental insurance
		meds	medications

Medsupp	Medicare supplemental insurance	N2O	nitrous oxide
mEq	milliequivalent	Na	sodium
mEq/l	milliequivalent per liter	NaCl	sodium chloride (salt)
MFD	minimum fatal dose	NAD	no appreciable disease
MFT	muscle function test	NAEHCA	National Association of Employers on Health Care Action
mg	milligram		
Mg	magnesium	NAHMOR	National Association of HMO Regulators
MHC	mental health clinic	NAIC	National Association of Insurance Commissioners
MH/CD	mental health/chemical dependency		
		NAT	nonaccidental trauma
MH/SA	mental health/substance abuse	NB	newborn
MI	myocardial infarction	NBICU	newborn intensive care unit
min	minimum, minimal, minute	NBT	nitroblue tetrazolium
misce.	miscellaneous	NCA	neurocirculatory asthenia
ML	midline	NCHS	National Center for Health Statistics
ml	milliliter		
MLC	midline catheter	NCPDP	National Council of Prescription Drug Programs
mm	millimeter		
mmHg	millimeters of mercury	NCPR	no cardiopulmonary resuscitation
MMPI	Minnesota Multiphasic Personality Inventory	NCQA	National Committee on Quality Assurance
MMRV	measles, mumps, rubella vaccine	NCR	no cardiac resuscitation
MOM	milk of magnesia	NCV	nerve conduction velocity
mono	monocyte/mononucleosis	NCVHS	National Committee on Vital Health Statistics
mor. dict.	in the manner directed		
MPD	maximum permissible dose	NDC	national drug code
MR	mitral regurgitation	NEC	necrotizing enterocolitis/not elsewhere classified
MRA	magnetic resonance angiography		
MRI	magnetic resonance imaging	neg.	negative
mRNA	messenger RNA	NF	National Formulary
MS	morphine sulfate/multiple sclerosis	NG	nasogastric
MSHJ	medical staff hospital joint venture	NGU	nongonococcal urethritis
MSLT	multiple sleep latency testing	NIDDM	non-insulin dependent diabetes mellitus
MSO	management service organization	NJ	nasojejunal
MSS	medical social services	NKA	no known allergies
MSW	masterís in social work	NKMA	no known medical allergies
MTD	right eardrum	NNR	new and nonofficial remedies
MTM	metamucil	noc.	Night
MTP	metatarsophalangeal	Non-par	Non-participating provider
MTS	left eardrum	NOS	not otherwise specified
multip.	multipara - pregnant woman who has more than one child	novem.	nine
		NP	neuropsychiatry/nurse practitioner
MVP	mitral valve prolapse	NPA	national prescription audit
MWS	Mickety-Wilson syndrome	NPA	Non-par approved
N	nitrogen		

NP-CPAP	nasopharyngeal continuous positive airway pressure
NPN	Non-par Not Approved/nonprotein nitrogen
n.p.o.	nothing by mouth
NPRM	Notice of Proposed Rule Making
npt	normal pressure and temperature
NS	normal saline/not significant
NSAID	nonsteroidal anti-inflammatory drug
NSD	nominal standard dose
NSR	normal sinus rhythm
NST	nonstress test
NSVB	normal spontaneous vaginal bleeding
NSVD	normal spontaneous vaginal delivery
NT	nasotracheal/nontender
NTE	neutral thermal environment
NTP	normal temperature and pressure
NUBC	National Uniform Billing Commission
N&V	nausea and vomiting
nyd	not yet diagnosed
o	no information
O	blood type/oxygen
O2	oxygen
OA	open access
OA	osteoarthritis
OAG	open angle glaucoma
OB	obstetrics
OB-GYN	obstetrics and gynecology
OC	open crib/oral contraceptive/ office call
OCT	ornithine carbamyl transterase/oxytocin challenge test
octo.	eight
o.d.	right eye
OFC	occipitofrontal circumference
oint	ointment
OJ	orange juice
o.m.	every morning/otitis media
omn. hor.	every hour
OMS	oralmaxillary surgery
OMT	osteopathic manipulation therapy
o.n.	every night
ONH	optic nerve head

OOA	out-of-area
OOB	out of bed
OOPs	out-of-pocket costs/expenses
O&P	ova and parasites
OPD	outpatient department
OPG	oculoplethysmography
ophth	ophthalmology
OPV	oral polio vaccine
OR	operating room
ORIF	open reduction internal fixation
ortho.	orthopedics
o.s.	left eye
os, oris	mouth
OSA	obstructive sleep apnea
OSHA	Occupational Safety and Health Administration
OST	oxytocin stress test
OT	occupational therapy
OTC	over-the-counter
OTD	organ tolerance dose
OTH	other routes of administration
o.u.	each eye, both eyes
ov.	ovum/office visit
OW	open ward
oz.	ounce
P	plan/after/pulse, phosphorus
P2	pulmonic 2nd sound
P& A	percussion and auscultation
P&T	pharmacy and therapeutics
PA	physician assistant/posteroanterior/pulmonary artery
PAB	premature atrial beats
PAC	pre-admission certification
PAC	premature atrial contraction
PACU	post anesthesia care unit
PAD	pulmonary artery diastolic
PAH	para-aminohippurate
PAP	Papanicolaou test or smear/pulmonary artery pressure
Par	participating provider
PAR	post anesthesia recovery/parenteral
para	along side of/number of pregnancies, as para 1, 2, 3, etc
PARR	post anesthesia recovery room
part. vic.	in divided doses

PAT	paroxysmal atrial tachycardia	PMG	primary medical group
path	pathology	PMHx	past medical history
PBI	protein-bound iodine	PMI	point of maximum intensity
PC	packed cells	PMPM	per member per month
p.c.	after eating	PMPY	per member per year
PCA	patient controlled analgesia	PMN	polymorphonuclear neutrophil leukocytes
PCD	polycystic disease		
PCG	phonocardiogram	PMS	premenstrual syndrome
PCN	penicillin	PNC	premature nodal contraction
PCN	primary care network	PND	paroxysmal nocturnal dyspnea/ post nasal drip
PCP	primary care physician		
PCPM	per contract per month	PNS	peripheral nervous system
PCR	physician contingency reserve/polymerase chain reaction	p/o	by mouth
		PO	(per os) by mouth/post operative
PCTA	percutaneous transluminal angioplasty	POD	post operative day
		polys	polymorphonuclear neutrophil leukocytes
PCV	packed cell volume		
PCW	pulmonary capillary wedge	POR	problem oriented record
PD	postural drainage/Parkinsonís disease	POS	place of service/point of service/point of sale
PDA	patent ductus arteriosus	pos.	positive
PE	physical examination/pulmonary embolism/pulmonary edema	post. cib.	after meals
		post or PM	postmortem exam or autopsy
PEC	pre-existing condition	PP	postprandial
Peds	pediatrics	p.p.	near point of visual accommodation
PEG	pneumoencephalogram		
PEN	parenteral and enteral nutrition	P+PD	percussion & postural drainage
PENS	percutaneous electrical nerve stimulation	PPD	percussion and postural drainage
		PPH	post partum hemorrhage
PERRLA	pupils equal, regular, reactive to light and accommodation	PPO	preferred provider organization
		PPP	protamine paracoagulation
PET	positron emission tomography	PPRC	physician payment review commission
PFC	persistent fetal circulation		
PFT	pulmonary function test	p.r.	far point of visual accommodation/through the rectum
PG	prostaglandin		
PH	past history	pr	per return
PharmD	Doctor of Pharmacy	PRBC	packed red blood cells
ph	potential of hydrogen	PREs	progressive resistive exercises
PHO	physician-hospital organization		
PI	present illness	preg	pregnant
PICC	peripherally inserted central catheter	previa	placenta previa
		primip	primipara - a woman having her first child
PID	pelvic inflammatory disease		
pk.	pack	p.r.n.	as needed for
PKU	phenylketonuria	PRO	professional (or peer) review organization
p.m.	after noon		
		PROM	premature rupture of membranes

ProPAC	prospective payment assessment commission	RATx	radiation therapy
		RBB	right bundle branch
PSA	prostate specific antigen	RBBB	right bundle branch block
PSP	phenolsulfonphthalein	RBC	red blood cell
PsyD	Doctor of Psychology	RBOW	ruptured bag of water
PT	physical therapy/prothrombin time	RBRVS	resource based relative value scale
Pt	patient/prothrombin time	RCD	relative cardiac dullness
PTA	prior to admission/percutaneous transluminal angioplasty	RDS	respiratory distress syndrome
		REM	rapid eye movement
PTB	patellar tendon bearing (cast)	RESA	radial cryosurgical ablation
PTCA	percutaneous transluminal coronary angioplasty	resp	respiration, respiratory
		Retro	retrospective rate derivation
PTH	parathyroid hormone	rev.	revise, revision
PTT	partial thromboplastin time	RFP	request for proposal
PUD	peptic ulcer disease	Rh	Rhesus
pulv.	powder	Rh neg	Rhesus factor negative
PVC	premature ventricular contraction	RHD	rheumatic heart disease
PVD	premature ventricular depolarization	RHF	right heart failure
		RIA	radioimmunoassay
PVL	paraventricular leukomalasia	RL	Ringer's lactate
Px	prognosis	RLE	right lower extremity
PZI	protamine zinc insulin	RLF	rentrolental fibroplasia
Q.	every	RLL	right lower lobe
q.2h	every two hours	rlq	right lower quadrant
QA	quality assurance	RMA	right mentum anterior position
q.a.m.	every morning	RMC	rating method code
q.d.	every day	RML	right middle lobe
q.h.	every hour	RMP	right mentum posterior position
q.h.s.	every night	RMT	right mentum transverse position
q.i.d.	four times daily	RN	registered nurse
QM	quality management	RNA	ribonucleic acid
QMB	qualified Medicare beneficiary	R/O	rule out
q.n.	every night	ROA	right occiput anterior position
qns	quantity not sufficient	ROM	range of motion
q.o.d.	every other day	ROP	right occiput posterior position
q.q.h.	every four hours	ROS	review of systems
qs	quantity sufficient	RPG	retrograde pyelogram
quattour	four	RPR	venereal disease report
quicdecem	fifteen	RR	recovery room
quinque	five	RRA	registered record administrator
quotid	daily	R,R,& E	round, regular, and equal
R	respiration/right atrium	RRR	regular rate and rhythm
r	roentgen units (x-rays)	RS	reducing substances
R&C	reasonable and customary	RSV	respiratory syncytial virus
RA	rheumatoid arthritis		

RT	recreational therapist/respiratory therapist/resting tracing/right	SOAP	subjective objective assessment plan
RTC	return to clinic	SOB	shortness of breath
RUL	right upper lobe	sol.	solution
ruq	right upper quadrant	SOP	standard operation procedure
RV	right ventricle	S.O.S.	if necessary (si opus sit)
Rx	take (prescription; treatment)	S/P	status post
RxN	reaction	SPD	summary plan description
s	without	SPIN	standard prescriber identification number
S& A	sugar and acetone		
SAH	subarachnoid hemorrhage	SpGr	specific gravity
SALT	serum alanine aminotransferase	SQ	status quo/subcutaneous
SAST	serum aspartate aminotransferase	SROM	spontaneous rupture of membranes
SB	sinus bradycardia	ss	half
SBFT	small bowel follow through	SSE	soap suds enema
s.c.	subcutaneous	ST	sinus tachycardia
S-C disease	sickle cell hemoglobin-c disease	staph	staphylococcus
SCI	spinal cord injury	stat	immediately
SCR	standard class rate	STD	sexually transmitted disease
sed rate	sedimentation rate of erythrocytes	STH	somatotrophic hormone
SEM	systolic ejection murmur	strep	streptococcus
Seno supp	Senokot suppository	STS	serology test for syphilis
septem	seven	STSG	split thickness skin graft
sex	six	STU	skin test unit
SG	Swan-Ganz	subcu	subcutaneous
SGA	small for gestational age	subind.	immediately after
SGOT	serum glutamic oxaloacetic acid	supp	suppository
SH	social history	Sv	scalp vein
SHBG	sex hormone binding globulin	SVC	service
SIADH	syndrome of inappropriate antidiuretic hormone	SVCS	superior vena cava syndrome
		Sx	sign/symptom
SIC	standard industry code	T	temperature/tender/thoracic vertebrae
SIDS	sudden infant death syndrome		
Sig.	write on label (Rx) or let it be labelled	T3	triiodothyronine
		T4	thyroxine
Sig. S. (Signa)	mark or write	T&A	tonsils and adenoids
sine	without	TA	tension by applanation/transactional analysis
SISI	short increment sensitivity index		
s.l.	under the tongue, sublingual	tab.	tablet (tabella)
SLE	systemic lupus erythematosus	TAH	total abdominal hysterectomy
SMI	supplementary medical insurance program	TAT	tetanus antitoxin/turnaround time
		Tb	tubercule bacillus
SMO	slip made out	TB	tuberculosis
SNF	skilled nursing facility	TBA	to be arranged
SNS	sympathetic nervous system	TBG	thyroxine/thyroid binding globulin
		TBI	total body irradiation

TBSA	total body surface area	TSD	Tay-Sachs disease
T&C	type and crossmatch	TSE	testicular self-exam
TC&DB	turn, cough, and deep breathe	TSH	thyroid stimulating hormone
Td	tetanus	TSS	toxic shock syndrome
t.d.s.	three times a day	TTN	transient tachypnea of newborn
TEFRA	Tax Equity and Fiscal Responsibility Act	TULIP	transurethral ultrasound guided laser induced prostate
temp	temperature	TUR	transurethral resection
TENS	transcutaneous electrical nerve stimulation	TURP	transurethral resection of prostate
TEVAP	transurethral electrovaporization of prostate	TWE or Tap/ H₂O/E	tap water enema
		Tx	treatment
TFT	transfer factor test	U	unit
THA	total hip arthroplasty	U/A	urinalysis
Thal	Thalassemia	UAC	umbilical artery catheter/catheterization
THC	tetrahydrocannabinol		
TI	tricuspid insufficiency	UB-92	Uniform Billing Code of 1992
TIA	transient ischemic attack	U&C	usual and customary
TIBC	total iron binding capacity	UC	unit clerk
t.i.d.	three times daily	UCHD	usual childhood diseases
tinct	tincture	UCR	usual, customary and reasonable
TKA	total knee arthroplasty	UE	upper extremity
TM	tympanic membrane	UFR	uroflowmetry
TMJ	temporomandibular joint	UGI	upper gastrointestinal
TNS	transcutaneous nerve stimulator/stimulation	UM	unit manager/utilization management
TO	telephone order	UMN	upper motor neuron
TOA	tubo-ovarian abscess	ung.	ointment
TORCH	Toxoplasmosis, Other (includes syphilis), Rubella, Cytomegalo virus, and Herpes virus	unus.	One
		UPIN	universal physician identification number
TP	total protein		
TPA	third party administrator	UPP	urethra pressure profile
TPAL	term pregnancies, premature infants, abortions, living children	ur.	Urine
		UR	utilization review
TPN	total parenteral nutrition	URAC	utilization review accreditation commission
TPR	temperature, pulse, respiration		
Tr	tinctura, tincture/trace	URI	upper respiratory infection
TRAM	transverse rectus abdominos musculocutaneous	URN	utilization review nurse
		UR/QA	utilization review/quality assurance
trans	transverse	US	unstable spine/ultrasound
tres	three	ut dict.	as directed
TRF	thyrotropin releasing factor	UTI	urinary tract infection
TRH	thyrotropin releasing hormone	UV	ultraviolet light
tRNA	transfer ribonucleic acid	UVC	umbilical vein catheter
Ts	tension by Schiotz	V Fib	ventricular fibrillation
TSA	tumor specific antigen	V tach	ventricular tachycardia

Abbreviations & Acronyms

Va	visual acuity
VA	Veterans Administration
VBAC	vaginal birth after cesarean
VC	vena cava
VCG	vectorcardiogram
VD	venereal disease
VDH	valvular disease of the heart
VDRL	venereal disease report
VE	voluntary effort
VEP	visual evoked potential
VF	visual field/ventricular fibrillation
VHA	Volunteer Hospital Association
VIP	vasoactive intestinal peptide
Vit	vitamin (followed by specific letter)
VO	verbal order
VO2	maximum oxygen consumption
VP	vasopressin/voiding pressure
VPC	ventricular premature contraction
VPRC	volume of packed red cells
VS	vital signs/vesicular sound
VSD	ventricular septal defect
vv	veins
WAK	wearable artificial kidney
WB	whole blood
WBC	white blood count
WC	wheelchair
WCC	well child care
WD	well developed
W-D	wet to dry (dressings)
WEDI	workgroup for electronic data interchange
WHO	World Health Organization
w/HSBH	warmed heelstick blood gas
WLS	wet lung syndrome
WN	well nourished
WNL	within normal limits
Wt	weight
x	except
XM	cross match
Y-O	year-old
YTD	year-to-date
ZIFT	zygote intrafallopian transfer

Prefixes & Suffixes

The uniquely efficient language of medicine is possible thanks to the prefixes and suffixes attached to roots. Changing prefixes and suffixes allows subtle and overt changes in meaning of the terms. The following prefixes and suffixes are paired with their meanings.

....

Prefixes

Prefixes are one half of the medical language equation and are attached to the beginning of words. For example, the prefix "eu-," meaning good or well, combined with the Greek word for death, "thanatos," produces euthanasia — a good death.

a-, an-	without, away from, not
ab-	from, away from, absent
acro-	extremity, top, highest point
ad-	indicates toward, adherence to, or increase
adeno-	relating to a gland
adip-	relating to fat (*also* adipo-)
aero-	relating to gas or air
all-	meaning another, other, or different
allo-	indicates difference or divergence from the norm
ambi-	both sides; about or around (*also* amphi-)
an-	without
angi-	relating to a vessel
aniso-	dissimilar, unequal, or asymmetrical
ankylo-	bent, crooked, or two parts growing together
ante-	in front of, before
antero-	before, front, anterior
anti-	in opposition to, against
antro-	relating to a chamber or cavity
arch-	beginning, first, principal (*also* arche-, archi-)
archo-	relating to the rectum or anus
arterio-	relating to an artery
arthro-	relating to a joint
astro-	star-like or shaped
atelo-	incomplete or imperfect
auto-	relating to the self
axio-	relating to an axis (*also* axo-)
balano-	relating to the glans penis or glans clitoridis
baro-	relating to weight or heaviness
basi-	relating to the base or foundation (*also* basio-)
bi-	double, twice, two
blasto-	relating to germs
blenn-	relating to mucus (*also* blenno-)
blepharo-	relating to the eyelid
brachi-	relating to the arm (*also* brachio-)
brachy-	short
brady-	meaning slow or prolonged
broncho-	relating to the trachea
cac-	meaning diseased or bad (*also* caci-, caco-)
cardio-	relating to the heart
carpo-	relating to the wrist
cata-	down from, down, according to
celo-	indicating a tumor or hernia; cavity
cervico-	relating to the neck or neck of an organ
chilo-	relating to the lip (*also* cheilo-)
chole-	relating to the gallbladder
cleido-	relating to the clavicle
cyst-	relating to the urinary bladder or a cyst (*also* cysto-)
cyto-	in relation to cell
dacry-	pertaining to the lacrimal glands
dactyl-	relating to the fingers or toes
demi-	half the amount
desmo-	relating to ligaments
deuter-	secondary or second
dextro-	meaning on or to the right
dorsi-	relating to the back (*also* dorso-)
dys-	painful, bad, disordered, difficult
echo-	reverberating sound
ecto-	external, outside

ectro-	congenital absence of something	lith-	relating to a hard or calcified substance (*also* litho-)
endo-	within, internal		
entero-	relating to the intestines	lumbo-	relating to the loin region
epi-	on, upon, in addition to	macro-	meaning oversized, large
eu-	well, healthy, good, normal	mal-	bad, poor, ill
exo-	outside of, without	melano-	dark or black in color
fibro-	relating to fibers or fibrous tissue	meningo-	relating to membranes covering the brain and spine
galacto-	relating to milk		
gastro-	relating to the stomach and abdominal region ·	mesio-	toward the middle; secondary (*also* meso-)
genito-	relating to reproduction	meta-	indicates a change
gono-	relating to the genitals, offspring, origination	mis-	bad, improper
		my-	relating to muscle (*also* myo-)
gyn-	relating to the female gender	myc-	relating to fungus (*also* myco-)
hema-	relating to blood (*also* hemato-)	myelo-	relating to bone marrow or the spinal cord
hemi-	half		
hepato-	relating to the liver	narco-	indicates insensate condition or numbness
histo-	relating to tissue		
homeo-	indicates resemblance or likeness (*also* homo-)	necro-	indicates death or dead tissue
		nephr-	relating to the kidney
hydro-	relating to fluid, water, or hydrogen	noci-	relating to injury or pain
		nycto-	relating to darkness or night
hyper-	excessive, above, exaggerated	odont-	relating to the teeth
hypo-	below, less than, under	oligo-	indicates few or small
hyster-	relating to either the womb or hysteria (*also* hystero-)	omo-	relating to the shoulder
		omphalo-	relating to the navel
idio-	distinct or individual characteristics	onco-	relating to a mass, tumor, or swelling
ileo-	relating to the ileum (part of the small intestine)	onycho-	relating to the finger- or toenails
		oophor-	relating to the ovaries
ilio-	relating to the pelvis	opistho-	indicates behind or backwards
infra-	meaning inferior to, beneath, under	orchi-	relating to the testicles (*also* orchido-)
irid-	relating to the iris	oscheo-	relating to the scrotum
ischio-	relating to the hip	osteo-	having to do with bone
iso-	equal	oto-	relating to the ear
jejuno-	relating to the jejunum (part of the small intestine)	pachy-	indicates heavy, large, or thick
		pali-	repetition, back again, recurring (*also* palin-)
juxta-	next to, near		
karyo-	relating to the nucleus of a cell	panto-	indicates the whole or all
kerato-	relating to the cornea or horny tissue	para-	indicates near, similar, beside, or past
laparo-	flank, loins; operations through the abdominal wall	patho-	indicates sensitivity, feeling, or suffering
laryngo-	relating to the larynx	ped-	relating to the foot (*also* pedi-)
lien-	relating to the spleen	peri-	about, around, or in the vicinity
lip-	relating to fat (*also* lipo-)	pero-	indicates being maimed or deformed

phaco-	relating to the lens of the eye
phago-	relating to eating and ingestion
pharyngo-	relating to the pharynx
phlebo-	relating to the vein
phreno-	relating to the diaphragm; head or mind
pimel-	relating to fat
platy-	indicates wide or broad
pleio-	more, additional
pleur-	relating to the side or ribs
pneum-	relating to respiration, air, the lungs
pod-	relating to the feet (*also* podo-)
poly-	indicates much or many
procto-	relating to the rectum and/or anus
proso-	indicates toward the front, anterior, forward
pseudo-	indicates false or imagined
pulmo-	relating to the lungs and respiration
pyelo-	relating to the pelvis
pygo-	relating to the buttocks or rump
pyle-	relating to an opening/orifice of the portal vein
pyloro-	relating to the pylorus, the stomach opening into the duodenum
pyo-	relating to pus
pyreto-	indicates a fever, heat
rachi-	relating to the spine (*also* rachio-)
recto-	meaning straight or relating to the rectum
retro-	indicates behind, backward, in a reverse direction
rheo-	indicates a flow or stream of fluid
rhino-	relating to the nose
sacro-	relating to the sacrum, the base of the vertebral column
salpingo-	relating to the fallopian or eustachian tubes
sarco-	relating to flesh
scapho-	indicates deformed condition, shaped like a boat
scapulo-	relating to the shoulder
schisto-	indicates cleft or split; a fissure
scoto-	relating to darkness; visual field gap
sial-	relating to saliva

sinistro-	meaning on or to the left
somato-	relating to the body
spheno-	relating to the sphenoid bone at the base of the skull
sphygmo-	relating to the pulse
splanch-	relating to the intestines; viscera
steato-	relating to fat
stetho-	relating to the chest
stomato-	relating to the mouth
sym-	indicates together with, along with, beside
syn-	indicates being joined together
tachy-	indicates swift or fast
tarso-	relating to the foot; margin of the eyelid
teleo-	indicates complete or perfectly formed
teno-	relating to tendons
terato-	indicates being seriously deformed, esp. a fetus
thalamo-	relating to the thalamus, origin of nerves in the brain
thanato-	relating to death
thoraco-	relating to the chest
thrombo-	relating to blood clots
thymo-	relating to the thymus
toco-	relating to birth
trachelo-	relating to the neck
trichi-	relating to hair; hair-like shape (*also* tricho-)
tympano-	relating to the eardrum
typhlo-	relating to the cecum; relating to blindness
vaso-	relating to blood vessels
ventro-	relating to the abdomen; anterior surface of the body
vesico-	relating to the bladder
viscero-	relating to the abdominal organs
xeno-	relating to a foreign substance
xero-	indicates a dry condition

Suffixes

Suffixes are the other half of the equation. These are attached to the ends of words.

-agra	indicating severe pain
-algia	pain

Prefixes & Suffixes

-ase	denoting an enzyme	-rhage	indicates bleeding or other fluid discharge (*also* -rhagia)
-blast	incomplete cellular development		
-centesis	puncture	-rhaphy	indicates a suture or seam joining two structures
-cephal	having to do with the head		
-cle	meaning small or little (*also* -cule)	-rrhagia	indicates an abnormal or excessive fluid discharge
-cyte	having to do with cells	-rrhexis	splitting or breaking
-dactyl	having to do with fingers	-spasm	contraction
-desis	binding or fusion	-taxy	arrangement, grouping (*also* -taxis)
-ectomy	excision, removal		
-ferous	produces, causes, or brings about	-tomy	indicates a cutting
-fuge	drive out or expel	-trophy	relating to food or nutrition
-genic	indicates production, causation, generation	-tropic	indicates an affinity for or turning toward
-gram	drawn, written, and recorded	-tropism	responding to an external stimulus
-graphic	written or drawn		
-ia	state of being, condition (abnormal)		
-iasis	condition		
-itis	inflammation		
-lysis	release, free, reduction of		
-metry	scientific measurement		
-odynia	indicates pain or discomfort		
-oid	indicates likeness or resemblance		
-ology	study of		
-oma	tumor		
-orraphy	suturing		
-oscopy	to examine		
-osis	condition, process		
-ostomy	indicates a surgically created artificial opening		
-otomy	indicates a cutting		
-pagus	indicates fixed or joined together		
-pathic	indicates a feeling, diseased condition, or therapy		
-penia	indicates a deficiency; less than normal		
-pexy	fixation		
-philia	inordinate love of or craving for something		
-phobia	abnormal fear of or aversion to something		
-plasty	indicates surgically formed or molded		
-plegia	indicates a stroke or paralysis		
-poietic	indicates producing or making		
-praxis	indicates activity, action, condition, or use		

Procedural Eponyms

The medical custom of honoring a popular procedure's originator by name may prove to be problematic for the coder, who may have no trouble coding a Marshall-Marchetti but be faced with choosing one of the many Campbell procedures.

The following list includes most of the procedures described by eponym in the CPT® book.

Adson test
95870   Needle electromyography; limited study of muscles in one extremity or non-limb (axial) muscles (unilateral or bilateral), other than thoracic paraspinal, cranial nerve supplied muscles, or sphincters

Test provides a physiological assessment for thoracic outlet syndrome.

Albarran test
89365   Water load test

Test screens for colibacilluria, a bacteria found in the intestine.

Alexander's operation
58400   Uterine suspension, with or without shortening of round ligaments, with or without shortening of sacrouterine ligaments; (separate procedure)
58410   with presacral sympathectomy

Uteral displacement is repaired by shortening round ligaments.

Altemeier procedure
45130   Excision of rectal procidentia, with anastomosis; perineal approach

Procedure removes a rectal prolapse through a perineal approach (45130), or through a combined abdominal and perineal approach (45135).

Amussat's operation
44025   Colotomy, for exploration, biopsy(s), or foreign body removal

Long transverse incision is made to expose the colon.

Anderson tibial lengthening
27715   Osteoplasty, tibia and fibula, lengthening or shortening

Tibia is severed and screws are affixed to plates supporting the bone across the gap in this technique to lengthen the patient's leg.

Aries-Pitanguy mammaplasty
19318   Reduction mammaplasty

Procedure reduces breast size.

Babcock operation
37730   Ligation and division and complete stripping of long and short saphenous veins

Varicose veins are eliminated using a long probe and tying the end of the vein to it to draw out the vein by invagination.

Baldy-Webster operation
58400   Uterine suspension, with or without shortening of round ligaments, with or without shortening of sacrouterine ligaments; (separate procedure)

Ligaments may be used to correct displacement of the uterus.

Barany caloric test
92533   Caloric vestibular test, each irrigation (binaural, bithermal stimulation constitutes four tests)

Extent of nystagmus is determined by irrigating the external auditory meatus with either hot or cold water.

Bardenheurer operation
37616   Ligation, major artery (eg, post-traumatic, rupture); chest

Arterial fistula in the chest is repaired by ligation and sutures.

Barkan's operation
65820   Goniotomy

Technique corrects glaucoma by opening Schlemm's canal.

Barker operation
28120   Partial excision (craterization, saucerization, sequestrectomy, or diaphysectomy) bone (eg, osteomyelitis or bossing); talus or calcaneus

Process involves incision of the dorsal area of the foot.

Barr procedure
27691   Transfer or transplant of single tendon (with muscle redirection or rerouting); deep (eg, anterior tibial or posterior tibial through interosseous space, flexor digitorum longus, flexor hallucis longus, or peroneal tendon to midfoot or hindfoot)

Procedure corrects talipes equinovarus that may result from polio, and includes the anterior transfer of the tibialis posterior tendon.

Barsky's procedure
26580   Repair cleft hand

Cleft hand is repaired by closing the cleft, bringing the ring and index fingers closer together, and correcting webbing between the fingers.

Bassett's operation
56630   Vulvectomy, radical, partial;
56631   with unilateral inguinofemoral lymphadenectomy
56632   with bilateral inguinofemoral lymphadenectomy
56633   Vulvectomy, radical, complete;
56634   with unilateral inguinofemoral lymphadenectomy
56637   with bilateral inguinofemoral lymphadenectomy
56640   Vulvectomy, radical, complete, with inguinofemoral, iliac, and pelvic lymphadenectomy

Dissection of the inguinal glands for a radical resection of the vulva.

Batch-Spittler-McFaddin operation
27598   Disarticulation at knee

Leg is severed at the knee joint, which offers an alternative to severing a long bone.

Battle's operation
44950   Appendectomy;
44960   for ruptured appendix with abscess or generalized peritonitis

Rectus muscle is temporarily retracted in this appendectomy.

Bender-Gestalt test
96100   Psychological testing (includes psychodiagnostic assessment of personality, psychopathology, emotionality, intellectual abilities, eg, WAIS-R, Rorschach, MMPI) with interpretation and report, per hour

Psychological test gauges perceptual-motor coordination to assess personality dynamics, review organic brain impairment, and measure neurological maturity.

Benedict test for dextrose
81005   Urinalysis; qualitative or semiquantitative, except immunoassays

Test using sodium or potassium citrate and sodium carbonate in a reagent determines dextrose content of urine.

Bevan's operation
54640   Orchiopexy, inguinal approach, with or without hernia repair

Procedure brings an undescended testicle down into the scrotum.

Biesenberger mammaplasty
19318   Reduction mammaplasty

Reduction procedure uses transposition of the nipple with excision of the side of the mammary gland and rotation of the remaining glandular pedicle to form a skin brassiere.

Billroth operation
43631   Gastrectomy, partial, distal; with gastroduodenostomy

Anastomosis of the stomach to the duodenum or jejunum.

Binet test
96100   Psychological testing (includes psychodiagnostic assessment of personality, psychopathology, emotionality, intellectual abilities, eg, WAIS-R, Rorschach, MMPI) with interpretation and report, per hour

Test gauges mental capacity among children and youth using a standard series of questions gauged on the capacity of normal intellect among the same age groups.

Bohler reduction
28405   Closed treatment of calcaneal fracture; with manipulation

Traction method treats a closed fracture of the heelbone.

Bristow procedure

23460 Capsulorrhaphy, anterior, any type; with bone block

Anterior capsulorrhaphy prevents chronic separation of the shoulder. In this procedure the bone block is affixed to the anterior glenoid rim with a screw.

Brock's operation

33470 Valvotomy, pulmonary valve, closed heart; transventricular
33471   via pulmonary artery
33472 Valvotomy, pulmonary valve, open heart; with inflow occlusion
33474   with cardiopulmonary bypass
33476 Right ventricular resection for infundibular stenosis, with or without commissurotomy

Valvulotime passed through the wall of the right ventricle into the pulmonary artery assists in the relief of pulmonary valvular stenosis.

Browne's operation

54324 One stage distal hypospadias repair (with or without chordee or circumcision); with urethroplasty by local skin flaps (eg, flip-flap, prepucial flap)

Hypospadias is repaired with a strip of epithelium left on the top of the penis to form a top of the urethra. Margins of the incision are used to form the bottom.

Burgess amputation

27880 Amputation, leg, through tibia and fibula;

Long posterior flap is preserved to cover the incision to amputate the leg below the knee.

Burrow's operation

14000 Adjacent tissue transfer or rearrangement, trunk; defect 10 sq cm or less

Triangles of skin at the base of the pedicle of a skin flap are excised to achieve advancement.

Callander knee disarticulation

27598 Disarticulation at knee

Patella is removed and the long anterior and posterior skin flaps of the tibia are retained to enhance healing.

Carpue's operation

30400 Rhinoplasty, primary; lateral and alar cartilages and/or elevation of nasal tip

Nose is repaired by folding a flap from the forehead and pedicle at the root of the nose around the area to be repaired.

Chiari osteotomy

27156 Osteotomy, iliac, acetabular or innominate bone; with femoral osteotomy and with open reduction of hip

Top of the femur is altered to correct a dislocated hip caused by congenital conditions or cerebral palsy. A plate and screws are often used.

Cotting's operation

11765 Wedge excision of skin of nail fold (eg, for ingrown toenail)

Physician removes part of the toe and the ingrown part of the toenail.

Dana rhizotomy

63185 Laminectomy with rhizotomy; one or two segments

Posterior nerve roots of the spine are severed to relieve chronic pain or spasms.

Dandy ventriculocisternostomy

62200 Ventriculocisternostomy, third ventricle;

Operation establishes an opening from the third ventricle to the interpeduncular cistern.

Daviel's operation

66830 Removal of secondary membranous cataract (opacified posterior lens capsule and/or anterior hyaloid) with corneo-scleral section, with or without iridectomy (iridocapsulotomy, iridocapsulectomy)

Cataract is extracted through a corneal incision.

Day test

82270 Blood, occult, by peroxidase activity (eg, guaiac), qualitative; feces, 1-3 simultaneous determinations

Test determines presence of blood in the feces.

Delorme pericardiectomy

33030 Pericardiectomy, subtotal or complete; without cardiopulmonary bypass

Method excises a diseased pericardium constricting the ventricle.

Denonvillier's operation

14060 Adjacent tissue transfer or rearrangement, eyelids, nose, ears and/or lips; defect 10 sq cm or less

Defective nasal ala is corrected using a triangular flap from the opposite side of the nose.

Procedural Eponyms

Dunn arthrodesis
28725   Arthrodesis; subtalar

Procedure fuses talus in the foot.

Dupuy-Dutemp reconstruction
67971   Reconstruction of eyelid, full thickness by transfer of tarsoconjunctival flap from opposing eyelid; up to two-thirds of eyelid, one stage or first stage

Skin from the opposing lid is used to reconstruct the other eyelid.

Dwyer instrumentation technique
22845   Anterior instrumentation; 2 to 3 vertebral segments
22846   4 to 7 vertebral segments
22847   8 or more vertebral segments

Anterior procedure using rods and attachments to straighten the spine.

Eggers procedure
27100   Transfer external oblique muscle to greater trochanter including fascial or tendon extension (graft)

Hamstring muscles of the knee and thigh area are transferred to a new position on the femoral condyle.

Emmet's operation
56800   Plastic repair of introitus
56810   Perineoplasty, repair of perineum, non-obstetrical (separate procedure)

Procedure involves: 1) Repair of perineum; 2) Repair of the cervix uteri.

Everbusch's operation
67904   Repair of blepharoptosis; (tarso) levator resection or advancement, external approach

Elevating the levator muscle corrects ptosis of the upper eyelid.

Farnsworth-Munsell color test
92283   Color vision examination, extended, eg, anomaloscope or equivalent

Test evaluates problems in depth perception.

Farr test
82784   Gammaglobulin; IgA, IgD, IgG, IgM, each
82785   IgE

Antibody reacts to radioactive antigen and precipitates, leaving a free antigen in solution. Radio markers tag the suspected antigen.

Frazier-Spiller procedure
61450   Craniectomy, subtemporal, for section, compression, or decompression of sensory root of gasserian ganglion

Sensory root of the gasserian ganglion is compressed or decompressed to relieve trigeminal neuralgia.

Frickman proctopexy
45550   Proctopexy combined with sigmoid resection, abdominal approach

To correct rectal prolapse, rectum is sutured to the anterior presacral fascia and attached to the sigmoid colon, which has been shortened to help suspend the rectum.

Fukala's operation
66840   Removal of lens material; aspiration technique, one or more stages

Physician removes the lens of the eye to treat near-sightedness.

Gol-Vernet pyelotomy
50120   Pyelotomy; with exploration

Calyces and renal pelvis of the kidney are explored.

Gonin's operation
67107   Repair of retinal detachment; scleral buckling (such as lamellar scleral dissection, imbrication or encircling procedure), with or without implant, with or without cryotherapy, photocoagulation, and drainage of subretinal fluid

Thermocautery of the fissure of a detached retina is performed through an incision in the sclera.

Graefe's operation
66830   Removal of secondary membranous cataract (opacified posterior lens capsule and/or anterior hyaloid) with corneo-scleral section, with or without iridectomy (iridocapsulotomy, iridocapsulectomy)

Cataracts are corrected by removing the lens, lacerating the capsule, and performing an iridectomy via the sclera.

Grice arthrodesis
28725   Arthrodesis; subtalar

Bone graft is planted in the lateral part of the subtalar joint.

Gritti amputation
27598   Disarticulation at knee

Leg is amputated through the knee, and kneecap is used as the flap over the wound.

Guthrie test
84030   Phenylalanine (PKU), blood

Bacterial inhibition assay measures serum phenylalanine; and is in widespread use for detection of phenylketonuria in newborn.

Halsted mastectomy
19200   Mastectomy, radical, including pectoral muscles, axillary lymph nodes

Radical mastectomy includes removal of the breast along with pectoral minor muscle.

Ham test
85475   Hemolysin, acid

Test checks for acidified serum.

Harii Procedure
25430   Insertion of vascular pedicle into carpal bone (eg, Harii procedure)

Procedure involves complex repair of an injury that affects the dorsal skin, subcutaneous fat, including the nerves and blood vessels and the covering immediately adjacent to the tendon.

Hartley-Krause
61450   Craniectomy, subtemporal, for section, compression, or decompression of sensory root of gasserian ganglion

Gasserion ganglion is removed to relieve trigeminal neuralgia.

Heaf test
86580   Skin test; tuberculosis, intradermal

Test checks for tuberculin antibodies.

Heine's operation
66700   Ciliary body destruction; diathermy

Ciliary body is destroyed to relieve glaucoma.

Hibb's fusion
22841   Internal spinal fixation by wiring of spinous processes

Physician fractures the spinous processes and presses each tip downward to rest in the fractured area of the process below it.

Hicks-Pitney test
85730   Thromboplastin time, partial (PTT); plasma or whole blood

Thromboplastin generation test measures the efficiency of plasma in forming thromboplastin.

Holten test
82575   Creatinine; clearance

Creatines are used to test renal efficiency.

Holter monitor procedure
93235   Electrocardiographic monitoring for 24 hours by continuous computerized monitoring and non-continuous recording, and real-time data analysis utilizing a device capable of producing intermittent full-sized waveform tracings, possibly patient activated; includes monitoring and real time data analysis with report, physician review and interpretation

Patient wears a portable instrument to chart long-term behavior of the heart.

Howard test
52005   Cystourethroscopy, with ureteral catheterization, with or without irrigation, instillation, or ureteropyelography, exclusive of radiologic service;

Both ureters are catheterized and urine is collected from each kidney to test renal function.

Huggins' orchiectomy
54520   Orchiectomy, simple (including subcapsular), with or without testicular prosthesis, scrotal or inguinal approach

Testes may be removed due to prostate cancer, among other diagnoses.

Hummelshein operation
67340   Strabismus surgery involving exploration and/or repair of detached extraocular muscle(s) (List separately in addition to code for primary procedure)

Correction of strabismus by adjusting the eye muscles.

Ishihara test
92283   Color vision examination, extended, eg, anomaloscope or equivalent

Color blindness test uses plates painted with dots depicting various figures.

Jannetta decompression

61458   Craniectomy, suboccipital; for exploration or
         decompression of cranial nerves

Microsurgery relieves pressure on the cranial nerves.

Keen laminectomy

63198   Laminectomy with cordotomy with section
         of both spinothalamic tracts, two stages
         within 14 days; cervical

*Physician removes sections of the posterior branches of
spinal nerves to affected muscles and spinal accessory
nerves to correct torticollis.*

Keitzer test

51772   Urethral pressure profile studies (UPP)
         (urethral closure pressure profile), any
         technique

*Sound is used to test the pressure of an external stream of
urine.*

Killian operation

31070   Sinusotomy frontal; external, simple
         (trephine operation)

*Wall of the frontal sinus is excised to remove diseased
tissue and create an opening through the nose.*

Knapp's operation

66160   Fistulization of sclera for glaucoma;
         sclerectomy with punch or scissors, with
         iridectomy

*Peripheral opening in the capsule is formed behind the
iris to remedy a cataract.*

Koop inguinal orchiopexy

54640   Orchiopexy, inguinal approach, with or
         without hernia repair

*Undescended testicle is retrieved from the abdomen via
an inguinal approach.*

Korte-Ballance anastomosis

64868   Anastomosis; facial-hypoglossal

Facial and hypoglossal nerves are joined.

Krause decompression

61450   Craniectomy, subtemporal, for section,
         compression, or decompression of sensory
         root of gasserian ganglion

*Gasserian ganglion is excised to relieve trigeminal
neuralgia.*

Krimer's palatoplasty

14040   Adjacent tissue transfer or rearrangement,
         forehead, cheeks, chin, mouth, neck, axillae,
         genitalia, hands and/or feet; defect 10 sq cm
         or less

*Physician sutures mucoperiosteal flaps from each side of
the palatal cleft at the medial line.*

Lambrinudi arthrodesis

28730   Arthrodesis, midtarsal or tarsometatarsal,
         multiple or transverse;

*Triple fusion prevents the foot drop that may result from
polio.*

Landboldt's operation

67971   Reconstruction of eyelid, full thickness by
         transfer of tarsoconjunctival flap from
         opposing eyelid; up to two-thirds of eyelid,
         one stage or first stage
67973   total eyelid, lower, one stage or first
                 stage
67974   total eyelid, upper, one stage or first
                 stage
67975   second stage

*Double pedicle or flap of eyelid skin is taken from the
upper lid to form a lower eyelid.*

Lane's operation

44150   Colectomy, total, abdominal, without
         proctectomy; with ileostomy or
         ileoproctostomy

*Fecal production is halted by dividing the ileum near the
cecum to close the distal portion of the colon. The
proximal end of the colon is anastomosized with the
upper part of the rectum or lower part of the sigmoid.*

Laroyenne operation

57010   Colpotomy; with drainage of pelvic abscess

*Douglas pouch is punctured to evacuate pus and to
facilitate drainage.*

Lempert's fenestration

69820   Fenestration semicircular canal

*Small window is drilled in the lateral semicircular canal
and a skin flap is placed over the fistula to remedy
otosclerosis.*

Leriche sympathectomy

64809   Sympathectomy, thoracolumbar

Procedure involves sympathetic denervation.

Longmire anastomosis

47765   Anastomosis, of intrahepatic ducts and gastrointestinal tract

Biliary obstruction is corrected with an intrahepatic cholangiojejunostomy and partial hepatectomy.

Lorenz's operation

27258   Open treatment of spontaneous hip dislocation (developmental, including congenital or pathological), replacement of femoral head in acetabulum (including tenotomy, etc);

Chronic dislocation of the hip is corrected by tying the head of the femur to the acetabulum to develop a socket.

Lowsley's operation

54380   Plastic operation on penis for epispadias distal to external sphincter;

Simple epispadias is corrected by closing the glandular cleft urethra, splitting the glans, and burying the repaired urethra deep into the soft tissue.

Luschka proctectomy

45111   Proctectomy; partial resection of rectum, transabdominal approach

Technique used to resect the rectum.

MacEwen hernia repair

49505   Repair initial inguinal hernia, age 5 years or over; reducible

Hernia sack is used to construct a closing ring in this radical cure of a hernia.

Madlener operation

58600   Ligation or transection of fallopian tube(s), abdominal or vaginal approach, unilateral or bilateral

In this sterilization method, a clamp crushes the middle portion of fallopian tube, which is then shut by suture.

Manchester colporrhaphy

58400   Uterine suspension, with or without shortening of round ligaments, with or without shortening of sacrouterine ligaments; (separate procedure)

Procedure attempts to preserve the uterus following prolapse by amputating the vaginal portion of the cervix, shortening the cardinal ligaments, and performing a colpoperineorrhaphy posteriorly.

Mantoux test

86585   Skin test; tuberculosis, tine test

Standard test checks for tuberculosis.

Maydl colostomy

45563   Exploration, repair, and presacral drainage for rectal injury; with colostomy

Procedure in which colon is drawn out through the wound and maintained in position by a glass rod until adhesions have formed.

Mayo hernia repair

49585   Repair umbilical hernia, age 5 years or over; reducible

Physician excises a hernia mass and overlaps the space with abdominal muscles.

McDonald cerclage

57700   Cerclage of uterine cervix, nonobstetrical

Opening of cervix is decreased via sutures around the bottom of the cervix

McIndoe vaginal construction

57291   Construction of artificial vagina; without graft

Physician constructs an artificial vagina without using a graft.

Meller's excision

68530   Removal of foreign body or dacryolith, lacrimal passages

Physician removes a tear sac obstructing the lacrimal passages.

Mikulicz resection

44320   Colostomy or skin level cecostomy; (separate procedure)

44322   with multiple biopsies (eg, for congenital megacolon) (separate procedure)

Procedure is done in stages and includes exteriorizing a section of intestine, usually the colon, resecting the exteriorized loop, and eliminating the fecal fistula by crushing the spur between the two barrels of the anastomosis. The fecal fistula is closed.

Procedural Eponyms

Miles' colectomy

44155   Colectomy, total, abdominal, with proctectomy; with ileostomy

Lower sigmoid colon and rectum are removed for treatment of cancer. Physician removes the pelvic colon, mesocolon, and adjacent lymph nodes and establishes a permanent colostomy.

Millen-Read

57288   Sling operation for stress incontinence (eg, fascia or synthetic)

Suprapubic approach is used in the procedure to remedy stress incontinence.

Mitrofanoff operation

50845   Cutaneous appendico-vesicostomy

Appendix is connected to the bladder and skin as an opening for urine.

Mosenthal test

81002   Urinalysis, by dip stick or tablet reagent for bilirubin, glucose, hemoglobin, ketones, leukocytes, nitrite, pH, protein, specific gravity, urobilinogen, any number of these constituents; non-automated, without microscopy

Urine test for kidney function that is taken while the patient prescribes to a general diet.

Moynihan test

74246   Radiological examination, gastrointestinal tract, upper, air contrast, with specific high density barium, effervescent agent, with or without glucagon; with or without delayed films, without KUB

Radiological test determines hourglass stomach, a condition marked by the inability of the stomach muscles to contract, consequently resulting in digestive problems.

Mumford procedure

29824   Arthroscopy, shoulder, surgical; distal claviculectomy including distal articular surface (Mumford procedure)

Physician removes part of the clavicle.

Naffziger operation

61330   Decompression of orbit only, transcranial approach

Lateral and superior orbital walls are removed to decompress the orbit in cases of severe malignant exophthalmos.

Noble intestinal plication

44680   Intestinal plication (separate procedure)

Procedure involves suturing the intestine.

Patey's mastectomy

19240   Mastectomy, modified radical, including axillary lymph nodes, with or without pectoralis minor muscle, but excluding pectoralis major muscle

Modified radical mastectomy includes removal of the breast and axillary lymph nodes with preservation of the pectoralis major muscle.

Patterson's test

84525   Urea nitrogen; semiquantitative (eg, reagent strip test)

Test using blood and a reagent detects urea. Blood turns green if positive.

Pean's amputation

27290   Interpelviabdominal amputation (hindquarter amputation)

Arteries and veins are ligated during each step to amputate the hip joint.

Pemberton osteotomy

27147   Osteotomy, iliac, acetabular or innominate bone; with open reduction of hip

Osteotomy is performed to position triradiate cartilage as a hinge for rotating the acetabular roof in cases of dysplasia of the hip in children.

Polya anastomosis

43632   Gastrectomy, partial, distal; with gastrojejunostomy

Anastomosis of the transected stomach to the side of the jejunum following gastrectomy.

Porter-Silber test

82528   Corticosterone

Test to determine corticosterone, a mineral important in sodium retention.

Prentice orchiopexy

54640   Orchiopexy, inguinal approach, with or without hernia repair

Inguinal incision is made to move undescended testicles to the scrotum.

Regnolli's excision

41140   Glossectomy; complete or total, with or without tracheostomy, without radical neck dissection

Partial or total surgical excision of the tongue.

Rehfuss' test

91055   Gastric intubation, washings, and preparing slides for cytology (separate procedure)

Gastric secretion is determined by drawing specimens of digestion every 15 minutes after eating.

Reinsch test

83015   Heavy metal (arsenic, barium, beryllium, bismuth, antimony, mercury); screen

Test determines level of heavy metals in body tissue.

Ridell sinusotomy

31080   Sinusotomy frontal; obliterative without osteoplastic flap, brow incision (includes ablation)

Physician destroys frontal sinus to eliminate tumors.

Salter osteotomy

27146   Osteotomy, iliac, acetabular or innominate bone;

Innominate bone of the hip is cut, removed, and repositioned to repair a congenital dislocation, subluxation, or deformity.

Shirodkar procedure

57700   Cerclage of uterine cervix, nonobstetrical

Nonabsorbent suture material is used for a cerclage involving purse-string suture of an incompetent cervical os.

Smith-Robinson arthrodesis

22808   Arthrodesis, anterior, for spinal deformity, with or without cast; 2 to 3 vertebral segments

Fusion procedure requires an anterior approach to remove cervical disks and use of a bone graft fashioned to replace the disks.

Stoffel rhizotomy

63185   Laminectomy with rhizotomy; one or two segments

Nerve roots are sectioned to relieve pain or spastic paralysis.

Strassman type

58540   Hysteroplasty, repair of uterine anomaly (Strassman type)

Plastic repair of a malformed uterus involves removing abnormal tissue, rearranging uterine walls, and suturing extensively.

Taarnhoj procedure

61450   Craniectomy, subtemporal, for section, compression, or decompression of sensory root of gasserian ganglion

The skull is opened at the temporal region and the gasserion ganglion nerve root is sectioned, decompressed, or compressed, depending on the patient's complaint.

Touroff ligation

37615   Ligation, major artery (eg, post-traumatic, rupture); neck

Neck is incised and an artery or a vein, damaged or ruptured by trauma, is isolated and tied off with sutures.

Tzank smear

87207   Smear, primary source with interpretation; special stain for inclusion bodies or intracellular parasites (eg, malaria, coccidia, microsporidia, cytomegalovirus, herpes viruses)

Test determines if there are altered epithelial cells (Tzank cells) in the fluid of the bullae of pemphigus vulgaris.

Valentine's test

81020   Urinalysis; two or three glass test

Another term for the three glass test which uses three vials of the same stream of urine to determine contents of the anterior urethra, bladder, ureters, and seminal vesicles.

Van Den Bergh test

82247   Bilirubin; total

Test involves comparing serum or plasma to bilirubin.

Van Slyke method

82131   Amino acids; single, quantitative, each specimen

Test checks for amino-acid nitrogen.

Walsh modified radical prostatectomy

55810   Prostatectomy, perineal radical;

Radical prostatectomy resects the rectum and surrounding tissue.

Procedural Eponyms

Wasserman test

86592   Syphilis test; qualitative (eg, VDRL, RPR, ART)

Wasserman is the original test for syphilis.

Wertheim hysterectomy

58210   Radical abdominal hysterectomy, with bilateral total pelvic lymphadenectomy and para-aortic lymph node sampling (biopsy), with or without removal of tube(s), with or without removal of ovary(s)

Radical operation for uterine carcinoma includes excising a portion of the vagina and lymph nodes.

Westergren test

85652   Sedimentation rate, erythrocyte; automated

Test determines the sedimentation rate of red blood cells in fluid blood by mixing venous blood with an aqueous solution of sodium citrate and allowing it to stand for measured periods of time.

Whitehead hemorrhoidectomy

46260   Hemorrhoidectomy, internal and external, complex or extensive;

Two circular incisions above and below hemorrhoidal veins pull down normal mucosa for suturing to anal skin.

Whitman astragalectomy

28130   Talectomy (astragalectomy)

Physician removes cartilage of the talus.

Surgical Terms

A special language is spoken in the surgical suite and written in the charts documenting procedures performed there. The following list includes many of the medical terms heard most often in the operating room.

ablation — surgical removal of a part

abrasion — removal of layers of skin

achalsia — failure of pylorus, cardia, sphincter muscles or other visceral openings to relax

acromioplasty — repair of the part of the shoulder blade that connects to the deltoid muscles and clavicle

advance — to move away from the starting point

allograft — transplanted tissue from the same species

amputation — removal of a limb or part of a limb

analysis — study of body section or parts

anastomosis — surgical connection of tubular structures

aneurysm — abnormal widening of an artery

angioplasty — reconstruction of blood vessel

antibody — immune or protective protein

antigen — substance inducing sensitivity

antrum — a chamber or cavity, typically with a small opening

appliance — device providing function to a body part

arthrocentesis — aspiration of fluid from joint with needle

arthrodesis — surgical fixation of a joint

arthroplasty — restoration of a joint

arthroscopy — endoscopic examination of a joint

arthrotomy — surgical incision into a joint

articulate — connect loosely to allow motion

aspiration — drawing in or out by suction

assay — a test of purity

astragalectomy — surgical excision of the talus (ankle) bone

augmentation — increasing the substance of

autograft — transplant of tissue from one part of the body to another part

avulse — to tear away from

benign — mild illness or nonmalignant neoplasm

biofeedback — technique allowing patient to control body function

biometry — statistical analysis of biological data

biopsy — excision and examination for diagnostic purposes

blood type — classification of blood by group

bougie — probe used to dilate or calibrate body part

brachytherapy — radiotherapy proximate to the organ being treated

bridge — a connection between two parts of an organ

brush — a tool used to gather cell samples or clean body part

bur — drill used to cut and shape bone

bursa — a cavity or sac containing fluid

bypass — an auxiliary flow

C-arm — portable x-ray machine for surgery

calculus — concretion of calcium, cholesterol, salts, or other substances that forms in any part of the body

cannula — tube inserted to facilitate passage

capsulorrhaphy — suture of a joint capsule

capsulotomy — opening of a joint capsule

cast — rigid encasement for therapeutic purposes

catheter — any of a number of tubes inserted in body parts

cauterize — heat or chemicals used to burn or cut

celiotomy — incision into the abdomen

cement — prosthesis glued to bone

centesis — puncture

cephalad — toward the head

cerclage — to loop an organ or tissue with wire or a ligature

chemodenervation — chemical destruction of nerves

chemosurgery — medication used to facilitate surgery

chemotherapy — treatment by chemical means or drugs

chisel — instrument for cutting or planing bone

chondral — pertaining to cartilage

chromotubation — medication injection into uterus and tubes

cicatricial — concerning a scar

ciliary — pertaining to the eyelid

circumcise — circular cutting around body part

clamp — tool used to grip, compress, join, or fasten body parts

closure — the suturing of an incision

clysis — fluids injected into the body

coctolabile — capable of being destroyed or altered when boiled

comminuted — a fracture type in which the bone is splintered or crushed

commissure — corner or angle of body part such of vagina or eye

complex — a composite of anatomical parts or surgical procedures

condyle — rounded end of a bone that forms an articulation

conization — a procedure of excision of a cone of tissue

constriction — therapeutic binding of a body part

contour — the act of shaping along desired lines

corpectomy — the removal of the body of a bone, such as a vertebra

correct — body part modification

craterization — the formation of a depression in body tissue

cross match — test for compatibility of donor's blood or organ

crus — 1) any body part resembling a leg; 2) the lower part of the leg

cryotherapy — therapeutic use of cold in a part of the body

culture — microorganisms grown in medium

curettage — removal of tissue by scraping

cutaneous — any procedure on the skin

cystotomy — incision into gallbladder or urinary bladder

debridement — the cleansing or removing of dead tissue from a wound

decompress — to relieve pressure

decubitus — 1) an ulcer often spawned by bedrest; 2) the patient's position in bed

dehiscence — a rupture or bursting open

deligation — closure by tying up; sutures, ligatures

depressor — tool used to push body tissue out of the way

dermabrasion — skin lesions removed by abrasive substance

destruction — tissue elimination

detection — search for presence of a tissue or material

diagnostic — an aid in diagnosis

dialysis — diffusion of body fluids to restore normal balance

diaphysis — central shaft of a long bone

diathermy — therapeutic use of heat in a part of the body

dilation — expansion or stretching an opening

dilution — concentration reduction of mixture or solution

disarticulation — amputation through a joint

diskectomy — removal of a intervertebral disk

dislocation — displacement of a body part

dissection — to expose during surgery

distension — the act of being stretched or dilated

diversion — diversion of body fluid to another channel

diverticulum — a pouch or sac in the walls of an organ or canal

division — separating into two or more parts

donor — person from whom tissues or organs are removed for transplantation

dorsum — upper or posterior part

dosimetry — determination of amount of radiation

drain — drawing of fluid from a cavity or site

drill — to make a hole in a bone or hard tissue

dynamic — motion in response to forces

echography — ultrasonography

ectopic — in an abnormal position

edentulous — toothless

electrocautery — instrument used to direct electrical energy through tissue for destructive or therapeutic reasons

elevator — a tool for lifting tissues or bone

elution — separation of one solid from another, usually by washing

embolism — obstruction of a blood vessel resulting from a clot or foreign substance

endoscopy — visual inspection of body using fiberoptic scope

enterostomy — an artificial anus in the abdominal wall

epiphyses — the ends of a long bone

epithelize — formation of epithelial cells over a surface

escharotomy — removal of the scab or crust resulting from a severe burn

esophagoscopy — endoscopic inspection of the esophagus

evacuation — removal of waste material

evisceration — removal of contents of cavity

examination — inspection made for diagnosis

exchange — substitution of one tissue for another

excise — to remove or cut out

exenteration — removal of organs or tissues

exfoliate — skin falling off in layers

exploration — examination for diagnostic purposes

exposure — displaying, revealing, or making accessible

expression — the squeezing out of tissue

exteriorize — to expose an organ temporarily for observation

external fixation — rods and pins connected in a lattice to secure bone

extract — condensed medication

fascia — sheet of fibrous tissue that envelopes organs, muscles, and groupings of muscles

fasciotomy — procedure of cutting through fascia

fenestration — openings in tissue or bandage

fibrosis — formation of fibrous tissue as part of restorative process

filiform — probe with woven-thread end

fissure — a deep furrow or groove in tissue structures

fistula — a tube-like passage between two cavities

fistulization — creation of fistula for therapeutic reasons

fit — attack of acute symptoms

fixate — to hold, suture, or fix in position

fixation — to attach tissue or material

flap — mass of flesh moved for grafting

fluoroscopy — examination of tissues by x-ray

follow-up — visits or treatment following a procedure

forceps — a tool for grasping or compressing tissue

fossa — an indentation or shallow depression

fragment — division into pieces

free graft — unattached tissue moved to another part of the body

frozen section — method of confirming the nature of tissue during a procedure

fulgurate — destruction by electric current

furuncle — cyst or boil

fusion — union of tissues, especially bone

Gigli saw — wire saw used for pubiotomy or craniotomy

graft — tissue implant from another part of the body or another person

guillotine — instrument for severing tonsil

halo — tool for stabilizing the head and spine

harvest — removal of a free graft from its native site

hematoma — localized mass of usually clotted blood

hemilaminectomy — excision of a portion of the vertebral lamina

hemiphalangectomy — excision of part of phalanx

hemostasis — stagnation of blood or cessation of bleeding

hemostat — tool for clamping vessels

hernia — protrusion of body structure through tissue

hidradenitis — infection of the apocrine glands

homograft — transplanted tissue from one member of species to another

hyperthermia — therapeutic raising of body temperature

hypertrophic — description of body part that has grown larger

hypophysectomy — destruction of pituitary gland

hypothermia — therapeutic lack of heat

identification — recognition of body part or tissue

imaging — x-ray, ultrasound, or magnetic resonance imagery

imbrication — overlapping of tissues during closure

immunotherapy — therapeutic use of serum or gamma globulin

implant — insertion of a material

impression — mark made by one organ on another

in situ — one position

incise — to cut open or into

incubation — culture cultivation under controlled conditions

infusion — introduction of substance into blood

inguinal — groin region

inject — introduction into body tissues

innervate — nerve fibers connected to a part

inseminate — injection of semen

insert — to put into

instillation — dropping of liquid on or into

instrumentation — use of tool or implement for therapeutic reasons

insufflation — to blow air or gas into a body cavity

interpretation — review of data with a written or verbal opinion by a professional

interstitial — spaces within tissue or organ

intracavitary — within a body cavity

intubate — insertion of tube into body canal or organ

inversion — to turn inward, inside out, or upside down

irrigate — washing out, lavage

kinetics — motion or movement

laminectomy — removal of a lamina

lance — incision with a lancet

lancet — a pointed surgical knife

laparoscopy — an endoscopic examination of abdomen

laparotomy — an opening of abdomen for therapy or diagnosis

laryngoscopy — examination of the larynx with an endoscope

laser — concentrated light used to cut or seal tissue

lateral — to the side

lavage — washing out of body cavity

lesion — any discontinuity of tissue

ligation — tying or binding

limited — bounded

lingual — relating to the tongue

lithotripsy — destruction of calcified substance in the gallbladder, urethra, or bladder (also litholapaxy)

localization — limitation to area

lysis — mobilizing of organ by freeing adhesions

manipulate — treatment by hand

manometric — measurement of gas pressure

marsupialization — creation of a pouch in an organ or tissue

mastectomy — removal of part or whole of breast

mastotomy — incision of breast

meatus — opening or passage

metatarsectomy — excision of metatarsus

microdissection — dissection of tissue using microscope

microrepair — repair of tissue using microscope

modification — changing of tissues

monitor — recording of events

motility — spontaneous movement

myotomy — division of muscle by surgeon

necropsy — autopsy

necrosis — death of cells

nephrotic — degeneration of renal epithelium

neurectomy — excision of a nerve

neurotomy — dissection of nerve

obliterate — destruction of tissue

observation — perception of events

obturate — to occlude an opening

obturator — any structure that closes an opening

occlusion — constriction or closure of a passage

open fracture — exposed fracture

orchiectomy — removal of testicle

osteophytes — bony outgrowth

osteoplasty — plastic repair of bone

osteoporotic — porous condition of bones

osteomyelitis — inflammation of bone and bone marrow

osteotome — tool used for cutting bone

osteotomy — bone incision

packing — material placed into a cavity

palpate — examination by hand

paring — reduction

paronychia — infection of nail structures

pedicle — a stem that is attached to a new growth

peduncle — connecting structures of brain

penetrate — pierce

percutaneous — through unbroken skin

periosteum — double-layered connective membrane on outer surface of bone

photocoagulation — use of laser to destroy tissue

pilonidal — growth of hair under skin or in cyst

pinning — bone fastening

plethysmography — measurement of changes in organ volume

pleurodesis — creation of adhesion

plication — placement of folds into an organ to reduce its size

portable — movable

probing — exploration with slender rod

procedure — conduct of operation

process — anatomical projection, usually bone

prone — lying face downward

prophylaxis — prevention of disease

prosthesis — man-made substitute for a missing body part

prostrate — to recline on one's front

pump — forcing gas or liquid from body part

puncture — to make a hole

pyelotomy — incision into kidney

radical — extensive surgery

radiograph — image made by an x-ray

radiopaque dye — medium injected into the body that is impenetrable by x-rays

ream — to shape or enlarge a hole

recess — a small empty cavity in a body part

reconstruct — tissue rebuilding

reduce — restoration to normal position or alignment

reduction — correction of fracture, dislocation, or hernia

refer — recommendation to another source

regulation — control of activity

reimplant — reinsertion of tissue

reinforce — the enhancement of strength

reinnervation — repair of nerve bundle

release — disconnection of a tendon or ligament

reoperation — repeat performance of operation

repair — correction of situation

replacement — insertion of new tissue or material in place of old one

reposition — to bring into position

resect — cutting of a portion of a bone, organ, or other structure

reservoir — storage of liquid in body cavity

response — reaction to stimulus

retraction — the sides of an incision pulled apart

revascularize — repairing of blood vessels

revision — re-ordering of tissue

rod — cylindrical metal instrument for therapeutics

rongeur — a tool for cutting tough tissue

routine — normal activity

sclerose — to become hard or firm

section — cut or division

selective — separation

sequestrectomy — excision of non-viable bone

seton — wire or gauze used to create fistula in tissues

sever — to cut

shunt — diversion or introduction of fluid via tube

sialolith — salivary calculus

sigmoidoscopy — endoscopy examination of part of the large intestines

smear — specimen for study

snare — tool for removal of polyps from body cavity

sound — long, curved tool for probing body cavity

spatulate — tissue cut into shape of spatula

speculum — tool to enlarge opening of any canal or cavity

spiculum — small spike

steal — diversion of blood to another channel

stenosis — narrowing or constriction of a passage

stent — mold to secure skin or tubes while healing

stereotaxis — method for precisely locating structures in the brain

stoma — an opening for elimination of waste

strapping — overlapping strips of plaster

stricture — narrowing of hollow structure

subluxation — partial or complete dislocation

suction — vacuum evacuation of fluid or tissue

supine — to recline on one's back

suppression — cessation of activity

suppurative — forming pus

survival — continued life

suspension — fixation of organ for support

suture — tissue stitching

symphysis — a fibro-cartilage unification of two bones

synchondrosis — two bones joined by hyaline cartilage or fibrocartilage

synovia — fluid lubricant of joints, bursae, tendon sheaths, etc.

talectomy — procedure of the ankle

tap — to withdraw fluid through a needle or trocar

technique — a manner of performance

teletherapy — x-ray therapy

tenodesis — stabilization of joint by anchoring tendons

tenolysis — release of a tendon from adhesions

therapeutic — treatment of disease

thoracentesis — puncture of the thoracic cavity

thoracotomy — incision in chest wall

thrombectomy — removal of venous occlusion (clot)

tomograph — method of precise x-ray

tracheostomy — creation of opening into trachea

traction — drawing or pulling during or after surgery or injury

tractor — instrument for pulling an organ

transcatheter — treatment via a catheter

transection — cut made across an axis

transfer — removal or moving body tissue

transplant — movement of organ or tissue from one person or site to another

transposition — removal from one side to another; change of position

treatment — management of patient

trephine — removal of a circular piece of bone from the skull

trocar — surgical instrument used to aspirate fluid from cavities

tube — hollow cylinder or pipe

ultrasound — imaging using ultra-high sound frequency

undiversion — restoration of continuity

urachus — a fibrous remnant of the umbilical cord stretching from the bladder to the navel

ureterocele — sacular formation of lower part of ureter, protruding into bladder

ureteropyelogram — x-ray study of ureter and bladder

ureostomy — the connection of the ureter to a stoma on the abdominal skin

valve — prosthesis to replace existing valve or to shunt body fluids

varices — enlarge, dilated, or tortured veins

vasectomy — removal of a segment of the vas deferens to facilitate sterility or prostectomy

vestigal — remains of a structure occurring in fetus

vomer — bone forming a portion of nasal septum

xenograft — graft taken from non-human animal

Syndromes

A syndrome is the composite of signs and symptoms that give a picture of the disease process. The symptoms may be singular or plural, specific or broadly outlined. Syndromes may be physical or behavioral, congenital or found later in life; and while syndromes are not diseases, they are used to describe diseases seen daily by health care givers. Commonly known diseases may be known by their accompanying syndromes, which complicates proper coding of ICD-9 codes.

ICD-9 contains a list of nearly 1500 syndromes cross-referenced under its numeric system. The following list contains most of those syndromes, explained and cross-referenced by number and name. Many syndromes carry a number of names, which are noted within parenthesis in each entry. Similar syndromes with negligible differences are also grouped together to ease use.

Look for the syndrome to find an explanation of what the syndrome means and what four or five-digit code is most appropriate. Syndromes for which there are a number of fourth- or fifth-digit codes are designated by the letter X.

13
758.1 (Patau's, trisomy D, D1) Variable symptoms of newborns with an extra chromosome in group D. Condition is usually fatal within two years and includes mental retardation and malformed ears, cardiac defects, convulsions, and others.

16-18 or E
758.2 (Edward's, trisomy E, E3) Congenital malformations in which extra chromosome is group E. Includes mental retardation, abnormal skull shape, malformed ears, small mandible, cardiac defects, short sternum, and other symptoms.

21 or 22
758.0 (Down, G, mongolism) Retardation with numerous markers varying from one person to another. Symptoms include retarded growth, flat face with short nose, epicanthic skin folds, protruding lower lip, rounded ears, thickened tongue, pelvic dysplasia, broad hands and feet, stubby fingers, and absence of Moro reflex.

Abercrombie's
277.3 One of a group of syndromes characterized by accumulation of insoluble fibrillar proteins in various organs and tissues of the body.

Achard-Thiers
255.2 Aranodactyly with small, receding mandible, broad skull, and laxity of joints in hands and feet.

Acid pulmonary aspiration
997.3 (Mendelson's) Pulmonary disorder resulting from aspirating the contents of stomach following vomiting or regurgitation.

Acquired immune deficiency
042 (AIDS) A contagious retroviral disease resulting from infection with human immunodeficiency virus (HIV) that can, in severe cases, suppress vital immunity. Several opportunistic infections, such as Kaposi's sarcoma and pneumocystitis pneumonia, are associated with this syndrome.

Acrocephalosyndactylism
755.55 (Aperts) A chromosomal condition with webbing of digits and a pointed head and variety of defects. Often associated with other chromosomal abnormalities.

Acute
293.0 Describes a mental health patient who chooses not to participate in day-to-day activities or therapy as a a result of emotional, organic, or chemical causes.

Adair-Dighton
756.51 (van der Hoeve's) Hereditary condition with symptoms including blue sclera, little growth, brittle bones, and deafness.

Adams-Stokes (-Morgagni)
426.9 (Stokes-Adams, Morgagni's disease, and Spens) Heart block often causing slow or absent pulse, vertigo, syncope, convulsions, and sometimes Cheyne-Stokes respiration.

Syndromes

Addisonian

255.4   (Bernard-Sergent) Acute adrenal insufficiency caused by illness, trauma, or large amounts of hormones used as therapy. Symptoms include hypotension, hyperthermia, hyponatremia, hyperkalemia, hypoglycemia, nausea, and vomiting.

Adie (-Holmes)

379.46   Paralysis of conjugate movement of eyes without paralysis of convergence. Caused by lesions of midbrain.

Adiposogenital

253.8   (Babinski-Frohlich, Frohlich) Obesity and hypogonadism in adolescent boys. Rare accompanying dwarfism is thought to indicate hypothyroidism.

Adrenogenital

255.2   (Achard-Thiers) Aranodactyly with small, receding mandible, broad skull, and joint laxity in hands and feet.

Adult maltreatment

995.8X   Maltreatment (abuse) of an adult with emotional or physical violence. Most often committed against spouses and elders.

Adult respiratory distress

518.5   Respiratory distress following surgery, shock, or trauma; similar to, but not caused by, adult respiratory distress system.

Affective NEC

293.83   (affective organic NEC) Organic disorder in which the patient exhibits a number of changes in personality such as amotivation, depression, outbursts, and poor social judgment.

Afferent loop NEC

537.89   (Gastrojejunal loop obstruction) Distended afferent loop with illness and pain caused by acute or chronic obstruction of the duodenum and jejunum proximal to a gastrojejunostomy.

African macroglobulinemia

273.3   (Waldenström's) Earmarked by an increase in macroglobulins in the blood with symptoms of hyperviscosity such as weakness, fatigue, bleeding disorders, and visual disturbances.

Ahumada-Del Castillo

253.1   (Argonz-Del Castillo) Lactation and amenorrhea not following pregnancy characterized by hyperprolactinemia and pituitary adenoma.

Albright (-Forbes)

275.4   (Martin-Albright, Seabright-Bantam) Similar to hypoparathyroidism and caused by a failure to respond to parathyroid hormone. Short stature, obesity, short metacarpals, and ectopic calcification.

Albright-McCune-Sternberg

756.59   (McCune-Albright, Albright's hereditary osteodystrophy) Patchy skin pigmentation, endocrine dysfunctions, and polyostotic fibrous dysplasia.

Alcohol withdrawal

291.81   (alcohol) Absence of alcohol in an alcohol-dependent individual with physiological and psychological symptoms. Severity may result in death.

Alcoholic amnestic

291.1   Physical and emotional symptoms resulting from profound ingestion of alcohol.

Alder's

288.2   Polymorphonuclear leukocytes, or white blood cells.

Aldrich (-Wiskott)

279.12   (Wiskott-Aldrich) Inherited immunodeficiency with eczema, thrombocyopenia, recurrent pyogenic infection, and increased susceptibility to infection with encapsulated bacteria.

Alibert-Bazin

202.1   Malignant neoplasm resembling a fungus and growing outside of the body.

Alice in Wonderland

293.89   Organic disorder with patient presenting an illusion of dreams, feelings of levitation, and alteration of passage of time. Associated with epilepsy, migraines, and other problems of the parietal part of brain.

Allen-Masters

620.6   Pelvic pain resulting from old laceration of broad ligament received during delivery.

Alligator baby
757.1   (Carini's) Scaling of skin similar to an alligator's or fish's that accompanies other congenital syndromes.

Alport's
759.89   Progressive sensorineural hearing loss, ocular defects, and glomerulonephritis, or pyelonephritis. Cause is inherited.

Alveolar capillary block
516.3   (Hamman-Rich) Chronic inflammation and progressive fibrosis of pulmonary alveolar walls, with progressive dyspnea leading to death by oxygen deprivation or right heart failure.

Amnestic
294.0   Amnestic dementia in which the patient has no short-term or long-term memories but is not delirious.

Amotivational
292.89   Patient who chooses not to participate in day-to-day activities or therapy as a a result of emotional, organic, or chemical causes.

Amyostatic
275.1   Accumulation of copper in the brain, cornea, kidney, liver, and other tissues causing cirrhosis of the liver and deterioration in the basal ganglia of the brain.

Angina
413.9   Acute, choking pain most notable in the pectoral region of the chest and implying the onset of a heart attack.

Angina cruris
443.9   (Charcot's) Number of symptoms in a moving limb including pain, tension, and weakness but absent at rest. Caused by occlusive arterial diseases of the limbs.

Antimongolism
758.3   Mental and growth retardation, hypertonia, high-arched palate, micrognathia, microcephaly and an anti-mongoloid obliquity of the palpebral fissures.

Apert's
755.55   Chromosomal condition with webbing of digits, a pointed head, and varieties of defects. Often associated with other chromosomal abnormalities.

Apert-Gallais
255.2   Type I acrocephalosyndactyly with a peaked head, fusion of digits (specifically the second through fifth digits), and severe acne vulgaris of forearms.

Aphasia-apraxia-alexia
784.69   (Bianchi's) Sensory aphasic condition with alexia and apraxia associated with lesions in the left parietal lobe.

Approximate answers
300.16   Psychotic-like condition (but without symptoms and signs of a traditional psychosis).

Arc-welders'
370.24   Temporary or permanent spot blindness resulting from observing bright light unprotected.

Arch
446.7   (Marorell-Fabre, Raed-Harbitz, Takayasu-Onishi) Progressive obliteration of brachiocephalic trunk and left subclavian and left common carotid arteries above their source in the aortic arch. Symptoms include ischemia, transient blindness, facial atrophy, and many others.

Arcuate ligament
447.4   Compression of the celiac artery by the median arcuate ligament in the diaphragm.

Argentaffin, argintaffinoma
259.2   (Bjorck-Thorson, Cassidy-Scholte, Hedinger's) Carcinoid tumors causing severe attacks of cyanotic flushing of the skin, diarrhea watery stools, bronchoconstrictive attacks, hypotension, edema, and ascites.

Argonz-Del Castillo
253.1   (Ahumada-Del Castillo) Lactation and amenorrhea not following pregnancy and characterized by hyperprolactinemia and pituitary adenoma.

Arm-shoulder
337.9   (Claude Bernard-Homer, Reilly's, Steinbrocker's) Disorder following a heart attack with pain and stiffness in the shoulder and swelling and pain in the hand.

Arnold-Chiari
741.0   Cerebellomedullary malformation syndrome. Displacement of the caudal spinal cord due to tethering with or without spina bifida and other problems such as meningomyelocele.

Arrillaga-Ayerza
416.0 (arteriosclerosis) Cyanosis and hypertension resulting from sclerosis of the pulmonary arteries.

Arteriomesenteric duodenum occlusion
537.89 (Gastrojejunal loop obstruction) Distended afferent loop with illness and pain caused by acute or chronic obstruction of the duodenum and jejunum proximal to a gastrojejunostomy.

Arteriosclerosis depressive
293.83 Organic disorder in which the patient exhibits changes in personality such as amotivation, depression, outbursts, poor social judgment, etc. Caused by constriction of the arteries to the brain.

Artery compression
447.4 Compression of the celiac artery by the median arcuate ligament in the diaphragm.

Artery entrapment
447.8 Malignant atrophic papulosis.

Artery, superior
557.1 (Wilkie's) Complete or partial block of the superior mesenteric artery with vomiting, pain, blood in the stool, distended abdomen, and resulting in bowel infarction.

Asherman's
621.5 Adhesions in the endometrial cavity causing amenorrhea and infertility.

Aspiration
770.1 Intrauterine fetal aspiration of amniotic fluid contaminated by meconium.

Ataxia-telangiectasia
334.8 (Boder-Sedgwick, Louis-Bar) Gonadal hypoplasia, insulin resistance and hyperglycemia, liver function problems, increased sensitivity to ionizing radiation, ataxia, and nystagmus.

Audry's
757.39 Increased thickening of the skin on extremities and face with clubbing of fingers and deformities in bone of the limb.

Auriculotemporal
350.8 (Frey's) Localized sweating and flushing of the cheek and ear in response to chewing.

Automatism
348.8 Infarction of the postero-inferior thalamus causing transient hemiparesis, severe loss of sensation with crude pain in the limbs, or vasomotor or trophic disturbances.

Avellis'
344.89 (Babinski-Nageotte, Benedikt's, Brown-Sequard, Cestan's, Cestan-Chenais, Foville's, Gubler-Millard, Jackson's, Weber-Leyden) Paraplegia and anesthesia over part of the body caused by lesions in the brain or spinal cord.

Axenfeld's
743.44 A dysgenesis of the eye marked through widened trabecular meshwork, large iridial bands, and glaucoma.

Ayerza (-Arrillaga)
416.0 Cyanosis and hypertension, resulting from sclerosis of the pulmonary arteries.

Baader's
695.1 Necrolysis of the skin caused by toxins.

Baastrup's
721.5 Kissing spine. Malformation of the spine in which kyphosis becomes so great nonadjacent vertebrae touch.

Babinski-Fröhlich
253.8 (Frölich) Obesity and hypogonadism in adolescent boys with rare accompanying dwarfism, thought to indicate hypothyroidism.

Babinski-Nageotte
344.89 (Avellis, Benedikt's, Brown-Sequard, Cestan's, Cestan-Chenais, Foville's, Gubler-Millard, Jackson's, Weber-Leyden) Paraplegia and anesthesia over part of the body caused by lesions in the brain or spinal cord.

Baby or child maltreatment
995.5 Maltreatment of a child (child abuse) through physical violence, emotional violence, or starvation.

Bagratuni's
446.5 (Horton's, giant cell arteritis) Temoral arteritis.

Bakwin-Krida
756.89 Overgrowth sclerosis of skull bones.

Balint's
368.16   (Balint's, Holmes', Riddoch's) Cortical paralysis of visual fixation, optic ataxia, and disturbance of visual attention with normal eye movements.

Ballantyne (-Runge)
766.2   Placental dysfunction occurring in postmature fetuses.

Ballooning posterior leaflet
424.0   (Barlow's) "Mid-late" systolic click of the heart due to massive protrusion of the mitral valvular leaflet in the left atrial cavity.

Bard-Pic's
157.0   Cancer of the pancreas.

Bardet-Biedl
759.89   Inherited mental retardation, pigmentary retinopathy, obesity, polydactyly, and hypogonadism.

Barlow (-Möller)
267   (Cheadle) Nutritionally-caused anemia, spongy gums, weakness, induration of leg muscles, and mucocutaneous hemorrhages.

Barlow's
424.0   "Mid-late" systolic click of the heart due to massive protrusion of the mitral valvular leaflet in the left atrial cavity.

Barré-Guillain
357.0   (Guillain-Barre, Landry, Fisher's, Strohl, Miller) Disorder of the immune system with paraplegia of limbs, flaccid paralysis, ophthalmoplegia, ataxia, and areflexia.

Barré-Liéou
723.2   Irritation of the nerve roots emanating from the posterior cervical spinal cord.

Barrett's
530.2   Gastrointestinal reflux in the esophagus associated heartburn and regurgitation caused by stricture constructed of epithelium.

Bársony-Polgár
530.5   (Barsony-Teschendorf) Strong, uncoordinated contraction of the esophagus evoked by deglutition in the elderly. Appears as a series of concentric narrows or as spiral on an x-ray.

Bársony-Teschendorf
530.XX   (Barsony-Polgar) Strong, uncoordinated contraction of the esophagus evoked by deglutition in the elderly. Appears as a series of concentric narrows or as spiral on an x-ray.

Bartter's
255.1   Found in children with hypokalemic alkalosis, elevated renin or angiotensin levels, low or normal blood pressure, no edema, and retarded growth.

Basedow's
242.0X   (Basedow, Parry's, Grave's disease) Fatigue, nervousness, emotional lability and irritability, heat intolerance and increased sweating, weight loss, palpitation, and tremor of hands and tongue. May be autoimmune in etiology.

Basilar artery
435.0   (Raymond-Cestan) Quadriplegia, anesthesia, and nystagmus. Due to obstruction of twigs of the basilar artery, causing lesions in the pontine region.

Basofrontal
377.04   (Foster-Kennedy, Gowers-Paton-Kennedy) Meningioma of the optic nerve, marked by central scotoma and contralateral choked disk.

Bassen-Kornzweig
272.5   Retinal pigmentary degeneration, malabsorption, engorgement of upper intestinal cells with triglycerides, neuromuscular abnormalities, and an absence from plasma of low density lipoproteins.

Batten-Steinert
359.2   Condition in which the peritoneal cover of the liver converts to a white mass resembling cake icing.

Baumgarten-Cruveilhier
571.5   Cirrhosis of the liver with patent paraumbilical, varicose periumbilical, or umbilical veins.

Bearn-Kunkel (-Slater)
571.49   Chronic hepatitis with autoimmune manifestations.

Beau's
429.1   Cardiac arrest.

Bechterew-Strümpell-Marie
720.0   Rheumatoid inflammation of the vertebrae.

Beck's
433.8X   Occlusion of the spinal artery as result of injury, disk damage, or cardiovascular disease.

Beckwith (-Wiedemann)
759.89   Congenital disorder with macroglossia, gigantism, dysplasia of the renal medulla, visceromegaly, adrenocortical cytomegaly, and exomphalos.

Bekhterev-Strümpell-Marie
720.0   Rheumatoid inflammation of the vertebrae.

Benedikt's
344.89   (Avellis, Babinski-Nageotte, Benedikt's, Brown-Sequard, Cestan's, Cestan-Chenais, Foville's, Gubler-Millard, Jackson's, Weber-Leyden) Paraplegia and anesthesia over part of the body caused by lesions in the brain or spinal cord.

Béquez César (-Steinbrinck-Chédiak-Higashi)
288.2   (Chediak-Higashi, Dohle body, Hegglin, Jordan's, May) Hepatosplenomegaly, lymphadenopathy, anemia, thrombocytopenia, with changes in the bones, cardiopulmonary system, skin, and psychomotor skills. Abnormalities of granulation and nuclear structure of white cells open the patient, who is often a child, to infection and result in death.

Bernard-Horner
337.9   Claude Bernard-Horner, Reilly's, Steinbrocker's) Disorder following a heart attack with pain and stiffness in the shoulder, and swelling and pain in the hand.

Bernard-Sergent
255.4   Acute adrenal insufficiency caused by illness or trauma or by large amounts of hormones used as therapy. Symptoms include hypotension, hyperthermia, hyponatremia, hyperkalemia, hypoglycemia, nausea, and vomiting.

Bernhardt-Roth
355.1   Tingling, formication, itching, and other symptoms on the outer side of the lower part of the thigh. Caused by lateral femoral cutaneous nerve.

Bernheim's
428.0   Right heart failure accompanied by enlarged liver, distended neck veins, and edema without pulmonary congestion, caused by hypertrophied septum.

Bertolotti's
756.15   Fusion of the bottom lumbar vertebra to the top sacral vertebra, making a sixth sacral vertebra accompanied by sciatica and scoliosis.

Besnier-Boeck-Schaumann
135   (Hutchinson-Boeck, Lofgren's, Schaumann's, Besnier-Boeck-Schaumann) Involves the lungs with resulting fibrosis, lymph nodes, skin, liver, eyes, spleen, phalangeal bones, and parotid glands. Identified by systemic granulomas composed of epithelioid and multinucleated giant cells.

Bianchi's
784.69   Sensory aphasic condition with alexia and apraxia and lesions in the left parietal lobe.

Biedl-Bardet
759.89   (Biemond's) Mental retardation, pigmentary retinopathy, obesity, polydactyly, and hypogonadism.

Biemond's
759.89   Mental retardation, pigmentary retinopathy, obesity, polydactyly, and hypogonadism.

Bifurcation
444.0   (Leriche's) Obstruction of the terminal aorta causing fatigue in the hips, thighs, or calves and pallor of lower extremities and impotence in exercising males.

Big Spleen
289.4   (hypersplenism) Enlarged spleen caused by cirrohsis of liver or portal or splenic vein thrombosis causing anemia, hyperplasia of marrow precursers of deficient cell type.

Bilateral polycystic ovarian
256.4   Acute adrenal insufficiency caused by illness, trauma, or by large amounts of hormones used as therapy with hypotension, hyperthermia, hyponatremia, hyperkalemia, hypoglycemia, nausea, and vomiting.

Biörck (-Thorson)

259.2 (Cassidy-Scholte, Hedinger's) Carcinoid tumors that cause cyanotic flushing of the skin, diarrhea watery stools, bronchoconstrictive attacks, hypotension, edema, and ascites.

Blackfan-Diamond

284.0 (Diamond-Blackfan, Fanconi, Kaznelson's) Congenital anemia that manifests during infancy and requires a number of blood transfusions to maintain life.

Blacklung

289.4 (coal miner's pneumoconiosis, anthracosis) Blockage of bronchioles by "coal machules" brought about by aspiration of coal dust.

Blind loop

579.2 Loop of small intestine detached surgically or detaching itself and, in the former case, becomes bacterial, and, in the latter case, accepts feces but cannot discharge it, becoming infected.

Bloch-Siemens

757.33 (Block-Sulzberger) Pigmented lesions appear in linear, zebra stripe, and other configurations and preceded by vesicles and bullae and followed by verrucal lesions.

Bloch-Sulzberger

757.33 (Block-Siemens) Pigmented lesions appear in linear, zebra stripe, and other configurations and preceded by vesicles and bullae and followed by verrucal lesions.

Bloom (-Machacek) (-Torre)

757.39 Butterfly-shaped lesions on the face and hands, dolichocephalic skull and narrow face, and dwarfism with normal body proportions.

Blount-Barber

732.4 Bow-legs in children.

Boder-Sedgwick

334.8 (Boder-Sedgwick, Louis-Bar) Gonadal hypoplasia, insulin resistance and hyperglycemia, liver function problems, increased sensitivity to ionizing radiation, ataxia, and nystagmus.

Body or sinus, carotid

337.0 (Charcot-Weiss-Baker, Sluder's) Stimulation of an overactive carotid sinus, causing a marked drop in blood pressure, which, in turn, may stop the heart.

Boerhaave's

530.4 Spontaneous rupture of esophagus either as result of defect or in response to stress.

Bonnevie-Ullrich

758.6 Short stature, webbed neck, congenital heart disease, and mental retardation.

Bonnier's

386.19 Ocular disturbances, deafness, nausea, thirst, anorexia, and symptoms resulting from a lesion of Deiters' nucleus and its connections.

Bouveret (-Hoffmann)

427.2 Rapid action of the heart with sudden onset and cessation.

Bowel

579.3 Hypoglycemia and malabsorption following surgery.

Bowel distress

564.1 Abdominal pain, watery stools, and gas.

Brachial plexus

353.0 (Naffziger's) Anesthesis and vascular contraction in extremities caused by pressure of brachial plexus and subclavian artery against first thoracic rib.

Brachman-de Lange

759.89 (de Lange) Impaired development, mental retardation, eyebrows growing across bridge of nose and hairline well down on forehead, uptilted tip of nose with depressed bridge of nose, and small head with low-set ears.

Bradycardia-tachycardia

427.81 Rapid action of the heart followed by protracted or transient stopping of the heart.

Brailsford-Morquio

277.5 Accumulation of mucopolysccharide sulfates affecting the eye, ear, skin, teeth, skeleton, joints, liver, spleen, cardiovascular system, respiratory system, and central nervous system.

Brandt's

686.8 (Danbolt) Zinc metabolism defect in young children with blisters, crusting, oozing eruptions, loss of hair, and diarrhea.

Syndromes

Brissaud-Meige
244.9 Hypothyroidism resulting from acquired injury of thyroid gland or presence of cretinism.

Brock's
518.0 Incomplete expansion of the right middle lobe of a lung with chronic pneumonitis.

Brown spot
756.59 (McCune-Albright, Albright's hereditary osteodystrophy) Patchy skin pigmentation, endocrine dysfunctions, and polyostotic fibrous dysplasia.

Brown's tendon sheath
378.61 Limited elevation of eye, marked by paresis of inferior oblique muscle.

Brown-Séquard
344.89 (Avellis, Babinski-Nageotte, Benedikt's, Cestan's, Cestan-Chenais, Foville's, Gubler-Millard, Jackson's, Weber-Leyden) Paraplegia and anesthesia over part of the body caused by lesions in the brain or spinal cord.

Brugsch's
757.39 Increased thickening of the skin on extremities and face with clubbing of fingers and deformities in bone of the limb.

Brugada
746.89 A congenital heart anamoly in which the hypertrophy (enlargement) is localized to the left ventricle.

Bruising
287.2 (Diamond-Gardner, Gardner-Diamond) Bruising occurring easily and large in women, involving surrounding tissues, resulting in pain, and spawning others.

Bubbly lung
770.7 Intrauterine fetal aspiration of amniotic fluid contaminated by meconium.

Buchem's
733.3 Multiple fractures and bowing of all extremities, thickening of skull bones, and osteoporosis beginning in childhood.

Budd-Chiari
453.0 Thrombosis of the hepatic vein with enlargement of the liver and severe hypertension.

Büdinger-Ludloff-Läwen
717.89 An old disruption of ligaments in the knee.

Bulbar
335.22 (Duchenne's) Paralysis-based symptoms from defects in the medulla oblongata.

Bundle of Kent
426.7 Muscular bundle forming a direct connection between the ventricle and atrial walls.

Bürger-Grütz
272.3 Abdominal pain, hepatosplenomegaly, pancreatitis, and eruptive zanthomas in a genetic condition.

Burke's
577.8 (Burke's, Clarke-Hadfield, Cystic Fibrosis) Obstruction of mucosal passageways, poor growth, chronic bronchitis, recurrent pneumonia, emphysema, clubbing of fingers, and salt depletion with abnormal secretions in exocrine glands.

Burnett's
999.9 Disorder of the kidneys induced by ingestion of large amounts of alkali and calcium in the therapy of a peptic ulcer. Reversible in the early stages, it can lead to renal failure.

Burnier's
253.3 (Levi, Lorain-Levi) Dwarfism resulting from malfunction of the pituitary gland.

Burning feet
266.2 (Gopalan's) Severe discomfort of the feet and other extremities with excessive sweating and elevated skin temperature, and believed to be caused by a riboflavin deficiency.

Bywaters'
958.5 Traumatic anuria following crushing, especially of kidneys.

Caffey's
756.59 Soft tissue swelling over the affected bones, irritability, and fever, and running periods of exacerbation and remission.

Calvé-Legg-Perthes
732.1 Disease of the growth centers, especially the top of the femur, in which the epiphyses is replaced by new calcification.

Caplan (-Colinet) syndrome

714.81 Multiple spherical nodular lesions with clearly demarcated borders found throughout lungs and associated with rheumatoid arthritis.

Carcinogenic thrombophlebitis

453.1 Spontaneous development of thromboses in the upper and lower limbs because of visceral neoplasm.

Carcinoid

259.2 (Bjorck-Thorson, Cassidy-Scholte, Hedinger's) Carcinoid tumors causing cyanotic flushing of the skin, diarrhea watery stools, bronchoconstrictive attacks, hypotension, edema, and ascites.

Cardiacos negros

416.0 (Arrilaga-Ayerza) Cyanosis and hypertension resulting from sclerosis of the pulmonary arteries.

Cardiopulmonary obesity

278.8 (Pickwick) Obesity, hypoventilation, somnolence, and erythrocytosis.

Cardiorespiratory distress (idiopathic), newborn

769 (Hyaline membrane) Respiratory distress resulting from reduced amounts of lung surfactant in premature infants. Frequently fatal.

Cardiovasorenal

272.7 Abnormal accumulations of neutral glycolipids in histiocytes in blood vessel walls, cornea verticillata, parasthesia in extremities, cataracts, and angioperatomas on the thighs, buttocks, and genitalia.

Carini's

757.1 Scaling of skin accompanying other congenital syndromes.

Carpal tunnel

354.0 Pain and tingling, numbness, or burning in the hand resulting from compression of the median nerve by tendons. Often called a repetitive motion injury.

Carpenter's

759.89 Small head with mental retardation as result of genetic disorder.

Cassidy (-Scholte)

259.2 (Bjorck-Thorson, Hedinger's) Carcinoid tumors that cause cyanotic flushing of the skin, diarrheal watery stools, bronchoconstrictive attacks, hypotension, edema, and ascites.

Cat-cry

758.3X (Cri-du-chat) Microcephaly, antimongoloid palpebral fissures, epicanthal folds, micrognathia, strabismus, mental and physical retardation, and a cat-like whine.

Cauda equina

344.60 Aching pain of the perineum, bladder, and sacrum, radiating in a sciatic fashion, due to compression of spinal nerve roots.

Cerebellomedullary malformation

741.0X (Arnold-Chiari) Displacement of the caudal spinal cord due to tethering with or without spina bifida and meningomyelocele.

Cerebral gigantism

253.0 (Soto's) Increased birth weight and length, accelerated growth rate for the first four or five years with no elevation of serum growth hormone levels, followed by revision to normal growth rate; antimongoloid slant; prognathism; hypertelorism; dolichocephalic skull; impaired coordination; and moderate mental retardation.

Cerebrohepatorenal

759.89 Craniofacial abnormalities, hypotonia, hepatomegaly, polycystic kidneys, jaundice, and death in infancy.

Cervical paralysis

337.0 (Charcot-Weiss-Baker, Sluder's) Overactive carotid sinus, causing a marked drop in blood pressure stopping or blocking the heart.

Cervical (root) (spine) NEC

723.8 Symptoms originating form the cervical spine.

Cervical sympathetic

723.2 (cervicocranial) Irritation of nerve roots emanating from posterior cervical spinal cord.

Cervicodorsal outlet

353.2 Pain or anesthesis affecting the neck and the upper back.

Céstan (-Raymond)

433.8X Quadriplegia, anesthesia, and nystagmus caused by obstruction of twigs of the basilar artery and lesions in the pontine region.

Céstan's

344.89 (Avellis, Babinski-Nageotte, Benedikt's, Brown-Sequard, Cestan-Chenais, Foville's, Gubler-Millard, Jackson's, Weber-Leyden) Paraplegia and anesthesia over part of the body caused by lesions in the brain or spinal cord.

Céstan-Chenais

344.89 (Avellis, Babinski-Nageotte, Benedikt's, Brown-Sequard, Cestan's, Foville's, Gubler-Millard, Jackson's, Weber-Leyden) Paraplegia and anesthesia over part of the body caused by lesions in the brain or spinal cord.

Chancriform

114.1 Symptoms resembling a chancre.

Charcot's

443.9 Pain, tension, and weakness in a moving limb but absent at rest and caused by occlusive arterial diseases of the limbs.

Charcot-Marie-Tooth

356.1 Pain across the shoulder and upper arm.

Charcot-Weiss-Baker

337.0 (Sluder's) Overactive carotid sinus, causing a marked drop in blood pressure stopping or blocking the heart.

Cheadle (-Möller) (-Barlow)

267 Anemia, spongy gums, weakness, induration of leg muscles, and mucocutaneous hemorrhages.

Chédiak-Higashi (-Steinbrinck)

288.2 (Chediak-Higashi, Dohle body, Hegglin, Jordan's, May) Hepatosplenomegaly, lymphadenopathy, anemia, thrombocytopenia and changes in the bones, cardiopulmonary system, skin, psychomotor skills, abnormalities of granulation, and nuclear structure of white cells open the patient to infection.

Chiari's

453.0 Thrombosis of the hepatic vein with enlargement of the liver and severe hypertension.

Chiari-Frommel

676.6X Unphysiological lactation and amenorrhea following pregnancy caused by hyperprolactinemia and a pituitary adenoma.

Chiasmatic

368.41 Impairment of vision, limitations of the field of vision, scotoma, headache, syncope, and vertigo.

Chilaiditi's

751.4 Interposition of the colon between the liver and diaphragm.

Child maltreatment

995.5 (child abuse) Maltreatment of a child through physical violence, emotional violence, or starvation.

Chondroectodermal dysplasia

756.55 (Ellis-van Creveld) Congenital dwarfism with defective development of the cardiac septum, skin, hair, and teeth.

Chorea-athetosis-agitans

275.1 Accumulation of copper in the brain, cornea, kidney, liver, and other tissues causing cirrhosis of the liver and deterioration in the basal ganglia of the brain.

Christian's

277.8 (Hand-Schuller-Christian) Multiple-system defects of the membranous bones, exophthalmos, diabetes insipidus, soft tissues, and bone involvement.

Chromosome 4 short arm deletion

758.3 (Cri-du-chat) Microcephaly, antimongoloid palpebral fissures, epicanthal folds, micrgnathia, strabismus, mental and physical retardation, and a cat-like whine.

Chronic

557.1 (Wilkie's) Complete or partial block of the superior mesenteric artery with symptoms of vomiting, pain, blood in the stool, and distended abdomen resulting in bowel infarction.

Chronic alcoholic

291.2 Numerous symptoms caused by constant, long-time ingestion of alcohol affecting the nervous and gastrointestinal systems.

Chronic fatigue
780.7 Persistent fatigue that significantly reduces daily activity with chronic sore throat, mild fever, muscle weakness, myalgia, headaches, and neurological problems.

Churg-Strauss
446.4 Form of systemic inflammation and cell death of vessels with prominent lung involvement, manifested by severe asthma, among other respiratory disorders.

Clarke-Hadfield
577.8 (Burke's, Cystic Fibrosis) Obstructions of mucosal passageways, poor growth, chronic bronchitis, recurrent pneumonia, emphysema, clubbing of fingers, salt depletion, and abnormal secretions of exocrine glands.

Claude Bernard-Horner
337.9 (Reilly's, Steinbrocker's) Disorder following a heart attack with pain and stiffness in the shoulder, and swelling and pain in the hand.

Clifford's
766.2 Placental dysfunction occurring in postmature fetuses.

Climacteric
627.2 Chills, depression, hot flashes, headache, and irritability in menopausal women.

Clouston's
757.31 Congenital thickened nails and sparse or absent scalp hair, often accompanied by keratoderma of the palms and soles.

Clumsiness
315.4 Dyspraxia disorder.

Coagulation-fibrinolysis (ICF)
286.6 (coagulopathy) Decrease of elements needed for coagulation of blood causing profuse bleeding.

Cockayne's
759.89 Dwarfism with deafness, retinal atrophy, mental retardation, and photo sensitivity.

Cockayne-Weber
757.39 Dwarfism with a precociously senile appearance, pigmentary degeneration of the retina, optic atrophy, deafness, sensitivity to sunlight, and mental retardation.

Cogan's
370.52 Abrupt onset of interstitial keratitis, tinnitus, and vertigo followed by deafness.

Cold injury (newborn)
778.2 Birth injury resulting from hypothermia.

Collet (-Sicard)
352.6 Unilateral lesions of the ninth, tenth, eleventh, and twelfth cranial nerves producing paralysis of the vagal, glossal, and other nerves and the tongue on the same side.

Compartment(al) (anterior) (deep) (posterior) (tibial)
958.8 Early complication of trauma.

Compression, cervical
721.1 Cervical spondylosis.

Compression, crushing
958.5 Traumatic anuria following crushing.

Concussion
310.2 Persistent personality disturbance following a blow to the head featuring affective instability, bursts of aggression, apathy and indifference, impaired social judgment, and suspiciousness or paranoid ideation.

Congenital muscle hypoplasia
756.89 Dysplasia of the fingernails and toenails, hypoplasia of the patella, iliac horns, thickening of the glomerular lamina densa, and a flask-shaped femur.

Congenital oculofacial paralysis
352.6 (Collet-Sicard) Unilateral lesions of the ninth, tenth, eleventh, and twelfth cranial nerves producing paralysis of the vagal, glossal, and other nerves and the tongue on the same side.

Conjunctivourethrosynovial
099.3 A symptom of Reiter's disease.

Conn (-Louis)
255.1 Headaches, nocturia, plyuria, fatigue, hypertension, hypokalemic alkalosis, potassium depletion, hyperfolemia, and decreased renin activity, caused by a benign pituitary tumor.

Conradi (-Hünermann)
756.59 Asymmetric shortening of the limbs and scoliosis. Caused by both genetic and maternal medication sources.

Conus medullaris
336.8 (Froin's) Cerebral spinal fluid of a yellowish hue signaling neoplastic or inflammatory obstruction.

Cooke-Apert-Gallais
255.2 Type I acrocephalosyndactyly with peak head and fusion of digits (specifically the second through fifth digits) and severe acne vulgaris of forearms.

Cornelia de Lange's
759.8X Mental retardation, eyebrows across bridge of nose, hairline well down on forehead, uptilted tip of nose with depressed bridge of nose, and small head with low-set ears.

Correct substance properly administered
695.1 Necrolysis of skin caused by administered toxins.

Corticosexual
255.2 (Apert-Gallais, Cooke) Type I acrocephalosyndactyly with peak head and fusion of digits, specifically the second through fifth digits fused and severe acne vulgaris of forearms.

Costen's (complex)
524.60 Otalgia, dizziness, headache, tinnitis or loss of hearing, and burning sensation of throat, tongue, and side of the nose originally thought to be dysfunction of mandibular joint, but now thought to be worsened by other causes as well.

Costochondral junction
733.6 (Tietze's) Painful swelling of costal cartilages, especially of the second rib and interpreted as coronary artery disease.

Costovertebral
253.0 Arthritis of spine accompanying acromegaly, resembling rheumatoid arthritis and progressing to bony ankylosis with lipping of vertebral margins.

Cotard's
297X Paranoia marked by sensory disturbances, delusions of negation, and suicidal ideations.

Craniovertebral
723.2 Nerve root irritation emanating from posterior cervical spinal cord.

Creutzfeldt-Jakob
046.1 Progressive destruction of the pyramidal and extrapyramidal systems with progressive dementia, wasting of muscles, tremor, and other symptoms leading to death.

Cri-du-chat
758.3 (Cat-cry) Microcephaly, antimongoloid palpebral fissures, epicanthal folds, micrgnathia, strabismus, mental and physical retardation, and a cat-like whine.

Crib death
798.0 (Sudden infant death) Unexpected death of healthy infant under 12 months old.

Crigler-Najjar
277.4 Nonhemolytic jaundice due to absence of hepatic enzyme glucuronsyltransferasen with excessive amounts of unconjugated bilirubin and disorders of nervous system.

Crocodile tears
351.8 (Melkersson-Rosenthal) Facial paralysis with dramatic lacrimation during eating prompted by lesion on the seventh cranial nerve, causing impulses to be misdirected from salivary glands to lacrimal glands.

Croup
464.4 Obstruction of the larynx caused by allergy, foreign body, infection, or new growth in infants and children.

CRST
710.1X Induration and thickening of the skin with circulatory and organ changes in the face and hands.

Cruveilhier-Baumgarten
571.5 Cirrhosis of the liver with patent paraumbilical, varicose periumbilical, or umbilical veins.

Cubital tunnel
354.2 Lesion of the ulnar nerve, affecting movement and feeling of hand.

Cuiffini-Pancoast
162.3 (Hare's) Neoplasm of upper lobe of lung.

Curschmann (-Batten) (-Steinert)

359.2 Condition in which the peritoneal cover of the liver converts into a white mass resembling cake icing.

Cushing's

255.0 Abdominal striae, acne, hypertension decreased carbohydrate tolerance, moon face, obesity, protein catabolism, and psychiatric disturbances resulting from increased adrenocortical secretion of cartisol caused by ACTH-dependent adrenocortical hyperplasia or tumor, or by effects of steriods.

Cutaneocerebral angioma

759.6 (Kalischer's) Formation of multiple angiomas in skin of head and scalp.

Cutaneous nerve of thigh

355.1 Tingling, formication, itching, and other symptoms on lower part of the thigh. Caused by lateral femoral cutaneous nerve.

Cyriax's

733.99 (Davies-Colley) Arthritis with degeneration of cartilage leading to collapse of the ears, nose, and tracheobronchial tree. Death may occur as the respiratory system is affected.

Cystic duct stump

576.0 Recurrence of gall bladder pain following removal of the organ.

D₁

758.1 (Patau's, trisomy D) Extra chromosome in group D. Condition is usually fatal within two years and includes mental retardation, malformed ears, cardiac defects, convulsions, and other symptoms.

Da Costa's

306.2X (cardiac neurosis) Cardiac disorder marked by neurocirculatory asthenia prompted by emotional problems.

Dameshek's

282.4 One of hemolytic anemias that share a common decreased rate of synthesis of hemoglobin polypeptide chains and classified according to chain involved.

Dana-Putnam

281.0 [336.2] Numbness, tingling, weakness, a sore tongue, dyspnea, faintness, pallor of the skin and mucous membranes, anorexia, diarrhea, loss of weight, and fever. Strikes in the fifth decade.

Danbolt (-Closs)

686.8 (Brandt's) Zinc metabolism defect in young children with blisters, crusting, oozing eruptions, loss of hair, and diarrhea.

Dandy-Walker

742.3 Hydrocephalus with atresia of the foramina of Luschka and Magendie.

Danlos'

756.83 (Meekeren, Ehlers) Group of congenital connective tissue diseases with overly elastic skin, hyperextensive joints, and fragility of blood vessels and arteries.

Davies-Colley

733.99 (Cyriax's) Arthritis with degeneration of cartilage leading to collapse of the ears, nose, and tracheobronchial tree. Death may occur as the respiratory system is affected.

De Lange's

759.89 Inherited deformity with impaired development, mental retardation, eyebrows growing across bridge of nose, hairline well down on forehead, uptilted tip of nose with depressed bridge of nose, and small head with low-set ears.

De Toni-Fanconi (-Debré)

270.0 (Harts) Renal tubular malfunction, including cytinosis and osteomalacia and caused by inherited disorders or resulting from multiple myeloma or proximal epithelial growth.

Dead fetus

641.3X Loss of non-clotting blood and lengthy retention of dead fetus following tachycardia and related symptoms.

Death, sudden (SIDS)

798.0 Unexpected death of healthy infant typically under 12 months old.

Debré

270.0 (Harts) Renal tubular malfunction, including cytinosis and osteomalacia and caused by inherited disorders or resulting from multiple myeloma or proximal epithelial growth.

Defeminization

255.2 Mature masculine somatic characteristics by prepubescent male, girl, or woman showing at birth or developing later as result of adrenocortical dysfunction.

Syndromes

Defibrination
286.6   Dilution of fibrin by enzyme action.

Deficiency
260   Any syndrome resulting from deficiencies in proteins, hormones, carolies, trace minerals, vitamins, and other chemicals necessary for function or growth.

Degos'
447.8   Malignant atrophic papulosis.

Deiters' nucleus
386.19   (Bonnier) Ocular disturbances, deafness, nausea, thirst, anorexia, and symptoms traced to vagus centers resulting from lesion of Deiters' nucleus and its connections.

Déjérine-Roussy
348.8X   Infarction of the postero-inferior thalamus causing transient hemiparesis, severe loss of superficial and deep sensation with crude pain in the limbs, and vasomotor or trophic disturbances.

Déjérine-Thomas
333.0   (Hallervorden-Spatz) Nerves between the striatum and pallidum are completely demyelinated.

Del Castillo's
606.0   Cessation of menses not associated with pregnancy.

Deletion chromosomes
758.3   General description of syndromes such as antimongolism and cat-cry in which chromosomes are missing rather than duplicated.

Delusional
293.81   Organic disorder including hallucinations, beliefs about being followed, being poisoned, etc., and not meeting criteria for schizophrenia.

Dementia-aphonia, of childhood
299.1X   Dementia in which child becomes mute.

Depersonalization
300.6   Patient feels detached from his or her body and experiences the feeling of being an automaton or in a dream-like state. Depersonalization must be a primary symptom and not part of schizophrenia or another disorder.

Depressive type
293.83   Organic disorder with changes in personality such as amotivation, depression, outbursts, poor social judgment, and others.

Dercum's
272.8   (Ander's) Deposits of painful symmetrical nodular or pendulous masses of fat in various body regions.

Diabetes mellitus in newborn infant
775.1   Diabetes mellitus

Diabetes mellitus-hypertension-nephrosis
250.4X   [581.81] High blood pressure and kidney failure resulting from diabetes in which carbohydrate utilization is reduced and lipid and protein use is enhanced.

Diabetes-dwarfism-obesity
258.1   Endocrine dysfunction causing diabetes and affecting growth and weight.

Diabetes-nephrosis
250.4X   [581.81] High blood pressure and kidney failure resulting from diabetes in which carbohydrate utilization is reduced and lipid and protein use is enhanced.

Diabetic amyotrophy
250.6X   [358.1] Muscular atrophy resulting from diabetes

Diamond-Blackfan
284.0   (Blackfan-Diamond, Fanconi, Kaznelson's) Congenital anemia of infancy requiring a number of blood transfusions to maintain life.

Diamond-Gardener
287.2   Bruising occuring easily and large, involving surrounding tissues, resulting in pain, and spawning others. Assumed to be a form of autoimmune problem.

Diaper
270.0   Infantile form of Fanconi's syndrome with cytinosis.

DIC
286.6   Decrease of elements needed for coagulation of blood causing profuse bleeding.

Diencephalohypophyseal
253.8   Problem with the thalamus or pituitary gland not otherwise specified.

DiGeorge's
279.11 Hypoplasia or aphasia of the thymus and parathyroid gland with congenital heart defects, anomalies of the great vessels, esophageal atresia, seizures, and facial deformities.

Dighton's
756.51 (van der Hoeve's) Blue sclera, little growth, brittle bones, and deafness.

Disseminated platelet thrombosis
446.6 Fatal disease with central nervous system involvement due to formation of fibrin or platelet thrombi in arterioles and capillaries in many organs.

Doan-Wiseman
288.0 (Kostmann's, Schultz, Shwachman) Inherited bronchiectasis and pancreatic insufficiency resulting in malnutrition, sinusitis, short stature, and bone abnormalities.

Döhle body
288.2 (Chediak-Higashi, Hegglin, Jordan's, May) Hepatosplenomegaly, lymphadenopathy, anemia, thrombocytopenia, changes in the bones, cardiopulmonary system, skin, and psychomotor skills. Granulation and nuclear structure of white cells opens patient to infection and results in death.

Donohue's
259.8 Slow physical and mental development, elfin facial features such as wide-set eyes and low-set ears, and severe endocrine disorders indicated by enlarged sexual organs. Rare and fatal.

Double whammy
360.81 Dislocation of eye ball.

Down's
758.0 (Trisomy 21) Retardation with numerous markers varying from one person to another. Symptoms include retarded growth, flat face with short nose, epicanthic skin folds, protruding lower lip, rounded ears, thickened tongue, pelvic dysplasia, broad hands and feet, stubby fingers, and absence of Moro reflex.

Dresbach's
282.1 Varying degrees of anemia and increased blood cell destruction caused by hereditary disorder in which the greater proportion of erythrocytes are elliptical in shape.

Dressler's
411.0 Fever, leukocytosis, chest pain, evidence of pericarditis, pleurisy, and pneumonia occurring days or weeks after a myocardial infarction.

Drug
292.0 A number of physical symptoms resulting from long-time ingestion of, and dependence on, therapeutic and illicit drugs.

Drug withdrawal, infant, of dependent mother
779.5 A number of physical symptoms suffered by newborns whose drug-dependent mothers allowed drugs to cross the placenta.

Drug-induced
292.84 Description of symptoms, physiological and psychological, produced by drug abuse or dependence.

Drum
381.02 Symptom of a number of syndromes affecting the ear.

Dry skin
701.1 Keratosis producing lesions appearing as dry skin.

DSAP
692.75 (Disseminated Superficial Actinic Porokeratosis) Skin disorder occurring on sun-exposed skin and characterized by numerous superficial, keratotic, brownish-red macules.

Duane's
378.71 (Still-Turk-Duane, Duane-Stilling-Turk) Simultaneous retraction of eye muscles causing an inability to abduct the affected eye with retraction of the globe.

Dubin-Johnson
277.4 (Dubin-Sprinz) Nonhemilitic jaundice thought as a defect in concentrated bilirubin and other organs causing a brown granular pigment in the hepatic duct.

Duchenne's
335.22 Paralysis symptoms caused by medulla oblongata.

Due to mesenteric artery insufficiency

557.1   (Wilkie's) Blocked superior mesenteric artery with vomiting, pain, blood in the stool, distended abdomen, and bowel infarction.

Dumping

564.2   Emptying of contents of jejunum with nausea, sweating, weakness, palpitation, syncope, warmth, and diarrhea. Occurs after eating in patients who have had partial gastrectomy and gastrojejunostomy.

Duplay's

726.2   Inflammation of subacromial or subdeltoid bursa.

Dupré's

781.6   Irritation of spinal cord and brain mimicking meningitis, but in which there is no swelling of membranes.

During labor

668.0X   (Mendelson's) Disorders of lung following vomiting and regurgitation by obstetric patients.

Dyke-Young

283.9   (Hayem-Widal) Anemia caused by exposure to trauma, poisons,and other causes.

Dyspraxia

315.4   Organic disorder affecting patient's ability to perform coordinated acts and not due to psychotic diagnosis.

Dyssynergia cerebellaris myoclonica

334.2   (Hunt's) Disorder marked by myoclonus epilepsy and muscular tremors associated with disturbance of muscle tone and coordination.

E₃

758.2   (Edward's, trisomy E) Congenital malformations in which extra chromosome is group E. Includes mental retardation, abnormal skull shape, malformed ears, small mandible, cardiac defects, short sternum, and other symptoms.

Eale's

362.18   Retinal vasculitis marked by phlebitis, arteritis, and endarteritis.

Eaton-Lambert

199.1   [358.1] (Lambert-Eaton) Progressive proximal muscle weakness resulting from antibodies directed against motor-nerve axon terminals.

Ebstein's

746.7   (Hypoplastic left heart) Hypoplasia or atresia of the left ventricle and aorta or mitral valve with respiratory distress and extreme cyanosis. Cardiac failure and death often result in early infancy.

Ectopic ACTH secretion

255.0   (Cushing) Abdominal striae, acne, hypertension decreased carbohydrate tolerance, moon face, obesity, protein catabolism, and psychiatric disturbances resulting from increased adrenocortical secretion of cortisol caused by ACTH-dependent adreocortical hyperplasia or tumor, or administration of steriods.

Eczema-thrombocytopenia

279.12   (Aldrich, Wiskott-Aldrich) Immunodeficiency shown by eczema, thrombocyopenia, and recurrent pyogenic infection with increased susceptibility to infection from encapsulated bacteria.

Eddowes'

756.51   (Ekman's, Spurway's) Blue sclera, little growth, brittle and malformed bones, and malformed teeth.

Edwards'

758.2   (E, trisomy E) Congenital malformations in which extra chromosome is group E. Includes mental retardation, abnormal skull shape, malformed ears, small mandible, cardiac defects, short sternum, and other symptoms.

Efferent loop

537.89   (Gastrojejunal loop obstruction) Distended efferent loop with illness and pain caused by acute or chronic obstruction of the duodenum and jejunum proximal to a gastrojejunostomy.

Ehlers-Danlos

756.83   (Meekeren, Ehlers, Danlos) Congenital connective tissue diseases with overly elastic skin, hyperextensive joints, and fragility of blood vessels and arteries.

Eisenmenger's
745.4 Pulmonary hypertension with congenital communication between two circulations so that a right to left shunt results.

Ekbom's
333.99 Sense of indescribable uneasiness, restlessness, insomnia, and twitching in the legs after going to bed caused by poor circulation or antipsychotic medications.

Ekman's
756.51 (Eddowes', Spurway's) Blue sclera, little growth, brittle and malformed bones, and malformed teeth.

Electric feet
266.2 (Gopalan's) Discomfort of feet and other extremities, excessive sweating, elevated skin temperature, and riboflavin deficiency.

Ellis-van Creveld
756.55 Dwarfism with defective development of cardiac septum, skin, hair, and teeth.

Ellison-Zollinger
251.5 (Zollinger-Ellison) Peptic ulceration with gastric hypersecretion, tumor of the pancreatic islets, and hypoglycemia.

Embryonic fixation
270.2 (Mendes, van der Hoeve-Halbertsma-Waardenburg, Waardenburg-Klein) Eyebrow or upper or lower eyelid sags.

Empty sella
253.8 Sella turcica containing no pituitary gland caused by herniating arachnoid, radiotherapy, or surgery.

Endocrine-hypertensive
255.3 (Schroeder's, Slocumb's) Disorder of adrenal medullary tissue with hypertension, attacks of palpitation, headache, nausea, dyspnea, anxiety, pallor, and profuse sweating.

Engel-von Recklinghausen
252.0 (Jaffe-Lichtenstein-Uehlinger) Osteitis with fibrous degeneration and formation of cysts with fibrous nodules on affected bones.

Enteroarticular
099.3 (Fiessinger-Leroy-Reiter) Association of arthritis, iredocyclitis, urethritis, and diarrhea.

Eosinophilia myalgia
710.5 Painful muscles resulting from accumulation of a large number of granular leukocytes.

Epidemic vomiting
078.82 (Winter's disease) Nausea and vomiting attacking a group of people suddenly without prior illness or malaise. Headache, vomiting, abdominal pain, and giddiness end quickly.

Erb (-Oppenheim) - Goldflam
358.0 (Goldflam, Erb, Hoppe) Myoneural conduction-caused progressive muscular weakness beginning in face and throat.

Erdheim's
253.0 Arthritis of spine accompanying acromegaly, resembling rheumatoid arthritis and progressing to bony ankylosis with lipping of vertebral margins.

Erlacher-Blount
732.4 Disease causing bow-legs in children.

Erythrocyte fragmentation
283.19 (Lederer-Brill) Fragmentation of red blood cells.

Evans'
287.3 Condition where number of platelets in circulating blood increases, causing bruising.

Exhaustion
300.5 Hypersomatic disorder.

Eye, dry
375.15 Lacrimal glands are unable to provide enough moisture to cover the eye.

Eye retraction
378.71 (Duane, Still-Turk-Duane) Retraction of eye muscles with inability to abduct the affected eye with retraction of the globe.

Eyelid-malar-mandible
756.0 (Franceschetti's) Malformations of derivatives of the first branchial arch, with pallpebral fissures sloping outward and downward with notches in the outer third of the lower lids, defects of malar bones and zygome, hypoplasia of the jawbone, high or cleft palate, low-set ears, unusual hair growth, and pits between mouth and ear.

Syndromes

Faber's

280.9   (Hayem-Faber) Central pallor in the red
         blood cells caused by lack of red cell
         hemoglobin in blood.

Fabry (-Anderson)

272.7   Neutral glycolipids in histiocytes in blood
         vessel walls, cornea verticillata, parasthesia
         in extremities, cataracts and angioperatomas
         on the thighs, buttocks, and genitalia. Death
         comes from cardiac, cerebrovascular, and
         renal complications.

Facial diplegia

352.6   (Collet-Sicard) Unilateral lesions of the
         ninth, tenth, eleventh, and twelfth cranial
         nerves producing paralysis of the vagal,
         glossal, other nerves, and the tongue on the
         same side. Most usually result of injury.

Fallot's

745.2   Also called tetralogy of Fallot. Congenital
         cardiac defects with pulmonary stenosis,
         intervetricular septal defect, dextroposeptum
         and venous as well as arterial blood, and
         right ventricular hypertrophy.

Familial acanthosis nigricans

701.2   Velvety acanthosis with gray, black, or
         brown pigmentation on axillae and other
         body folds. In adults, it results from internal
         carcinoma. In children, it results from
         obesity-producing endocrine disturbance.

Familial eczema-thrombocytopenia

279.12   (Aldrich, Wiskott-Aldrich) Eczema,
         thrombocyopenia, and recurrent pyogenic
         infection with increased susceptibility to
         infection from encapsulated bacteria.

Fanconi

759.81   Rounded face, almond-shaped eyes,
         strabismus, low forehead, hypogonadism,
         hypotomia, mental retardation, and an
         insatiable appetite.

Fanconi (-de Toni) (-Debré)

270.0   (Harts) Renal tubular malfunction, including
         cytinosis and osteomalacia caused by
         inherited disorders, the result of multiple
         myeloma, or proximal epithelial growth.

Fanconi's

284.0   (Blackfan-Diamond, Kaznelson's) Anemia of
         infancy requiring a number of blood
         transfusions to maintain life.

Farber (-Uzman)

272.8   Swollen joints, lymphadenopathy,
         subcutaneous nodules, and accumulation in
         lyosomes of affected cells of PAS-positive
         lipid consisting of ceramide. Begins soon
         after birth and caused by deficiency of
         ceramidase.

Fatigue NEC

300.5   Hypersomatic disorder with no identifiable
         pathology.

FDH

757.39   Linear areas of dermal hyperplasia with soft
         yellow nodules of fat. Areas are widely
         distributed and resemble striae distensae.

Feet, burning

266.2   (Gopalan's) Severe discomfort of feet and
         other extremities associated with excessive
         sweating and elevated skin temperature;
         believed to be caused by a riboflavin
         deficiency.

Feil-Klippel

756.16   Shorter than average neck and a low
         hairline. Caused by fewer than average
         cervical vertebrae or fusion of hemivertebrae
         into one bony mass.

Felty's

714.1   Splenomegaly, leukopenia, arthritis,
         hypersplenism, anemia and other symptoms.

Feminizing

255.2   (Achard-Thiers) Aranodactyly with small,
         receding mandible, broad skull, and joint
         laxity in hands and feet.

Fertile eunuch

257.2   Hypogonadism with gynecomastia,
         hypospadias, and pospubertal testicular
         atrophy. Caused by an inherited defect of
         androgen receptors and insensitivity to
         testosterone.

Fetal alcohol

760.71   Growth deficiency, craniofacial anomalies,
         and limb defects among offspring of mothers
         who are chronic alcoholics.

Fiedler's

422.91   Isolated infection of heart muscle.

Fiessinger-Leroy (-Reiter)
099.3   (Fiessinger-Leroy-Reiter) An association of arthritis, iredocyclitis, and urethritis, sometimes with diarrhea. While symptoms may recur, the arthritis is constant.

Fiessinger-Rendu
695.1   Necrolysis of the skin caused by toxins.

First arch
756.0   (Franceschetti's) Malformations of the first branchial arch with pallpebral fissures sloping outward and downward with notches in the outer third of the lower lids, defects of malar bones and zygoma, hypoplasia of the jawbone, high or cleft palate, low-set ears, unusual hair growth, and pits between mouth and ear.

Fisher's
357.0   (Guillain-Barre, Landry, Strohl, Miller) Paraplegia of limbs, flaccid paralysis, ophthalmoplegia, ataxia, and areflexia caused by disorder of immune system.

Fitz's
577.0   Acute infection of the pancreas with the formation of necrotic areas, bleeding in the gland, fever, leukocytosis, nausea, and pain.

Flajani (-Basedow)
242.XX   (Basedow, Parry's, Grave's disease) Fatigue, nervousness, emotional lability and irritability, heat intolerance and increased sweating, weight loss, palpitation, and tremor of hands and tongue caused by excess thyroidal hormones.

Flush
259.2   (Bjorck-Thorson, Cassidy-Scholte, Hedinger's) Carcinoid tumors causing severe attacks of cyanotic flushing of the skin, diarrheal watery stools, bronchoconstrictive attacks, hypotension, edema, and ascites.

Foix-Alajouanine
336.1   Ophthalmoplegia, paresis of the sympathetic nerves, and neuroparalytic keratitis from compression of lateral wall of the cavernous sinus.

Following crush injury
958.5   Traumatic anuria following crushing by a heavy object.

Following delivery
674.8X   Hepatorenal syndrome, cardiomyopathy, uterine hypertrophy, and other symptoms following childbirth.

Fong's
756.89   Dysplasia of the fingernails and toenails, hypoplasia of patella, iliac horns, thickening of the glomerular lamina densa, and a flask-shaped femur.

Foramen magnum
348.4   Compression of brain from the space above.

Forbes-Albright
253.1   Persistent lactation and amenorrhea caused by pituitary tumor, marked by secretion of excessive amounts of prolactin.

Fossa compression
348.4   Compression of brain from the fossa underneath.

Foster-Kennedy
377.04   (Gowers-Paton-Kennedy) Meningioma of optic nerve with central scotoma and contralateral choked disk.

Foville's
344.89   (Avellis, Babinski-Nageotte, Benedikt's, Brown-Sequard, Cestan's, Cestan-Chenais, Gubler-Millard, Jackson's, Weber-Leyden) Paraplegia and anesthesia over part of the body caused by lesions in the brain or spinal cord.

Fragile X
759.83   Mental retardation, enlarged testes, big jaw, high forehead, and long ears in males. In females, fragile X presents mild retardation and heterozygous sexual structures. In some families, males have shown no symptoms but carry the gene.

Franceschetti's
756.0   Malformations of derivatives of the first branchial arch, marked by pallpebral fissures sloping outward and downward with notches in the outer third of the lower lids, defects of malar bones and zygome, hypoplasia of the jawbone, high or cleft palate, low-set ears, unusual hair growth, and pits between mouth and ear.

Fraser's

759.89   Cyptophthalmus with ear malformations, cleft palate, laryngeal deformity, displacement of umbilicus and nipples, digital malformation, separation of symphysis pubis, maldeveloped kidneys, and masculine female genitals.

Freeman-Sheldon

759.89   (Whistling face syndrome) Deviation of hands and face with protrusion of lips as in whistling, sunken eyes, and small nose.

Frey's

350.8   Localized sweating and flushing of cheek and ear in response to chewing.

Friderichsen-Waterhouse

036.3   Fulminating meningococcal septicemia in children below 10 years of age with vomiting, cyanosis, diarrhea, purpura, convulsions, circulatory collapse, meningitis, and hemorrhaging into the adrenal glands.

Friedrich-Erb-Arnold

757.39   Thickening of skin on extremities and face with clubbing of fingers and deformities in bone of the limb.

Fröhlich's

253.8   (Babinski-Frohlich, Launois-Cleret, Renon-Delille) Obesity and hypogonadism in adolescent boys. Dwarfism indicates hypothyroidism.

Froin's

336.8   (Froin's) Alteration in the cerebral spinal fluid resulting in a yellowish hue and indictive of neoplastic or inflammatory obstruction.

Frommel-Chiari

676.6X   Hyperprolactinemia and a pituitary adenoma causing unphysiological lactation and amenorrhea following pregnancy.

Frontal Lobe Syndrome

310.0   Changes in behavior following damage to the frontal areas of the brain including reduction in self-control, foresight, creativity, spontaneity, emotional vivaciousness, and empathy.

Fuller Albright's

756.59   (McCune-Albright; Albright's hereditary osteodystrophy) Patchy skin pigmentation, endocrine dysfunctions, and polyostotic fibrous dysplasia.

Functional, hyperinsulinism

251.1   (Harris', organic hyperinsulinism) Hyperinsulinism due to organic endogenous factors with hypoglycemia, weakness, perspiration, jitteriness, tachycardia, mental confusion, and vision disturbances.

G

758.0   A congenital retardation with numerous markers, which may vary from one person to another. Common symptoms include retarded growth, flat face with short nose, epicanthic skin folds, protruding lower lip, rounded ears, thickened tongue, pelvic dysplasia, broad hands, stubby fingers, and absence of Moro reflex in newborns.

Gaisböck's

289.0   Associated with hypertension, but without hyposplenomegaly.

Ganser's, hysterical

300.16   Psychotic-like condition (but without symptoms and signs of a traditional psychosis) occurring in prisoners who feign insanity or who suffer head injury.

Gardner-Diamond

287.2   Bruising occurring easily and large, involving surrounding tissues, resulting in pain, and spawning others. Assumed to be a form of autoimmune deficiency.

Gastrojejunal loop obstruction

537.89   (Gastrojejunal loop obstruction) A distended afferent loop marked by illness and pain. Caused by acute or chronic obstruction of the duodenum and jejunum proximal to a gastrojejunostomy.

Gayet-Wernicke's

265.1   Thiamine deficiency, disturbances in ocular motility, pulpillary alterations, nystagmus, ataxia with tremors, and co-existing organic toxic psychosis. Most often due to alcoholism.

Gee-Herter-Heubner

579.0   Catarrhal dysentery. Malabsortion syndrome of all ages precipitated by gluten-containing foods. Wasting and fatigue in both adults and children. Children suffer growth retardation and irritability. Adults suffer difficulty in breathing and clubbing of fingers.

Gélineau's
347   Narcolepsy, a form of epilepsy where the patient abruptly falls asleep rather than suffering grand or petite mals.

Geniculate ganglion
053.11   (Hunt's) Facial paralysis, otalgia, and herpes zoster caused by viral infection in seventh cranial nerve and genticulate ganglion.

Gerhardt's
478.30   Paralysis of vocal cords causing inspiratory dyspnea.

Gerstmann's
784.69   Right-left disorientation, finger agnosia, agraphia, and constructional apraxia, due to lesion in the angular gyrus of the dominant hemisphere of the brain.

Gilbert's
277.4   Benign elevation of unconjugated bilirubin with no liver damage or other deformities.

Gilford (-Hutchinson)
259.8   (Hutchinson-Gilford) Precocious senility with death from coronary artery disease occurring before 10 years of age.

Gilles de la Tourette's
307.23   Motor and vocal tics occurring many times a day beginning before age 21 and in which the type of tic changes over time.

Gillespie's
759.89   Congenital dysplasia of the eyes, teeth, and extremities.

Glénard's
569.89   Bloating, gas, pain, and fullness experienced in left upper abdominal quadrant with pain sometimes radiating up into left chest. Downward displacement of viscera may cause bulging of abdomen and other symptoms.

Glinski-Simmonds
253.2   Wasting of pituitary gland as result of some other condition or affliction.

Glucuronyl transferase
277.4   Benign elevation of unconjugated bilirubin with no liver damage or other deformities.

Glue ear
381.20   Painless secretion of mucoid fluid in the middle ear, stopping up the eustachian tube and causing hearing loss.

Goldberg (-Maxwell) (-Morris)
257.8   (Morris, hairless women, Goldberg-Maxwell) Male pseudohermaphroditism with incompletely developed vagina with rudimentary uterus and fallopian tubes, scanty or absent axillary/public hair, and amenorrhea.

Goldenhar's
756.0   Epibulbar dermoid cysts, preauricular appendages, micrognathia, and vertebral anomalies.

Goldflam-Erb
358.0   (Goldflam, Erb, Hoppe) Progressive muscular weakness beginning in face and throat caused by a defect in myoneural conduction.

Goltz-Gorlin
757.39   Irregular linear streaks of skin atrophy, skeletal malformations, papillomas of the lips and labia, and occassional alopecia.

Goodpasture's
446.21   Renal condition where nephritis progresses rapidly to death, leaving lungs showing extensive hemosiderosis or bleeding.

Gopalan's
266.2   Severe discomfort of the feet and other extremities associated with excessive sweating and elevated skin temperature; believed to be caused by a riboflavin deficiency.

Gorlin-Chaudhry-Moss
759.89   Congenital lesion of the basal cells.

Gougerot (-Houwer) - Sjögren
710.2   (Sicca) Complex of symptoms of unknown source in middle aged women in which following triad exists: keratoconjunctivitis sicca, zerostomia, and connective tissue disease (usually rheumatoid arthritis but sometimes systemic lupus erythematosus). Cause may be abnormal immune response.

Gougerot-Blum
709.1   Purpuric skin eruption seen on the legs, thighs, and lower trunk of men 40 to 60 years of age and characterized by minute rust-colored papules that fuse into plaques.

Syndromes

Gougerot-Carteaud

701.8   Benign neoplasm producing fingerlike projections from epithelial surface in girls nearing puberty. Papillas begin on back and between breasts, eventually spreading over the torso and throughout the body.

Gowers'

780.2   Fall in blood pressure, slow pulse, and convulsions. Believed to be sudden stimulation of vagal nerve by receptors in heart, carotid sinus, or aortic arch.

Gowers-Paton-Kennedy

377.04   (Foster-Kennedy, Gowers-Paton-Kennedy) Meningioma of optic nerve with central scotoma and contralateral choked disk.

Gradenigo's

383.02   Localized meningitis in fifth and sixth cranial nerves, causing paralysis and pain in the temporal region.

Gray or grey

779.4   Effects of chloramphenicol taken by mother during gestation on the newborn.

Greig's

756.0   Abnormal increase in the interorbital distance with cleidcranial or craniofacial malformations, along with occasional mental deficiencies.

Gubler-Millard

344.89   (Avellis, Babinski-Nageotte, Benedikt's, Brown-Sequard, Cestan's, Cestan-Chenais, Foville's, Jackson's, Weber-Leyden) Paraplegia and anesthesia over half or part of the body caused by lesions in the brain or spinal cord.

Guérin-Stern

754.89   Congenital immobility of most joints, fixed in various postures, with little muscle development and growth.

Guillain-Barré (-Strohl)

357.0   (Landry, Fisher's, Strohl, Miller) Often follows viral infections and may be a disorder of immune system with paraplegia of limbs, flaccid paralysis, ophthalmoplegia, ataxia, and areflexia.

Gunn's

742.8   (jaw-winking) Eyelids widen during chewing, sometimes with an elevation of the upper lid when the mouth is open and closing of the lid when the mouth is closed.

Günther's

277.1   Cutaneous photosensitivity leading to mutilating skin lesions, homlytic anemia and splenomegaly, and greatly increased urinary excretion of uroporphyrin.

Gustatory sweating

350.8   (Frey's) Localized sweating and flushing of cheek and ear in response to chewing.

H30

759.81   Rounded face, almond-shaped eyes, strabismus, low forehead, hypogonadism, hypotomia, mental retardation, and an insatiable appetite.

Hadfield-Clarke

577.8   (Burke's, Clarke-Hadfield, Cystic Fibrosis) Abnormal secretions of exocrine glands, obstructions of mucosal passageways, poor growth, chronic bronchitis, recurrent pneumonia, emphysema, clubbing of fingers, and salt depletion.

Haglund-Läwen-Fründ

717.89   Traumatic separation of the cartilage of the patella with fissures.

Hairless women

257.8   (Morris, Goldberg, Goldberg-Maxwell) Male pseudohermaphroditism with incompletely developed vagina, rudimentary uterus and fallopian tubes, scanty or absent axillary/public hair, and amenorrhea.

Hallermann-Streiff

756.0   Congenital dyscephaly with parrot nose, mandibular hypoplasia, congenital cataracts, and microthalmia.

Hallervorden-Spatz

333.0   (Dejerine-Thomas) Nerves between the striatum and pallidum are completely demyelated.

Hallucinatory type

293.82   (hallucinosis) Organic disorder in which the patient exhibits chronic hallucinations not occuring during the course of delirium.

Hamman's

518.1   Pneumothorax or pneumopericardium resulting from presence of air or gas in the mediastinum beginning spontaneously or from trauma or disease. Sometimes induced to aid in diagnosis.

Hamman-Rich
516.3　Chronic inflammation, progressive fibrosis of the pulmonary alveolar walls, and progressive dyspnea leading to death by oxygen deprivation or right heart failure.

Hand-foot
282.61　(Herrick's) Sickle cell anemia.

Hand-Schüller-Christian
277.8　(Christian) Histiocytosis with an occasional accumulation of cholesterol, defects of the membranous bones, exophthalmos, diabetes insipidus, and multiple-system, soft tissue, and bone involvement.

Hanot-Chauffard (-Troisier)
275.0　Hypertrophic cirrhosis with pigmentation and diabetes mellitus.

Hare's
162.3　(Cuiffini-Pancoast) Neoplasm of upper lobe of lung.

Harkavy's
446.0　(MCLS) Fever, conjunctival injection reddening of the oral cavity, ulcerative gingivitis, cervical lymph nodes, and skin eruptions that cover the hands and feet. Skin becomes puffy and sloughs off.

Harris'
251.1　Hyperinsulinism due to organic endogenous factors, hypoglycemia, weakness, perspiration, jitteriness, tachycardia, mental confusion, and vision disturbances.

Hart's
270.0　Renal tubular malfunction, cytinosis, and osteomalacia caused by inherited disorders or the result of multiple myeloma or proximal epithelial growth.

Hayem-Faber
280.9　(Faber) Central pallor in red blood cells caused by lack of red cell hemoglobin in blood.

Hayem-Widal
283.9　(Dyke-Young, Widal) One of a group of anemic syndromes caused by exposures to trauma, poisons, and other causes that decreases the number of red blood cells.

Heat exhaustion or prostration
992.4　Salt depletion following exposure to sunlight and heat, causing heat exhaustion.

Heberden's
413.9　(angina pectoris) Severe pain in the chest caused by ischemia of the heart prompted by coronary artery disease.

Hedinger's
259.2　(Bjorck-Thorson, Cassidy-Scholte) Carcinoid tumors causing severe attacks of cyanotic flushing of skin, diarrheal watery stools, bronchoconstrictive attacks, hypotension, edema, and ascites.

Hegglin's
288.2　(Chediak-Higashi, Dohle body, Jordan's, May) Hepatosplenomegaly, lymphadenopathy, anemia, thrombocytopenia, and changes in the bones, cardopulmonary system, skin, and psychomotor skills. Abnormalities of granulation and nuclear structure of white cells open patients to infection and result in death.

Heller's
299.1X　Dementia in which a child becomes mute with irritability, tantrums, and other behavioral disorders.

Hemoglobinuria
283.2　(Marchiafava-Micheli) Acquired blood cell dysplasis in which there are many clones of stem cells producing red blood cells, platelets, and granulocytes.

Hemolytic-uremic
283.11　Enlargement of liver and spleen and many erythroblasts in circulation.

Hemorrhage
036.3　(Friderichsen-Waterhouse, Waterhouse, 036.3) Fulminating meningococcal septicemia occurring in children below 10 years of age with vomiting, cyanosis, diarrhea, purpura, convulsions, circulatory collapse, meningitis, and hemorrhaging into adrenal glands.

Hench-Rosenberg
719.3X　Repeated episodes of arthritis and periarthritis without fever or changes in joints.

Henoch-Schönlein
287.0　Eruption of purpuric lesions with joint pain and swelling, colic, passage of bloody stools, and glomerulonephritis in young children.

Syndromes

Hepatic flexure
569.89 Bloating, gas, pain, and fullness experienced in left upper abdominal quadrant with pain sometimes radiating up into left chest.

Hepatorenal
572.4 (Heyd's, hepatourologic) Acute renal failure in patients with disease of the biliary or liver tract. Caused by decreased renal blood flow, damaging both organs.

Hercules
255.2 (Apert-Gallais, Cooke) Type I acrocephalosyndactyly with peaked head, fusion of digits (specifically the second through fifth digits), and severe acne vulgaris of forearms.

Herpetic geniculate ganglionitis
053.11 (Hunt's) Facial paralysis, otalgia, and herpes zoster caused by viral infection in seventh cranial nerve and genticulate ganglion.

Herrick's
282.61 Sickle cell anemia.

Herter (-Gee)
579.0 (Heubner-Herter) Catarrhal dysentery. Inherited malabsortion syndrome of all ages precipitated by gluten-containing foods with wasting and fatigue. Children suffer growth retardation and irritability. Adults suffer difficulty in breathing and clubbing of fingers.

Heyd's
572.4 Acute renal failure with disease of the biliary or liver tract. Cause is decreased renal blood flow, damaging both organs.

HHHO
759.81 (H3O) Rounded face, almond-shaped eyes, strabismus, low forehead, hypogonadism, hypotomia, mental retardation, and an insatiable appetite.

Hoffa (-Kastert)
272.8 Traumatic proliferation of fatty tissue on knee joint.

Hoffmann's
244.9 [359.5] Hypothyroidism beginning during infancy as result of acquired injury of thyroid gland or presence of cretinism.

Hoffmann-Bouveret
427.2 Rapid action of the heart having sudden onset and cessation.

Holländer-Simons
272.6 Loss of subcutanious fat of the upper torso, the arms, the neck, and face but with an increase in fat on and below the pelvis.

Holmes'
368.16 (Balint's, Riddoch's) Corical paralysis of visual fixation, optic ataxia, and disturbance of visual attention. Eye movements are normal.

Holmes-Adie
379.46 (Adie, Holmes, Markus, Saenger's) Pathological reaction in which the pupil does not react to changes in light and changes if focus is changed. Cause is certain tendon deficiency.

Hoppe-Goldflam
358.0 (Goldflam, Erb, Hoppe) Progressive muscular weakness beginning in face and throat caused by a defect in myoneural conduction.

Horner's
337.9 (Claude Bernard-Homer, Reilly's, Steinbrocker's) Pain and stiffness in the shoulder, with puffy swelling and pain in the hand following a heart attack.

Hospital addiction
301.51 (Multiple operations, Munchhausen) Description of psychoxomatic behavior with physical symptoms exhibited by some patients with histrionic personality disorder.

Hunt's
053.11 (Ramsey-Hunt) Facial paralysis, otalgia, and herpes zoster caused by viral infection in seventh cranial nerve and genticulate ganglion.

Hunter (-Hurler)
277.5 Mucopolysccharide sulfates affecting the eye, ear, skin, teeth, skeleton, joints, liver, spleen, cardiovascular system, respiratory system, and central nervous system.

Hutchinson-Boeck
135 (Lofgren's, Schaumann's, Besnier-Boeck-Schaumann) Disorder with fibrosis, lymph nodes, skin, enlarged liver, eyes, enlarged spleen, phalangeal bones, parotid glands, and systemic granulomas composed of epithelioid and multinucleated giant cells.

Hutchinson-Gilford
259.8   (Gilford) Precocious senility with death from coronary artery disease occurring before 16 years of age.

Hyperabduction
447.8   Malignant atrophic papulosis.

Hyperactive bowel
564.1   Abdominal pain, watery stools, and gas.

Hyperaldosteronism with hypokalemic alkalosis
255.1   (Bartter's) Low or normal blood pressure, no edema, retarded growth, hypokalemic alkalosis, and elevated renin or angiotensin levels.

Hypercalcemic
275.4   (Albright-Martin, Seabright-Bantam) Similar to hypoparthyroidism, Failure to repond to parathyroid hormone causing short stature, obesity, short metacarpals, and ectopic calcification.

Hypersomnia-bulimia
349.89   (Kleine-Levin, Parry-Romberg) Hypersomnia associated with bulimia and occurring in males between 10 to 25 years of age. Ravenous appetite is followed by prolonged sleep, along with behavioral disturbances, impaired thought processes, and hallucinations.

Hypersympathetic
337.9   (Claude Bernard-Homer, Reilly's, Steinbrocker's) Pain and stiffness in the shoulder and swelling and pain in the hand following heart attack.

Hypertransfusion, newborn
776.4   Polycythemia of newborn resulting from blood flow from mother.

Hyperviscosity
273.3   Increase in macroglobulins in the blood, hyperviscosity, weakness, fatigue, bleeding disorders, and visual disturbances.

Hypoglycemic
251.2   (idiopathic familial hypoglycemia) Hypoglycemia described as unspecified

Hypoperfusion
769   (Hyaline membrane) Respiratory distress in premature neonates associated with reduced amounts of lung surfactant. Frequently fatal.

Hypophyseal
253.8   Relating to hyphysis.

Hypophyseothalamic
253.8   Relating to thalamis.

Hypopituitarism
253.2   Decreasing production of pituitary hormones caused by lessening activity of of the anterior lobe of the hypophysis.

Hypoplastic left heart
746.7   Hypoplasia or atresia of the left ventricle and aorta or mitral valve with respiratory distress and extreme cyanosis. Cardiac failure and death often result in early infancy.

Hypotension, maternal
669.2X   Significantly reduced blood pressure during pregnancy.

Hypotonia-hypomentia-hypogonadism-obesity
759.81   (Prader-Willi) Rounded face, almond-shaped eyes, strabismus, low forehead, hypogonadism, hypotomia, mental retardation, and an insatiable appetite.

ICF
286.6   Decrease of elements needed for coagulation of blood and profuse bleeding.

Idiopathic cardiorespiratory distress, newborn
769   (Hyaline membrane, respiratory distress) Respiratory distress in premature neonates associated with reduced amounts of lung surfactant. Frequently fatal.

Idiopathic nephrotic
581.9   Affects the kidneys of a child with unknown cause.

Imerslund (-Gräsbeck)
281.1   (Other vitamin B12 deficiency anemia) Anemias in which the body fails to utilize vitamin B12 causing skeletal malformation, mongoloid features, cardiac enlargement, and severe anemia.

Immobility
728.3   Paralysis of legs and lower part of body.

Syndromes

Inappropriate secretion of antidiuretic hormone

253.6   (Schwartz-Bartter) Low or normal blood pressure, no edema, and retarded growth found in children with hypokalemic alkalosis and elevated renin or angiotensin levels.

Induced by drug

292.11   Description of symptoms, physiological and psychological, produced by drug abuse or dependence.

Infantilism

253.3   Profound retardation of mental and physical development

Inferior vena cava

459.2   Obstruction of the vena cava.

Inspissated bile, newborn

774.4   Biliary obstruction in newborn resulting from plugging of outflow tract.

IRDS (infant reflex distress)

769   (Hyaline membrane) Respiratory distress in premature neonates associated with reduced amounts of lung surfactant. Frequently fatal.

Itsenko-Cushing

255.0   (Cushing) Increased adrenocortical secretion of cortisol caused by ACTH-dependent adrenocortical hyperplasia or tumor with abdominal striae, acne, hypertension decreased carbohydrate tolerance, moon face, obesity, protein catabolism, and psychiatric disturbances.

IVC (intravascular coagulopathy)

286.6   Decrease of elements needed for coagulation of blood. Later stages are marked by profuse bleeding.

Ivemark's

759.0   Organs of left side of the body are a mirror image of organs on right side. Splenic agenisis and cardiac malformation are associated.

Jaccoud's

714.4   Post rheumatic fever arthritis with fibrous changes in the joint capsules and tendons. Malformation of the joints resembles rheumatoid arthritis.

Jackson's

344.89   (Avellis, Babinski-Nageotte, Benedikt's, Brown-Sequard, Cestan's, Cestan-Chenais, Foville's, Gubler-Millard, Weber-Leyden) Paraplegia and anesthesia over part of the body. Caused by lesions in the brain or spinal cord.

Jadassohn-Lewandowski

757.5   Abnormal thickness and elevation of nail plates with palmar and plantar hyperkeratosis. The tongue is whitish.

Jaffe-Lichtenstein (-Uehlinger)

252.0   (Engel-von Recklinghausen) Osteitis with fibrous degeneration and formation of cysts, along with fibrous nodules on affected bones due to misfunctioning parathyroid gland.

Jahnke's

759.6   Angioma in trigeminal nerve, homolateral meningeal angioma with intracranial calcification, and/or angioma of choroid.

Jakob-Creutzfeldt

046.1   Progressive dementia, wasting of muscles, tremor, and other symptoms. Communicable, rare spongiform encephalopathy occurring in middle life with progressive destruction of the pyramidal and extrapyramidal systems to death.

Jaw-winking

742.8   Eyelids widen during chewing, sometimes with an elevation of upper lid when mouth is open and closing of the lid when mouth is closed.

Jejunal

564.2   (dumping) Emptying of contents of jejunum with nausea, sweating, weakness, palpitation, syncope, warmth, and diarrhea occurring after eating in patients who have had partial gastrectomy and gastrojejunostomy.

Jet lag

307.45   Imbalance of the normal circadian rhythm resulting from airplane travel through a number of time zones. Leads to fatigue, irritability, and other consitutional disturbances.

Jeune's

756.4   (ATD) Pelvis and phalanges are malformed, and cartilage of rib cage is unable to support breath action, leading to asphyxia.

Job's
288.1 Autosomal disorder of neutrophils with abnormal or absent chemotactic responses, eczema, and staphylococcal abcesses on the skin. Patients tend to be females with fair skin and red hair.

Jordan's
288.2 (Chediak-Higashi, Dohle body, Hegglin, May) Hepatosplenomegaly, lymphadenopathy, anemia, and thrombocytopenia with changes in the bones, cardiopulmonary system, skin, and psychomotor skills. Abnormalities of granulation and nuclear structure of white cells opens patient to infection and results in death.

Joseph-Diamond-Blackfan
284.0 (Fanconi's, Blackfan-Diamond, Kaznelson's) Congenital anemia of infancy requiring a number of blood transfusions to maintain life.

Jugular foramen
352.6 (Collet-Sicard) Unilateral lesions of the ninth, tenth, eleventh, and twelfth cranial nerves producing paralysis of the vagal, glossal, and other nerves and the tongue on the same side resulting from injury.

Kahler's
203.0X Malignant neoplasm associated with anemia, hemorrhages, recurrent infections, and weakness that originates in bone marrow.

Kalischer's
759.6 Multiple angiomas in skin of head and scalp.

Kallmann's
253.4 Failure of sexual development resulting from inadequate secretion of pituitary gonadotropines. Associated with anosmia due to agenisis of the olfactory lobes in the brain, a product of X-linked inheritance.

Kanner's
299.0X Marked lack of awareness of existence and feelings of others, absence of or abnormal seeking of comfort in times of distress, no imitation of adults, abnormal social play, and no attempt to make peer friendships.

Kartagener's
759.3 Reversal of the position or location of organs or viscera.

Kasabach-Merritt
287.3 Small number of platelets in circulating blood, causing bruising.

Kast's
756.4 (Maffucci's) Benign cartilaginous growths in bones with bleeding in viscera and skin.

Kaznelson's
284.0 (Diamond-Blackfan, Fanconi's, Joseph) Congenital anemia of infancy and requiring a number of blood transfusions to maintain life.

Kelly's
280.8 (Paterson-Brown-Kelly, Plummer-Vinson) Condition in middle-aged women with hypochronic anemia, cracks or fissures at the corners of the mouth, painful tongue, and dysphagia due to esophageal stenosis or webs.

Kimmelstiel-Wilson
250.4X [581.81] High blood pressure and kidney failure resulting from a form of diabetes in which carbohydrate utilization is reduced and lipid and protein enhanced.

Klauder's
695.1 Necrolysis of skin caused by toxins.

Klein-Waardenburg
270.2 (Mendes, van der Hoeve-Halbertsma-Waardenburg, Waardenburg-Klein) Eyebrow or upper or lower eyelid sags.

Kleine-Levin
349.89 (Parry-Romberg) Hypersomnia with bulimia occurring in males between 10 to 25 years of age. Ravenous appetite is followed by prolonged sleep, along with behavioral disturbances, impaired thought processes, and hallucinations.

Klinefelter's
758.7 (XXY) Male in development, but with seminal tube dysgenisis, gynecomastia, and urinary gonadotropins.

Klippel-Feil
756.16 Shorter than average neck and a low hairline caused by fewer than average cervical vertebrae or fusion of hemivertebrae into one bony mass.

Syndromes

Klippel-Trenaunay
759.89 One extremity with hypertrophy of bone and soft tissues, hemangiomas on the skin, and port-wine stain over the bone.

Klumpke (-Déjérine)
767.6 Atrophic paralysis of forearm and hand as result of birth trauma to brachial plexus.

Klüver-Bucy (-Terzian)
310.0 Bilateral temporal lobe ablation with psychic hyperreactivity to visual stimuli or blindness, increased oral and sexual activity, and depressed drive and emotional reactions.

Köhler-Pellegrini-Stieda
726.62 Calcification of medial collateral ligament of the knee.

König's
564.8 Alternating constipation and diarrhea with pain meterorism and gurgling sounds in the right illiac fossa.

Korsakoff (-Wernicke)
294.0 Amnestic dementia in which the patient cannot remember short-term or long-term memories but is not delirious.

Kostmann's
288.0 (Doan-Wiseman, Schultz, Schwachman) Bronchiectasis and pancreatic insufficiency, resulting in malnutrition, sinusitis, short stature, and bone abnormalities.

Kunkel
571.49 (lupid hepatitis) Chronic hepatitis with autoimmune manifestations.

Langdon Down
758.0 (mongolism) Congenital retardation with retarded growth, flat face with short nose, epicanthic skin folds, protruding lower lip, rounded ears, thickened tongue, pelvic dysplasia, broad hands and feet, stubby fingers, and absence of Moro reflex.

Larsen's
755.8 Numerous congenital dislocations with anomalies of the bones and flattened facial features.

Late effect
760.71 Late effects of fetal malformation resulting among offspring of mothers who are chronic alcoholics. Symptoms include growth deficiency, craniofacial anomalies, and limb defects.

Launois'
253.0 Pituitary secretions causing gigantism beginning before puberty with eosinophilic cell hyperplasia, eosinophilic adenoma, or chromophobe adenoma.

Launois-Cléret
253.8 (Babinski-Frolich, Renon-Delille) Marked by obesity and hypogonadism in adolescent boys with dwarfism indicating hypothyroidism.

Laurence-Moon (-Bardet) - Biedl
759.89 Retardation, pigmentary retinopathy, obesity, polydactyly, and hypogonadism.

Lawford's
759.6 (Kalischer's) Formation of multiple angiomas in skin of head and scalp.

Lederer-Brill
283.19 Anemic syndrome noted for fragmentation of red blood cells.

Legg-Calvé-Perthes
732.1 Disease of children in growth centers, especially at top of femur, in which the epiphyses is replaced by new calcification.

Lennox's
345.0 Childhood epilepsy with slow brain waves.

Lenticular
275.1 Accumulation of copper in the brain, cornea, kidney, liver, and other tissues causing cirrhosis of the liver and deterioration in the basal ganglia of the brain.

Lepore hemoglobin
282.4 Cardiac defects, coarse facial features, multiple lentigines, pulmonary stenosis, abnormalities of the genitalia, sensorineural deafness, and skeletal changes.

Léri-Weill
756.59 Dorsal dislocation of the distal ulna and carpal bones, bowing of the radius, and mesomelic dwarfism.

Leriche's
444.0   Obstruction of the terminal aorta causing fatigue in the hips, thighs, and calves; pallor of lower extremities; and impotence of exercising males.

Lermoyez's
386.00   Vertigo, nausea, vomiting, tinnitus, and progressive deafness caused by endolymphatic hydrops.

Lesch-Nyhan
277.2   Physical and mental retardation, compulsive self-mutilation of the lips and fingers through biting, impaired renal function, choreoathetosis, spastic cerebral palsy, and purine synthesis and consequent hyperuricemia and uricaciduria.

Leukocyte
288.0   (Doan-Wiseman, Schultz, Schachman) Bronchiectasis and pancreatic insufficiency, resulting in malnutrition, sinusitis, short stature, and bone abnormalities.

Lev's
426.0   (Rytand-Lipstitch) Bundle branch block in patient with normal coronary arteries and myocardium resulting from calcification of the conducting system.

Levi's
253.3   (Burnier, Lorain-Levi) (pituitary dwarfism) Dwarfism resulting from the absence of functional anterior pituitary gland.

Lichtheim's
281.0   [336.2] Numbness and tingling, weakness, a sore tongue, dyspnea, faintness, pallor of the skin and mucous membranes, anorexia, diarrhea, loss of weight, and fever. Most often strikes in the fifth decade.

Lightwood's
588.8   Variety of syndromes resulting from metabolic acidosis springing from renal misfunction.

Likoff's
413.9   Severe pain in the chest caused by ischemia of heart prompted by coronary artery disease.

Liver-kidney
572.4   (Heyd's) Acute renal failure in patients with disease of biliary or liver tract. Cause seems to be decreased renal blood flow, damaging both organs.

Lloyd's
258.1   Endocrine dysfunction causing diabetes and affecting growth and weight.

Lobe (lung) (right)
518.0   (Brock) Incomplete expansion of right middle lobe of lung with chronic pneumonitis.

Lobectomy behavior
310.0   Symptomatic description of Kluver-Bucy syndrome.

Löffler's
518.3   Transient infiltrations of lungs by eosinophilia resulting in coughing, fever, and dyspnea.

Löfgren's
135   (Hutchinson-Boeck, Schaumann's, Besnier-Boeck-Schaumann) Involves fibrosis in lungs, lymph nodes, skin, liver, eyes, spleen, phalangeal bones, and parotid glands. Identified by systemic granulomas composed of epithelioid and multinucleated giant cells.

Long arm 18 or 21 deletion
758.3   Autosomal deletion causing a variety of symptoms.

Looser (-Debray) - Milkman
268.2   (Milkman) Osteoporosis with frequent fractures striking middle-aged women.

Lorain-Levi
253.3   (Burnier, Levi) Dwarfism resulting from absence of functional anterior pituitary gland.

Louis-Bar
334.8   (Boder-Sedgwick) Gonadal hypoplasia, insulin resistance and hyperglycemia, liver function problems, ataxia, nystagmus, and increased sensitivity to ionizing radiation.

Lowe's
270.8   (Lowe-Terrey-MacLachlan) Aminoaciduria, cataracts, mental retardation, hydrophthalmia, rickets, and reduced ammonia production by the kidney.

Lower radicular, newborn
767.4   Damage of nerve root during birth.

Syndromes

Lown (-Ganong)-Levine
426.81   Electrocardiographic disorder indicated by a short P-R interval with normal duration of the QRS complex.

Lucey-Driscoll
774.30   Retention jaundice in newborn infants resulting from defective bilirubin conjugation, a product of a steroid in mother's blood being transferred to the infant.

Lung
518.5   Respiratory distress following surgery, shock or trauma, similar to but not caused by, adult respiratory distress system.

Lutembacher's
745.5   Atrial septal defect associated with mitral stenosis.

Lyell's
695.1   Necrolysis of skin caused by toxins.

MacLeod's
492.8   (Swyer-James) Acquired unilateral hyperlucent lung with severe airway obstruction during expiration.

Macrogenitosomia praecox
259.8   1) Excessive bodily development with unusual growth of sexual organs; 2) a description of symptoms indicating Donohue's and other syndromes.

Macroglobulinemia
273.3   (Waldenström's) Earmarked by increase in macroglobulins in the blood. Has symptoms of hyperviscosity such as weakness, fatigue, bleeding disorders, and visual disturbances.

Maffucci's
756.4   (Maffucci's) Benign cartilaginous growths in bones with bleeding in viscera and skin.

Magnesium-deficiency
781.7   Tetany. Any number of syndromes affecting newborns and others. Hyperexcitability of nerve and muscles due to decrease in concentration of extracellular ionized calcium, resulting in calcium and magnesium deficiency.

Malabsorption
579.9   A number of syndromes in which the body does not adequately absorb dietary constituents and loses nonabsorbed substances in the stool. Due to muscle, digestive, or lymphactic defect.

Malignant carcinoid
259.2   (Bjorck-Thorson, Cassidy-Scholte, Hedinger's) Carcinoid tumors causing cyanotic flushing of skin, diarrheal watery stools, bronchoconstrictive attacks, hypotension, edema, and ascites.

Mallory-Weiss
530.7   A tear in esophagus following several hours or days of vomiting, marked by vomiting of blood.

Mandibulofacial
756.0   (Franceschetti's, mandibulofacial dysostosis) Malformations of derivatives of the first branchial arch, marked by pallpebral fissures sloping outward and downward with notches in the outer third of the lower lids, defects of malar bones and zygome, hypoplasia of the jawbone, high or cleft palate, low-set ears, unusual hair growth, and pits between mouth and ear.

Manic depression
296.80   (bipolar) Alternating major depressive and manic periods.

Mankowsky's
731.2   (Pierre Marie-Bamberger) Symmetrical osteitis of limbs localized to phalanges and terminal epiphyses of the long bones of forearm and leg. Symptoms include kyphosis of spine and affection of joints.

Maple syrup
270.3   Anomaly in amino acid metabolism marked by urine and perspiration odor, hypertonicity, convulsions, coma, and death.

Marable's
447.4   Compression of celiac artery by median arcuate ligament in diaphragm.

Marchesani (-Weill)
759.89   Short stature, heavy musculature, reduced joint mobility, myopic, glaucoma, and many other symptoms.

Marchiafava-Micheli
283.2   Acquired blood cell dysplasia in which there are many clones of stem cells producing red blood cells, platelets, and granulocytes.

Marcus Gunn's
742.8   (jaw-winking) Eyelids widen during chewing, sometimes with elevation of upper lid when the mouth is open and closing of lid when mouth is closed.

Marfan's
759.82   Unusually long extremities, subluxation of the lens, dilation of the aorta, and other symptoms.

Marie's
253.0   Secondary to chronic conditions in lung and heart, localized to phalanges and terminal epiphyses of long bones of arm and leg, and accompanied by kyphosis. Caused by pituitary disorder.

Markus-Adie
379.46   Paralysis of conjugate movement of eyes without paralysis of convergence. Caused by lesions of midbrain.

Maroteaux-Lamy
277.5   Accumulation of mucopolysaccharide sulfates affecting eye, ear, skin, teeth, skeleton, joints, liver, spleen, cardiovascular system, respiratory system, and central nervous system.

Martin-Albright
275.4   (Albright-Martin, Seabright-Bantam) Short stature, obesity, short metacarpals, and ectopic calcification. Similar to hypoparathyroidism and caused by failure to repond to parathyroid hormone.

Martorell-Fabré
446.7   (Marorell-Fabre, Raed-Harbitz, Takayasu-Onishi) Ischemia, transient blindness, facial atrophy, and many others. Progressive obliteration of the brachiocephalic trunk and the left subclavian and common carotid arteries above their source in the aortic arch.

Massive aspiration of newborn
770.1   Intrauterine aspiration of amniotic fluid contaminated by meconium.

Masters-Allen
620.6   Pelvic pain resulting from old laceration of broad ligament received during delivery.

Mastocytosis
757.33   Inherited disorder of skin (and sometimes other structures) in which pigmented lesions appear in linear, zebra stripe, and other configurations and are preceded by vesicles and bullae and followed by verrucal lesions.

Maternal hypotension
669.2X   Significantly reduced blood pressure during pregnancy.

Maternal obesity
646.1X   Edema or excessive weight gain in pregnancy with no hypertension.

May (-Hegglin)
288.2   (Chediak-Higashi, Dohle body, Hegglin, Jordan's, May) Hepatosplenomegaly, lymphadenopathy, anemia, thrombocytopenia, along with changes in the bones, cardiopulmonary system, skin, and psychomotor skills. Abnormalities of granulation and nuclear structure of white cells open child to infection and result in death.

McArdle (-Schmid) (-Pearson)
271.0   Glucose-6-phosphatase deficiency due to inherited defects of glycogen metabolism resulting in excess accumulation of glycogen in muscle, characterized by myopathies and hepatorenal effects.

McCune-Albright
756.59   (Albright's hereditary osteodystrophy) Patchy skin pigmentation, endocrine dysfunctions, and polyostotic fibrous dysplasia.

McQuarrie's
251.2   Hypoglycemia described as primary and unspecified, reactive, or spontaneous.

Median arcuate ligament
447.4   Compression of celiac artery by median arcuate ligament in diaphragm.

Meekeren-Ehlers-Danlos
756.83   (Meekeren, Ehlers, Danlos) Group of congenital connective tissue diseases with overly elastic skin, hyperextensive joints, and fragility of blood vessels and arteries.

Meige
757.0   (Nonne-Milroy-Meige) Lymphatic edema of the legs (and face and arms in severe cases) caused by obstruction of lymphatic ducts.

Syndromes

Melkersson (-Rosenthal)

351.8   (crocodile tears) Facial paralysis with dramatic lacrimation during eating. Caused by lesion on seventh cranial nerve, prompting impulses to be misdirected from salivary glands to lacrimal glands.

Mende's (ptosis-epicanthus)

270.2   (Mendes, van der Hoeve-Halbertsma-Waardenburg, Waardenburg-Klein) Eyebrow or upper or lower eyelid sags.

Mendelson's

997.3   Pulmonary disorders caused by aspirating of lung following vomiting or regurgitation during medical procedure.

Ménétrier's

535.2X   Giant hypertrophy of gastric mucosa.

Ménière's

386.00   Vertigo, nausea, vomiting, tinnitus, and progressive deafness caused by endolymphatic hydrops.

Meningo-eruptive

047.1   Enteric cytopathogenic human orphan (ECHO) virus. Common form of virus (which has many variations) is meningo-eruptive, with fever and aseptic meningitis.

Meningococcic

036.3   (Friderichsen-Waterhouse, Waterhouse,) Acute fulminating meningococcal septicemia occurring in children below 10 years of age with vomiting, cyanosis, diarrhea, purpura, convulsions, circulatory collapse, meningitis, and hemorrhaging into adrenal glands.

Menkes'

759.89   Congenital abnormality in copper absorption characterized by severe cerebral degeneration and arterial changes resulting in death in infancy.

Menopause

627.2   Chills, depression, hot flashes, headache, and irritability.

Menstruation

625.4   (Premenstrual, PMS) Monthly physiological and emotional distress during the several days preceding menses with symptoms of nervousness, fluid retention, weight gain, and depression.

Mesenteric artery

557.1   (Wilkie's) Complete or partial block of the superior mesenteric artery with symptoms of vomiting, pain, blood in the stool, and distended abdomen. Results in bowel infarction.

Metastatic carcinoid

259.2   (Bjorck-Thorson, Cassidy-Scholte, Hedinger's) Carcinoid tumors that causes cyanotic flushing of skin, diarrheal watery stools, bronchoconstrictive attacks, hypotension, edema, and ascites.

Meyenburg-Altherr-Uehlinger

733.99   Arthritis with degeneration of cartilage leading to collapse of ears, nose, and tracheobronchial tree. Death may occur as respiratory system is affected.

Meyer-Schwickerath and Weyers

759.89   Abnormally small nose with anteverted nostrils, dental anomalies, and missing phalanges of toes.

Micheli-Rietti

282.4   Hemolytic anemias that share a common decreased rate of synthesis of one or more hemoglobin polypeptide chains and are classified according to the chain involved.

Michotte's

721.5   Kissing spine. Malformation of spine in which kyphosis becomes so great nonadjacent vertebrae touch.

Micrognathia-glossoptosis

756.0   Description of anomalies of face and skull.

Microphthalmos

759.89   Reduction in the size of the eye, opacities of the cornea and lens, and scarring of the retina.

Midbrain

348.8   Infarction of postero-inferior thalamus causing transient hemiparesis, severe loss of superficial and deep sensation with crude pain in the hypalgic limbs, vasomotor, or trophic disturbances.

Mieten's

759.89   Affects multiple systems.

Mikity-Wilson

770.7 Symptoms include hypercapnia and cyanosis of rapid onset during first month of life and frequently result in death. Rare pulmonary insufficiency in newborn babies, especially those with low birth weight.

Mikulicz's

527.1 Complex of lacrimal and salivary gland swelling, which may include enlargement associated with other syndromes, such as Sjogren's.

Milk alkali

999.9 (Burnett's) (milk drinkers) Disorder of kidneys induced by ingestion of large amounts of alkali and calcium in therapy of a peptic ulcer. While reversable in the early stages, it can lead to renal failure.

Milkman (-Looser-Debray)

268.2 Osteoporosis striking middle-aged women with frequent fractures.

Millard-Gubler

344.89 (Avellis, Babinski-Nageotte, Benedikt's, Brown-Sequard, Cestan's, Cestan-Chenais, Foville's, Gubler-Millard, Jackson's, Weber-Leyden) Paraplegia and anesthesia over half or part of the body. Caused by lesions in brain or spinal cord.

Miller Fisher's

357.0 (Guillain-Barre, Landry, Fisher's, Strohl, Miller) Often follows viral infections and may be a disorder of the immune system with symptoms of paraplegia of limbs, flaccid paralysis, ophalmoplegia, ataxia, and areflexia.

Milles'

759.6 (Kalischer's) Formation of multiple angiomas in skin of head and scalp.

Milroy

757.0 (Nonne-Milroy-Meige) Lymphatic edema of the legs (and face and arms in severe cases) caused by obstruction of lymphatic ducts.

Minkowski-Chauffard

282.0 Hemolytic anemia with spherocytosis, fragility of erthrocytes, splenomegaly, and jaundice.

Mirizzi's

576.2 Stone in cystic duct and chronic cystitis leading to spasms and scarring of connective tissue and obstruction of hepatic ducts.

Mohr's

759.89 (Oral-Facial-Digital) Cranial, facial, lingual, mandibular, digital, and palatal abnormalities.

Monofixation

378.34 Strabismus of slight degree.

Moore's

345.5 Epilepsy with unilateral clonic movements starting in one group of muscles and spreading to adjacent groups, following the movement of the epilepsy through the contralateral motor cortex.

Morel-Moore

733.3 (Morel-Morgagni, -Stewart-Morel) Thickening of the inner table of the frontal bone related to obesity in women nearing menopause.

Morgagni-Adams-Stokes

426.9 (Stokes-Adams; Morgagni's disease; and Spens) Heart block causing slow or absent pulse, vertigo, syncope, convulsions, and Cheyne-Stokes respiration.

Morquio (-Brailsford) (-Ullrich)

277.5 Accumulation of mucopolysccharide sulfates affecting the eye, ear, skin, teeth, skeleton, joints, liver, spleen, cardiovascular system, respiratory system, and central nervous system.

Morris

257.8 (Morris, hairless women, Goldberg, Goldberg-Maxwell) Male pseudohermaphroditism with incompletely developed vagina, rudimentary uterus, fallopian tubes, scanty or absent axillary/public hair, and amenorrhea.

Morton's

355.6 Pain in the forefoot caused by a lesion of the plantar nerve.

Moschcowitz (-Singer-Symmers)

446.6 Central nervous system involvement due to formation of fibrin or platelet thrombi in arterioles and capillaries in many organs.

Mounier-Kuhn

494 Tracheobronchomegaly.

Mucha-Haberman

696.2   Chronic dermatosis of unknown origin with scaling lesions that produce small pox-like scars. Recurrence of attacks are common, but disease is self-limiting.

Mucocutaneous lymph node

446.1   (Harkavy) Fever, conjunctival injection reddening of the oral cavity, ulcerative gingivitis, cervical lymph nodes, skin eruptions that cover the hands and feet, and skin becoming puffy and sloughs off.

Munchhausen's

301.51   (Hospital addiction, Multiple operations) Emotional condidtion in which patient exhibits physical, but psychosomatic, symptoms.

Münchmeyer's

728.11   Diffuse progressive ossifying polymyositis.

Muscle deficiency

756.7   (Prune Belly, Eagle-Barrett) Absence of muscles of abdomen and genitourinary anomalies. Intestinal outlines are visible on patient's skin.

Myelodysplastic

238.7   Neoplasm of lymphatic and hematopoietic tissues, affecting the spinal cord.

Myeloproliferative

238.7   Unusual proliferation of myelopoietic tissue.

Naffziger's

353.0   Raynaud-like symptoms of vascular contractions caused by pressure of brachial plexus and subclavian artery against first thoracic rib.

Nager-de Reynier

756.0   Franceschetti's syndrome with limb deformities consisting of absence of the radius, radioulnar synostosis, and hypoplasia or absence of thumbs.

Nail-patella

756.89   Dysplasia of the fingernails and toenails, hypoplasia of the patella, iliac horns, thickening of the glomerular lamina densa, and a flask-shaped femur.

Nebécourt's

253.3   (Burnier, Lorain-Levi) Dwarfism resulting from absence of functional anterior pituitary gland.

Neill-Dingwall

759.89   Small head and dwarfism. One of many syndromes affecting several body systems, but not elsewhere specified.

Nerve compression

354.8   Pain in upper and posterior part of the shoulder radiating into neck and occiput, down the arm, and around the chest. Caused by abnormal positioning between the scapula and thorax, pain includes tingling in the fingers.

Netherton's

757.1   Scaling of skin showing a peripheral double margin in and around the vagina.

Neurocutaneous

759.6   Occurance of nevi and skeletal deformities as result of gliosis and abiotrophy of central nervous system.

Neuroleptic malignant

333.92   Description of the effects of antipsychotic drugs on behavior and cognition.

Newborn distress

770.6   Intrauterine fetal aspiration of amniotic fluid contaminated by meconium.

Nezelof's

279.13   Immunodeficiency syndromes with profoundly deficient cellular immunity and varying degrees of humoral immunodeficiency. Patients easily catch life-threatening infections.

Niemann-Pick

272.7   Accumulation of phospholipid in histiocytes in the bone marrow, liver, lymph nodes, and spleen, cerebral involvement, and red macular spots similar to Tay-Sachs disease. Most commonly found in Jewish infants.

Nonne-Milroy-Meige

757.0   (Milroy) Lymphatic edema of the legs (and face and arms in severe cases) caused by obstruction of lymphatic ducts.

Nonpsychotic

310.2   Persistent personality disturbance of nonpsychotic origin following blow to the head with affective instability, bursts of aggression, apathy and indifference, impaired social judgment, and suspiciousness or paranoid ideation.

Noonan's
759.89 (Ulrich-Turner) Ptosis, hypogonadism webbed, neck, congenital heart disease, short stature; once diagnosed as Turner's syndrome until this female component was identified.

Nucleus ambiguous-hypoglossal
352.6 (Collet-Sicard) Unilateral lesions of the ninth, tenth, eleventh, and twelfth cranial nerves producing paralysis of vagal, glossal, other nerves, and tongue on the same side. Most usually result of injury.

OAV (oculoauriulovertebral dysplasia)
756.0 (Goldenhar's) Number of anomalies, including epibulbar dermoids, preauricular appendages, micrognathia, and vertebral.

Oculocutaneous
364.24 (Vogt-Koyanagi) Uveomeningitis with patchy depigmentation of hair, eyebrows, and lashes; retinal detatchment, deafness, and tinnitus may also result.

Oculoglandular
372.02 Syndrome of the eyes and glands.

Oculomotor
378.81 (Parinaud's) Paralysis of conjugate movement of the eyes without paralysis of convergence. Caused by lesions of the midbrain.

Of diabetic mother
775.0 Maternal diabetes mellitus affecting fetus or newborn with hypoglycemia.

Ogilvie's
560.89 Colonic obstruction with symptoms of persistent contraction of intestinal musculature. Caused by defect in sympathetic nerve supply.

Ophthalmica
053.19 Any symptoms of herpes arising in eye.

Ophthalmoplegia-cerebellar ataxia
378.52 Paralysis of one or more optic muscles or failure to control muscles.

Ophthalmoplegic migraine
346.8X Migraine headache accompanied by amblyopia and other visual disturbances.

Oppenheim-Urbach
250.8X [709.3] Diabetes with skin disorder.

Oral-facial-digital
759.89 (Papillon-Leage and Psaume) Defects of the oral cavity, face, and hands including bifid tongue, cleft palate, missing teeth, pug-nose, depressed nasal bridge, mental retardation, and others. Syndrome is lethal in males.

Organic affective
293.83 Patient may exhibit a number of changes in personality such as amotivation, depression, outbursts, poor social judgment, and others.

Organic personality
310.1 Persistent personality disturbance of nonpsychotic origin featuring affective instability, bursts of aggression, apathy and indifference, impaired social judgment, and suspiciousness or paranoid ideation.

Ormond's
593.4 (Ormond's) Retroperitoneal structures involving and often obstructing ureters sometimes following certain types of chemical treatment; there is no identified cause.

Orthostatic hypotensive-dysautonomic dyskinetic
333.0 (Hallervorden-Spatz, Dejerine-Thomas) Nerves between the striatum and pallidum are completely demyelated.

Osler-Weber-Rendu
448.0 A post-pubescent disorder with small telangiectasia and dilated venules developing slowly on the skin and mucus membranes of the lips, nasopharynx, and tongue.

Osteodermopathic hyperostosis
757.39 Irregular linear streaks of skin atrophy, skeletal malformations, and papillomas of lips.

Osteoporosis-osteomalacia
268.2 (Milkman, Looser, Debray) Osteoporosis striking middle-aged women with frequently-suffered fractures.

Österreicher-Turner
756.89 Dysplasia of the fingernails and toenails, hypoplasia of the patella, iliac horns, thickening of the glomerular lamina densa, and a flask-shaped femur.

Ostrum-Furst
756.59 Deformities of neck, platybasia, and Sprengel's neck.

Otolith

386.19 (Bonnier) Ocular disturbances, deafness, nausea, thirst, anorexia, and symptoms traced to vagus centers as result of a lesion of Deiters nucleus and its connections.

Otopalatodigital

759.89 Defects of ear, oral cavity, face, and hands.

Outlet

353.0 (Naffziger's) Vascular contractions of the digits similar to Raynaud's, caused by pressure of brachial plexus and subclavian artery against first thoracic rib.

Ovarian remnant

620.8 Pelvic pain typically occurring several weeks or several months following surgical removal of the ovaries, often due to the survival of an ovarian fragment after the operation.

Ovarian vein

593.4 (Ormond's) Retroperitoneal structures involving and often obstructing the ureters following certain types of chemical treatment; there is no identified cause.

Owren's

286.3 (Stewart-Prower) Deficiencies of clotting factors noticable from birth.

P-R interval

426.81 (Lown-Ganong) Electrocardiographic disorder indicated by a short P-R interval with normal duration of the QRS complex.

Pacemaker

429.4 Functional deficiency following heart surgery in which the triggering mechanism of the heart may be irregular.

Paget-Schroetter

453.8 Stress thrombosis of subclavian or axillary vein.

Pancoast's

162.3 (Hare's, Cuiffini) Neoplasm of upper lobe of the lung.

Panhypopituitary

253.2 Secretion of all anterior pituitary hormones is inadequate or absent after childbirth.

Papillon-Léage and Psaume

759.89 Defects of the oral cavity, face, and hands including bifid tongue, cleft palate, missing teeth, pug-nose, depressed nasal bridge, mental retardation, and others. Syndrome is lethal in males.

Parabiotic (transfusion) donor (twin)

772.0 Transfusion of blood from one fetus to another.

Parabiotic (transfusion) recipient (twin)

776.4 Polycythemia of newborn as result of blood flow from mother.

Paranoid type

293.81 Organic disorder with hallucinations, beliefs about being followed, being poisoned, etc.; and not meeting criteria for schizophrenia.

Parinaud's

378.81 Paralysis of conjugate movement of eyes without paralysis of convergence caused by lesions of the midbrain.

Parkes Weber and Dimitri

759.6 (Kalischer's) Formation of multiple angiomas in skin of head and scalp.

Parry's

242.0X (Basedow, Grave's disease) Fatigue, nervousness, emotional lability and irritability, heat intolerance and increased sweating, weight loss, palpitation, and tremor of hands and tongue. Autoimmune in etiology and caused by excess thyroidal hormones.

Parry-Romberg

349.89 (Kleine-Levin) Hypersomnia associated with bulimia and occurring in males between 10 to 25 years of age with ravenous appetite followed by prolonged sleep, along with behavioral disturbances, impaired thought processes, and hallucinations.

Parsonage-Aldren-Turner

353.5 Paroxysmal pain extending length of one of many nerves.

Patau's

758.1 (Patau's, trisomy D) Variety of symptoms in newborns with extra chromosome in group D and number of symptoms, including mental retardation and malformed ears, cardiac defects, convulsions, and others.

Paterson (-Brown) (-Kelly)

280.8 (Kelly, Plummer-Vinson) Condition in middle-aged women with hypochronic anemia of cracks or fissures at the corners of the mouth, painful tongue, and dysphagia due to esophageal stenosis or webs.

Payr's

569.89 Bloating, gas, pain, and fullness experienced left upper abdominal quadrant with pain sometimes radiating up into left chest.

Pectoral girdle

447.8 Malignant atrophic papulosis.

Pelger-Huët

288.2 (Chediak-Higashi, Dohle body, Hegglin, Jordan's, May) Patients present hepatosplenomegaly, lymphadenopathy, anemia, thrombocytopenia, along with changes in bones, cardopulmonary system, skin, and psychomotor skills. Abnormalities of granulation and nuclear structure of white cells open child to infection and result in death.

Pellagra-cerebellar ataxia-renal aminoaciduria

270.0 (Harts, Toni, Fanconi, Debre) Renal tubular malfunction, including cytinosis and osteomalacia, caused by inherited disorders or the result of multiple myeloma or proximal epithelial growth.

Pellagroid

265.2 Resembling pellagra or a description of pellagra.

Pellegrini-Stieda

726.62 (Kohler-Pellegrini-Stieda) Calcification of medial collateral ligament of knee.

Pellizzi's

259.8 Precocious development of external sexual organs, precocious development of long bones, and hydrocephalus indicating lesion of pineal body.

Pendred's

243 Familial goiter paired with congenital nerve deafness due to defective organic binding of iodine in the thyroid.

Penfield's

345.5X Epilepsy with unilateral clonic movements starting in one group of muscles and spreading to adjacent groups, following the movement of the epilepsy through the contralateral motor cortex.

Penta X

758.81 Pentasomy. Presence of three additional chromosomes of one type.

Perabduction

447.8 Malignant atrophic papulosis.

Periurethral fibrosis

593.4 (Ormond's) Retroperitoneal structures involving and often obstructing the ureters.

Petges-Cléjat

710.3 (Unverricht-Wagner) Polymyositis occurring with characteristic skin changes including rash on upper eyelids with edema, a rash on the forehead, neck, shoulders, trunk, and arms, and papules on knuckles.

Peutz-Jeghers

759.6 Formation of multiple hematomas.

Phantom limb

353.6 Itching, dull ache, or sharp, shooting pains mimicking the nerves of amputated limb.

Pharyngeal pouch

279.11 (DiGeorge's) Hypoplasia or aphasia of the thymus and prathyroid gland with congenital heart defects, anomalies of the great vessels, esophageal atresia, and facial deformities result from aphasia or hypoplasia of thymus and parathyroid glands. Seizures may accompany most severe cases.

Pick-Herxheimer

701.8 Atrophy of skin throughout body and of unknown cause.

Pickwickian

278.8 Obesity, hypoventilation, somnolence, and erythrocytosis. After Pickwick, Dicken's character.

PIE

518.3 (Loffler's) Transient infiltrations of lungs by eosinophilia, resulting in coughing, fever, and dyspnea.

Pierre Marie-Bamberger

731.2 (Mankowsky's) Symmetrical osteitis of limbs localized to phalanges, terminal epiphyses of long bones of forearm and leg, kyphosis of the spine, and affection of the joints.

Syndromes

Pierre Mauriac's
258.1 Endocrine dysfunction causing diabetes and affecting growth and weight.

Pierre Robin
756.0 Brachygnathia and cleft palate, upward displacement of larynx, and angulation of manubrium sterni. May be paired with others or sole hyperplasia.

Pigment dispersion, iris
364.53 Lack of pigment in iris.

Pineal
259.8 (Pellizi's) Precocious development of external sexual organs, precocious development of long bones, and hydrocephalus indicating lesion of pineal body.

Pink puffer
492.8 (Swyer-James) Acquired unilateral hyperlucent lung with severe airway obstruction during expiration, oligemia, and a small hilum.

Pituitary
253.0 Excessive pituitary secretions causing gigantism and beginning before puberty.

Placental dysfunction
762.2 (placental insufficiency) Fetal hypoxia and malnutrition resulting from lack of nutrition and oxygen transferred from mother. Due to degeneration of placenta and identified by yellow vernix.

Placental transfusion
762.3 Birth of one anemic twin and one plethoric twin due to forcing of blood of one twin into other.

Plantar fascia
728.71 Disorder of the fascia at the bottom of the foot.

Plug (newborn) NEC
777.1 Meconium obstruction of newborn's intestines, resulting from unusually thick or hard meconium.

Plummer-Vinson
280.8 (Kelly, Paterson-Brown-Vinson) Condition in middle-aged women with hypochronic anemia, marked by cracks or fissures at the corners of mouth, painful tongue, and dysphagia due to esophageal stenosis or webs.

Polycythemic
289.0 Gaisbock's syndrome.

Polysplenia
759.0 Organs of left side of body are mirror image of organs on right side. Splenic agenisis and cardiac malformation are associated.

Pontine
433.8X Quadriplegia, anesthesia, and nystagmus due to the obstruction of twigs of the basilar artery, causing lesions in pontine region.

Post-gastric surgery
564.2 (Dumping) Emptying of contents of jejunum with nausea, sweating, weakness, palpitation, syncope, warmth, and diarrhea. Occurs after eating in patients who have had partial gastrectomy and gastrojejunostomy.

Postartificial
627.4 Menopausal symptoms suffered by some women following destruction of their ovaries, including chills, depression, hot flashes, headache, and irritability.

Postcholecystectomy
576.0 Recurrence of gall bladder pain following removal of organ.

Postconcussional
310.2 (postcontusional, postencephalitic) Persistent personality disturbance of nonpsychotic origin following blow to head and featuring affective instability, bursts of aggression, apathy and indifference, impaired social judgment, and suspiciousness or paranoid ideation.

Posthepatitis
780.7 Chronic Fatigue Syndrome. Marked by persistent or relapsing fatigue not resolved by bed rest that significantly reduces daily activity. Other symptoms include chronic sore throat, mild fever, muscle weakness, myalgia, headaches, and neurological problems. Patients are primarily women. The syndrome arises sporadically with no confirmed etiology but is known to occur in clusters.

Postherpetic
053.19 Description of any symptoms of herpes arising in parts of body.

Postinfarction
411.0 (Dressler) Fever, leukocytosis, chest pain, evidence of pericarditis, pleurisy and pneumonia occurring days or weeks after a myocardial infarction.

Postinfluenza
780.7 Chronic Fatigue Syndrome. Persistent or relapsing fatigue not resolved by bed rest that significantly reduces daily activity. Other symptoms include chronic sore throat, mild fever, muscle weakness, myalgia, headaches, and neurological problems. Patients are primarily women. Arises sporadically with no confirmed etiology but is known to occur in clusters.

Postleukotomy
310.0 Kluver-Bucy or postlobotomy syndrome.

Postmastectomy lymphedema
457.0 Edema of arms and hands following a mastectomy requiring removal of adjacent lymph nodes.

Postmature
766.2 Placental dysfunction occurring in postmature fetuses.

Postmyocardial infarction
411.0 (Dressler) Fever, leukocytosis, chest pain, evidence of pericarditis, pleurisy, and pneumonia occurring days or weeks after myocardial infarction.

Postpartum panhypopituitary
253.2 Secretion of all anterior pituitary hormones is inadequate or absent after childbirth.

Postphlebitic
459.1 Deep vein thrombosis with edema, pain, purpua, and increased cutaneous pigmentation, eczema dermatitis, pruritus, ulceration, and cellulitis.

Postpolio
138 Inflammation of spinal cord following polio. Symptoms vary.

Postsurgical
579.3 Hypoglycemia and malabsorption following surgery.

Posttraumatic
294.0 Amnestic dementia in which patient cannot remember short-term or long-term memories but is not delirious.

Postvagotomy
564.2 (dumping) Emptying of contents of jejunum with nausea, sweating, weakness, palpitation, syncope, warmth, and diarrhea. Occurs after eating in patients who have had partial gastrectomy and vagotomy.

Potain's
536.1 Dilation of stomach with indigestion.

Potassium intoxication
276.7 (potassium overload) Excessive potassium, causing a number of symptoms.

Potter's
753.0 Renal agenesis with hypoplastic lungs and associated neonatal respiratory distress, hemodynamic instability, acidosis, cyanosis, edema, and characteristic facial features. Death usually occurs from lack of oxygen.

Pre-ulcer
536.8 (Reichmann's) Excessive secretion of gastric juice either constantly or during digestion only.

Premenstrual tension
625.4 (Premenstrual, PMS) Monthly physiological and emotional distress during the days preceding menses with symptoms of nervousness, fluid retention, weight gain, and depression.

Primary or idiopathic
757.39 Increased thickening of skin on extremities and face with clubbing of fingers and deformities in bone of limb.

Prinzmetal
786.52 Chest pain secondary to large vessel spasm that may interfere with breathing.

Profichet's
729.9 Calcareous nodules in the subcutaneous tissues primarily around larger joints. The nodules ulcerate and exhibit nervous symptoms.

Progeria
259.8 (Hutchinson-Gilford) Precocious senility with death from coronary artery disease occurring before 10 years of age.

Syndromes

Progressive pallidal degeneration

333.0   (Hallervorden-Spatz, Dejerine-Thomas) Condition in which the nerves between the striatum and pallidum are completely demyelated.

Prolonged gestation

766.2   Gestation beyond the standard number of weeks.

Prune belly

756.7   Congenital absence of muscles of abdomen and genitourinary anomalies. Intestinal outlines are visible on skin.

Prurigo-asthma

691.8   Several itchy skin eruptions of unknown cause accompanying asthma.

Pseudo-Turner's

759.89   (Bonnevie-Ullrich) Congenital disorder with short stature, mental retardation, and a webbed neck but, unlike Turner's, patients can be of either sex and have normal chromosomes and no renal abnormalities.

Pseudocarpal tunnel

354.0   Pain and tingling, numbness, or burning in the hand as result of compression of median nerve by tendons.

Pseudohermaphroditism-virilism-hirsutism

255.2   Possession of mature masculine somatic characteristics by a prepubescent male, girl, or woman. This syndrome may show at birth or develop later as result of adrenocortical dysfunction.

Pseudoparalytica

358.0   (Goldflam, Erb, Hoppe) Progressive muscular weakness beginning in face and throat and caused by a defect in myoneural conduction.

Pterygolymphangiectasia

758.6   (XO) Congenital disorder characterized by short stature and webbed neck. Patients of either sex suffer congenital heart disease, mental retardation, and other symptoms.

Ptosis-epicanthus

270.2   (Mendes, van der Hoeve-Halbertsma-Waardenburg, Waardenburg-Klein) Eyebrow or upper or lower eyelid sags.

Pulmonary sulcus

162.3   (Cuiffini-Pancoast, Hare's) Neoplasm of upper lobe of lung.

Putnam-Dana

281.0   [336.2] Numbness and tingling, weakness, a sore tongue, dyspnea, faintness, pallor of the skin and mucous membranes, anorexia, diarrhea, loss of weight, and fever. Strikes in fifth decade.

Pyloroduodenal

537.89   (Gastrojejunal loop obstruction) Distended efferent loop causing illness and pain with acute or chronic obstruction of the duodenum and jejunum proximal to a gastrojejunostomy.

Pyriformis

355.0   Lesion on the sciatica nerve causing a pear shaped area of pain and parasthesia.

Q-T interval prolongation

794.31   (Romano-Ward) Prolonged Q-T interval and syncope, sometimes leading to ventricular fibrillation and sudden death.

Radicular

353.0   (Naffziger's) A disorder presenting symptoms similar to Raynaud's, caused by pressure of brachial plexus and subclavian artery against first thoracic rib.

Raeder-Harbitz

446.7   (Marorell-Fabre, Takayasu-Onishi) Progressive obliteration of brachiocephalic trunk and left subclavian and left common carotid arteries above their source in the aortic arch. Symptoms include ischemia, transient blindness, facial atrophy, and many others.

Rapid time-zone change

307.45   (jet lag) Imbalance of normal circadian rhythm resulting from airplane travel through a number of time zones. Leads to fatigue, irritability, and other consitutional disturbances.

Raymond (-Céstan)

433.8X   Identified through symptoms of quadriplegia, anesthesia, and nystagmus due to the obstruction of twigs of the basilar artery, causing lesions in the pontine region.

Raynaud's

443.0 (Patriots disease) Constriction of the arteries of the digits caused by cold or emotion. Temperature drops in extremities as much as 30 degrees Farenheit, and skin turns white with red and blue mottling. Caused by nerve or arterial damage and can be prompted by stress.

RDS

769 (Hyaline membrane) Reduced amounts of lung surfactant in premature neonates with respiratory distress. Frequently fatal.

Recipient twin

776.4 Polycythemia of newborn as result of blood flow from mother.

Refsum's

356.3 Deafness, retinitis pigmentosa, polyneuritis, nystagmus, and cerebellar signs.

Reichmann's

536.8 Excessive secretion of gastric juice either constantly or during digestion only.

Reifenstein's

257.2 Hypogonadism with gynecomastia, hypospadias, and pospubertal testicular atrophy. Caused by inherited defect of androgen receptors and insensitivity to testosterone.

Reilly's

337.9 (Claude Bernard-Homer, Steinbrocker's) Pain and stiffness in the shoulder, with puffy swelling and pain in the hand following a heart attack.

Reiter's

099.3 (Fiessinger-Leroy-Reiter) Arthritis, iredocyclitis, and urethritis, sometimes with diarrhea. While symptoms may recur, arthritis is constant.

Renal

446.21 (Goodpasture's) Renal condition in which nephritis progresses rapidly to death, with lungs showing extensive hemosiderosis or bleeding.

Renal glomerulohyalinosis-diabetic

250.4X [581.81] High blood pressure and kidney failure resulting from a form of diabetes in which carbohydrate utilization is reduced and that of lipid and protein enhanced.

Rendu-Osler-Weber

448.0 Post-pubescent disorder with small telagiectases and dilated venules developing slowly on skin and mucus membranes of lips, tongue, nasopharynx, tongue, and face.

Renofacial

753.0 Renal agenesis with hypoplastic lungs and associated neonatal respiratory distress, hemodynamic instability, acidosis, cyanosis, edema, and characteristic facial features. Death usually occurs from lack of oxygen.

Rénon-Delille

253.8 (Babinski-Frolich, Launois-Cleret) Obesity and hypogonadism in adolescent boys. Rare accompanying dwarfism is thought to indicate hypothyroidism.

Respiratory distress

769 (Hyaline membrane) Premature neonates with respiratory distress and associated with reduced amounts of lung surfactant. Frequently fatal.

Restless leg

333.99 (Ekborn's) Indescribable uneasiness, restlessness, or twitching in the legs after going to bed. Often caused by poor circulation or antipsychotic medications, it can lead to insomnia.

Retraction

378.71 (Still-Turk-Duane) Simultaneous retraction of eye muscles causing an inability to abduct the affected eye with retraction of the globe.

Retroperitoneal fibrosis

593.4 (Ormond's) Retroperitoneal structures obstructing ureters following certain types of chemical treatment; there is no identified cause.

Rett's

330.8 Progressive disease affecting grey matter of the brain, where infant females present ataxia, autism, dementia, seizures, loss of purposeful use of the hands, and cerebral atrophy.

Reye's

331.81 Condition of childhood spawned by a spirochetic or viral disease of the upper respiratory system. Symptoms include recurrent vomiting, brain swelling, disturbances of consciousness, and seizures. Often fatal. Can be prompted by use of aspirin.

Syndromes

Reye-Sheehan's
253.2 (Sheehan's) Secretion of all anterior pituitary hormones is inadequate or absent presenting after childbirth.

Riddoch's
368.16 (Balint's, Holmes', Riddoch's) Corical paralysis of visual fixation, optic ataxia, and disturbance of visual attention. Eye movements are normal.

Ridley's
428.1 Left heart failure marked by acute edema of lung.

Rieger's
743.44 Dysgenesis of eye marked through widened trabecular meshwork, large iridial bands, and glaucoma.

Rietti-Greppi-Micheli
282.4 One of a group of hemolytic anemias sharing a common decreased rate of synthesis of one or more hemoglobin polypeptide chains and are classified according to chain involved.

Riley-Day
742.8 Eyelids widen during chewing, sometimes with an elevation of the upper lid when mouth is open and closing of lid when mouth is closed.

Robin's
756.0 (Pierre Robin's) Brachygnathia and cleft palate, upward displacement of the larynx, and angulation of the manubrium sterni. May be paired with others or the sole hyperplasia.

Rokitansky-Kuster-Hauser
752.49 Absence of vagina and uterus with normal karyotype and ovaries. Amenorrhea.

Romano-Ward
794.31 Prolonged Q-T interval and syncope, sometimes leading to ventricular fibrillation and sudden death.

Romberg's
349.89 (Kleine-Levin, Parry-Romberg) Hypersomnia associated with bulimia and occurring in males between 10 to 25 years of age. Ravenous appetite following prolonged sleep, along with behavioral disturbances, impaired thought processes, and hallucinations.

Rosen-Castleman-Liebow
516.0 Chronic disease of lungs marked by chest pain, weakness, hemoptysis, dyspnea, and productive cough. Ventilation of affected areas is prevented by a proteinaceous material.

Roth's
355.1 Feeling of tingling, formication, itching, and other symptoms on the outer side of the lower part of the thigh caused by lateral femoral cutaneous nerve.

Rothmund's
757.33 Pigmentation and atrophy of the skin, along with cataracts, saddle nose, bone defects, disturbance of hair growth, and hypogonadism.

Rotor's
277.4 Nonhemolytic jaundice differing from Dubin-Johnson syndrome in that it does not produce liver pigmentation.

Rubella
771.0 Developmental abnormalities of newborn baby as resulting from transplacental transference of rubella during the first trimester of pregnancy. Symptoms include ocular and cardiac lesions, deafness, microcephaly, mental retardation, hepatitis, encephalitis, and others.

Rubinstein-Taybi's
759.89 Congenital defects including broad thumb and great toe, antimongloid slant to the eyes, beaked nose, prominent forehead, low set ears, high arched palate, mental retardation, and cardiac defects.

Rud's
759.89 Dwarfism, hypogonadism, and epilepsy with scaly skin as result of inherited disorder.

Ruiter-Pompen (-Wyers)
272.7 (Fabry's) Corneal opacities; burning pain in palms, soles, and abdomen; chronic paresthesia on hands and feet; cardiopulmonary involvement; edema of the legs; osteoporosis; retarded growth; and delayed puberty. Patients die of renal, cardiac, or cerebrovascular failure.

Runge's
766.2 (Ballantyne) Placental dysfunction occurring in postmature fetuses.

Russell (-Silver)
759.89 Suprasellar lesions in anterior third ventricle, hampering a child's ability to thrive. Despite elevated growth hormones, child is emaciated and looses body fat.

Rytand-Lipsitch
426.0 (Lev's) Bundle branch block in a patient with normal coronary arteries and myocardium resulting from calcification of conducting system.

Sacralization-scoliosis-sciatica
756.15 (Bertolotti's) Fusion of bottom lumbar vertebra to top sacral vertebra, making a sixth sacral vertebra. Other symptoms include sciatica and scoliosis.

Saenger's
379.46 Paralysis of conjugate movement of eyes without paralysis of convergence. Caused by lesions of midbrain.

Sanfilippo's
277.5 Results from accumulation of mucopolysaccharide sulfates affecting the eye, ear, skin, teeth, skeleton, joints, liver, spleen, cardiovascular system, respiratory system, and central nervous system.

Scaglietti-Dagnini
253.0 Arthritis of spine accompanying acromegaly, resembling rheumatoid arthritis, and progressing to bony ankylosis with lipping of vertebral margins.

Scalded skin
695.1 Necrolysis of skin caused by toxins.

Scalenus anticus
353.0 (Naffziger's) A disorder presenting symptoms similar to Raynaud's, caused by pressure of brachial plexus and subclavian artery against first thoracic rib.

Scapulocostal
354.8 Pain in upper and posterior part of the shoulder radiating into neck and occiput, down the arm, and around the chest. Caused by abnormal positioning between scapula and thorax, pain can include tingling in the fingers.

Scapuloperoneal
359.1 A position of fetus in which the scapula rests closest to the perineal area.

Schaumann's
135 (Hutchinson-Boeck, Lofgren's, Besnier-Boeck-Schaumann) Involves the lungs with resulting fibrosis, lymph nodes, skin, liver, eyes, spleen, phalangeal bones, and parotid glands. Identified by systemic granulomas composed of epithelioid and multinucleated giant cells.

Scheie's
277.5 Accumulation of mucopolysaccharide sulfates affecting the eye, ear, skin, teeth, skeleton, joints, liver, spleen, cardiovascular system, respiratory system, and central nervous system.

Scheuthauer-Marie-Sainton
755.59 Defective bone formation in skull, often associated with other symptoms.

Schirmer's
759.6 (Kalischer's) Formation of multiple angiomas in skin of the head and scalp.

Schizophrenic, of childhood
299.9X Description of schizophrenia occurring in childhood.

Schneider's
047.9 Viral meningitis that is unspecified.

Scholte's
259.2 (Bjorck-Thorson, Cassidy-Scholte, Hedinger's) Carcinoid tumors causing cyanotic flushing of skin, diarrheal watery stools, bronchoconstrictive attacks, hypotension, edema, and ascites.

Scholz (-Bielschowsky-Henneberg)
330.0 Metachromatic leukodystrophy, a disturbance of white substance of brain.

Schroeder's
255.3 (Slocumb's) Disorder of adrenal medullary tissue resulting in hypertension accompanied with attacks of palpitation, headache, nausea, dyspnea, anxiety, pallor, and profuse sweating.

Schüller-Christian
277.8 (Hand-Schuller-Christian) Histiocytosis with occasional accumulation of cholesterol. Symptoms include defects of the membranous bones, exophthalmos and diabetes insipidus. There is often also a multiple-system, soft tissue, and skeletal involvement.

Schultz's
288.0 (Doan-Wiseman, Kostmann, Schwachman) Bronchiectasis and pancreatic insufficiency, resulting in malnutrition, sinusitis, short stature, and bone abnormalities.

Schwartz (-Jampel)
756.89 Dysplasia of fingernails and toenails, hypoplasia of patella, iliac horns, thickening of glomerular lamina densa, and flask-shaped femur.

Schwartz-Bartter
253.6 Found in children with hypokalemic alkalosis and elevated renin or angiotensin levels with low or normal blood pressure, no edema, and retarded growth.

Scimitar
747.49 Venous drainage of right lung into the inferior vena cava with hypoplasia of the right lung. Name comes from the convex shadow of the anomalous vein to the right of the lower border of the heart in an x-ray.

Sclera
756.51 (van der Hoeve's) Blue sclera, little growth, brittle bones, and deafness.

Sclerocystic ovary
256.4 (Stein, Stein-Leventhal) Oligomenorrhea or amenorrhea, anovulation and infertility, and hirsutism. Most often caused by bilateral polycystic ovaries.

Sea-blue histiocyte
272.7 (Ruiter-Pompen-Wyers, Fabry's) Corneal opacities; burning pain in palms, soles, and abdomen; chronic paresthesia of hands and feet; cardiopulmonary involvement; edema of the legs; osteoporosis; retarded growth; and delayed puberty. Patients die of renal, cardiac, or cerebrovascular failure.

Seabright-Bantam
275.4 (Albright-Martin, Martin-Albright) Similar to hypoparathyroidism, caused by failure to repond to parathyroid hormone with short stature, obesity, short metacarpals, and ectopic calcification.

Seckel's
759.89 Dwarfism with low birth weight, microcephaly, large eyes, beaked nose, receding mandible, and moderate mental retardation.

Secondary
731.2 Symmetrical osteitis of limbs localized to phalanges and terminal epiphyses of long bones of forearm and leg. Symptoms include kyphosis of the spine and affection of joints.

Secretan's
782.3 Traumatic, recurrent edema or hemorrhage of the back of the hand.

Secretoinhibitor
710.2 (Gougerot-Houwer, Sjogren) Complex of symptoms of unknown source in middle aged women in which the following triad exists: keratoconjunctivitis sicca, zerostomia, and connective tissue disease (usually rheumatoid arthritis but sometimes systemic lupus erythematosus. Cause may be an abnormal immune response.

Senear-Usher
694.4 Eruption of the skin on the face, scalp, and trunk with lesions scaling erthymatosus.

Senilism
259.8 Progeria syndrome which includes marked senility by 10 years of age.

Serous meningitis
348.2 Meningitis with serious inflammation in subarachnoid and ventricle spaces and little change in cerebrospinal fluid.

Sertoli cell
606.0 Congenital germinal epithelium absence of the testes.

Shaver's
503 Condition resulting from the ingestion of bauxite fumes and fine particles of alumina and silica in the aluminum mining and manufacturing process. Symptoms include pulmonary emphysema and pneumothorax.

Sheehan's
253.2 (Reye-Sheehan) Secretion of all anterior pituitary hormones is inadequate or absent; presenting after childbirth.

Shoulder-arm
337.9 (Claude Bernard-Homer, Reilly's, Steinbrocker's, shoulder-hand) Clinical disorder following a heart attack, marked by pain and stiffness in the shoulder, with puffy swelling and pain in the hand.

Shwachman's
288.0 (Doan-Wiseman, Kostmann, Schultz) Bronchiectasis and pancreatic insufficiency, resulting in malnutrition and sinusitis. Other symptoms include short stature and bone abnormalities.

Shy-Drager
333.0 (Hallervorden-Spatz, Dejerine-Thomas) Condition in which the nerves between the striatum and pallidum are completely demyelated.

Sicard's
352.6 (Collet-Sicard) Unilateral lesions of ninth, tenth, eleventh, and twelfth cranial nerves producing paralysis of the vagal, glossal, and other nerves and tongue on same side. Usually result of injury.

Sicca
710.2 (Gougerot-Houwer, Sjogren) Complex of symptoms of unknown source in middle-aged women in which the following triad exists: keratoconjunctivitis sicca, zerostomia, and connective tissue disease (usually rheumatoid arthritis but sometimes systemic lupus erythematosus). Cause may be an abnormal immune response.

Sideropenic
280.8 Eczema, thrombocyopenia, and recurrent pyogenic infection. Patients suffer an increased susceptibility to infection with encapsulated bacteria.

Siemens' ectodermal dysplasia
757.31 Congenitally absent sweat glands, smooth finely wrinkled skin, sunken nose, malformed teeth, sparse hair, and deformed nails. Sometimes absent breast tissue, mental retardation, or syndactyly.

Siemens' keratosis follicularis spinulosa
757.39 Inherited condition in which the hair follicles are replaced by keratosis.

Silfverskiöld's
756.50 A dominant inherited disease with skeletal changes in extremities.

Silver's
759.89 Dwarfism marked by late closure of anterior fontanel, bilateral body asymmetry, low birth weight, clinodactyly of the fifth fingers, triangular facial shape, and carp mouth.

Silvestroni-Bianco
282.4 One of a group of hemolytic anemias that shares common decreased rate of synthesis of one or more hemoglobin polypeptide chains and are classified according to chain involved.

Simons'
272.6 (Hollander-Simons) Characterized by loss of subcutaneous fat of upper torso, the arms, the neck, and the face but with an increase in fat on and below the pelvis.

Sinus tarsi
355.5 Caused by posterior tibial nerve at ankle, syndrome can produce significant neuropathy.

Sinusitis-bronchiectasis-situs inversus
759.3 (Kartagener's) Transposition or misplacement of organs or viscera.

Sipple's
193 Familial endocrine adenomatosis

Sjögren (-Gougerot)
710.2 (Gougerot-Houwer) Complex of symptoms of unknown source in middle aged women in which the following triad exists: keratoconjunctivitis sicca, zerostomia, and connective tissue disease (usually rheumatoid arthritis but sometimes systemic lupus erythematosus). Cause may be an abnormal immune response.

Sjögren-Larsson
757.1 Congenital malformation of the skin with scaling and spastic paraplegia.

Slocumb's
255.3 (Schroeder's) Disorder of adrenal medullary tissue resulting in hypertension accompanied with attacks of palpitation, headache, nausea, dyspnea, anxiety, pallor, and profuse sweating.

Sluder's
337.0 (Charcot-Weiss-Baker) Stimulation of an overactive carotid sinus, causing a marked drop in blood pressure, which, in turn, may stop or block the heart.

Smith-Lemli-Opitz
759.89 Mental retardation, small stature, ptosis, male genital anomalies, anteverted nostrils, and syndactyly of the second and third toes.

Syndromes

Sneddon-Wilkinson
694.1   Non-inflammatory intimal hyperplasia of medium-sized vessels.

Sotos'
253.0   Increased birth weight and length, accelerated growth rate for the first four or five years with no elevation of serum growth hormone levels, followed by revision to normal growth rate, antimongoloid slant, prognathism, hypertelorism, dolichocephalic skull, impaired coordination, and moderate mental retardation may be present.

Specified focal (partial)
310.8   Persistent personality disturbance of nonpsychotic origin with one of the following symptoms: affective instability, bursts of aggression, apathy and indifference, impaired social judgment, and suspiciousness or paranoid ideation.

Spens'
426.9   (Stokes-Adams; Morgagni's disease) Heart block often causing slow or absent pulse, vertigo, syncope, convulsions, and Cheyne-Stokes respiration.

Sphallo-pharyngo-laryngeal hemiplegia
352.6   (Collet-Sicard) Unilateral lesions of the ninth, tenth, eleventh, and twelfth cranial nerves producing paralysis of the vagal, glossal, and other nerves and the tongue on the same side. Most usually result of injury.

Spherophakia-brachymorphia
759.89   (Weill-Marchesani) Abnormally round and small lens of the eyes, short stature, and brachydactyly.

Spinal artery
433.8X   (Beck's) Occlusion of spinal artery as result of injury, disk damage, or cardiovascular disease.

Splenic agenesis
759.0   Congenital disorder in which organs of left side of body are a mirror image of the organs on the right side. Splenic agenesis and cardiac malformation are associated.

Splenic flexure
569.89   Bloating, gas, pain, and fullness experienced in left upper abdominal quadrant with pain sometimes radiating up into left chest.

Splenic neutropenia
288.0   Inherited disorder with bronchiectasis and pancreatic insufficiency, resulting in malnutrition, sinusitis, short stature, and bone abnormalities.

Spousal abuse
995.8X   Maltreatment (abuse) of spouses and elders with emotional or physical violence.

Spurway's
756.51   (Ekman's, Eddowes') Blue sclera, little growth, brittle and malformed bones, and malformed teeth.

Staphylococcal scalded skin
695.1   Necrolysis of skin caused by toxins.

Steal
435.1   A number of symptoms in a moving limb including pain, tension, and weakness but absent at rest. Caused by occlusive arterial diseases of limbs.

Stein's
256.4   (Stein-Leventhal) Oligomenorrhea or amenorrhea, anovulation and infertility, and hirsutism. Most often caused by bilateral polycystic ovaries.

Steinbrocker's
337.9   (Claude-Bernard-Homer, Reilly's) Pain and stiffness in the shoulder with puffy swelling and pain in the hand following a heart attack.

Stevens-Johnson
695.1   Necrolysis of skin caused by toxins.

Stewart-Morel
733.3   Thickening of inner table of the frontal bone associated with obesity in women nearing menopause.

Stiff-man
333.91   Increasing but fluctuating rigidity of upper limb and axial muscles and increasing cerebral and spinal disease but with increased electrical activity.

Still-Felty
714.1   Splenomegaly, leukopenia, arthritis, hypersplenism, anemia and other symptoms.

Stilling-Türk-Duane

378.71   (Duane) Simultaneous retraction of eye
muscles causing an inability to abduct
affected eye with retraction of globe.

Stokes (-Adams)

426.9   (Morgagni's disease, and Spens) Heart block
often causing slow or absent pulse, vertigo,
syncope, convulsions, and Cheyne-Stokes
respiration.

Straight-back

756.19   Loss of the anterior concavity in the upper
thoracic vertebrae causing spine to move
forward and compress the heart between
sternum and vertebral body.

Sturge-Kalischer-Weber

759.6   Subclavian steal

Subclavian-carotid obstruction

446.7   (Marorell-Fabre, Raed-Harbitz, Takayasu-
Onishi) Occurs in the brachiocephalic trunk
and the left subclavian and left common
carotid arteries above their source in the
aortic arch. Symptoms include ischemia,
transient blindness, facial atrophy, and many
others.

Subcoracoid-pectoralis minor

447.8   Malignant atrophic papulosis.

Subperiosteal hematoma

267   (Barlow, Moller, Cheadle) Anemia, spongy
gums, weakness, induration of leg muscles,
and mucocutaneous hemorrhages.

Subphrenic interposition

751.4   Interposition of colon between liver and
diaphragm.

Sudden infant death

798.0   (crib death) Unexpected death of healthy
infant typically under 12 months old.

Sudeck's

733.7   (Sudeck-Leriche) Post-traumatic
osteoporosis associated with vasospasm.

Suprarenal cortical

255.3   (Schroeder's, Slocumb's) Disorder of adrenal
medullary tissue resulting in hypertension
with attacks of palpitation, headache,
nausea, dyspnea, anxiety, pallor, and profuse
sweating.

Supraspinatus

726.10   Pain on abduction of shoulder and
tenderness upon deep pressure of
supraspinatus tendon.

Swallowed blood

777.3   Swallowed blood syndrome in the newborn,
causing hematemesis and melena.

Sweet

695.89   Disease of women marked by plaque-like
lesions on face, neck, and upper extremities
and conjunctivitis, mucosal lesion, malaise,
fever, and arthralgia.

Swyer-James

492.8   (MacLeod's) Acquired unilateral hyperlucent
lung with severe airway obstruction during
expiration, oligemia, and a small hilum.

Symonds'

348.2   (Symonds') Meningitis with serious
inflammation in subarachnoid and ventricle
spaces and little change in the cerebrospinal
fluid.

Sympathetic paralysis

337.0   (Charcot-Weiss-Baker, Sluder's) Stimulation
of overactive carotid sinus, causing a marked
drop in blood pressure, which, in turn, may
stop or block the heart.

Syndactylic oxycephaly

755.55   (Aperts) Chromosomal condition with
primary symptoms including webbing of
digits and a pointed head with variations of
defects. Often associated with other
chromosomal abnormalities.

Systemic fibrosclerosing

710.8   Widespread formation of fibrous tissue.

Tachycardia-bradycardia

427.81   Rapid action of heart followed by protracted
or transient stopping of heart.

Takayasu (-Onishi)

446.7   (Marorell-Fabre, Raed-Harbitz)
Brachiocephalic trunk and the left
subclavian and left common carotid arteries
above their source in the aortic arch.
Symptoms include ischemia, transient
blindness, facial atrophy, and many others.

Syndromes

Tapia's
352.6 (Collet-Sicard) Unilateral lesions of ninth, tenth, eleventh, and twelfth cranial nerves producing paralysis of vagal, glossal, and other nerves and tongue on the same side. Most usually result of injury.

Tarsal tunnel
355.5 Caused by posterior tibial nerve at the ankle, syndrome can produce significant neuropathy.

Taussig-Bing
745.11 Complete transposition of aorta, with major vessels transposed, high septral ventricular defect, and other symptoms.

Taybi's
759.89 Condition affecting ears, palate, mouth, and fingers.

Teething
520.7 Eruption of teeth in small child.

Tegmental
344.89 (Avellis, Babinski-Nageotte, Benedikt's, Brown-Sequard, Cestan's, Cestan-Chenais, Foville's, Gubler-Millard, Jackson's, Weber-Leyden) Paraplegia and anesthesia over part of the body. Caused by lesions in the brain or spinal cord.

Telangiectasis-pigmentation-cataract
757.33 (Rothmund's) An inherited disorder marked by pigmentation and atrophy of skin, along with cataracts, saddle nose, bone defects, disturbance of hair growth, and hypogonadism.

Temporal
383.02 (Gradenigo's) Localized meningitis in fifth and sixth cranial nerves, causing paralysis and pain in temporal region.

Temporomandibular joint-pain-dysfunction [TMJ]
524.60 Headache, dizziness, tinnitis, and other symptoms resulting from dysfunction of the mandibular joint.

Terry's
362.21 Retinopathy occurring in premature infants treated with high amounts of oxygen. Retina converts into a fibrous mass stunting growth of eye, resulting in blindness.

Testicular feminization
257.8 (Morris, hairless women, Goldberg, Goldberg-Maxwell, testis, nonvirilizing) Male pseudohermaphroditism marked by female external genitalia. This includes incompletely developed vagina with rudimentary uterus and fallopian tubes, scanty or absent axillary/public hair, and amenorrhea.

Tethered (spinal) cord
742.59 Adhesions distorting spinal cord in the caudal area and associated with Arnold-Chiari syndrome and spina bifida.

Thalamic
348.8 Infarction of postero-inferior thalamus causing transient hemiparesis and severe loss of superficial and deep sensation with crude pain in the limbs. Limbs frequently have vasomotor or trophic disturbances.

Thibierge-Weissenbach
710.1 Systemic disorder of connective tissue marked by induration and thickening of the skin, with circulatory and organ changes. May reside in the face and hands for some time. Also includes Raynaud's phenomenon and, in some cases, esophageal problems.

Thoracic outlet
353.0 (Naffziger's) Disorder presenting symptoms similar to Raynaud's, caused by pressure of brachial plexus and subclavian artery against first thoracic rib.

Thoracogenous rheumatic
731.2 (Mankowsky's, Pierre Marie-Bamberger) Symmetrical osteitis of the limbs localized to the phalanges and terminal epiphyses of the long bones of the forearm and leg. Symptoms include kyphosis of the spine and affection of the joints.

Thorson-Biörck
259.2 (Cassidy-Scholte, Hedinger's) Carcinoid tumors causing cyanotic flushing of skin, diarrheal watery stools, bronchoconstrictive attacks, hypotension, edema, and ascites.

Thrombopenia-hemangioma
287.3 Small number of platelets in circulating blood, causing bruising.

Thyroid-adrenocortical insufficiency
258.1 Insufficient production of hormones by the pituitary and thyroid glands.

Tibial
958.8   Early complication of trauma.

Tietze's
733.6   Painful swelling of unknown origin of one or more costal cartilages, especially of second rib. Patients may interpret chest pain as coronary artery disease.

Time-zone
307.45   (jet lag) Imbalance of the normal circadian rhythm resulting from airplane travel through a number of time zones. Leads to fatigue, irritability, and other consitutional disturbances.

Tobias'
162.3   (Cuiffini-Pancoast, Hare's) Neoplasm of the upper lobe of the lung.

Tolosa-Hunt
378.55   Cavernous sinus syndrome produced by idiopathic granuloma.

Toni-Fanconi
270.0   (Harts) Renal tubular malfunction, including cytinosis and osteomalacia that may be caused by inherited disorders or may be the result of multiple myeloma or proximal epithelial growth.

Touraine's
756.89   Dysplasia of the fingernails and toenails, hypoplasia of the patella, iliac horns, thickening of the glomerular lamina densa, and a flask-shaped femur.

Touraine-Solente-Golé
757.39   Thickening of the skin on extremities and face with clubbing of fingers and deformities in bone of limb.

Toxic oil
710.5   Pain in muscles as a result of accumulation of a large number of granular leukocytes.

Toxic shock
040.89   Staphylococci producing an endotoxin, presenting a high fever, vomiting and diarrhea, decreasing blood pressure, a skin rash, and shock. Hyperemia of several mucous membranes also occurs.

Transfusion donor
772.0   Transfusion of fetus's blood across the placenta to mother's blood supply.

Transfusion recipient
776.4   Polycythemia of newborn as result of blood flow from mother.

Traumatic (acute)
847.0   Acute cervical sprain caused by hyperextension of the neck (C4-C5) during an accident, usually in an automobile.

Traumatic shock
958.4   Particularly dangerous state of shock following a traumatic injury.

Treacher Collins'
756.0   (Franceschetti's) Malformations of derivatives of the first branchial arch, marked by palpebral fissures sloping outward and downward with notches in the outer third of the lower lids, defects of malar bones and zygome, hypoplasia of the jawbone, high or cleft palate, low-set ears, unusual hair growth, and pits between mouth and ear.

Trigeminal plate
259.8   Progeria, which includes marked senility by 10 years of age.

Triplex X female
758.81   Three X chromosomes where the only confirmed symptom is the occurrence of twin Barr bodies in a typical cell.

Troisier-Hanot-Chauffard
275.0   Hypertrophic cirrhosis with pigmentation and diabetes mellitus.

Trousseau's
453.1   Spontaneous development of thromboses in upper and lower limbs as a result of visceral neoplasm.

Türk's
378.71   (Duane, Still-Turk-Duane) Simultaneous retraction of eye muscles causing an inability to abduct affected eye with retraction of the globe.

Turner's
758.6   (XO, Turner-Varny) Congenital disorder characterized by short stature, webbed neck, congenital heart disease, mental retardation, and other symptoms.

Syndromes

Twin-to-twin transfusion
762.3   The birth of one anemic twin and one plethoric twin due to the forcing of blood of one twin into the other.

Type I
348.4   Brain damage as result of compression.

Uehlinger's
757.39   Thickening of skin on extremities and face with clubbing of fingers and deformities in bone of limb.

Ullrich (-Bonnevie) (-Turner)
758.6   (XO, Turner-Varny) Congenital disorder characterized by short stature, webbed neck, congenital heart disease, mental retardation, and other symptoms.

Ullrich-Feichtiger
759.89   Congenital abnormalities, depressed nose, small eyes, hypertelorism, and protuberant ears.

Universal joint, cervix
620.6   (Allen-Masters, Masters-Allen) Pelvic pain resulting from old laceration of broad ligament received during delivery.

Unverricht-Wagner
710.3   (Petges-Clejat) Polymyositis occurring with characteristic skin changes that include a rash on upper eyelids with edema, a rash on the forehead, neck, shoulders, trunk, and arms, and papules on the knuckles.

Upward gaze
378.81   (Parinaud's) Paralysis of conjugate movement of eyes without paralysis of convergence. Caused by lesions of the midbrain.

Urbach-Oppenheim
250.8X   [709.3] Diabetes with skin disorder.

Urbach-Wiethe
272.8   Deposition of hyaline material in the skin and mucosa of mouth, pharynx, hypopharynx, and larynx. Skin lesions as pustules on faces and exposed surfaces of arms and legs, which heal and form scars.

Urethro-oculoarticular
099.3   (Fiessinger-Leroy-Reiter, urethro-oculosynovial) Association of arthritis, iridocyclitis, and urethritis, sometimes with diarrhea. While symptoms may recur, the arthritis is constant.

Urohepatic
572.4   (Heyd's) Acute renal failure in patients with disease of biliary or liver tract. Cause seems to be decreased renal blood flow, damaging both organs.

Uveocutaneous
364.24   (Vogt-Koyanagi) Uveomeningitis marked by patchy depigmentation of hair, eyebrows, and lashes. Retinal detatchment, deafness, and tinnitus may also result.

Vagoaccessory
352.6   (Collet-Sicard, vagohypoglossal) Unilateral lesions of the ninth, tenth, eleventh, and twelfth cranial nerves producing paralysis of the vagal, glossal, and other nerves and the tongue on the same side. Most usually result of injury.

Valve prolapse
424.0   (Barlow's) "Mid-late" systolic click due to massive protrusion of mitral valvular leaflet in left atrial cavity.

Van Buchem's
733.3   Multiple fractures and bowing of all extremities, thickening of skull bones, and osteoporosis.

Van der Hoeve's
756.51   Blue sclera, little growth, brittle bones, and deafness.

Van der Hoeve-Halbertsma-Waardenburg
270.2   (Mendes, Waardenburg-Kleinvan, der Hoeve-Waardenburg-Gualdi, ptosis-epicanthus) Eyebrow or upper or lower eyelid sags.

Van Neck-Odelberg
732.1   Disease of growth centers, especially at the top of the femur, in which the epiphyses is replaced by new calcification.

Vascular insufficiency
557.1   (Wilkie's) Complete or partial block of the superior mesenteric artery with symptoms of vomiting, pain, blood in the stool, and distended abdomen. Results in bowel infarction.

Vascular splanchnic
557.0   Visceral circulation syndrome.

Vasomotor
443.9 (Charcot's) Symptoms in a moving limb including pain tension, and weakness but absent at rest. Caused by occlusive arterial diseases of the limbs.

Vasomotor acroparesthesia
443.89 (Nothnagels Type) Parasthesia of the tips of the extremities or attacks of tingling resulting from nerve compression at several levels, and cyanosis. May result in gangrene of the affected areas.

Vasovagal
780.2 (Gower's) Fall in blood pressure, slow pulse, and convulsions. Believed to be sudden stimulation of the vagal nerve by receptors in the heart, carotid sinus, or aortic arch.

VATER
759.89 Vertebral defects, anal atresia, tracheoesophageal fistula with esophageal atresia, and radial and renal anomalies.

Vena cava
459.2 Obstruction of the vena cava.

Verbiest's
435.1 (Charcot's) Symptoms in a moving limb including pain, tension, and weakness but absent at rest. Caused by occlusive arterial diseases of the limbs.

Vernet's
352.6 (Collet-Sicard) Unilateral lesions of the ninth, tenth, eleventh, and twelfth cranial nerves producing paralysis of the vagal, glossal, and other nerves and the tongue on the same side. Most usually result of injury.

Video display tube
723.8 (VDT) Chronic neck and back pain developing from sitting at a computer.

Villaret's
352.6 (Collet-Sicard) Unilateral lesions of the ninth, tenth, eleventh, and twelfth cranial nerves producing paralysis of the vagal, glossal, and other nerves and the tongue on the same side. Most usually result of injury.

Vinson-Plummer
280.8 (Kelly, Plummer-Vinson, Paterson-Brown-Vinson) Condition in middle-aged women with hypochromic anemia, marked by cracks or fissures at the corners of the mouth, painful tongue, and dysphagia due to esophageal stenosis or webs.

Virilism
255.2 (virilizing adrenocortical hyperplasia, congenital) Mature masculine somatic characteristics by a prepubescent male, girl, or woman. This syndrome may show at birth or develop later as result of adrenocortical dysfunction.

Visceral larval migrans
128.0 Prolonged migration of nematode larvae in the viscera, which can cause hyperosinophilia, hepatomegaly, and pneumonitis.

Visual disorientation
368.16 (Balint's, Holmes', Riddoch's) ACorical paralysis of visual fixation, optic ataxia, and disturbance of visual attention. Eye movements are normal.

Vitamin B6 deficiency
266.1 Pellagra, a deficiency-caused syndrome exhibiting gastrointestinal disturbance, erythema, nervous disorders, and mental disturbances.

Vogt's
333.7 Spastic diplegia with athetosis and pseudobulbar paralysis found with a lesion of the caudate nucleus and putamen.

Vogt-Koyanagi
364.24 Uveomeningitis marked by patchy depigmentation of hair, eyebrows, and lashes. Retinal detatchment, deafness, and tinnitus may also result.

Von Bechterew-Strümpell
720.0 Rheumatoid infllammation of vertebrae.

Von Graefe's
378.72 Progressive external ophthalmoplegia, a slowly progressive bilateral myopathy only affecting the muscles around the eye, including lids. Paralysis of the muscles around the eye results.

Von Hippel-Lindau
759.6 Formation of multiple angiomas on the retina.

Von Schroetter's
453.8 Stress thrombosis of the subclavian or axillary vein.

Syndromes

Waardenburg-Klein

270.2 (Mendes, van der Hoeve-Halbertsma-Waardenburg) Eyebrow or upper or lower eyelid sags.

Wagner (-Unverricht)

710.3X (Petges-Clegat, Unverricht-Wagner) Polymyositis occurring with characteristic skin changes that include a rash on the upper eyelids with edema, a rash on the forehead, neck, shoulders, trunk, and arms, and papules on the knuckles.

Waldenström's

273.3 Increase in macroglobulins in the blood. Has symptoms of hyperviscosity such as weakness, fatigue, bleeding disorders, and visual disturbances.

Waldenström-Kjellberg

280.8 (Kelly, Plummer-Vinson, Paterson-Brown-Vinson) Condition in middle-aged women with hypochronic anemia, marked by cracks or fissures at the corners of the mouth, painful tongue, and dysphagia due to esophageal stenosis or webs.

Water retention

276.6 Fluid overload caused by electrolyte and acid-base imbalance.

Waterhouse (-Friderichsen)

036.3 Acute fulminating meningococcal septicemia occurring in children below 10 years of age. Symptoms include vomiting, cyanosis, diarrhea, purpura, convulsions, and circulatory collapse. The patient will often display meningitis and hemorrhaging into the adrenal glands.

Weakness

300.5 Hypersomatic disorder with no idenfiable pathology.

Web

756.89 Dysplasia of the fingernails and toenails, hypoplasia of the patella, iliac horns, thickening of the glomerular lamina densa, and a flask-shaped femur.

Weber's

344.89 (Avellis, Babinski-Nageotte, Benedikt's, Brown-Sequard, Cestan's, Cestan-Chenais, Foville's, Gubler-Millard, Jackson's, Weber-Leyden) Paraplegia and anesthesia over half or part of the body. Caused by lesions in the brain or spinal cord.

Weber-Christian

729.30 Relapsing febrile nodular nonsuppurative panniculitis with development of nodules that spread centrifugally with erythematous borders and clearing centrally to form pigmented plaques.

Weber-Cockayne

757.39 Dwarfism with a precociously senile appearance, pigmentary degeneration of the retina, optic atrophy, deafness, sensitivity to sunlight, and mental retardation.

Weber-Dimitri

759.6 (Kalischer's) Formation of multiple angiomas in the skin of the head and scalp.

Weber-Gubler

344.89 (Avellis, Babinski-Nageotte, Benedikt's, Brown-Sequard, Cestan's, Cestan-Chenais, Foville's, Gubler-Millard, Jackson's, Weber-Leyden) Paraplegia and anesthesia over half or part of the body. Caused by lesions in the brain or spinal cord.

Weber-Osler

448.0 Small telagiectases and dilated venules that develop slowly on the skin and mucus membranes of the lips, tongue, nasopharynx, tongue, and the face.

Wegener's

446.4 Necrotizing granulomatous vasculitis involving the upper and lower respiratory tracts, which is thought to be a hypersensitivity to unknown antigens.

Weill-Marchesani

759.89 Abnormally round and small lens, short stature, and brachydactyly.

Weingarten's

518.3 Transient infiltrations of lungs by eosinophilia, resulting in night coughing, fever, and dyspnea.

Weiss-Baker

337.0 (Charcot-Weiss-Baker, Sluder's) Stimulation of an overactive carotid sinus, causing a marked drop in blood pressure, which, in turn, may stop or block the heart.

Weissenbach-Thibierge
710.1   Systemic disorder of the connective tissue marked by induration and thickening of the skin, with circulatory and organ changes. May reside in the face and hands for some time. Also includes Raynaud's phenomenon and, in some cases, esophageal problems.

Werlhof-Wichmann
287.3   Small number of platelets in circulating blood, causing bruising.

Wermer's
258.0   Tumors in more than one endocrine gland, including the pancreatic islets and parathyroid glands. Syndrome is inherited.

Werner's
259.8   Premature aging in the adult as result of genetic trait and characterized by sclerodermal skin changes, cataracts, muscular atrophy, diabetes mellitus, baldness, and high incidence of neoplasm.

Wernicke's
265.1   (Gayet-Wernicke) Thiamine deficiency, disturbances in ocular motility, pupillary alterations, nystagmus, and ataxia with tremors. Organic toxic psychosis often co-exists. Most often due to alcoholism.

Wernicke-Korsakoff
294.0   Amnestic dementia where the patient cannot remember short-term or long-term memories but is not delirious.

Westphal-Strümpell
275.1   (Wilson) Defect in the metabolism of copper. Marked by accumulation of copper in the brain, cornea, kidney, liver, and other tissues causing cirrhosis of the liver and deterioration in the basal ganglia of the brain.

Wet brain
303.9X   Description of chronic alcoholism.

Wet feet
991.4   (immersion foot, trench foot) Blotchy cyanosis, increased sweating, parasthesia, and edema. Caused by hypothermia.

Whiplash
847.0   Acute cervical sprain caused by hyperextension of the neck (C4-C5) during an accident, usually in an automobile.

Whipple's
040.2   Radical removal of the head of the pancreas, duodenum, and distal third of the stomach. Jejunum is connected to the stomach, pancreas, and bile duct.

"Whistling face"
759.89   (Freeman-Sheldon) Deviation of hands and face, with protrusion of lips as in whistling, sunken eyes, and small nose.

Widal (-Abrami)
283.9   (Dyke-Young, Hayem-Widal) One of anemic syndromes caused by exposures to trauma, poisons, and other causes that decreases the number of red blood cells.

Wilkie's
557.1   Complete or partial block of the superior mesenteric artery with symptoms of vomiting, pain, blood in the stool, and distended abdomen. Results in bowel infarction.

Wilkinson-Sneddon
694.1   Non-inflammatory intimal hyperplasia of medium sized vessels.

Willan-Plumbe
696.1   Eruption of circumscribed, discrete, reddish, silvery-scaled maculopapules on the knees, elbows, scalp, and trunk.

Willi-Prader
759.81   Rounded face, almond-shaped eyes, strabismus, low forehead, hypogonadism, hypotomia, mental retardation, and an insatiable appetite.

Wilson's
275.1   (Westphal-Strumpell) Defect in the metabolism of copper with accumulation of copper in the brain, cornea, kidney, liver, and other tissues causing cirrhosis of the liver and deterioration in the basal ganglia of the brain.

Wilson-Mikity
770.7   Pulmonary insufficiency in newborn babies, especially those with low birth weight with hypercapnia and cyanosis of rapid onset during the first month of life and resulting frequently in death.

Winking
307.20   Tic motor disorder not otherwise specified.

Syndromes

Wiskott-Aldrich
279.12 Immunodeficiency shown by eczema, thrombocytopenia, and recurrent pyogenic infection. Patients suffer an increased susceptibility to infection with encapsulated bacteria.

With neurogenic bladder
344.61 Aching pain of the perineum, bladder, and sacrum, radiating in a sciatic fashion, due to compression of spinal nerve roots. Symptoms include paralysis of organs and limbs served by those roots, including the bladder.

With spina bifida
741.0X (Arnold-Chiari) Displacement of the caudal spinal cord due to tethering with or without spina bifida and other problems such as meningomyelocele.

Woake's
471.1 (polypoid sinus degeneration) Polyp-like growths that hamper sinus function.

XO
758.6 (Turner's) Short stature, webbed neck, congenital heart disease, mental retardation, and other symptoms.

Yellow vernix
656.7 (placental dysfunction) Marked by placental dysfunction, infarction, and insufficiency.

Zahorsky's
074.0 (herpangina) Vesicular pharyngitis caused by Coxsackie virus.

Ziere's
571.1 Acute hepatitis or cirrhosis of the liver associated with alcoholism.

Zollinger-Ellison
251.5 (Ellison-Zollinger) Peptic ulceration with gastric hypersecretion, tumor of the pancreatic islets, and hypoglycemia.

Zuelzer-Ogden
281.2 Folate-deficiency anemia caused by a drug, congenital, dietary, or other reason.

Anatomy Charts

Body Planes and Movements

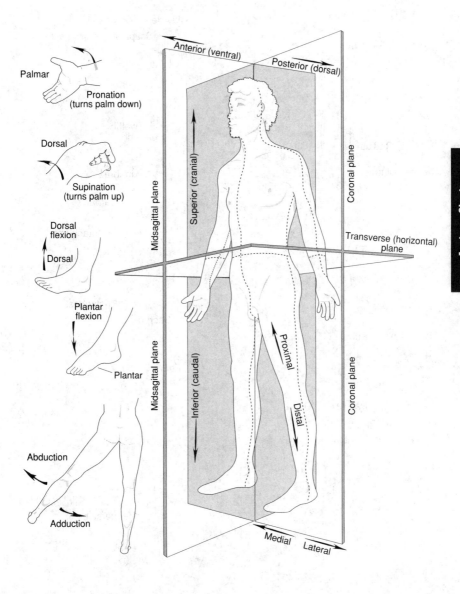

Skeletal System

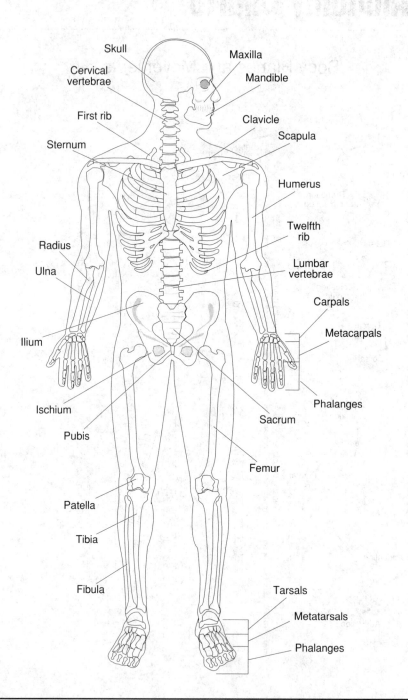

Skull

Maxilla

Cervical vertebrae

Mandible

First rib

Clavicle

Sternum

Scapula

Humerus

Twelfth rib

Radius

Lumbar vertebrae

Ulna

Carpals

Metacarpals

Ilium

Phalanges

Ischium

Sacrum

Pubis

Femur

Patella

Tibia

Fibula

Tarsals

Metatarsals

Phalanges

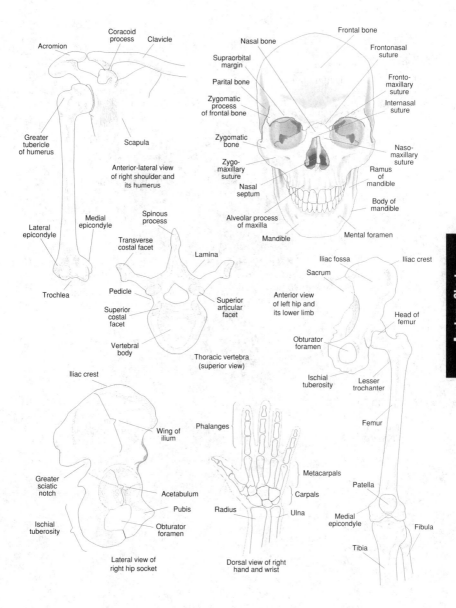

Coracoid process
Acromion
Clavicle

Greater tubericle of humerus
Scapula

Anterior-lateral view of right shoulder and its humerus

Lateral epicondyle
Medial epicondyle

Trochlea

Nasal bone
Supraorbital margin
Parital bone
Zygomatic process of frontal bone
Zygomatic bone
Zygo-maxillary suture
Nasal septum
Alveolar process of maxilla
Mandible

Frontal bone
Frontonasal suture
Fronto-maxillary suture
Internasal suture
Naso-maxillary suture
Ramus of mandible
Body of mandible
Mental foramen

Spinous process
Transverse costal facet
Lamina
Pedicle
Superior articular facet
Superior costal facet
Vertebral body
Thoracic vertebra (superior view)

Iliac fossa
Sacrum
Iliac crest
Anterior view of left hip and its lower limb
Head of femur
Obturator foramen
Ischial tuberosity
Lesser trochanter

Iliac crest
Wing of ilium
Phalanges
Greater sciatic notch
Acetabulum
Pubis
Ischial tuberosity
Obturator foramen
Radius
Metacarpals
Carpals
Ulna
Femur
Patella
Medial epicondyle
Fibula
Tibia

Lateral view of right hip socket
Dorsal view of right hand and wrist

Anatomy Charts

Lymphatic Systems

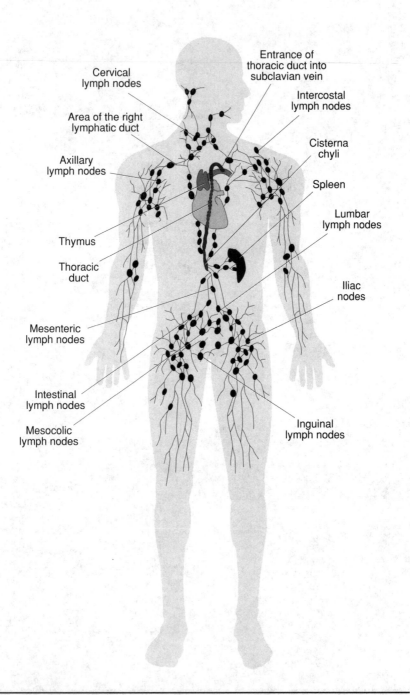

Cervical
lymph nodes

Entrance of
thoracic duct into
subclavian vein

Intercostal
lymph nodes

Area of the right
lymphatic duct

Cisterna
chyli

Axillary
lymph nodes

Spleen

Lumbar
lymph nodes

Thymus

Thoracic
duct

Iliac
nodes

Mesenteric
lymph nodes

Intestinal
lymph nodes

Mesocolic
lymph nodes

Inguinal
lymph nodes

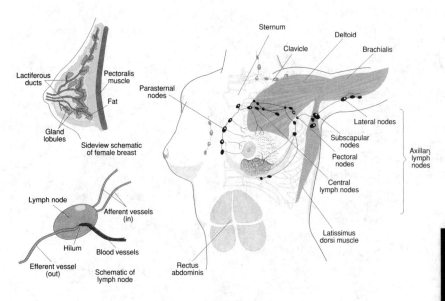

Lactiferous ducts

Pectoralis muscle

Fat

Gland lobules

Sideview schematic of female breast

Parasternal nodes

Sternum

Clavicle

Deltoid

Brachialis

Lateral nodes

Subscapular nodes

Pectoral nodes

Central lymph nodes

Axillary lymph nodes

Latissimus dorsi muscle

Rectus abdominis

Lymph node

Afferent vessels (in)

Hilum

Blood vessels

Efferent vessel (out)

Schematic of lymph node

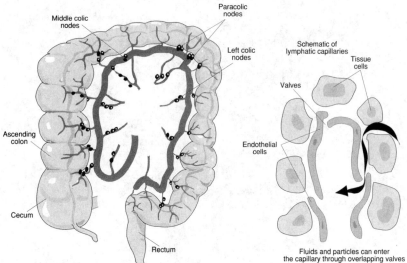

Middle colic nodes

Paracolic nodes

Left colic nodes

Ascending colon

Cecum

Rectum

Lymphatic drainage of the colon follows blood supply

Schematic of lymphatic capillaries

Tissue cells

Valves

Endothelial cells

Fluids and particles can enter the capillary through overlapping valves

Endocrine System

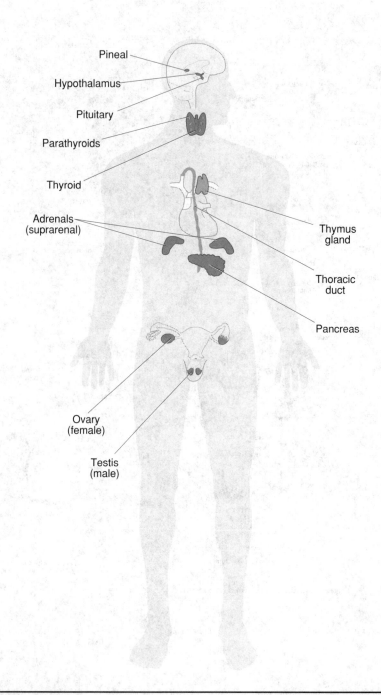

Pineal

Hypothalamus

Pituitary

Parathyroids

Thyroid

Adrenals
(suprarenal)

Thymus
gland

Thoracic
duct

Pancreas

Ovary
(female)

Testis
(male)

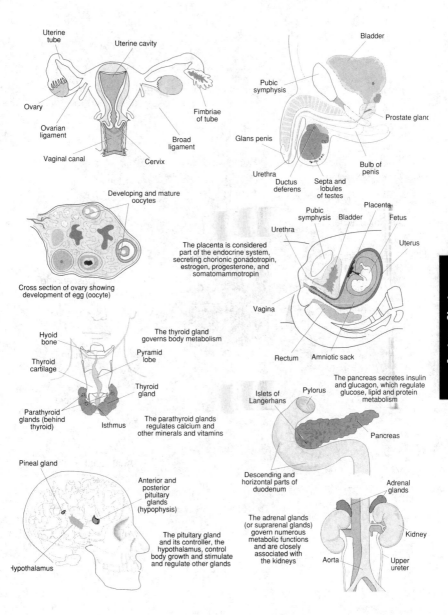

Uterine tube

Uterine cavity

Ovary

Ovarian ligament

Vaginal canal

Fimbriae of tube

Broad ligament

Cervix

Bladder

Pubic symphysis

Prostate gland

Glans penis

Urethra

Ductus deferens

Septa and lobules of testes

Bulb of penis

Developing and mature oocytes

Cross section of ovary showing development of egg (oocyte)

The placenta is considered part of the endocrine system, secreting chorionic gonadotropin, estrogen, progesterone, and somatomammotropin

Pubic symphysis

Bladder

Placenta

Fetus

Urethra

Uterus

Vagina

Rectum

Amniotic sack

Hyoid bone

The thyroid gland governs body metabolism

Thyroid cartilage

Pyramid lobe

Thyroid gland

Parathyroid glands (behind thyroid)

Isthmus

The parathyroid glands regulates calcium and other minerals and vitamins

Islets of Langerhans

Pylorus

The pancreas secretes insulin and glucagon, which regulate glucose, lipid and protein metabolism

Pancreas

Descending and horizontal parts of duodenum

Pineal gland

Anterior and posterior pituitary glands (hypophysis)

The pituitary gland and its controller, the hypothalamus, control body growth and stimulate and regulate other glands

Hypothalamus

The adrenal glands (or suprarenal glands) govern numerous metabolic functions and are closely associated with the kidneys

Adrenal glands

Kidney

Aorta

Upper ureter

Digestive Tract

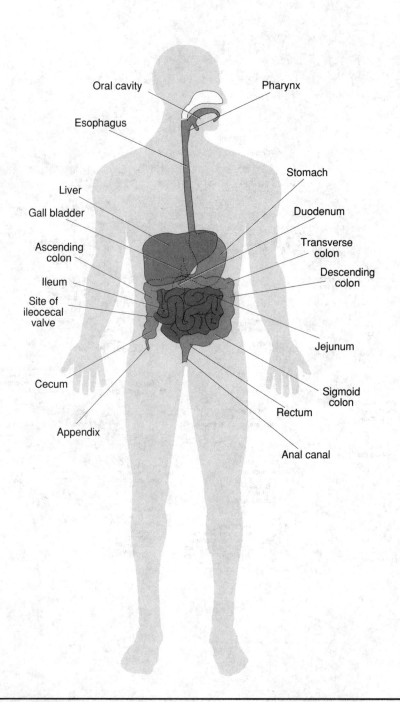

Oral cavity

Pharynx

Esophagus

Liver

Gall bladder

Ascending colon

Ileum

Site of ileocecal valve

Cecum

Appendix

Stomach

Duodenum

Transverse colon

Descending colon

Jejunum

Sigmoid colon

Rectum

Anal canal

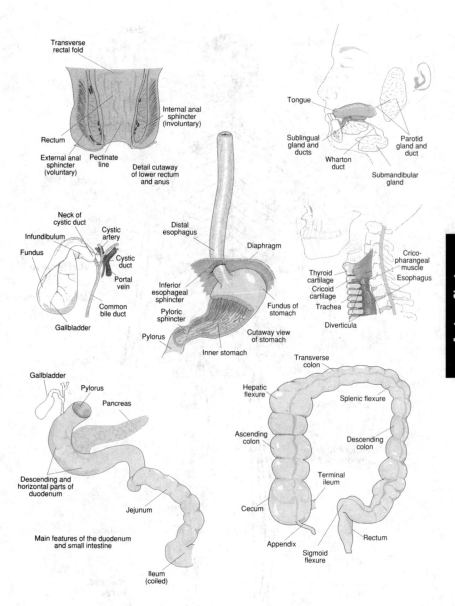

Transverse rectal fold

Rectum

External anal sphincter (voluntary)

Pectinate line

Internal anal sphincter (involuntary)

Detail cutaway of lower rectum and anus

Tongue

Sublingual gland and ducts

Wharton duct

Parotid gland and duct

Submandibular gland

Neck of cystic duct

Infundibulum

Fundus

Cystic artery

Cystic duct

Portal vein

Common bile duct

Gallbladder

Distal esophagus

Inferior esophageal sphincter

Pyloric sphincter

Pylorus

Inner stomach

Diaphragm

Fundus of stomach

Cutaway view of stomach

Thyroid cartilage

Cricoid cartilage

Trachea

Diverticula

Crico-pharangeal muscle

Esophagus

Gallbladder

Pylorus

Pancreas

Descending and horizontal parts of duodenum

Jejunum

Main features of the duodenum and small intestine

Ileum (coiled)

Transverse colon

Hepatic flexure

Ascending colon

Cecum

Appendix

Splenic flexure

Descending colon

Terminal ileum

Sigmoid flexure

Rectum

Nervous System

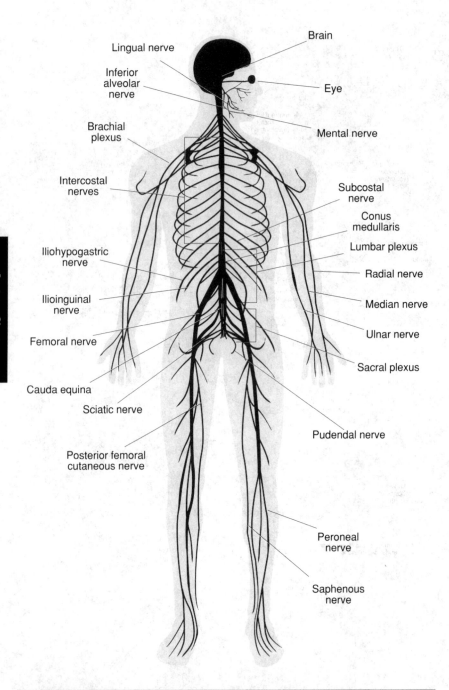

Lingual nerve

Inferior alveolar nerve

Brachial plexus

Intercostal nerves

Iliohypogastric nerve

Ilioinguinal nerve

Femoral nerve

Cauda equina

Sciatic nerve

Posterior femoral cutaneous nerve

Brain

Eye

Mental nerve

Subcostal nerve

Conus medullaris

Lumbar plexus

Radial nerve

Median nerve

Ulnar nerve

Sacral plexus

Pudendal nerve

Peroneal nerve

Saphenous nerve

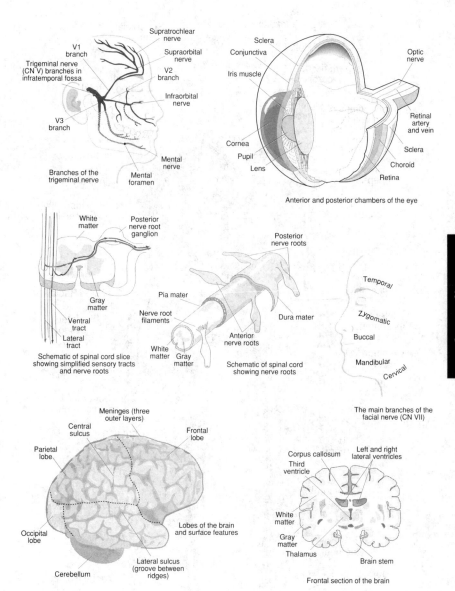

Branches of the trigeminal nerve

Supratrochlear nerve
V1 branch
Trigeminal nerve (CN V) branches in infratemporal fossa
Supraorbital nerve
V2 branch
Infraorbital nerve
V3 branch
Mental nerve
Mental foramen

Anterior and posterior chambers of the eye

Sclera
Conjunctiva
Iris muscle
Cornea
Pupil
Lens
Optic nerve
Retinal artery and vein
Sclera
Choroid
Retina

Schematic of spinal cord slice showing simplified sensory tracts and nerve roots

White matter
Posterior nerve root ganglion
Gray matter
Ventral tract
Lateral tract
White matter
Gray matter

Schematic of spinal cord showing nerve roots

Posterior nerve roots
Pia mater
Nerve root filaments
Dura mater
Anterior nerve roots

The main branches of the facial nerve (CN VII)

Temporal
Zygomatic
Buccal
Mandibular
Cervical

Lobes of the brain and surface features

Meninges (three outer layers)
Central sulcus
Frontal lobe
Parietal lobe
Occipital lobe
Cerebellum
Lateral sulcus (groove between ridges)

Frontal section of the brain

Corpus callosum
Third ventricle
Left and right lateral ventricles
White matter
Gray matter
Thalamus
Brain stem

Circulatory System: Arterial

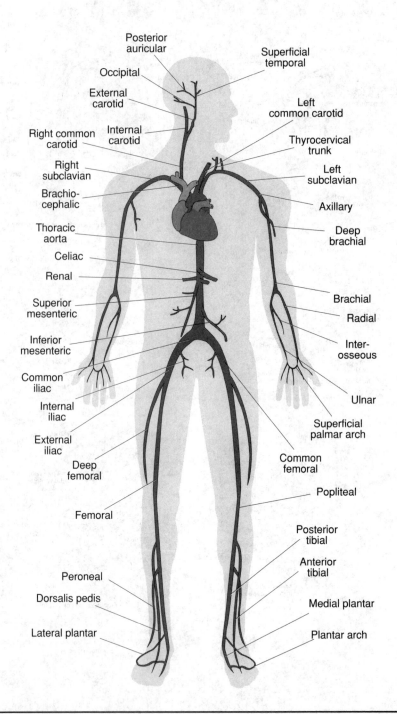

Posterior auricular

Superficial temporal

Occipital

External carotid

Left common carotid

Right common carotid

Internal carotid

Thyrocervical trunk

Right subclavian

Left subclavian

Brachio-cephalic

Axillary

Thoracic aorta

Deep brachial

Celiac

Renal

Superior mesenteric

Brachial

Radial

Inferior mesenteric

Inter-osseous

Common iliac

Internal iliac

Ulnar

External iliac

Superficial palmar arch

Deep femoral

Common femoral

Femoral

Popliteal

Posterior tibial

Anterior tibial

Peroneal

Dorsalis pedis

Medial plantar

Lateral plantar

Plantar arch

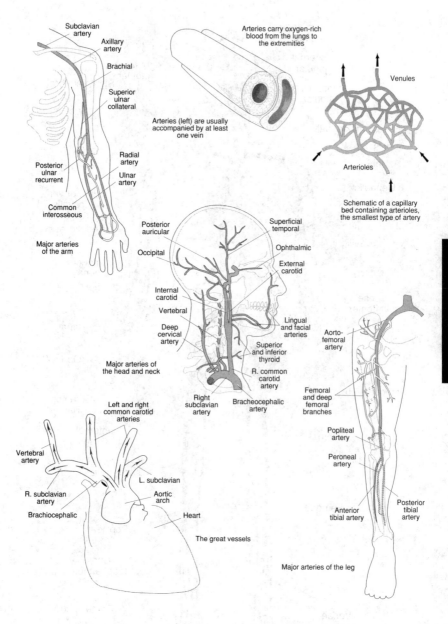

Subclavian artery

Axillary artery

Brachial

Superior ulnar collateral

Posterior ulnar recurrent

Radial artery

Ulnar artery

Common interosseous

Major arteries of the arm

Arteries carry oxygen-rich blood from the lungs to the extremities

Arteries (left) are usually accompanied by at least one vein

Venules

Arterioles

Schematic of a capillary bed containing arterioles, the smallest type of artery

Posterior auricular

Occipital

Internal carotid

Vertebral

Deep cervical artery

Major arteries of the head and neck

Superficial temporal

Ophthalmic

External carotid

Lingual and facial arteries

Superior and inferior thyroid

R. common carotid artery

Right subclavian artery

Bracheocephalic artery

Aorto-femoral artery

Femoral and deep femoral branches

Popliteal artery

Peroneal artery

Anterior tibial artery

Posterior tibial artery

Major arteries of the leg

Left and right common carotid arteries

Vertebral artery

R. subclavian artery

Brachiocephalic

L. subclavian

Aortic arch

Heart

The great vessels

Anatomy Charts

Circulatory System: Venous

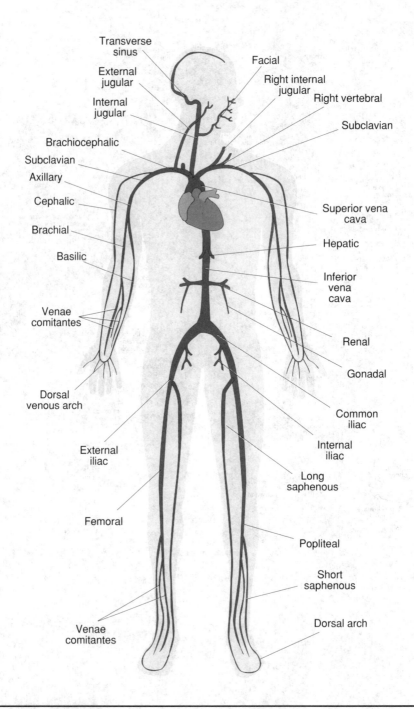

Transverse sinus

External jugular

Internal jugular

Facial

Right internal jugular

Right vertebral

Subclavian

Brachiocephalic

Subclavian

Axillary

Cephalic

Brachial

Basilic

Venae comitantes

Dorsal venous arch

External iliac

Femoral

Venae comitantes

Superior vena cava

Hepatic

Inferior vena cava

Renal

Gonadal

Common iliac

Internal iliac

Long saphenous

Popliteal

Short saphenous

Dorsal arch

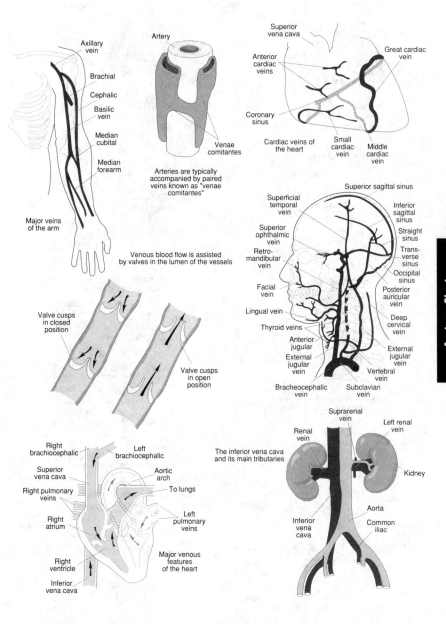

Axillary vein

Brachial

Cephalic

Basilic vein

Median cubital

Median forearm

Major veins of the arm

Artery

Venae comitantes

Arteries are typically accompanied by paired veins known as "venae comitantes"

Venous blood flow is assisted by valves in the lumen of the vessels

Valve cusps in closed position

Valve cusps in open position

Superior vena cava

Anterior cardiac veins

Coronary sinus

Cardiac veins of the heart

Great cardiac vein

Small cardiac vein

Middle cardiac vein

Superior sagittal sinus

Superficial temporal vein

Superior ophthalmic vein

Retro-mandibular vein

Facial vein

Lingual vein

Thyroid veins

Anterior jugular

External jugular vein

Bracheocephalic vein

Inferior sagittal sinus

Straight sinus

Trans-verse sinus

Occipital sinus

Posterior auricular vein

Deep cervical vein

External jugular vein

Vertebral vein

Subclavian vein

Right brachiocephalic

Superior vena cava

Right pulmonary veins

Right atrium

Right ventricle

Inferior vena cava

Left brachiocephalic

Aortic arch

To lungs

Left pulmonary veins

Major venous features of the heart

The inferior vena cava and its main tributaries

Suprarenal vein

Renal vein

Left renal vein

Kidney

Aorta

Inferior vena cava

Common iliac

Anatomy Charts

Urogenital Tract

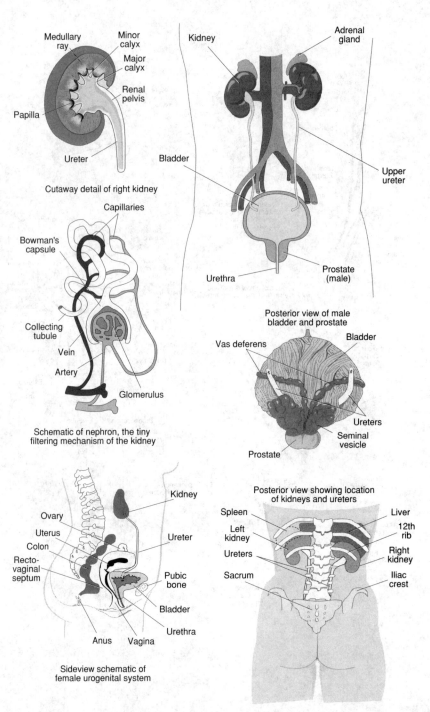

Medullary ray

Minor calyx

Major calyx

Renal pelvis

Papilla

Ureter

Cutaway detail of right kidney

Kidney

Adrenal gland

Bladder

Upper ureter

Urethra

Prostate (male)

Capillaries

Bowman's capsule

Collecting tubule

Vein

Artery

Glomerulus

Schematic of nephron, the tiny
filtering mechanism of the kidney

Posterior view of male
bladder and prostate

Vas deferens

Bladder

Ureters

Seminal vesicle

Prostate

Kidney

Ovary

Uterus

Colon

Recto-
vaginal
septum

Ureter

Pubic bone

Bladder

Urethra

Anus

Vagina

Sideview schematic of
female urogenital system

Posterior view showing location
of kidneys and ureters

Spleen

Left kidney

Ureters

Sacrum

Liver

12th rib

Right kidney

Iliac crest

Anatomy Charts

Respiratory system

The bronchi (dark below) branch further into bronchioles and then into alveolar sacs where venous blood is aerated

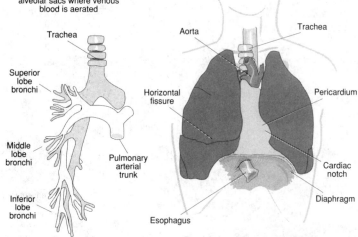

Trachea

Superior lobe bronchi

Middle lobe bronchi

Inferior lobe bronchi

Pulmonary arterial trunk

The pulmonary arteries (white above) deliver venous blood to the lungs where it is oxygenated and converted into arterial blood

Aorta

Trachea

Horizontal fissure

Pericardium

Cardiac notch

Diaphragm

Esophagus

The right lung is larger and heavier than its counterpart due to space lost to the bulge of the heart at the cardiac notch

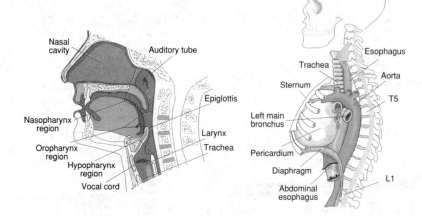

Nasal cavity

Auditory tube

Epiglottis

Nasopharynx region

Larynx

Oropharynx region

Trachea

Hypopharynx region

Vocal cord

Esophagus

Trachea

Sternum

Aorta

T5

Left main bronchus

Pericardium

Diaphragm

Abdominal esophagus

L1

Rule of Nines for Burns

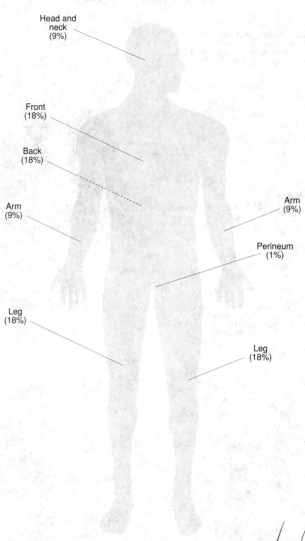

Head and neck (9%)

Front (18%)

Back (18%)

Arm (9%)

Arm (9%)

Perineum (1%)

Leg (18%)

Leg (18%)

First-degree burns involve surface layers only and tissue destruction is minimal.

Second-degree burns damage deeper epidermal layers and upper layers of the dermis; damage to sweat glands, hair follicles, and sebaceous glands may occur.

Third-degree burns include destruction of both epidermis and dermis and tissue death extends below the hair follicles and sweat glands.

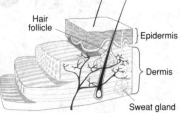

Hair follicle

Epidermis

Dermis

Sweat gland

Anatomy Charts

Anesthesia Crosswalk

Accurate coding of anesthesia is paramount to full reimbursement. Often, more than one CPT® anesthesia code may apply to a procedure; the challenge is selecting the proper code for each case.

The following CPT® surgery to CPT® anesthesia crosswalk includes anesthesia codes for procedures in which palliative care may be necessary. As a result, not all surgical codes are included and not all anesthesia codes are ideal for each case. Inclusion in this list also does not mean an anesthesia code is necessary if anesthesia was not provided in a patient's particular case.

The crosswalk is based on Medicode's own database of 450 million cases. Each surgical code is listed with applicable anesthesia codes below it.

0001T–0002T
00880 Anesthesia for procedures on major lower abdominal vessels; not otherwise specified

0009T
00940 Anesthesia for vaginal procedures (including biopsy of labia, vagina, cervix or endometrium); not otherwise specified

0012T–0013T
01382 Anesthesia for arthroscopic procedures of knee joint

0014T
01400 Anesthesia for open procedures on knee joint; not otherwise specified

01953
01953 Anesthesia for second and third degree burn excision or debridement with or without skin grafting, any site, for total body surface area (TBSA) treated during anesthesia and surgery; each additional nine percent total body surface area or part thereof (List separately in addition to code for primary procedure)

10061–10080
00300 Anesthesia for all procedures on the integumentary system, muscles and nerves of head, neck, and posterior trunk, not otherwise specified

00400 Anesthesia for procedures on the integumentary system on the extremities, anterior trunk and perineum; not otherwise specified

00920 Anesthesia for procedures on male genitalia (including open urethral procedures); not otherwise specified

10140
00300 Anesthesia for all procedures on the integumentary system, muscles and nerves of head, neck, and posterior trunk, not otherwise specified

00400 Anesthesia for procedures on the integumentary system on the extremities, anterior trunk and perineum; not otherwise specified

00920 Anesthesia for procedures on male genitalia (including open urethral procedures); not otherwise specified

00940 Anesthesia for vaginal procedures (including biopsy of labia, vagina, cervix or endometrium); not otherwise specified

11010
00300 Anesthesia for all procedures on the integumentary system, muscles and nerves of head, neck, and posterior trunk, not otherwise specified

00400 Anesthesia for procedures on the integumentary system on the extremities, anterior trunk and perineum; not otherwise specified

11011
00402 Anesthesia for procedures on the integumentary system on the extremities, anterior trunk and perineum; reconstructive procedures on breast (eg, reduction or augmentation mammoplasty, muscle flaps)

00700 Anesthesia for procedures on upper anterior abdominal wall; not otherwise specified

00730 Anesthesia for procedures on upper posterior abdominal wall

00800 Anesthesia for procedures on lower anterior abdominal wall; not otherwise specified

00820 Anesthesia for procedures on lower posterior abdominal wall

01170 Anesthesia for open procedures involving symphysis pubis or sacroiliac joint

01250 Anesthesia for all procedures on nerves, muscles, tendons, fascia, and bursae of upper leg

01320   Anesthesia for all procedures on nerves, muscles, tendons, fascia, and bursae of knee and/or popliteal area

01470   Anesthesia for procedures on nerves, muscles, tendons, and fascia of lower leg, ankle, and foot; not otherwise specified

01610   Anesthesia for all procedures on nerves, muscles, tendons, fascia, and bursae of shoulder and axilla

01710   Anesthesia for procedures on nerves, muscles, tendons, fascia, and bursae of upper arm and elbow; not otherwise specified

01810   Anesthesia for all procedures on nerves, muscles, tendons, fascia, and bursae of forearm, wrist, and hand

11012

00190   Anesthesia for procedures on facial bones or skull; not otherwise specified

00450   Anesthesia for procedures on clavicle and scapula; not otherwise specified

00470   Anesthesia for partial rib resection; not otherwise specified

01120   Anesthesia for procedures on bony pelvis

01170   Anesthesia for open procedures involving symphysis pubis or sacroiliac joint

01230   Anesthesia for open procedures involving upper 2/3 of femur; not otherwise specified

01360   Anesthesia for all open procedures on lower 1/3 of femur

01392   Anesthesia for all open procedures on upper ends of tibia, fibula, and/or patella

01400   Anesthesia for open procedures on knee joint; not otherwise specified

01480   Anesthesia for open procedures on bones of lower leg, ankle, and foot; not otherwise specified

01630   Anesthesia for open procedures on humeral head and neck, sternoclavicular joint, acromioclavicular joint, and shoulder joint; not otherwise specified

01740   Anesthesia for open procedures on humerus and elbow; not otherwise specified

01830   Anesthesia for open procedures on radius, ulna, wrist, or hand bones; not otherwise specified

11040

00300   Anesthesia for all procedures on the integumentary system, muscles and nerves of head, neck, and posterior trunk, not otherwise specified

00400   Anesthesia for procedures on the integumentary system on the extremities, anterior trunk and perineum; not otherwise specified

00920   Anesthesia for procedures on male genitalia (including open urethral procedures); not otherwise specified

00940   Anesthesia for vaginal procedures (including biopsy of labia, vagina, cervix or endometrium); not otherwise specified

11041–11042

00300   Anesthesia for all procedures on the integumentary system, muscles and nerves of head, neck, and posterior trunk, not otherwise specified

00400   Anesthesia for procedures on the integumentary system on the extremities, anterior trunk and perineum; not otherwise specified

00920   Anesthesia for procedures on male genitalia (including open urethral procedures); not otherwise specified

00940   Anesthesia for vaginal procedures (including biopsy of labia, vagina, cervix or endometrium); not otherwise specified

11043

00402   Anesthesia for procedures on the integumentary system on the extremities, anterior trunk and perineum; reconstructive procedures on breast (eg, reduction or augmentation mammoplasty, muscle flaps)

00700   Anesthesia for procedures on upper anterior abdominal wall; not otherwise specified

00730   Anesthesia for procedures on upper posterior abdominal wall

00800   Anesthesia for procedures on lower anterior abdominal wall; not otherwise specified

00820   Anesthesia for procedures on lower posterior abdominal wall

00920   Anesthesia for procedures on male genitalia (including open urethral procedures); not otherwise specified

01250   Anesthesia for all procedures on nerves, muscles, tendons, fascia, and bursae of upper leg

01320   Anesthesia for all procedures on nerves, muscles, tendons, fascia, and bursae of knee and/or popliteal area

01470   Anesthesia for procedures on nerves, muscles, tendons, and fascia of lower leg, ankle, and foot; not otherwise specified

01610   Anesthesia for all procedures on nerves, muscles, tendons, fascia, and bursae of shoulder and axilla

01710   Anesthesia for procedures on nerves, muscles, tendons, fascia, and bursae of upper arm and elbow; not otherwise specified

01810   Anesthesia for all procedures on nerves, muscles, tendons, fascia, and bursae of forearm, wrist, and hand

11044

00160   Anesthesia for procedures on nose and accessory sinuses; not otherwise specified

00190   Anesthesia for procedures on facial bones or skull; not otherwise specified

00450	Anesthesia for procedures on clavicle and scapula; not otherwise specified
00470	Anesthesia for partial rib resection; not otherwise specified
01120	Anesthesia for procedures on bony pelvis
01170	Anesthesia for open procedures involving symphysis pubis or sacroiliac joint
01210	Anesthesia for open procedures involving hip joint; not otherwise specified
01230	Anesthesia for open procedures involving upper 2/3 of femur; not otherwise specified
01360	Anesthesia for all open procedures on lower 1/3 of femur
01392	Anesthesia for all open procedures on upper ends of tibia, fibula, and/or patella
01400	Anesthesia for open procedures on knee joint; not otherwise specified
01480	Anesthesia for open procedures on bones of lower leg, ankle, and foot; not otherwise specified
01630	Anesthesia for open procedures on humeral head and neck, sternoclavicular joint, acromioclavicular joint, and shoulder joint; not otherwise specified
01740	Anesthesia for open procedures on humerus and elbow; not otherwise specified
01742	Anesthesia for open procedures on humerus and elbow; osteotomy of humerus
01830	Anesthesia for open procedures on radius, ulna, wrist, or hand bones; not otherwise specified

11400–11406

00300	Anesthesia for all procedures on the integumentary system, muscles and nerves of head, neck, and posterior trunk, not otherwise specified
00400	Anesthesia for procedures on the integumentary system on the extremities, anterior trunk and perineum; not otherwise specified

11420–11426

00300	Anesthesia for all procedures on the integumentary system, muscles and nerves of head, neck, and posterior trunk, not otherwise specified
00400	Anesthesia for procedures on the integumentary system on the extremities, anterior trunk and perineum; not otherwise specified
00940	Anesthesia for vaginal procedures (including biopsy of labia, vagina, cervix or endometrium); not otherwise specified
00920	Anesthesia for procedures on male genitalia (including open urethral procedures); not otherwise specified

11440–11446

00300	Anesthesia for all procedures on the integumentary system, muscles and nerves of head, neck, and posterior trunk, not otherwise specified

11450–11471

00400	Anesthesia for procedures on the integumentary system on the extremities, anterior trunk and perineum; not otherwise specified

11600–11606

00300	Anesthesia for all procedures on the integumentary system, muscles and nerves of head, neck, and posterior trunk, not otherwise specified
00400	Anesthesia for procedures on the integumentary system on the extremities, anterior trunk and perineum; not otherwise specified

11620–11626

00300	Anesthesia for all procedures on the integumentary system, muscles and nerves of head, neck, and posterior trunk, not otherwise specified
00400	Anesthesia for procedures on the integumentary system on the extremities, anterior trunk and perineum; not otherwise specified
00920	Anesthesia for procedures on male genitalia (including open urethral procedures); not otherwise specified
00940	Anesthesia for vaginal procedures (including biopsy of labia, vagina, cervix or endometrium); not otherwise specified

11640–11646

00300	Anesthesia for all procedures on the integumentary system, muscles and nerves of head, neck, and posterior trunk, not otherwise specified

11719–11730

00400	Anesthesia for procedures on the integumentary system on the extremities, anterior trunk and perineum; not otherwise specified

11740–11765

00400	Anesthesia for procedures on the integumentary system on the extremities, anterior trunk and perineum; not otherwise specified

11770–11772

00300	Anesthesia for all procedures on the integumentary system, muscles and nerves of head, neck, and posterior trunk, not otherwise specified

Anesthesia Crosswalk

11960–11971

00300   Anesthesia for all procedures on the integumentary system, muscles and nerves of head, neck, and posterior trunk, not otherwise specified

00400   Anesthesia for procedures on the integumentary system on the extremities, anterior trunk and perineum; not otherwise specified

00920   Anesthesia for procedures on male genitalia (including open urethral procedures); not otherwise specified

12001–12007

00400   Anesthesia for procedures on the integumentary system on the extremities, anterior trunk and perineum; not otherwise specified

00920   Anesthesia for procedures on male genitalia (including open urethral procedures); not otherwise specified

00940   Anesthesia for vaginal procedures (including biopsy of labia, vagina, cervix or endometrium); not otherwise specified

00300   Anesthesia for all procedures on the integumentary system, muscles and nerves of head, neck, and posterior trunk, not otherwise specified

12011–12018

00300   Anesthesia for all procedures on the integumentary system, muscles and nerves of head, neck, and posterior trunk, not otherwise specified

12031–12037

00300   Anesthesia for all procedures on the integumentary system, muscles and nerves of head, neck, and posterior trunk, not otherwise specified

00400   Anesthesia for procedures on the integumentary system on the extremities, anterior trunk and perineum; not otherwise specified

12041–12047

00300   Anesthesia for all procedures on the integumentary system, muscles and nerves of head, neck, and posterior trunk, not otherwise specified

00400   Anesthesia for procedures on the integumentary system on the extremities, anterior trunk and perineum; not otherwise specified

00920   Anesthesia for procedures on male genitalia (including open urethral procedures); not otherwise specified

00940   Anesthesia for vaginal procedures (including biopsy of labia, vagina, cervix or endometrium); not otherwise specified

12051–12057

00300   Anesthesia for all procedures on the integumentary system, muscles and nerves of head, neck, and posterior trunk, not otherwise specified

13100–13101

00400   Anesthesia for procedures on the integumentary system on the extremities, anterior trunk and perineum; not otherwise specified

00300   Anesthesia for all procedures on the integumentary system, muscles and nerves of head, neck, and posterior trunk, not otherwise specified

13120–13121

00300   Anesthesia for all procedures on the integumentary system, muscles and nerves of head, neck, and posterior trunk, not otherwise specified

00400   Anesthesia for procedures on the integumentary system on the extremities, anterior trunk and perineum; not otherwise specified

13131–13132

00400   Anesthesia for procedures on the integumentary system on the extremities, anterior trunk and perineum; not otherwise specified

00300   Anesthesia for all procedures on the integumentary system, muscles and nerves of head, neck, and posterior trunk, not otherwise specified

00920   Anesthesia for procedures on male genitalia (including open urethral procedures); not otherwise specified

00940   Anesthesia for vaginal procedures (including biopsy of labia, vagina, cervix or endometrium); not otherwise specified

13150–13152

00300   Anesthesia for all procedures on the integumentary system, muscles and nerves of head, neck, and posterior trunk, not otherwise specified

14000–14021

00400   Anesthesia for procedures on the integumentary system on the extremities, anterior trunk and perineum; not otherwise specified

00300   Anesthesia for all procedures on the integumentary system, muscles and nerves of head, neck, and posterior trunk, not otherwise specified

14040–14041
00400 Anesthesia for procedures on the integumentary system on the extremities, anterior trunk and perineum; not otherwise specified

00940 Anesthesia for vaginal procedures (including biopsy of labia, vagina, cervix or endometrium); not otherwise specified

00300 Anesthesia for all procedures on the integumentary system, muscles and nerves of head, neck, and posterior trunk, not otherwise specified

00920 Anesthesia for procedures on male genitalia (including open urethral procedures); not otherwise specified

14060–14061
00300 Anesthesia for all procedures on the integumentary system, muscles and nerves of head, neck, and posterior trunk, not otherwise specified

14350
00400 Anesthesia for procedures on the integumentary system on the extremities, anterior trunk and perineum; not otherwise specified

15000
00300 Anesthesia for all procedures on the integumentary system, muscles and nerves of head, neck, and posterior trunk, not otherwise specified

00400 Anesthesia for procedures on the integumentary system on the extremities, anterior trunk and perineum; not otherwise specified

00920 Anesthesia for procedures on male genitalia (including open urethral procedures); not otherwise specified

15050
00300 Anesthesia for all procedures on the integumentary system, muscles and nerves of head, neck, and posterior trunk, not otherwise specified

00400 Anesthesia for procedures on the integumentary system on the extremities, anterior trunk and perineum; not otherwise specified

00920 Anesthesia for procedures on male genitalia (including open urethral procedures); not otherwise specified

15100
00400 Anesthesia for procedures on the integumentary system on the extremities, anterior trunk and perineum; not otherwise specified

00300 Anesthesia for all procedures on the integumentary system, muscles and nerves of head, neck, and posterior trunk, not otherwise specified

15120
00300 Anesthesia for all procedures on the integumentary system, muscles and nerves of head, neck, and posterior trunk, not otherwise specified

00920 Anesthesia for procedures on male genitalia (including open urethral procedures); not otherwise specified

00940 Anesthesia for vaginal procedures (including biopsy of labia, vagina, cervix or endometrium); not otherwise specified

00400 Anesthesia for procedures on the integumentary system on the extremities, anterior trunk and perineum; not otherwise specified

15200
00400 Anesthesia for procedures on the integumentary system on the extremities, anterior trunk and perineum; not otherwise specified

00300 Anesthesia for all procedures on the integumentary system, muscles and nerves of head, neck, and posterior trunk, not otherwise specified

15220
00300 Anesthesia for all procedures on the integumentary system, muscles and nerves of head, neck, and posterior trunk, not otherwise specified

00400 Anesthesia for procedures on the integumentary system on the extremities, anterior trunk and perineum; not otherwise specified

15240
00300 Anesthesia for all procedures on the integumentary system, muscles and nerves of head, neck, and posterior trunk, not otherwise specified

00920 Anesthesia for procedures on male genitalia (including open urethral procedures); not otherwise specified

00940 Anesthesia for vaginal procedures (including biopsy of labia, vagina, cervix or endometrium); not otherwise specified

00400 Anesthesia for procedures on the integumentary system on the extremities, anterior trunk and perineum; not otherwise specified

15260
00300 Anesthesia for all procedures on the integumentary system, muscles and nerves of head, neck, and posterior trunk, not otherwise specified

Anesthesia Crosswalk

15342–15343

00300 Anesthesia for all procedures on the integumentary system, muscles and nerves of head, neck, and posterior trunk, not otherwise specified

00400 Anesthesia for procedures on the integumentary system on the extremities, anterior trunk and perineum; not otherwise specified

15350

00920 Anesthesia for procedures on male genitalia (including open urethral procedures); not otherwise specified

00940 Anesthesia for vaginal procedures (including biopsy of labia, vagina, cervix or endometrium); not otherwise specified

00300 Anesthesia for all procedures on the integumentary system, muscles and nerves of head, neck, and posterior trunk, not otherwise specified

00400 Anesthesia for procedures on the integumentary system on the extremities, anterior trunk and perineum; not otherwise specified

15400

00300 Anesthesia for all procedures on the integumentary system, muscles and nerves of head, neck, and posterior trunk, not otherwise specified

00400 Anesthesia for procedures on the integumentary system on the extremities, anterior trunk and perineum; not otherwise specified

00920 Anesthesia for procedures on male genitalia (including open urethral procedures); not otherwise specified

00940 Anesthesia for vaginal procedures (including biopsy of labia, vagina, cervix or endometrium); not otherwise specified

15570–15572

00400 Anesthesia for procedures on the integumentary system on the extremities, anterior trunk and perineum; not otherwise specified

00300 Anesthesia for all procedures on the integumentary system, muscles and nerves of head, neck, and posterior trunk, not otherwise specified

15574

00300 Anesthesia for all procedures on the integumentary system, muscles and nerves of head, neck, and posterior trunk, not otherwise specified

00920 Anesthesia for procedures on male genitalia (including open urethral procedures); not otherwise specified

00400 Anesthesia for procedures on the integumentary system on the extremities, anterior trunk and perineum; not otherwise specified

00940 Anesthesia for vaginal procedures (including biopsy of labia, vagina, cervix or endometrium); not otherwise specified

15576

00300 Anesthesia for all procedures on the integumentary system, muscles and nerves of head, neck, and posterior trunk, not otherwise specified

15600–15610

00400 Anesthesia for procedures on the integumentary system on the extremities, anterior trunk and perineum; not otherwise specified

00300 Anesthesia for all procedures on the integumentary system, muscles and nerves of head, neck, and posterior trunk, not otherwise specified

15620

00300 Anesthesia for all procedures on the integumentary system, muscles and nerves of head, neck, and posterior trunk, not otherwise specified

00920 Anesthesia for procedures on male genitalia (including open urethral procedures); not otherwise specified

00400 Anesthesia for procedures on the integumentary system on the extremities, anterior trunk and perineum; not otherwise specified

00940 Anesthesia for vaginal procedures (including biopsy of labia, vagina, cervix or endometrium); not otherwise specified

15630

00300 Anesthesia for all procedures on the integumentary system, muscles and nerves of head, neck, and posterior trunk, not otherwise specified

15732

00300 Anesthesia for all procedures on the integumentary system, muscles and nerves of head, neck, and posterior trunk, not otherwise specified

15734

00400 Anesthesia for procedures on the integumentary system on the extremities, anterior trunk and perineum; not otherwise specified

00300 Anesthesia for all procedures on the integumentary system, muscles and nerves of head, neck, and posterior trunk, not otherwise specified

15736

01610   Anesthesia for all procedures on nerves, muscles, tendons, fascia, and bursae of shoulder and axilla

01710   Anesthesia for procedures on nerves, muscles, tendons, fascia, and bursae of upper arm and elbow; not otherwise specified

01810   Anesthesia for all procedures on nerves, muscles, tendons, fascia, and bursae of forearm, wrist, and hand

15738

01250   Anesthesia for all procedures on nerves, muscles, tendons, fascia, and bursae of upper leg

01320   Anesthesia for all procedures on nerves, muscles, tendons, fascia, and bursae of knee and/or popliteal area

01470   Anesthesia for procedures on nerves, muscles, tendons, and fascia of lower leg, ankle, and foot; not otherwise specified

15740–15750

00300   Anesthesia for all procedures on the integumentary system, muscles and nerves of head, neck, and posterior trunk, not otherwise specified

00400   Anesthesia for procedures on the integumentary system on the extremities, anterior trunk and perineum; not otherwise specified

00920   Anesthesia for procedures on male genitalia (including open urethral procedures); not otherwise specified

15756–15757

00300   Anesthesia for all procedures on the integumentary system, muscles and nerves of head, neck, and posterior trunk, not otherwise specified

00400   Anesthesia for procedures on the integumentary system on the extremities, anterior trunk and perineum; not otherwise specified

15758

01250   Anesthesia for all procedures on nerves, muscles, tendons, fascia, and bursae of upper leg

01320   Anesthesia for all procedures on nerves, muscles, tendons, fascia, and bursae of knee and/or popliteal area

01470   Anesthesia for procedures on nerves, muscles, tendons, and fascia of lower leg, ankle, and foot; not otherwise specified

01610   Anesthesia for all procedures on nerves, muscles, tendons, fascia, and bursae of shoulder and axilla

01710   Anesthesia for procedures on nerves, muscles, tendons, fascia, and bursae of upper arm and elbow; not otherwise specified

01810   Anesthesia for all procedures on nerves, muscles, tendons, fascia, and bursae of forearm, wrist, and hand

15760

00300   Anesthesia for all procedures on the integumentary system, muscles and nerves of head, neck, and posterior trunk, not otherwise specified

15770

00300   Anesthesia for all procedures on the integumentary system, muscles and nerves of head, neck, and posterior trunk, not otherwise specified

00400   Anesthesia for procedures on the integumentary system on the extremities, anterior trunk and perineum; not otherwise specified

00700   Anesthesia for procedures on upper anterior abdominal wall; not otherwise specified

00730   Anesthesia for procedures on upper posterior abdominal wall

00800   Anesthesia for procedures on lower anterior abdominal wall; not otherwise specified

00820   Anesthesia for procedures on lower posterior abdominal wall

15775–15781

00300   Anesthesia for all procedures on the integumentary system, muscles and nerves of head, neck, and posterior trunk, not otherwise specified

15782

00300   Anesthesia for all procedures on the integumentary system, muscles and nerves of head, neck, and posterior trunk, not otherwise specified

00400   Anesthesia for procedures on the integumentary system on the extremities, anterior trunk and perineum; not otherwise specified

15788–15789

00300   Anesthesia for all procedures on the integumentary system, muscles and nerves of head, neck, and posterior trunk, not otherwise specified

15792–15793

00300   Anesthesia for all procedures on the integumentary system, muscles and nerves of head, neck, and posterior trunk, not otherwise specified

00400 Anesthesia for procedures on the integumentary system on the extremities, anterior trunk and perineum; not otherwise specified

15819
00300 Anesthesia for all procedures on the integumentary system, muscles and nerves of head, neck, and posterior trunk, not otherwise specified

15820–15823
00103 Anesthesia for reconstructive procedures of eyelid (eg, blepharoplasty, ptosis surgery)

15824–15829
00300 Anesthesia for all procedures on the integumentary system, muscles and nerves of head, neck, and posterior trunk, not otherwise specified

15831
00802 Anesthesia for procedures on lower anterior abdominal wall; panniculectomy

15832–15834
00400 Anesthesia for procedures on the integumentary system on the extremities, anterior trunk and perineum; not otherwise specified

15835
00300 Anesthesia for all procedures on the integumentary system, muscles and nerves of head, neck, and posterior trunk, not otherwise specified

15836–15837
00400 Anesthesia for procedures on the integumentary system on the extremities, anterior trunk and perineum; not otherwise specified

15838
00300 Anesthesia for all procedures on the integumentary system, muscles and nerves of head, neck, and posterior trunk, not otherwise specified

15840–15845
00300 Anesthesia for all procedures on the integumentary system, muscles and nerves of head, neck, and posterior trunk, not otherwise specified

15876
00300 Anesthesia for all procedures on the integumentary system, muscles and nerves of head, neck, and posterior trunk, not otherwise specified

15877
00400 Anesthesia for procedures on the integumentary system on the extremities, anterior trunk and perineum; not otherwise specified

00300 Anesthesia for all procedures on the integumentary system, muscles and nerves of head, neck, and posterior trunk, not otherwise specified

15878–15879
00400 Anesthesia for procedures on the integumentary system on the extremities, anterior trunk and perineum; not otherwise specified

15920–15922
01120 Anesthesia for procedures on bony pelvis

15931
00300 Anesthesia for all procedures on the integumentary system, muscles and nerves of head, neck, and posterior trunk, not otherwise specified

15933
01120 Anesthesia for procedures on bony pelvis

15934
00300 Anesthesia for all procedures on the integumentary system, muscles and nerves of head, neck, and posterior trunk, not otherwise specified

15935
01120 Anesthesia for procedures on bony pelvis

15936
00300 Anesthesia for all procedures on the integumentary system, muscles and nerves of head, neck, and posterior trunk, not otherwise specified

15937
01120 Anesthesia for procedures on bony pelvis

15940
00300 Anesthesia for all procedures on the integumentary system, muscles and nerves of head, neck, and posterior trunk, not otherwise specified

15941
01120 Anesthesia for procedures on bony pelvis

15944
00300 Anesthesia for all procedures on the integumentary system, muscles and nerves of head, neck, and posterior trunk, not otherwise specified

15945–15946
01120   Anesthesia for procedures on bony pelvis

15950
00400   Anesthesia for procedures on the integumentary system on the extremities, anterior trunk and perineum; not otherwise specified

15951
01230   Anesthesia for open procedures involving upper 2/3 of femur; not otherwise specified

15952
00400   Anesthesia for procedures on the integumentary system on the extremities, anterior trunk and perineum; not otherwise specified

15953
01230   Anesthesia for open procedures involving upper 2/3 of femur; not otherwise specified

15956
00400   Anesthesia for procedures on the integumentary system on the extremities, anterior trunk and perineum; not otherwise specified

15958
01230   Anesthesia for open procedures involving upper 2/3 of femur; not otherwise specified

16010
01951   Anesthesia for second and third degree burn excision or debridement with or without skin grafting, any site, for total body surface area (TBSA) treated during anesthesia and surgery; less than four percent total body surface area

16015
01952   Anesthesia for second and third degree burn excision or debridement with or without skin grafting, any site, for total body surface area (TBSA) treated during anesthesia and surgery; between four and nine percent of total body surface area

01953   Anesthesia for second and third degree burn excision or debridement with or without skin grafting, any site, for total body surface area (TBSA) treated during anesthesia and surgery; each additional nine percent total body surface area or part thereof (List separately in addition to code for primary procedure)

16035
00300   Anesthesia for all procedures on the integumentary system, muscles and nerves of head, neck, and posterior trunk, not otherwise specified

00400   Anesthesia for procedures on the integumentary system on the extremities, anterior trunk and perineum; not otherwise specified

00920   Anesthesia for procedures on male genitalia (including open urethral procedures); not otherwise specified

16036
00300   Anesthesia for all procedures on the integumentary system, muscles and nerves of head, neck, and posterior trunk, not otherwise specified

00400   Anesthesia for procedures on the integumentary system on the extremities, anterior trunk and perineum; not otherwise specified

17106–17250
00300   Anesthesia for all procedures on the integumentary system, muscles and nerves of head, neck, and posterior trunk, not otherwise specified

00920   Anesthesia for procedures on male genitalia (including open urethral procedures); not otherwise specified

00940   Anesthesia for vaginal procedures (including biopsy of labia, vagina, cervix or endometrium); not otherwise specified

00400   Anesthesia for procedures on the integumentary system on the extremities, anterior trunk and perineum; not otherwise specified

17260–17266
00400   Anesthesia for procedures on the integumentary system on the extremities, anterior trunk and perineum; not otherwise specified

00300   Anesthesia for all procedures on the integumentary system, muscles and nerves of head, neck, and posterior trunk, not otherwise specified

17270–17276
00400   Anesthesia for procedures on the integumentary system on the extremities, anterior trunk and perineum; not otherwise specified

00920   Anesthesia for procedures on male genitalia (including open urethral procedures); not otherwise specified

00300   Anesthesia for all procedures on the integumentary system, muscles and nerves of head, neck, and posterior trunk, not otherwise specified

00940   Anesthesia for vaginal procedures (including biopsy of labia, vagina, cervix or endometrium); not otherwise specified

17280–17286

00300   Anesthesia for all procedures on the integumentary system, muscles and nerves of head, neck, and posterior trunk, not otherwise specified

19000

00400   Anesthesia for procedures on the integumentary system on the extremities, anterior trunk and perineum; not otherwise specified

19020–19125

00400   Anesthesia for procedures on the integumentary system on the extremities, anterior trunk and perineum; not otherwise specified

19140–19160

00400   Anesthesia for procedures on the integumentary system on the extremities, anterior trunk and perineum; not otherwise specified

19162

00404   Anesthesia for procedures on the integumentary system on the extremities, anterior trunk and perineum; radical or modified radical procedures on breast

19180–19182

00400   Anesthesia for procedures on the integumentary system on the extremities, anterior trunk and perineum; not otherwise specified

19200

00404   Anesthesia for procedures on the integumentary system on the extremities, anterior trunk and perineum; radical or modified radical procedures on breast

19220

00406   Anesthesia for procedures on the integumentary system on the extremities, anterior trunk and perineum; radical or modified radical procedures on breast with internal mammary node dissection

19240

00404   Anesthesia for procedures on the integumentary system on the extremities, anterior trunk and perineum; radical or modified radical procedures on breast

19260

00470   Anesthesia for partial rib resection; not otherwise specified

19271

00472   Anesthesia for partial rib resection; thoracoplasty (any type)

19272

00540   Anesthesia for thoracotomy procedures involving lungs, pleura, diaphragm, and mediastinum (including surgical thoracoscopy); not otherwise specified

19290

00400   Anesthesia for procedures on the integumentary system on the extremities, anterior trunk and perineum; not otherwise specified

19316–19325

00402   Anesthesia for procedures on the integumentary system on the extremities, anterior trunk and perineum; reconstructive procedures on breast (eg, reduction or augmentation mammoplasty, muscle flaps)

19328–19330

00400   Anesthesia for procedures on the integumentary system on the extremities, anterior trunk and perineum; not otherwise specified

19340

00402   Anesthesia for procedures on the integumentary system on the extremities, anterior trunk and perineum; reconstructive procedures on breast (eg, reduction or augmentation mammoplasty, muscle flaps)

19342–19355

00400   Anesthesia for procedures on the integumentary system on the extremities, anterior trunk and perineum; not otherwise specified

19357–19380

00402   Anesthesia for procedures on the integumentary system on the extremities, anterior trunk and perineum; reconstructive procedures on breast (eg, reduction or augmentation mammoplasty, muscle flaps)

20100

00320   Anesthesia for all procedures on esophagus, thyroid, larynx, trachea and lymphatic system of neck; not otherwise specified

20150

01210   Anesthesia for open procedures involving hip joint; not otherwise specified

01230   Anesthesia for open procedures involving upper 2/3 of femur; not otherwise specified

01360   Anesthesia for all open procedures on lower 1/3 of femur

01400 Anesthesia for open procedures on knee joint; not otherwise specified

01480 Anesthesia for open procedures on bones of lower leg, ankle, and foot; not otherwise specified

01830 Anesthesia for open procedures on radius, ulna, wrist, or hand bones; not otherwise specified

01740 Anesthesia for open procedures on humerus and elbow; not otherwise specified

20200

00170 Anesthesia for intraoral procedures, including biopsy; not otherwise specified

01810 Anesthesia for all procedures on nerves, muscles, tendons, fascia, and bursae of forearm, wrist, and hand

01710 Anesthesia for procedures on nerves, muscles, tendons, fascia, and bursae of upper arm and elbow; not otherwise specified

01610 Anesthesia for all procedures on nerves, muscles, tendons, fascia, and bursae of shoulder and axilla

01470 Anesthesia for procedures on nerves, muscles, tendons, and fascia of lower leg, ankle, and foot; not otherwise specified

01320 Anesthesia for all procedures on nerves, muscles, tendons, fascia, and bursae of knee and/or popliteal area

01250 Anesthesia for all procedures on nerves, muscles, tendons, fascia, and bursae of upper leg

00940 Anesthesia for vaginal procedures (including biopsy of labia, vagina, cervix or endometrium); not otherwise specified

00920 Anesthesia for procedures on male genitalia (including open urethral procedures); not otherwise specified

00840 Anesthesia for intraperitoneal procedures in lower abdomen including laparoscopy; not otherwise specified

00820 Anesthesia for procedures on lower posterior abdominal wall

00800 Anesthesia for procedures on lower anterior abdominal wall; not otherwise specified

00730 Anesthesia for procedures on upper posterior abdominal wall

00300 Anesthesia for all procedures on the integumentary system, muscles and nerves of head, neck, and posterior trunk, not otherwise specified

00700 Anesthesia for procedures on upper anterior abdominal wall; not otherwise specified

00400 Anesthesia for procedures on the integumentary system on the extremities, anterior trunk and perineum; not otherwise specified

20205

00140 Anesthesia for procedures on eye; not otherwise specified

00170 Anesthesia for intraoral procedures, including biopsy; not otherwise specified

00400 Anesthesia for procedures on the integumentary system on the extremities, anterior trunk and perineum; not otherwise specified

00730 Anesthesia for procedures on upper posterior abdominal wall

00820 Anesthesia for procedures on lower posterior abdominal wall

00800 Anesthesia for procedures on lower anterior abdominal wall; not otherwise specified

01810 Anesthesia for all procedures on nerves, muscles, tendons, fascia, and bursae of forearm, wrist, and hand

01710 Anesthesia for procedures on nerves, muscles, tendons, fascia, and bursae of upper arm and elbow; not otherwise specified

01610 Anesthesia for all procedures on nerves, muscles, tendons, fascia, and bursae of shoulder and axilla

01470 Anesthesia for procedures on nerves, muscles, tendons, and fascia of lower leg, ankle, and foot; not otherwise specified

01320 Anesthesia for all procedures on nerves, muscles, tendons, fascia, and bursae of knee and/or popliteal area

01250 Anesthesia for all procedures on nerves, muscles, tendons, fascia, and bursae of upper leg

00940 Anesthesia for vaginal procedures (including biopsy of labia, vagina, cervix or endometrium); not otherwise specified

00920 Anesthesia for procedures on male genitalia (including open urethral procedures); not otherwise specified

00840 Anesthesia for intraperitoneal procedures in lower abdomen including laparoscopy; not otherwise specified

00700 Anesthesia for procedures on upper anterior abdominal wall; not otherwise specified

00300 Anesthesia for all procedures on the integumentary system, muscles and nerves of head, neck, and posterior trunk, not otherwise specified

20220

01340 Anesthesia for all closed procedures on lower 1/3 of femur

01390 Anesthesia for all closed procedures on upper ends of tibia, fibula, and/or patella

01620 Anesthesia for all closed procedures on humeral head and neck, sternoclavicular joint, acromioclavicular joint, and shoulder joint

01820 Anesthesia for all closed procedures on radius, ulna, wrist, or hand bones

01730 Anesthesia for all closed procedures on humerus and elbow

01462 Anesthesia for all closed procedures on lower leg, ankle, and foot

Anesthesia Crosswalk

01120   Anesthesia for procedures on bony pelvis

00470   Anesthesia for partial rib resection; not otherwise specified

20225

01230   Anesthesia for open procedures involving upper 2/3 of femur; not otherwise specified

01220   Anesthesia for all closed procedures involving upper 2/3 of femur

00630   Anesthesia for procedures in lumbar region; not otherwise specified

00620   Anesthesia for procedures on thoracic spine and cord; not otherwise specified

20240

00470   Anesthesia for partial rib resection; not otherwise specified

01220   Anesthesia for all closed procedures involving upper 2/3 of femur

01120   Anesthesia for procedures on bony pelvis

20245

01230   Anesthesia for open procedures involving upper 2/3 of femur; not otherwise specified

01360   Anesthesia for all open procedures on lower 1/3 of femur

01740   Anesthesia for open procedures on humerus and elbow; not otherwise specified

20250

00620   Anesthesia for procedures on thoracic spine and cord; not otherwise specified

20251

00600   Anesthesia for procedures on cervical spine and cord; not otherwise specified

00630   Anesthesia for procedures in lumbar region; not otherwise specified

20520–20525

01250   Anesthesia for all procedures on nerves, muscles, tendons, fascia, and bursae of upper leg

01320   Anesthesia for all procedures on nerves, muscles, tendons, fascia, and bursae of knee and/or popliteal area

01470   Anesthesia for procedures on nerves, muscles, tendons, and fascia of lower leg, ankle, and foot; not otherwise specified

01710   Anesthesia for procedures on nerves, muscles, tendons, fascia, and bursae of upper arm and elbow; not otherwise specified

01810   Anesthesia for all procedures on nerves, muscles, tendons, fascia, and bursae of forearm, wrist, and hand

01610   Anesthesia for all procedures on nerves, muscles, tendons, fascia, and bursae of shoulder and axilla

00300   Anesthesia for all procedures on the integumentary system, muscles and nerves of head, neck, and posterior trunk, not otherwise specified

20650

01120   Anesthesia for procedures on bony pelvis

01820   Anesthesia for all closed procedures on radius, ulna, wrist, or hand bones

01620   Anesthesia for all closed procedures on humeral head and neck, sternoclavicular joint, acromioclavicular joint, and shoulder joint

01462   Anesthesia for all closed procedures on lower leg, ankle, and foot

01390   Anesthesia for all closed procedures on upper ends of tibia, fibula, and/or patella

01340   Anesthesia for all closed procedures on lower 1/3 of femur

01220   Anesthesia for all closed procedures involving upper 2/3 of femur

20660–20661

00190   Anesthesia for procedures on facial bones or skull; not otherwise specified

20662

01120   Anesthesia for procedures on bony pelvis

20663

01220   Anesthesia for all closed procedures involving upper 2/3 of femur

20664

00190   Anesthesia for procedures on facial bones or skull; not otherwise specified

20665–20670

01462   Anesthesia for all closed procedures on lower leg, ankle, and foot

01220   Anesthesia for all closed procedures involving upper 2/3 of femur

01390   Anesthesia for all closed procedures on upper ends of tibia, fibula, and/or patella

01340   Anesthesia for all closed procedures on lower 1/3 of femur

01120   Anesthesia for procedures on bony pelvis

01620   Anesthesia for all closed procedures on humeral head and neck, sternoclavicular joint, acromioclavicular joint, and shoulder joint

01820   Anesthesia for all closed procedures on radius, ulna, wrist, or hand bones

20680

00600   Anesthesia for procedures on cervical spine and cord; not otherwise specified

01230   Anesthesia for open procedures involving upper 2/3 of femur; not otherwise specified

01392   Anesthesia for all open procedures on upper ends of tibia, fibula, and/or patella

01360	Anesthesia for all open procedures on lower 1/3 of femur
01830	Anesthesia for open procedures on radius, ulna, wrist, or hand bones; not otherwise specified
01740	Anesthesia for open procedures on humerus and elbow; not otherwise specified
01630	Anesthesia for open procedures on humeral head and neck, sternoclavicular joint, acromioclavicular joint, and shoulder joint; not otherwise specified
01480	Anesthesia for open procedures on bones of lower leg, ankle, and foot; not otherwise specified
01400	Anesthesia for open procedures on knee joint; not otherwise specified
01210	Anesthesia for open procedures involving hip joint; not otherwise specified
00620	Anesthesia for procedures on thoracic spine and cord; not otherwise specified
00630	Anesthesia for procedures in lumbar region; not otherwise specified
01170	Anesthesia for open procedures involving symphysis pubis or sacroiliac joint
01120	Anesthesia for procedures on bony pelvis

20910
| 00470 | Anesthesia for partial rib resection; not otherwise specified |

20912
| 00160 | Anesthesia for procedures on nose and accessory sinuses; not otherwise specified |

20955
| 01480 | Anesthesia for open procedures on bones of lower leg, ankle, and foot; not otherwise specified |

20956
| 01120 | Anesthesia for procedures on bony pelvis |

20957
| 01480 | Anesthesia for open procedures on bones of lower leg, ankle, and foot; not otherwise specified |

20970
| 01120 | Anesthesia for procedures on bony pelvis |

20972
| 01480 | Anesthesia for open procedures on bones of lower leg, ankle, and foot; not otherwise specified |

20973
| 01480 | Anesthesia for open procedures on bones of lower leg, ankle, and foot; not otherwise specified |

21010
| 00190 | Anesthesia for procedures on facial bones or skull; not otherwise specified |

21015
| 00300 | Anesthesia for all procedures on the integumentary system, muscles and nerves of head, neck, and posterior trunk, not otherwise specified |

21025–21044
| 00190 | Anesthesia for procedures on facial bones or skull; not otherwise specified |

21045
| 00192 | Anesthesia for procedures on facial bones or skull; radical surgery (including prognathism) |

21050–21070
| 00190 | Anesthesia for procedures on facial bones or skull; not otherwise specified |

21100
| 00190 | Anesthesia for procedures on facial bones or skull; not otherwise specified |

21110
| 00170 | Anesthesia for intraoral procedures, including biopsy; not otherwise specified |

21120–21137
| 00190 | Anesthesia for procedures on facial bones or skull; not otherwise specified |

21138–21208
| 00192 | Anesthesia for procedures on facial bones or skull; radical surgery (including prognathism) |

21209–21230
| 00190 | Anesthesia for procedures on facial bones or skull; not otherwise specified |

21235
| 00160 | Anesthesia for procedures on nose and accessory sinuses; not otherwise specified |
| 00120 | Anesthesia for procedures on external, middle, and inner ear including biopsy; not otherwise specified |

21240–21244
| 00190 | Anesthesia for procedures on facial bones or skull; not otherwise specified |

21245–21260
| 00192 | Anesthesia for procedures on facial bones or skull; radical surgery (including prognathism) |

21261–21263
00210 Anesthesia for intracranial procedures; not otherwise specified

21267
00192 Anesthesia for procedures on facial bones or skull; radical surgery (including prognathism)

21268
00210 Anesthesia for intracranial procedures; not otherwise specified

21270
00190 Anesthesia for procedures on facial bones or skull; not otherwise specified

21275
00192 Anesthesia for procedures on facial bones or skull; radical surgery (including prognathism)

21280–21282
00300 Anesthesia for all procedures on the integumentary system, muscles and nerves of head, neck, and posterior trunk, not otherwise specified

21295
00190 Anesthesia for procedures on facial bones or skull; not otherwise specified

21296
00170 Anesthesia for intraoral procedures, including biopsy; not otherwise specified

21310–21340
00160 Anesthesia for procedures on nose and accessory sinuses; not otherwise specified

21343–21360
00190 Anesthesia for procedures on facial bones or skull; not otherwise specified

21365–21366
00192 Anesthesia for procedures on facial bones or skull; radical surgery (including prognathism)

21385–21422
00190 Anesthesia for procedures on facial bones or skull; not otherwise specified

21423
00192 Anesthesia for procedures on facial bones or skull; radical surgery (including prognathism)

21431
00190 Anesthesia for procedures on facial bones or skull; not otherwise specified

21432–21436
00192 Anesthesia for procedures on facial bones or skull; radical surgery (including prognathism)

21440–21490
00190 Anesthesia for procedures on facial bones or skull; not otherwise specified

21494–21495
00300 Anesthesia for all procedures on the integumentary system, muscles and nerves of head, neck, and posterior trunk, not otherwise specified

21497
00170 Anesthesia for intraoral procedures, including biopsy; not otherwise specified

21501
00300 Anesthesia for all procedures on the integumentary system, muscles and nerves of head, neck, and posterior trunk, not otherwise specified

21502–21510
00470 Anesthesia for partial rib resection; not otherwise specified

21550–21557
00300 Anesthesia for all procedures on the integumentary system, muscles and nerves of head, neck, and posterior trunk, not otherwise specified

21600–21620
00470 Anesthesia for partial rib resection; not otherwise specified

21627
00550 Anesthesia for sternal debridement

21630–21632
00474 Anesthesia for partial rib resection; radical procedures (eg, pectus excavatum)

21700
00300 Anesthesia for all procedures on the integumentary system, muscles and nerves of head, neck, and posterior trunk, not otherwise specified

21705
00470 Anesthesia for partial rib resection; not otherwise specified

21720–21725
00300 Anesthesia for all procedures on the integumentary system, muscles and nerves of head, neck, and posterior trunk, not otherwise specified

21740

00474 Anesthesia for partial rib resection; radical procedures (eg, pectus excavatum)

21750

00540 Anesthesia for thoracotomy procedures involving lungs, pleura, diaphragm, and mediastinum (including surgical thoracoscopy); not otherwise specified

00400 Anesthesia for procedures on the integumentary system on the extremities, anterior trunk and perineum; not otherwise specified

21805

00470 Anesthesia for partial rib resection; not otherwise specified

21810

00472 Anesthesia for partial rib resection; thoracoplasty (any type)

21825

00472 Anesthesia for partial rib resection; thoracoplasty (any type)

21920–21935

00300 Anesthesia for all procedures on the integumentary system, muscles and nerves of head, neck, and posterior trunk, not otherwise specified

22100

00600 Anesthesia for procedures on cervical spine and cord; not otherwise specified

22101

00620 Anesthesia for procedures on thoracic spine and cord; not otherwise specified

22102

00630 Anesthesia for procedures in lumbar region; not otherwise specified

22110

00600 Anesthesia for procedures on cervical spine and cord; not otherwise specified

22112

00620 Anesthesia for procedures on thoracic spine and cord; not otherwise specified

22114

00630 Anesthesia for procedures in lumbar region; not otherwise specified

22210

00600 Anesthesia for procedures on cervical spine and cord; not otherwise specified

22212

00620 Anesthesia for procedures on thoracic spine and cord; not otherwise specified

22214

00630 Anesthesia for procedures in lumbar region; not otherwise specified

22220

00600 Anesthesia for procedures on cervical spine and cord; not otherwise specified

22222

00620 Anesthesia for procedures on thoracic spine and cord; not otherwise specified

22224

00630 Anesthesia for procedures in lumbar region; not otherwise specified

22315

00620 Anesthesia for procedures on thoracic spine and cord; not otherwise specified

00600 Anesthesia for procedures on cervical spine and cord; not otherwise specified

00630 Anesthesia for procedures in lumbar region; not otherwise specified

22318–22319

00600 Anesthesia for procedures on cervical spine and cord; not otherwise specified

22325

00630 Anesthesia for procedures in lumbar region; not otherwise specified

22326

00600 Anesthesia for procedures on cervical spine and cord; not otherwise specified

22327

00620 Anesthesia for procedures on thoracic spine and cord; not otherwise specified

22505

00600 Anesthesia for procedures on cervical spine and cord; not otherwise specified

00620 Anesthesia for procedures on thoracic spine and cord; not otherwise specified

00630 Anesthesia for procedures in lumbar region; not otherwise specified

22520–22521

01905 Anesthesia for myelography, diskography, vertebroplasty

22548

00670 Anesthesia for extensive spine and spinal cord procedures (eg, spinal instrumentation or vascular procedures)

22554
00600 Anesthesia for procedures on cervical spine and cord; not otherwise specified

22556
00620 Anesthesia for procedures on thoracic spine and cord; not otherwise specified

22558
00630 Anesthesia for procedures in lumbar region; not otherwise specified

22590–22600
00600 Anesthesia for procedures on cervical spine and cord; not otherwise specified

22610
00620 Anesthesia for procedures on thoracic spine and cord; not otherwise specified

22612
00630 Anesthesia for procedures in lumbar region; not otherwise specified

22630
00630 Anesthesia for procedures in lumbar region; not otherwise specified

22800–22855
00670 Anesthesia for extensive spine and spinal cord procedures (eg, spinal instrumentation or vascular procedures)

22900
00700 Anesthesia for procedures on upper anterior abdominal wall; not otherwise specified
00800 Anesthesia for procedures on lower anterior abdominal wall; not otherwise specified

23000–23031
01610 Anesthesia for all procedures on nerves, muscles, tendons, fascia, and bursae of shoulder and axilla

23035–23044
01630 Anesthesia for open procedures on humeral head and neck, sternoclavicular joint, acromioclavicular joint, and shoulder joint; not otherwise specified

23065
00400 Anesthesia for procedures on the integumentary system on the extremities, anterior trunk and perineum; not otherwise specified

23066
01610 Anesthesia for all procedures on nerves, muscles, tendons, fascia, and bursae of shoulder and axilla

23075
00400 Anesthesia for procedures on the integumentary system on the extremities, anterior trunk and perineum; not otherwise specified

23076–23077
01610 Anesthesia for all procedures on nerves, muscles, tendons, fascia, and bursae of shoulder and axilla

23100–23107
01630 Anesthesia for open procedures on humeral head and neck, sternoclavicular joint, acromioclavicular joint, and shoulder joint; not otherwise specified

23120
00450 Anesthesia for procedures on clavicle and scapula; not otherwise specified

23125
00452 Anesthesia for procedures on clavicle and scapula; radical surgery

23130
01630 Anesthesia for open procedures on humeral head and neck, sternoclavicular joint, acromioclavicular joint, and shoulder joint; not otherwise specified

23140–23146
00450 Anesthesia for procedures on clavicle and scapula; not otherwise specified

23150–23156
01740 Anesthesia for open procedures on humerus and elbow; not otherwise specified

23170–23172
00450 Anesthesia for procedures on clavicle and scapula; not otherwise specified

23174
01630 Anesthesia for open procedures on humeral head and neck, sternoclavicular joint, acromioclavicular joint, and shoulder joint; not otherwise specified

23180–23182
00450 Anesthesia for procedures on clavicle and scapula; not otherwise specified

23184
01740 Anesthesia for open procedures on humerus and elbow; not otherwise specified

23190
00450 Anesthesia for procedures on clavicle and scapula; not otherwise specified

23195

01630 Anesthesia for open procedures on humeral head and neck, sternoclavicular joint, acromioclavicular joint, and shoulder joint; not otherwise specified

23200–23210

00452 Anesthesia for procedures on clavicle and scapula; radical surgery

23220–23222

01632 Anesthesia for open procedures on humeral head and neck, sternoclavicular joint, acromioclavicular joint, and shoulder joint; radical resection

23330

00400 Anesthesia for procedures on the integumentary system on the extremities, anterior trunk and perineum; not otherwise specified

23331–23332

01650 Anesthesia for procedures on arteries of shoulder and axilla; not otherwise specified

23395–23397

01610 Anesthesia for all procedures on nerves, muscles, tendons, fascia, and bursae of shoulder and axilla

23400

00450 Anesthesia for procedures on clavicle and scapula; not otherwise specified

23405–23415

01610 Anesthesia for all procedures on nerves, muscles, tendons, fascia, and bursae of shoulder and axilla

23420

01630 Anesthesia for open procedures on humeral head and neck, sternoclavicular joint, acromioclavicular joint, and shoulder joint; not otherwise specified

23430

01716 Anesthesia for procedures on nerves, muscles, tendons, fascia, and bursae of upper arm and elbow; tenodesis, rupture of long tendon of biceps

23440

01610 Anesthesia for all procedures on nerves, muscles, tendons, fascia, and bursae of shoulder and axilla

23450–23466

01630 Anesthesia for open procedures on humeral head and neck, sternoclavicular joint, acromioclavicular joint, and shoulder joint; not otherwise specified

23470–23472

01638 Anesthesia for open procedures on humeral head and neck, sternoclavicular joint, acromioclavicular joint, and shoulder joint; total shoulder replacement

23480–23490

00450 Anesthesia for procedures on clavicle and scapula; not otherwise specified

23491

01630 Anesthesia for open procedures on humeral head and neck, sternoclavicular joint, acromioclavicular joint, and shoulder joint; not otherwise specified

23505–23515

00450 Anesthesia for procedures on clavicle and scapula; not otherwise specified

23520–23525

01620 Anesthesia for all closed procedures on humeral head and neck, sternoclavicular joint, acromioclavicular joint, and shoulder joint

23530–23532

01630 Anesthesia for open procedures on humeral head and neck, sternoclavicular joint, acromioclavicular joint, and shoulder joint; not otherwise specified

23540–23545

01620 Anesthesia for all closed procedures on humeral head and neck, sternoclavicular joint, acromioclavicular joint, and shoulder joint

23550–23552

01630 Anesthesia for open procedures on humeral head and neck, sternoclavicular joint, acromioclavicular joint, and shoulder joint; not otherwise specified

23570–23585

00450 Anesthesia for procedures on clavicle and scapula; not otherwise specified

23600–23605

01620 Anesthesia for all closed procedures on humeral head and neck, sternoclavicular joint, acromioclavicular joint, and shoulder joint

Anesthesia Crosswalk

23615–23616

01630   Anesthesia for open procedures on humeral head and neck, sternoclavicular joint, acromioclavicular joint, and shoulder joint; not otherwise specified

23620–23625

01620   Anesthesia for all closed procedures on humeral head and neck, sternoclavicular joint, acromioclavicular joint, and shoulder joint

23630

01630   Anesthesia for open procedures on humeral head and neck, sternoclavicular joint, acromioclavicular joint, and shoulder joint; not otherwise specified

23655

01620   Anesthesia for all closed procedures on humeral head and neck, sternoclavicular joint, acromioclavicular joint, and shoulder joint

23660

01630   Anesthesia for open procedures on humeral head and neck, sternoclavicular joint, acromioclavicular joint, and shoulder joint; not otherwise specified

23665

01620   Anesthesia for all closed procedures on humeral head and neck, sternoclavicular joint, acromioclavicular joint, and shoulder joint

23670

01630   Anesthesia for open procedures on humeral head and neck, sternoclavicular joint, acromioclavicular joint, and shoulder joint; not otherwise specified

23675

01620   Anesthesia for all closed procedures on humeral head and neck, sternoclavicular joint, acromioclavicular joint, and shoulder joint

23680

01630   Anesthesia for open procedures on humeral head and neck, sternoclavicular joint, acromioclavicular joint, and shoulder joint; not otherwise specified

23700

01620   Anesthesia for all closed procedures on humeral head and neck, sternoclavicular joint, acromioclavicular joint, and shoulder joint

23800–23802

01630   Anesthesia for open procedures on humeral head and neck, sternoclavicular joint, acromioclavicular joint, and shoulder joint; not otherwise specified

23900

01636   Anesthesia for open procedures on humeral head and neck, sternoclavicular joint, acromioclavicular joint, and shoulder joint; interthoracoscapular (forequarter) amputation

23920

01634   Anesthesia for open procedures on humeral head and neck, sternoclavicular joint, acromioclavicular joint, and shoulder joint; shoulder disarticulation

23921

00400   Anesthesia for procedures on the integumentary system on the extremities, anterior trunk and perineum; not otherwise specified

23930

01740   Anesthesia for open procedures on humerus and elbow; not otherwise specified

23931

01710   Anesthesia for procedures on nerves, muscles, tendons, fascia, and bursae of upper arm and elbow; not otherwise specified

23935–24006

01740   Anesthesia for open procedures on humerus and elbow; not otherwise specified

24065

00400   Anesthesia for procedures on the integumentary system on the extremities, anterior trunk and perineum; not otherwise specified

24066

01710   Anesthesia for procedures on nerves, muscles, tendons, fascia, and bursae of upper arm and elbow; not otherwise specified

24075

00400   Anesthesia for procedures on the integumentary system on the extremities, anterior trunk and perineum; not otherwise specified

24076

01710   Anesthesia for procedures on nerves, muscles, tendons, fascia, and bursae of upper arm and elbow; not otherwise specified

24077

00400   Anesthesia for procedures on the integumentary system on the extremities, anterior trunk and perineum; not otherwise specified

24100–24102

01740   Anesthesia for open procedures on humerus and elbow; not otherwise specified

24105

01710   Anesthesia for procedures on nerves, muscles, tendons, fascia, and bursae of upper arm and elbow; not otherwise specified

24110–24116

01758   Anesthesia for open procedures on humerus and elbow; excision of cyst or tumor of humerus

24120–24126

01740   Anesthesia for open procedures on humerus and elbow; not otherwise specified

24130

01830   Anesthesia for open procedures on radius, ulna, wrist, or hand bones; not otherwise specified

24134

01740   Anesthesia for open procedures on humerus and elbow; not otherwise specified

24136–24138

01830   Anesthesia for open procedures on radius, ulna, wrist, or hand bones; not otherwise specified

24140

01740   Anesthesia for open procedures on humerus and elbow; not otherwise specified

24145–24147

01830   Anesthesia for open procedures on radius, ulna, wrist, or hand bones; not otherwise specified

24149–24153

01756   Anesthesia for open procedures on humerus and elbow; radical procedures

24155–24160

01740   Anesthesia for open procedures on humerus and elbow; not otherwise specified

24164

01830   Anesthesia for open procedures on radius, ulna, wrist, or hand bones; not otherwise specified

24200

00400   Anesthesia for procedures on the integumentary system on the extremities, anterior trunk and perineum; not otherwise specified

24201

01710   Anesthesia for procedures on nerves, muscles, tendons, fascia, and bursae of upper arm and elbow; not otherwise specified

24220–24300

01730   Anesthesia for all closed procedures on humerus and elbow

24301–24305

01710   Anesthesia for procedures on nerves, muscles, tendons, fascia, and bursae of upper arm and elbow; not otherwise specified

24310

01712   Anesthesia for procedures on nerves, muscles, tendons, fascia, and bursae of upper arm and elbow; tenotomy, elbow to shoulder, open

24320–24331

01714   Anesthesia for procedures on nerves, muscles, tendons, fascia, and bursae of upper arm and elbow; tenoplasty, elbow to shoulder

24332–24354

01710   Anesthesia for procedures on nerves, muscles, tendons, fascia, and bursae of upper arm and elbow; not otherwise specified

24356–24362

01740   Anesthesia for open procedures on humerus and elbow; not otherwise specified

24363

01760   Anesthesia for open procedures on humerus and elbow; total elbow replacement

24365–24366

01740   Anesthesia for open procedures on humerus and elbow; not otherwise specified

24400–24420

01742   Anesthesia for open procedures on humerus and elbow; osteotomy of humerus

24430–24435

01744   Anesthesia for open procedures on humerus and elbow; repair of nonunion or malunion of humerus

Anesthesia Crosswalk

24470
01740 Anesthesia for open procedures on humerus and elbow; not otherwise specified

24495
01810 Anesthesia for all procedures on nerves, muscles, tendons, fascia, and bursae of forearm, wrist, and hand

24498
01740 Anesthesia for open procedures on humerus and elbow; not otherwise specified

24500–24505
01730 Anesthesia for all closed procedures on humerus and elbow

24515–24516
01740 Anesthesia for open procedures on humerus and elbow; not otherwise specified

24530–24538
01730 Anesthesia for all closed procedures on humerus and elbow

24545–24546
01740 Anesthesia for open procedures on humerus and elbow; not otherwise specified

24560–24566
01730 Anesthesia for all closed procedures on humerus and elbow

24575
01740 Anesthesia for open procedures on humerus and elbow; not otherwise specified

24576–24577
01730 Anesthesia for all closed procedures on humerus and elbow

24579
01740 Anesthesia for open procedures on humerus and elbow; not otherwise specified

24582
01730 Anesthesia for all closed procedures on humerus and elbow

24586–24587
01740 Anesthesia for open procedures on humerus and elbow; not otherwise specified

24605
01730 Anesthesia for all closed procedures on humerus and elbow

24615
01740 Anesthesia for open procedures on humerus and elbow; not otherwise specified

24620
01730 Anesthesia for all closed procedures on humerus and elbow

24635
01740 Anesthesia for open procedures on humerus and elbow; not otherwise specified

24640
01730 Anesthesia for all closed procedures on humerus and elbow

24650
01820 Anesthesia for all closed procedures on radius, ulna, wrist, or hand bones

24655
01730 Anesthesia for all closed procedures on humerus and elbow

24665–24666
01830 Anesthesia for open procedures on radius, ulna, wrist, or hand bones; not otherwise specified

24670–24675
01820 Anesthesia for all closed procedures on radius, ulna, wrist, or hand bones

24685–24802
01830 Anesthesia for open procedures on radius, ulna, wrist, or hand bones; not otherwise specified

24900–24920
01756 Anesthesia for open procedures on humerus and elbow; radical procedures

24925
00400 Anesthesia for procedures on the integumentary system on the extremities, anterior trunk and perineum; not otherwise specified

24930–24931
01756 Anesthesia for open procedures on humerus and elbow; radical procedures

24935
00400 Anesthesia for procedures on the integumentary system on the extremities, anterior trunk and perineum; not otherwise specified
01810 Anesthesia for all procedures on nerves, muscles, tendons, fascia, and bursae of forearm, wrist, and hand
01740 Anesthesia for open procedures on humerus and elbow; not otherwise specified
01710 Anesthesia for procedures on nerves, muscles, tendons, fascia, and bursae of upper arm and elbow; not otherwise specified

24940

01710 Anesthesia for procedures on nerves, muscles, tendons, fascia, and bursae of upper arm and elbow; not otherwise specified

01740 Anesthesia for open procedures on humerus and elbow; not otherwise specified

01810 Anesthesia for all procedures on nerves, muscles, tendons, fascia, and bursae of forearm, wrist, and hand

25000–25031

01810 Anesthesia for all procedures on nerves, muscles, tendons, fascia, and bursae of forearm, wrist, and hand

25035–25040

01830 Anesthesia for open procedures on radius, ulna, wrist, or hand bones; not otherwise specified

25065

00400 Anesthesia for procedures on the integumentary system on the extremities, anterior trunk and perineum; not otherwise specified

25066

01810 Anesthesia for all procedures on nerves, muscles, tendons, fascia, and bursae of forearm, wrist, and hand

25075

00400 Anesthesia for procedures on the integumentary system on the extremities, anterior trunk and perineum; not otherwise specified

25076

01810 Anesthesia for all procedures on nerves, muscles, tendons, fascia, and bursae of forearm, wrist, and hand

25077

00400 Anesthesia for procedures on the integumentary system on the extremities, anterior trunk and perineum; not otherwise specified

25085

01810 Anesthesia for all procedures on nerves, muscles, tendons, fascia, and bursae of forearm, wrist, and hand

25100–25107

01830 Anesthesia for open procedures on radius, ulna, wrist, or hand bones; not otherwise specified

25110–25118

01810 Anesthesia for all procedures on nerves, muscles, tendons, fascia, and bursae of forearm, wrist, and hand

25119–25240

01830 Anesthesia for open procedures on radius, ulna, wrist, or hand bones; not otherwise specified

25246

01820 Anesthesia for all closed procedures on radius, ulna, wrist, or hand bones

25248

01810 Anesthesia for all procedures on nerves, muscles, tendons, fascia, and bursae of forearm, wrist, and hand

25250–25251

01830 Anesthesia for open procedures on radius, ulna, wrist, or hand bones; not otherwise specified

25259

01820 Anesthesia for all closed procedures on radius, ulna, wrist, or hand bones

25260–25320

01810 Anesthesia for all procedures on nerves, muscles, tendons, fascia, and bursae of forearm, wrist, and hand

25332–25445

01830 Anesthesia for open procedures on radius, ulna, wrist, or hand bones; not otherwise specified

25446

01832 Anesthesia for open procedures on radius, ulna, wrist, or hand bones; total wrist replacement

25447–25492

01830 Anesthesia for open procedures on radius, ulna, wrist, or hand bones; not otherwise specified

25500–25505

01820 Anesthesia for all closed procedures on radius, ulna, wrist, or hand bones

25515

01830 Anesthesia for open procedures on radius, ulna, wrist, or hand bones; not otherwise specified

25520

01820 Anesthesia for all closed procedures on radius, ulna, wrist, or hand bones

25525–25526
01830 Anesthesia for open procedures on radius, ulna, wrist, or hand bones; not otherwise specified

25530–25535
01820 Anesthesia for all closed procedures on radius, ulna, wrist, or hand bones

25545
01830 Anesthesia for open procedures on radius, ulna, wrist, or hand bones; not otherwise specified

25560–25565
01820 Anesthesia for all closed procedures on radius, ulna, wrist, or hand bones

25574–25575
01830 Anesthesia for open procedures on radius, ulna, wrist, or hand bones; not otherwise specified

25600–25611
01820 Anesthesia for all closed procedures on radius, ulna, wrist, or hand bones

25620
01830 Anesthesia for open procedures on radius, ulna, wrist, or hand bones; not otherwise specified

25622–25624
01820 Anesthesia for all closed procedures on radius, ulna, wrist, or hand bones

25628
01830 Anesthesia for open procedures on radius, ulna, wrist, or hand bones; not otherwise specified

25630–25635
01820 Anesthesia for all closed procedures on radius, ulna, wrist, or hand bones

25645
01830 Anesthesia for open procedures on radius, ulna, wrist, or hand bones; not otherwise specified

25650
01820 Anesthesia for all closed procedures on radius, ulna, wrist, or hand bones

25651–25652
01830 Anesthesia for open procedures on radius, ulna, wrist, or hand bones; not otherwise specified

25660
01820 Anesthesia for all closed procedures on radius, ulna, wrist, or hand bones

25670–25671
01830 Anesthesia for open procedures on radius, ulna, wrist, or hand bones; not otherwise specified

25675
01820 Anesthesia for all closed procedures on radius, ulna, wrist, or hand bones

25676
01830 Anesthesia for open procedures on radius, ulna, wrist, or hand bones; not otherwise specified

25680
01820 Anesthesia for all closed procedures on radius, ulna, wrist, or hand bones

25685
01830 Anesthesia for open procedures on radius, ulna, wrist, or hand bones; not otherwise specified

25690
01820 Anesthesia for all closed procedures on radius, ulna, wrist, or hand bones

25695–25905
01830 Anesthesia for open procedures on radius, ulna, wrist, or hand bones; not otherwise specified

25907
00400 Anesthesia for procedures on the integumentary system on the extremities, anterior trunk and perineum; not otherwise specified

25909–25920
01830 Anesthesia for open procedures on radius, ulna, wrist, or hand bones; not otherwise specified

25922
00400 Anesthesia for procedures on the integumentary system on the extremities, anterior trunk and perineum; not otherwise specified

25924–25927
01830 Anesthesia for open procedures on radius, ulna, wrist, or hand bones; not otherwise specified

25929

00400   Anesthesia for procedures on the integumentary system on the extremities, anterior trunk and perineum; not otherwise specified

25931

01830   Anesthesia for open procedures on radius, ulna, wrist, or hand bones; not otherwise specified

26010–26011

00400   Anesthesia for procedures on the integumentary system on the extremities, anterior trunk and perineum; not otherwise specified

26020–26030

01810   Anesthesia for all procedures on nerves, muscles, tendons, fascia, and bursae of forearm, wrist, and hand

26034

01830   Anesthesia for open procedures on radius, ulna, wrist, or hand bones; not otherwise specified

26035

01830   Anesthesia for open procedures on radius, ulna, wrist, or hand bones; not otherwise specified

00400   Anesthesia for procedures on the integumentary system on the extremities, anterior trunk and perineum; not otherwise specified

26037–26060

01810   Anesthesia for all procedures on nerves, muscles, tendons, fascia, and bursae of forearm, wrist, and hand

26070–26110

01830   Anesthesia for open procedures on radius, ulna, wrist, or hand bones; not otherwise specified

26115

00400   Anesthesia for procedures on the integumentary system on the extremities, anterior trunk and perineum; not otherwise specified

26116

01810   Anesthesia for all procedures on nerves, muscles, tendons, fascia, and bursae of forearm, wrist, and hand

26117

01830   Anesthesia for open procedures on radius, ulna, wrist, or hand bones; not otherwise specified

00400   Anesthesia for procedures on the integumentary system on the extremities, anterior trunk and perineum; not otherwise specified

26121–26123

01810   Anesthesia for all procedures on nerves, muscles, tendons, fascia, and bursae of forearm, wrist, and hand

26130–26180

01810   Anesthesia for all procedures on nerves, muscles, tendons, fascia, and bursae of forearm, wrist, and hand

26185–26320

01830   Anesthesia for open procedures on radius, ulna, wrist, or hand bones; not otherwise specified

26340

01820   Anesthesia for all closed procedures on radius, ulna, wrist, or hand bones

26350–26520

01810   Anesthesia for all procedures on nerves, muscles, tendons, fascia, and bursae of forearm, wrist, and hand

26525–26536

01830   Anesthesia for open procedures on radius, ulna, wrist, or hand bones; not otherwise specified

26540–26545

01810   Anesthesia for all procedures on nerves, muscles, tendons, fascia, and bursae of forearm, wrist, and hand

26546

01830   Anesthesia for open procedures on radius, ulna, wrist, or hand bones; not otherwise specified

26548–26550

01810   Anesthesia for all procedures on nerves, muscles, tendons, fascia, and bursae of forearm, wrist, and hand

26551–26554

01840   Anesthesia for procedures on arteries of forearm, wrist, and hand; not otherwise specified

26555

01830   Anesthesia for open procedures on radius, ulna, wrist, or hand bones; not otherwise specified

Anesthesia Crosswalk

26556

01840   Anesthesia for procedures on arteries of forearm, wrist, and hand; not otherwise specified

26560–26561

00400   Anesthesia for procedures on the integumentary system on the extremities, anterior trunk and perineum; not otherwise specified

26562–26590

01830   Anesthesia for open procedures on radius, ulna, wrist, or hand bones; not otherwise specified

26591–26593

01810   Anesthesia for all procedures on nerves, muscles, tendons, fascia, and bursae of forearm, wrist, and hand

26596

01830   Anesthesia for open procedures on radius, ulna, wrist, or hand bones; not otherwise specified

26597

01810   Anesthesia for all procedures on nerves, muscles, tendons, fascia, and bursae of forearm, wrist, and hand

26600–26608

01820   Anesthesia for all closed procedures on radius, ulna, wrist, or hand bones

26615

01830   Anesthesia for open procedures on radius, ulna, wrist, or hand bones; not otherwise specified

26641–26650

01820   Anesthesia for all closed procedures on radius, ulna, wrist, or hand bones

26665

01830   Anesthesia for open procedures on radius, ulna, wrist, or hand bones; not otherwise specified

26675–26676

01820   Anesthesia for all closed procedures on radius, ulna, wrist, or hand bones

26685–26686

01830   Anesthesia for open procedures on radius, ulna, wrist, or hand bones; not otherwise specified

26705–26706

01820   Anesthesia for all closed procedures on radius, ulna, wrist, or hand bones

26715

01830   Anesthesia for open procedures on radius, ulna, wrist, or hand bones; not otherwise specified

26720–26727

01820   Anesthesia for all closed procedures on radius, ulna, wrist, or hand bones

26735

01830   Anesthesia for open procedures on radius, ulna, wrist, or hand bones; not otherwise specified

26740–26742

01820   Anesthesia for all closed procedures on radius, ulna, wrist, or hand bones

26746

01830   Anesthesia for open procedures on radius, ulna, wrist, or hand bones; not otherwise specified

26750–26756

01820   Anesthesia for all closed procedures on radius, ulna, wrist, or hand bones

26765

01830   Anesthesia for open procedures on radius, ulna, wrist, or hand bones; not otherwise specified

26775–26776

01820   Anesthesia for all closed procedures on radius, ulna, wrist, or hand bones

26785–26860

01830   Anesthesia for open procedures on radius, ulna, wrist, or hand bones; not otherwise specified

26862

01830   Anesthesia for open procedures on radius, ulna, wrist, or hand bones; not otherwise specified

26910–26952

01830   Anesthesia for open procedures on radius, ulna, wrist, or hand bones; not otherwise specified

26990

01210   Anesthesia for open procedures involving hip joint; not otherwise specified

26991

01250   Anesthesia for all procedures on nerves, muscles, tendons, fascia, and bursae of upper leg

26992

01120   Anesthesia for procedures on bony pelvis
01210   Anesthesia for open procedures involving hip joint; not otherwise specified

27000–27025

01250   Anesthesia for all procedures on nerves, muscles, tendons, fascia, and bursae of upper leg

27030–27033

01210   Anesthesia for open procedures involving hip joint; not otherwise specified

27035

01250   Anesthesia for all procedures on nerves, muscles, tendons, fascia, and bursae of upper leg

27036

01210   Anesthesia for open procedures involving hip joint; not otherwise specified

27040–27047

00400   Anesthesia for procedures on the integumentary system on the extremities, anterior trunk and perineum; not otherwise specified

27048

01210   Anesthesia for open procedures involving hip joint; not otherwise specified

27049

01150   Anesthesia for radical procedures for tumor of pelvis, except hindquarter amputation

27050

01170   Anesthesia for open procedures involving symphysis pubis or sacroiliac joint

27052–27054

01210   Anesthesia for open procedures involving hip joint; not otherwise specified

27060–27062

01250   Anesthesia for all procedures on nerves, muscles, tendons, fascia, and bursae of upper leg

27065–27071

01120   Anesthesia for procedures on bony pelvis

27075

01170   Anesthesia for open procedures involving symphysis pubis or sacroiliac joint

27076–27079

01150   Anesthesia for radical procedures for tumor of pelvis, except hindquarter amputation

27080

01120   Anesthesia for procedures on bony pelvis

27086–27087

00300   Anesthesia for all procedures on the integumentary system, muscles and nerves of head, neck, and posterior trunk, not otherwise specified
00400   Anesthesia for procedures on the integumentary system on the extremities, anterior trunk and perineum; not otherwise specified

27090–27091

01210   Anesthesia for open procedures involving hip joint; not otherwise specified

27095

01200   Anesthesia for all closed procedures involving hip joint

27097–27111

01250   Anesthesia for all procedures on nerves, muscles, tendons, fascia, and bursae of upper leg

27120–27122

01210   Anesthesia for open procedures involving hip joint; not otherwise specified

27125–27132

01214   Anesthesia for open procedures involving hip joint; total hip arthroplasty

27134–27138

01215   Anesthesia for open procedures involving hip joint; revision of total hip arthroplasty

27140–27156

01210   Anesthesia for open procedures involving hip joint; not otherwise specified

27158

01120   Anesthesia for procedures on bony pelvis

27161–27170

01230   Anesthesia for open procedures involving upper 2/3 of femur; not otherwise specified

27175

01200   Anesthesia for all closed procedures involving hip joint

27176–27177

01210   Anesthesia for open procedures involving hip joint; not otherwise specified

27178

01200   Anesthesia for all closed procedures involving hip joint

27179–27181
01230   Anesthesia for open procedures involving upper 2/3 of femur; not otherwise specified

27185
01210   Anesthesia for open procedures involving hip joint; not otherwise specified

27187
01230   Anesthesia for open procedures involving upper 2/3 of femur; not otherwise specified

27193
01120   Anesthesia for procedures on bony pelvis

27194–27216
01120   Anesthesia for procedures on bony pelvis

27217–27218
01170   Anesthesia for open procedures involving symphysis pubis or sacroiliac joint

27220–27222
01200   Anesthesia for all closed procedures involving hip joint

27226–27228
01210   Anesthesia for open procedures involving hip joint; not otherwise specified

27230–27235
01220   Anesthesia for all closed procedures involving upper 2/3 of femur

27236
01230   Anesthesia for open procedures involving upper 2/3 of femur; not otherwise specified

27238–27240
01220   Anesthesia for all closed procedures involving upper 2/3 of femur

27244–27245
01230   Anesthesia for open procedures involving upper 2/3 of femur; not otherwise specified

27246
01220   Anesthesia for all closed procedures involving upper 2/3 of femur

27248
01230   Anesthesia for open procedures involving upper 2/3 of femur; not otherwise specified

27252
01200   Anesthesia for all closed procedures involving hip joint

27253–27254
01210   Anesthesia for open procedures involving hip joint; not otherwise specified

27257
01200   Anesthesia for all closed procedures involving hip joint

27258–27259
01210   Anesthesia for open procedures involving hip joint; not otherwise specified

27266–27275
01200   Anesthesia for all closed procedures involving hip joint

27280–27282
01170   Anesthesia for open procedures involving symphysis pubis or sacroiliac joint

27284–27286
01210   Anesthesia for open procedures involving hip joint; not otherwise specified

27290
01140   Anesthesia for interpelviabdominal (hindquarter) amputation

27295
01212   Anesthesia for open procedures involving hip joint; hip disarticulation

27301
01250   Anesthesia for all procedures on nerves, muscles, tendons, fascia, and bursae of upper leg

27303
01230   Anesthesia for open procedures involving upper 2/3 of femur; not otherwise specified
01400   Anesthesia for open procedures on knee joint; not otherwise specified
01360   Anesthesia for all open procedures on lower 1/3 of femur
01390   Anesthesia for all closed procedures on upper ends of tibia, fibula, and/or patella

27305–27307
01250   Anesthesia for all procedures on nerves, muscles, tendons, fascia, and bursae of upper leg

27310
01400   Anesthesia for open procedures on knee joint; not otherwise specified

27315
01250   Anesthesia for all procedures on nerves, muscles, tendons, fascia, and bursae of upper leg

27320
01320   Anesthesia for all procedures on nerves, muscles, tendons, fascia, and bursae of knee and/or popliteal area

27323

00400   Anesthesia for procedures on the integumentary system on the extremities, anterior trunk and perineum; not otherwise specified

27324

01320   Anesthesia for all procedures on nerves, muscles, tendons, fascia, and bursae of knee and/or popliteal area

27327

00400   Anesthesia for procedures on the integumentary system on the extremities, anterior trunk and perineum; not otherwise specified

27328–27329

01320   Anesthesia for all procedures on nerves, muscles, tendons, fascia, and bursae of knee and/or popliteal area

27330–27334

01400   Anesthesia for open procedures on knee joint; not otherwise specified

27340–27345

01320   Anesthesia for all procedures on nerves, muscles, tendons, fascia, and bursae of knee and/or popliteal area

27347

01400   Anesthesia for open procedures on knee joint; not otherwise specified

27350

01392   Anesthesia for all open procedures on upper ends of tibia, fibula, and/or patella

27355–27357

01230   Anesthesia for open procedures involving upper 2/3 of femur; not otherwise specified
01360   Anesthesia for all open procedures on lower 1/3 of femur

27360

01230   Anesthesia for open procedures involving upper 2/3 of femur; not otherwise specified
01480   Anesthesia for open procedures on bones of lower leg, ankle, and foot; not otherwise specified
01360   Anesthesia for all open procedures on lower 1/3 of femur
01392   Anesthesia for all open procedures on upper ends of tibia, fibula, and/or patella

27365

01230   Anesthesia for open procedures involving upper 2/3 of femur; not otherwise specified
01360   Anesthesia for all open procedures on lower 1/3 of femur

01390   Anesthesia for all closed procedures on upper ends of tibia, fibula, and/or patella
01400   Anesthesia for open procedures on knee joint; not otherwise specified

27370

01380   Anesthesia for all closed procedures on knee joint

27372–27400

01320   Anesthesia for all procedures on nerves, muscles, tendons, fascia, and bursae of knee and/or popliteal area

27403–27418

01400   Anesthesia for open procedures on knee joint; not otherwise specified

27420–27422

01320   Anesthesia for all procedures on nerves, muscles, tendons, fascia, and bursae of knee and/or popliteal area

27424

01392   Anesthesia for all open procedures on upper ends of tibia, fibula, and/or patella

27425–27427

01320   Anesthesia for all procedures on nerves, muscles, tendons, fascia, and bursae of knee and/or popliteal area

27428–27429

01400   Anesthesia for open procedures on knee joint; not otherwise specified

27430–27435

01320   Anesthesia for all procedures on nerves, muscles, tendons, fascia, and bursae of knee and/or popliteal area

27437–27441

01392   Anesthesia for all open procedures on upper ends of tibia, fibula, and/or patella

27442–27446

01400   Anesthesia for open procedures on knee joint; not otherwise specified

27447

01402   Anesthesia for open procedures on knee joint; total knee arthroplasty

27448–27450

01230   Anesthesia for open procedures involving upper 2/3 of femur; not otherwise specified
01360   Anesthesia for all open procedures on lower 1/3 of femur

27454

01230   Anesthesia for open procedures involving upper 2/3 of femur; not otherwise specified

Anesthesia Crosswalk

27455–27457
01392 Anesthesia for all open procedures on upper ends of tibia, fibula, and/or patella

27465–27468
01360 Anesthesia for all open procedures on lower 1/3 of femur

27470–27472
01230 Anesthesia for open procedures involving upper 2/3 of femur; not otherwise specified
01360 Anesthesia for all open procedures on lower 1/3 of femur

27475
01360 Anesthesia for all open procedures on lower 1/3 of femur

27477
01392 Anesthesia for all open procedures on upper ends of tibia, fibula, and/or patella

27479
01360 Anesthesia for all open procedures on lower 1/3 of femur

27485
01360 Anesthesia for all open procedures on lower 1/3 of femur
01392 Anesthesia for all open procedures on upper ends of tibia, fibula, and/or patella

27486–27488
01402 Anesthesia for open procedures on knee joint; total knee arthroplasty

27495
01230 Anesthesia for open procedures involving upper 2/3 of femur; not otherwise specified
01360 Anesthesia for all open procedures on lower 1/3 of femur

27496–27499
01250 Anesthesia for all procedures on nerves, muscles, tendons, fascia, and bursae of upper leg
01320 Anesthesia for all procedures on nerves, muscles, tendons, fascia, and bursae of knee and/or popliteal area

27500
01220 Anesthesia for all closed procedures involving upper 2/3 of femur

27501
01340 Anesthesia for all closed procedures on lower 1/3 of femur

27502
01220 Anesthesia for all closed procedures involving upper 2/3 of femur

27503
01340 Anesthesia for all closed procedures on lower 1/3 of femur

27506
01220 Anesthesia for all closed procedures involving upper 2/3 of femur
01360 Anesthesia for all open procedures on lower 1/3 of femur

27507
01230 Anesthesia for open procedures involving upper 2/3 of femur; not otherwise specified

27508–27510
01340 Anesthesia for all closed procedures on lower 1/3 of femur

27511–27514
01360 Anesthesia for all open procedures on lower 1/3 of femur

27516–27517
01340 Anesthesia for all closed procedures on lower 1/3 of femur

27519
01360 Anesthesia for all open procedures on lower 1/3 of femur

27520
01390 Anesthesia for all closed procedures on upper ends of tibia, fibula, and/or patella

27524
01392 Anesthesia for all open procedures on upper ends of tibia, fibula, and/or patella

27530–27532
01390 Anesthesia for all closed procedures on upper ends of tibia, fibula, and/or patella

27535–27536
01392 Anesthesia for all open procedures on upper ends of tibia, fibula, and/or patella

27538
01390 Anesthesia for all closed procedures on upper ends of tibia, fibula, and/or patella

27540
01392 Anesthesia for all open procedures on upper ends of tibia, fibula, and/or patella

27552
01380 Anesthesia for all closed procedures on knee joint

27556–27558
01400 Anesthesia for open procedures on knee joint; not otherwise specified

27562
01390 Anesthesia for all closed procedures on upper ends of tibia, fibula, and/or patella

27566
01392 Anesthesia for all open procedures on upper ends of tibia, fibula, and/or patella

27570
01380 Anesthesia for all closed procedures on knee joint

27580
01400 Anesthesia for open procedures on knee joint; not otherwise specified

27590–27592
01232 Anesthesia for open procedures involving upper 2/3 of femur; amputation

27594
00400 Anesthesia for procedures on the integumentary system on the extremities, anterior trunk and perineum; not otherwise specified

27596
01232 Anesthesia for open procedures involving upper 2/3 of femur; amputation

27598
01404 Anesthesia for open procedures on knee joint; disarticulation at knee

27600–27602
01470 Anesthesia for procedures on nerves, muscles, tendons, and fascia of lower leg, ankle, and foot; not otherwise specified

27603
00400 Anesthesia for procedures on the integumentary system on the extremities, anterior trunk and perineum; not otherwise specified

27604
01470 Anesthesia for procedures on nerves, muscles, tendons, and fascia of lower leg, ankle, and foot; not otherwise specified

27606
01470 Anesthesia for procedures on nerves, muscles, tendons, and fascia of lower leg, ankle, and foot; not otherwise specified

27607–27612
01480 Anesthesia for open procedures on bones of lower leg, ankle, and foot; not otherwise specified

27613
00400 Anesthesia for procedures on the integumentary system on the extremities, anterior trunk and perineum; not otherwise specified

27614–27615
01470 Anesthesia for procedures on nerves, muscles, tendons, and fascia of lower leg, ankle, and foot; not otherwise specified

27618–27619
00400 Anesthesia for procedures on the integumentary system on the extremities, anterior trunk and perineum; not otherwise specified

27620–27626
01480 Anesthesia for open procedures on bones of lower leg, ankle, and foot; not otherwise specified

27630
01470 Anesthesia for procedures on nerves, muscles, tendons, and fascia of lower leg, ankle, and foot; not otherwise specified

27635–27641
01480 Anesthesia for open procedures on bones of lower leg, ankle, and foot; not otherwise specified

27645–27647
01482 Anesthesia for open procedures on bones of lower leg, ankle, and foot; radical resection (including below knee amputation)

27648
01462 Anesthesia for all closed procedures on lower leg, ankle, and foot

27650–27654
01472 Anesthesia for procedures on nerves, muscles, tendons, and fascia of lower leg, ankle, and foot; repair of ruptured Achilles tendon, with or without graft

27656–27675
01470 Anesthesia for procedures on nerves, muscles, tendons, and fascia of lower leg, ankle, and foot; not otherwise specified

27676
01484 Anesthesia for open procedures on bones of lower leg, ankle, and foot; osteotomy or osteoplasty of tibia and/or fibula

27680–27686
01470 Anesthesia for procedures on nerves, muscles, tendons, and fascia of lower leg, ankle, and foot; not otherwise specified

27687

01474 Anesthesia for procedures on nerves, muscles, tendons, and fascia of lower leg, ankle, and foot; gastrocnemius recession (eg, Strayer procedure)

27690–27691

01470 Anesthesia for procedures on nerves, muscles, tendons, and fascia of lower leg, ankle, and foot; not otherwise specified

27695–27698

01470 Anesthesia for procedures on nerves, muscles, tendons, and fascia of lower leg, ankle, and foot; not otherwise specified

27700

01480 Anesthesia for open procedures on bones of lower leg, ankle, and foot; not otherwise specified

27702–27703

01486 Anesthesia for open procedures on bones of lower leg, ankle, and foot; total ankle replacement

27704

01480 Anesthesia for open procedures on bones of lower leg, ankle, and foot; not otherwise specified

27705–27715

01484 Anesthesia for open procedures on bones of lower leg, ankle, and foot; osteotomy or osteoplasty of tibia and/or fibula

27720–27740

01480 Anesthesia for open procedures on bones of lower leg, ankle, and foot; not otherwise specified

27742

01392 Anesthesia for all open procedures on upper ends of tibia, fibula, and/or patella

27745

01462 Anesthesia for all closed procedures on lower leg, ankle, and foot
01480 Anesthesia for open procedures on bones of lower leg, ankle, and foot; not otherwise specified

27750–27752

01462 Anesthesia for all closed procedures on lower leg, ankle, and foot

27756–27759

01480 Anesthesia for open procedures on bones of lower leg, ankle, and foot; not otherwise specified

27760–27762

01462 Anesthesia for all closed procedures on lower leg, ankle, and foot

27766

01480 Anesthesia for open procedures on bones of lower leg, ankle, and foot; not otherwise specified

27780–27781

01462 Anesthesia for all closed procedures on lower leg, ankle, and foot

27784

01480 Anesthesia for open procedures on bones of lower leg, ankle, and foot; not otherwise specified

27786–27788

01462 Anesthesia for all closed procedures on lower leg, ankle, and foot

27792

01480 Anesthesia for open procedures on bones of lower leg, ankle, and foot; not otherwise specified

27808–27810

01462 Anesthesia for all closed procedures on lower leg, ankle, and foot

27814

01480 Anesthesia for open procedures on bones of lower leg, ankle, and foot; not otherwise specified

27816–27818

01462 Anesthesia for all closed procedures on lower leg, ankle, and foot

27822–27823

01480 Anesthesia for open procedures on bones of lower leg, ankle, and foot; not otherwise specified

27824–27825

01462 Anesthesia for all closed procedures on lower leg, ankle, and foot

27826–27829

01480 Anesthesia for open procedures on bones of lower leg, ankle, and foot; not otherwise specified

27831

01462 Anesthesia for all closed procedures on lower leg, ankle, and foot

27832
01480 Anesthesia for open procedures on bones of lower leg, ankle, and foot; not otherwise specified

27842
01462 Anesthesia for all closed procedures on lower leg, ankle, and foot

27846–27848
01480 Anesthesia for open procedures on bones of lower leg, ankle, and foot; not otherwise specified

27860
01462 Anesthesia for all closed procedures on lower leg, ankle, and foot

27870–27871
01480 Anesthesia for open procedures on bones of lower leg, ankle, and foot; not otherwise specified

27880–27886
01482 Anesthesia for open procedures on bones of lower leg, ankle, and foot; radical resection (including below knee amputation)

27888–27889
01480 Anesthesia for open procedures on bones of lower leg, ankle, and foot; not otherwise specified

27892–27894
01470 Anesthesia for procedures on nerves, muscles, tendons, and fascia of lower leg, ankle, and foot; not otherwise specified

28001–28003
01470 Anesthesia for procedures on nerves, muscles, tendons, and fascia of lower leg, ankle, and foot; not otherwise specified

28005
01480 Anesthesia for open procedures on bones of lower leg, ankle, and foot; not otherwise specified

28008–28011
01470 Anesthesia for procedures on nerves, muscles, tendons, and fascia of lower leg, ankle, and foot; not otherwise specified

28020–28024
01480 Anesthesia for open procedures on bones of lower leg, ankle, and foot; not otherwise specified

28030–28035
01470 Anesthesia for procedures on nerves, muscles, tendons, and fascia of lower leg, ankle, and foot; not otherwise specified

28043
00400 Anesthesia for procedures on the integumentary system on the extremities, anterior trunk and perineum; not otherwise specified

28045–28046
01470 Anesthesia for procedures on nerves, muscles, tendons, and fascia of lower leg, ankle, and foot; not otherwise specified

28050–28054
01480 Anesthesia for open procedures on bones of lower leg, ankle, and foot; not otherwise specified

28060–28092
01470 Anesthesia for procedures on nerves, muscles, tendons, and fascia of lower leg, ankle, and foot; not otherwise specified

28100–28160
01480 Anesthesia for open procedures on bones of lower leg, ankle, and foot; not otherwise specified

28171–28175
01482 Anesthesia for open procedures on bones of lower leg, ankle, and foot; radical resection (including below knee amputation)

28190
00400 Anesthesia for procedures on the integumentary system on the extremities, anterior trunk and perineum; not otherwise specified

28192–28280
01470 Anesthesia for procedures on nerves, muscles, tendons, and fascia of lower leg, ankle, and foot; not otherwise specified

28285–28312
01480 Anesthesia for open procedures on bones of lower leg, ankle, and foot; not otherwise specified

28313–28322
01470 Anesthesia for procedures on nerves, muscles, tendons, and fascia of lower leg, ankle, and foot; not otherwise specified

28340
01470 Anesthesia for procedures on nerves, muscles, tendons, and fascia of lower leg, ankle, and foot; not otherwise specified

28341–28344
01480 Anesthesia for open procedures on bones of lower leg, ankle, and foot; not otherwise specified

28345
00400 Anesthesia for procedures on the integumentary system on the extremities, anterior trunk and perineum; not otherwise specified

28360
01480 Anesthesia for open procedures on bones of lower leg, ankle, and foot; not otherwise specified

28400–28406
01462 Anesthesia for all closed procedures on lower leg, ankle, and foot

28415–28420
01480 Anesthesia for open procedures on bones of lower leg, ankle, and foot; not otherwise specified

28430–28436
01462 Anesthesia for all closed procedures on lower leg, ankle, and foot

28445
01480 Anesthesia for open procedures on bones of lower leg, ankle, and foot; not otherwise specified

28450–28456
01462 Anesthesia for all closed procedures on lower leg, ankle, and foot

28465
01480 Anesthesia for open procedures on bones of lower leg, ankle, and foot; not otherwise specified

28470–28476
01462 Anesthesia for all closed procedures on lower leg, ankle, and foot

28485
01480 Anesthesia for open procedures on bones of lower leg, ankle, and foot; not otherwise specified

28490–28496
01462 Anesthesia for all closed procedures on lower leg, ankle, and foot

28505
01480 Anesthesia for open procedures on bones of lower leg, ankle, and foot; not otherwise specified

28510–28515
01462 Anesthesia for all closed procedures on lower leg, ankle, and foot

28525
01480 Anesthesia for open procedures on bones of lower leg, ankle, and foot; not otherwise specified

28530
01462 Anesthesia for all closed procedures on lower leg, ankle, and foot

28531
01480 Anesthesia for open procedures on bones of lower leg, ankle, and foot; not otherwise specified

28545–28546
01462 Anesthesia for all closed procedures on lower leg, ankle, and foot

28555
01480 Anesthesia for open procedures on bones of lower leg, ankle, and foot; not otherwise specified

28575–28576
01462 Anesthesia for all closed procedures on lower leg, ankle, and foot

28585
01480 Anesthesia for open procedures on bones of lower leg, ankle, and foot; not otherwise specified

28605–28606
01462 Anesthesia for all closed procedures on lower leg, ankle, and foot

28615
01480 Anesthesia for open procedures on bones of lower leg, ankle, and foot; not otherwise specified

28635–28636
01462 Anesthesia for all closed procedures on lower leg, ankle, and foot

28645
01480 Anesthesia for open procedures on bones of lower leg, ankle, and foot; not otherwise specified

28665–28666
01462 Anesthesia for all closed procedures on lower leg, ankle, and foot

28675–28825
01480   Anesthesia for open procedures on bones of lower leg, ankle, and foot; not otherwise specified

29000–29046
01130   Anesthesia for body cast application or revision

29049
01680   Anesthesia for shoulder cast application, removal or repair; not otherwise specified

29055
01682   Anesthesia for shoulder cast application, removal or repair; shoulder spica

29058–29065
01680   Anesthesia for shoulder cast application, removal or repair; not otherwise specified

29075–29086
01860   Anesthesia for forearm, wrist, or hand cast application, removal, or repair

29105
01680   Anesthesia for shoulder cast application, removal or repair; not otherwise specified

29125–29131
01860   Anesthesia for forearm, wrist, or hand cast application, removal, or repair

29260–29280
01860   Anesthesia for forearm, wrist, or hand cast application, removal, or repair

29305–29325
01130   Anesthesia for body cast application or revision

29345–29365
01420   Anesthesia for all cast applications, removal, or repair involving knee joint

29405–29425
01490   Anesthesia for lower leg cast application, removal, or repair

29435
01420   Anesthesia for all cast applications, removal, or repair involving knee joint

29445
01420   Anesthesia for all cast applications, removal, or repair involving knee joint

29450
01490   Anesthesia for lower leg cast application, removal, or repair

29505
01420   Anesthesia for all cast applications, removal, or repair involving knee joint

29515
01490   Anesthesia for lower leg cast application, removal, or repair

29520
01200   Anesthesia for all closed procedures involving hip joint

29700
01130   Anesthesia for body cast application or revision

29705
01420   Anesthesia for all cast applications, removal, or repair involving knee joint

29710
01680   Anesthesia for shoulder cast application, removal or repair; not otherwise specified

29715–29720
01130   Anesthesia for body cast application or revision

29730–29740
01130   Anesthesia for body cast application or revision

01860   Anesthesia for forearm, wrist, or hand cast application, removal, or repair

01682   Anesthesia for shoulder cast application, removal or repair; shoulder spica

01420   Anesthesia for all cast applications, removal, or repair involving knee joint

01680   Anesthesia for shoulder cast application, removal or repair; not otherwise specified

01490   Anesthesia for lower leg cast application, removal, or repair

29750
01490   Anesthesia for lower leg cast application, removal, or repair

29800–29804
00190   Anesthesia for procedures on facial bones or skull; not otherwise specified

29805–29826
01622   Anesthesia for arthroscopic procedures of shoulder joint

29830–29838
01732   Anesthesia for arthroscopic procedures of elbow joint

29840–29847
01820   Anesthesia for all closed procedures on radius, ulna, wrist, or hand bones

Anesthesia Crosswalk

29848
01810　Anesthesia for all procedures on nerves, muscles, tendons, fascia, and bursae of forearm, wrist, and hand

29850–29851
01400　Anesthesia for open procedures on knee joint; not otherwise specified

29855–29856
01392　Anesthesia for all open procedures on upper ends of tibia, fibula, and/or patella

29860–29863
01202　Anesthesia for arthroscopic procedures of hip joint

29870–29887
01382　Anesthesia for arthroscopic procedures of knee joint

29888–29889
01400　Anesthesia for open procedures on knee joint; not otherwise specified

29891–29892
01464　Anesthesia for arthroscopic procedures of ankle joint

29893
01470　Anesthesia for procedures on nerves, muscles, tendons, and fascia of lower leg, ankle, and foot; not otherwise specified

29894–29898
01464　Anesthesia for arthroscopic procedures of ankle joint

29900–29902
01820　Anesthesia for all closed procedures on radius, ulna, wrist, or hand bones

30000–30020
00160　Anesthesia for procedures on nose and accessory sinuses; not otherwise specified

30100
00164　Anesthesia for procedures on nose and accessory sinuses; biopsy, soft tissue

30110–30140
00160　Anesthesia for procedures on nose and accessory sinuses; not otherwise specified

30150–30160
00162　Anesthesia for procedures on nose and accessory sinuses; radical surgery

30200–30220
00160　Anesthesia for procedures on nose and accessory sinuses; not otherwise specified

30310–30930
00160　Anesthesia for procedures on nose and accessory sinuses; not otherwise specified

31000–31020
00160　Anesthesia for procedures on nose and accessory sinuses; not otherwise specified

31030–31032
00162　Anesthesia for procedures on nose and accessory sinuses; radical surgery

31040–31225
00160　Anesthesia for procedures on nose and accessory sinuses; not otherwise specified

31230
00162　Anesthesia for procedures on nose and accessory sinuses; radical surgery

31231–31294
00160　Anesthesia for procedures on nose and accessory sinuses; not otherwise specified

31300–31420
00320　Anesthesia for all procedures on esophagus, thyroid, larynx, trachea and lymphatic system of neck; not otherwise specified

31502–31595
00320　Anesthesia for all procedures on esophagus, thyroid, larynx, trachea and lymphatic system of neck; not otherwise specified

31600–31615
00320　Anesthesia for all procedures on esophagus, thyroid, larynx, trachea and lymphatic system of neck; not otherwise specified

31622–31656
00520　Anesthesia for closed chest procedures; (including bronchoscopy) not otherwise specified

31700
00320　Anesthesia for all procedures on esophagus, thyroid, larynx, trachea and lymphatic system of neck; not otherwise specified

31710
00520　Anesthesia for closed chest procedures; (including bronchoscopy) not otherwise specified

31715
00320　Anesthesia for all procedures on esophagus, thyroid, larynx, trachea and lymphatic system of neck; not otherwise specified

31717
00520   Anesthesia for closed chest procedures; (including bronchoscopy) not otherwise specified

31730–31755
00320   Anesthesia for all procedures on esophagus, thyroid, larynx, trachea and lymphatic system of neck; not otherwise specified

31760–31775
00548   Anesthesia for thoracotomy procedures involving lungs, pleura, diaphragm, and mediastinum (including surgical thoracoscopy); intrathoracic procedures on the trachea and bronchi

31780
00320   Anesthesia for all procedures on esophagus, thyroid, larynx, trachea and lymphatic system of neck; not otherwise specified

31781
00548   Anesthesia for thoracotomy procedures involving lungs, pleura, diaphragm, and mediastinum (including surgical thoracoscopy); intrathoracic procedures on the trachea and bronchi

31785
00320   Anesthesia for all procedures on esophagus, thyroid, larynx, trachea and lymphatic system of neck; not otherwise specified

31786
00548   Anesthesia for thoracotomy procedures involving lungs, pleura, diaphragm, and mediastinum (including surgical thoracoscopy); intrathoracic procedures on the trachea and bronchi

31800
00320   Anesthesia for all procedures on esophagus, thyroid, larynx, trachea and lymphatic system of neck; not otherwise specified

31805
00548   Anesthesia for thoracotomy procedures involving lungs, pleura, diaphragm, and mediastinum (including surgical thoracoscopy); intrathoracic procedures on the trachea and bronchi

31820–31825
00320   Anesthesia for all procedures on esophagus, thyroid, larynx, trachea and lymphatic system of neck; not otherwise specified

31830
00300   Anesthesia for all procedures on the integumentary system, muscles and nerves of head, neck, and posterior trunk, not otherwise specified

32000
00524   Anesthesia for closed chest procedures; pneumocentesis

32002
00520   Anesthesia for closed chest procedures; (including bronchoscopy) not otherwise specified

32005
00524   Anesthesia for closed chest procedures; pneumocentesis

32020
00520   Anesthesia for closed chest procedures; (including bronchoscopy) not otherwise specified

32035–32151
00540   Anesthesia for thoracotomy procedures involving lungs, pleura, diaphragm, and mediastinum (including surgical thoracoscopy); not otherwise specified

32160
00560   Anesthesia for procedures on heart, pericardial sac, and great vessels of chest; without pump oxygenator

32200–32215
00540   Anesthesia for thoracotomy procedures involving lungs, pleura, diaphragm, and mediastinum (including surgical thoracoscopy); not otherwise specified

32220–32225
00542   Anesthesia for thoracotomy procedures involving lungs, pleura, diaphragm, and mediastinum (including surgical thoracoscopy); decortication

32310
00544   Anesthesia for thoracotomy procedures involving lungs, pleura, diaphragm, and mediastinum (including surgical thoracoscopy); pleurectomy

32320
00542   Anesthesia for thoracotomy procedures involving lungs, pleura, diaphragm, and mediastinum (including surgical thoracoscopy); decortication

32400
00522 Anesthesia for closed chest procedures; needle biopsy of pleura

32402
00540 Anesthesia for thoracotomy procedures involving lungs, pleura, diaphragm, and mediastinum (including surgical thoracoscopy); not otherwise specified

32405
00522 Anesthesia for closed chest procedures; needle biopsy of pleura

32420
00524 Anesthesia for closed chest procedures; pneumocentesis

32440
00540 Anesthesia for thoracotomy procedures involving lungs, pleura, diaphragm, and mediastinum (including surgical thoracoscopy); not otherwise specified

32442
00548 Anesthesia for thoracotomy procedures involving lungs, pleura, diaphragm, and mediastinum (including surgical thoracoscopy); intrathoracic procedures on the trachea and bronchi

32445–32500
00540 Anesthesia for thoracotomy procedures involving lungs, pleura, diaphragm, and mediastinum (including surgical thoracoscopy); not otherwise specified

32520–32525
00546 Anesthesia for thoracotomy procedures involving lungs, pleura, diaphragm, and mediastinum (including surgical thoracoscopy); pulmonary resection with thoracoplasty

32540
00540 Anesthesia for thoracotomy procedures involving lungs, pleura, diaphragm, and mediastinum (including surgical thoracoscopy); not otherwise specified

32601–32606
00528 Anesthesia for closed chest procedures; mediastinoscopy and diagnostic thoracoscopy

32650
00540 Anesthesia for thoracotomy procedures involving lungs, pleura, diaphragm, and mediastinum (including surgical thoracoscopy); not otherwise specified

32651–32652
00542 Anesthesia for thoracotomy procedures involving lungs, pleura, diaphragm, and mediastinum (including surgical thoracoscopy); decortication

32653–32655
00540 Anesthesia for thoracotomy procedures involving lungs, pleura, diaphragm, and mediastinum (including surgical thoracoscopy); not otherwise specified

32656
00544 Anesthesia for thoracotomy procedures involving lungs, pleura, diaphragm, and mediastinum (including surgical thoracoscopy); pleurectomy

32657
00540 Anesthesia for thoracotomy procedures involving lungs, pleura, diaphragm, and mediastinum (including surgical thoracoscopy); not otherwise specified

32658–32661
00560 Anesthesia for procedures on heart, pericardial sac, and great vessels of chest; without pump oxygenator

32662–32665
00540 Anesthesia for thoracotomy procedures involving lungs, pleura, diaphragm, and mediastinum (including surgical thoracoscopy); not otherwise specified

32800–32810
00472 Anesthesia for partial rib resection; thoracoplasty (any type)

32815
00548 Anesthesia for thoracotomy procedures involving lungs, pleura, diaphragm, and mediastinum (including surgical thoracoscopy); intrathoracic procedures on the trachea and bronchi

32820
00472 Anesthesia for partial rib resection; thoracoplasty (any type)

32850
01990 Physiological support for harvesting of organ(s) from brain-dead patient

32851–32854
00580 Anesthesia for heart transplant or heart/lung transplant

32900
00470 Anesthesia for partial rib resection; not otherwise specified

32905–32906
00472   Anesthesia for partial rib resection; thoracoplasty (any type)

32940
00540   Anesthesia for thoracotomy procedures involving lungs, pleura, diaphragm, and mediastinum (including surgical thoracoscopy); not otherwise specified

32960
00524   Anesthesia for closed chest procedures; pneumocentesis

32997
00520   Anesthesia for closed chest procedures; (including bronchoscopy) not otherwise specified

33010–33011
00520   Anesthesia for closed chest procedures; (including bronchoscopy) not otherwise specified

33015–33030
00560   Anesthesia for procedures on heart, pericardial sac, and great vessels of chest; without pump oxygenator

33031
00562   Anesthesia for procedures on heart, pericardial sac, and great vessels of chest; with pump oxygenator

00563   Anesthesia for procedures on heart, pericardial sac, and great vessels of chest; with pump oxygenator with hypothermic circulatory arrest

33050
00560   Anesthesia for procedures on heart, pericardial sac, and great vessels of chest; without pump oxygenator

33120
00562   Anesthesia for procedures on heart, pericardial sac, and great vessels of chest; with pump oxygenator

00563   Anesthesia for procedures on heart, pericardial sac, and great vessels of chest; with pump oxygenator with hypothermic circulatory arrest

33130–33140
00560   Anesthesia for procedures on heart, pericardial sac, and great vessels of chest; without pump oxygenator

33200–33201
00560   Anesthesia for procedures on heart, pericardial sac, and great vessels of chest; without pump oxygenator

33206–33208
00530   Anesthesia for permanent transvenous pacemaker insertion

33210–33214
00560   Anesthesia for procedures on heart, pericardial sac, and great vessels of chest; without pump oxygenator

33216–33217
00534   Anesthesia for transvenous insertion or replacement of pacing cardioverter-defibrillator

33218–33220
00560   Anesthesia for procedures on heart, pericardial sac, and great vessels of chest; without pump oxygenator

33222–33223
00400   Anesthesia for procedures on the integumentary system on the extremities, anterior trunk and perineum; not otherwise specified

33233
00560   Anesthesia for procedures on heart, pericardial sac, and great vessels of chest; without pump oxygenator

33234–33235
00520   Anesthesia for closed chest procedures; (including bronchoscopy) not otherwise specified

33236–33237
00560   Anesthesia for procedures on heart, pericardial sac, and great vessels of chest; without pump oxygenator

33238
00540   Anesthesia for thoracotomy procedures involving lungs, pleura, diaphragm, and mediastinum (including surgical thoracoscopy); not otherwise specified

33240–33241
00534   Anesthesia for transvenous insertion or replacement of pacing cardioverter-defibrillator

33243
00560   Anesthesia for procedures on heart, pericardial sac, and great vessels of chest; without pump oxygenator

33244
00534   Anesthesia for transvenous insertion or replacement of pacing cardioverter-defibrillator

33245-33246

00540   Anesthesia for thoracotomy procedures involving lungs, pleura, diaphragm, and mediastinum (including surgical thoracoscopy); not otherwise specified

33249

00534   Anesthesia for transvenous insertion or replacement of pacing cardioverter-defibrillator

33250-33253

00537   Anesthesia for cardiac electrophysiologic procedures including radiofrequency ablation

33261

00537   Anesthesia for cardiac electrophysiologic procedures including radiofrequency ablation

00563   Anesthesia for procedures on heart, pericardial sac, and great vessels of chest; with pump oxygenator with hypothermic circulatory arrest

33282-33300

00560   Anesthesia for procedures on heart, pericardial sac, and great vessels of chest; without pump oxygenator

33305

00562   Anesthesia for procedures on heart, pericardial sac, and great vessels of chest; with pump oxygenator

00563   Anesthesia for procedures on heart, pericardial sac, and great vessels of chest; with pump oxygenator with hypothermic circulatory arrest

33310

00560   Anesthesia for procedures on heart, pericardial sac, and great vessels of chest; without pump oxygenator

33315

00562   Anesthesia for procedures on heart, pericardial sac, and great vessels of chest; with pump oxygenator

00563   Anesthesia for procedures on heart, pericardial sac, and great vessels of chest; with pump oxygenator with hypothermic circulatory arrest

33320

00560   Anesthesia for procedures on heart, pericardial sac, and great vessels of chest; without pump oxygenator

33321-33322

00562   Anesthesia for procedures on heart, pericardial sac, and great vessels of chest; with pump oxygenator

00563   Anesthesia for procedures on heart, pericardial sac, and great vessels of chest; with pump oxygenator with hypothermic circulatory arrest

33330

00560   Anesthesia for procedures on heart, pericardial sac, and great vessels of chest; without pump oxygenator

33332

00563   Anesthesia for procedures on heart, pericardial sac, and great vessels of chest; with pump oxygenator with hypothermic circulatory arrest

33335-33417

00563   Anesthesia for procedures on heart, pericardial sac, and great vessels of chest; with pump oxygenator with hypothermic circulatory arrest

00562   Anesthesia for procedures on heart, pericardial sac, and great vessels of chest; with pump oxygenator

33420

00560   Anesthesia for procedures on heart, pericardial sac, and great vessels of chest; without pump oxygenator

33422-33468

00562   Anesthesia for procedures on heart, pericardial sac, and great vessels of chest; with pump oxygenator

00563   Anesthesia for procedures on heart, pericardial sac, and great vessels of chest; with pump oxygenator with hypothermic circulatory arrest

33470-33471

00560   Anesthesia for procedures on heart, pericardial sac, and great vessels of chest; without pump oxygenator

33472-33500

00562   Anesthesia for procedures on heart, pericardial sac, and great vessels of chest; with pump oxygenator

00563   Anesthesia for procedures on heart, pericardial sac, and great vessels of chest; with pump oxygenator with hypothermic circulatory arrest

33501-33503

00560   Anesthesia for procedures on heart, pericardial sac, and great vessels of chest; without pump oxygenator

33504

00562   Anesthesia for procedures on heart, pericardial sac, and great vessels of chest; with pump oxygenator

00563   Anesthesia for procedures on heart, pericardial sac, and great vessels of chest; with pump oxygenator with hypothermic circulatory arrest

33505–33506
00560   Anesthesia for procedures on heart, pericardial sac, and great vessels of chest; without pump oxygenator

33510–33516
00566   Anesthesia for direct coronary artery bypass grafting without pump oxygenator

00562   Anesthesia for procedures on heart, pericardial sac, and great vessels of chest; with pump oxygenator

00563   Anesthesia for procedures on heart, pericardial sac, and great vessels of chest; with pump oxygenator with hypothermic circulatory arrest

33517–33523
00566   Anesthesia for direct coronary artery bypass grafting without pump oxygenator

33533–33536
00566   Anesthesia for direct coronary artery bypass grafting without pump oxygenator

00562   Anesthesia for procedures on heart, pericardial sac, and great vessels of chest; with pump oxygenator

00563   Anesthesia for procedures on heart, pericardial sac, and great vessels of chest; with pump oxygenator with hypothermic circulatory arrest

33542–33545
00566   Anesthesia for direct coronary artery bypass grafting without pump oxygenator

33600–33641
00562   Anesthesia for procedures on heart, pericardial sac, and great vessels of chest; with pump oxygenator

00563   Anesthesia for procedures on heart, pericardial sac, and great vessels of chest; with pump oxygenator with hypothermic circulatory arrest

33645
00560   Anesthesia for procedures on heart, pericardial sac, and great vessels of chest; without pump oxygenator

33647–33688
00562   Anesthesia for procedures on heart, pericardial sac, and great vessels of chest; with pump oxygenator

00563   Anesthesia for procedures on heart, pericardial sac, and great vessels of chest; with pump oxygenator with hypothermic circulatory arrest

33690
00560   Anesthesia for procedures on heart, pericardial sac, and great vessels of chest; without pump oxygenator

33692–33732
00562   Anesthesia for procedures on heart, pericardial sac, and great vessels of chest; with pump oxygenator

00563   Anesthesia for procedures on heart, pericardial sac, and great vessels of chest; with pump oxygenator with hypothermic circulatory arrest

33735
00560   Anesthesia for procedures on heart, pericardial sac, and great vessels of chest; without pump oxygenator

33736–33737
00562   Anesthesia for procedures on heart, pericardial sac, and great vessels of chest; with pump oxygenator

00563   Anesthesia for procedures on heart, pericardial sac, and great vessels of chest; with pump oxygenator with hypothermic circulatory arrest

33750–33767
00560   Anesthesia for procedures on heart, pericardial sac, and great vessels of chest; without pump oxygenator

33770–33786
00562   Anesthesia for procedures on heart, pericardial sac, and great vessels of chest; with pump oxygenator

00563   Anesthesia for procedures on heart, pericardial sac, and great vessels of chest; with pump oxygenator with hypothermic circulatory arrest

33788–33813
00560   Anesthesia for procedures on heart, pericardial sac, and great vessels of chest; without pump oxygenator

33814
00562   Anesthesia for procedures on heart, pericardial sac, and great vessels of chest; with pump oxygenator

00563   Anesthesia for procedures on heart, pericardial sac, and great vessels of chest; with pump oxygenator with hypothermic circulatory arrest

33820–33852
00560   Anesthesia for procedures on heart, pericardial sac, and great vessels of chest; without pump oxygenator

33853-33870
00562   Anesthesia for procedures on heart, pericardial sac, and great vessels of chest; with pump oxygenator

00563   Anesthesia for procedures on heart, pericardial sac, and great vessels of chest; with pump oxygenator with hypothermic circulatory arrest

33875-33877
00563   Anesthesia for procedures on heart, pericardial sac, and great vessels of chest; with pump oxygenator with hypothermic circulatory arrest

00560   Anesthesia for procedures on heart, pericardial sac, and great vessels of chest; without pump oxygenator

00562   Anesthesia for procedures on heart, pericardial sac, and great vessels of chest; with pump oxygenator

33910
00563   Anesthesia for procedures on heart, pericardial sac, and great vessels of chest; with pump oxygenator with hypothermic circulatory arrest

00562   Anesthesia for procedures on heart, pericardial sac, and great vessels of chest; with pump oxygenator

33915
00560   Anesthesia for procedures on heart, pericardial sac, and great vessels of chest; without pump oxygenator

33916
00562   Anesthesia for procedures on heart, pericardial sac, and great vessels of chest; with pump oxygenator

00563   Anesthesia for procedures on heart, pericardial sac, and great vessels of chest; with pump oxygenator with hypothermic circulatory arrest

33917-33918
00560   Anesthesia for procedures on heart, pericardial sac, and great vessels of chest; without pump oxygenator

33919
00562   Anesthesia for procedures on heart, pericardial sac, and great vessels of chest; with pump oxygenator

00563   Anesthesia for procedures on heart, pericardial sac, and great vessels of chest; with pump oxygenator with hypothermic circulatory arrest

33920
00560   Anesthesia for procedures on heart, pericardial sac, and great vessels of chest; without pump oxygenator

33922
00562   Anesthesia for procedures on heart, pericardial sac, and great vessels of chest; with pump oxygenator

00563   Anesthesia for procedures on heart, pericardial sac, and great vessels of chest; with pump oxygenator with hypothermic circulatory arrest

33930
01990   Physiological support for harvesting of organ(s) from brain-dead patient

33935
00580   Anesthesia for heart transplant or heart/lung transplant

33940
01990   Physiological support for harvesting of organ(s) from brain-dead patient

33945
00580   Anesthesia for heart transplant or heart/lung transplant

33967-33971
01270   Anesthesia for procedures involving arteries of upper leg, including bypass graft; not otherwise specified

33973-33980
00560   Anesthesia for procedures on heart, pericardial sac, and great vessels of chest; without pump oxygenator

34001
00350   Anesthesia for procedures on major vessels of neck; not otherwise specified

34051
00560   Anesthesia for procedures on heart, pericardial sac, and great vessels of chest; without pump oxygenator

34101
01772   Anesthesia for procedures on arteries of upper arm and elbow; embolectomy

34111
01840   Anesthesia for procedures on arteries of forearm, wrist, and hand; not otherwise specified

34151
00770   Anesthesia for all procedures on major abdominal blood vessels

34201
01274   Anesthesia for procedures involving arteries of upper leg, including bypass graft; femoral artery embolectomy

34203

01502 Anesthesia for procedures on arteries of lower leg, including bypass graft; embolectomy, direct or with catheter

34401

00880 Anesthesia for procedures on major lower abdominal vessels; not otherwise specified

34421

01260 Anesthesia for all procedures involving veins of upper leg, including exploration

34451

00880 Anesthesia for procedures on major lower abdominal vessels; not otherwise specified

34471

00350 Anesthesia for procedures on major vessels of neck; not otherwise specified

34490

01670 Anesthesia for all procedures on veins of shoulder and axilla

34501

01270 Anesthesia for procedures involving arteries of upper leg, including bypass graft; not otherwise specified

34502–34520

01260 Anesthesia for all procedures involving veins of upper leg, including exploration

34530

01430 Anesthesia for procedures on veins of knee and popliteal area; not otherwise specified

34800–34804

00770 Anesthesia for all procedures on major abdominal blood vessels

34812

01270 Anesthesia for procedures involving arteries of upper leg, including bypass graft; not otherwise specified

34820

00880 Anesthesia for procedures on major lower abdominal vessels; not otherwise specified

34825

00770 Anesthesia for all procedures on major abdominal blood vessels

34830–34832

00770 Anesthesia for all procedures on major abdominal blood vessels

35001–35005

00350 Anesthesia for procedures on major vessels of neck; not otherwise specified

35011–35013

01652 Anesthesia for procedures on arteries of shoulder and axilla; axillary-brachial aneurysm

35021–35022

00560 Anesthesia for procedures on heart, pericardial sac, and great vessels of chest; without pump oxygenator

35045

01840 Anesthesia for procedures on arteries of forearm, wrist, and hand; not otherwise specified

35081–35092

00770 Anesthesia for all procedures on major abdominal blood vessels

35102–35103

00880 Anesthesia for procedures on major lower abdominal vessels; not otherwise specified

35111–35122

00770 Anesthesia for all procedures on major abdominal blood vessels

35131–35132

00880 Anesthesia for procedures on major lower abdominal vessels; not otherwise specified

35141–35142

01270 Anesthesia for procedures involving arteries of upper leg, including bypass graft; not otherwise specified

35151–35152

01444 Anesthesia for procedures on arteries of knee and popliteal area; popliteal excision and graft or repair for occlusion or aneurysm

35180

01770 Anesthesia for procedures on arteries of upper arm and elbow; not otherwise specified

01780 Anesthesia for procedures on veins of upper arm and elbow; not otherwise specified

35182

00880 Anesthesia for procedures on major lower abdominal vessels; not otherwise specified

35184

01770 Anesthesia for procedures on arteries of upper arm and elbow; not otherwise specified

Anesthesia Crosswalk

01780   Anesthesia for procedures on veins of upper arm and elbow; not otherwise specified

01432   Anesthesia for procedures on veins of knee and popliteal area; arteriovenous fistula

01840   Anesthesia for procedures on arteries of forearm, wrist, and hand; not otherwise specified

35188

01770   Anesthesia for procedures on arteries of upper arm and elbow; not otherwise specified

01780   Anesthesia for procedures on veins of upper arm and elbow; not otherwise specified

35189

00880   Anesthesia for procedures on major lower abdominal vessels; not otherwise specified

35190

01770   Anesthesia for procedures on arteries of upper arm and elbow; not otherwise specified

01780   Anesthesia for procedures on veins of upper arm and elbow; not otherwise specified

01432   Anesthesia for procedures on veins of knee and popliteal area; arteriovenous fistula

01840   Anesthesia for procedures on arteries of forearm, wrist, and hand; not otherwise specified

35201

00350   Anesthesia for procedures on major vessels of neck; not otherwise specified

35206

01650   Anesthesia for procedures on arteries of shoulder and axilla; not otherwise specified

01770   Anesthesia for procedures on arteries of upper arm and elbow; not otherwise specified

01840   Anesthesia for procedures on arteries of forearm, wrist, and hand; not otherwise specified

01850   Anesthesia for procedures on veins of forearm, wrist, and hand; not otherwise specified

01780   Anesthesia for procedures on veins of upper arm and elbow; not otherwise specified

01670   Anesthesia for all procedures on veins of shoulder and axilla

35207

01840   Anesthesia for procedures on arteries of forearm, wrist, and hand; not otherwise specified

35211

00562   Anesthesia for procedures on heart, pericardial sac, and great vessels of chest; with pump oxygenator

00563   Anesthesia for procedures on heart, pericardial sac, and great vessels of chest; with pump oxygenator with hypothermic circulatory arrest

35216

00560   Anesthesia for procedures on heart, pericardial sac, and great vessels of chest; without pump oxygenator

35221

00770   Anesthesia for all procedures on major abdominal blood vessels

35226

01260   Anesthesia for all procedures involving veins of upper leg, including exploration

01500   Anesthesia for procedures on arteries of lower leg, including bypass graft; not otherwise specified

01440   Anesthesia for procedures on arteries of knee and popliteal area; not otherwise specified

01520   Anesthesia for procedures on veins of lower leg; not otherwise specified

01270   Anesthesia for procedures involving arteries of upper leg, including bypass graft; not otherwise specified

01430   Anesthesia for procedures on veins of knee and popliteal area; not otherwise specified

35231

00350   Anesthesia for procedures on major vessels of neck; not otherwise specified

35236

01650   Anesthesia for procedures on arteries of shoulder and axilla; not otherwise specified

01770   Anesthesia for procedures on arteries of upper arm and elbow; not otherwise specified

01840   Anesthesia for procedures on arteries of forearm, wrist, and hand; not otherwise specified

01850   Anesthesia for procedures on veins of forearm, wrist, and hand; not otherwise specified

01780   Anesthesia for procedures on veins of upper arm and elbow; not otherwise specified

01670   Anesthesia for all procedures on veins of shoulder and axilla

35241

00562   Anesthesia for procedures on heart, pericardial sac, and great vessels of chest; with pump oxygenator

00563   Anesthesia for procedures on heart, pericardial sac, and great vessels of chest; with pump oxygenator with hypothermic circulatory arrest

35246

00560   Anesthesia for procedures on heart, pericardial sac, and great vessels of chest; without pump oxygenator

35251

00770   Anesthesia for all procedures on major abdominal blood vessels

35256

01260   Anesthesia for all procedures involving veins of upper leg, including exploration

01440   Anesthesia for procedures on arteries of knee and popliteal area; not otherwise specified

01520   Anesthesia for procedures on veins of lower leg; not otherwise specified

01500   Anesthesia for procedures on arteries of lower leg, including bypass graft; not otherwise specified

01430   Anesthesia for procedures on veins of knee and popliteal area; not otherwise specified

01270   Anesthesia for procedures involving arteries of upper leg, including bypass graft; not otherwise specified

35261

00350   Anesthesia for procedures on major vessels of neck; not otherwise specified

35266

01650   Anesthesia for procedures on arteries of shoulder and axilla; not otherwise specified

01670   Anesthesia for all procedures on veins of shoulder and axilla

01780   Anesthesia for procedures on veins of upper arm and elbow; not otherwise specified

01850   Anesthesia for procedures on veins of forearm, wrist, and hand; not otherwise specified

01840   Anesthesia for procedures on arteries of forearm, wrist, and hand; not otherwise specified

01770   Anesthesia for procedures on arteries of upper arm and elbow; not otherwise specified

35271

00562   Anesthesia for procedures on heart, pericardial sac, and great vessels of chest; with pump oxygenator

00563   Anesthesia for procedures on heart, pericardial sac, and great vessels of chest; with pump oxygenator with hypothermic circulatory arrest

35276

00560   Anesthesia for procedures on heart, pericardial sac, and great vessels of chest; without pump oxygenator

35281

00770   Anesthesia for all procedures on major abdominal blood vessels

35286

01260   Anesthesia for all procedures involving veins of upper leg, including exploration

01430   Anesthesia for procedures on veins of knee and popliteal area; not otherwise specified

01500   Anesthesia for procedures on arteries of lower leg, including bypass graft; not otherwise specified

01520   Anesthesia for procedures on veins of lower leg; not otherwise specified

01440   Anesthesia for procedures on arteries of knee and popliteal area; not otherwise specified

01270   Anesthesia for procedures involving arteries of upper leg, including bypass graft; not otherwise specified

35301

00350   Anesthesia for procedures on major vessels of neck; not otherwise specified

35311

00560   Anesthesia for procedures on heart, pericardial sac, and great vessels of chest; without pump oxygenator

35321

01650   Anesthesia for procedures on arteries of shoulder and axilla; not otherwise specified

35331–35341

00770   Anesthesia for all procedures on major abdominal blood vessels

35351–35355

00880   Anesthesia for procedures on major lower abdominal vessels; not otherwise specified

35361–35363

00770   Anesthesia for all procedures on major abdominal blood vessels

35371–35372

01270   Anesthesia for procedures involving arteries of upper leg, including bypass graft; not otherwise specified

35381

01270   Anesthesia for procedures involving arteries of upper leg, including bypass graft; not otherwise specified

01442   Anesthesia for procedures on arteries of knee and popliteal area; popliteal thromboendarterectomy, with or without patch graft

Anesthesia Crosswalk

35450

00770   Anesthesia for all procedures on major abdominal blood vessels

35452

00560   Anesthesia for procedures on heart, pericardial sac, and great vessels of chest; without pump oxygenator

35454

00880   Anesthesia for procedures on major lower abdominal vessels; not otherwise specified

35456

01270   Anesthesia for procedures involving arteries of upper leg, including bypass graft; not otherwise specified

35458

01650   Anesthesia for procedures on arteries of shoulder and axilla; not otherwise specified

35459

01500   Anesthesia for procedures on arteries of lower leg, including bypass graft; not otherwise specified

35460

01430   Anesthesia for procedures on veins of knee and popliteal area; not otherwise specified

01670   Anesthesia for all procedures on veins of shoulder and axilla

01850   Anesthesia for procedures on veins of forearm, wrist, and hand; not otherwise specified

01780   Anesthesia for procedures on veins of upper arm and elbow; not otherwise specified

01520   Anesthesia for procedures on veins of lower leg; not otherwise specified

01260   Anesthesia for all procedures involving veins of upper leg, including exploration

35480

00770   Anesthesia for all procedures on major abdominal blood vessels

35481

00560   Anesthesia for procedures on heart, pericardial sac, and great vessels of chest; without pump oxygenator

35482

00880   Anesthesia for procedures on major lower abdominal vessels; not otherwise specified

35483

01270   Anesthesia for procedures involving arteries of upper leg, including bypass graft; not otherwise specified

35484

01650   Anesthesia for procedures on arteries of shoulder and axilla; not otherwise specified

35485

01500   Anesthesia for procedures on arteries of lower leg, including bypass graft; not otherwise specified

35490

00770   Anesthesia for all procedures on major abdominal blood vessels

35491–35492

00880   Anesthesia for procedures on major lower abdominal vessels; not otherwise specified

35493

01270   Anesthesia for procedures involving arteries of upper leg, including bypass graft; not otherwise specified

35494

01650   Anesthesia for procedures on arteries of shoulder and axilla; not otherwise specified

35495

01500   Anesthesia for procedures on arteries of lower leg, including bypass graft; not otherwise specified

35501–35515

00350   Anesthesia for procedures on major vessels of neck; not otherwise specified

35516–35518

01654   Anesthesia for procedures on arteries of shoulder and axilla; bypass graft

35521

01656   Anesthesia for procedures on arteries of shoulder and axilla; axillary-femoral bypass graft

35526

00560   Anesthesia for procedures on heart, pericardial sac, and great vessels of chest; without pump oxygenator

35531

00770   Anesthesia for all procedures on major abdominal blood vessels

35533

01656   Anesthesia for procedures on arteries of shoulder and axilla; axillary-femoral bypass graft

35536

00770   Anesthesia for all procedures on major abdominal blood vessels

35541–35551
00880   Anesthesia for procedures on major lower abdominal vessels; not otherwise specified

35556–35558
01270   Anesthesia for procedures involving arteries of upper leg, including bypass graft; not otherwise specified

35560
00770   Anesthesia for all procedures on major abdominal blood vessels

35563–35565
00880   Anesthesia for procedures on major lower abdominal vessels; not otherwise specified

35566
01270   Anesthesia for procedures involving arteries of upper leg, including bypass graft; not otherwise specified

35571
01500   Anesthesia for procedures on arteries of lower leg, including bypass graft; not otherwise specified

35582
00770   Anesthesia for all procedures on major abdominal blood vessels

35583–35585
01270   Anesthesia for procedures involving arteries of upper leg, including bypass graft; not otherwise specified

35587
01500   Anesthesia for procedures on arteries of lower leg, including bypass graft; not otherwise specified

35601–35612
00350   Anesthesia for procedures on major vessels of neck; not otherwise specified

35616
01654   Anesthesia for procedures on arteries of shoulder and axilla; bypass graft

35621
01656   Anesthesia for procedures on arteries of shoulder and axilla; axillary-femoral bypass graft

35623
01654   Anesthesia for procedures on arteries of shoulder and axilla; bypass graft

35626
00560   Anesthesia for procedures on heart, pericardial sac, and great vessels of chest; without pump oxygenator

35631–35636
00770   Anesthesia for all procedures on major abdominal blood vessels

35641
00880   Anesthesia for procedures on major lower abdominal vessels; not otherwise specified

35642–35645
00350   Anesthesia for procedures on major vessels of neck; not otherwise specified

35646–35647
00880   Anesthesia for procedures on major lower abdominal vessels; not otherwise specified

35650
01654   Anesthesia for procedures on arteries of shoulder and axilla; bypass graft

35651
00880   Anesthesia for procedures on major lower abdominal vessels; not otherwise specified

35654
01656   Anesthesia for procedures on arteries of shoulder and axilla; axillary-femoral bypass graft

35656–35661
01270   Anesthesia for procedures involving arteries of upper leg, including bypass graft; not otherwise specified

35663–35665
00880   Anesthesia for procedures on major lower abdominal vessels; not otherwise specified

35666
01270   Anesthesia for procedures involving arteries of upper leg, including bypass graft; not otherwise specified

35671
01440   Anesthesia for procedures on arteries of knee and popliteal area; not otherwise specified

35691–35695
00350   Anesthesia for procedures on major vessels of neck; not otherwise specified

35701
00350   Anesthesia for procedures on major vessels of neck; not otherwise specified

35721

01270 Anesthesia for procedures involving arteries of upper leg, including bypass graft; not otherwise specified

35741

01440 Anesthesia for procedures on arteries of knee and popliteal area; not otherwise specified

35761

00350 Anesthesia for procedures on major vessels of neck; not otherwise specified

01770 Anesthesia for procedures on arteries of upper arm and elbow; not otherwise specified

01840 Anesthesia for procedures on arteries of forearm, wrist, and hand; not otherwise specified

01650 Anesthesia for procedures on arteries of shoulder and axilla; not otherwise specified

01270 Anesthesia for procedures involving arteries of upper leg, including bypass graft; not otherwise specified

01440 Anesthesia for procedures on arteries of knee and popliteal area; not otherwise specified

01500 Anesthesia for procedures on arteries of lower leg, including bypass graft; not otherwise specified

00880 Anesthesia for procedures on major lower abdominal vessels; not otherwise specified

35800

00350 Anesthesia for procedures on major vessels of neck; not otherwise specified

35820

00560 Anesthesia for procedures on heart, pericardial sac, and great vessels of chest; without pump oxygenator

35840

00770 Anesthesia for all procedures on major abdominal blood vessels

35870

00770 Anesthesia for all procedures on major abdominal blood vessels

35875–35876

00350 Anesthesia for procedures on major vessels of neck; not otherwise specified

01270 Anesthesia for procedures involving arteries of upper leg, including bypass graft; not otherwise specified

00452 Anesthesia for procedures on clavicle and scapula; radical surgery

00840 Anesthesia for intraperitoneal procedures in lower abdomen including laparoscopy; not otherwise specified

35879–35881

01440 Anesthesia for procedures on arteries of knee and popliteal area; not otherwise specified

01500 Anesthesia for procedures on arteries of lower leg, including bypass graft; not otherwise specified

35901

00350 Anesthesia for procedures on major vessels of neck; not otherwise specified

35903

01270 Anesthesia for procedures involving arteries of upper leg, including bypass graft; not otherwise specified

35905

00452 Anesthesia for procedures on clavicle and scapula; radical surgery

35907

00840 Anesthesia for intraperitoneal procedures in lower abdomen including laparoscopy; not otherwise specified

36011–36012

00532 Anesthesia for access to central venous circulation

36013–36015

00560 Anesthesia for procedures on heart, pericardial sac, and great vessels of chest; without pump oxygenator

36100

00350 Anesthesia for procedures on major vessels of neck; not otherwise specified

36120

01650 Anesthesia for procedures on arteries of shoulder and axilla; not otherwise specified

36140

01270 Anesthesia for procedures involving arteries of upper leg, including bypass graft; not otherwise specified

01440 Anesthesia for procedures on arteries of knee and popliteal area; not otherwise specified

01500 Anesthesia for procedures on arteries of lower leg, including bypass graft; not otherwise specified

01770 Anesthesia for procedures on arteries of upper arm and elbow; not otherwise specified

01840 Anesthesia for procedures on arteries of forearm, wrist, and hand; not otherwise specified

36145
01844   Anesthesia for vascular shunt, or shunt revision, any type (eg, dialysis)

36160
00770   Anesthesia for all procedures on major abdominal blood vessels

36200
00560   Anesthesia for procedures on heart, pericardial sac, and great vessels of chest; without pump oxygenator

00770   Anesthesia for all procedures on major abdominal blood vessels

36215–36217
00350   Anesthesia for procedures on major vessels of neck; not otherwise specified

00560   Anesthesia for procedures on heart, pericardial sac, and great vessels of chest; without pump oxygenator

00210   Anesthesia for intracranial procedures; not otherwise specified

36245–36247
00770   Anesthesia for all procedures on major abdominal blood vessels

00880   Anesthesia for procedures on major lower abdominal vessels; not otherwise specified

01270   Anesthesia for procedures involving arteries of upper leg, including bypass graft; not otherwise specified

01440   Anesthesia for procedures on arteries of knee and popliteal area; not otherwise specified

01500   Anesthesia for procedures on arteries of lower leg, including bypass graft; not otherwise specified

36260–36262
00532   Anesthesia for access to central venous circulation

36469
00300   Anesthesia for all procedures on the integumentary system, muscles and nerves of head, neck, and posterior trunk, not otherwise specified

36500
00532   Anesthesia for access to central venous circulation

36530–36535
00532   Anesthesia for access to central venous circulation

36800
01850   Anesthesia for procedures on veins of forearm, wrist, and hand; not otherwise specified

36810–36821
01844   Anesthesia for vascular shunt, or shunt revision, any type (eg, dialysis)

36822
00560   Anesthesia for procedures on heart, pericardial sac, and great vessels of chest; without pump oxygenator

36823–36833
01844   Anesthesia for vascular shunt, or shunt revision, any type (eg, dialysis)

36834
01770   Anesthesia for procedures on arteries of upper arm and elbow; not otherwise specified

01780   Anesthesia for procedures on veins of upper arm and elbow; not otherwise specified

36835
01844   Anesthesia for vascular shunt, or shunt revision, any type (eg, dialysis)

36870
01844   Anesthesia for vascular shunt, or shunt revision, any type (eg, dialysis)

37140–37181
00770   Anesthesia for all procedures on major abdominal blood vessels

37200
00216   Anesthesia for intracranial procedures; vascular procedures

01440   Anesthesia for procedures on arteries of knee and popliteal area; not otherwise specified

01650   Anesthesia for procedures on arteries of shoulder and axilla; not otherwise specified

01840   Anesthesia for procedures on arteries of forearm, wrist, and hand; not otherwise specified

01770   Anesthesia for procedures on arteries of upper arm and elbow; not otherwise specified

01500   Anesthesia for procedures on arteries of lower leg, including bypass graft; not otherwise specified

01270   Anesthesia for procedures involving arteries of upper leg, including bypass graft; not otherwise specified

00350   Anesthesia for procedures on major vessels of neck; not otherwise specified

00880   Anesthesia for procedures on major lower abdominal vessels; not otherwise specified

00770   Anesthesia for all procedures on major abdominal blood vessels

37203

00216	Anesthesia for intracranial procedures; vascular procedures
01840	Anesthesia for procedures on arteries of forearm, wrist, and hand; not otherwise specified
01770	Anesthesia for procedures on arteries of upper arm and elbow; not otherwise specified
00880	Anesthesia for procedures on major lower abdominal vessels; not otherwise specified
01270	Anesthesia for procedures involving arteries of upper leg, including bypass graft; not otherwise specified
01440	Anesthesia for procedures on arteries of knee and popliteal area; not otherwise specified
01650	Anesthesia for procedures on arteries of shoulder and axilla; not otherwise specified
01500	Anesthesia for procedures on arteries of lower leg, including bypass graft; not otherwise specified
00770	Anesthesia for all procedures on major abdominal blood vessels
00350	Anesthesia for procedures on major vessels of neck; not otherwise specified

37204

00770	Anesthesia for all procedures on major abdominal blood vessels
01440	Anesthesia for procedures on arteries of knee and popliteal area; not otherwise specified
01650	Anesthesia for procedures on arteries of shoulder and axilla; not otherwise specified
01840	Anesthesia for procedures on arteries of forearm, wrist, and hand; not otherwise specified
01770	Anesthesia for procedures on arteries of upper arm and elbow; not otherwise specified
01500	Anesthesia for procedures on arteries of lower leg, including bypass graft; not otherwise specified
00880	Anesthesia for procedures on major lower abdominal vessels; not otherwise specified
01270	Anesthesia for procedures involving arteries of upper leg, including bypass graft; not otherwise specified

37205

00216	Anesthesia for intracranial procedures; vascular procedures
00880	Anesthesia for procedures on major lower abdominal vessels; not otherwise specified
01440	Anesthesia for procedures on arteries of knee and popliteal area; not otherwise specified
01650	Anesthesia for procedures on arteries of shoulder and axilla; not otherwise specified

01840	Anesthesia for procedures on arteries of forearm, wrist, and hand; not otherwise specified
01770	Anesthesia for procedures on arteries of upper arm and elbow; not otherwise specified
01500	Anesthesia for procedures on arteries of lower leg, including bypass graft; not otherwise specified
01270	Anesthesia for procedures involving arteries of upper leg, including bypass graft; not otherwise specified
00350	Anesthesia for procedures on major vessels of neck; not otherwise specified
00770	Anesthesia for all procedures on major abdominal blood vessels

37207

00216	Anesthesia for intracranial procedures; vascular procedures
01270	Anesthesia for procedures involving arteries of upper leg, including bypass graft; not otherwise specified
01500	Anesthesia for procedures on arteries of lower leg, including bypass graft; not otherwise specified
01770	Anesthesia for procedures on arteries of upper arm and elbow; not otherwise specified
01840	Anesthesia for procedures on arteries of forearm, wrist, and hand; not otherwise specified
01650	Anesthesia for procedures on arteries of shoulder and axilla; not otherwise specified
01440	Anesthesia for procedures on arteries of knee and popliteal area; not otherwise specified
00880	Anesthesia for procedures on major lower abdominal vessels; not otherwise specified
00350	Anesthesia for procedures on major vessels of neck; not otherwise specified
00770	Anesthesia for all procedures on major abdominal blood vessels

37209

00216	Anesthesia for intracranial procedures; vascular procedures
01650	Anesthesia for procedures on arteries of shoulder and axilla; not otherwise specified
01840	Anesthesia for procedures on arteries of forearm, wrist, and hand; not otherwise specified
01770	Anesthesia for procedures on arteries of upper arm and elbow; not otherwise specified
01500	Anesthesia for procedures on arteries of lower leg, including bypass graft; not otherwise specified
00770	Anesthesia for all procedures on major abdominal blood vessels
00880	Anesthesia for procedures on major lower abdominal vessels; not otherwise specified

01440   Anesthesia for procedures on arteries of knee and popliteal area; not otherwise specified

01270   Anesthesia for procedures involving arteries of upper leg, including bypass graft; not otherwise specified

00350   Anesthesia for procedures on major vessels of neck; not otherwise specified

37565–37606

00352   Anesthesia for procedures on major vessels of neck; simple ligation

37609–37615

00352   Anesthesia for procedures on major vessels of neck; simple ligation

37616

00560   Anesthesia for procedures on heart, pericardial sac, and great vessels of chest; without pump oxygenator

37617

00770   Anesthesia for all procedures on major abdominal blood vessels

37618

01270   Anesthesia for procedures involving arteries of upper leg, including bypass graft; not otherwise specified

01650   Anesthesia for procedures on arteries of shoulder and axilla; not otherwise specified

01840   Anesthesia for procedures on arteries of forearm, wrist, and hand; not otherwise specified

01770   Anesthesia for procedures on arteries of upper arm and elbow; not otherwise specified

01440   Anesthesia for procedures on arteries of knee and popliteal area; not otherwise specified

01500   Anesthesia for procedures on arteries of lower leg, including bypass graft; not otherwise specified

37620

00882   Anesthesia for procedures on major lower abdominal vessels; inferior vena cava ligation

37650

01260   Anesthesia for all procedures involving veins of upper leg, including exploration

37660

00882   Anesthesia for procedures on major lower abdominal vessels; inferior vena cava ligation

37700

01260   Anesthesia for all procedures involving veins of upper leg, including exploration

37720

01260   Anesthesia for all procedures involving veins of upper leg, including exploration

01430   Anesthesia for procedures on veins of knee and popliteal area; not otherwise specified

01520   Anesthesia for procedures on veins of lower leg; not otherwise specified

37730–37760

01260   Anesthesia for all procedures involving veins of upper leg, including exploration

01520   Anesthesia for procedures on veins of lower leg; not otherwise specified

01430   Anesthesia for procedures on veins of knee and popliteal area; not otherwise specified

37780

01430   Anesthesia for procedures on veins of knee and popliteal area; not otherwise specified

37785

01260   Anesthesia for all procedures involving veins of upper leg, including exploration

01430   Anesthesia for procedures on veins of knee and popliteal area; not otherwise specified

01520   Anesthesia for procedures on veins of lower leg; not otherwise specified

37788–37790

00920   Anesthesia for procedures on male genitalia (including open urethral procedures); not otherwise specified

38100–38101

00790   Anesthesia for intraperitoneal procedures in upper abdomen including laparoscopy; not otherwise specified

38115–38120

00790   Anesthesia for intraperitoneal procedures in upper abdomen including laparoscopy; not otherwise specified

38200

00790   Anesthesia for intraperitoneal procedures in upper abdomen including laparoscopy; not otherwise specified

38230

01120   Anesthesia for procedures on bony pelvis

38380

00320   Anesthesia for all procedures on esophagus, thyroid, larynx, trachea and lymphatic system of neck; not otherwise specified

38381

00540   Anesthesia for thoracotomy procedures involving lungs, pleura, diaphragm, and mediastinum (including surgical thoracoscopy); not otherwise specified

38382

00790   Anesthesia for intraperitoneal procedures in upper abdomen including laparoscopy; not otherwise specified

38510–38520

00320   Anesthesia for all procedures on esophagus, thyroid, larynx, trachea and lymphatic system of neck; not otherwise specified

38525

01610   Anesthesia for all procedures on nerves, muscles, tendons, fascia, and bursae of shoulder and axilla

38530

00540   Anesthesia for thoracotomy procedures involving lungs, pleura, diaphragm, and mediastinum (including surgical thoracoscopy); not otherwise specified

38542

00320   Anesthesia for all procedures on esophagus, thyroid, larynx, trachea and lymphatic system of neck; not otherwise specified

38550–38555

00320   Anesthesia for all procedures on esophagus, thyroid, larynx, trachea and lymphatic system of neck; not otherwise specified

01610   Anesthesia for all procedures on nerves, muscles, tendons, fascia, and bursae of shoulder and axilla

38562

00840   Anesthesia for intraperitoneal procedures in lower abdomen including laparoscopy; not otherwise specified

38564

00860   Anesthesia for extraperitoneal procedures in lower abdomen, including urinary tract; not otherwise specified

38570–38572

00840   Anesthesia for intraperitoneal procedures in lower abdomen including laparoscopy; not otherwise specified

38700–38724

00320   Anesthesia for all procedures on esophagus, thyroid, larynx, trachea and lymphatic system of neck; not otherwise specified

38740–38475

01610   Anesthesia for all procedures on nerves, muscles, tendons, fascia, and bursae of shoulder and axilla

38760–38770

00840   Anesthesia for intraperitoneal procedures in lower abdomen including laparoscopy; not otherwise specified

38780

00860   Anesthesia for extraperitoneal procedures in lower abdomen, including urinary tract; not otherwise specified

39000

00528   Anesthesia for closed chest procedures; mediastinoscopy and diagnostic thoracoscopy

39010–39220

00540   Anesthesia for thoracotomy procedures involving lungs, pleura, diaphragm, and mediastinum (including surgical thoracoscopy); not otherwise specified

39400

00528   Anesthesia for closed chest procedures; mediastinoscopy and diagnostic thoracoscopy

39501

00540   Anesthesia for thoracotomy procedures involving lungs, pleura, diaphragm, and mediastinum (including surgical thoracoscopy); not otherwise specified

39502

00790   Anesthesia for intraperitoneal procedures in upper abdomen including laparoscopy; not otherwise specified

39503–39531

00540   Anesthesia for thoracotomy procedures involving lungs, pleura, diaphragm, and mediastinum (including surgical thoracoscopy); not otherwise specified

39540–39541

00540   Anesthesia for thoracotomy procedures involving lungs, pleura, diaphragm, and mediastinum (including surgical thoracoscopy); not otherwise specified

00756   Anesthesia for hernia repairs in upper abdomen; transabdominal repair of diaphragmatic hernia

39545

00540   Anesthesia for thoracotomy procedures involving lungs, pleura, diaphragm, and mediastinum (including surgical thoracoscopy); not otherwise specified

00790   Anesthesia for intraperitoneal procedures in upper abdomen including laparoscopy; not otherwise specified

39560–39561
00540   Anesthesia for thoracotomy procedures involving lungs, pleura, diaphragm, and mediastinum (including surgical thoracoscopy); not otherwise specified

40490–40654
00300   Anesthesia for all procedures on the integumentary system, muscles and nerves of head, neck, and posterior trunk, not otherwise specified

40700–40761
00102   Anesthesia for procedures on plastic repair of cleft lip

40800–40845
00170   Anesthesia for intraoral procedures, including biopsy; not otherwise specified

41000
00170   Anesthesia for intraoral procedures, including biopsy; not otherwise specified

41006–41010
00170   Anesthesia for intraoral procedures, including biopsy; not otherwise specified

41015–41018
00300   Anesthesia for all procedures on the integumentary system, muscles and nerves of head, neck, and posterior trunk, not otherwise specified

41100–41113
00170   Anesthesia for intraoral procedures, including biopsy; not otherwise specified

41115–41130
00170   Anesthesia for intraoral procedures, including biopsy; not otherwise specified

41135–41155
00176   Anesthesia for intraoral procedures, including biopsy; radical surgery

41250–41520
00170   Anesthesia for intraoral procedures, including biopsy; not otherwise specified

41800–41874
00170   Anesthesia for intraoral procedures, including biopsy; not otherwise specified

42000–42182
00170   Anesthesia for intraoral procedures, including biopsy; not otherwise specified

42200–42225
00172   Anesthesia for intraoral procedures, including biopsy; repair of cleft palate

42226–42260
00170   Anesthesia for intraoral procedures, including biopsy; not otherwise specified

42281
00170   Anesthesia for intraoral procedures, including biopsy; not otherwise specified

42300–42305
00100   Anesthesia for procedures on salivary glands, including biopsy

42310–42340
00170   Anesthesia for intraoral procedures, including biopsy; not otherwise specified

42400–42405
00100   Anesthesia for procedures on salivary glands, including biopsy

42408–42409
00170   Anesthesia for intraoral procedures, including biopsy; not otherwise specified

42410–42425
00100   Anesthesia for procedures on salivary glands, including biopsy

42426
00320   Anesthesia for all procedures on esophagus, thyroid, larynx, trachea and lymphatic system of neck; not otherwise specified

42440
00100   Anesthesia for procedures on salivary glands, including biopsy

42450–42505
00170   Anesthesia for intraoral procedures, including biopsy; not otherwise specified

42507–42510
00100   Anesthesia for procedures on salivary glands, including biopsy

42600
00100   Anesthesia for procedures on salivary glands, including biopsy

42665
00170   Anesthesia for intraoral procedures, including biopsy; not otherwise specified

42700–42809
00170   Anesthesia for intraoral procedures, including biopsy; not otherwise specified

Anesthesia Crosswalk

42810–42815

00300 Anesthesia for all procedures on the integumentary system, muscles and nerves of head, neck, and posterior trunk, not otherwise specified

42820–42836

00170 Anesthesia for intraoral procedures, including biopsy; not otherwise specified

42842–42845

00176 Anesthesia for intraoral procedures, including biopsy; radical surgery

42860–42870

00170 Anesthesia for intraoral procedures, including biopsy; not otherwise specified

42890–42894

00176 Anesthesia for intraoral procedures, including biopsy; radical surgery

42900–42950

00170 Anesthesia for intraoral procedures, including biopsy; not otherwise specified

42953

00320 Anesthesia for all procedures on esophagus, thyroid, larynx, trachea and lymphatic system of neck; not otherwise specified

42955

00300 Anesthesia for all procedures on the integumentary system, muscles and nerves of head, neck, and posterior trunk, not otherwise specified

42962

00170 Anesthesia for intraoral procedures, including biopsy; not otherwise specified

42971–42972

00170 Anesthesia for intraoral procedures, including biopsy; not otherwise specified

43020–43030

00320 Anesthesia for all procedures on esophagus, thyroid, larynx, trachea and lymphatic system of neck; not otherwise specified

43045

00500 Anesthesia for all procedures on esophagus

43100

00320 Anesthesia for all procedures on esophagus, thyroid, larynx, trachea and lymphatic system of neck; not otherwise specified

43101–43123

00500 Anesthesia for all procedures on esophagus

43124

00320 Anesthesia for all procedures on esophagus, thyroid, larynx, trachea and lymphatic system of neck; not otherwise specified

00500 Anesthesia for all procedures on esophagus

43130

00320 Anesthesia for all procedures on esophagus, thyroid, larynx, trachea and lymphatic system of neck; not otherwise specified

43135

00500 Anesthesia for all procedures on esophagus

43200–43272

00740 Anesthesia for upper gastrointestinal endoscopic procedures, endoscope introduced proximal to duodenum

43280

00790 Anesthesia for intraperitoneal procedures in upper abdomen including laparoscopy; not otherwise specified

43300–43305

00320 Anesthesia for all procedures on esophagus, thyroid, larynx, trachea and lymphatic system of neck; not otherwise specified

43310–43330

00500 Anesthesia for all procedures on esophagus

43331

00500 Anesthesia for all procedures on esophagus

43340

00790 Anesthesia for intraperitoneal procedures in upper abdomen including laparoscopy; not otherwise specified

43341

00500 Anesthesia for all procedures on esophagus

43350

00790 Anesthesia for intraperitoneal procedures in upper abdomen including laparoscopy; not otherwise specified

43351

00500 Anesthesia for all procedures on esophagus

43352

00320 Anesthesia for all procedures on esophagus, thyroid, larynx, trachea and lymphatic system of neck; not otherwise specified

43360–43401

00500 Anesthesia for all procedures on esophagus

43405
00790 Anesthesia for intraperitoneal procedures in upper abdomen including laparoscopy; not otherwise specified

43410
00320 Anesthesia for all procedures on esophagus, thyroid, larynx, trachea and lymphatic system of neck; not otherwise specified

43415
00500 Anesthesia for all procedures on esophagus

43420
00320 Anesthesia for all procedures on esophagus, thyroid, larynx, trachea and lymphatic system of neck; not otherwise specified

43425–43496
00500 Anesthesia for all procedures on esophagus

43500–43520
00790 Anesthesia for intraperitoneal procedures in upper abdomen including laparoscopy; not otherwise specified

43605–43634
00790 Anesthesia for intraperitoneal procedures in upper abdomen including laparoscopy; not otherwise specified

43638–43653
00790 Anesthesia for intraperitoneal procedures in upper abdomen including laparoscopy; not otherwise specified

43750
00700 Anesthesia for procedures on upper anterior abdominal wall; not otherwise specified

43760
00700 Anesthesia for procedures on upper anterior abdominal wall; not otherwise specified

43800–43840
00790 Anesthesia for intraperitoneal procedures in upper abdomen including laparoscopy; not otherwise specified

43842–43848
00797 Anesthesia for intraperitoneal procedures in upper abdomen including laparoscopy; gastric restrictive procedure for morbid obesity

43850–43880
00790 Anesthesia for intraperitoneal procedures in upper abdomen including laparoscopy; not otherwise specified

44005
00790 Anesthesia for intraperitoneal procedures in upper abdomen including laparoscopy; not otherwise specified
00840 Anesthesia for intraperitoneal procedures in lower abdomen including laparoscopy; not otherwise specified

44010
00790 Anesthesia for intraperitoneal procedures in upper abdomen including laparoscopy; not otherwise specified

44020–44050
00840 Anesthesia for intraperitoneal procedures in lower abdomen including laparoscopy; not otherwise specified

44055
00790 Anesthesia for intraperitoneal procedures in upper abdomen including laparoscopy; not otherwise specified

44110–44120
00840 Anesthesia for intraperitoneal procedures in lower abdomen including laparoscopy; not otherwise specified

44125–44127
00840 Anesthesia for intraperitoneal procedures in lower abdomen including laparoscopy; not otherwise specified

44130
00840 Anesthesia for intraperitoneal procedures in lower abdomen including laparoscopy; not otherwise specified

44132
01990 Physiological support for harvesting of organ(s) from brain-dead patient

44133
00840 Anesthesia for intraperitoneal procedures in lower abdomen including laparoscopy; not otherwise specified

44135
01990 Physiological support for harvesting of organ(s) from brain-dead patient

44136
00840 Anesthesia for intraperitoneal procedures in lower abdomen including laparoscopy; not otherwise specified

44140–44202
00840 Anesthesia for intraperitoneal procedures in lower abdomen including laparoscopy; not otherwise specified

Anesthesia Crosswalk

44204–44205
00840   Anesthesia for intraperitoneal procedures in lower abdomen including laparoscopy; not otherwise specified

44300
00840   Anesthesia for intraperitoneal procedures in lower abdomen including laparoscopy; not otherwise specified

44310
00840   Anesthesia for intraperitoneal procedures in lower abdomen including laparoscopy; not otherwise specified

44312
00800   Anesthesia for procedures on lower anterior abdominal wall; not otherwise specified

44314–44322
00840   Anesthesia for intraperitoneal procedures in lower abdomen including laparoscopy; not otherwise specified

44340
00800   Anesthesia for procedures on lower anterior abdominal wall; not otherwise specified

44345–44346
00840   Anesthesia for intraperitoneal procedures in lower abdomen including laparoscopy; not otherwise specified

44360–44397
00810   Anesthesia for lower intestinal endoscopic procedures, endoscope introduced distal to duodenum

44602–44700
00840   Anesthesia for intraperitoneal procedures in lower abdomen including laparoscopy; not otherwise specified

44800–44850
00840   Anesthesia for intraperitoneal procedures in lower abdomen including laparoscopy; not otherwise specified

44900
00840   Anesthesia for intraperitoneal procedures in lower abdomen including laparoscopy; not otherwise specified

44901
00800   Anesthesia for procedures on lower anterior abdominal wall; not otherwise specified

44950
00840   Anesthesia for intraperitoneal procedures in lower abdomen including laparoscopy; not otherwise specified

44960–44970
00840   Anesthesia for intraperitoneal procedures in lower abdomen including laparoscopy; not otherwise specified

45000–45108
00902   Anesthesia for; anorectal procedure

45110
00844   Anesthesia for intraperitoneal procedures in lower abdomen including laparoscopy; abdominoperineal resection

45111
00840   Anesthesia for intraperitoneal procedures in lower abdomen including laparoscopy; not otherwise specified

45112–45114
00844   Anesthesia for intraperitoneal procedures in lower abdomen including laparoscopy; abdominoperineal resection

45116
00904   Anesthesia for; radical perineal procedure

45119–45121
00844   Anesthesia for intraperitoneal procedures in lower abdomen including laparoscopy; abdominoperineal resection

45123
00902   Anesthesia for; anorectal procedure

45126
00848   Anesthesia for intraperitoneal procedures in lower abdomen including laparoscopy; pelvic exenteration

45130
00902   Anesthesia for; anorectal procedure

45135
00844   Anesthesia for intraperitoneal procedures in lower abdomen including laparoscopy; abdominoperineal resection

45136
00840   Anesthesia for intraperitoneal procedures in lower abdomen including laparoscopy; not otherwise specified

45150–45321
00902   Anesthesia for; anorectal procedure

45327
00810   Anesthesia for lower intestinal endoscopic procedures, endoscope introduced distal to duodenum

45330–45339
00902   Anesthesia for; anorectal procedure

45341–45387
00810   Anesthesia for lower intestinal endoscopic procedures, endoscope introduced distal to duodenum

45500–45520
00902   Anesthesia for; anorectal procedure

45540
00840   Anesthesia for intraperitoneal procedures in lower abdomen including laparoscopy; not otherwise specified

45541
00902   Anesthesia for; anorectal procedure

45550
00844   Anesthesia for intraperitoneal procedures in lower abdomen including laparoscopy; abdominoperineal resection

45560–45562
00902   Anesthesia for; anorectal procedure

45563–45825
00840   Anesthesia for intraperitoneal procedures in lower abdomen including laparoscopy; not otherwise specified

45900–45915
00902   Anesthesia for; anorectal procedure

46020–46211
00902   Anesthesia for; anorectal procedure

46220
00400   Anesthesia for procedures on the integumentary system on the extremities, anterior trunk and perineum; not otherwise specified

46221–46716
00902   Anesthesia for; anorectal procedure

46730–46748
00904   Anesthesia for; radical perineal procedure

46750–46762
00902   Anesthesia for; anorectal procedure

46900–46917
00400   Anesthesia for procedures on the integumentary system on the extremities, anterior trunk and perineum; not otherwise specified

46922–46946
00902   Anesthesia for; anorectal procedure

47000
00702   Anesthesia for procedures on upper anterior abdominal wall; percutaneous liver biopsy

47010–47100
00790   Anesthesia for intraperitoneal procedures in upper abdomen including laparoscopy; not otherwise specified

47120–47130
00792   Anesthesia for intraperitoneal procedures in upper abdomen including laparoscopy; partial hepatectomy or management of liver hemorrhage (excluding liver biopsy)

47133
01990   Physiological support for harvesting of organ(s) from brain-dead patient

47134
00792   Anesthesia for intraperitoneal procedures in upper abdomen including laparoscopy; partial hepatectomy or management of liver hemorrhage (excluding liver biopsy)

47135–47136
00796   Anesthesia for intraperitoneal procedures in upper abdomen including laparoscopy; liver transplant (recipient)

47300
00790   Anesthesia for intraperitoneal procedures in upper abdomen including laparoscopy; not otherwise specified

47350–47361
00792   Anesthesia for intraperitoneal procedures in upper abdomen including laparoscopy; partial hepatectomy or management of liver hemorrhage (excluding liver biopsy)

47362–47371
00790   Anesthesia for intraperitoneal procedures in upper abdomen including laparoscopy; not otherwise specified

47380–47382
00790   Anesthesia for intraperitoneal procedures in upper abdomen including laparoscopy; not otherwise specified

47400–47500
00790   Anesthesia for intraperitoneal procedures in upper abdomen including laparoscopy; not otherwise specified

47510–47511
00702   Anesthesia for procedures on upper anterior abdominal wall; percutaneous liver biopsy

Anesthesia Crosswalk

47525–47530
00700   Anesthesia for procedures on upper anterior abdominal wall; not otherwise specified

47552
00700   Anesthesia for procedures on upper anterior abdominal wall; not otherwise specified

47553–47556
00740   Anesthesia for upper gastrointestinal endoscopic procedures, endoscope introduced proximal to duodenum

47556
00740   Anesthesia for upper gastrointestinal endoscopic procedures, endoscope introduced proximal to duodenum

47560–47570
00790   Anesthesia for intraperitoneal procedures in upper abdomen including laparoscopy; not otherwise specified

47600–47620
00790   Anesthesia for intraperitoneal procedures in upper abdomen including laparoscopy; not otherwise specified

47630
00700   Anesthesia for procedures on upper anterior abdominal wall; not otherwise specified

47700–47900
00790   Anesthesia for intraperitoneal procedures in upper abdomen including laparoscopy; not otherwise specified

48000–48100
00790   Anesthesia for intraperitoneal procedures in upper abdomen including laparoscopy; not otherwise specified

48102
00702   Anesthesia for procedures on upper anterior abdominal wall; percutaneous liver biopsy

48120
00790   Anesthesia for intraperitoneal procedures in upper abdomen including laparoscopy; not otherwise specified

48140–48146
00794   Anesthesia for intraperitoneal procedures in upper abdomen including laparoscopy; pancreatectomy, partial or total (eg, Whipple procedure)

48148
00790   Anesthesia for intraperitoneal procedures in upper abdomen including laparoscopy; not otherwise specified

48150–48160
00794   Anesthesia for intraperitoneal procedures in upper abdomen including laparoscopy; pancreatectomy, partial or total (eg, Whipple procedure)

48180
00790   Anesthesia for intraperitoneal procedures in upper abdomen including laparoscopy; not otherwise specified

48500–48510
00790   Anesthesia for intraperitoneal procedures in upper abdomen including laparoscopy; not otherwise specified

48511
00700   Anesthesia for procedures on upper anterior abdominal wall; not otherwise specified

48520–48547
00790   Anesthesia for intraperitoneal procedures in upper abdomen including laparoscopy; not otherwise specified

48550
01990   Physiological support for harvesting of organ(s) from brain-dead patient

48554–48556
00790   Anesthesia for intraperitoneal procedures in upper abdomen including laparoscopy; not otherwise specified

49000–49020
00840   Anesthesia for intraperitoneal procedures in lower abdomen including laparoscopy; not otherwise specified

49021
00800   Anesthesia for procedures on lower anterior abdominal wall; not otherwise specified

49040
00790   Anesthesia for intraperitoneal procedures in upper abdomen including laparoscopy; not otherwise specified

49041
00700   Anesthesia for procedures on upper anterior abdominal wall; not otherwise specified

49060
00840   Anesthesia for intraperitoneal procedures in lower abdomen including laparoscopy; not otherwise specified

49061
00820   Anesthesia for procedures on lower posterior abdominal wall

49062

00840   Anesthesia for intraperitoneal procedures in lower abdomen including laparoscopy; not otherwise specified

49080–49081

00800   Anesthesia for procedures on lower anterior abdominal wall; not otherwise specified

49085

00840   Anesthesia for intraperitoneal procedures in lower abdomen including laparoscopy; not otherwise specified

49180

00800   Anesthesia for procedures on lower anterior abdominal wall; not otherwise specified

00820   Anesthesia for procedures on lower posterior abdominal wall

49200–49201

00840   Anesthesia for intraperitoneal procedures in lower abdomen including laparoscopy; not otherwise specified

49215

01150   Anesthesia for radical procedures for tumor of pelvis, except hindquarter amputation

49220

00790   Anesthesia for intraperitoneal procedures in upper abdomen including laparoscopy; not otherwise specified

49250–49323

00840   Anesthesia for intraperitoneal procedures in lower abdomen including laparoscopy; not otherwise specified

49400–49422

00800   Anesthesia for procedures on lower anterior abdominal wall; not otherwise specified

49423–49424

00800   Anesthesia for procedures on lower anterior abdominal wall; not otherwise specified

00820   Anesthesia for procedures on lower posterior abdominal wall

49425–49429

00790   Anesthesia for intraperitoneal procedures in upper abdomen including laparoscopy; not otherwise specified

49491–49525

00830   Anesthesia for hernia repairs in lower abdomen; not otherwise specified

49540

00752   Anesthesia for hernia repairs in upper abdomen; lumbar and ventral (incisional) hernias and/or wound dehiscence

49550–49557

00830   Anesthesia for hernia repairs in lower abdomen; not otherwise specified

49560–49566

00752   Anesthesia for hernia repairs in upper abdomen; lumbar and ventral (incisional) hernias and/or wound dehiscence

00832   Anesthesia for hernia repairs in lower abdomen; ventral and incisional hernias

49570–49590

00750   Anesthesia for hernia repairs in upper abdomen; not otherwise specified

49600–49611

00754   Anesthesia for hernia repairs in upper abdomen; omphalocele

49650–49651

00840   Anesthesia for intraperitoneal procedures in lower abdomen including laparoscopy; not otherwise specified

49900

00752   Anesthesia for hernia repairs in upper abdomen; lumbar and ventral (incisional) hernias and/or wound dehiscence

49906

00790   Anesthesia for intraperitoneal procedures in upper abdomen including laparoscopy; not otherwise specified

50010–50020

00862   Anesthesia for extraperitoneal procedures in lower abdomen, including urinary tract; renal procedures, including upper 1/3 of ureter, or donor nephrectomy

50021

00860   Anesthesia for extraperitoneal procedures in lower abdomen, including urinary tract; not otherwise specified

50040–50081

00862   Anesthesia for extraperitoneal procedures in lower abdomen, including urinary tract; renal procedures, including upper 1/3 of ureter, or donor nephrectomy

50100–50135

00880   Anesthesia for procedures on major lower abdominal vessels; not otherwise specified

Anesthesia Crosswalk

50200

00860   Anesthesia for extraperitoneal procedures in lower abdomen, including urinary tract; not otherwise specified

50205–50280

00862   Anesthesia for extraperitoneal procedures in lower abdomen, including urinary tract; renal procedures, including upper 1/3 of ureter, or donor nephrectomy

50290

00860   Anesthesia for extraperitoneal procedures in lower abdomen, including urinary tract; not otherwise specified

50300

01990   Physiological support for harvesting of organ(s) from brain-dead patient

50320–50340

00862   Anesthesia for extraperitoneal procedures in lower abdomen, including urinary tract; renal procedures, including upper 1/3 of ureter, or donor nephrectomy

50360–50365

00868   Anesthesia for extraperitoneal procedures in lower abdomen, including urinary tract; renal transplant (recipient)

50370

00862   Anesthesia for extraperitoneal procedures in lower abdomen, including urinary tract; renal procedures, including upper 1/3 of ureter, or donor nephrectomy

50380

00868   Anesthesia for extraperitoneal procedures in lower abdomen, including urinary tract; renal transplant (recipient)

50390–50393

00860   Anesthesia for extraperitoneal procedures in lower abdomen, including urinary tract; not otherwise specified

50395

00860   Anesthesia for extraperitoneal procedures in lower abdomen, including urinary tract; not otherwise specified

50398

00820   Anesthesia for procedures on lower posterior abdominal wall

50400–50500

00862   Anesthesia for extraperitoneal procedures in lower abdomen, including urinary tract; renal procedures, including upper 1/3 of ureter, or donor nephrectomy

50520

00860   Anesthesia for extraperitoneal procedures in lower abdomen, including urinary tract; not otherwise specified

50525

00862   Anesthesia for extraperitoneal procedures in lower abdomen, including urinary tract; renal procedures, including upper 1/3 of ureter, or donor nephrectomy

50526

00540   Anesthesia for thoracotomy procedures involving lungs, pleura, diaphragm, and mediastinum (including surgical thoracoscopy); not otherwise specified

50540

00862   Anesthesia for extraperitoneal procedures in lower abdomen, including urinary tract; renal procedures, including upper 1/3 of ureter, or donor nephrectomy

50541–50544

00790   Anesthesia for intraperitoneal procedures in upper abdomen including laparoscopy; not otherwise specified

50545

00862   Anesthesia for extraperitoneal procedures in lower abdomen, including urinary tract; renal procedures, including upper 1/3 of ureter, or donor nephrectomy

50546

00790   Anesthesia for intraperitoneal procedures in upper abdomen including laparoscopy; not otherwise specified

50547

00862   Anesthesia for extraperitoneal procedures in lower abdomen, including urinary tract; renal procedures, including upper 1/3 of ureter, or donor nephrectomy

50548

00790   Anesthesia for intraperitoneal procedures in upper abdomen including laparoscopy; not otherwise specified

50551–50561

00820   Anesthesia for procedures on lower posterior abdominal wall

50570–50580

00860   Anesthesia for extraperitoneal procedures in lower abdomen, including urinary tract; not otherwise specified

50590

00872   Anesthesia for lithotripsy, extracorporeal shock wave; with water bath

50600–50610

00862   Anesthesia for extraperitoneal procedures in lower abdomen, including urinary tract; renal procedures, including upper 1/3 of ureter, or donor nephrectomy

50620–50650

00860   Anesthesia for extraperitoneal procedures in lower abdomen, including urinary tract; not otherwise specified

50660

00862   Anesthesia for extraperitoneal procedures in lower abdomen, including urinary tract; renal procedures, including upper 1/3 of ureter, or donor nephrectomy

50688

00860   Anesthesia for extraperitoneal procedures in lower abdomen, including urinary tract; not otherwise specified

50700–50715

00862   Anesthesia for extraperitoneal procedures in lower abdomen, including urinary tract; renal procedures, including upper 1/3 of ureter, or donor nephrectomy

50722

00860   Anesthesia for extraperitoneal procedures in lower abdomen, including urinary tract; not otherwise specified

50725

00862   Anesthesia for extraperitoneal procedures in lower abdomen, including urinary tract; renal procedures, including upper 1/3 of ureter, or donor nephrectomy

50727–50728

00860   Anesthesia for extraperitoneal procedures in lower abdomen, including urinary tract; not otherwise specified

50740–50770

00862   Anesthesia for extraperitoneal procedures in lower abdomen, including urinary tract; renal procedures, including upper 1/3 of ureter, or donor nephrectomy

50780–50830

00860   Anesthesia for extraperitoneal procedures in lower abdomen, including urinary tract; not otherwise specified

50840

00862   Anesthesia for extraperitoneal procedures in lower abdomen, including urinary tract; renal procedures, including upper 1/3 of ureter, or donor nephrectomy

50845

00840   Anesthesia for intraperitoneal procedures in lower abdomen including laparoscopy; not otherwise specified

50860–50940

00860   Anesthesia for extraperitoneal procedures in lower abdomen, including urinary tract; not otherwise specified

50945

00840   Anesthesia for intraperitoneal procedures in lower abdomen including laparoscopy; not otherwise specified

50947

00860   Anesthesia for extraperitoneal procedures in lower abdomen, including urinary tract; not otherwise specified

50948

00860   Anesthesia for extraperitoneal procedures in lower abdomen, including urinary tract; not otherwise specified

50951–50961

00820   Anesthesia for procedures on lower posterior abdominal wall

50970–50980

00860   Anesthesia for extraperitoneal procedures in lower abdomen, including urinary tract; not otherwise specified

51000–51010

00800   Anesthesia for procedures on lower anterior abdominal wall; not otherwise specified

51020–51045

00860   Anesthesia for extraperitoneal procedures in lower abdomen, including urinary tract; not otherwise specified

51050

00870   Anesthesia for extraperitoneal procedures in lower abdomen, including urinary tract; cystolithotomy

51060–51565

00860   Anesthesia for extraperitoneal procedures in lower abdomen, including urinary tract; not otherwise specified

51570–51596

00864   Anesthesia for extraperitoneal procedures in lower abdomen, including urinary tract; total cystectomy

51597

00848   Anesthesia for intraperitoneal procedures in lower abdomen including laparoscopy; pelvic exenteration

51600–51700

00910   Anesthesia for transurethral procedures (including urethrocystoscopy); not otherwise specified

51705–51710

00800   Anesthesia for procedures on lower anterior abdominal wall; not otherwise specified

51715–51726

00910   Anesthesia for transurethral procedures (including urethrocystoscopy); not otherwise specified

51772

00910   Anesthesia for transurethral procedures (including urethrocystoscopy); not otherwise specified

51800–51920

00860   Anesthesia for extraperitoneal procedures in lower abdomen, including urinary tract; not otherwise specified

51925

00840   Anesthesia for intraperitoneal procedures in lower abdomen including laparoscopy; not otherwise specified

51940–51980

00860   Anesthesia for extraperitoneal procedures in lower abdomen, including urinary tract; not otherwise specified

51990–51992

00840   Anesthesia for intraperitoneal procedures in lower abdomen including laparoscopy; not otherwise specified

52000–52224

00910   Anesthesia for transurethral procedures (including urethrocystoscopy); not otherwise specified

52234–52240

00912   Anesthesia for transurethral procedures (including urethrocystoscopy); transurethral resection of bladder tumor(s)

52250–52260

00910   Anesthesia for transurethral procedures (including urethrocystoscopy); not otherwise specified

52270–52318

00910   Anesthesia for transurethral procedures (including urethrocystoscopy); not otherwise specified

52320–52325

00918   Anesthesia for transurethral procedures (including urethrocystoscopy); with fragmentation, manipulation and/or removal of ureteral calculus

52327–52351

00910   Anesthesia for transurethral procedures (including urethrocystoscopy); not otherwise specified

52352–52353

00918   Anesthesia for transurethral procedures (including urethrocystoscopy); with fragmentation, manipulation and/or removal of ureteral calculus

52354

00910   Anesthesia for transurethral procedures (including urethrocystoscopy); not otherwise specified

52355

00912   Anesthesia for transurethral procedures (including urethrocystoscopy); transurethral resection of bladder tumor(s)

52400–52510

00910   Anesthesia for transurethral procedures (including urethrocystoscopy); not otherwise specified

52601

00914   Anesthesia for transurethral procedures (including urethrocystoscopy); transurethral resection of prostate

52606

00916   Anesthesia for transurethral procedures (including urethrocystoscopy); post-transurethral resection bleeding

52612–52648

00914   Anesthesia for transurethral procedures (including urethrocystoscopy); transurethral resection of prostate

52700

00910   Anesthesia for transurethral procedures (including urethrocystoscopy); not otherwise specified

53000–53010

00942   Anesthesia for vaginal procedures (including biopsy of labia, vagina, cervix or endometrium); colpotomy, vaginectomy, colporrhaphy, and open urethral procedures

00920 Anesthesia for procedures on male genitalia (including open urethral procedures); not otherwise specified

53020

00940 Anesthesia for vaginal procedures (including biopsy of labia, vagina, cervix or endometrium); not otherwise specified

00942 Anesthesia for vaginal procedures (including biopsy of labia, vagina, cervix or endometrium); colpotomy, vaginectomy, colporrhaphy, and open urethral procedures

53025–53220

00942 Anesthesia for vaginal procedures (including biopsy of labia, vagina, cervix or endometrium); colpotomy, vaginectomy, colporrhaphy, and open urethral procedures

00920 Anesthesia for procedures on male genitalia (including open urethral procedures); not otherwise specified

53230

00942 Anesthesia for vaginal procedures (including biopsy of labia, vagina, cervix or endometrium); colpotomy, vaginectomy, colporrhaphy, and open urethral procedures

53235

00920 Anesthesia for procedures on male genitalia (including open urethral procedures); not otherwise specified

53240–53405

00920 Anesthesia for procedures on male genitalia (including open urethral procedures); not otherwise specified

00942 Anesthesia for vaginal procedures (including biopsy of labia, vagina, cervix or endometrium); colpotomy, vaginectomy, colporrhaphy, and open urethral procedures

53410–53425

00910 Anesthesia for transurethral procedures (including urethrocystoscopy); not otherwise specified

53430

00942 Anesthesia for vaginal procedures (including biopsy of labia, vagina, cervix or endometrium); colpotomy, vaginectomy, colporrhaphy, and open urethral procedures

53431

00942 Anesthesia for vaginal procedures (including biopsy of labia, vagina, cervix or endometrium); colpotomy, vaginectomy, colporrhaphy, and open urethral procedures

00920 Anesthesia for procedures on male genitalia (including open urethral procedures); not otherwise specified

53440

00920 Anesthesia for procedures on male genitalia (including open urethral procedures); not otherwise specified

53442–53460

00920 Anesthesia for procedures on male genitalia (including open urethral procedures); not otherwise specified

00942 Anesthesia for vaginal procedures (including biopsy of labia, vagina, cervix or endometrium); colpotomy, vaginectomy, colporrhaphy, and open urethral procedures

53502

00942 Anesthesia for vaginal procedures (including biopsy of labia, vagina, cervix or endometrium); colpotomy, vaginectomy, colporrhaphy, and open urethral procedures

53505–53520

00920 Anesthesia for procedures on male genitalia (including open urethral procedures); not otherwise specified

53605–53665

00910 Anesthesia for transurethral procedures (including urethrocystoscopy); not otherwise specified

53675

00910 Anesthesia for transurethral procedures (including urethrocystoscopy); not otherwise specified

53850–53852

00914 Anesthesia for transurethral procedures (including urethrocystoscopy); transurethral resection of prostate

53853

00910 Anesthesia for transurethral procedures (including urethrocystoscopy); not otherwise specified

54000–54065

00920 Anesthesia for procedures on male genitalia (including open urethral procedures); not otherwise specified

54100

00400 Anesthesia for procedures on the integumentary system on the extremities, anterior trunk and perineum; not otherwise specified

54105–54120

00920 Anesthesia for procedures on male genitalia (including open urethral procedures); not otherwise specified

Anesthesia Crosswalk

54125

00932 Anesthesia for procedures on male genitalia (including open urethral procedures); complete amputation of penis

54130

00934 Anesthesia for procedures on male genitalia (including open urethral procedures); radical amputation of penis with bilateral inguinal lymphadenectomy

54135

00936 Anesthesia for procedures on male genitalia (including open urethral procedures); radical amputation of penis with bilateral inguinal and iliac lymphadenectomy

54152–54235

00920 Anesthesia for procedures on male genitalia (including open urethral procedures); not otherwise specified

54300–54385

00920 Anesthesia for procedures on male genitalia (including open urethral procedures); not otherwise specified

54390

00860 Anesthesia for extraperitoneal procedures in lower abdomen, including urinary tract; not otherwise specified

54400–54405

00938 Anesthesia for procedures on male genitalia (including open urethral procedures); insertion of penile prosthesis (perineal approach)

54406

00920 Anesthesia for procedures on male genitalia (including open urethral procedures); not otherwise specified

54407

00938 Anesthesia for procedures on male genitalia (including open urethral procedures); insertion of penile prosthesis (perineal approach)

54408

00920 Anesthesia for procedures on male genitalia (including open urethral procedures); not otherwise specified

54409–54411

00938 Anesthesia for procedures on male genitalia (including open urethral procedures); insertion of penile prosthesis (perineal approach)

54415

00920 Anesthesia for procedures on male genitalia (including open urethral procedures); not otherwise specified

54416–54417

00938 Anesthesia for procedures on male genitalia (including open urethral procedures); insertion of penile prosthesis (perineal approach)

54420–54522

00920 Anesthesia for procedures on male genitalia (including open urethral procedures); not otherwise specified

54530

00926 Anesthesia for procedures on male genitalia (including open urethral procedures); radical orchiectomy, inguinal

54535

00928 Anesthesia for procedures on male genitalia (including open urethral procedures); radical orchiectomy, abdominal

54550

00924 Anesthesia for procedures on male genitalia (including open urethral procedures); undescended testis, unilateral or bilateral

54560

00860 Anesthesia for extraperitoneal procedures in lower abdomen, including urinary tract; not otherwise specified

54600–54620

00920 Anesthesia for procedures on male genitalia (including open urethral procedures); not otherwise specified

54640–54650

00930 Anesthesia for procedures on male genitalia (including open urethral procedures); orchiopexy, unilateral or bilateral

54660–54680

00920 Anesthesia for procedures on male genitalia (including open urethral procedures); not otherwise specified

54690–54692

00840 Anesthesia for intraperitoneal procedures in lower abdomen including laparoscopy; not otherwise specified

54700–55200

00920 Anesthesia for procedures on male genitalia (including open urethral procedures); not otherwise specified

55250

00869 Anesthesia for extraperitoneal procedures in lower abdomen, including urinary tract; vasectomy, unilateral/bilateral

55300–55400

00920 Anesthesia for procedures on male genitalia (including open urethral procedures); not otherwise specified

55450

00869 Anesthesia for extraperitoneal procedures in lower abdomen, including urinary tract; vasectomy, unilateral/bilateral

55500–55530

00920 Anesthesia for procedures on male genitalia (including open urethral procedures); not otherwise specified

55535

00840 Anesthesia for intraperitoneal procedures in lower abdomen including laparoscopy; not otherwise specified

55540

00830 Anesthesia for hernia repairs in lower abdomen; not otherwise specified

55550

00840 Anesthesia for intraperitoneal procedures in lower abdomen including laparoscopy; not otherwise specified

55600–55680

00922 Anesthesia for procedures on male genitalia (including open urethral procedures); seminal vesicles

55700–55725

00400 Anesthesia for procedures on the integumentary system on the extremities, anterior trunk and perineum; not otherwise specified

55801

00908 Anesthesia for; perineal prostatectomy

55810–55815

00904 Anesthesia for; radical perineal procedure

55821–55845

00865 Anesthesia for extraperitoneal procedures in lower abdomen, including urinary tract; radical prostatectomy (suprapubic, retropubic)

55859

00400 Anesthesia for procedures on the integumentary system on the extremities, anterior trunk and perineum; not otherwise specified

55860–55865

00860 Anesthesia for extraperitoneal procedures in lower abdomen, including urinary tract; not otherwise specified

55870

00902 Anesthesia for; anorectal procedure

55873

00910 Anesthesia for transurethral procedures (including urethrocystoscopy); not otherwise specified

55970–55980

00904 Anesthesia for; radical perineal procedure

56405–56605

00940 Anesthesia for vaginal procedures (including biopsy of labia, vagina, cervix or endometrium); not otherwise specified

56620–56625

00906 Anesthesia for; vulvectomy

56630–56640

00904 Anesthesia for; radical perineal procedure

56700–56805

00940 Anesthesia for vaginal procedures (including biopsy of labia, vagina, cervix or endometrium); not otherwise specified

56810

00400 Anesthesia for procedures on the integumentary system on the extremities, anterior trunk and perineum; not otherwise specified

57000–57010

00942 Anesthesia for vaginal procedures (including biopsy of labia, vagina, cervix or endometrium); colpotomy, vaginectomy, colporrhaphy, and open urethral procedures

57022–57105

00940 Anesthesia for vaginal procedures (including biopsy of labia, vagina, cervix or endometrium); not otherwise specified

57106–57107

00942 Anesthesia for vaginal procedures (including biopsy of labia, vagina, cervix or endometrium); colpotomy, vaginectomy, colporrhaphy, and open urethral procedures

57109
00940   Anesthesia for vaginal procedures (including biopsy of labia, vagina, cervix or endometrium); not otherwise specified

57110–57111
00942   Anesthesia for vaginal procedures (including biopsy of labia, vagina, cervix or endometrium); colpotomy, vaginectomy, colporrhaphy, and open urethral procedures

57112
00940   Anesthesia for vaginal procedures (including biopsy of labia, vagina, cervix or endometrium); not otherwise specified

57120
00942   Anesthesia for vaginal procedures (including biopsy of labia, vagina, cervix or endometrium); colpotomy, vaginectomy, colporrhaphy, and open urethral procedures

57130–57135
00940   Anesthesia for vaginal procedures (including biopsy of labia, vagina, cervix or endometrium); not otherwise specified

57155
00940   Anesthesia for vaginal procedures (including biopsy of labia, vagina, cervix or endometrium); not otherwise specified

57200–57210
00942   Anesthesia for vaginal procedures (including biopsy of labia, vagina, cervix or endometrium); colpotomy, vaginectomy, colporrhaphy, and open urethral procedures

57220–57230
00940   Anesthesia for vaginal procedures (including biopsy of labia, vagina, cervix or endometrium); not otherwise specified

57240–57268
00942   Anesthesia for vaginal procedures (including biopsy of labia, vagina, cervix or endometrium); colpotomy, vaginectomy, colporrhaphy, and open urethral procedures

57270–57282
00840   Anesthesia for intraperitoneal procedures in lower abdomen including laparoscopy; not otherwise specified

57284–57289
00942   Anesthesia for vaginal procedures (including biopsy of labia, vagina, cervix or endometrium); colpotomy, vaginectomy, colporrhaphy, and open urethral procedures

57291–57292
00904   Anesthesia for; radical perineal procedure

57300
00902   Anesthesia for; anorectal procedure

57305–57307
00840   Anesthesia for intraperitoneal procedures in lower abdomen including laparoscopy; not otherwise specified

57308
00904   Anesthesia for; radical perineal procedure

57310–57320
00940   Anesthesia for vaginal procedures (including biopsy of labia, vagina, cervix or endometrium); not otherwise specified

57330
00860   Anesthesia for extraperitoneal procedures in lower abdomen, including urinary tract; not otherwise specified

57335–57530
00940   Anesthesia for vaginal procedures (including biopsy of labia, vagina, cervix or endometrium); not otherwise specified

57531
00846   Anesthesia for intraperitoneal procedures in lower abdomen including laparoscopy; radical hysterectomy

57540–57545
00840   Anesthesia for intraperitoneal procedures in lower abdomen including laparoscopy; not otherwise specified

57550
00940   Anesthesia for vaginal procedures (including biopsy of labia, vagina, cervix or endometrium); not otherwise specified

57555–57556
00942   Anesthesia for vaginal procedures (including biopsy of labia, vagina, cervix or endometrium); colpotomy, vaginectomy, colporrhaphy, and open urethral procedures

57700
00948   Anesthesia for vaginal procedures (including biopsy of labia, vagina, cervix or endometrium); cervical cerclage

57720
00942   Anesthesia for vaginal procedures (including biopsy of labia, vagina, cervix or endometrium); colpotomy, vaginectomy, colporrhaphy, and open urethral procedures

57800–58120
00940   Anesthesia for vaginal procedures (including biopsy of labia, vagina, cervix or endometrium); not otherwise specified

58140
00840   Anesthesia for intraperitoneal procedures in lower abdomen including laparoscopy; not otherwise specified

58145
00940   Anesthesia for vaginal procedures (including biopsy of labia, vagina, cervix or endometrium); not otherwise specified

58150–58200
00840   Anesthesia for intraperitoneal procedures in lower abdomen including laparoscopy; not otherwise specified

58210
00846   Anesthesia for intraperitoneal procedures in lower abdomen including laparoscopy; radical hysterectomy

58240
00848   Anesthesia for intraperitoneal procedures in lower abdomen including laparoscopy; pelvic exenteration

58260–58285
00944   Anesthesia for vaginal procedures (including biopsy of labia, vagina, cervix or endometrium); vaginal hysterectomy

58300–58322
00940   Anesthesia for vaginal procedures (including biopsy of labia, vagina, cervix or endometrium); not otherwise specified

58340–58345
00952   Anesthesia for vaginal procedures (including biopsy of labia, vagina, cervix or endometrium); hysteroscopy and/or hysterosalpingography

58346
00940   Anesthesia for vaginal procedures (including biopsy of labia, vagina, cervix or endometrium); not otherwise specified

58350
00952   Anesthesia for vaginal procedures (including biopsy of labia, vagina, cervix or endometrium); hysteroscopy and/or hysterosalpingography

58353
00940   Anesthesia for vaginal procedures (including biopsy of labia, vagina, cervix or endometrium); not otherwise specified

58400–58551
00840   Anesthesia for intraperitoneal procedures in lower abdomen including laparoscopy; not otherwise specified

58555–58563
00952   Anesthesia for vaginal procedures (including biopsy of labia, vagina, cervix or endometrium); hysteroscopy and/or hysterosalpingography

58600–58605
00851   Anesthesia for intraperitoneal procedures in lower abdomen including laparoscopy; tubal ligation/transection

58615
00851   Anesthesia for intraperitoneal procedures in lower abdomen including laparoscopy; tubal ligation/transection

58660–58662
00840   Anesthesia for intraperitoneal procedures in lower abdomen including laparoscopy; not otherwise specified

58670–58671
00851   Anesthesia for intraperitoneal procedures in lower abdomen including laparoscopy; tubal ligation/transection

58672–58673
00840   Anesthesia for intraperitoneal procedures in lower abdomen including laparoscopy; not otherwise specified

58700–58770
00840   Anesthesia for intraperitoneal procedures in lower abdomen including laparoscopy; not otherwise specified

58800
00940   Anesthesia for vaginal procedures (including biopsy of labia, vagina, cervix or endometrium); not otherwise specified

58805
00840   Anesthesia for intraperitoneal procedures in lower abdomen including laparoscopy; not otherwise specified

58820
00940   Anesthesia for vaginal procedures (including biopsy of labia, vagina, cervix or endometrium); not otherwise specified

58822
00840   Anesthesia for intraperitoneal procedures in lower abdomen including laparoscopy; not otherwise specified

58823

00940   Anesthesia for vaginal procedures (including biopsy of labia, vagina, cervix or endometrium); not otherwise specified

58825–58950

00840   Anesthesia for intraperitoneal procedures in lower abdomen including laparoscopy; not otherwise specified

58951–58952

00846   Anesthesia for intraperitoneal procedures in lower abdomen including laparoscopy; radical hysterectomy

58953–58970

00840   Anesthesia for intraperitoneal procedures in lower abdomen including laparoscopy; not otherwise specified

58974

00940   Anesthesia for vaginal procedures (including biopsy of labia, vagina, cervix or endometrium); not otherwise specified

58976

00840   Anesthesia for intraperitoneal procedures in lower abdomen including laparoscopy; not otherwise specified

59012–59015

00842   Anesthesia for intraperitoneal procedures in lower abdomen including laparoscopy; amniocentesis

59100–59136

00840   Anesthesia for intraperitoneal procedures in lower abdomen including laparoscopy; not otherwise specified

59140

00940   Anesthesia for vaginal procedures (including biopsy of labia, vagina, cervix or endometrium); not otherwise specified

59150–59151

00840   Anesthesia for intraperitoneal procedures in lower abdomen including laparoscopy; not otherwise specified

59160

00940   Anesthesia for vaginal procedures (including biopsy of labia, vagina, cervix or endometrium); not otherwise specified

59300

00940   Anesthesia for vaginal procedures (including biopsy of labia, vagina, cervix or endometrium); not otherwise specified

59320

00948   Anesthesia for vaginal procedures (including biopsy of labia, vagina, cervix or endometrium); cervical cerclage

59325–59350

00840   Anesthesia for intraperitoneal procedures in lower abdomen including laparoscopy; not otherwise specified

59409

01960   Anesthesia for; vaginal delivery only

59514

01961   Anesthesia for; cesarean delivery only

59612

01960   Anesthesia for; vaginal delivery only

59620

01961   Anesthesia for; cesarean delivery only

59812–59841

01964   Anesthesia for; abortion procedures

59850–59851

00940   Anesthesia for vaginal procedures (including biopsy of labia, vagina, cervix or endometrium); not otherwise specified

59852

00840   Anesthesia for intraperitoneal procedures in lower abdomen including laparoscopy; not otherwise specified

59855–59856

00940   Anesthesia for vaginal procedures (including biopsy of labia, vagina, cervix or endometrium); not otherwise specified

59857–59866

00840   Anesthesia for intraperitoneal procedures in lower abdomen including laparoscopy; not otherwise specified

59870

00940   Anesthesia for vaginal procedures (including biopsy of labia, vagina, cervix or endometrium); not otherwise specified

59871

01964   Anesthesia for; abortion procedures

60000

00300   Anesthesia for all procedures on the integumentary system, muscles and nerves of head, neck, and posterior trunk, not otherwise specified

60001–60100
00322   Anesthesia for all procedures on esophagus, thyroid, larynx, trachea and lymphatic system of neck; needle biopsy of thyroid

60200–60260
00320   Anesthesia for all procedures on esophagus, thyroid, larynx, trachea and lymphatic system of neck; not otherwise specified

60270
00540   Anesthesia for thoracotomy procedures involving lungs, pleura, diaphragm, and mediastinum (including surgical thoracoscopy); not otherwise specified

60271–60502
00320   Anesthesia for all procedures on esophagus, thyroid, larynx, trachea and lymphatic system of neck; not otherwise specified

60505
00540   Anesthesia for thoracotomy procedures involving lungs, pleura, diaphragm, and mediastinum (including surgical thoracoscopy); not otherwise specified

60520
00320   Anesthesia for all procedures on esophagus, thyroid, larynx, trachea and lymphatic system of neck; not otherwise specified

60521–60522
00540   Anesthesia for thoracotomy procedures involving lungs, pleura, diaphragm, and mediastinum (including surgical thoracoscopy); not otherwise specified

60540–60545
00866   Anesthesia for extraperitoneal procedures in lower abdomen, including urinary tract; adrenalectomy

60600
00320   Anesthesia for all procedures on esophagus, thyroid, larynx, trachea and lymphatic system of neck; not otherwise specified

60605
00350   Anesthesia for procedures on major vessels of neck; not otherwise specified

60650
00840   Anesthesia for intraperitoneal procedures in lower abdomen including laparoscopy; not otherwise specified

61000–61050
00212   Anesthesia for intracranial procedures; subdural taps

61105–61210
00214   Anesthesia for intracranial procedures; burr holes, including ventriculography

61215
00400   Anesthesia for procedures on the integumentary system on the extremities, anterior trunk and perineum; not otherwise specified

61250–61253
00214   Anesthesia for intracranial procedures; burr holes, including ventriculography

61304
00210   Anesthesia for intracranial procedures; not otherwise specified

61305
00218   Anesthesia for intracranial procedures; procedures in sitting position

61312–61313
00210   Anesthesia for intracranial procedures; not otherwise specified

61314–61315
00218   Anesthesia for intracranial procedures; procedures in sitting position

61320
00210   Anesthesia for intracranial procedures; not otherwise specified

61321
00218   Anesthesia for intracranial procedures; procedures in sitting position

61330–61340
00210   Anesthesia for intracranial procedures; not otherwise specified

61343–61345
00218   Anesthesia for intracranial procedures; procedures in sitting position

61440–61350
00210   Anesthesia for intracranial procedures; not otherwise specified

61458
00218   Anesthesia for intracranial procedures; procedures in sitting position

61460–61516
00210   Anesthesia for intracranial procedures; not otherwise specified

61518–61524
00218   Anesthesia for intracranial procedures; procedures in sitting position

61526
00210 Anesthesia for intracranial procedures; not otherwise specified

61530
00218 Anesthesia for intracranial procedures; procedures in sitting position

61531–61608
00210 Anesthesia for intracranial procedures; not otherwise specified

61613
00216 Anesthesia for intracranial procedures; vascular procedures

61615–61619
00210 Anesthesia for intracranial procedures; not otherwise specified

61624
00210 Anesthesia for intracranial procedures; not otherwise specified
00216 Anesthesia for intracranial procedures; vascular procedures
00600 Anesthesia for procedures on cervical spine and cord; not otherwise specified
00630 Anesthesia for procedures in lumbar region; not otherwise specified
00620 Anesthesia for procedures on thoracic spine and cord; not otherwise specified

61626
00210 Anesthesia for intracranial procedures; not otherwise specified
00350 Anesthesia for procedures on major vessels of neck; not otherwise specified
00216 Anesthesia for intracranial procedures; vascular procedures

61680–61711
00216 Anesthesia for intracranial procedures; vascular procedures

61720
00210 Anesthesia for intracranial procedures; not otherwise specified

61735
00214 Anesthesia for intracranial procedures; burr holes, including ventriculography

61750–61760
00210 Anesthesia for intracranial procedures; not otherwise specified

61770
00214 Anesthesia for intracranial procedures; burr holes, including ventriculography

61790–61791
00222 Anesthesia for intracranial procedures; electrocoagulation of intracranial nerve

61850
00214 Anesthesia for intracranial procedures; burr holes, including ventriculography

61860–61880
00210 Anesthesia for intracranial procedures; not otherwise specified

61885–61888
00300 Anesthesia for all procedures on the integumentary system, muscles and nerves of head, neck, and posterior trunk, not otherwise specified

62000–62005
00215 Anesthesia for intracranial procedures; cranioplasty or elevation of depressed skull fracture, extradural (simple or compound)

62010–62115
00210 Anesthesia for intracranial procedures; not otherwise specified

62116
00215 Anesthesia for intracranial procedures; cranioplasty or elevation of depressed skull fracture, extradural (simple or compound)

62117
00210 Anesthesia for intracranial procedures; not otherwise specified

62120
00215 Anesthesia for intracranial procedures; cranioplasty or elevation of depressed skull fracture, extradural (simple or compound)

62121
00210 Anesthesia for intracranial procedures; not otherwise specified

62140–62141
00215 Anesthesia for intracranial procedures; cranioplasty or elevation of depressed skull fracture, extradural (simple or compound)

62142–62145
00210 Anesthesia for intracranial procedures; not otherwise specified

62146–62147
00215 Anesthesia for intracranial procedures; cranioplasty or elevation of depressed skull fracture, extradural (simple or compound)

62180–62230
00220 Anesthesia for intracranial procedures; cerebrospinal fluid shunting procedures

62256–62258
00220 Anesthesia for intracranial procedures; cerebrospinal fluid shunting procedures

62268–62269
00620 Anesthesia for procedures on thoracic spine and cord; not otherwise specified
00630 Anesthesia for procedures in lumbar region; not otherwise specified
00600 Anesthesia for procedures on cervical spine and cord; not otherwise specified

62350–62355
00630 Anesthesia for procedures in lumbar region; not otherwise specified

62360–62362
00300 Anesthesia for all procedures on the integumentary system, muscles and nerves of head, neck, and posterior trunk, not otherwise specified

62365
00630 Anesthesia for procedures in lumbar region; not otherwise specified

63001
00600 Anesthesia for procedures on cervical spine and cord; not otherwise specified

63003
00620 Anesthesia for procedures on thoracic spine and cord; not otherwise specified

63005–63012
00630 Anesthesia for procedures in lumbar region; not otherwise specified

63015
00600 Anesthesia for procedures on cervical spine and cord; not otherwise specified

63016
00620 Anesthesia for procedures on thoracic spine and cord; not otherwise specified

63017
00630 Anesthesia for procedures in lumbar region; not otherwise specified

63020
00600 Anesthesia for procedures on cervical spine and cord; not otherwise specified

63030
00630 Anesthesia for procedures in lumbar region; not otherwise specified

63040
00600 Anesthesia for procedures on cervical spine and cord; not otherwise specified
00604 Anesthesia for procedures on cervical spine and cord; procedures with patient in the sitting position

63042
00630 Anesthesia for procedures in lumbar region; not otherwise specified

63045
00600 Anesthesia for procedures on cervical spine and cord; not otherwise specified

63046
00620 Anesthesia for procedures on thoracic spine and cord; not otherwise specified

63047
00630 Anesthesia for procedures in lumbar region; not otherwise specified

63055
00620 Anesthesia for procedures on thoracic spine and cord; not otherwise specified

63056
00630 Anesthesia for procedures in lumbar region; not otherwise specified

63064
00620 Anesthesia for procedures on thoracic spine and cord; not otherwise specified

63075
00600 Anesthesia for procedures on cervical spine and cord; not otherwise specified

63077
00620 Anesthesia for procedures on thoracic spine and cord; not otherwise specified

63081
00600 Anesthesia for procedures on cervical spine and cord; not otherwise specified

63085
00620 Anesthesia for procedures on thoracic spine and cord; not otherwise specified

63087
00620 Anesthesia for procedures on thoracic spine and cord; not otherwise specified
00630 Anesthesia for procedures in lumbar region; not otherwise specified

63090
00630 Anesthesia for procedures in lumbar region; not otherwise specified

Anesthesia Crosswalk

63170

00600   Anesthesia for procedures on cervical spine and cord; not otherwise specified

00630   Anesthesia for procedures in lumbar region; not otherwise specified

00604   Anesthesia for procedures on cervical spine and cord; procedures with patient in the sitting position

00620   Anesthesia for procedures on thoracic spine and cord; not otherwise specified

63172–63173

00670   Anesthesia for extensive spine and spinal cord procedures (eg, spinal instrumentation or vascular procedures)

63180–63182

00600   Anesthesia for procedures on cervical spine and cord; not otherwise specified

63185–63190

00630   Anesthesia for procedures in lumbar region; not otherwise specified

63191–63194

00600   Anesthesia for procedures on cervical spine and cord; not otherwise specified

63195

00620   Anesthesia for procedures on thoracic spine and cord; not otherwise specified

63196

00600   Anesthesia for procedures on cervical spine and cord; not otherwise specified

63197

00620   Anesthesia for procedures on thoracic spine and cord; not otherwise specified

63198

00600   Anesthesia for procedures on cervical spine and cord; not otherwise specified

63199

00620   Anesthesia for procedures on thoracic spine and cord; not otherwise specified

63200

00630   Anesthesia for procedures in lumbar region; not otherwise specified

63250–63252

00670   Anesthesia for extensive spine and spinal cord procedures (eg, spinal instrumentation or vascular procedures)

63265

00600   Anesthesia for procedures on cervical spine and cord; not otherwise specified

63266

00620   Anesthesia for procedures on thoracic spine and cord; not otherwise specified

63267–63268

00630   Anesthesia for procedures in lumbar region; not otherwise specified

63270

00600   Anesthesia for procedures on cervical spine and cord; not otherwise specified

63271

00620   Anesthesia for procedures on thoracic spine and cord; not otherwise specified

63272–63273

00630   Anesthesia for procedures in lumbar region; not otherwise specified

63275

00600   Anesthesia for procedures on cervical spine and cord; not otherwise specified

63276

00620   Anesthesia for procedures on thoracic spine and cord; not otherwise specified

63277–63278

00630   Anesthesia for procedures in lumbar region; not otherwise specified

63280

00600   Anesthesia for procedures on cervical spine and cord; not otherwise specified

63281

00620   Anesthesia for procedures on thoracic spine and cord; not otherwise specified

63282

00630   Anesthesia for procedures in lumbar region; not otherwise specified

63283

01120   Anesthesia for procedures on bony pelvis

63285

00600   Anesthesia for procedures on cervical spine and cord; not otherwise specified

63286

00620   Anesthesia for procedures on thoracic spine and cord; not otherwise specified

63287

00630   Anesthesia for procedures in lumbar region; not otherwise specified

63300
00600 Anesthesia for procedures on cervical spine and cord; not otherwise specified

63301–63302
00620 Anesthesia for procedures on thoracic spine and cord; not otherwise specified

63303
00630 Anesthesia for procedures in lumbar region; not otherwise specified

63304
00600 Anesthesia for procedures on cervical spine and cord; not otherwise specified

63305–63306
00620 Anesthesia for procedures on thoracic spine and cord; not otherwise specified

63307
00630 Anesthesia for procedures in lumbar region; not otherwise specified

63600
00630 Anesthesia for procedures in lumbar region; not otherwise specified

00600 Anesthesia for procedures on cervical spine and cord; not otherwise specified

63610
00630 Anesthesia for procedures in lumbar region; not otherwise specified

63615
00600 Anesthesia for procedures on cervical spine and cord; not otherwise specified

00630 Anesthesia for procedures in lumbar region; not otherwise specified

00620 Anesthesia for procedures on thoracic spine and cord; not otherwise specified

63650
00630 Anesthesia for procedures in lumbar region; not otherwise specified

63660
00630 Anesthesia for procedures in lumbar region; not otherwise specified

63685
00400 Anesthesia for procedures on the integumentary system on the extremities, anterior trunk and perineum; not otherwise specified

63688
00300 Anesthesia for all procedures on the integumentary system, muscles and nerves of head, neck, and posterior trunk, not otherwise specified

63700–63746
00630 Anesthesia for procedures in lumbar region; not otherwise specified

64573
00300 Anesthesia for all procedures on the integumentary system, muscles and nerves of head, neck, and posterior trunk, not otherwise specified

64575
01250 Anesthesia for all procedures on nerves, muscles, tendons, fascia, and bursae of upper leg

01320 Anesthesia for all procedures on nerves, muscles, tendons, fascia, and bursae of knee and/or popliteal area

01810 Anesthesia for all procedures on nerves, muscles, tendons, fascia, and bursae of forearm, wrist, and hand

01470 Anesthesia for procedures on nerves, muscles, tendons, and fascia of lower leg, ankle, and foot; not otherwise specified

01610 Anesthesia for all procedures on nerves, muscles, tendons, fascia, and bursae of shoulder and axilla

01710 Anesthesia for procedures on nerves, muscles, tendons, fascia, and bursae of upper arm and elbow; not otherwise specified

64577
00400 Anesthesia for procedures on the integumentary system on the extremities, anterior trunk and perineum; not otherwise specified

00300 Anesthesia for all procedures on the integumentary system, muscles and nerves of head, neck, and posterior trunk, not otherwise specified

64580
01250 Anesthesia for all procedures on nerves, muscles, tendons, fascia, and bursae of upper leg

01320 Anesthesia for all procedures on nerves, muscles, tendons, fascia, and bursae of knee and/or popliteal area

01710 Anesthesia for procedures on nerves, muscles, tendons, fascia, and bursae of upper arm and elbow; not otherwise specified

01810 Anesthesia for all procedures on nerves, muscles, tendons, fascia, and bursae of forearm, wrist, and hand

01610 Anesthesia for all procedures on nerves, muscles, tendons, fascia, and bursae of shoulder and axilla

01470 Anesthesia for procedures on nerves, muscles, tendons, and fascia of lower leg, ankle, and foot; not otherwise specified

Anesthesia Crosswalk

64581

00300   Anesthesia for all procedures on the integumentary system, muscles and nerves of head, neck, and posterior trunk, not otherwise specified

64702–64704

01470   Anesthesia for procedures on nerves, muscles, tendons, and fascia of lower leg, ankle, and foot; not otherwise specified

01810   Anesthesia for all procedures on nerves, muscles, tendons, fascia, and bursae of forearm, wrist, and hand

64708

01250   Anesthesia for all procedures on nerves, muscles, tendons, fascia, and bursae of upper leg

01470   Anesthesia for procedures on nerves, muscles, tendons, and fascia of lower leg, ankle, and foot; not otherwise specified

01810   Anesthesia for all procedures on nerves, muscles, tendons, fascia, and bursae of forearm, wrist, and hand

01710   Anesthesia for procedures on nerves, muscles, tendons, fascia, and bursae of upper arm and elbow; not otherwise specified

01320   Anesthesia for all procedures on nerves, muscles, tendons, fascia, and bursae of knee and/or popliteal area

64712

01250   Anesthesia for all procedures on nerves, muscles, tendons, fascia, and bursae of upper leg

64713

01610   Anesthesia for all procedures on nerves, muscles, tendons, fascia, and bursae of shoulder and axilla

64714

00630   Anesthesia for procedures in lumbar region; not otherwise specified

64716

00300   Anesthesia for all procedures on the integumentary system, muscles and nerves of head, neck, and posterior trunk, not otherwise specified

64718

01710   Anesthesia for procedures on nerves, muscles, tendons, fascia, and bursae of upper arm and elbow; not otherwise specified

64719–64721

01810   Anesthesia for all procedures on nerves, muscles, tendons, fascia, and bursae of forearm, wrist, and hand

64726

01470   Anesthesia for procedures on nerves, muscles, tendons, and fascia of lower leg, ankle, and foot; not otherwise specified

64732–64736

00300   Anesthesia for all procedures on the integumentary system, muscles and nerves of head, neck, and posterior trunk, not otherwise specified

64738–64740

00170   Anesthesia for intraoral procedures, including biopsy; not otherwise specified

64742–64746

00300   Anesthesia for all procedures on the integumentary system, muscles and nerves of head, neck, and posterior trunk, not otherwise specified

64752

00540   Anesthesia for thoracotomy procedures involving lungs, pleura, diaphragm, and mediastinum (including surgical thoracoscopy); not otherwise specified

64755–64760

00790   Anesthesia for intraperitoneal procedures in upper abdomen including laparoscopy; not otherwise specified

64761–64763

01180   Anesthesia for obturator neurectomy; extrapelvic

64766

01190   Anesthesia for obturator neurectomy; intrapelvic

64771

00210   Anesthesia for intracranial procedures; not otherwise specified

64776

01470   Anesthesia for procedures on nerves, muscles, tendons, and fascia of lower leg, ankle, and foot; not otherwise specified

01810   Anesthesia for all procedures on nerves, muscles, tendons, fascia, and bursae of forearm, wrist, and hand

64782

01810   Anesthesia for all procedures on nerves, muscles, tendons, fascia, and bursae of forearm, wrist, and hand

64786

01250   Anesthesia for all procedures on nerves, muscles, tendons, fascia, and bursae of upper leg

64802–64804
00600 Anesthesia for procedures on cervical spine and cord; not otherwise specified

64809
00622 Anesthesia for procedures on thoracic spine and cord; thoracolumbar sympathectomy

64818
00632 Anesthesia for procedures in lumbar region; lumbar sympathectomy

64820
01470 Anesthesia for procedures on nerves, muscles, tendons, and fascia of lower leg, ankle, and foot; not otherwise specified
01810 Anesthesia for all procedures on nerves, muscles, tendons, fascia, and bursae of forearm, wrist, and hand

64821–64823
01810 Anesthesia for all procedures on nerves, muscles, tendons, fascia, and bursae of forearm, wrist, and hand

64831
01470 Anesthesia for procedures on nerves, muscles, tendons, and fascia of lower leg, ankle, and foot; not otherwise specified
01810 Anesthesia for all procedures on nerves, muscles, tendons, fascia, and bursae of forearm, wrist, and hand

64834
01470 Anesthesia for procedures on nerves, muscles, tendons, and fascia of lower leg, ankle, and foot; not otherwise specified
01810 Anesthesia for all procedures on nerves, muscles, tendons, fascia, and bursae of forearm, wrist, and hand

64835–64836
01810 Anesthesia for all procedures on nerves, muscles, tendons, fascia, and bursae of forearm, wrist, and hand

64840
01470 Anesthesia for procedures on nerves, muscles, tendons, and fascia of lower leg, ankle, and foot; not otherwise specified

64856–64857
01250 Anesthesia for all procedures on nerves, muscles, tendons, fascia, and bursae of upper leg
01810 Anesthesia for all procedures on nerves, muscles, tendons, fascia, and bursae of forearm, wrist, and hand
01320 Anesthesia for all procedures on nerves, muscles, tendons, fascia, and bursae of knee and/or popliteal area

01710
Anesthesia for procedures on nerves, muscles, tendons, fascia, and bursae of upper arm and elbow; not otherwise specified

01470
Anesthesia for procedures on nerves, muscles, tendons, and fascia of lower leg, ankle, and foot; not otherwise specified

64858
00400 Anesthesia for procedures on the integumentary system on the extremities, anterior trunk and perineum; not otherwise specified

64861
01610 Anesthesia for all procedures on nerves, muscles, tendons, fascia, and bursae of shoulder and axilla

64862
00630 Anesthesia for procedures in lumbar region; not otherwise specified

64864
01470 Anesthesia for procedures on nerves, muscles, tendons, and fascia of lower leg, ankle, and foot; not otherwise specified
01810 Anesthesia for all procedures on nerves, muscles, tendons, fascia, and bursae of forearm, wrist, and hand

64865
00210 Anesthesia for intracranial procedures; not otherwise specified

64866–64870
00300 Anesthesia for all procedures on the integumentary system, muscles and nerves of head, neck, and posterior trunk, not otherwise specified

64885–64886
00300 Anesthesia for all procedures on the integumentary system, muscles and nerves of head, neck, and posterior trunk, not otherwise specified

64890–64891
01470 Anesthesia for procedures on nerves, muscles, tendons, and fascia of lower leg, ankle, and foot; not otherwise specified
01810 Anesthesia for all procedures on nerves, muscles, tendons, fascia, and bursae of forearm, wrist, and hand

64892–64893
01610 Anesthesia for all procedures on nerves, muscles, tendons, fascia, and bursae of shoulder and axilla
01470 Anesthesia for procedures on nerves, muscles, tendons, and fascia of lower leg, ankle, and foot; not otherwise specified

Anesthesia Crosswalk

01810   Anesthesia for all procedures on nerves, muscles, tendons, fascia, and bursae of forearm, wrist, and hand

01710   Anesthesia for procedures on nerves, muscles, tendons, fascia, and bursae of upper arm and elbow; not otherwise specified

01320   Anesthesia for all procedures on nerves, muscles, tendons, fascia, and bursae of knee and/or popliteal area

01250   Anesthesia for all procedures on nerves, muscles, tendons, fascia, and bursae of upper leg

64895–64896

01470   Anesthesia for procedures on nerves, muscles, tendons, and fascia of lower leg, ankle, and foot; not otherwise specified

01810   Anesthesia for all procedures on nerves, muscles, tendons, fascia, and bursae of forearm, wrist, and hand

64897

01610   Anesthesia for all procedures on nerves, muscles, tendons, fascia, and bursae of shoulder and axilla

01810   Anesthesia for all procedures on nerves, muscles, tendons, fascia, and bursae of forearm, wrist, and hand

01250   Anesthesia for all procedures on nerves, muscles, tendons, fascia, and bursae of upper leg

01470   Anesthesia for procedures on nerves, muscles, tendons, and fascia of lower leg, ankle, and foot; not otherwise specified

01710   Anesthesia for procedures on nerves, muscles, tendons, fascia, and bursae of upper arm and elbow; not otherwise specified

64898

01610   Anesthesia for all procedures on nerves, muscles, tendons, fascia, and bursae of shoulder and axilla

01250   Anesthesia for all procedures on nerves, muscles, tendons, fascia, and bursae of upper leg

01320   Anesthesia for all procedures on nerves, muscles, tendons, fascia, and bursae of knee and/or popliteal area

01470   Anesthesia for procedures on nerves, muscles, tendons, and fascia of lower leg, ankle, and foot; not otherwise specified

01710   Anesthesia for procedures on nerves, muscles, tendons, fascia, and bursae of upper arm and elbow; not otherwise specified

01810   Anesthesia for all procedures on nerves, muscles, tendons, fascia, and bursae of forearm, wrist, and hand

65091–65175

00140   Anesthesia for procedures on eye; not otherwise specified

65210–65222

00140   Anesthesia for procedures on eye; not otherwise specified

65235

00142   Anesthesia for procedures on eye; lens surgery

65260–65426

00140   Anesthesia for procedures on eye; not otherwise specified

65435–65600

00140   Anesthesia for procedures on eye; not otherwise specified

65710–65755

00144   Anesthesia for procedures on eye; corneal transplant

65760

00140   Anesthesia for procedures on eye; not otherwise specified

65765

00144   Anesthesia for procedures on eye; corneal transplant

65767

00140   Anesthesia for procedures on eye; not otherwise specified

65770

00144   Anesthesia for procedures on eye; corneal transplant

65771–66130

00140   Anesthesia for procedures on eye; not otherwise specified

66150–66160

00147   Anesthesia for procedures on eye; iridectomy

66165–66505

00140   Anesthesia for procedures on eye; not otherwise specified

66600–66635

00147   Anesthesia for procedures on eye; iridectomy

66680–66740

00140   Anesthesia for procedures on eye; not otherwise specified

66761–66762

00147   Anesthesia for procedures on eye; iridectomy

66770

00140   Anesthesia for procedures on eye; not otherwise specified

66820–66986

00142   Anesthesia for procedures on eye; lens surgery

67005–67027

00145   Anesthesia for procedures on eye; vitreoretinal surgery

67028

00140   Anesthesia for procedures on eye; not otherwise specified

67030–67040

00145   Anesthesia for procedures on eye; vitreoretinal surgery

67101–67107

00140   Anesthesia for procedures on eye; not otherwise specified

67108

00145   Anesthesia for procedures on eye; vitreoretinal surgery

67110

00140   Anesthesia for procedures on eye; not otherwise specified

67112

00145   Anesthesia for procedures on eye; vitreoretinal surgery

67115–67221

00140   Anesthesia for procedures on eye; not otherwise specified

67227–67255

00140   Anesthesia for procedures on eye; not otherwise specified

67311–67318

00140   Anesthesia for procedures on eye; not otherwise specified

67343–67350

00140   Anesthesia for procedures on eye; not otherwise specified

67400–67415

00140   Anesthesia for procedures on eye; not otherwise specified

67420–67450

00190   Anesthesia for procedures on facial bones or skull; not otherwise specified

67550–67570

00140   Anesthesia for procedures on eye; not otherwise specified

67700–67715

00300   Anesthesia for all procedures on the integumentary system, muscles and nerves of head, neck, and posterior trunk, not otherwise specified

67808–67810

00300   Anesthesia for all procedures on the integumentary system, muscles and nerves of head, neck, and posterior trunk, not otherwise specified

67825–67875

00300   Anesthesia for all procedures on the integumentary system, muscles and nerves of head, neck, and posterior trunk, not otherwise specified

67880–67882

00140   Anesthesia for procedures on eye; not otherwise specified

67900

00300   Anesthesia for all procedures on the integumentary system, muscles and nerves of head, neck, and posterior trunk, not otherwise specified

67901–67915

00140   Anesthesia for procedures on eye; not otherwise specified

67916–67917

00103   Anesthesia for reconstructive procedures of eyelid (eg, blepharoplasty, ptosis surgery)

67921–67922

00140   Anesthesia for procedures on eye; not otherwise specified

67923–67924

00103   Anesthesia for reconstructive procedures of eyelid (eg, blepharoplasty, ptosis surgery)

67930–67935

00140   Anesthesia for procedures on eye; not otherwise specified

67938

00300   Anesthesia for all procedures on the integumentary system, muscles and nerves of head, neck, and posterior trunk, not otherwise specified

67950–67975

00140   Anesthesia for procedures on eye; not otherwise specified

Anesthesia Crosswalk

68020–68362
00140 Anesthesia for procedures on eye; not otherwise specified

68400–68850
00140 Anesthesia for procedures on eye; not otherwise specified

69000–69020
00120 Anesthesia for procedures on external, middle, and inner ear including biopsy; not otherwise specified

69100–69150
00120 Anesthesia for procedures on external, middle, and inner ear including biopsy; not otherwise specified

69155
00320 Anesthesia for all procedures on esophagus, thyroid, larynx, trachea and lymphatic system of neck; not otherwise specified

69205–69210
00124 Anesthesia for procedures on external, middle, and inner ear including biopsy; otoscopy

69220–69320
00120 Anesthesia for procedures on external, middle, and inner ear including biopsy; not otherwise specified

69400–69401
00160 Anesthesia for procedures on nose and accessory sinuses; not otherwise specified

69405–69410
00120 Anesthesia for procedures on external, middle, and inner ear including biopsy; not otherwise specified

69420–69424
00126 Anesthesia for procedures on external, middle, and inner ear including biopsy; tympanotomy

69436–69711
00120 Anesthesia for procedures on external, middle, and inner ear including biopsy; not otherwise specified

69714–69718
00190 Anesthesia for procedures on facial bones or skull; not otherwise specified

69720–69745
00120 Anesthesia for procedures on external, middle, and inner ear including biopsy; not otherwise specified

69801–69930
00120 Anesthesia for procedures on external, middle, and inner ear including biopsy; not otherwise specified

69950
00210 Anesthesia for intracranial procedures; not otherwise specified

69955–69960
00120 Anesthesia for procedures on external, middle, and inner ear including biopsy; not otherwise specified

69970
00210 Anesthesia for intracranial procedures; not otherwise specified

85095
01120 Anesthesia for procedures on bony pelvis

85102
01120 Anesthesia for procedures on bony pelvis

90870
00104 Anesthesia for electroconvulsive therapy

90871
00104 Anesthesia for electroconvulsive therapy

92018
00148 Anesthesia for procedures on eye; ophthalmoscopy

92019
00148 Anesthesia for procedures on eye; ophthalmoscopy

92502
00124 Anesthesia for procedures on external, middle, and inner ear including biopsy; otoscopy

92511
00160 Anesthesia for procedures on nose and accessory sinuses; not otherwise specified

92960
00410 Anesthesia for procedures on the integumentary system on the extremities, anterior trunk and perineum; electrical conversion of arrhythmias

92961
00410 Anesthesia for procedures on the integumentary system on the extremities, anterior trunk and perineum; electrical conversion of arrhythmias

93318
00740   Anesthesia for upper gastrointestinal endoscopic procedures, endoscope introduced proximal to duodenum

93600
00537   Anesthesia for cardiac electrophysiologic procedures including radiofrequency ablation

93602
00537   Anesthesia for cardiac electrophysiologic procedures including radiofrequency ablation

93603
00537   Anesthesia for cardiac electrophysiologic procedures including radiofrequency ablation

93607
00537   Anesthesia for cardiac electrophysiologic procedures including radiofrequency ablation

93609
00537   Anesthesia for cardiac electrophysiologic procedures including radiofrequency ablation

93610
00537   Anesthesia for cardiac electrophysiologic procedures including radiofrequency ablation

93612
00537   Anesthesia for cardiac electrophysiologic procedures including radiofrequency ablation

93615
00537   Anesthesia for cardiac electrophysiologic procedures including radiofrequency ablation

93616
00537   Anesthesia for cardiac electrophysiologic procedures including radiofrequency ablation

93618
00537   Anesthesia for cardiac electrophysiologic procedures including radiofrequency ablation

93619
00537   Anesthesia for cardiac electrophysiologic procedures including radiofrequency ablation

93620
00537   Anesthesia for cardiac electrophysiologic procedures including radiofrequency ablation

93621
00537   Anesthesia for cardiac electrophysiologic procedures including radiofrequency ablation

93622
00537   Anesthesia for cardiac electrophysiologic procedures including radiofrequency ablation

93623
00537   Anesthesia for cardiac electrophysiologic procedures including radiofrequency ablation

93624
00537   Anesthesia for cardiac electrophysiologic procedures including radiofrequency ablation

93631
00537   Anesthesia for cardiac electrophysiologic procedures including radiofrequency ablation

93640
00537   Anesthesia for cardiac electrophysiologic procedures including radiofrequency ablation

93641
00537   Anesthesia for cardiac electrophysiologic procedures including radiofrequency ablation

93642
00537   Anesthesia for cardiac electrophysiologic procedures including radiofrequency ablation

93650
00537   Anesthesia for cardiac electrophysiologic procedures including radiofrequency ablation

93651
00537   Anesthesia for cardiac electrophysiologic procedures including radiofrequency ablation

93652
00537   Anesthesia for cardiac electrophysiologic procedures including radiofrequency ablation

Anesthesia Crosswalk

96440

00524   Anesthesia for closed chest procedures;
        pneumocentesis

96445

00840   Anesthesia for intraperitoneal procedures in
        lower abdomen including laparoscopy; not
        otherwise specified

99170

00400   Anesthesia for procedures on the
        integumentary system on the extremities,
        anterior trunk and perineum; not otherwise
        specified
00902   Anesthesia for; anorectal procedure
00950   Anesthesia for vaginal procedures (including
        biopsy of labia, vagina, cervix or
        endometrium); culdoscopy

Anesthesia Crosswalk

CPT® Lay Descriptions

CPT® descriptions are written for people with medical training but may not offer the details needed to choose a code based on a patient's chart or an operative report. The following overview of the procedures listed in CPT® describe the most common methods of each in general terms. Where possible, descriptions are in lay terms for coders' use. Key words used in the operative report are included to facilitate coding.

Unlisted procedures are generally excluded from this chapter. Be aware that insurance payers review unlisted procedure codes manually, increasing processing time and the need for documentation.

Because some consecutive codes describe similar procedures, their descriptions have been combined under one heading, which indicates the range of codes described. If a satisfactory code description cannot be matched with the patient's chart, consult the physician.

0001T–0002T

Endovascular repair or dissection of an infrarenal aortic aneurysm requires the skills of both a vascular surgeon and a radiologist. General anesthesia is typically used. In endovascular repair, a small incision is made in the groin over one femoral artery or both femoral arteries through which the endovascular devices are inserted. If contralateral femoral access is necessary, a percutaneous sheath may be placed. Under separately reported fluoroscopy, a synthetic stent graft contained inside a plastic holding capsule is thread through the arteries to the site of the infrarenal aneurysm. Once the stent is in place, the holding capsule is removed. The stent graft is anchored into place with a modular bifurcated prosthesis with two docking limbs that are pulled down and released into the appropriate axis (0001T). Alternatively, under separate fluoroscopy, the aorto-uni-iliac or aorto-unifemoral prosthetic fabric graft device (0002T), which is supported along its entire length by a series of metal rings sutured to the graft, is brought through the opening to the site of the infrarenal aneurysm. The endograft is held in place by the radial force applied by the rings to the patient's aorta. Once in place, the arteriotomy site is closed.

0003T

Cervicography is a system of cervical cancer screening that uses a static photographic image of the ectocervix, taken with a specially designed camera for evaluation purposes and to provide photo documentation. The physician inserts a speculum for visualization of the cervix. A Pap smear is obtained and the cervix is cleaned using an acetic acid solution; any bleeding is stopped and discharge removed from the posterior fornix. The physician views the cervix through the camera, noting obstructions and observing the acetic acid effect on the epithelium. A second application of acetic acid solution is applied. Adjustments are made and obstructions are removed, including blood, mucus, hair, or excessive pooling of the acetic acid in the posterior fornix. Two images are taken within 30 seconds of the second application of the acetic acid solution. If the acetic acid effect wears off, the physician reapplies the solution and takes the remaining images. A negative evaluation means that no lesion was visible to the evaluator and if a lesion does exist, it may be in the endocervical canal.

0005T–0006T

Duplex examination of the extracranial cerebral arteries is initially performed (reported separately) to identify stenosis, occlusion, dissection, fibromuscular dysplasias, aneurysm, carotid body tumors, kinking, and subclavian steal syndrome. The patient is placed under general anesthesia. The procedure is performed percutaneously from an arterial approach. A stent is loaded into a delivery pod that is advanced up to the narrowing artery from the groin through a standard catheter. Once in position, the stent is advanced out of the pod until its arms partially extrude from the sheath. The stent expands to open the narrowing. The position is confirmed both by angiocardiography and by transthoracic echocardiography. Category III code 0005T reports the placement of the stent in the initial vessel and 0006T is used to report each additional vessel for the separately reported primary procedure.

0007T

The patient is placed under general anesthesia. The procedure is performed percutaneously from an arterial approach. A stent is loaded into a delivery pod that is advanced up to the narrowing artery from the groin through a standard catheter. Once in position, the stent is advanced out of the pod until its arms partially extrude from the sheath. The stent expands to open the narrowing. The position is confirmed both by angiocardiography and by transthoracic echocardiography. This code reports the radiological supervision and interpretation only for this procedure, each vessel.

0008T

The physician uses an endoscope to examine the upper gastrointestinal tract and performs suturing of the esophagogastric junction. The physician passes an endoscope through the patient's mouth into the esophagus. The entire esophagus, stomach, duodenum, and sometimes the jejunum are examined. The scope is withdrawn to the level of the esophagogastric junction. Using a special suturing system inserted through the scope, the physician places a series of stitches in the esophagogastric junction, essentially pleating the sphincter to prevent the backflow of stomach acid into the esophagus. The suturing instrument and scope are removed.

0009T

The physician performs a sterile prep of the vagina and inserts a speculum for visualization of the cervix. A numbing block is placed in the cervix. The ultra thin cryoablation device is inserted through the cervix and the uterus is frozen via a 5.5 mm probe with a tip that is cooled through conductive heat transfer from the coolant-charged control unit. The instrument is withdrawn following completion of the procedure. Ultrasound provides visualization of probe placement and real-time monitoring of the ice ball growth.

0010T

This tuberculosis test uses whole blood for detecting cell-mediated immune responses. The test is based on lymphocytes in the blood that maintain a memory for certain antigens. Adding an antigen to blood results in restimulation of antigen-specific and memory T cells along with the release of the cytokine Interferon-gamma (IFN-gamma), a specific marker for a cellular immune response. Samples of whole blood are incubated overnight with controls. After overnight incubation, samples of plasma are used for IFN-gamma quantification in a single-step enzyme linked immunoabsorbent assay (ELISA). Plasma samples react to antibodies in the solution. Any unbound material is removed by washing. Enzyme substrate is added and after 30 minutes the amount of color development is estimated by spectrophotometer.

0012T–0013T

The physician harvests small circular autogenous grafts (4.5 mm in diameter and 15-20 mm deep) from the non-weight bearing regions of the knee and the grafts are transplanted in a mosaic pattern until the osteochondral defect is filled in a process called Mosaicplasty. Typically, the grafts are harvested from the periphery of the supero-lateral trochlea, but often, the superomedial portion, with drill tunnels 1.0 millimeter apart. The osteochondral graft is fixed by wire. Fibrocartilage fills in the residual defects. Report 0013T if allografts are used to treat the articular surface defects.

0014T

The physician performs meniscal transplantation using an allograft (transplant) from a cadaver donor. The procedure may be performed by an arthrotomy or arthroscopy approach. The patient is placed under anesthesia. The physician makes an incision in the knee and carries dissection down to the joint, or the physician inserts an arthroscope and other ports (to pass instruments) into the joint. Once in the joint capsule, the physician prepares the surface for the transplant. The appropriately sized and shaped frozen, freeze-dried, or cryopreserved transplant is fitted in the correct anatomical position and sutured in place. The incision is closed.

0016T

Transpupillary thermotherapy is a subthreshold laser photocoagulation technique that can result in closure of choroidal neovascularization (CNV) while sparing the neurosensory retina. Treatment is typically done without retrobulbar anesthesia, though topical anesthesia may be applied. The laser aiming beam is set at low to moderate intensity and the ophthalmologist bisects the retina by a moderate-to-high slit beam to visualize the retina and the RPE. Treatment is stopped at the first sign of retinal color change. Settings for treatment of occult CNV (in lightly pigmented fundi) are 800 mW for one minute for a 3-mm spot size. Classic CNV generally requires less power.

0017T

Laser treatment in patients with dry, age-related macular degeneration (AMD) has been shown to cause resorption of drusen, which may benefit the natural course of the disease. There are ongoing clinical trials that utilize "sub-threshold" diode laser treatment that minimizes damage to the retina and is not perceptible to the patient or to the clinician. The method consists of placing a grid of 48 ophthalmoscopically invisible diode laser spots around the macula. The ophthalmologist administers photocoagulation as a grid in four concentric rings that spares the fovea. The dose for threshold is determined by placing a test spot on the nasal retina using a 200-msec pulse duration and increasing the power to produce a barely visible gray lesion.

0018T

Transcranial magnetic stimulation (TMS) is a technique to stimulate the brain by electromagnetic induction with a coil placed on the scalp. For direct stimulation to cortical neurons, a strong magnetic field pulse is generated over the patient's scalp to activate cortical neurons in the brain. This procedure has been applied to activate neuronal processes and to disturb the normal operation of the brain.

0019T–0020T

Extracorporeal shock wave therapy involves the application of pressure waves that travel through fluid and soft tissue, with effects of the therapy occurring at sites where there is a change in impedence, such as the bone-soft tissue interface. The clinician can deliver the therapy in various ways: piezoelectric, electromagnetic, and electrohydraulic. The piezoelectric system utilizes a crystalline material, which when stimulated with high voltage electricity can expand or contract to initiate a pressure wave in the surrounding fluid. The electromagnetic mechanism has coils that create opposite magnetic fields when an electric current is applied to them causing a submerged membrane to move, starting a pressure wave within the fluid. The electrohydraulic method uses a high voltage spark gap. The spark generates a plasma bubble that compresses the liquid, initiating the pressure wave. Each mechanism creates a characteristic waveform and energy density. Extracorporeal shock wave therapy is used in Europe to treat common orthopedic conditions (i.e., plantar calcaneal spurs, epicondylopathic humeri radialis) because of the therapy's stimulatory effect on bone formation. The Food and Drug Administration (FDA) is currently studying the feasibility for similar use in the United States. Other potential uses of osteogenesis by extracorporeal shock wave therapy include bone marrow hypoxia; subperiosteal hemorrhage; increased regional blood flow; and activation of osteogenic factors such as bone morphogenic protein, direct cellular effects, and mechanical effects as a result of strain gradients.

0021T

Oximetry is a method of monitoring intrapartum fetal oxygen saturation (FSpO2) and can be used as an adjunct to fetal heart rate monitoring in the presence of a non-reassuring fetal heart rate pattern. It is used after maternal membranes have ruptured and on a fetus in vertex presentation with gestational age greater than or equal to 36 weeks. The fetal sensor is designed for use in the intrauterine environment. The physician inserts the distal end of the sensor beyond the cervix, to where the sensor is captured between the fetal head and the uterus, with the cable traveling under the cervix and exiting through the birth canal. The sensor does not penetrate the fetal skin. The fulcrum is a smooth and flexible lever arm on the most distal end of the sensor that helps hold the sensor down against the fetal skin. It does this by taking up any remaining space between the fetal head and the adjacent uterine wall. The fulcrum flexes as the spacing between the fetus and the uterus varies to assure continuous contact between the sensor and the skin. Contact electrodes located on the front of the sensor are used to determine if the sensor is in positive contact with the tissue bed. The system determines fetal oxygen saturation by measuring the change in light levels caused by the pulsing arterial blood volume in the tissue. To verify that the system is monitoring oxygen saturation from fetal arterial pulses, the physician can check fetal heart rate by auscultation and palpating the maternal pulse.

0023T

This Category III code describes a test that directly and quantitatively measures resistance of a patient's HIV to antiviral drugs in order to help physicians select appropriate drugs for their HIV patients. The test uses nucleic acid amplification to derive HIV protease (PR) and reverse transcriptase (RT) sequences from a patient plasma sample. A resistance test vector (RTV) is constructed by incorporating the patient-derived segment into a viral vector with an indicator gene, firefly luciferase, inserted within a deleted portion of the HIV envelope gene. Since HIV exists in infected patients as mixtures of genetic variants, RTVs are prepared as large pools of sequences that accurately represent the viral population present in the patient at the time of sample collection. The assay is performed by introducing RTVs into host cells (transfection), collecting virus particles after transfection, and using the particles to infect target cells. The completion of a single round of viral replication results in the production of luciferase. Serial concentrations of PR inhibitors are added at the transfection step and RT inhibitors at the infection step. Drug susceptibility is measured by comparing luciferase activity produced in the presence and absence of drugs. Susceptible viruses produce low levels of luciferase activity in the presence of PR and/or RT inhibitors, whereas viruses with reduced susceptibility to these drugs produce higher levels of luciferase activity.

0024T

Hypertrophic obstructive cardiomyopathy leads to left ventricular outflow tract obstruction. Alternatively dual chamber pacing alters LV contractile pattern and results in reduction in outflow gradient. The physician identifies septal branches of the left anterior descending (LAD) artery, which supply blood to the thickened septum, and injects a small amount of absolute alcohol into the septal branch of the left anterior descending artery that supplies the culprit hypertrophied portion of the interventricular septum. The injection of alcohol results in a controlled myocardial infarction, reducing obstruction and improving symptoms. Controlled injury is produced to the interventricular septum and gradient is reduced thus avoiding overload in the left ventricle.

0025T

Corneal optical pachymetry is the measurement of the thickness of the optical cross section of the cornea viewed in a slit lamp. The slit lamp using oblique illumination observes an oblique slice of cornea. The ophthalmologist makes a physical measurement by rotating the top image (front surface) and aligning it to the bottom image (back surface) and moving an optical marker from the front to the back of the cornea. The optical pachymeter produces two images of the oblique section. The cornea thickness equals the oblique optical section divided by the sine of the observation angle. The measurement technique has several uses, including a parameter that can differentiate a good fitting contact lens from a poor fitting contact lens and corneal health of a transplanted cornea after surgery.

0026T

Remnant lipoproteins are byproducts of chylomicrons, very low-density lipoproteins (VLDL), or both and research indicates that they may be an important risk factor for coronary artery disease. The most typical findings are high triglyceride (Tg) concentrations, low levels of HDL cholesterol (HDLc), and normal or slightly increased IDL cholesterol. To check the levels, blood samples are obtained after an overnight fast and left at room temperature for 30 minutes before separating the serum by centrifugation. Total cholesterol (Tc), Tg, HDLc, and apo(B) are immediately analyzed from total serum. For lipoprotein analysis, a preservative solution is added. Tc and Tg are measured by commercial enzymatic methods in an analyzer. HDLc is measured by a commercial direct method, without precipitation. Intermediate density lipoproteins are calculated by Friedenwald's formula.

10021–10022

Fine needle aspiration (FNA) is a percutaneous procedure that uses a fine gauge needle (22 or 25 gauge) and a syringe to sample fluid from a cyst or remove clusters of cells from a solid mass. First, the skin is cleansed. If a lump can be felt, the radiologist or surgeon guides a needle into the area by palpating the lump. If the lump is non-palpable, the FNA procedure is performed under image guidance using fluoroscopy, ultrasound, or computerized axial tomography (CAT), with the patient positioned according to the area of concern. In fluoroscopic guidance, intermittent fluoroscopy guides the advancement of the needle. Ultrasonography-guided aspiration biopsy involves inserting an aspiration catheter needle device through the accessory channel port of the echoendoscope; the needle is placed into the area to be sampled under endoscopic ultrasonographic guidance. After the needle is placed into the region of the lesion, a vacuum is created and multiple in and out needle motions are performed. Several needle insertions are usually required to ensure that an adequate tissue sample is taken. CAT image-guidance allows computer-assisted targeting of the area to be sampled. At the completion of the procedure, the needle is withdrawn and a small bandage is placed over the area. Report 10021 if fine needle aspiration is performed without image guidance. Report 10022 if image guidance is used to assist in the location of the lump.

10040

The physician makes a small incision through the skin overlying the lesion. The skin over the lesion is removed. The lesion is opened with a surgical instrument and the fluid is drained for secondary

healing. The lesion may be removed. No sutures are needed. Do not bill benign lesion excision code (11400–11446) and chemical exfoliation for acne (17360) on same date of service with code 10040.

10060–10061

The physician makes a small incision through the skin overlying an abscess or cyst. The abscess or cyst is opened with a surgical instrument, allowing the contents to drain. The lesion may be cureted and irrigated. The physician leaves the surgical wound open to allow for continued drainage. For complicated or multiple cysts in 10061, the physician may place either a Penrose latex drain or gauze strip packing to allow continued drainage. Complicated cysts may require later surgical closure. Report 10061 if the repair is complicated or involves multiple lesions.

10080–10081

Pilonidal cysts are entrapped epithelial tissue located in the sacrococcygeal region around the buttocks. The cyst may produce fluid or exudate into the cystic lining. These cysts may be associated with ingrown hair. The physician first shaves the hair adjacent to the cysts. An incision is made to allow drainage of cystic fluid or exudate. Curettage is performed to remove the cystic epithelial lining. The wound heals secondarily relying on local wound care. Report 10081 if the procedure is more complicated and requires excision of tissue, primary closure, and/or Z-plasty.

10120–10121

A foreign body becomes embedded in the subcutaneous tissues. The physician makes a simple incision in the skin overlying the foreign body. The foreign body is retrieved using hemostats or forceps. The skin may be sutured or allowed to heal secondarily. Report 10121 if the procedure is more complicated, requiring dissection of underlying tissues.

10140

The physician makes an incision in the skin to decompress and drain a collection of fluid. A hemostat bluntly penetrates the fluid pockets, allowing the fluid to evacuate. A latex drain or gauze packing may be placed into the incision site. This will allow the escape of any fluids that may continue to enter the pocket. A pressure dressing may be placed over the region. Any drain or packing is removed within 48 hours. The incision can be closed primarily or may be left to granulate without closure.

10160

A palpable collection of fluid is located subcutaneously. The physician cleanses the overlying skin and introduces a large bore needle on a syringe into the fluid space. The fluid is aspirated into the syringe, decompressing the fluid space. A pressure dressing may be placed over the fluid site.

10180

This procedure treats an infected surgical site. An incision and drainage is necessary to remove this fluid to allow the surgical wound to heal. The physician either removes the surgical sutures or staples or make additional incisions into the skin. The wound is drained of infected fluid. Necrotic tissue is removed from the surgical site. The wound is irrigated. The wound may either be sutured closed or packed open with sterile gauze to allow additional drainage. If closed, the surgical site may have suction or latex drains placed into the wound. If packed open, the wound may be sutured again during a later procedure.

11000–11001

The physician surgically removes damaged or necrotic skin. The skin may be of eczematous nature possessing erythema, vesicles, and scales. Bacteria of fungus may be causing a skin infection. Wet compresses are used initially to remove scaly skin. Abrasive techniques may be employed to remove remaining scales. A scalpel may be used to decompress vesicles and excise dead skin. After debridement, topical lubricants and antibiotic preparations are placed on the skin. Report 11000 for up to 10 percent of the body surface; report 11001 once for each additional 10 percent of the body surface, in addition to the primary procedure.

11010

The physician manually or surgically removes foreign matter and contaminated or devitalized skin and/or subcutaneous tissues in and around the site of an open fracture (where bone has been exposed to the air by breaking through the skin and subcutaneous tissues) and/or the area of a dislocated joint.

11011

The physician manually or surgically removes foreign matter and contaminated or devitalized skin, subcutaneous tissues, muscle fascia, and/or muscle in and around the site of an open fracture (where bone has been exposed to the air by breaking through the skin and subcutaneous tissues) and/or the area of a dislocated joint.

11012

The physician manually or surgically removes foreign matter and contaminated or devitalized skin, subcutaneous tissues, muscle fascia, muscle and/or bone in and around the site of an open fracture (where bone has been exposed to the air by breaking through the skin and subcutaneous tissues) and/or the area of a dislocated joint.

11040–11042

The physician surgically removes partially necrotic or dead skin. The physician uses a scalpel or dermatome to remove a superficial layer of affected skin. The epidermal layer is removed with the underlying dermis remaining intact. The partial thickness of skin is excised until viable, bleeding tissue is encountered. A topical antibiotic is placed on the wound. Either a gauze dressing or an occlusive dressing may be placed over the surgical site. Report 11041 if full thickness; report 11042 if debridement includes subcutaneous tissue.

11043–11044

The physician surgically removes necrotic skin, underlying tissue, and muscle. The physician uses a scalpel to excise the affected tissue into the muscle layer. The dissection is continued until viable, bleeding tissue is encountered. Depending on wound size, closure may be immediate or delayed. The wound may be packed open with sterile gauze and require immediate or delayed reconstruction. Report 11044 if bone is also debrided.

11055–11057

The physician removes a benign skin lesion such as a corn or callus by cutting, clipping, or paring. Report 11055 when one lesion is removed, and 11056 is used when two to four lesions are removed. Report 11057 when more than four lesions are removed.

11100–11101

The physician removes skin and/or mucous membrane for separately reportable histologic study under a microscope. A portion of a single lesion is excised in 11100. Report 11101 for each separate additional lesion biopsied in addition to the primary procedure. Some normal tissue adjacent to the diseased mucosa is also removed for comparison purposes. The excision site may be closed primarily or may be allowed to granulate without closure.

11200–11201

The physician removes skin tag lesions. Skin tags are common benign tumors found on many body regions and most frequently around the axilla, inguinal, and head and neck. The physician removes the skin tags with or without local anesthesia. The physician uses sharp excision with scissors or scalpel. Skin tags may also be removed by using chemical cautery, electrical cautery, or by ligature strangulation. Report 11200 for up to 15 lesions; report 11201 for each additional ten lesions.

11300–11303

The physician removes an elevated skin lesion from the trunk, arm or legs by shave excision. Local anesthesia is injected beneath the lesion. A scalpel blade is placed against the skin adjacent to the lesion. The physician uses a sawing motion to excise the lesion from its base. Electrocautery may be used to smooth the edges. Both electrocautery or chemical cautery may be used to control bleeding. report 11300 for a lesion diameter 0.5 cm or less. Report 11301 for

0.6 cm to 1.0 cm; 11302 for 1.21 cm to 2.0 cm; and 11303 for lesions greater than 2.0 cm.

11305–11308

The physician removes an elevated skin lesion from the scalp, neck, hands, feet or genitalia by shave excision. Local anesthesia is injected beneath the lesion. A scalpel blade is placed against the skin adjacent to the lesion. The physician uses a sawing motion to excise the lesion from its base. Electrocautery may be used to smooth the edges. Both electrocautery or chemical may be used to control bleeding. Report 11305 for a lesion diameter 0.5 cm or less; 11306 for 0.6 cm to 1.0 cm; 11307 for 1.1 cm to 2.0 cm; and 11308 for lesions greater than 2.0 cm.

11310–11313

The physician removes a single lesion from the face, ears, eyelids, lips, nose, or mucous membrane. The lesion diameter is 0.5 cm or less for 11310, from 0.6 cm to 1.0 cm for 11311, from 1.1 cm to 2.0 cm for 11312, or over 2.0 cm for 11313. The physician "shaves" through the outer layer of skin, or deeper into the dermis (partial thickness), with a transverse or horizontal cut. The wound does not require suturing and bleeding is controlled by chemical or electrical cauterization.

11400–11406

The physician excises a benign lesion, except a skin tag, on the trunk, arms or legs. The lesion diameter is 0.5 cm or less. The physician excises the lesion with a scalpel. The physician may suture the wound simply. Report 11401 if the lesion diameter is 0.6 cm to 1.0 cm; report 11402 if the lesion diameter is 1.1 cm to 2.0 cm; report 11403 if the lesion diameter is 2.1 cm to 3.0 cm; report 11404 if the lesion diameter is 3.1 cm to 4.0 cm; and report 11406 if the lesion diameter is over 4.0 cm.

11420–11426

The physician excises a benign lesion, except a skin tag, on the scalp, neck, hands, feet, and genitalia. The lesion diameter is 0.5 cm or less. The physician excises the lesion with a scalpel. The physician may suture the wound simply. Report 11421 if the lesion diameter is 0.6 cm to 1.0 cm; report 11422 if the lesion diameter is 1.1 cm to 2.0 cm; report 11423 if the lesion diameter is 2.1 cm to 3.0 cm; report 11424 if the lesion diameter is 3.1 cm to 4.0 cm; and report 11426 if the lesion diameter is over 4.0 cm.

11440–11446

The physician removes a benign (noncancerous) lesion from the eyelids, ears, face, lips, nose or mucous membrane. The lesion diameter is up to 0.5 cm for 11440, from 0.6 cm to 1.0 cm for 11441, or from 1.1 cm to 2.0 cm for 11442. The lesion diameter is from 2.1 cm to 3.0 cm for 11443, from 3.1 cm to 4.0 cm for 11444, or over 4.0 cm for 11446. The physician makes an incision through the skin, usually in an elliptical shape, around and under the lesion, and removes it. The skin incision is sutured. The physician makes an elliptical incision through the skin (full thickness) around and under the lesion. The lesion is removed. The skin incision is then sutured simply.

11450–11451

Hidradenitis is chronic suppurative disease that produces scarring of the skin and subcutaneous tissue. Clinically visible are at least two blackheads with several surface openings, subcutaneous communication, and subsequent abscess formation in the axillary region. The abscesses lead to extensive scarring of the dermis. The physician performs a wide excision of the abscess. The excision site is left open to heal by granulation or may be sutured in layers. Report 11451 if complex repair requires local pedicle flap coverage or skin graft.

11462–11463

Hidradenitis is chronic suppurative disease that produces scarring of the skin and subcutaneous tissue. Clinically visible are at least two blackheads with several surface openings, subcutaneous communication, and subsequent abscess formation in the inguinal region. The abscesses lead to extensive scarring of the dermis. The physician performs a wide excision of the abscess. The excision site is left open to heal by granulation or may be sutured in layers. Report 11463 if complex repair requires local pedicle flap coverage or skin graft.

11470–11471

Hidradenitis is chronic suppurative disease that produces scarring of the skin and subcutaneous tissue. Clinically visible are at least two blackheads with several surface openings, subcutaneous communication, and subsequent abscess formation in the perianal, perineal, or umbilical regions. The abscesses lead to extensive scarring of the dermis. The physician performs a wide excision of the abscess. The excision site is left open to heal by granulation or may be sutured in layers. Report 11471 if complex repair requires local pedicle flap coverage or skin graft.

11600–11606

The physician removes a malignant lesion from the trunk, arms, or legs. The lesion diameter is up to 0.5 cm for 11600, from 0.6 cm to 1.0 cm for 11601, or from 1.1 cm to 2.0 cm for 11602. The lesion diameter is from 2.1 cm to 3.0 cm for 11603, from 3.1 cm to 4.0 cm for 11604, or over 4.0 cm for 11606. The physician makes an incision through the skin, usually in an elliptical shape, around and under the lesion, and removes it. The skin incision is then sutured simply. The physician makes an elliptical incision through the skin (full thickness) around and under the lesion. The lesion is removed. The skin incision is sutured simply. Small wounds may be closed simply.

Immediate reconstruction with local flaps (separately reported) may be necessary.

11620–11626

The physician removes a malignant lesion from the scalp, neck, hands, feet, or genitalia. The lesion diameter is up to 0.5 cm for 11620, from 0.6 cm to 1.0 cm for 11621, or from 1.1 cm to 2.0 cm for 11622, The lesion diameter is from 2.1 cm to 3.0 cm for 11623, from 3.1 cm to 4.0 cm for 11624, or over 4.0 cm for 11626. The physician makes an incision through the skin, usually in an elliptical shape, around and under the lesion, and removes it. The skin incision is sutured simply. Small wounds may be closed simply. Immediate reconstruction with local flaps (separately reported) may be necessary.

11640–11642

The physician removes a malignant lesion from the face, ears, eyelids, nose or lips. The lesion diameter is up to 0.5 cm for 11640, from 0.6 cm to 1.0 cm for 11641, or from 1.1 cm to 2.0 cm for 11642. The physician makes an elliptical incision through the skin (full thickness) around and under the lesion. The lesion and a rim of normal tissue is removed. The skin incision is sutured simply. Small wounds may be closed simply. Immediate reconstruction with local flaps (separately reported) may be necessary.

11643–11646

The physician removes a malignant (cancerous) lesion from the face, ears, eyelids, nose, or lips. The lesion diameter is from 2.1 cm to 3.0 cm for 11643, from 3.1 cm to 4.0 cm for 11644, or over 4.0 cm for 11646. The physician makes an incision through the skin, usually in an elliptical shape. The lesion and a rim of normal tissue is removed. The skin incision is sutured simply. Small wounds may be closed simply. Immediate reconstruction with local flaps (separately reported) may be necessary.

11719

A physician trims a fingernail or toenail usually with scissors, nail cutters, or other instruments. This code is used when the nails are not defective from nutritional or metabolic abnormalities. It is used for one or more nails.

11720–11721

The physician cleans up to five fingernails or toenails, including tops and exposed undersides. The cleaning is performed manually with cleaning solutions, abrasive materials, and tools. The nails are shortened and shaped. Report 11721 for each group of up to five nails beyond the initial five.

11730–11732

The physician enlarges and removes all or part of a fingernail or toenail. A digital nerve block is used to numb the top of the digit. The physician bluntly dissects the nail plate from the nail bed. Any bleeding is cauterized. The digit is bandaged. Report 11730 if only one nail is removed. Report 11732 for each additional nail plate removed. Small wounds may be closed simply. Immediate reconstruction with local flaps (separately reported) may be necessary.

11740

The physician evacuates blood from a hematoma located beneath a fingernail or toenail. The physician uses an electrocautery needle to pierce the nail plate so a hematoma can drain. Pressure may be applied to the nail bed to force the blood from beneath the nail plate. A loose dressing is applied so the area can continue to drain.

11750–11752

The physician removes all or part of a fingernail or toenail, including the nail plate and matrix. In 11750, the physician bluntly dissects the nail plate away from the nail bed. The germ matrix is destroyed using electrocautery or excision. Bleeding is stopped with electrocautery and the wound is dressed. In 11752, the entire tuft of the distal phalanx is removed.

11755

The physician removes a portion of the nail unit for separately reportable biopsy. Sections may be taken from the hard nail itself, the nail bed, lateral skin, or underlying soft tissue. The specimen is excised by clippers or with a scalpel.

11760

The physician repairs a damaged nail bed. The physician removes the damaged and surrounding nail from the nail bed. The nail bed is sutured into correct position. Bleeding is controlled through electrocautery and the wound is dressed.

11762

The physician repairs a damaged nail bed using a skin graft. The physician cleans the nail bed and prepares it for the graft. The graft is obtained and sutured into place. Hemostasis is achieved and a dressing is applied.

11765

The physician excises restrictive skin to free an ingrown nail. The physician performs a wedge excision of the skin overlapping the lateral nail. The nail is examined and trimmed to encourage straight growth. The wound is dressed.

11770

A pilonidal cyst or sinus is entrapped epithelial tissue. These lesions may be associated with ingrown hair. A sinus cavity is present and may have a fluid producing cystic lining. With a small sinus, the physician uses a scalpel to completely excise the involved tissue. The wound is sutured in a single layer.

11771

A pilonidal cyst or sinus is entrapped epithelial tissue. These lesions may be associated with ingrown hair. A sinus cavity is present and may have a fluid producing cystic lining. The sinus is superficial to the underlying fascia but has subcutaneous extensions. The physician uses a scalpel to completely excise this lesion. The wound is sutured in several layers.

11772

A pilonidal cyst or sinus is entrapped epithelial tissue. These lesions may be associated with ingrown hair. A large sinus cavity is present and may have a fluid producing cystic lining. The sinus is superficial to the underlying fascia having many subcutaneous extensions. The physician uses a scalpel to completely excise the involved tissue. Local soft tissue flaps (i.e. z-plasty) are required for closure of the large defect. The wound is closed in several layers.

11900

The physician uses a syringe to inject a pharmacologic agent underneath or into seven or fewer skin lesions. The lesion may be any healed skin lesion including post-laceration and post-surgical scar bands. The physician may inject steroids or anesthetics into these lesions.

11901

The physician uses a syringe to inject a pharmacologic agent underneath or into more than seven skin lesions. The lesion may be any healed skin lesion including post-laceration and post-surgical scar bands. The physician may inject steroids or anesthetics into these lesions.

11920–11922

The physician uses a marking pen to outline the area to be tattooed, then injects dye into the skin. The dye is injected with a pneumatic tattooing instrument for the purpose of creating an artificial pigmentation area that approximates the appearance of normal skin tissue. Code 11920 reports a tattoo area of 6.0 sq cm or less; 11921 reports 6.1 to 20.0 sq cm. Each additional 20.0 sq cm is reported with 11922. Report 11922 in conjunction with 11921.

11950–11954

The physician uses an injectable dermal implant to correct small soft tissue deformities. This technique is used to treat facial wrinkles, post-surgical defects, and acne scars. The injectable filling material can be either autologous fat, synthetic surgical compound, or a commercially produced collagen preparation. The physician uses a syringe to inject the selected material into the dermis of the skin. The injection will augment the dermal layer and alleviate the soft tissue depression. Report 11950 for an injection of 1.0 cc or less; report 11951 for an injection of 1.1 to 5.0 cc; report 11952 if 5.1 to 10.0 cc; report 11954 if over 10.0 cc.

11960

The physician uses a tissue expander to distend contracted skin and soft tissue prior to definitive reconstruction. These expanders are balloon-type devices that stretch the skin and enhance epithelial and collagen expansion. The physician makes an incision into the skin. The subcutaneous layer is identified. Blunt dissection is then used to separate the skin and subcutaneous layers. The tissue expander is then placed into the prepared site. The wound is sutured. The expander is inflated. During the post-operative visits, greater volume is placed into the expander stretching the skin. The expander remains in place until the final reconstruction is performed.

11970

The physician removes a subcutaneous tissue expander and places a permanent prosthesis for final reconstruction. Initially, the tissue expander is deflated. The physician then uses a scalpel to make an incision. Blunt dissection is used to remove the tissue expander. The permanent prosthesis is placed into the recipient bed. The prosthesis may be an autologous graft or a commercially prepared synthetic material. The graft prosthesis may require stabilization with sutures, wires, or screws. The incision is closed with sutures.

11971

The physician removes a subcutaneous tissue expander. Final reconstruction is not performed at this surgery. Initially, the tissue expander is deflated. The physician uses a scalpel to make an incision. Blunt dissection is used to remove the tissue expander. A surgical drain may be placed in the wound. The incision is closed with sutures.

11975

The physician makes a small incision in the skin on the inside of the upper arm and, using a trocar, inserts six 3.0 cm capsules subdermally. The trocar is a sharp-tipped metal tube through which the capsules are passed. The incision is then closed.

11976

The physician makes a small incision in the skin on the inside of the upper arm and removes six 3 cm contraceptive capsules previously implanted subdermally. The incision is then closed.

11977

The physician makes a small incision in the skin on the inside of the upper arm and removes six 3.0 cm contraceptive capsules previously implanted subdermally. New capsules are inserted in their place or into a new site. The incision is then closed.

11980

Biodegradable time-release medication pellets are implanted subcutaneously beneath the skin for the slow delivery of hormones. The physician makes a small incision in the skin with a scalpel. A trocar and cannula are inserted into the incised area. Hormone pellets are inserted through the cannula, and the cannula is withdrawn. Pressure is applied to the incised area until any bleeding is stopped, and the incision is closed with steri-strips. The time-release medication has been used for women who require hormone replacement during menopause. One method is to implant pellets of testosterone or a combination of that hormone with estrogen (taken in conjunction with progesterone) in the fatty tissue of the buttocks. This relatively painless procedure is performed routinely on an outpatient basis. New pellets are added every six to nine months, or whenever symptoms recur because the pellet has been used up.

11981

Non-biodegradable drug implant delivers a therapeutic dose of the drug continuously at a predetermined rate of continuous release. The system works via a semipermeable membrane at one end of the subcutaneous cylinder that permits the entrance of water; the drug is delivered from a port at the other end of the cylinder at a controlled rate appropriate to the specific therapeutic agent. The physician injects local anesthesia and makes a small incision in the skin with a scalpel to insert the miniature drug-containing titanium cylinder, which is held in place by suture and tied by a knot or secured by a single running suture. The wound is closed with sutures.

11982

Non-biodegradable drug implant delivers a therapeutic dose of the drug continuously at a predetermined rate of continuous release. The system works via a semipermeable membrane at one end of the subcutaneous cylinder that permits the entrance of water; the drug is delivered from a port at the other end of the cylinder at a controlled rate appropriate to the specific therapeutic agent. The physician injects local anesthesia and makes a small incision in the skin with a scalpel to remove a previously implanted miniature drug-containing titanium cylinder, which is held in place by suture and tied by aknot or secured by a single running suture. The wound is closed with sutures.

11983

Non-biodegradable drug implant delivers a therapeutic dose of the drug continuously at a predetermined rate of continuous release. The system works via a semipermeable membrane at one end of the subcutaneous cylinder that permits the entrance of water; the drug is delivered from a port at the other end of the cylinder at a controlled rate appropriate to the specific therapeutic agent. The physician injects local anesthesia and makes a small incision in the skin with a scalpel to remove a previously implanted miniature drug-containing titanium cylinder, which is held in place by suture and tied by a knot or secured

by a single running suture. A replacement cylinder is inserted. The wound is closed with sutures.

12001–12007

The physician sutures superficial lacerations of the scalp, neck, axillae, external genitalia, trunk, or extremities. Up to 7.5 cm for 12002, from 7.5 cm to 12.5 cm for 12004, or from 12.6 cm to 20.0 cm for 12005 in total length. Also code 12006 for 20.1 cm to 30.0 cm, 12007 for over 30.0 cm. With multiple wounds of the same complexity and in the same anatomical area, the length of all wounds sutured is summed and reported as one total length. The physician performs a simple, one-layer repair of the epidermis, dermis, or subcutaneous tissues with sutures.

12011–12018

The physician sutures superficial lacerations of the face, ears eyelids, nose, lips, and/or mucous membranes up to 2.5 cm for 12011, from 2.6 cm to 5.0 cm for 12013, or from 5.1 cm to 7.5 cm for 12014 in total length. Report 12015 if 7.6 cm to 12.5 cm in length, report 12016 if 12.6 cm to 20.0 cm in total length, report 12017 if 20.1 cm to 30.0 cm, and report 12018 if over 30.0 cm. A local anesthetic is injected around the laceration and the wound is thoroughly cleansed, explored, and often irrigated with a saline solution. The physician performs a simple, one-layer repair of the epidermis, dermis, or subcutaneous tissue with sutures. Bleeding may be controlled by simple ligation of vessels or by chemical or electrical cautery.

12020

There has been a breakdown of the healing skin either before or after suture removal. The skin margins have opened. There is no evidence of infection. The physician cleanses the wound with irrigation and antimicrobial solutions. The skin margins may be trimmed to initiate bleeding surfaces. The wound is sutured in a single layer.

12021

There has been a breakdown of the healing skin either before or after suture removal. The skin margins have opened. Infection is evident with presence of pus. The physician cleanses the wound with irrigation and antimicrobial solutions. The wound is left open and packed with gauze strips. This allows infection to drain from the wound. The skin closure will be delayed until the wound is no longer infected.

12031–12037

The physician repairs lacerations of the scalp, axillae, trunk and/or extremities (except hands and feet) of 2.5 cm or less in 12031, 2.6 cm to 7.5 cm in 12032, 7.6 cm to 12.5 cm in 12034, 12.6 cm to 20.0 cm in 12035, 20.1 cm to 30.0 cm in 12036, and over 30.0 cm in 12037. Due to deeper or more complex lacerations, subcutaneous or layered suturing techniques are required. The physician sutures tissue layers under the skin with dissolvable sutures before suturing the skin. Extensive cleaning of the wound prior to suturing may also be required.

12041–12047
The physician repairs lacerations of the neck, hands, feet and/or external genitalia of 2.5 cm or less in 12041, 2.6 cm to 7.5 cm in 12042, 7.6 cm to 12.5 cm in 12044, 12.6 cm to 20.0 cm in 12045, 20.1 to 30.0 cm in 12046, and over 30.0 cm in 12047. Due to deeper or more complex lacerations, subcutaneous or layered suturing techniques are required. The physician sutures tissue layers under the skin with dissolvable sutures before suturing the skin. Extensive cleaning of the wound prior to suturing may also be required.

12051–12057
The physician repairs lacerations of the face, ears, eyelids, nose, lips, and/or mucous membranes up to 2.5 cm for 12051, from 2.6 cm to 5.0 cm for 12052, from 5.1 cm to 7.5 cm for 12053, or from 7.6 cm to 12.5 cm for 12054 in total length. Report 12055 for 12.6 cm to 20.0 cm, 12056 for 20.1 cm to 30.0 cm wounds, and report 12057 for more than 30 wounds. Due to deeper or more complex lacerations, subcutaneous or layered suturing techniques are required. The physician sutures tissue layers under the skin with dissolvable sutures before suturing the skin. Extensive cleaning of the wound prior to suturing may also be required.

13100–13102
The physician repairs complex wounds of the trunk from 1.1 cm to over 7.5 cm. The physician performs complex layered suturing of torn, crushed, or deeply lacerated tissue. The physician debrides the wound by removing foreign material or damaged tissue. Irrigation of the wound is performed and antimicrobial solutions are used to decontaminate and cleanse the wound. The physician may trim skin margins with a scalpel or scissors to allow for proper closure. The wound is closed in layers. Reconstructive procedures such as utilization of local flaps may also be performed. Report 13100 for wounds 1.1 cm to 2.5 cm, 13101 for wounds 2.6 cm to 7.5 cm, and 13102 for each additional 5 cm.

13120–13122
The physician repairs complex wounds of the scalp, arms, and/or legs from 1.1 cm to over 7.5 cm. The physician performs complex layered suturing of torn, crushed, or deeply lacerated tissue. The physician debrides the wound by removing foreign material or damaged tissue. Irrigation of the wound is performed and antimicrobial solutions are used to decontaminate and cleanse the wound. The physician may trim skin margins with a scalpel or scissors to allow for proper closure. The wound is closed in layers. Reconstructive procedures such as utilization of local flaps may also

be performed. Report 13120 for wounds 1.1 cm to 2.5 cm; 13121 for wounds 2.6 cm to 7.5 cm; and 13122 for each additional 5 cm.

13131–13133
The physician repairs complex wounds of the feet from 1.1 cm to 2.5 cm in 13131; from 2.6 cm to 7.5 cm in 13132; and each additional 5.0 cm or less in 13133. The physician performs complex layered suturing of torn, crushed, or deeply lacerated tissue of the feet. The physician uses irrigation and antimicrobial solutions to cleanse the wound. The physician may trim skin margins with a scalpel or scissors. The wound is closed in layers. Reconstructive procedures, such as removal of foreign material or damaged tissue, utilization of local flaps, and scar revision, may also be performed.

13150–13153
The physician repairs complex wounds of the eyelids, nose, ears and/or lips from 1.1 cm to over 7.5 cm. The physician performs complex layered suturing of torn, crushed, or deeply lacerated tissue. The physician debrides the wound by removing foreign material or damaged tissue. Irrigation of the wound is performed and antimicrobial solutions are used to decontaminate and cleanse the wound. The physician may trim skin margins with a scalpel or scissors to allow for proper closure. The wound is closed in layers. Reconstructive procedures such as utilization of local flaps may also be performed. Report 13150 for wounds 1.0 cm or less, 13151 for wounds 1.1 cm to 2.5 cm; 13152 for wounds 2.6 cm to 7.5 cm; and 13153 for each additional 5 cm.

13160
The physician secondarily repairs a surgical skin closure after an infectious breakdown of the healing skin. After resolution of the infection, the wound is now ready for closure. The physician uses a scalpel to excise granulation and scar tissue. Skin margins are trimmed to bleeding edges. The wound is sutured in several layers.

14000
The physician transfers or rearranges adjacent tissue to repair traumatic or surgical wounds of the trunk. This applies to wounds that are 10.0 sq cm or less. This includes, but is not limited to, such rearrangement procedures as Z-plasty, W-plasty, ZY-plasty, or tissue transfers such as rotational or advancement flaps.

14001
The physician transfers or rearranges adjacent tissue to repair traumatic or surgical wounds of the trunk. This applies to wounds from 10.1 sq cm to 30.0 sq cm. This includes, but is not limited to, such rearrangement procedures as Z-plasty, W-plasty, ZY-plasty, or tissue transfers such as rotational or advancement flaps.

14020

The physician transfers or rearranges adjacent tissue to repair traumatic or surgical wounds of the scalp, arms, and/or legs. This applies to wounds that are 10.0 sq cm or less. This includes, but is not limited to, such rearrangement procedures as Z-plasty, W-plasty, ZY-plasty, or tissue transfers such as rotational or advancement flaps.

14021

The physician transfers or rearranges adjacent tissue to repair traumatic or surgical wounds of the scalp, arms, and/or legs. This applies to wounds from 10.1 sq cm to 30.0 sq cm. This includes, but is not limited to, such rearrangement procedures as Z-plasty, W-plasty, ZY-plasty, or tissue transfers such as rotational or advancement flaps.

14040–14041

The physician transfers or rearranges adjacent tissue to repair traumatic or surgical wounds on the forehead, cheeks, chin, mouth, neck, axillae, genitalia, hands and/or feet. This applies to wounds of 10.0 sq cm or less in 14040 or 10.1 sq cm to 30.0 sq cm in 14041. This includes, but is not limited to, such rearrangement procedures as Z-plasty, W-plasty, ZY-plasty, or tissue transfers such as rotational flaps, advancement flaps, or double pedicle flaps.

14060–14061

The physician transfers or rearranges adjacent tissue to repair traumatic or surgical wounds. This applies to wounds of the eyelids, nose, ears, and/or lips of 10.0 sq cm or less for 14060 or from 10.1 to 30.0 sq cm for 14061. This includes, but is not limited to, such rearrangement procedures as Z-plasty, W-plasty, ZY-plasty, or tissue transfers such as rotational flaps or advancement flaps.

14300

The physician transfers or rearranges adjacent tissue to repair traumatic or surgical wounds. This applies to wounds greater than 30.0 sq cm. This includes, but is not limited to, such rearrangement procedures as Z-plasty, W-plasty, ZY-plasty, or tissue transfers such as rotational flaps, or advancement flaps.

14350

The physician creates a filleted finger or toe flap to repair a large deficit on the hand or foot. The physician makes a bilateral longitudinal incision and dissects the tissue away from the bone, protecting vascular integrity. The recipient site is prepared and the flap is rotated into place. Excess tissue is excised and the wound is closed in sutured layers.

15000–15001

The physician prepares tissue, first 100 sq cm or one percent of body area of infants and children, to receive a free skin graft needed to close or repair a defect. Skin, subcutaneous tissue, scars, or lesions are excised

to provide a healthy, vascular tissue bed (where new vessels have been formed) onto which a skin graft will be placed. Simple debridement of granulations or of recent avulsion is included. Report 15001 for each additional 100 sq cm of graft area or each additional 1 percent of surface body area in infants and children. For appropriate skin grafts, see 15050–15261.

15050

The physician obtains one or more pinch grafts to cover a 2.0 cm or less open area. The physician incises the skin to obtain a split thickness skin graft. The donor site is closed. The recipient site is cleaned and prepared. The graft is sewn into place.

15100–15101

The physician harvests a split thickness skin graft. Only the epidermis or top layer of skin is taken. The dermis or bottom layer is left behind and will regenerate new skin. This graft is then applied to an area on the trunk, arms or legs, first 100.0 sq cm or less in adults or less than 1 percent of the total body area of infants and children. Report 15101 for each additional 100.0 sq cm or each 1 percent of the total body area in infants and children. Use 15101 in conjunction with code 15100.

15120–15121

The physician takes skin from one area of the body and grafts it to an area needing repair. This procedure is performed when direct wound closure or adjacent tissue transfer is not possible. A split thickness graft is used. This is a graft using only the top layers of the skin, rather than the full thickness of the skin, leaving the deeper layers intact. The physician uses a dermatome to harvest the split thickness graft in one cut. The tissue is then sutured or stapled onto the recipient bed. The tissue may also be meshed prior to placement. This procedure (e.g., 15120) applies to split thickness skin grafts to the face, scalp, eyelids, neck, ears, orbits, mouth, genitalia, hands, feet and/or multiple digits of 100.0 sq cm or less and each of 1 percent of total body area of infants and children. For each additional 100.0 sq cm and each additional 1 percent of total body area of infants and children, or part thereof (e.g. 15121) a larger tissue harvest is needed. Use 15121 in conjunction with 15120.

15200–15201

The physician harvests a full thickness skin graft, which is removing both layers of skin (epidermis and dermis). The resulting surgical wound is closed by lifting the remaining skin edges and placing sutures to close directly. The graft is then used to cover a defect of the trunk of no more than 20.0 sq cm. Report 15201 for each additional 20.0 sq cm. Use 15201 in conjunction with 15200.

15220–15221

The physician harvests a full thickness skin graft, which is removing both layers of skin (epidermis and

CPT ® Lay Descriptions

dermis). The resulting surgical wound is closed by lifting the remaining skin edges and placing sutures to close directly. The graft is used to cover a defect of the scalp, arms, and/or legs of no more than 20.0 sq cm. Report 15221 for each additional 20.0 sq cm. Use 15221 in conjunction with 15220.

15240–15241

The physician takes skin from one area of the body and grafts it onto an area needing repair. This procedure is performed when direct wound closure or adjacent tissue transfer is not possible. A full thickness graft is used. This is a graft using the deeper layers of skin. The physician uses a scalpel to harvest the full thickness graft. Fat is removed from the graft and the tissue is then sutured onto the recipient bed. The procedure applies to full thickness skin grafts to the forehead, cheeks, chin, mouth, neck, axillae, genitalia, hands, and/or feet of 20.0 sq cm or less. Report 15241 for each additional 20.0 sq cm. Use 15241 in conjunction with 15240.

15260–15261

The physician harvests full-thickness skin from the patient and grafts it elsewhere. Using a scalpel to harvest the full-thickness graft, the physician then sutures or staples the tissue onto the recipient bed in the nose, ears, eyelids, and/or lips. Code 15260 reports a graft up to 20.0 sq cm or 1 percent of total body area of infants and children. For each additional 20.0 sq cm or each additional 1 percent of total body area of infants and children, report 15261. The donor site is usually closed directly with sutures after undermining the skin edge. Use 15261 in conjunction with 15260.

15342–15343

The physician applies a skin substitute/neodermis to a burn site. In a separately reportable procedure the physician excises a full-thickness or partial-thickness thermal injury (burn wound) to viable tissue. After the burn wound is excised the physician covers the site with a skin substitute (artificial skin). The skin substitute closes the excised wounds until skin autografts can be placed. Some skin substitutes interact with the body and promote wound healing; they help control the moisture loss that occurs with full-thickness or deep partial-thickness dermal injury. Skin substitutes serve as a template to generate neodermis, a dermal-like tissue that readily accepts a thin epidermal autograft. Report 15342 for the application of a skin substitute up to and including 25 square centimeters. Report 15343 for the application of a skin substitute for each additional 25 square centimeters.

15350–15351

The physician applies a donor graft to cover a wound on the patient. The tissue may be from a genetically matched living person or may be tissue harvested from a cadaver and processed to make it sterile by a tissue bank. Report 15351 for each additional 100.0 sq cm of graft area. Use 15351 in conjunction with 15350.

15400–15401

The physician applies a xenograft to cover a wound on the patient, 100.0 sq cm or less.. The tissue is harvested from a non-human species and used to cover a skin defect in a living human. For example, the physician may use processed skin from a pig to cover wounds on the patient. The physician applies a xenograft to cover a wound on the patient. Report 15401 for each additional 100.0 sq cm of graft. Use 15401 in conjunction with 15400.

15570–15576

The physician uses a direct or tubed pedicle flap to reconstruct traumatic defects of the trunk. A full thickness flap is developed in the scalp and rotated to the defect area. The pedicle retains its supporting blood vessels and is sutured to the recipient bed in multiple layers. The physician closes the harvest region in layers or covers it with a split thickness skin graft. Other exposed regions, including portions of the pedicle, may also be covered with a split thickness skin graft. Once the recipient site has healed, a second surgery will detach the pedicle and return the unused flap to its anatomic location. Report 15572 for pedicle on scalp, arms, or legs; report 15574 if applied to forehead cheeks, chin, mouth, neck, axillae, genitalia, hands, or feet; report 15576 if applied to eyelids, nose, ears, lips, or intraoral.

15600–15630

The physician sections the direct or tubed pedicle flap several weeks following reconstruction of traumatic defects. Blood flow is now established in the recipient area. The unused portion of the flap is detached and prepared for reinsertion into its original anatomic site. Previous skin grafts are removed from the donor beds. The returned flap is sutured in layers to the harvest site. Any exposed subcutaneous tissue is closed primarily or covered with a split thickness skin graft. Report 15610 if performed on scalp, arms, or legs; report 15620 if performed on forehead, cheeks, chin, neck, axillae, genitalia, hands, or feet; report 15630 if performed on eyelids nose, ears, or lips.

15650

A previously placed flap has been in position long enough to receive a good blood supply from the recipient area. As an intermediate step the physician releases the flap from its donor attachment and moves it completely to a new location. This same tissue may be moved further along the body in a similar manner at a later date. This is known as "walking" the flap or "walk up" procedure.

15732–15738

The physician repairs an area of the head or neck using a muscle, a muscle and skin, or a fascia and skin flap. The physician rotates the flap from the donor area to the site needing repair, suturing the flap in place. The donor area is closed primarily. Report 15734 if performed on the trunk; 15736 if performed on an upper extremity; and 15738 if performed on a lower extremity.

15740–15750
The physician forms an island pedicle flap. A defect is being covered by elevation of a flap of skin and subcutaneous tissue. The flap is rotated into a nearby but not immediately adjacent defect. Often this flap will be transferred through a tunnel underneath the skin and sutured into its new position. The donor site is closed directly. Report 15750 if neurovascular pedicle.

15756
The physician implants a free muscle flap with or without skin with microvascular anastomosis. With the patient under general anesthesia, the physician prepares and irrigates the wound. The new muscle is removed from the donor site and prepared. The physician inserts the new muscle and uses half-mattress sutures to secure the section. Using microscopy, the physician joins the vessels, uniting the new muscle to the site. Before all are joined, the physician may inject fluorescein dye in the vascular system and check the area for fluorescence under an ultraviolet light. Adjustments and corrections to the vascular connections are made, and the physician sutures the skin. Light dressing is applied; and, in many cases, the flap is splinted to help prevent shrinkage. The donor site is sutured and covered with a light dressing.

15757
The physician implants a free skin flap with microvascular astomosis. With the patient under general anesthesia, the physician prepares and irrigates the wound. The new skin is removed from the donor site and prepared. The physician inserts the new skin and uses half-mattress sutures to secure the section. Using microscopy, the physician joins the vessels and nerves uniting the new skin to the site. Before all are joined, the physician may inject fluorescein dye in the vascular system and check the area for fluorescence under an ultraviolet light. Adjustments and corrections to the vascular connections are made, and the physician sutures the skin. Light dressing is applied; and, in many cases, the flap is splinted to help prevent shrinkage. The donor site is sutured and covered with a light dressing.

15758
The physician implants a free fascial flap with microvascular anastomosis. With the patient under general anesthesia, the physician prepares and irrigates the wound. The new fascia is removed from the donor site and prepared. The physician inserts the new fascia and uses sutures to secure the section.

Using microscopy, the physician joins the vessels and nerves uniting the new fascia to the site. The physician sutures the skin. Light dressing is applied; and, in many cases, the flap is splinted to help prevent shrinkage. The donor site is sutured and covered with a light dressing.

15760–15770
The physician takes a full thickness graft with subcutaneous tissue. This is a graft using the deeper layers of the skin. The physician uses a scalpel to harvest the full thickness graft. The tissue is then sutured onto the recipient bed. The incision is closed with layered sutures. Report 15770 if derma, fat, or fascia is used.

15775–15776
The physician performs a punch graft for hair transplant. The physician uses a punch tool to remove a small segment of scalp containing hair and hair follicles. This is then transferred and inset into a non-hair bearing area. Report 15775 for one to 15 punch grafts; report 15776 for more than 15 punch grafts.

15780–15783
The physician performs dermabrasion of the total face. The physician uses a powered rotary instrument to "sand down" or smooth scarred or wrinkled areas. The physician lowers raised lesions or thins thickened tissue to regenerate skin with a smoother appearance. Report 15781 for a dermabrasion performed on a segment of the face. Report 15782 for regional dermabrasion, other than the face. Report 15783 for superficial dermabrasion on any site.

15786–15787
The physician uses abrasive techniques to smooth down or remove an isolated lesion even as one scar or skin thickening secondary to sun damage. Report 15786 for single lesion; report 15787 for each additional four lesions or less. Use 15787 in conjunction with 15786.

15788–15793
The physician performs a chemical peel of the epidermal layer of the face. The physician uses chemical agents such as glycolic acid or phenol to remove fine facial wrinkles or areas of abnormal pigmentation. The treatment is localized to surface layers of skin only. Report 15789 for chemical facial peel of the dermal layer. Report 15792 for epidermal chemical peel other than facial. Report 15793 for dermal chemical peel other than facial.

15810–15811
The physician applies a concentrated saline solution to the skin as a chemical irritant. Code with caution: this procedure has largely been replaced with dermabrasion or laser therapy. Report 15810 if the treatment area is 20.0 sq cm or less; report 15811 if the treatment area is over 20.0 sq cm.

15819

The physician removes excess skin from the neck area. The physician marks the area to be removed. The skin is incised and the excess tissues are resected. The skin is reapproximated and closed in sutured layers.

15820–15821

Through an incision beneath the eyelash line, the physician dissects the skin of the lower eyelid to the subcutaneous/muscle fascial layers. The skin is pulled tight and excess skin is excised. Muscle fascia may be sutured to support sagging muscles. In 15821, excess fat is removed from the tissues. The incision is closed with multiple layers.

15822–15823

Through an incision usually in the crease of the upper eyelid, the physician dissects the skin of the upper eyelid to the subcutaneous/muscle fascial layers. The skin is pulled tight and excess skin is excised. Muscle fascia may be sutured to support sagging muscles. In 15823, excess fat is removed from the tissues. The incision is closed with multiple layers.

15824

The physician performs a rhytidectomy of the forehead. The physician excises a portion of skin in order to eliminate wrinkles in the forehead. Most commonly an incision is made in the hairline and a subcutaneous dissection is carried down to the level of the eyebrow. The excess skin is then removed and the forehead is elevated and sutured into the new position. Incisions are repaired in multiple layers.

15825

The physician performs a rhytidectomy of the neck. The physician makes an incision usually in front of the ear. Tension is increased in the facial muscles by freeing the superficial musculoaponeurotic system (SMAS) (facial muscles are interlinked by the SMAS). The physician trims and tightens the SMAS by securing it with sutures to tissues in front of the ear. An additional incision below the chin is necessary to correct the platysma muscle. The physician makes an incision through the platysma muscle, creating a flap which is moved up and back. The muscle is tightened, trimmed and secured with layered sutures. The skin incisions are closed with layered sutures.

15826

The physician makes an incision in a crease or wrinkle of the cheek, chin and neck. Tension is increased by removing excess skin and fat. An additional incision in front of the ear may be necessary to increase tension of the facial muscles. The incision is closed with layered sutures.

15828–15829

The physician makes an incision in a crease or wrinkle of the cheek, chin or neck. Tension is

increased by removing excess skin and fat. An additional incision in front of the ear may be necessary to increase tension of the facial muscles. The incision is closed with layered sutures. Tension is increased in the facial muscles by freeing the superficial musculoaponeurotic system (SMAS) (facial muscles are interlinked by the SMAS). The physician trims and tightens the SMAS by securing it with sutures to tissues in front of the ear. Report 15829 for SMAS flap.

15831–15839

The physician removes excessive skin. The physician makes an incision traversing the abdomen below the belly button in a horizontal fashion. Excessive skin and subcutaneous tissue are elevated off the abdominal wall and excess tissue and fat are excised. The flaps are then brought together and sutured in at least three layers. The physician may also suture the rectus abdomini muscles together in the midline to reinforce the area. Report 15832 for thigh; 15833 for leg; 15834 for hip; 15835 for buttock; 15836 for arm; 15837 for forearm or hand; report 15838 for submental fat pad; and report 15839 for any other area.

15840–15845

The physician harvests a graft for facial nerve paralysis. The physician removes connective tissue (fascia) from a predetermined location of the body (often fascia lata from the leg). This graft is then transplanted to the face and sutured into place underneath the skin in order to partially suspend or reanimate previously paralyzed areas of the face. Report 15841 if free muscle graft; report 15842 if free muscle graft by microsurgical technique; and report 15845 if regional muscle transfer is performed.

15850–15851

The physician who completed the surgery on the patient now removes sutures on that patient with the aid of sedation or general anesthesia. Report 15851 for removal of sutures by another surgeon.

15852

The physician places the patient under sedation or general anesthesia to change a dressing. This is common for severe crush injuries where serial tissue debridement is required, also for certain types of infection.

15860

The physician injects a dye such as fluorescein or methylene blue to test the viability of a flap or sutured vessel. The agent is injected intravenously.

15876–15879

The physician performs a lipectomy of the head and neck. The physician makes small incisions inside the mouth or in the skin of the chin overlying an area of fat deposits. A liposuction cannula is inserted through the incision. The physician moves the cannula through the fat deposits, creating tunnels and removing excess deposits. A separate incision behind the ear may be necessary to remove additional fat deposits. The incisions are closed simply. Report 15877 if performed on trunk, 15878 if on upper extremity, and 15879 if on lower extremity.

15920

The physician excises a coccygeal pressure ulcer. The patient is positioned prone. The physician makes a 15.0 cm elliptical incision over the coccyx (tailbone) removing the strip of skin that contains the pressure sore. After freeing the coccyx from the surrounding soft tissues it is separated from the sacrum and removed. The soft tissue is then brought back together and the wound is closed with sutures.

15922

The physician excises a coccygeal pressure ulcer. The patient is positioned prone. The physician makes a 15.0 cm elliptical incision over the coccyx (tailbone) removing the strip of skin that contains the pressure sore. After freeing the coccyx from the surrounding soft tissues it is separated from the sacrum and removed. The soft tissue is then brought back together and the wound is closed with sutures. The wound is closed using a skin flap from the scapula, groin or other donor site. The flap is sutured in place and covered with mesh petroleum gauze and loose bandages.

15931

The physician excises a sacral pressure ulcer. The patient is positioned prone. The physician makes an elliptical incision over the sacrum removing the strip of skin that contains the pressure sore. The wound is irrigated, the soft tissue is then brought back together and closed with sutures.

15933

The physician excises a sacral pressure ulcer. The patient is positioned prone. The physician makes a 15.0 cm elliptical incision over the sacrum removing the strip of skin that contains the pressure sore. Bone below the wound is removed. The soft tissue is then brought back together and the wound is closed with sutures. A bone graft may be inserted in the bone wound. The wound is irrigated and the soft tissue is then brought back together and the wound is closed with sutures.

15934

The physician excises a sacral pressure ulcer. The patient is positioned prone. The physician makes a 15.0 cm elliptical incision over the sacrum removing the strip of skin that contains the pressure sore. Bone below the wound is removed. The soft tissue is then brought back together and the wound is closed with sutures. A bone graft may be inserted in the bone wound. The wound is irrigated and the soft tissue is

then brought back together and the wound is closed with sutures.

15935

The physician excises a sacral pressure ulcer. The patient is positioned prone. The physician makes a 15.0 cm elliptical incision over the sacrum removing the strip of skin that contains the pressure sore. Bone below the wound is removed. The soft tissue is then brought back together and the wound is closed with sutures. A bone graft may be inserted in the bone wound. The wound is irrigated and the soft tissue is then brought back together and the wound is closed with sutures.

15936–15937

The physician excises a sacral ulcer to prepare for muscle or myocutaneous flap or skin graft closure. The physician makes an incision around the pressure sore that lies over the sacrum. The infected wound is removed and the area is irrigated. The space that remains is filled with a muscle flap graft, usually taken from the latissimus dorsi muscle and the overlying skin. The donor site is prepared and the incision is made for the appropriate size of graft to be taken. Once the portion of the muscle is removed, the overlying skin is removed and the wound is sutured closed. The graft is sutured in place and a soft dressing is applied. Report 15937 if the underlying bone is removed.

15940–15941

The physician excises a ischial pressure ulcer. An incision is made around the wound over the ischial tuberosity to remove the infected pressure sore. The remaining healthy tissues are irrigated and the wound is closed with sutures and a soft dressing is applied. Report 15941 if a portion of the ischium bone is removed during the procedure.

15944–15945

The physician excises a ischial pressure ulcer. An incision is made around the wound over the ischial tuberosity in order to remove the infected pressure sore. The infected tissue is removed, however, the wound is large enough to require a graft of skin from another part of the body to completely close the area. Two common skin flap donor sites are the scapular region and the groin area at the front of the hip. The physician takes an appropriate size graft from the donor area and sutures it in place following the removal of the infected tissue. The donor site is sutured closed and soft dressings are used to cover the wounds. Report 15945 if the procedure requires an ostectomy.

15946

The physician excises an ischial pressure ulcer and performs an ostectomy to prepare for muscle or myocutaneous flap of skin graft closure. The infected wound is removed and the area is irrigated. The space

CPT® Lay Descriptions

that remains is filled with a muscle flap graft, usually taken from the latissimus dorsi muscle and the overlying skin. The donor site is prepared and the incision is made for the appropriate size of graft to be taken. Once the portion of the muscle is removed, the overlying skin is removed and the wound is sutured closed. The graft is sutured in place and a soft dressing is applied.

15950–15951

The physician excises a trochanteric pressure ulcer. The physician makes an elliptical shaped incision around the wound which is located over the outer hip bone. The infected tissues are removed and the wound is irrigated. The soft tissues are sutured and the skin is closed with sutures. A soft dressing is applied. Report 15951 if a portion of the underlying bone is removed because of the extent of the infection.

15952–15953

The physician excises a trochanteric pressure ulcer. An incision is made around the wound over the trochanter (outer hip bone) in order to remove the infected pressure sore. The infected tissue is removed, however the wound is large enough to require a graft of skin from another part of the body to completely close the area. Two common skin flap donor sites are the scapular region (upper back over the shoulder blade) and the groin area at the front of the hip. The physician takes an appropriate size graft from the donor area and sutures it in place following the removal of the infected tissue. The donor site is sutured closed and soft dressings are used to cover the wounds. Report 15953 if both skin grafting and bone removal is required.

15956–15958

The physician excises a trochanteric pressure ulcer to prepare for muscle or myocutaneous flap of skin graft closure. The physician makes an incision around the pressure sore that lies over the trochanter (hip bone). The wound may be of substantial size where muscle and skin grafting are necessary to fill the space left by the removal of the infected tissues. The infected wound is removed and the area is irrigated. The space that remains is filled with a muscle flap graft, usually taken from the latissimus dorsi muscle and the overlying skin. The donor site is prepared and the incision is made for the appropriate size of graft to be taken. Once the portion of the muscle is removed, the overlying skin is removed and the wound is sutured closed. The graft is sutured in place and a soft dressing is applied. Report 15958 if a portion of the trochanter is removed.

16000

The physician treats a first degree burn. The physician performs a simple cleaning and applies an ointment or dressing.

16010–16030

The patient who suffers burns requires frequent changes of bandages or dressings and debridement of tissues. With the patient under anesthesia, diseased tissue is removed, the wound is cleansed and a new dressing is applied. Report 16015 if performed medium or large, or with major debridement; report 16020 if without anesthesia, office or hospital small; report 16025 without anesthesia, medium; and report 16030 if without anesthesia, large.

16035–16036

The physician performs an escharotomy. Eschar is a leathery slough provided by thermal burns. The physician makes an incision through the area of Eschar and undermines it. With adequate incision of the Eschar the physician achieves release of movement for the underlying tissue. Report 16035 for the initial incision and 16036 for each additional incision.

17000–17003

The physician uses a laser, electrosurgery, cryosurgery, chemical treatment, or other methods to obliterate abnormal tissue. The physician destroys benign, premalignant, or malignant lesions and premalignant lesions other than cutaneous vascular proliferative lesions, including local anesthesia. Report 17000 when one lesion is destroyed. Report 17003 for second through 14 lesions, each. For destruction of flat warts, molluscum contagiosum, or milia, use 17110–17111.

17004

The physician uses a laser, electrosurgery, crysurgery, chemical treatment, or other methods to obliterate abnormal tissue. The physician destroys benign, premalignant or malignant lesions and premalignant lesions other than cutaneous vascular proliferative lesions, including local anesthesa. Report 17004 for 15 or more lesions. Do not report 17004 in conjunction with 17000–17003.

17106–17108

The physician destroys a collection of abnormal blood vessels within the skin. The treated area totals less than 10.0 sq cm for 17106 and 10.0 sq cm to 50.0 sq cm for 17107. To complete this procedure, the physician may apply laser or electrocautery in a technique similar to painting the skin. This destroys the vessels, creating scar tissue that eventually fades. No incision is made and no tissue is removed.

17110–17111

The physician uses a laser, electrosurgery, cryosurgery, chemical treatment, or other methods to obliterate or vaporize flat (plane, juvenile) warts, molluscum contagiosum, or milia. Use 17110 to report up to 14 lesions; use 17111 to report 15 or more lesions. For destruction of condylomata, papillomata, herpetic lesions, common and plantar warts, or other benign, premalignant, or malignant lesions, use 17000–17004.

17250

The physician destroys a form of exuberant/excessive healing tissue known as granulation tissue or "proud flesh." The physician destroys the tissue with chemicals such as silver nitrate.

17260–17266

The physician destroys a malignant lesion of the trunk, arm, or legs. The lesion diameter is up to 0.5 cm for 17260, from 0.6 cm to 1.0 cm for 17261, from 1.1 cm to 2.0 cm for 17262, from 2.1 cm to 3.0 cm for 17263, from 3.1 cm to 4.0 cm for 17264, and over 4.0 cm for 17266. Destruction may be accomplished by using a laser or electrosurgery to burn the lesion, cryotherapy to freeze the lesion, or chemicals to destroy the lesion.

17270–17276

The physician destroys a malignant lesion of the scalp, neck, hands, feet, or genitalia. The lesion diameter is up to 0.5 cm for 17270, from 0.6 cm to 1.0 cm for 17271, or from 1.1 cm to 2.0 cm for 17272, from 2.1 cm to 3.0 cm for 17273, from 3.1 cm to 4.0 cm for 17274, and over 4.0 cm for 17276. Destruction may be accomplished by using a laser or electrosurgery to burn the lesion, cryotherapy to freeze the lesion, or chemicals to destroy the lesion.

17280–17286

The physician destroys a malignant lesion of the face, ears, eyelids, nose, lips, or mucous membranes.. The lesion diameter is up to 0.5 cm for 17280, from 0.6 cm to 1.0 cm for 17281, or from 1.1 cm to 2.0 cm for 17282, from 2.1 cm to 3.0 cm for 17283, from 3.1 cm to 4.0 cm for 17284, and over 4.0 cm for 17286. Destruction may be accomplished by using a laser or electrosurgery to burn the lesion, cryotherapy to freeze the lesion, or chemicals to destroy the lesion.

17304–17310

The physician performs chemosurgery using Moh's micrographic technique. The physician places a chemical agent on the lesion prior to excision. This chemical acts as a tissue fixative. The lesion is then excised via serial tangential cuts, allowing the physician to more closely assess wound margins and extent of tumor. Report 17305 for second stage, fixed or fresh tissue, up to five specimens; report 17306 for third stage, fixed or fresh tissue, up to five specimens; report 17307 for additional stages, each stage; report 17310 for more than five specimens, any stage.

17340

The physician performs cryotherapy for acne. The physician freezes the area of acne with a chemical such as liquid nitrogen by applying a soaked cotton tip application to the lesion for a short period of time. This leads to scabbing and healing.

17360

The physician destroys the area of acne with a chemical such as acne paste or acid by applying a soaked cotton tip applicator to the lesion for a short period of time (commonly 30 seconds). This leads to formation of eventual eschar and healing.

17380

The physician uses electrolysis to remove hair. This code is used to report a 30 minute session. The physician inserts the electroneedle into the hair follicle and applies electrical current, killing the follicle. The electroneedle is removed.

19000–19001

The physician punctures with a syringe needle the skin of the breast overlying a cyst. The needle is inserted into the cyst and fluid is evacuated into the syringe, thus reducing the size of the cyst. The physician withdraws the needle and applies pressure to the puncture wound to stop the bleeding. This process may be repeated for additional lumps in the same breast (e.g., 19001).

19020

The physician makes an incision in the skin of the breast over the site of an abscess or suspicious tissue. The infected cavity is accessed, and specimens for culture are taken before the cavity is irrigated with warm saline solution. Bleeding vessels may be tied or cauterized. If no abscess or suspicious tissue is found, the wound is closed with sutures. In the case of an abscess, the wound is usually loosely packed with gauze to promote free drainage rather than being closed with sutures.

19030

The physician performs an injection procedure for mammary ductogram or galactogram. A cannula or needle is inserted into the duct of the breast. Contrast media is introduced into the breast duct for the purpose of radiographic study. A dissecting microscope may be used to aid placing the cannula. The needle and cannula are removed once the study has been completed.

19100

The physician inserts a large gauge needle through the skin of the breast and into the suspect breast tissue. The needle is removed along with a core of breast tissue. Pressure is applied to the puncture site to stop any bleeding.

19101

The physician makes an incision in the skin of the breast near the site of the suspect mass. The mass is identified and a small tissue specimen is removed. This specimen is often examined immediately. If the lesion is benign, the wound is repaired with a layered closure. If malignant, the incision may be closed pending a separate, more extensive surgical session.

19102–19103

The physician performs a breast biopsy using a percutaneous needle core, automated vacuum assisted or rotating biopsy device, using image guidance. In 19102, under image guidance the physician inserts a large gauge (e.g., 14 gauge), hallow core biopsy needle through the skin of the breast and into the suspicious breast tissue. The physician takes five or more cores of tissue, to obtain a sufficient amount of tissue for diagnosis. In 19103, under image guidance an automated vacuum assisted or rotating biopsy device is inserted through the skin into the suspicious breast tissue, and a core of suspect tissue is removed for biopsy. The needle, automated vacuum assisted or rotating biopsy device is withdrawn. Pressure applied to the puncture site is sufficient to stop any bleeding present. A bandage is applied.

19110

The physician makes an incision at the edge of the areola near the site of the suspect duct. The duct is dissected from surrounding tissue and examined. Surrounding ducts and tissue are also examined. The suspect duct may be excised. Bleeding vessels may be controlled with electrocautery or ligated with sutures. The incision is sutured in a layered closure and a light pressure dressing is applied.

19112

The physician makes an incision around the abnormal opening on the skin of the fistula. The fistula is dissected down to the lactiferous duct. The duct, fistula and skin opening are all excised. The remaining portion of the duct may be ligated. The wound is irrigated with warm sterile saline and closed in layers.

19120

The physician makes an incision in the skin of the breast overlying the site of the mass. Skin and tissue is dissected from the site of the lesion. The lesion and a rim of surrounding apparently normal tissue is excised. Bleeding vessels may be controlled with electrocautery or ligated with sutures. This procedure is often referred to as a lumpectomy or tylectomy. A drain may be inserted into the wound. The incision is sutured in a layered closure and a light pressure dressing is applied.

19125–19126

The physician makes an incision in the skin of the breast over the site of the marked lesion. The lesion, marker, and a rim of surrounding apparently normal tissue is excised. Bleeding vessels may be controlled with electrocautery or ligated with sutures. A drain may be inserted into the wound. The incision is sutured in a layered closure and a light dressing is applied. Additional lesions (e.g., for 19126) may be removed during the same surgical session. Use 19126 in conjunction with code 19125.

19140

The physician makes a circular incision in the skin of the breast at the edge of the areola or in the inframammary fold. Extraneous fat and breast tissue is dissected from the pectoral fascia and removed. Bleeding vessels are ligated with electrocautery or sutures. The incision is sutured in a layered closure and a light pressure dressing is applied.

19160

The physician makes an incision through the skin and fascia over the breast tumor and clamps any lymphatic and blood vessels. The physician excises the tumor mass and a margin of surrounding normal tissue. A drainage tube may be placed through a separate stab incision to enhance drainage from the wound. This procedure is often referred to as a "segmental mastectomy" or a "quadrantectomy." The incision is repaired with a layered closure and a dressing is applied.

19162

The physician makes an incision through the skin and fascia over the breast tumor and clamps any lymphatic and blood vessels. The physician excises the tumor mass and a margin of surrounding normal tissue. The lymph nodes between the pectoralis major and the pectoralis minor muscles, and the nodes in the axilla, are removed through a separate incision. A tube may be placed through a separate stab incision to enhance drainage from the lymphatic system. The incisions are repaired with layered closures and dressings are applied.

19180

The physician makes an elliptical incision that includes the tail of Spence. The skin is separated from the breast tissue, which is dissected from the pectoral fascia and sternum. The breast tissue is removed along with a portion of skin including the nipple. The physician ligates any bleeding vessels. A closed wound drainage catheter may be inserted and the edges of skin are approximated and sutured. A light pressure dressing is applied.

19182

The physician makes an incision in the inframammary crease. The breast is dissected from the pectoral fascia and from the skin. The breast tissue is removed, but the skin and pectoral fascia remain. The physician may ligate any bleeding vessels. The nipple and areola may be examined by a pathologist and retained if free of disease. If no prosthesis is to be inserted, a closed wound suction catheter may be inserted. The wound is closed, and a light pressure dressing is applied.

19200

The physician makes an elliptical incision that includes the nipple and the tail of Spence. The breast, along with the overlying skin, the pectoralis major and minor muscles, and the lymph nodes in the axilla, are removed as a single specimen. Bleeding vessels are ligated or electrocauterized. In large-breasted patients, adequate skin may be available for primary closure. Patients with insufficient skin for coverage may require skin grafts or myocutaneous flaps. If no prosthesis is to be inserted, a closed wound suction catheter may be inserted. The wound is closed, and a pressure dressing is applied.

19220

The physician makes an elliptical skin incision that includes the nipple and the tail of Spence. The breast is dissected from the pectoral fascia and removed. All tissue within the parameters of the sternum, the rectus fascia, the latissimus dorsi muscle, and the clavicle are removed. Bleeding vessels are ligated or electrocauterized. In large-breasted patients, adequate skin may be available for primary closure. Patients with insufficient skin for coverage may require skin grafts or myocutaneous flaps. If no prosthesis is to be inserted, a closed wound suction catheter may be inserted. The wound is closed, and a pressure dressing is applied.

19240

The physician makes an elliptical incision that includes the nipple and the tail of Spence. The breast and the pectoral fascia are removed from the pectoral muscle. The pectoralis minor may be resected to facilitate the axillary dissection. Bleeding vessels are ligated or electrocauterized. The breast tissue and axillary tissue is removed en bloc. The wound is irrigated and closed tube suction drainage is placed. Adequate skin is usually available for primary closure. Patients with insufficient skin for coverage may require skin grafts or myocutaneous flaps. If no prosthesis is to be inserted, a closed wound suction catheter may be inserted. The wound is closed, and a pressure dressing is applied.

19260

The physician makes an incision in the skin of the chest overlying the site of the tumor. The tumor and surrounding tissue is excised. This tissue includes at least one adjacent rib above and below the tumor site and all intervening intercostal muscles. It may also include an en bloc resection of muscles including the pectoralis minor or major, the serratus anterior or the latissimus dorsi. The physician ligates or cauterizes bleeding vessels. A chest tube may be placed to re-expand the lung. The incision is repaired with a layered closure and a pressure dressing is applied to the wound.

19271

The physician makes an incision in the skin of the chest overlying the site of the tumor. The tumor and surrounding tissue is excised. This tissue includes at least one adjacent rib above and below the tumor site and all intervening intercostal muscles. It may also include an en bloc resection of muscles including the

pectoralis minor or major, the serratus anterior or the latissimus dorsi. The physician ligates or cauterizes bleeding vessels. A chest tube may be placed to re-expand the lung. Reconstruction is required, and may involve rib grafts and/or a myocutaneous flap. A pressure dressing is applied to the wound.

19272

The physician makes an incision in the skin of the chest overlying the tumor. This tissue includes at least one adjacent rib above and below the tumor site and all intervening intercostal muscles. It may also include an en bloc resection of muscles including the pectoralis minor or major, the serratus anterior or the latissimus dorsi. Lymphatic tissue lying in the mediastinum is also removed. The physician ligates or cauterizes bleeding vessels as necessary. A chest tube may be placed to re-expand the lung. Reconstruction is required, and may involve rib grafts and/or a myocutaneous flap. A pressure dressing is applied to the wound.

19290–19291

Needle placement is performed to assist in operative identification of the suspect tissue. The physician punctures the skin overlying a breast mass and inserts a needle threaded with a guidance wire. Using radiological guidance to facilitate placement, the physician inserts the wire into the mass. Sometimes dye is also injected into the suspect tissue. The wire will help identify a nonpalpable mass that is to be removed from the patient during a separate session. Use 19291 for each additional lesion. Use 19291 in conjunction with 19290.

19295

The physician places a metallic clip prior to a breast biopsy. Using image guidance the physician places a metallic clip adjacent to a breast lesion to mark the site for a separately reportable percutaneous, needle core breast biopsy.

19316

The physician performs a breast lift, relocating the nipple and areola to a higher position and removing excess skin below the nipple and above the lower breast crease. The physician makes a skin incision above the nipple, in the location to which the nipple will be elevated. Another skin incision is made around the circumference of the nipple. Two skin incisions are made from the circular cut above the nipple to the fold beneath the breast, one on either side of the nipple, forming a "keyhole" shaped skin incision. This skin is cut away from the breast tissue and removed. The physician elevates the breast to its new position and closes the incision, excising any redundant skin in the fold beneath the breast. The incision is repaired with a layered closure.

CPT® Lay Descriptions

19318

The physician reduces the size of the breast, removing wedges of skin and breast tissue from the patient. The physician makes a circular skin incision above the nipple, in the position to which the nipple will be elevated. Another skin incision is made around the circumference of the nipple. Two incisions are made from the circular cut above the nipple to the fold beneath the breast, one on either side of the nipple, creating a "key hole" shaped skin and breast incision. Wedges of skin and breast tissue are removed. Bleeding vessels may be ligated or cauterized. The physician elevates the nipple and its pedicle of subcutaneous tissue to its new position and sutures the nipple pedicle with a layered closure. The remaining incision is repaired with a layered closure.

19324

The physician increases the size of the breast, rearranging existing fat and mammary tissue of the patient. The physician makes a skin incision in the fold beneath the breast or in a circular cut around the areola. This skin is cut away from the breast tissue and the breast tissue is rearranged. The physician may excise redundant skin to augment the breast's appearance. The incision or incisions are repaired with a layered closure.

19325

The physician makes an incision in the fold under the breast, and dissects the breast tissue and muscle layer free from the chest wall to accommodate a prosthesis positioned under the muscle. As an alternative, the prosthesis may also be positioned between the muscle and the existing breast tissue or skin. The incision is repaired with a layered closure.

19328

The physician makes an incision in the fold under the breast, around the nipple, or at the site of an existing mastectomy incision and dissects muscle, fat and breast tissue from the existing implant. The intact implant is removed. Any infection is irrigated. The physician repairs the incision with a layered closure.

19330

The physician makes an incision in the fold under the breast or around the nipple and dissects muscle, fat and breast tissue from the existing implant. The leaking implant is removed. Surrounding tissue is closely examined for adhesions or deposits of leaking implant material. The implant material and any affected tissue are excised. The physician repairs the incision with a layered closure.

19340

The physician dissects the breast tissue and muscle layer free from the chest wall to accommodate a prosthesis positioned under the muscle in a patient who has undergone mastopexy, mastectomy or a reconstructive process during this same surgical

session. The same surgical skin incisions are most often used. As an alternative, the prosthesis may also be positioned between the muscle and the existing breast tissue or skin. The incision is repaired with a layered closure.

19342

The physician makes an incision in the fold under the breast or along a previous surgical incision, and dissects the tissue and muscle layer free from the chest wall to accommodate a prosthesis positioned under the muscle. As an alternative, the prosthesis may also be positioned between the muscle and the existing breast tissue or skin. The incision is repaired with a layered closure.

19350

The physician excises graft skin, usually from the inner thigh, behind the ear, or a section excised from the patient's existing areola. The donor site is repaired with sutures. To create a new nipple, the physician excises the lower section of tissue from the patient's existing nipple, or removes tissue from the ear, or from labia. This donor site is repaired with sutures. A thin, circular layer of surface skin is removed from the breast at the site of the graft. The areola skin graft is positioned and sutured to the breast, and the nipple graft is sutured to a small, circular incision in the areola's center.

19355

The physician makes two or more radial incisions in the areola and elevates the inverted nipple into an everted position. Ductal channels and fibrous bands may be transected to accomplish this. Tissue may be removed. The nipple is secured with sutures and incisions into the areola are closed.

19357

The physician makes an incision in the skin of a patient who has undergone a mastectomy. A pocket is created using an existing chest wall muscle and an expandable implant is placed into it at the site of mastectomy. In some cases, the implant's button-shaped portal may be brought out through the skin so it is accessible by needle. Usually, the portal remains beneath the surface of the skin. The physician injects saline into the access portal to expand the implant. These injections continue until the implant has stretched the surrounding tissue to a size slightly larger than the patient's existing breast. In some cases, the expander remains a permanent prosthesis and small amount of fluid is aspirated until it duplicates the size of the existing breast. In other cases, a second surgery (reported separately) excises the implant and replaces it with a permanent breast prosthesis.

19361

The physician transfers skin and muscle from the patient's back to the breast area to correct defects created from a previous modified radical mastectomy or radical mastectomy. The physician makes a skin incision in the back and dissects a portion of the latissimus muscle and attached, overlying skin from surrounding structures. The muscle-skin flap remains attached to a main artery. In preparation for the transfer, the mastectomy scar is excised. The muscle flap is rotated to the front of the chest through a tunnel under the armpit so that it extends through to the mastectomy incision. The incision in the back is repaired with a layered closure. The physician adjusts the flap for the most aesthetic appearance and secures it with sutures to the chest wall, adjacent muscles, and skin. A breast implant may be positioned under the muscle. The incision is repaired with sutures.

19364

The physician excises a flap of skin, fat, and muscle from another site on the patient for use in the reconstruction of the breast following a modified radical or radical mastectomy. The free flap is excised with careful dissection of a major artery and vein, commonly from the thigh or buttocks, and the operative wound is sutured in a layered repair. In preparation for the graft, the mastectomy scar is excised and an artery and vein dissected in preparation for the graft. The free flap is transferred to the mastectomy site where the artery and vein are connected to a local artery and vein. The physician adjusts the flap for the most aesthetic appearance and secures it with sutures to the chest wall, adjacent muscles, and skin. If the free flap does not have sufficient fat, a breast implant may be required. The chest incision is repaired with sutures.

19366

The physician excises skin, fat, and/or muscle from another site on the patient for use in the reconstruction of the breast following a modified radical or radical mastectomy. The tissue is excised and the operative wound is sutured in a layered repair. In preparation for the graft, any mastectomy scar is excised. The tissue is transferred to the mastectomy site. The physician adjusts the flap for the most aesthetic appearance and secures it with sutures to the chest wall, adjacent muscles, and skin. If the tissue does not have sufficient bulk, a breast implant may be required. The chest incision is repaired with sutures.

19367–19369

The physician performs a transverse rectus abdominus myocutaneous flap (TRAM) procedure. The physician first designs then cuts a skin island flap on the lower abdominal wall. A superior skin, fat flap is elevated off the rectus abdominis muscle. A transverse incision is then made in the rectus sheath and the muscle is divided and elevated keeping the superior epigastric arteries intact for blood supply. Once the muscle is elevated the physician makes an incision through chest skin. This is also elevated creating a pocket for the muscle flap. A connecting tunnel is made between the elevated chest skin and the inferiorly positioned flap. The flap is then carefully passed superiorly under the tunnel of tissue, placed into its new position and sutured after contouring a breast. The abdominal wall is then closed by reapproximating remaining anterior rectus muscle to the remaining lateral muscle and sheath. Skin edges are then brought together and sutured in layers. The physician will also place suction drains. Report 19368 if microvascular anastomosis is used. Report 19369 if the muscle/skin complex has two pedicles or both sides of rectus abdominus are elevated (bilateral or hemiflaps).

19370

The physician makes an incision in the skin of the breast, either at the site of a mastectomy scar or in the skin fold beneath the breast or around the nipple. The physician uses a cautery knife to cut into the area of fibrous scarring associated with a breast implant. The scar (capsular contraction) is cut radically around its circumference to enlarge the pocket in which the prosthesis is placed. No tissue is removed. The incision is repaired with a layered closure.

19371

The physician makes an incision in the skin of the breast, either at the site of a mastectomy scar or in the skin fold beneath the breast or around the nipple. The physician uses a cautery knife to cut into the area of fibrous scarring associated with a breast implant. The scar (capsular contraction) is excised from the breast tissue. The incision is repaired with a layered closure.

19380

Usually to correct a problem with asymmetry of the reconstructed breast, the physician makes an incision in the breast skin along the areola or at the fold under the breast or in prior surgical incisions. Tissue therein may be rearranged or secured with sutures to revise the shape of the reconstructed breast. An existing breast prosthesis may be replaced with a prosthesis of a different configuration. Excess skin or tissue from the reconstructed breast may be removed. Once the breast has been revised to its desired shape, the physician repairs the incision with a layered closure.

19396

The physician creates a custom breast implant model that closely resembles the remaining breast configuration of a mastectomy patient. From this a custom breast implant will be created.

20000–20005

The physician makes an incision through skin directly over an abscessed area. The abscess cavity is explored, debrided, and drained with the use of forceps dissection. The physician then evaluates the underlying bone. Depending on the appearance of the area, the physician may remove dead bone and place a drain or packing after copious irrigation of the area. Report 20005 if deep or complicated.

20100–20103

The physician explores a penetrating wound in the operating room, sometimes in diagnostic studies (reported separately) to help identify damaged structures. Nerve, organ, and blood vessel integrity is assessed. Debridement, removal of foreign bodies, ligation or coagulation of minor subcutaneous/or muscular blood vessels, subcutaneous tissues, fascia, and muscle are also included in this range of codes. Damaged tissues are debrided and repaired when possible. The wound is closed (if clean) or packed open if contaminated by the penetrating body. Report 20100 for exploration of a neck wound. Report 20101 for exploration of a chest wound. Report 20102 for exploration of an abdomen, flank, or back wound. Report 20103 for exploration of a wound to an extremity.

20150

Excision of the epiphyseal bar is a procedure performed to treat a partial epiphyseal arrest in a patient with significant remaining growth in the femur, tibia, or both caused, in many cases, by an injury or infection involving the epiphyseal plate (growth plate). The patient is placed in the supine position and a tourniquet is applied to the proximal thigh and raised to the appropriate pressure. For excision of the distal femur or proximal tibia, the knee is extended on a radiolucent operating table with the intention of resecting two rectangular areas, one on the medial side and one on the lateral side of the bone. Under fluoroscopic image intensification, a stab wound incision is made laterally or medially at the level of the growth plate. One side at a time, an osteotome is driven to a depth of 1 centimeter into the growth plate and rotated 180° to create an opening in the epiphysis. An oval curette is directed through the hole to a depth of about one-third the width of the growth plate. The physician sweeps the curette across the growth plate to remove the rectangular area. If an excision of the epiphyseal bar of the proximal tibia or fibula is performed, the peroneal nerve must be protected. The proximal growth plate of the fibula is approached through an incision anterior to the fibula and exposed anteriorly by subcutaneous blunt dissection. The growth plate is identified by subperiosteal elevation and a rectangular area is removed with a curette. The tourniquet is released, and hemostasis is achieved. A piece of autogenous fat from the subcutaneous tissue (though the same incision) or an inert substance may be interpositioned in the cavity allowing growth to continue in the epiphysis. The wound is closed with suture and the knee is wrapped with compressive dressing to reduce the formation of a hematoma. The limb is placed in a knee immobilizer.

20200–20205

The physician secures a sample of tissue from a superficial muscle for biopsy. The physician incises the overlying skin and bluntly dissects to the suspect muscle. The muscle tissue is obtained. Bleeding is controlled and the wound is closed in sutured layers. Report 20200 if the muscle site sampled is superficial and 20205 if the muscle site sampled is deep.

20206

The physician removes a sample of muscle tissue using a percutaneous needle. The physician applies a local anesthetic to the skin. The physician uses a bore needle to pierce the skin, fascia, and muscle, obtaining a sample of muscle tissue. The needle is withdrawn. No repair is usually necessary. Radiologic supervision, if necessary, is reported separately.

20220–20225

The physician usually performs a biopsy on the spinal process or vertebral body to confirm a suspected growth, disease, or infection. The physician normally uses local anesthesia; however, general anesthesia may be used. Different approaches are taken based on differing levels of vertebrae. The top three cervical vertebrae are approached from a pharyngeal or anterior approach. The lower four cervical vertebrae are approached from a lateral direction. Thoracic and lumbar vertebra are approached from behind and to the right to avoid major arteries. The physician places a large needle into the spinous process or other superficial bone in code 20220; or into the vertebral body, or other deep bone, in 20225 by using an Ottlenghi bar and a preset angle appropriate for the spinal level. An exploring needle is then passed through the larger needle to the desired depth and a piece of tissue is removed for testing. Radiographs are sometimes used to confirm the placement of the needle. Once the needles and frames are removed, the patient is moved to the recovery area.

20240–20245

The physician usually performs a superficial biopsy on the spinous process or other superficial spinal bone to confirm a suspected growth, disease, or infection. The physician performs the procedure with the patient under general anesthesia. The patient is placed in a prone position and an incision is made overlying the vertebrae. The incision is carried down through the tissue to the level of the spinous process or other superficial vertebral process. A piece of bone tissue is removed and sent for examination. The wound is sutured closed and the patient is moved to the recovery area. Report 20240 if the biopsy is superficial; report 20245 if it is deep.

20250–20251

This procedure is used to confirm a suspected growth, disease, or infection. The patient is placed in a prone position. A midline incision is made overlying the vertebrae to be biopsied. The incision is carried down and the fascia is incised. Paravertebral muscles are retracted and the vertebral area to be biopsied is identified. A piece of tissue is then excised or a needle is used to extract a sample of tissue for evaluation. The paravertebral muscles are replaced in their anatomical position and the incision is closed in layers. Report 20250 for thoracic biopsy, 20251 for a lumbar or cervical biopsy.

20500

A physician injects a sinus tract (a canal or passage leading to an abscess) with a therapeutic agent using Betadine as a chemical irritant or antibiotics to clear infection in an abscess or a cyst. X-rays are reported separately.

20501

The physician injects a sinus tract (a canal or passage leading to an abscess) with a radiopaque agent, to determine the existence, nature, or size of an abscess or cyst. X-rays are reported separately.

20520–20525

The physician removes a foreign body in a muscle or tendon sheath. The physician incises the skin and dissects to the muscle or sheath. The foreign body is isolated by palpation or radiographic imagery (separately reported) and removed. The incision may be closed if clean or packed if contaminated by the object. Report 20520 if the removal is simple; report 20525 if removal of the foreign object requires a deep or complicated procedure.

20526

A physician administers a single injection of corticosteroid, four centimeters proximal to the wrist crease between the tendons of the radial flexor and the long palmar muscles on the lateral side of the forearm. This procedure is performed for therapeutic relief of the persistent symptoms of carpal tunnel syndrome.

20550–20553

The physician injects a therapeutic agent into a tendon sheath, ligament, or ganglion cyst in 20550, and into a tendon origin/insertion in 20551. The physician identifies the injection site by palpation or radiographs (reported separately), marks the injection site, and inserts the needle. After withdrawing the needle, the patient is monitored for reactions to the therapeutic agent. Report 20552 for the injection of a therapeutic agent into a single trigger point or multiple trigger points of one or two muscle groups. Report 20553 for the injection of a therapeutic agent into a single trigger point or multiple trigger points of three or more muscle groups.

20600–20610

After administering a local anesthetic, the physician inserts a needle through the skin and into a small joint, bursa or ganglion cyst. A fluid sample may be removed from the joint or a fluid may be injected for lavage or drug therapy. The needle is withdrawn and pressure applied to stop any bleeding. Report 20605 if an intermediate joint, bursa or ganglion cyst is injected. Report 20610 if major joint or bursa is injected.

20615

After administering a local anesthetic, the physician inserts a needle through the skin and into a cyst. A fluid sample may be removed from the joint or a fluid may be injected for lavage or drug therapy. The needle is withdrawn and pressure applied to stop any bleeding.

20650

The physician makes a small skin incision on the lateral or medial distal femur or proximal tibia. A Steinmann pin is drilled transversely through the bone so that an end protrudes from either side. An apparatus with a weight is attached to the pin, providing a traction force to reduce (reposition) and align the fracture as a temporary measure to stabilize it until the fracture itself can be addressed.

20660

The physician uses cranial tongs, a caliper, or a stereotactic frame to stabilize an injured cervical spine for radiography, a stretch test, surgery, or spinal realignment. The physician places the patient supine with the head supported just over the end of the table. The physician applies Betadine solution with sponges to the hair above the ears. The physician separates or removes hair 1.0 cm above ears slightly posterior to mid lateral line. A local anesthetic is injected into the areas selected for pin insertion. Tongs are held in the appropriate position while both skull pins are inserted simultaneously, keeping the tongs equidistant from the skull on either side. The pins are advanced until the indicator button on one pin protrudes 2.0 mm to 3.0 mm. Lock nuts are applied and the pins are checked every two to three hours for proper tightness.

20661–20663

The physician uses a halo to stabilize an injured cervical spine for radiography, traction, or to facilitate surgery. The physician places the patient supine (lying on the back) with the head supported just over the end of the stretcher. Skin and scalp are sterilized with a povidone-iodine solution. The halo is positioned about the patient's head below the area of greatest skull diameter. A local anesthetic is injected into the areas selected for frame pin insertion. The anterior pins are inserted first, followed by the posterior pins. Two diagonally opposed pins are tightened simultaneously until all four engage the skin and bone. Using a torque screwdriver, all are tightened and secured with nuts or set screws before attachment to a traction set up or to a halo vest or cast. Report 20662 for pelvic and 20663 for femoral procedures.

20664

The physician places a cranial halo on the skull of a child whose skull is unusually thin because of a congenital or developmental problem. With the patient soothed by general anesthesia, the physician sterilizes skin and scalp with a povidone-iodine solution. The halo is positioned on the patient's head and pins are advanced until firm, but not to the tension allowed by a normal skull. Diagonally opposed pins are tightened simultaneously. All are secured with nuts. This code includes the removal of the halo.

20665

The physician removes tongs or a halo applied by another physician. Maintaining alignment of the cervical spine, the physician unscrews the frame pins from the skull and removes the tongs or halo. Bone wax may be applied to the wounds to promote healing of the skull. Dressing may be applied to the skin wounds, and the skin may be sutured.

20670

The physician makes a small incision overlying the site of the implant. The implant is located. The physician removes the implant by pulling or unscrewing it. The incision is closed with sutures and/or Steri-strips.

20680

The physician makes an incision overlying the site of the implant. Deep dissection is carried down to visualize the implant, which is usually below the muscle level and within bone. The physician uses instruments to remove the implant from the bone. The incision is repaired in multiple layers using sutures, staples, and/or Steri-strips.

20690–20692

The physician applies an external fixation system to help a fracture or joint injury heal. This procedure is performed in addition to a coded treatment of fracture or joint injury unless listed as part of the basic procedure. This procedure involves the use of an external fixator to stabilize an injury such as a simple fracture. One or more pins or wires may by used. Small stab incisions are made in the skin and a drill is used to make a hole in to the bone. Each pin or wire is inserted into the bone through the drill holes and secured to an external fixation device. This holds the fracture or joint in a stable position. Report 20690 if uniplane fixation is applied and 20692 if multiplane fixation is applied.

20693

The physician performs adjustment or revision of external fixation to allow for healing, development of neurovascular problems, infections, loosening of pins, or failure of the bone fracture to heal. The physician places the patient under anesthesia. If additional pins are needed or must be moved, the physician drills a hole through the bone and inserts the pin, which is attached to external frame devices.

20694

The physician removes the external fixation frame and pulls pins out manually while the patient is under anesthesia. Incisions are closed with sutures and Steri-strips.

20802

The physician replants an arm following a complete amputation. The physician reattaches the upper extremity at a level between the elbow and shoulder. With the patient under anesthesia, the physician identifies the severed neurovascular structures, muscles, bone, and tendons. Each tissue is systematically reattached using sutures, wires, plates, or other fixation devices. Dead tissue is debrided. The skin is joined and closed with sutures after thorough cleaning and irrigation.

20805

The physician reattaches a severed forearm at a level between the wrist and the elbow. With the patient under anesthesia, the physician identifies each structure that has been cut or separated. The nerves, blood vessels, tendons, and bone are each reattached using sutures, wires, plates or other fixation devices. Dead tissue is debrided. The skin is joined and closed with sutures after thorough cleaning and irrigation.

20808

The physician reattaches a hand that has been completely severed from the forearm between the wrist and the fingers. With the patient under anesthesia, the physician identifies the nerves, blood vessels, tendon, and bones. Each structure is reattached in a systematic fashion with debridement of dead tissue. Sutures, wires, plates, or other devices may be used. Copious irrigation is required. The overlying soft tissues and skin are joined with sutures in layers.

20816

The physician reattaches one of the four fingers, excluding the thumb, that has been completely severed from the hand at or near its articulation with its specific metacarpal bone. With the patient under anesthesia, the physician identifies the nerves, tendons, and bones. Dead tissue is debrided and the wound is irrigated thoroughly. Each tissue is systematically reattached using sutures, wires, plates, or other devices. Skin is joined and sutured closed.

20822

The physician reattaches one of the four fingers, excluding the thumb, that has been completely severed from the hand at a level between the fingertip and the attachment of the finger to the hand itself. With the patient under anesthesia, the physician identifies severed structures, including nerves, blood vessels, tendons, and bones. Dead tissue is debrided and the wound is thoroughly irrigated. Each tissue is reattached using sutures, wires, plates, or other devices. Skin is joined in layers with sutures.

20824

The physician reattaches the thumb that has been completely severed from the hand at the attachment of the thumb to the hand itself. With the patient under anesthesia, the physician identifies severed structures, including nerves, blood vessels, tendons, and bones. Dead tissue is debrided and the wound is thoroughly irrigated. Each tissue is reattached using sutures, wires, plates, or other devices. Skin is joined in layers with sutures.

20827

The physician reattaches a thumb that has been completely severed from the hand at a point distal to where the thumb attaches to the hand. With the patient under anesthesia, the physician carefully identifies severed tissues, including nerves, blood vessels, tendons, and bones. Dead tissue is debrided and the wound is thoroughly irrigated. Each tissue is reattached using sutures, wires, plates, or other devices. Skin is joined in layers with sutures.

20838

The physician reattaches a foot that has been completely amputated at or near the ankle. With the patient under anesthesia, the physician carefully identifies severed structures, including blood vessels, nerves, tendons, and bones. Dead tissue is debrided and the wound is thoroughly irrigated. Each tissue is reattached using sutures, wires, plates, pins, or other devices. Skin is joined in layers with sutures.

20900–20902

Bone grafts offer physicians excellent building blocks when repairing skeletal problems. The physician makes an incision overlying the rib, ilium, fibula, or other site from which the autograft will be harvested. Fascia and muscles are incised and retracted. A knife, chisel, cutter, or saw may be used to obtain the bone graft, which will be prepared as needed for implantation of the graft. Cancellous bone chips may be obtained, as well. The incision is closed with sutures. Report 20900 if the graft is small; report 20902 if the graft is larger than a dowel or a button.

20910–20912

The physician takes a cartilage graft from the rib for later use in reconstructing areas of the lower face such as the temporomandibular joint (TMJ). The physician makes a small incision in the skin through the pectoralis muscle and dissects adjacent tissues away near the sternum. The rib is exposed where the bone and cartilage meet. The cartilage is then removed. After the cartilage is harvested, the donor site is closed with layered sutures. Report 20912 if the graft is taken from the nasal septum.

20920

The physician harvests fascia lata by making a small incision over the lateral aspect of the lower thigh. A stripper instrument is advanced upward underneath the fascia as the physician maintains downward pressure on the cut end of fascia lata. Once the desired graft length is obtained, the cutting mechanism on the stripper is used to release the fascia from above. The stripper and graft are then removed together and the wound is sutured. A compressive dressing is also applied.

20922

Fascia lata is a thick band of connective tissue lying underneath the skin of the thigh. It is also called the external invessing fascia. To obtain a portion to use for a graft the physician incises skin and subcutaneous tissue, then elevates the flap of off the fascia lata. The amount of connective tissue is then acquired by incising and elevating the fascia of the thigh musculature. A small strip or patch may be obtained in this manner. The wound is closed primarily.

20924

The physician decides on a donor site then makes a cut down to the desired tendon. The tendon is severed and one end held with a hemostat. Dissection is then carried to the muscular origin and the tendon is removed. A pressure dressing is applied.

20926

The physician obtains a paratenon, fat, or dermis graft. The physician incises the skin and retracts the skin flap to expose the underlying connective tissue. The tissue is incised to the required layer. The graft is lifted and implanted in the recipient site in a separately reportable procedure. The donor site is closed in sutured layers.

20930–20931

The physician obtains a bone graft from a cadaver donor that is frozen or freeze dried until used. The physician prepares and inserts the allograft in a separately reportable spinal procedure. In 20930, the allograft may be prepared as cancellous chips (morselized), or in 20931 it is prepared in a bicortical or tricortical shape for structural use.

20936

During a vertebral fusion or other spinal procedure, the physician may choose to use bone fragments taken from the vertebral bodies adjacent to the affected disk, from the spinous process, or laminar fragment(s). Some of these may have been removed during the surgery or as part of the surgical approach. Local grafts prevent extra morbidity caused by obtaining an iliac or tibial graft and lessen the possibility of cadaver-borne transmittable diseases. When grafts are harvested, they are obtained through the use of power tools or special chisels. The grafts may be morselized, carved into pegs, or shaped as bars. This code is listed in addition to the primary procedure.

20937–20938

Bone grafts offer physicians excellent building blocks when repairing vertebral problems. The physician makes an incision over the ilium, fibula, or other site from which the autograft will be obtained. Fascia and muscles are incised and retracted. A knife, chisel, cutter, or saw may be used to obtain the autograft, which will be prepared as needed for implantation of the graft. In 20937, cancellous bone chips (morselized) are obtained. In 20938, structural bicortical or tricortical grafts are obtained. The incision is closed with sutures.

20950

The physician inserts an interstitial fluid pressure monitoring device into a muscle compartment using a wick catheter, needle, or other method. The physician checks the monitoring device for escalation of pressure, which indicates developing compartment syndrome and tissue ischemia. Once the data has been gathered, the catheter or needle is removed.

20955–20962

The physician takes a bone graft from the fibula for later reconstruction of the lower face. The physician makes an incision in the skin overlying the fibula. The bone is isolated and dissected away from adjacent structures with the small blood vessels that supply blood to the bone attached. The bone is then grafted to the face to eliminate a defect. The small blood vessels are sutured to blood vessels at the recipient site to provide blood flow to the grafted bone. After the graft is complete, the skin incision is closed with layered sutures. Report 20956 if iliac crest, 20957 if metatarsal, and 20962 if other than than fibula, iliac crest, or metatarsal.

20969

The physician makes an incision in the skin overlying the area of harvest. The physician includes a portion of the overlying skin to be removed along with bone. The skin lives by being supplied blood from vessels coming from the bone. This allows the surgeon to reconstruct defect of bone and skin.

20970–20973

The physician harvests a portion of the iliac crest along with overlying skin and dissection of all other bones. The physician makes an incision in the skin overlying the iliac crest. The bone is isolated and dissected away from adjacent structures with the small blood vessels that supply blood to the bone attached. In this case the surgeon usually includes the deep circumflex iliac artery. The wound is closed, suction drains placed and a pressure dressing applied. Report 20972 if performed at the metatarsal; report 20973 if performed on the great toe with web space.

20974–20975

The physician performs electrical stimulation of bone. The physician places electrodes over skin surface along the region of a fracture or defect and then administers a low voltage current. This is a non-surgical technique used to stimulate bone healing. Report 20975 if invasive.

20979

A rehabilitation specialist or physical therapist applies low-intensity ultrasound to a bone by placing a transducer on the skin to stimulate bone healing.

21010

The physician makes an incision in the skin overlying the temporomandibular joint (TMJ). The physician may use several incisional patterns, including the preauricular approach, making an incision through the skin anterior to the contour of the ear. The physician may also approach the TMJ through an incision inside or behind the ear. The physician dissects the tissue layers away until the TMJ is exposed. The skin incision is closed with sutures.

21015

The physician removes from the face a malignant soft tissue tumor not involving bone. The physician excises the tumor and any adjacent tissue where the tumor may have spread. The surgical wound is then repaired by intermediate or complex closure, adjacent tissue transfer, or graft.

21025

The physician removes infected or dead bone tissue from the mandible. This procedure can be performed intraorally through the mucosa or extraorally through a skin incision. If only a small amount of bone is affected, the physician may saucerize the area by grinding the dead bone away with drills and osteotomes. Healthy bone and the continuity of the mandible are left intact. Antibiotic-impregnated acrylic beads may be implanted into the surgical site to stop infection after the removal of bone. These beads are removed at a later time. Extensive bone removal in large sections or blocks may require a separate bone harvesting/grafting procedure to repair continuity defects. The incisions are closed simply.

21026

The physician removes dead bone from midfacial bones. A transoral incision in the maxillary buccal vestibule is the most frequent approach. Facial incisions would only be used for very large lesions or for additional surgical access. The physician reflects the overlying mucosa, exposing the dead bone. Drills, saws, and osteotomes are used to remove the bone. The transoral incisions are closed in a single layer. Any cutaneous incision is closed in multiple layers.

21029

The physician removes excessive bone from midfacial bones. A transoral incision is made in the maxillary buccal vestibule. The physician reflects the overlying mucosa, exposing the excessive bone. Rotary burs, files, and osteotomes are used to remove this bone. The transoral incision is closed in a single layer.

21030

The physician removes a benign tumor or cyst from midfacial bones. Transoral incisions (gingival and maxillary buccal vestibular) are made. Facial incisions would only be used for very large lesions or for additional surgical access. The physician reflects the overlying mucosa, exposing the tumor or cyst in the bone. Drills, saws, and osteotomes are used to remove the lesion from the bone. The physician may use a curet to remove any remaining contents of the tumor or cyst. The transoral incisions are closed in a single layer. Any facial incision is closed in multiple layers.

21031

The physician removes a benign outgrowth of bone (torus mandibularis) most commonly from the lingual (tongue) side of the mandible. Using an intraoral approach, the physician makes an incision in the mucosa overlying the outgrowth of bone and reflects the tissue. The excess bone is removed with a drill or osteotome. The mucosal incision is then closed with sutures.

21032

The physician makes an incision through the mucosa overlying a torus palatinus (a bony protuberance), usually found at the junction of the intermaxillary and transverse palatine structures. The torus is exposed. Drills, osteotomes, or files are used to remove and contour the bone. The tissue is then sutured directly over the bone. Some soft tissue may be excised prior to closure for adaptation over the newly contoured bone.

21034

The physician removes a malignant tumor from the bones of the midface. Incisions include transoral (e.g., maxillary buccal vestibular) and facial (e.g., Weber-Ferguson). The bony mass is excised with the use of drills, saws, and osteotomes. The tumor is removed to "free margins" as determined with intraoperative tissue specimens sent to the pathologist for immediate microscopic examination. The physician may remove teeth and overlying mucosa. Some surgical defects may require immediate soft tissue reconstruction (e.g., myocutaneous flaps). Transoral incisions are closed in a single layer and facial incisions are closed in layers. Intraoral surgical splints may be used.

21040–21041

The physician removes a cyst or benign tumor from the mandible. Using an intraoral approach, the physician incises and reflects a mucosal flap of the

tissue overlying the tumor. In an extraoral approach, the physician approaches the defect through a skin incision. The tumor is identified and removed from the mandible. Removal of overlying bone with a drill or osteotome may be required. The mucosal flap is then sutured primarily. Additional bone removal (e.g., 21041) may also be necessary. With large tumors, the surgical wounds may be packed and sutured, or reconstructive procedures such as harvest of bone may be needed, depending on the size of the surgical wound. The incisions are closed with layered sutures.

21044

The physician removes a malignant tumor from the mandible. Through an intraoral and /or extraoral approach, the physician isolates and dissects the mandibular tumor. The tumor and surrounding tissues are removed. The tissues are then closed with layered sutures, or may be packed and left open. A separately reportable reconstructive procedure, such as bone harvesting, may be necessary.

21045

The physician removes a malignant tumor from the mandible. An intraoral and/or extraoral approach is used. The tumor and surrounding tissues are removed. Resection or removal of a part or all of the mandible is performed. Immediate or delayed reconstruction with bone grafts, tissue rearrangement, flaps, or prosthetic devices is sometimes required. The skin incisions are closed with layered sutures.

21050

The physician removes the condyle of the mandible. An incision is usually made in the skin anterior to the contour of the ear. The physician dissects the tissue layers until the condyle is exposed. The condyle is cut with drills or saws from the mandible and removed. An additional incision just under the angle of the mandible may be required. The area can be reconstructed with bone and cartilage, or a prosthetic condyle may be inserted. The skin incision is closed with layered sutures and a pressure dressing may be applied.

21060

The physician removes part or all of the meniscus (articular disc) of the temporomandibular joint. An incision is usually made in the skin anterior to the contour of the ear. The physician dissects the tissue layers until the meniscus is exposed. The meniscus is then clamped and removed. The joint may be left without a disc, or the disc may be replaced with tissue grafted from other areas of the body or an artificial disc. The skin incision is then closed with layered sutures and a pressure dressing may be applied.

21070

The physician removes the diseased or fractured coronoid process of the mandible. The physician makes an incision intraorally along the external oblique ridge of the mandible. The tissue is then reflected from the bone, exposing the coronoid process. Using drills and/or osteotomes, the coronoid process is clamped and sectioned from the mandible. The muscle attachments are cut from the coronoid process and will retract, forming scar tissue. The coronoid process is removed. The mucosal incision is closed primarily.

21076

The physician fabricates a custom obturator prosthesis to separate the mouth from other structures of the face and skull while performing surgery or allowing facial injuries to heal. The physician identifies the extent of the patient's injures and determines the type of prosthesis that is required. Impressions of the mouth are taken to make models. A custom obturator prosthesis for that particular patient is prepared from the models.

21077

The physician fabricates a custom orbital prosthesis for the orbit of the eye for the purpose of protecting surrounding structures while surgery is performed or for the healing of facial and skull injuries. The physician identifies the extent of the patient's injuries or disease to determine the exact nature of the required prosthesis. Impressions of the orbit of the eye are taken and used to make models. A custom prosthesis for the particular patient is made from the models.

21079–21080

The physician fabricates an obturator to provide a separation between the mouth and the surgical site and/or protect the surgical site while assisting the patient's ability to talk and chew. Impressions are made of the mouth. The impressions are then used to make models from which a custom obturator is fabricated. The physician makes an interim or temporary obturator (21079) while waiting for a definitive obturator. A definitive obturator (21080) separates the nasal and sinus complex from the mouth.

21081

The physician fabricates a prosthesis used in a mandibular resection procedure. Impressions are made of the mandible. The impression is fashioned into a cast model which the physician uses to construct an external prosthetic device.

21082

The physician fabricates a prosthesis used to augment the palate. Impressions are made of the maxilla and palate. The impression is then fashioned into a cast model. The prosthesis is then fabricated from this cast.

21083

The physician fabricates a palatal lift prosthesis for the patient requiring the prosthesis to maintain velopharyngeal competence. Impressions are made of the maxilla and palate. The impression is then fashioned into a cast model. A customized prosthesis is then fabricated from this cast.

21084

The physician fabricates a prosthesis used to aid speech. An impression is made of the affected area and the physician customizes a prosthetic device from a cast model of the impression.

21085

The physician fabricates a splint used in an oral surgical procedure. An impression is made of the area and the physician customizes the splint from the cast model of the impression. These splints may be used in orthognathic reconstructive jaw surgery (repositioning of jaws), for repair of traumatic injuries, or in ablative tumor surgery with or without jaw resection.

21086

The physician designs and prepares a prosthesis for the auricle (pinna, or external ear). An impression is taken, from which a cast is made, and the prosthesis is fabricated from this mold. The mold is then shaped and honed to fit.

21087

The physician makes a nasal prosthesis after resection of part or all of the nose. A full face impression or moulage is taken before or after removal of the nose. A stone cast of the patient's face is made from the moulage. Presurgical photographs of the patient are also used as a guide. A customized nasal prosthesis is fabricated on the face cast. The prosthesis is made of latex and is painted to match the color of the patient's skin. This artificial nose is placed and maintained with skin adhesive glue.

21088

The physician makes a facial prosthesis after resection of part or all of the face. A full face impression or moulage is taken before or after removal of the nose. A stone cast of the patient's face is made from the moulage. Presurgical photographs of the patient are also used as a guide. A customized nasal prosthesis is fabricated on the face cast. The prosthesis is made of latex and is painted to match the color of the patient's skin. This artificial face is placed and maintained with skin adhesive glue.

21100

With the patient's eyes closed, the physician places the halo over the patient's head and tightens four screws. Now in place, the halo is connected to interdental fixation (wires the jaws together). Arch bars, ivy loops, or other wires are attached to the teeth then wired together. For edentulous (without teeth), or partially edentulous patients, dentures or splints may be wired to the jaws and then wired together to provide intermaxillary fixation. Orthodontic appliances may also be used.

21110

The physician applies interdental fixation (wires the jaws together). Arch bars, ivy loops, or other wires are attached to the teeth then wired together. For edentulous (without teeth), or partially edentulous patients, dentures or splints may be wired to the jaws and then wired together to provide intermaxillary fixation. Orthodontic appliances may also be used.

21116

The physician injects a radiopaque dye into the temporomandibular joint. The physician or radiologist threads a small catheter into the temporomandibular joint by inserting a needle through the skin and into the superior and/or inferior joint spaces. Dye is then injected. Separately reported radiographs are taken to study the soft tissue anatomy of the joint, such as the articular disc or ligaments.

21120–21123

The physician places an implant or a graft onto the chin to augment or enlarge it. Various materials can be used, including tissue grafted from the patient's own body or taken from a tissue bank. Prosthetic devices may also be used. This procedure is most commonly performed from an intraoral approach. The physician makes an incision in the mandibular labial vestibule inside the lower lip. The mucosa is then reflected from the chin and the implanted material placed between the mucosa and the bone. A skin incision may also be made under the chin. The implant may be secured to the bone using wires or screws, or may be left to be held in place by the surrounding tissue. The mucosa is then sutured simply. Report 21121 if a sliding osteotomy is performed; report 21122 if two or more osteotomies are performed; and report 21123 if interpositional bone grafts are included.

21125

The physician uses prosthetic material to augment the body or angle of the mandible. The physician may use an intraoral approach or may make skin incisions extraorally below the body or angle of the mandible. The physician dissects tissues away and the bone of the body or angle is exposed. A synthetic material is placed on the mandible to augment the contours. The material is secured with screws or wires. The incisions are sutured simply.

21127

The physician uses a bone graft to augment the body or angle of the mandible. The physician harvests bone from another site on the patient's body, most commonly the rib, hip, or skull, and repairs the surgically created wound of the harvest site. The

physician may use an intraoral approach or skin incisions. The physician dissects adjacent structures away and the body or angle of the mandible is exposed. The graft is placed on an area of the body or angle to augment the contours. The graft may also be placed between portions of bone of the body or angle (interpositional grafting). The graft is secured with screws or wires. The intraoral incisions are sutured simply. The extraoral incisions are closed with layered sutures.

21137

The physician performs surgery on the forehead to correct a skeletal deformity. With the patient under anesthesia, the physician makes an incision in the hairline to expose the forehead of the skull. The deformity in the bone is identified and fully exposed. The physician uses a variety of surgical instruments to reshape the bone to make it follow a more normal contour. The wound is thoroughly irrigated and closed in layers.

21138

The physician performs surgery on the forehead to correct a skeletal deformity using the application of prostheses or bone grafts to obtain a more normal contour. With the patient under anesthesia, the physician makes an incision in the hairline to expose the forehead of the skull. The deformity in the bone is identified and fully exposed. The physician uses a variety of surgical instruments to reshape the bone to make it follow a more normal contour. Prostheses may be applied and/or autografts may be harvested and applied as part of the procedure. The wounds are thoroughly irrigated and closed in layers.

21139

The physician corrects a skeletal deformity of the frontal sinus or repairs the anterior frontal sinus wall. An incision is made either at the forehead hairline or the eyebrows. The forehead is exposed directly over the frontal sinus wall. The deformity or deficit is identified. Soft tissue is debrided. The physician reshapes the anterior wall of the sinus. If the wall is prominent or badly misshapen, the physician elevates it from the forehead and then resets it in the appropriate anatomic and cosmetic position. Fixation devices such as wires may be required to maintain the repaired wall. The wound is irrigated and closed in layers. A soft dressing is applied.

21141–21143

The physician performs surgery on the midface to repair a single fracture with movement in any direction and without using a bone graft. X-rays and computerized tomography scans (reported separately) are obtained to identify the nature of the fracture. With the patient under anesthesia, the physician exposes the fracture usually from inside the mouth. Surgical instruments are used to manipulate the fragments into an acceptable reduction. The physician uses any of several interfixation devices to maintain stability. The may include arch bars, plates and screws, and various wire techniques. The fracture site is thoroughly irrigated with antibiotic solution and the oral mucosa is closed as needed. Wires placed around the teeth are rechecked for sharp edges. Report 21141 if a single piece is repaired during the procedure. Report 21142 if two pieces are repaired. Report 21143 if three or more pieces are repaired.

21145–21147

The physician performs surgery on the midface to repair a single fracture with movement in any direction and using a bone graft. Separately reportable x-rays and computerized tomography scans are obtained to identify the nature of the fracture. With the patient under anesthesia, the physician exposes the fracture usually from inside the mouth. Surgical instruments are used to manipulate the fragments into an acceptable reduction. Bone grafts are harvested and applied. The physician uses any of several interfixation devices to maintain stability. The may include arch bars, plates and screws, and various wire techniques. The fracture site is thoroughly irrigated with antibiotic solution and the oral mucosa is closed as needed. Wires placed around the teeth are rechecked for sharp edges. Report 21145 if a single piece is repaired. Report 21146 if two pieces are repaired. Report 21147 if three or more pieces are repaired.

21150

The physician reconstructs the midface to correct developmental skeletal deformities. The physician may use a variety of incisions, including a bicoronal scalp flap, lower eyelid, and transoral incisions. Through these incisions the nasofrontal junction, inferior orbital rims, and maxilla are exposed. Osteotomies of the pyramidal midface (LeFort II) are performed with saws, burs, or osteotomes. The midface is down-fractured from the stable bone. The physician removes excess bone at fracture sites and repositions the midface. The midface is then reduced with wires, plates, and/or screws. The transoral incision is closed in a single layer. Lower eyelid and scalp incisions are closed in multiple layers. Intermaxillary fixation may or may not be applied.

21151

The physician reconstructs the midface to correct developmental skeletal deformities. The physician may use a variety of incisions, including a bicoronal scalp flap, lower eyelid, and transoral incisions. Through these incisions the physician exposes the nasofrontal junction, inferior orbital rims, and maxilla. Osteotomies of the pyramidal midface (LeFort II) are performed with saws, burs, or osteotomes. The midface is down-fractured from the stable bone and placed with precise measurement into a new position. The physician then reduces the midface with wires, plates, and/or screws. Through a

separate incision, the physician may harvest a bone graft from the patient's hip, rib, or skull and close the surgically created wound. The interpositional bone grafts may be placed between the bony interfaces of the midface. The transoral incisions are closed in a single layer. Lower eyelid and scalp incisions are closed in multiple layers. Intermaxillary fixation may be applied.

21154

The physician reconstructs the midface to correct developmental skeletal deformities. The physician uses a variety of incisions, including a bicoronal scalp flap, lower eyelid, and transoral incisions. Complete separation of the midface (LeFort III) from the cranial base is necessary. Surgical fractures are made through the zygomas, orbits, and bones of the nasofrontal region. Osteotomies of the complete midface are performed with saws, burs, or osteotomes. The midface is down-fractured from the stable bone and placed with precise measurement into presurgically predicted sites. The physician reduces the midface with wires, plates, and/or screws. Through a separate incision, the physician may harvest a bone graft from the patient's hip, rib, or skull and close the surgically created wound. The interpositional bone grafts may be placed between the bony interfaces of the midface. The transoral incisions are closed in a single layer. Lower eyelid and scalp incisions are closed in multiple layers. Intermaxillary fixation may be applied.

21155

The physician reconstructs both the midface and the maxilla to correct developmental skeletal deformities. The physician uses a variety of incisions, including a bicoronal scalp flap, lower eyelid, and transoral incisions. Complete separation of the midface (LeFort III) from the cranial base is necessary. Additionally, horizontal down-fracture of the maxilla may be necessary to correct alignment of the teeth. Surgical fractures are made through the zygomas, orbits, and bones of the nasofrontal region with saws, burs, or osteotomes. The physician also makes a horizontal osteotomy, separating the maxilla from the midface. The midface is down-fractured from the stable cranial base and the maxilla is down-fractured from the midface. Both the midface and maxilla are placed into new positions and reduced with wires, plates, and/or screws. Through a separate incision, the physician may harvest bone grafts from the patient's hip, rib, or skull and close the surgically created wound. The interpositional bone grafts may be placed between the bony interfaces of the maxilla and midface. The transoral incisions are closed in a single layer. Lower eyelid and scalp incisions are closed in multiple layers. Intermaxillary fixation may or may not be applied.

21159

The physician reconstructs the midface with the forehead to correct developmental skeletal deformities. Surgical fractures are made through the zygomas, frontal bone, and orbits. Complete separation of the midface with the frontal bone from the cranial base is necessary. The physician uses a variety of incisions, including a bicoronal scalp flap, eyelid, and transoral incisions. Osteotomies of the complete midface with the frontal bone are performed with saws, burs, or osteotomes. The midface with the frontal bone is down-fractured from the stable cranial base. The midface and frontal bone are placed with precise measurement into new positions and reduced with wires, plates, and/or screws. Through a separate incision, the physician may harvest bone grafts from the patient's hip, rib, or skull and close the surgically created wound. The interpositional bone grafts may be placed between the bony interfaces of the maxilla and midface. The transoral incisions are closed in a single layer. Eyelid and scalp incisions are closed in multiple layers. Intermaxillary fixation may be applied.

21160

The physician reconstructs both the midface with the forehead and the maxilla to correct developmental skeletal deformities. Complete separation of the midface with the frontal bone from the cranial base and horizontal down-fracture of the maxilla are necessary. Surgical fractures are made through zygomas, frontal bone, and orbits. The physician uses a variety of incisions, including a bicoronal scalp flap, eyelid, and transoral incisions. Through the incisions, the physician performs osteotomies of the complete midface, frontal bone, and maxilla with saws, burs, or osteotomes. The midface and frontal bone are down-fractured from the stable cranial base and the maxilla is down-fractured from the midface. The midface, frontal bone and maxilla are placed into new positions and reduced with wires, plates, and/or screws. Through a separate incision, the physician may harvest bone grafts from the patient's hip, rib, or skull and close the surgically created wound. The interpositional bone grafts may be placed between the bony interfaces of the maxilla and midface. The transoral incisions are closed in a single layer. Eyelid and scalp incisions are closed in multiple layers. Intermaxillary fixation may be applied.

21172

The physician performs reconstructive surgery on the lower forehead and superior-lateral orbit of the eye to correct skeletal abnormalities, with or without grafts. The physician may use a variety of incisions, including through the eyelids and scalp, to obtain access to the site. Through those incisions, the physician performs osteotomies of the forehead and orbit as needed. The bones are manipulated and realigned to the desired position. Through a separate incision, the physician may obtain bone grafts that

can be placed to augment the forehead and orbit reconstruction. The bones are held in place with the use of wires, plates, or screws (reported separately). The wounds are irrigated and each closed in layers.

21175

The physician performs reconstructive surgery on the lower forehead and both superior lateral orbital rims to correct skeletal abnormalities of the cranium. The physician utilizes a variety of incisions about the eyes, forehead, and scalp to gain access to these bones. The soft tissues are carefully dissected as needed. The physician identifies the bones through exposure. Several osteotomies are made so that the deformity can be corrected. Through a separate incision, the physician may obtain bone grafts to augment the reconstruction. The bones are manipulated, contoured, and shifted as needed to place them in the desired positions. Various internal fixation devices are employed, such as wires, pins, plates, or screws, to hold the reduction. Bone graft is used as needed. The wounds are thoroughly irrigated, debrided, and closed in layers.

21179–21180

The physician performs reconstructive surgery of the entire forehead and the supraorbital rims of both eyes to correct skeletal deformities of the cranium. With the patient under anesthesia, the physician uses any of a variety of incisions to access the sites. These may include multiple scalp and eyelid sites. The incisions are carried deep to the bones and the deformities are identified and exposed. The physician performs osteotomies of the bones in multiple places so the bones can be shifted and manipulated to the desired position. The bones are shaped as needed. In 21179, the physician utilizes allografts or synthetic prosthetic material to augment the reconstruction. In 21180, the physician employs autografts. Pins wire, plates, and screws are used to hold the bones and graft stable. The wounds are irrigated thoroughly and closed in layers.

21181

The physician performs surgery to correct distortion expansion or deformity of a cranial bone caused by a benign extracranial lesion. The physician utilizes any of a variety of incisions to expose the site. The incisions are carried deep to the bone and the lesions are identified and exposed. The physician uses surgical instruments to debride, reshape, or contour the cranial bone to conform to its normal anatomic position and profile. The bone and wounds are thoroughly irrigated and closed in layers.

21182–21184

The physician performs reconstructive surgery of the cranial bones including the orbits, forehead, and nasoethmoid complex following the excision of benign tumors from within and without the cranium. The physician utilizes a variety of incisions through intraoral, eyelid, and scalp sites to gain access to these bones. The incisions are carried deep to the bones that are individually identified and exposed. The physician performs osteotomies as needed to manipulate the bones into their desired and acceptable positions. This may require advancement of the forehead. Through a separate incision, the physician harvests bone grafts from a site such as the hip. Multiple grafts may be required to augment and stabilize the reconstructed bones. The physician also uses internal fixation devices such as wires, plates, and screws to hold the reduction. The incisions are all thoroughly irrigated and closed in layers. Report 21182 if the total area of bone grafting is less than 40.0 sq cm. Report 21183 if the total area of bone grafting is greater than 40.0 sq cm but less than 80.0 sq cm; report 21184 if the total area of bone grafting is greater than 80.0 sq cm.

21188

The physician reconstructs the midface to correct developmental or traumatic skeletal deformities. Reconstruction includes both osteotomies and bone grafts. The physician may use a variety of incisions, including a bicoronal scalp flap, eyelid, and transoral incisions. Through the incisions, the physician performs osteotomies of the midface with saws, burs, or osteotomes. The midfacial bones are down-fractured from the stable cranial base. The midface is placed with precise measurement into a new position. Through a separate incision, the physician may harvest bone grafts from the patient's hip, rib, or skull and close the surgically created wound. The interpositional bone grafts may be placed between the bony interfaces of the maxilla and midface. The transoral incisions are closed in a single layer. Eyelid and scalp incisions are closed in multiple layers. Intermaxillary fixation may or may not be applied.

21193

The physician reconstructs the ramus of the mandible using various osteotomies (bone cuts) to correct mandibular deformities. Vertical ramus, horizontal, L, inverted L, and C osteotomies are used. The type of osteotomy refers to the shape and direction of the bone cuts. The physician makes a skin incision below the angle of the mandible. Vertical ramus and horizontal osteotomies may also be accomplished from an intraoral approach. The tissue is dissected to the mandible and the bone of the mandibular ramus is exposed. Bone cuts are made in various shapes according to the type of osteotomy using drills, saws, or osteotomes. The physician moves part of the separated mandible into a new position. The osteotomy cuts are stabilized with wires, screws, or plates. The incision is then sutured. No bone grafts are used.

21194

The physician reconstructs the ramus of the mandible using various osteotomies (bone cuts) to correct

mandibular deformities. Vertical ramus, horizontal, L, inverted L, and C osteotomies are used. The type of osteotomy refers to the shape and direction of the bone cuts. The physician harvests bone from another site on the patient's body, most commonly the rib, hip, or skull, and repairs the surgically created wound. The physician makes a skin incision below the angle of the mandible. Vertical ramus and horizontal osteotomies can be accomplished from an intraoral approach. The tissue is dissected to the mandible and the bone of the mandibular ramus is exposed. Bone cuts are made in various shapes according to the type of osteotomy using drills, saws, or osteotomes. The physician moves part of the separated mandible into a new position. A harvested bone is grafted along the osteotomy cuts to aid in the reconstruction and healing process. The osteotomy cuts are stabilized with wires, screws, or plates. The incision is then sutured with a layered closure.

21195

The physician reconstructs the mandibular ramus to lengthen, set back, or rotate the mandible. Using an intraoral approach, the physician makes an incision overlying the external oblique ridge and through the mucosa near the second mandibular molars. The mandibular ramus is then exposed by reflecting the tissue from both sides of the ramus. Drills, saws, and/or osteotomes are used to cut the mandible along the inside, top, and outside surfaces of the bone, but not completely through. The physician uses osteotomes and/or other instruments to pry the mandible apart along the bone cuts in a sagittal plane. Once separated, the physician moves the mandible into the desired position and stabilizes the bone cuts using wires. The mucosal incisions are then sutured primarily.

21196

The physician reconstructs the mandibular ramus to lengthen, set back, or rotate the mandible. Using an intraoral approach, the physician makes an incision over the external oblique ridge and through the mucosa near the second mandibular molars. The mandibular ramus is then exposed by reflecting the tissue from both sides of the ramus. Drills or saws are used to cut the mandible along the inside, top, and outside surfaces of the bone, but not completely through. The physician uses osteotomes and/or other instruments to pry the mandible apart along the bone cuts in a sagittal plane. Once separated, the physician moves the mandible into the desired position and stabilizes the bone cuts using screws or plates placed in or on the bone. The physician may also make small 0.5 cm skin incisions near the mandibular angle, through which instruments place the plates or screws. Intermaxillary fixation may be placed. The mucosa and skin incisions are then closed with sutures.

21198–21199

The physician performs an osteotomy on a segment of the mandible to correct a localized deformity. The teeth are moved within a segment or block of bone. Using an intraoral approach, the physician makes an incision in the mucosa to expose the segment of bone to be moved. Drills, saws, and/or osteotomes are used to cut a section of the alveolar bone. These cuts do not extend entirely through the mandible, but include only a segment above the inferior border. The segment is moved into the desired position and stabilized with wires, screws, or plates. The segment may also be held in place by a preformed acrylic interocclusal splint. The mucosa is then sutured simply and intermaxillary fixation may or may not be placed. Report 21198 when a segmental osteotomy of the mandible is performed. Report 21199 when a segmental osteotomy of the mandible is performed and the genioglossus (primary tongue muscle) is advanced.

21206

The physician performs an osteotomy on a segment of the maxilla to correct a localized deformity. The teeth are moved within a segment or block of bone. Using a circumvestibular incision, the physician exposes the segment of bone to be moved. Drills, saws, and/or osteotomes are used to cut a section of the alveolar bone. These cuts do not extend entirely through the maxilla, but include only a segment. The segment is moved into the desired position and stabilized with wires, screws, or plates. The segment may also be held in place by a preformed acrylic interocclusal splint. The mucosa is then sutured simply and intermaxillary fixation may or may not be placed.

21208

The physician augments the maxilla with implanted grafts or prosthetic devices, altering the contours of the face. The physician may use an intraoral approach. The tissue is dissected, exposing the bone of the maxilla. A bone graft is taken from another part of the body, such as the hip or rib, and grafted onto the maxilla to contour the face. Other materials such as prosthetic implants or donor bone may also be used. The implant is secured to the maxilla using screws, wires, or plates. The mucosa is then sutured simply.

21209

The physician removes bone of the maxilla, reducing the contours of the face. The physician may make a circumvestibular incision. The tissue is dissected, exposing the bone of the maxilla. A reciprocation saw or drill is used to cut and remove the bone, reducing its contours. The mucosal incision is sutured simply.

21210

The physician harvests bone from the patient's hip, rib, or skull. Incisions are made overlying the harvest site. Tissues are dissected away to the desired bone.

The physician then removes the bone. After the bone is harvested, the donor site is repaired in multiple layers.

21215

The physician reconstructs the mandible to correct defects due to injury, infection, or tumor resection. The procedure may also be performed to augment atrophic or thin mandibles, or to aid in healing fractures. The physician harvests bone from another site on the patient's body, most commonly the rib, hip, or skull, and repairs the surgically created wound. The physician makes facial skin incisions to expose the mandible and place the graft from the donor site. Occasionally, intraoral incisions are used. The graft is stabilized with wires, plates, or screws. The physician may or may not place the patient in intermaxillary fixation. The incisions are then sutured with a layered closure.

21230–21235

The physician reconstructs an area of the midface with a cartilage graft harvested from the rib. The physician makes a small incision near the sternum through the pectoralis muscle exposing the rib where the bone and cartilage meet. Cartilage is removed from the area and the donor site is closed directly. The physician makes circumvestibular or lower eyelid incisions to expose the area of the midface and place the graft. The graft is stabilized with wires, plates, or screws. The physician may place the patient in intermaxillary fixation. The incisions are then sutured with a layered closure. Report 21235 if ear cartilage is used on the nose or ear.

21240

The physician repairs or reconstructs the temporomandibular joint. An incision is made through the skin anterior to the contour of the ear or within the ear. The tissues are dissected and the joint is exposed. Once the joint is exposed, a variety of repairs may be performed. The articular disc may be repositioned or the ligaments may be repaired or shortened. The condylar head may be smoothed or recontoured, or the articular disc may be removed. If removed, tissue may be taken from another part of the body to replace the articular disc. The tissue may be fascia from nearby muscles such as the temporalis muscle, cartilage from the ear, dermis, or other tissues. The incisions are then closed directly.

21242

The physician repairs or reconstructs the temporomandibular joint. An incision is made through the skin anterior to the contour of the ear or within the ear. The tissues are dissected and the joint is exposed. Once the joint is exposed, a variety of repairs may be performed. Donor tissue (allograft material) may replace the articular disc or other parts of the joint. The incisions are then closed directly.

21243

The physician partially or totally replaces the diseased or injured temporomandibular joint with a prosthetic joint. An incision is made through the skin anterior to the contour of the ear or within the ear. An additional skin incision just beneath the angle of the mandible may also be necessary. An artificial fossa can be placed above the condyle and secured with screws. If the condyle needs replacement, it is removed and a prosthetic condyle is secured to the remaining condylar neck, typically using screws. Both the fossa and the condyle may need to be replaced. The incisions are then closed directly.

21244

The physician inserts a bone plate with posts that extend through the lower border of the mandible and into the mouth. The posts can be used to retain dentures in an atrophic or thin mandible. The physician makes an incision through the skin under the chin and dissects the tissues to the bone. Holes are drilled upward through the bone and into the mouth. The posts of the plate are placed through the holes and into the mouth. The plate is then secured to the mandible with screws and the incision is closed with layered sutures.

21245–21246

The physician places a metal framework between the mucosa and the bone of the maxilla. The metal framework has posts which extend vertically and protrude through the mucosa into the mouth. The posts are used to retain an upper denture when teeth are missing. Intraoral surgery is performed in one or two sessions. The physician makes an incision along the crest of the edentulous area (without teeth) and exposes as much of the bone as possible. If performed in two sessions, the physician makes impressions of the exposed bone and sutures the mucosa closed. The impression in used to make models for custom framework. At the second surgical session, the physician removes the sutures and again exposes the bone. The metal framework, with the attached posts, is placed on the bone. The mucosa and periosteum are sutured over the framework and around the protruding posts. Scarring, which occurs with healing, keeps the framework in place. If performed in one session, a CT scan is used to make a plastic model of the mandible from which the framework and posts are fabricated. A single surgical session is used to insert the framework as described above. Incisions are closed simply with sutures. Report 21245 for partial reconstruction. Report 21246 for complete reconstruction.

21247

The physician reconstructs the temporomandibular joint (TMJ) and mandibular condyle using bone and cartilage taken from the rib. The physician makes facial skin incisions using an extraoral approach. The physician harvests the rib by making a small incision through the pectoralis major muscle, and dissecting through the tissue to the rib. Part of the rib and the cartilage near the sternum is removed. The donor site is closed with layered sutures. The physician then makes incisions through the skin anterior to the contour of the ear and dissects tissue to the TMJ site. Another incision is often made beneath the angle of the mandible and the tissue is dissected to the bone. The bone is exposed superiorly as far as possible. The rib graft is then inserted through the lower incision with the cartilaginous end placed upward into the joint, replacing the condyle. Through both incisions, the rib is manipulated into the proper position and secured to the mandible using plates, screws, or wires. The incisions are then closed with layered sutures. Intermaxillary fixation may be placed.

21248–21249

The physician places metal implants into the bone of the maxilla. Metal posts attached to the implants protrude through the mucosa into the mouth. Artificial teeth or dentures are attached to the roots to replace missing teeth. These implants may be cylindrical or thin blades. The physician makes incisions through the mucosa to expose the bone using an intraoral approach. Precision holes are then drilled in the bone where the implants are to be placed. With blade style implants, the posts are already attached to the implant and the mucosa is sutured simply around the post. With cylindrical implants, the mucosa is sutured over the top of the implant and is allowed to heal while buried under the mucosa. The incisions are then closed simply. A second procedure is performed three to eight months later. The implant is exposed again and the abutment connectors are attached. Report 21248 for partial reconstruction. Report 21249 for complete reconstruction.

21255

The physician reconstructs the zygomatic arch and glenoid fossa. Bone and cartilage grafts are used in reconstruction. Through a separate incision, the physician harvests bone grafts from the patient's hip, rib, or skull and closes the surgically created wound. Costal cartilage grafts are most frequently used. The physician makes a hemicoronal incision with a preauricular (in front of the ear) extension. The reconstructed arch and fossa are stabilized with internal fixation of sutures, wires, plates, and/or screws. The incision is closed in layers.

21256

The physician increases both the size of the bone structure and outline of the bony orbit. The physician uses a variety of incisions to access the surgical site including bicoronal, lower eyelid, eyebrow, and maxillary vestibular incisions. Cuts are made in the orbital rims using drills or saws. The bone is advanced to desired positions and secured with wires, plates, and/or screws. The physician harvests bone from the patient's hip, rib, or skull and closes the surgically created graft donor site. These bone grafts are fashioned by the physician to augment bone or replace congenitally absent bone. The grafts are secured with wires, plates, and/or screws. Incisions through skin are repaired with a layered closure. Intraoral incisions are closed in a single layer.

21260

The physician moves one orbit closer to the other. The physician uses a variety of incisions to access the surgical site including bicoronal, lower eyelid, eyebrow, and maxillary vestibular incisions. Cuts are made 360 degrees around the orbit with drills or saws. Bony cuts are made in the nasal and ethmoid bones and portions of these bones are removed. The bony orbits are realigned to desired positions and secured with wires, plates, and/or screws. The physician harvests bone from the patient's hip, rib, or skull and then closes the surgically created graft donor site. These bone grafts are fashioned by the physician to augment the bone and recontour facial shapes. Small, separate bone grafts may be placed directly on bony step defects. Large grafts are secured with wires, plates, and/or screws. Incisions through skin are repaired with a layered closure. Intraoral incisions are closed in a single layer.

21261

The physician moves one orbit closer to the other. The physician uses a variety of incisions to access the surgical site including bicoronal, lower eyelid, eyebrow, and maxillary vestibular incisions. To gain complete access to the orbits, a frontal craniotomy is performed temporarily removing a portion of the frontal bone, retracting the brain, and making orbital osteotomy cuts from the inside of the skull. Cuts are then made 360 degrees around the orbit using drills or saws. Bony cuts are made in the nasal and ethmoidal bones and portions of these bones are removed. The bony orbits are realigned to desired positions and secured with wires, plates, and/or screws. The physician harvests bone from the patient's hip, rib, or skull and then closes the surgically created graft donor site. Small, separate bone grafts may be fashioned by the physician and placed directly on bony step defects. Large grafts are secured with wires, plates, and/or screws. The frontal bone is again placed in its anatomic location and secured with wires, plates, and/or screws. Incisions through skin are repaired with a layered closure. Intraoral incisions are closed in a single layer.

21263

The physician moves one orbit closer to the other and advances the frontal bone to increase forehead contours. The physician uses a variety of incisions to access the surgical site including bicoronal, lower eyelid, eyebrow, and maxillary vestibular incisions. To gain complete access to the orbits, a frontal craniotomy is performed temporarily removing a

portion of the frontal bone, retracting the brain, and making orbital cuts from the inside of the skull. Cuts are then made 360 degrees around the orbit using drills or saws. Bony cuts are made in the nasal and ethmoidal bones and portions of these bones are removed. The bony orbits are realigned to desired positions and secured with wires, plates, and/or screws. The physician harvests bone from the patient's hip, rib, or skull and then closes the surgically created graft donor site. These bone grafts are fashioned by the physician to augment bone and recontour facial shapes. Small, separate bone grafts may be placed directly on bony defects. Large grafts are fixated with wires, plates, and/or screws. The frontal bone is advanced to its desired location and secured with wires, plates, and/or screws. Incisions through skin are repaired with a layered closure. Intraoral incisions are closed in a single layer.

21267

The physician increases both the size of the bone structure and outline of the bony orbit. The physician uses a variety of incisions to access the surgical site including bicoronal, lower eyelid, eyebrow, and maxillary vestibular incisions. Cuts are made in the orbital rims using drills or saws. The bony orbit is realigned to the desired position and secured with wires, plates, and/or screws. The physician harvests bone from the patient's hip, rib, or skull and then closes the surgically created graft donor site. These bone grafts are fashioned by the physician to augment bone, replace congenitally absent bone, and recontour facial shapes. Small separate bone grafts may be placed directly on bony step defects. Large grafts are fashioned and secured with wires, plates, and/or screws. Incisions through skin are repaired with a layered closure. Intraoral incisions are closed in a single layer.

21268

The physician increases both the size of the bone structure and the outline of the bony orbit. The physician uses a variety of incisions to access the surgical site including bicoronal, lower eyelid, eyebrow, and maxillary vestibular incisions. To gain complete access to the orbit, a frontal craniotomy is performed, temporarily removing a portion of the frontal bone, retracting the brain, and making cuts from the inside of the skull. Cuts are made in the orbital rims using drills and saws. The bony orbit is realigned to the desired position and secured with wires, plates, and/or screws. The physician harvests bone from the patient's hip, rib, or skull and closes the surgically created graft donor site. These bone grafts are fashioned by the physician to augment bone, replace congenitally absent bone, and recontour facial shapes. Small, separate bone grafts may be placed directly on bony step defects. Large grafts are secured with wires, plates, and/or screws. The frontal bone is replaced in its anatomic location and secured with wires, plates, and/or screws. Incisions through skin are repaired with a layered closure. Intraoral incisions are closed in a single layer.

21270

The physician augments the malar prominence with prosthetic material. Incisions are made through the lower eyelids and maxillary buccal vestibule to expose the malar defect. The prosthetic implant is fixated on the malar prominence with wires, plates, and/or screws. The eyelid incisions are closed in layers. The oral vestibular incision is closed in a single layer.

21275

The physician performs a second procedure to continue corrections of skeletal deformities of the orbits and face. The physician uses a variety of incisions to access the surgical site including bicoronal, lower eyelid, eyebrow, and maxillary vestibular incisions. Revision cuts are made using drills and saws. Bone is realigned to the desired positions and secured with wires, plates, and/or screws. The physician may harvest bone from the patient's hip, rib, or skull and then close the surgically created graft donor site. Bone grafts are fashioned by the physician and secured with wires, plates, and/or screws. Incisions through skin are repaired with a layered closure. Intraoral incisions are closed in a single layer.

21280

The physician reattaches the medial canthal ligament. The medial canthal ligament is attached medially to nasal-orbital bones and laterally to the orbital fascia, the upper eyelid, and the lower eyelid. The ligament is isolated either through a bicoronal incision or through skin incisions placed beside the ligament. After locating the ligament, stainless steel suture or wire is placed through the ligament. A hole is made in nasal bones of the opposite side with a drill or awl. Then the suture or wire is passed under the nasal complex to the opposite side through the bony hole. The suture or wire is then ligated to the bone. A bicoronal incision is repaired with a layered closure and any skin incisions are closed in a single layer.

21282

The physician reattaches the lateral canthal ligament to correct soft tissue structures of the lateral aspect of the eye and eyelids. The lateral canthal ligament is attached laterally to the orbital aspect of the zygoma and medially to the orbital fascia, the upper eyelid, and the lower eyelid. The ligament is isolated through a horizontal skin incision placed beside the ligament. After locating the ligament, the physician places stainless steel suture or wire through the ligament. A hole is made in the zygoma with a drill. The physician then passes the suture or wire through the bony hole. The suture or wire is then ligated to the bone. Skin incisions are repaired with a layered closure.

21295–21296

The physician reduces the size of the masseter muscle, and bone, if necessary, when the muscle has become hypertrophic (overly enlarged). The physician makes skin incisions in the neck just beneath the angle of the mandible. The tissues are dissected to expose the masseter muscle and mandible. The physician removes appropriate amounts of muscle and may use drills, saws, or osteotomes to remove bone in the area of the angle to produce the desired contour. The incision is then repaired with a layered closure and pressure dressings are placed on the site. Report 21295 for extraoral approach. Report 21296 for intraoral approach.

21300

The physician treats a skull fracture without surgical intervention. X-rays and computerized tomography (CT) scans (reported separately) demonstrate a skull fracture in which the fracture fragments are in acceptable positions. The physician elects to treat this in a closed fashion by limiting the patient's activities and monitoring the fracture until healing is complete.

21310

The physician treats a stable, non-displaced nasal fracture. No physical manipulation of the nasal bones or stabilization from splints is necessary. Treatment includes external agents (i.e., ice therapy) and prescribing pharmacologic agents.

21315

The physician treats a displaced nasal fracture by manipulating the fractured bones. The physician places nasal elevators or forceps into the nose and realigns the nasal bones. After the bones are realigned, they are stable and require no additional stabilization with splints.

21320

The physician treats a displaced nasal fracture by manipulating the nasal bones. The physician places nasal elevators or forceps into the nose and realigns the nasal bones. After the bones are realigned, they remain slightly mobile and require additional stabilization with splints. External splinting may consist of a cast taped to the reduced nose. Internal splinting consists of supporting the nasal septum by splints or packing with gauze strips.

21325

The physician treats a displaced nasal fracture. After unsatisfactory results with closed manipulation of the fractured bones, the physician makes an incision. Open reductions allow the physician to visualize the fracture. Lacerations may be present, allowing direct visualization. Incisions are made inside the nose to expose the nasal septum and portions of the nasal bones. The physician realigns the fractured bones using nasal elevators and forceps. It may be necessary to remove small segments of bone for adequate realignment. Intranasal incisions are closed in single layers. Any lacerated skin areas are closed in layers. After the bones are realigned, they remain slightly mobile and require additional stabilization with splints. External splinting may consist of a cast taped to the reduced nose. Internal splinting consists of supporting the nasal septum by splints or packing with gauze strips.

21330

The physician treats a displaced nasal fracture. After unsatisfactory results with closed manipulation of the fractured bones, the physician makes an incision. Open reductions allow the physician to visualize the fracture. Lacerations may be present, allowing direct visualization. Incisions are made inside the nose to expose the nasal septum and portions of the nasal bones. Additionally, bicoronal or other local skin incisions may be used to expose the fractured nasal bones. The physician then realigns the fractured bones using nasal elevators and forceps. The bones are stabilized with wires, plates, and/or screws. Intranasal incisions are closed in single layers. Lacerations and other skin incisions repaired with a layered closure. After the bones are realigned, they remain slightly mobile and require additional stabilization with splints. External splinting may consist of a cast taped to the reduced nose. Internal splinting consists of supporting the nasal septum by splints or packing with gauze strips.

21335

The physician makes an incision to treat a displaced nasal fracture and also repair the fractured nasal septum. Open treatment is necessary after unsatisfactory results with closed manipulation of the fractured bones and allows the physician to visualize the fractures. Lacerations overlying the fractures may allow direct visualization. Incisions may be made inside the nose to expose the nasal septum and portions of the nasal bones. Additionally, bicoronal and other local skin incisions may be used to expose the fractured nasal bones. The nasal septum is exposed and portions of the fractured cartilaginous and bony septum are removed. The physician then realigns the nasal bones using nasal elevators and forceps. The bones are stabilized using wires, plates, and/or screws. Transseptal sutures are placed to prevent formation of a septal hematoma. Intranasal incisions are closed in single layers. Lacerations and other skin incisions are repaired with a layered closure. After the bones are realigned, they remain slightly mobile and require additional stabilization with splints. External splinting may consist of a cast taped to the reduced nose. Internal splinting consists of supporting the nasal septum by splints or packing with gauze strips.

21336

The physician makes an incision to repair a nasal septal fracture. Open treatment is necessary after

unsatisfactory results with closed manipulation of the fractured septum and allows the physician to visualize the septal fracture. Incisions are made inside the nose. The nasal septum is exposed and portions of the fractured cartilaginous and bony septum are removed. Transseptal sutures are placed to prevent formation of a septal hematoma. Intranasal incisions are closed in single layers. Internal splinting consists of supporting the nasal septum by splints or packing with gauze strips.

21337

The physician repairs a fracture of the nasal septum. No intranasal incisions are made. The physician uses nasal elevators and forceps to realign the septal fracture. Internal stabilization may be used to support the septum during healing. Internal splints or packing with gauze strips are used for stabilization.

21338

The physician repairs fractures of the nasoethmoid region, which includes nasal and ethmoid bones and the medial wall of the orbit. Lacerations may be present allowing direct visualization. The physician may use bicoronal, local skin, and lower eyelid incisions to expose the fractured bones. The medial canthal ligaments are examined, and if detached, are repaired in a separately reportable procedure with transnasal stainless steel sutures or wire. The physician realigns the fractured bones with internal wires, plates, and/or screws. Any lacerated skin areas are closed in layers. Other skin incisions are repaired with a layered closure. After the bones are realigned, they may remain slightly mobile and require additional stabilization with splints. External splinting may consist of a cast taped to the reduced nasal complex. Internal splinting may be used for additional support consisting of intranasal splints or packing with gauze strips.

21339

The physician repairs fractures of the nasoethmoid region, which includes nasal and ethmoid bones and the medial wall of the orbit. Lacerations may be present allowing direct visualization. The physician may use bicoronal, local skin, and lower eyelid incisions to expose the fractured bones. The medial canthal ligaments are examined, and if detached, are repaired in a separately reportable procedure with transnasal stainless steel sutures or wire. The physician realigns the fractured bones with internal wires, plates, and/or screws. External pin fixation may be used to support grossly depressed fractures. Any lacerated skin areas are repaired with a layered closure. Other skin incisions are closed in multiple layers. After the bones are realigned, they may remain slightly mobile and require additional stabilization with splints. External splinting may consist of a cast taped to the reduced nasal complex. Internal splinting may be used for additional support consisting of intranasal splints or packing with gauze strips.

21340

The physician repairs fractures of the nasoethmoid region with percutaneous (through the skin) approaches. Percutaneous pins or screws are placed into stable bone. External fixation, splints, or headcaps may suspend the complex aiding reduction of the fractures. If the medial canthal ligaments are detached, they are repaired through a percutaneous approach with awls or K-wires and transnasal stainless steel sutures or wire. Injuries of the nasolacrimal complex are repaired without incisions using non-resorbable sutures and polyethylene tubing.

21343

The physician realigns a depressed frontal bone fracture overlying the frontal sinus. This fracture does not involve injury to the nasofrontal duct drainage of the frontal sinus. The physician may access the frontal bone with a bicoronal incision or local skin incisions overlying the fracture. Sinus mucosa may be removed. The bone is realigned and stabilized with wires, plates, and/or screws. The incisions are repaired with a layered closure.

21344

The physician realigns a complicated frontal bone fracture and obliterates the frontal sinus. This fracture injures the duct drainage of the frontal sinus and requires obliteration of the nasofrontal duct to prevent postoperative sinus complications. The physician may access the frontal bone with a bicoronal incision or local skin incisions overlying the fracture. Sinus mucosa is removed from the frontal sinus. If the posterior wall of the sinus is fractured, the bony wall may be removed, thus cranializing the sinus. The nasofrontal duct is plugged (i.e., bone) and obliterating material (i.e., fat, muscle) is placed into the sinus cavity. The frontal bone is realigned and stabilized with wires, plates, and/or screws. The incisions are repaired with a layered closure.

21345

The physician realigns a pyramidal fracture (LeFort II) of the nasal and maxillary complex without making incisions. The fractured bones can be realigned without internal fixation. Intermaxillary fixation is used to realign the fracture. Arch bars placed on the patient's teeth may provide interdental fixation. For edentulous patients, a splint or the patient's dentures can be modified to provide fixation to the mandible. Skeletal wire fixation placed over the zygomatic arches may be used to stabilize the intermaxillary fixation.

21346

The physician realigns a pyramidal (LeFort II) midface fracture of the nasomaxillary complex. An incision is made through the maxillary buccal vestibule (cheek side) to expose the bony maxilla. The nasomaxillary complex is manipulated, realigning the fracture. The physician uses wires, plates, and/or

screws to stabilize the fracture. The mucosal incision is closed in a single layer. Intermaxillary fixation may be applied.

21347

The physician realigns a complex pyramidal (LeFort II) midface fracture of the nasomaxillary complex. Multiple incisions are made to expose the fracture sites. These incisions include the bicoronal scalp flap, lower eyelid, and transoral incisions. The nasomaxillary complex is manipulated, realigning the fractured bones. The fracture is stabilized with wires, plates, and/or screws. The transoral incision is closed in a single layer. The scalp and lower eyelid incisions are repaired with a layered closure. Intermaxillary fixation may be applied.

21348

The physician realigns a complex pyramidal (LeFort II) midface fracture of the nasomaxillary complex. Multiple incisions include the bicoronal scalp flap, lower eyelid, and transoral incisions. The pyramidal fracture is exposed and the complex is manipulated, realigning the fractured bones. Comminution of bone (e.g., nasofrontal region, orbital floors) requires bone grafting of these areas. The physician then uses wires, plates, and/or screws to stabilize the fracture. Through a separate incision, the physician may harvest a bone graft from the patient's hip, rib, or skull and close the surgically created wound. The physician reconstructs areas of bony defect. The transoral incision is then closed in a single layer. The scalp and lower eyelid incisions are repaired with a layered closure. Intermaxillary fixation may be used to additionally stabilize the fracture.

21355

The physician reduces a fracture of the malar area, including the zygomatic arch. A stab incision is made through the skin overlying the fracture area. Without soft tissue dissection, an instrument (e.g., bone hook, Carroll-Girard screw) is inserted and then used to lift and reduce the fracture. The stab incision is closed in a single layer.

21356

The physician reduces a fracture of the zygomatic arch. A facial incision (e.g., Gilles approach) is made in the scalp extending beneath the temporalis fascia. An instrument is inserted through the incision following underneath the fascia and taken to the middle surface of the zygomatic arch. A transoral incision (e.g., Keen approach) is made in the posterior buccal sulcus. An instrument is inserted through the incision and taken to the middle surface of the zygomatic arch, avoiding damage to branches of the facial nerve passing beside the arch. The arch is then lifted laterally to its correct anatomic position. The facial incision is closed in layers. The transoral incision is closed in a single layer.

21360

The physician reduces a fracture of the malar complex. No internal fixation is used. The physician makes facial incisions through the scalp, eyebrow, and/or lower eyelid. A transoral incision is also made through the maxillary buccal vestibule. The fracture sites are exposed. Instruments may be inserted into the bone (e.g., Carroll-Girard screw) or beneath the complex to lift the fracture. The fractured malar complex is reduced manually. The facial incisions are closed in layers. The transoral incision is closed in a single layer.

21365

The physician reduces a complicated fracture of the malar area. Internal fixation is necessary for fracture stability. The physician makes multiple incisions to expose and explore the fracture. Facial incisions are made through the scalp, eyebrow, and/or lower eyelid. A transoral incision is made though the maxillary buccal vestibule. Instruments may be inserted into the bone (e.g., Carroll-Girard screw) or beneath the complex to lift the fracture. The fractured malar complex is reduced and fixated with wires, plates, and/or screws. The facial incisions are closed in layers. The transoral incision is closed in a single layer.

21366

The physician reduces a complicated fracture of the malar area. Bone grafting is necessary to reconstruct bony defects (e.g., orbital floor, anterior maxillary wall). Internal fixation is necessary for fracture stability. The physician makes multiple incisions to expose and explore the fracture. Facial incisions are made through the scalp, eyebrow, and/or lower eyelid. A transoral incision is made though the maxillary buccal vestibule. Instruments may be inserted into the bone (e.g., Carroll-Girard screw) or beneath the malar complex to lift the fracture. The fractured complex is reduced and fixated with wires, plates, and/or screws. Through a separate incision, the physician harvests a bone graft from the patient's hip, rib, or skull and closes the surgically created wound. The graft is placed on the malar area and may be stabilized with sutures, wires, plates, and/or screws. The facial incisions are closed in layers. The transoral incision is closed in a single layer.

21385

The physician repairs a fracture of the orbital floor. A maxillary vestibular incision is made on the side of the orbital fracture. In the maxillary bone, a window opening is made into the maxillary sinus, using a drill and bone forceps. The orbital floor is visualized from inside the maxillary sinus. The fractured orbital floor is realigned and supported from inside the maxillary sinus with lubricated gauze packing or a ballooned catheter. The physician sutures the end portion of the gauze or catheter to the maxillary mucosa. Most of the intraoral incision is sutured in a single layer. The

exposed gauze or catheter remains in place and is removed after adequate healing.

21386

The physician repairs a fracture of the orbital floor. Lower eyelid incisions are made to expose and explore this fracture. A lower eyelid incision allows the physician to inspect the floor, infraorbital rim, and medial/lateral orbital walls. The physician realigns the fractured orbital floor by gentle manipulation. The realigned orbital floor is stable or the fracture is very small, not requiring an implant or bone graft. The lower eyelid incision is closed in layers.

21387

The physician repairs a fracture of the orbital floor. The physician makes both eyelid and intraoral incisions to expose and explore this fracture. A lower eyelid incision allows the physician to inspect the infraorbital rim and floor. Additionally, the orbital floor is visualized from inside the maxillary sinus by a maxillary vestibular incision. The physician realigns the fractured orbital floor by manipulation from either access. The realigned orbital floor may be supported from inside the maxillary sinus with lubricated gauze packing or a ballooned catheter. The physician sutures the end portion of the gauze or catheter to the maxillary mucosa. Then most of the intraoral incision is sutured in a single layer. The lower eyelid incision is closed in layers. The exposed gauze or catheter remains in place intraorally and is removed after adequate healing.

21390

The physician repairs a fracture of the orbital floor using lower eyelid incisions. A lower eyelid incision allows the physician to inspect the floor, infraorbital rim, and medial/lateral orbital walls. The physician elevates the orbital soft tissue from the bone, exposing the fracture. Small fragments of fractured bone may be removed and the remaining fractured bone is realigned by gentle manipulation. A bony hole remains in the orbital floor, requiring an implant to prevent orbital soft tissue from entering the maxillary sinus below. The physician fashions an alloplastic implant material to cover the hole. The physician then places the implant over the bony hole. The lower eyelid incision is closed in layers.

21395

The physician repairs a fracture of the orbital floor using lower eyelid incisions. A lower eyelid incision allows the physician to inspect the floor, infraorbital rim, and medial/lateral orbital walls. The physician elevates the orbital soft tissue from the bone, exposing the fracture. Small fragments of fractured bone may be removed and the remaining fractured bone is realigned by gentle manipulation. A bony hole remains in the orbital floor and will require an implant to prevent orbital soft tissue from entering the maxillary sinus below. The physician harvests bone from the patient's hip, rib, or skull, and closes the surgically created graft donor site. The harvested bone is fashioned to cover the hole. The physician places the bone graft over the bony hole and may secure it to the infraorbital rim with wire or sutures. The lower eyelid incision is repaired with a layered closure.

21400

The physician treats orbital fractures other than floor fractures. Incisions and bony manipulation are not necessary. These are non-displaced or minimally displaced fractures of the orbital rims or walls that can be identified on x-ray.

21401

The physician treats orbital fractures other than floor fractures. No incisions are necessary. These are minimally displaced fractures of the orbital rims or walls that can be identified on x-ray. The physician realigns the fracture bones by using manual manipulation or with bone hooks and Carroll-Girard screws. The realigned bones are stable and no internal fixation is necessary.

21406

The physician treats orbital fractures other than floor fractures. These are displaced fractures of the orbital rims or walls which can be identified on x-ray. The physician makes periorbital incisions to expose the fractures. The fractured bones are realigned and stabilized with wires, plates, and/or screws. No sizable bony holes that would require coverage remain in the orbit. The incisions are closed in both single and multiple layers.

21407

The physician treats orbital fractures other than floor fractures. These are displaced fractures of the orbital rims or walls which can be identified on x-ray. The physician makes periorbital incisions to expose the fractures. The fractured bones are realigned and stabilized with wires, plates, and/or screws. After realignment, bony holes remain in the orbit which require coverage to prevent orbital soft tissue from entering into these holes. These holes are usually found in the medial or lateral walls of the orbit. An alloplastic implant is selected, shaped, and placed over the bony hole. The incisions are closed in both single and multiple layers.

21408

The physician treats orbital fractures other than floor fractures. These are displaced fractures of the orbital rims or walls which can be identified on x-ray. The physician makes periorbital incisions to expose the fractures. The fractured bones are realigned and may be stabilized with wires, plates, and/or screws. After realignment, bony holes remain in the orbit, requiring coverage to prevent orbital soft tissue from entering these holes. The holes are usually found in the medial

or lateral walls of the orbit. The physician harvests bone from the patient's hip, rib, or skull, and closes the surgically created graft donor site. The bone graft is shaped and placed over the bony hole. The incisions are closed in both single and multiple layers.

21421

The physician treats a palatal or maxillary fracture by applying interdental (intermaxillary) fixation for stabilization. No incisions are made with this technique. The physician may wire arch bars to the teeth or use other wiring techniques to provide the fixation. Edentulous patients may have dentures or custom-made acrylic splints wired to the jaws. The jaws are then wired together to provide intermaxillary fixation.

21422

The physician repositions and stabilizes a palatal or maxillary fracture. Transoral incisions are made in the maxillary buccal vestibule (cheek part of vestibule) to expose the maxillary fracture. The fracture is repositioned and stabilized with plates, screws, and/or wires. The transoral mucosal incision is closed in a single layer. Intermaxillary fixation may or may not be applied. A customized acrylic palatal splint may be wired to the maxillary teeth to stabilize the palatal fracture.

21423

The physician repositions and stabilizes a complicated palatal or maxillary fracture. Transoral incisions are made in the maxillary buccal vestibule to expose the maxillary fracture. Additional lower eyelid or skin incisions may be necessary to assist repair of the fracture. The maxilla is repositioned and stabilized with plates, screws, and/or wires. The infraorbital nerve may need to be repositioned. The anterior maxillary walls may need bone grafting to support the infraorbital nerve. The transoral mucosal incision is closed in a single layer. Any skin or eyelid incisions are closed in multiple layers. Intermaxillary fixation may be applied. A customized acrylic palatal splint may be wired to the maxillary teeth to stabilize a palatal fracture.

21431

The physician treats a craniofacial separation without surgically opening the fracture but with the use of interdental wiring of denture or splint. The physician uses surgical instruments intranasally and intraorally to reduce the separation without the need to open it surgically. Arch bands and wires are applied to the teeth for immobilization until healing is complete.

21432–21436

The physician performs surgery to treat a craniofacial separation. The physician uses any of a variety of incisions, including intraoral and lateral eyebrow incisions. Surgical instruments are utilized to reduce the separation. The physician uses wire, plates, and screws to hold the bones in their acceptable anatomic positions for healing. The wounds are thoroughly irrigated and closed in layers. Report 21433 if the procedure is complicated, using multiple surgical approaches; report 21435 if the procedure is complicated, utilizing internal and/or external fixation techniques; and report 21436 if the procedure is complicated, using multiple surgical approaches and internal fixation with bone grafting.

21440

The physician stabilizes and repairs a fracture of the mandibular or maxillary alveolar bone without making incisions. The physician moves the fractured bone into the desired position manually. The fracture is stabilized by wiring both involved teeth and adjacent stable teeth to an arch bar. Another technique utilizes dental composite bonding of both involved and stable teeth to a heavy, stainless steel wire. A customized acrylic splint may be used to stabilize the teeth. Intermaxillary fixation may also be applied.

21445

The physician stabilizes and reduces a fracture of the mandibular or maxillary alveolar bone. Intraoral incisions are made in the buccal vestibule to expose the fracture. The physician moves the fractured bone into the desired position manually. The fracture is stabilized by wiring both involved teeth and adjacent stable teeth to an arch bar. A customized acrylic splint may be used to stabilize the teeth. The fractured alveolar bone may be reduced by wires, plates, and/or screws. Intermaxillary fixation may also be applied. The intraoral incision is closed in a single layer.

21450–21451

The physician treats a mandibular fracture with no direct manipulation or stabilization. Close observation, a soft diet, or other restrictions of activity are examples of treatment. A minimally or non-displaced fracture of the condylar head or neck (e.g., 21450) is an example of a fracture that may be treated in this way. The physician may reposition a mandibular fracture with some manipulation (e.g., 21451) to relocate the bone. The physician moves the fractured bone into the desired position manually. No incisions are made with this technique.

21452

The physician treats a mandibular fracture by applying external fixation. Intermaxillary fixation (wiring jaws together) is often applied to stabilize the fracture before any incisions are made. The physician makes 0.5 cm incisions in the skin at several points near the inferior border of the mandible on both sides of the fracture. The physician then dissects the tissues to the bone. Holes are drilled at the inferior border of the mandible. Threaded rods or pins are screwed into the holes. A metal or acrylic bar is connected to the protruding posts in a horizontal fashion, stabilizing

the fracture. Intermaxillary fixation may be left in place.

21453

The physician treats a mandibular fracture by applying intermaxillary fixation (wiring jaws together) for stabilization. No incisions are made with this technique. The physician may wire arch bars to the teeth or use other wiring techniques to provide the intermaxillary fixation. Edentulous (without teeth) patients may have dentures or custom-made acrylic splints wired to the jaws. The jaws are then wired together to provide intermaxillary fixation.

21454

The physician treats a mandibular fracture by applying external fixation. An intraoral approach may be used or a skin incision may be made extraorally overlying the area to expose and reposition the fracture directly. The fracture may also be approached through traumatic lacerations. Once the fracture is moved to the desired position, the physician makes 0.5 cm incisions in the skin at several points near the inferior border of the mandible on both sides of the fracture. The physician then dissects the tissues to the bone. Holes are drilled at the inferior border of the mandible. Threaded rods or pins are screwed into the holes. A metal or acrylic bar is connected to the protruding posts in a horizontal fashion, stabilizing the fracture. Intermaxillary fixation may be placed.

21461–21462

The physician repositions and stabilizes a mandibular fracture(s). Incisions are made either in the skin overlying the fractured area or intraorally through the mucosa. The tissue is dissected to the bone and the fracture exposed. The fracture is repositioned and stabilized with plates, screws, or wires. The incisions are then closed with sutures. Intermaxillary fixation is not applied in this procedure. For 21462, intermaxillary fixation is applied.

21465

The physician repositions and/or stabilizes a fracture of the mandibular condyle. An incision is made through the skin anterior to the contour of the ear or through the ear. An intraoral approach is used on occasion. The tissues are dissected to the temporomandibular joint and the fractured condyle is exposed. Depending on the location of the fracture, a second skin incision below the angle of the mandible may be necessary to move the fracture to the desired position. The fractured condyle is then repositioned, either manually or with instruments. The fracture is stabilized with wires, screws, or plates, or may be left without internal fixation. The incision is then closed with layered sutures. Intermaxillary fixation may be placed.

21470

The physician repositions and/or stabilizes a complicated fracture of the mandible. Multiple incisions are made through the skin and/or mucosa intraorally to approach and treat the fracture(s). The fracture is stabilized with wires, screws, plates, or various forms of interdental fixation. The mucosal incisions are sutured simply and the skin incisions are closed with layered sutures.

21480

The physician repositions a dislocation of the temporomandibular joint. No incisions are made and no intermaxillary fixation is used. The physician corrects the dislocation manually to rearticulate the joint.

21485

The physician repositions a dislocation of the temporomandibular joint. The physician corrects the dislocation manually to rearticulate the joint. Intermaxillary fixation is required because of a complicated or persistent dislocation.

21490

The physician surgically repositions a dislocation of the temporomandibular joint. The physician exposes the joint by making an incision anterior to the contour of the ear or through the ear. Tissues are dissected to expose the joint. The condyle and disc are then moved into normal position using instruments. The ligaments may be repaired. The incision is then closed with layered sutures.

21493-21494

The physician treats a fracture of the hyoid bone without the need for manipulation of the fracture pieces or any surgical intervention in 21493. The physician obtains separately reportable x-rays of the neck that demonstrate a fractured hyoid bone in which the pieces are still in acceptable position and alignment. The patient is often treated by placement in a collar or brace until the fracture heals. In 21494, manipulation is performed as part of the procedure. The physician, based on x-rays (reported separately) of the neck, repositions the fragments of the hyoid bone and places the patient in a collar or brace until the fracture heals.

21495

The physician treats a fracture of the hyoid bone by open surgery. The physician obtains x-rays (reported separately) that demonstrate a fracture of the hyoid bone, leaving it in an unstable or unsatisfactory position. With the patient under anesthesia, the physician makes an incision in the neck overlying the hyoid bone. Tissues are carefully dissected deep to the bone and the fracture is identified. Using internal fixation devices, the physician manipulations the fracture fragments in position. The wound is irrigated and closed in layers.

21497

The physician treats conditions other than fractures by applying intermaxillary fixation (wiring jaws together) for stabilization. No incisions are made with this technique. The physician may wire arch bars to the teeth, or use other wiring techniques to provide the intermaxillary fixation. For edentulous (without teeth) patients, dentures or custom made acrylic splints are wired to the jaws. The jaws are then wired together.

21501-21502

The physician performs surgery to remove or drain an abscess or hematoma from the deep soft tissues of the neck or thorax. With the patient under anesthesia, the physician makes an incision in the skin overlying the site. Subcutaneous and fascial layers are dissected. The incision is carried deep in to the muscles of the neck or thorax and the abscess or hematoma is identified. The physician uses sharp and blunt dissection techniques to ascertain the extent of the mass and to drain its contents. Copious irrigation is applied and debridement is needed. Surgical drains are usually inserted. The wound may be closed in layers over the drains or left open for secondary closure. Report 21502 if a partial rib ostectomy is performed during this procedure.

21510

The physician performs surgery to debride and drain infection from an area of infected bone within the thorax. With the patient under anesthesia, the physician makes an incision in the skin overlying the site. The incision is carried deep to the bone dissecting and debriding tissue as needed. The bone is identified, exposed, and explored. The physician opens the bone through an osteotomy. The inside of the bone and surrounding tissues are irrigated and debrided. Any necrotic or infected tissue is removed. Surgical drains are typically inserted. The bony cortex may be closed or left open. The incision also may be closed in layers over the drains or left open for later secondary closure.

21550

The physician performs a biopsy of the area of the neck or thorax. With the patient under anesthesia, the physician identifies the mass through palpitation and x-ray (reported separately), if needed. An excision is made over the site and dissection is taken down to the area of soft tissue (muscle). A portion of the tissue (mass) is excised and submitted for pathology. The area is irrigated and the incision is closed with layered sutures.

21555

The physician removes a tumor from the area of the neck or chest that is located in the subcutaneous layer. With the patient under anesthesia, the physician makes an incision in the skin overlying the tumor. The extent of the tumor is identified and a dissection is undertaken all the way around the tumor. Irrigation is employed and the surrounding tissues are dissected free from the tumor. The tumor is removed in one piece or in multiple pieces. The wound is irrigated and sutured closed in layers.

21556

The physician removes a tumor from the area of the neck or chest that is deep, subfascial, and intramuscular. With the patient under anesthesia, the physician makes an incision in the skin overlying the tumor and dissects to the tumor. The extent of the tumor is identified and a dissection is undertaken all the way around the tumor. Irrigation is employed and the surrounding tissues are dissected free from the tumor. The tumor is removed in one piece or in multiple pieces. The wound is irrigated and sutured closed in layers.

21557

The physician removes a tumor from the soft tissue of the neck or thorax that requires extensive debridement of surrounding tissues. With the patient under anesthesia, the physician makes a long incision overlying the tumor. The tumor is dissected free from surrounding tissues in multiple pieces. Adjacent muscles, fascia, and other tissues are also removed in a large area completely surrounding the entire tumor. Large resections may be needed. The wound is thoroughly irrigated and the remaining tissues are approximated. The closure is sutured in layers.

21600

The physician removes part of one rib. With the patient under anesthesia, the physician makes an incision in the skin of the chest overlying the rib. The tissues are dissected deep to the rib itself. The rib is identified. The physician removes the desired part of the rib using a saw and other instruments. The remaining pieces of the rib and the wound itself are irrigated and debrided. The incision is sutured in layers.

21610

The physician resects the costovertebral joint. The physician makes a posterior incision overlying the joint. The tissues are dissected from the joint and the transverse process is cut from the vertebral body. The physician removes all or a portion of the adjacent rib. The incision is closed in sutured layers.

21615–21616

The physician performs surgery to remove the first rib and/or an extraneous cervical rib. With the patient under anesthesia, the physician makes an incision in the skin just above the clavicle on the affected side. Tissues are dissected deep to the rib. The rib is identified and the attached soft tissues are carefully debrided. The physician excises the rib using a saw and other surgical instruments. The rib is freed from its articulation and removed. The wound is irrigated

thoroughly and closed in layers. A dressing is applied. Report 21616 if a sympathectomy is performed during the procedure.

21620

The physician removes a portion of the sternum from the chest. With the patient under anesthesia, the physician makes an incision in the skin overlying the sternum. This is carried deep through the subcutaneous tissues to the bone. The sternum is identified and soft tissues are debrided. The physician marks the portion of the sternum to be removed. The bone is cut in the appropriate places using a saw and other surgical instruments. The remaining portion of the bone is irrigated and smoothed as needed. The wound is closed in layers and a dressing is applied.

21627

The physician performs a debridement of the sternum. With the patient under anesthesia, the physician makes an incision in the skin overlying the sternum. The incision is carried deep to the bone. The sternum is debrided as warranted using any of a variety of hand or powered surgical instruments. Irrigation is used so that debridement can be completed as extensively as indicated. The wound is closed in layers and a dressing is applied.

21630–21632

The physician removes most or all of the sternum from the chest. With the patient under anesthesia, the physician makes a long incision overlying the sternum and anterior chest. This is carried deep to the bone. Dissection is performed around the sternum. Ribs are disarticulated as needed, and thorough debridement is accomplished. Using saws and other surgical instruments, the physician removes the bone. Internal fixation devices (reported separately) are often needed to support the ribs and chest wall. The wound is thoroughly irrigated and closed in layers. Report 21632 if a mediastinal lymphadenectomy is performed during the procedure.

21700–21705

The physician performs a surgical procedure where the scalenus anticus muscle is divided usually for the purpose of treating thoracic outlet syndrome. With the patient under anesthesia, the physician makes an incision overlying the scalene muscle. This incision is carried deep to the muscle. The muscle is exposed and identified. A sclerotomy or discission of the muscle is performed in line of the fibers. This relieves the pressure on the neurovascular structures. The wound is thoroughly irrigated and closed in layers. Report 21700 if the procedure does not include resection of the cervical rib. Report 21705 if resection of the cervical rib is performed during the procedure.

21720

Torticollis is a dysfunction of the neck with congenital or traumatic onset. The head becomes inclined toward the affected side and the face toward the opposite side. The physician makes an incision 5.0 cm long above and parallel to the medial end of the collar bone to access the tendons of the sternocleidomastoid muscle. A blunt instrument is placed behind the tendons to protect vital structures in neck. The muscle's tendons attach just behind the ear and to the collar bone. The physician splits the tendons further up the muscle to release the restriction. The physician probes the wound with a finger to identify remaining tight muscles or fascia, which is cut until full motion is obtained. The physician closes the incision with sutures and Steri-strips. A cervical collar is applied for six weeks.

21725

Torticollis is a dysfunction of the neck with congenital or traumatic onset. The head becomes inclined toward the affected side and the face toward the opposite side. The physician makes an incision 5.0 cm long above and parallel to the medial end of the collar bone to access the tendons of the sternocleidomastoid muscle. A blunt instrument is placed behind the tendons to protect vital structures in neck. The muscle's tendon attach just behind the ear and to the collar bone. The physician splits the tendons further up the muscle to release the restriction. The physician probes the wound with a finger to identify remaining tight muscles or fascia, which is cut until full motion is obtained. The physician closes the incision with sutures and Steri-strips. A cast is applied to hold the neck in place.

21740

The physician performs surgery on the anterior chest to correct pectus excavatum (a depression in the chest wall) or pectus carinatum (a forward projection of the chest wall). With the patient under anesthesia, the physician makes an incision overlying the anterior sternum. This is carried deep to the bone. The costal cartilages are exposed and deformed rib ends are freed from their sternal attachments. The sternum is mobilized and restored to its normal position. Internal fixation devices are employed to hold the sternum in corrected alignment. The physician irrigates the wound and closes it in layers with sutures.

21750

The physician performs surgery on the sternum bone to put the bone back together following previous surgical separation. With the patient under anesthesia, the physician makes an incision overlying the sternum. The incision is carried deep to the bone and the separated pieces are identified. The physician may debride soft tissue or bone. The bony fragments are manipulated back together and held in place. The physician uses wire or other internal fixation devices to maintain the bone in appropriate position. The wound is thoroughly irrigated and closed in layers.

21800

Separately reportable x-rays are used to identify if a fracture of the rib is present. If the fracture is non-displaced and stable, closed treatment is initiated. Braces or splints are not used. The patient's activity is modified while the fracture heals.

21805

The physician performs surgery on a fractured rib without the need for any internal or external fixation devices. With the patient under anesthesia, the physician makes an incision overlying the fractured rib. This is carried deep to the bone. The fracture is found and the pieces are identified. Dead tissue is debrided as needed. The physician manipulates the fracture fragments into an acceptable position and alignment. The wound is irrigated thoroughly and closed in layers.

21810

The physician treats a rib fracture that results in a so-called "flail chest" using external fixation devices. A flail chest inhibits proper pulmonary function. With the patient under anesthesia, the physician makes an incision overlying the fractured rib. The physician identifies the rib involved. Using external fixation and other devices such as pins, screws, sandbags, the physician stabilizes the rib fracture and the chest wall. The wound is closed with layered sutures.

21820

Separately reportable x-rays are used to identify if a fracture of the sternum is present. If the fracture is non-displaced and stable, closed treatment is initiated. Braces or splints are not used. The patient's activity is modified while the fracture heals.

21825

Separately reportable x-rays are used to identify if a fracture is present. If the fracture is not stable, an open reduction may be needed. The patient is positioned supine on the operating table. A longitudinal incision is made along the midportion of the sternum. Dissection is carried down to expose the sternum. The surgeon then reduces the fracture. If fixation is needed to keep the fracture stable, the physician drills holes on either side of the fracture. Wire is passed through the holes and around the fracture and the wire ends twists together to stabilize the fracture. The incision is repaired in layers with sutures, staples, or Steri-strips.

21920–21925

The patient is positioned sidelying or prone and an incision is made over the tumor or cyst. Dissection is carried down to the superficial layer of fascia so that the tumor or cyst is exposed. An incision is made in the capsule surrounding the tumor or cyst and a small sample of tissue is removed. Report 21925 if the tumor or cyst is within or below the muscles and a drain tube is considered. The capsule is then sutured together. The incision is closed with sutures, staples, or Steri-strips.

21930

The patient is positioned sidelying or prone. An incision is made over the tumor and carried down to the tumor. The entire tumor, including the surrounding capsule, is removed. A portion of surrounding soft tissue may also be removed to ensure adequate removal of all tumor tissue. A drain may be inserted, and the incision is repaired with multiple layers of sutures, staples, or Steri-strips.

21935

The patient is positioned sidelying or prone. An incision is made over the tumor. Dissection is carried down to expose the tumor, and the entire tumor and capsule are removed. Since the malignancy can spread along fascial planes and muscles, the physician may remove surrounding affected soft tissue to complete adequate resection. The physician may also need to repair muscle layers or fascial planes with sutures. One or two drain tubes may be inserted. The incision is repaired in multiple layers with sutures, staples, or Steri-strips.

22100–22103

The physician removes spurs, other growths, or bone disease by partial resection of a posterior vertebral component such as spinous process, lamina, or facet. The patient is placed prone and an incision is made overlying the affected vertebra and taken down to the level of the fascia. The fascia is incised and the paravertebral muscles are retracted. The physician removes the affected part of the spinous process, lamina, or facet. Paravertebral muscles are repositioned and the tissue and skin is closed with layered sutures. Use 22101 to report the procedure when performed on the thoracic vertebrae; use 22102 for the lumbar vertebrae. Report 22103 for each additional segment (list separately in addition to code for primary procedure).

22110–22116

The physician makes an anterior incision with the patient stabilized by a halo or cranial tongs. Lower cervical vertebrae are approached above the clavicle, dividing the superficial muscles and fascia and then retracting the trachea, esophagus, and thyroid medially. After blunt division of the deep fascia and paravertebral muscles, the anterior aspect of the cervical spine is exposed. The bony lesion is identified and excised from the affected vertebral body. Once the lesion is removed, a drain is placed and the incision is closed in layered sutures. The halo or tongs are attached to a body jacket to assure stabilization of the spine. Report 22110 for cervical segment; report 22112 if the site is thoracic; report 22114 if the site is lumbar; report 22116 for each additional segment (list separately in addition to code for primary procedure).

22210–22216

This procedure is performed to correct spinal deformities. The patient is placed in a sitting position with the head supported by a halo. In 22210, a posterior midline incision is made over the cervicothoracic junction. The physician exposes the spine from C5 to T1. The posterior elements of C7 are removed as are the caudal half of C6 and cephalad half of T1. The osteotomy continues laterally. The patient is placed under general anesthesia and the forward parts of the vertebrae are fractured. The resected bone is placed laterally and the muscles are reattached with sutures. The wound is closed with layered sutures. The angle of the neck is adjusted using the halo and a halo vest. Report 22210 if the site is cervical; report 22212 if the site is thoracic; report 22214 if the site is lumbar; report 22216 for each additional segment (list separately in addition to code for primary procedure).

22220–22226

The physician makes incisions overlying more than one section of spine and retracts the fascia, paraspinal muscles, and vertebral ligaments, depending on the approach needed. A wedge of bone is removed from the vertebrae above and below, and the spine is extended. Several levels may be corrected at once. Separately reportable bone grafts are placed in the wedges and instrumentation (e.g., Harrington, Cotrel-Dubosset) is placed to maintain the newly straightened spine. The muscles are sutured together over the instrumentation and the incision is closed with layered sutures. This procedure is often performed in conjunction with gradual halo-gravity traction. Report 22222 if the site is thoracic. Report 22224 if the site is lumbar. Report 22226 for additional segments (list separately in addition to code for primary procedure).

22305–22310

Closed treatment of a vertebral process fracture is only indicated if the spine is stable and the type of fracture does not require surgical intervention. In the case of the cervical spine, the physician initially immobilizes the patient's neck and spine with sandbags or a cervical collar as necessary. Report 22305 if the fracture is located in the vertebral processes; report 22310 if the fracture is located in the vertebral body, without manipulation, requiring and including casting or bracing.

22315

Following traumatic or pathological fracture of the vertebrae, the physician immobilizes the vertebrae and decompresses the spine. In the case of the cervical spine, the physician will initially immobilize the patient's neck and spine with sandbags or a cervical collar as necessary. Tongs or a halo are affixed to the patient, who is lying supine on a table with the head extending beyond the top. Dislocation requires spinal alignment by manipulation or skeletal traction. As the

CPT® Lay Descriptions

traction is increased in stages, the physician assures that there is no additional neurological deficit by checking the patient.

22318–22319

The physician performs an open treatment and/or reduction of odontoid fracture(s) and/or dislocation(s) including the os odontoideum. The odontoid/os odontoideum (dens) is the tooth-like process located on the second cervical vertebra in the neck. The patient is placed in a supine position and the fracture(s)/dislocation(s)is reduced with skeletal traction. The physician then makes an anterior 6–7 cm transverse skin incision at the level of the C5–6 disc space. Dissection is carried down to the odontoid process by longitudinally splitting the muscle and by blunt careful dissection of the space between the carotid, trachea, and esophagus; a retractor is placed and the anterior longitudinal ligament is incised. The superior thyroid artery may be ligated. Using imaging intensification, guidewires are inserted into an area of the dens and screws are placed over the wires. In 22319 bone graft(s) are placed to stabilize the fracture(s)/disclocation(s). When the procedure is completed a drain may be placed and the wound is closed with layered sutures.

22325–22328

The patient is placed prone and the skin, fascia, and paravertebral muscles are incised and retracted. The proper rod (e.g., Harrington, Edwards) is selected and anatomic or C-shaped hooks are placed on vertebrae above and below the injury. The rod is inserted in the hooks and the spine is aligned. If fusion is desired, the physician may place separately reportable grafts between the vertebrae or place sleeves on the rod and position them to stabilize the injured vertebrae. The incision is closed by layered sutures. Report 22325 if the site is the lumbar; report 22326 if the site is cervical; report 22327 if the site is thoracic; report 22328 for each addtional fractured vertebrae or dislocated segment (list separately in addition to code for primary procedure).

22505

Fracture or dislocation of the spine often requires manipulation. The patient is placed supine with a halo or tongs affixed to the skull. General anesthesia is administered. Traction is applied to the feet and the halo or tongs, decompressing the vertebrae. The patient remains under anesthesia until desired correction of the spine is accomplished. Traction is removed and the patient is immobilized in a halo cast, Stryker bed, or circular bed.

22520–22522

A local anesthetic is administered. In a separately reportable procedure, the radiologist uses imaging techniques, such as CT scanning and fluoroscopy, to guide percutaneous placement of the needle during the procedure and to monitor the injection procedure.

Sterile biomaterial (e.g., methyl methacrylate) is injected into the spine to reinforce the fractured or collapsed vertebra. The compound quickly hardens inside the vertebra, restoring strength to the fractured or collapsed vertebral body. The procedure does not restore the original shape to the vertebra, but it does stabilize the bone preventing further fracture or collapse. Following the procedure, the patient may experience significant, almost immediate, pain relief. Report 22520 for percutaneous vertebroplasty of one vertebral body at the thoracic level; 22521 for percutaneous vertebroplasty of one vertebral body at the lumbar level; and 22522 for each additional thoracic or lumbar vertebral body treated.

22548

This procedure may use arthrodesis techniques for herniated disk surgery but is much more commonly used for fractures and dislocations to stabilize the spine. Skull tong traction is applied. Avoiding the esophagus, pharynx, or esophageal nerve, the physician may incise the back of the throat, but most often enters from the outside of the neck, left of the throat. The jawbone may be dislocated. Retractors separate the intervertebral muscles. A drill is inserted in the affected vertebrae and the location confirmed by x-ray. The physician incises a trough in the front of the vertebrae with a drill or saw. The physician cleans out the intervertebral disk spaces with a rongeur and removes the cartilaginous plates above and below the vertebrae to be fused. The physician obtains and packs separately reportable grafts of iliac bone into the spaces and trims them. Traction is gradually decreased to maintain the graft in its bed. The fascia is sutured. A drain is placed in the incision and the incision is sutured.

22554–22585

This procedure may use arthrodesis techniques for herniated disk surgery but is much more commonly used for fractures and dislocations to stabilize the spine. Skull tong traction is applied. Retractors separate the intervertebral muscles. A drill is inserted in the affected vertebrae and the location is confirmed by separately reportable x-ray. The physician incises a trough in the front of the vertebrae with a drill or saw. The physician cleans out the intervertebral disk spaces with a rongeur and removes the cartilaginous plates above and below the vertebrae to be fused. The physician obtains and packs separately reportable grafts of iliac or donor bone into the spaces and trims them. Traction is gradually decreased to maintain the graft in its bed. The fascia is sutured. A drain is placed and the incision is sutured. Report 22556 if the site is thoracic. Report 22558 if the site is lumbar. Report 22585 for each additional segment (list separately in addition to code for primary procedure).

22590

The physician performs this procedure because of degenerative, traumatic, and/or congenital lesions of the spine. The patient is placed in a Stryker frame with a previously applied halo vest. The physician incises the skin from the occiput to the C3 vertebra, opens the fascia, and retracts the paravertebral muscles. A horizontal hole is drilled in the occiput using a burr. A second hole is drilled in the base of C2. The physician places wires through these holes. A third wire is placed around the ring of C1. Separately reportable bone grafts are obtained from the iliac crest; they are prepared, drilled, and tied in place using the wires. The retractors are removed and the incision is closed over a drain.

22595

The physician performs this procedure because of degenerative, traumatic, and/or congenital lesions of the spine. The patient is placed in a prone on a Stryker frame with a halo or tong in place. The physician makes an incision from the occiput to the fourth or fifth vertebra. The physician exposes the posterior arch of the atlas and laminae of C2 and removes all soft tissue from bony surfaces. The upper arch of the C1 is exposed and a wire loop is brought from below upward under the arch of the atlas and sutured. The physician passes the free ends through the loop, grasping the arch of the C1. A graft taken from the iliac crest is placed against the lamina of the C2 and the arch of C1 beneath the wire. The physician then passes one end of the wire through the spinous process of C2 and twists it securely into place. The retractors are removed and the incision is closed over a drain.

22600–22614

In 22600, the physician makes an incision overlying the vertebrae, separates the fascia, and divides the supraspinous ligaments in line with the skin incision. The physician prepares the vertebrae and lifts ligaments and muscles out of the way. A chisel elevator is used to strip away the capsules of lateral articulations. The physician frees the top layer of the ligamentum flavum. A gouge is used to cut chips from the fossa and denude it of cortical bone. Separately reportable chips from the laminae and ilium are used to join the laminae. Tissues are sutured to secure the chips. Skin is closed with sutures, as well. Report 22610 for thoracic arthrodesis; 22612 for lumbar arthrodesis; and 22614 for each additional vertebral segment (list separately in addition to code for primary procedure).

22630–22632

The patient is placed prone. The physician makes a midline incision, separates the fascia, and divides the supraspinous ligaments in line with the skin incision. The physician prepares the vertebrae and lifts ligaments and muscles of the way. A chisel elevator is used to strip away the capsules of lateral articulations. The physician frees the top layer of the ligamentum flavum. A gouge is used to cut chips from the fossa and denude it of cortical bone. Part of the lamina may

be removed on one side to allow access to the spinal cord. In addition, part of the disk may be removed to facilitate preparation of the interspace for fusion. Separately reportable chips from the laminae and ilium are used to laterally join the laminae. Paravertebral muscles and fascia are sutured to secure the chips. Skin is closed with sutures as well. Report 22632 for each additional interspace (list separately in addition to code for primary procedure).

22800–22804

The patient is placed prone. A midline incision is made overlying the affected vertebra. The fascia and the paravertebral muscles are incised and retracted. The physician uses a curet and rongeur to clean interspinous ligaments, and one of several techniques may be used. In one, the spinous processes are split and removed, and a curet is used to cut into the lateral articulations. Thin slices of separately reportable iliac bone graft are placed in these slots. Grafts are obtained from the iliac crest, prepared, and packed with separately reportable bone chips on both sides of the spinal curve, with more bone chips on the concave sides. Separately reportable instrumentation may be affixed to the spine. The incision is closed with layered sutures. A cast may or may not be applied to stabilize the spine. Report 22802 for fusion of seven to 12 vertebral segments. Report 22804 for 13 or more vertebral segments.

22808–22812

An anterior spinal fusion is a procedure often performed in conjunction with separately reportable spinal instrumentation and/or a posterior spinal fusion to correct a scoliotic deformity or prevent further deformity. The approach is anterior with the patient sidelying in the case of a thoracolumbar curve. The dissection is carried out through the abdominal muscles to the tenth rib, which is resected to allow entry to the chest. Dissection continues until the vertebral bodies are exposed and the disks are resected. Osteotomes and rongeurs may be used to prepare the disk space for a separately reportable bone graft. After the bone grafting, a chest tube is inserted and the wound is closed in layered sutures. Report 22802 if three or fewer vertebrae are fused; report 22810 if four to seven vertebrae are fused; report 22812 if eight or more are repaired.

22818–22819

The physician performs this procedure for spinal deformities such as kyphosis and scoliosis. The patient is placed prone. The physician makes a posterior midline incision, superior to the spinal abnormality, and past the lateral bony ridges. Dissection is carried down into the lamina, until the foramina are exposed on both sides of the spine. The nerve, artery, and vein within the foramina are divided, and cauterized exposing the dural sac. Any bleeding is controlled with bone wax and electrocautery. The sac is entered, and the dura is closed with suture, leaving the sac remnant. Affected vertebral body(s) and posterior elements are removed until the kyphosis is corrected. The sac remnant that was left is used to cover the site of the resected vertebrae. Removed vertebral bodies are morselized; and, along with allograft material, are used for bone grafting. Rod instrumentation is applied and segmental wires are used to hold the rod in place. The wound is irrigated and closed with layered sutures over suction drains. A body jacket is applied. If a single or two segment kyphectomy is performed, report 22818, if three or more segments, report 22819.

22830

The physician explores an existing fusion to diagnose and correct problems. The patient is placed in various positions depending on how the original fusion was performed (e.g. anterior, posteral, posterolateral). The physician makes an incision overlying the fused vertebrae. Fascia and paravertebral muscles are incised and retracted. The physician explores previous instrumentation, grafts, and wires. Any or all may be partially replaced, or adjusted during the exploration. When the exploration is complete, the fascia and vertebral muscles are repaired and returned to their anatomical positions. The incision is closed with layered sutures.

22840–22844

The physician performs these procedures to correct a defect of the spine caused by disease, trauma, or congenital anomaly. In 22840, the patient is placed in a prone position. The physician makes a midline incision in the skin, fascia, and paravertebral muscles over the affected vertebrae. The lower hook is introduced in the pedicle. The site for the upper hook is prepared by removing a small piece of the inferior facet to allow the hook to be more securely seated. A sharp-edged hook is inserted and withdrawn to guarantee there is enough room for the permanent hook, a dull-flanged hook. Once seated, the hooks are tested for purchase in their sites. The most inferior hook is placed in a lumbar vertebra with the help of a spreader. The space for the rod (e.g., Harrington) is prepared and a rod of proper length is selected. With the help of an assistant, the rod is placed in the inferior hook and in the superior hook on the convex side of the spine. An outrigger attached to the hooks is used to distract and correct the spine. At the correct level of distraction, a C washer is placed behind the upper hook to prevent it from slipping. The wound is closed with layered sutures. Report 22841 when internal spinal fixation is accomplished by wiring of the spinous processes. Report 22842, 22843 or 22844 if segmental fixation of the spine is performed. Segmental fixation differs in that at least one additional hook or wire is placed between the proximal and distal bony attachment devices.

22845–22847

Separately reportable anterior instrumentation is used primarily to correct a spinal deformity such as scoliosis. Several methods and types are available (e.g., Dwyer, Zielke, Scottish Rite) but all are based on a rod and some method of fixation, such as screws, wires, or hooks. Approach differs with level of spine being corrected and the configuration is unique to each case. Report 22845 for two to three vertebral segments; report 22846 for four to seven vertebral segments; and report 22847 for eight or more vertebral segments.

22848

This procedure, usually called the "Galveston technique," often accompanies a procedure for scoliosis, myelomeningocele, or paralytic spinal defects where sacral fixation is not desirable. The physician joins axial connectors to a rod configured to fit along the flat of the sacrum and impacted longitutudinally between the cornices of the ilium just above the greater sciatic notch. The rod is driven through the ilium and negates the need for anterior instrumentation. Report this in addition to the primary procedure.

22849

This code describes the procedures used following failure of a wire, instrumentation, or plate. The patient is placed in the position dictated by the failure. The physician makes a midline incision overlying the damaged section. The fascia, paravertebral muscles, and ligaments are retracted. A number of reparative techniques may be used, depending on the device and point of failure. In most cases, the device must be replaced. The physician closes the muscles, fascia, and skin with layered sutures.

22850

Instrumentation is sometimes removed when correction is complete and stable, when the patient is a growing juvenile, or when the instrumentation causes complications, such as infection or pain. The patient is placed prone. The physician makes an incision overlying the affected area through the skin, fascia, and paravertebral muscles. Bone and collagen are removed. The instrumentation is exposed and the superior hook or screw is loosened. Using forceps, the superior hook is disconnected from the vertebra. The inferior hook is disconnected from the vertebrae. The hardware is removed.

22851

This procedure is performed to replace a vertebral body or partial vertebral body resected due to destruction by disease, trauma, or other processes. Once the vertebral body has been removed by a separately identifiable procedure, a hole is cored out of the vertebral bodies above and below the removed vertebrae to secure a biomechanical device (ceramic block, metal/synthetic cage, threaded bone dowel, methylmethacrylate). The physician selects the biomechanical device best suited to the location and type of deformity being corrected. For example, to correct a deformity caused by a malignancy, the physician may elect to inject methylmethacrylate into the area and allow it to dry to replace the excised vertebral body. Screws, wires or plates may be used to secure the device. Muscles are allowed to fall back into place and the wound is closed over a drain with layered sutures.

22852

Instrumentation is sometimes removed when correction is complete and stable or when the patient is a growing juvenile. The patient is placed prone. The physician makes a midline incision overlying the affected area through the skin, fascia, and paravertebral muscles. Collagen is removed. The instrumentation is exposed. Using forceps, the superior hook is disconnected from the vertebra. The inferior and segmental hooks are disconnected from the vertebrae. The hardware is removed. The incision is closed with layered sutures.

22855

Instrumentation is sometimes removed when correction is complete and stable or when the patient is a growing juvenile. The patient is placed supine. The physician makes an incision overlying the affected area through the skin, fascia, and paravertebral muscles. Collagen is removed. The instrumentation is exposed and the superior hook or screw is loosened. Using forceps, the superior hook or screw is disconnected from the vertebra. The inferior and segmental hooks or screws are disconnected from the vertebrae. The hardware is removed. The incision is closed with layered sutures.

22900

The physician removes a tumor most frequently occurring in the anterior abdominal wall. The patient is positioned supine on the operating table. A longitudinal incision is made over the tumor. Dissection is carried down to expose the affected muscle and tumor. Because these tumors are prone to recur, the tumor, surrounding tissue, and muscle are excised. The incision is then repaired in multiple layers with sutures, staples, or Steri-strips.

23000

The physician makes a small incision over the deltoid muscle to expose the rotator cuff tendons. The raised area over the calcium deposits is incised in line with the axis of the fibers. A large cavity is made in the tendon with a curet to remove all damaged tissue. The opening is then closed with side-to-side sutures. Once the tendon is repaired, the skin incision is closed and a soft dressing is applied.

23020

This procedure is not commonly performed unless the shoulder is fixed in marked internal rotation and adduction. (In this position the arm is unable to move away from the body.) The physician makes an incision at the front of the shoulder where the deltoid meets the pectoral muscle. The subscapularis tendon is removed from the glenoid rim. The anterior capsule is left intact. The pectoralis major tendon is severed from its attachment on the humerus. The skin incision is closed and soft dressing is applied. The arm is positioned in abduction (arm elevated out to the side of the body).

23030–23031

A small skin incision is made over the abscess or hematoma. The soft tissues are reflected to expose the area requiring drainage. The area is irrigated and treated with antibiotics if necessary. A drainage tube may be placed in the region and the skin loosely sutured over the drains. Once the drains are removed the skin is closed with sutures or Steri strips. Report 23031 if treating an infected bursa.

23035

A longitudinal incision is made through the skin and the underlying muscles are divided to expose the bone. The periosteum is spilt and reflected back from the bone overlying the infected area. A curet is used to scrape the abscess or infected portion from the bone down to healthy bony tissue. The area is irrigated and the periosteum is closed over the bone and the soft tissues are closed with sutures. A soft dressing is applied.

23040–23044

The physician performs an arthrotomy of the glenohumeral joint in 23040 or of the acromioclavicular joint in 23044. An incision may be made overlying the shoulder joint. Tissues are dissected down to the joint. The joint is explored, drained, and any foreign bodies are removed. The incision may be repaired in multiple layers.

23065–23066

A biopsy is performed to take a sample of the tissue for further testing. A small incision is made overlying the area to be biopsied. The skin is reflected to expose the soft tissue to be tested. A small portion of the soft tissue is removed and saved for testing. Report 23066 if the sample is taken from a deeper part of the bone.

23075–23076

The physician makes an incision through the skin and reflects it back to expose the tumor. The tumor is removed leaving healthy, normal tissue around the circumference. The area is irrigated and the soft tissues are sutured. A soft dressing is applied. Report 23076 if the procedure is deep, subfascial, or intramuscular.

23077

The physician removes a malignant soft tissue tumor not invading bone from the shoulder. The physician excises the tumor and any adjacent tissue where the tumor may have spread. The physician may perform marginal margin resection, marginal resection, local wide resection, or radical margin resection, depending on the stage of the lesion. The surgical wound is repaired by complex closure, adjacent tissue transfer, or graft.

23100

The physician makes an incision over the shoulder joint. Incisions are made through the soft tissues to gain access to the glenohumeral joint. A sample of the joint tissue is removed and saved for testing (biopsy). The wound is repaired in layered sutures.

23101

The physician makes an incision overlying the shoulder joint. An incision is made through the skin and the underlying muscle is divided to gain access to the joint capsule of the acromioclavicular or sternoclavicular. Once the capsule is penetrated the torn cartilage is identified and a specimen is removed for biopsy. The torn cartilage also may be removed. The joint is irrigated the capsule is closed and the soft tissues are sutured closed. A soft dressing is applied.

23105–23106

With the patient in a sidelying position and the arm suspended in traction, the physician makes an incision overlying the shoulder. The instruments are properly placed into the shoulder and the synovium is removed with motorized synovial resectors. Following completion, the shoulder is irrigated and the incision closed with sutures or Steri-strips. Report 23106 if the procedure includes the sternoclavicular joint. Biopsy of the tissue can be taken in the same manner.

23107

The physician performs an arthrotomy of the glenohumeral joint. An incision is made overlying the shoulder joint. Tissues are dissected down to the joint. The joint is explored and any loose or foreign bodies are identified and removed. The incision may be repaired in multiple layers. After identification the loose body is divided and removed. The joint is irrigated and the incisions are closed.

23120–23125

Removal of the clavicle (collar bone) is successfully performed without significant loss of function to the upper extremity. An incision is made horizontally along the portion of the bone to be removed. The skin is reflected back and the bone is divided with an osteotome and rounded at the end to eliminate the rough edge. The ligament that connects the clavicle to the adjacent bone is divided to allow disarticulation of the joint and the bone is removed. The wound is

closed with Steri-strips and a soft dressing is applied. Report 23120 if partial, 23125 if total.

23130

This procedure is commonly performed during repair to the rotator cuff in effort to increase the space below the acromion where the cuff tendons traverse toward their insertion on the humerus. An incision is made overlying the area. Dissection is carried down to the acromion. Acromioplasty involves the division of the acromioclavicular ligament followed by a bur that is used to cut away the under surface of the acromion. During acromionectomy, the distal portion of the acromion is removed. The acromionial ligament may be released. The joint is irrigated and the incisions are closed with sutures or Steri-strips.

23140–23146

The physician makes an incision overlying the clavicle and scapula. The skin and underlying soft tissues are reflected back to expose the periosteum where it is separated from the bone. The benign tumor or cyst is removed by scraping or osteotome. Once healthy bone tissue is present the periosteum is repositioned and the skin is closed with sutures and a soft dressing is applied. Report 23145 if with autograft; report 23146 if allograft is used.

23150–23156

A longitudinal incision is made toward the top of the arm and the underlying deltoid muscle is divided. The periosteum is split and divided from the bone. The growth is identified and removed from the humerus by scraping with a curet until healthy bone is exposed. The periosteum is repositioned and the deltoid sutured if necessary. The skin is closed with sutures and a soft dressing and sling are applied. Report 23155 if an autograft is used; report 23156 if an allograft is used.

23170–23174

The physician removes infected portions of the clavicle due to osteomyelitis. Often this infection leaves open sinus tracts in the bone that require removal. The physician makes an incision overlying the clavicle. Once the skin and soft tissues are reflected, a small window is cut into the bone to gain access to the sequestra. Purulent material and scarred and necrotic tissue are removed. The remaining space is filled with surrounding soft tissues or free tissue transfer. The area is irrigated and antibiotic is used to prevent further infection. The wound is closed loosely over drains if possible. The arm is positioned in a sling or splint and protected to prevent fracture of the clavicle. Report 23172 if this procedure performed on the scapula; report 23174 if this procedure is performed on the humeral head to surgical neck.

23180

The physician makes a horizontal incision inferior to the clavicle overlying the infection. The skin is

between the humeral head and glenoid. In this case the remaining stump of the tendon can be removed by a motorized shaver. A simultaneous subacromial decompression may be performed. Debridement of the frayed portion of the tendon may be performed.

23440

The tendon of the long head of the biceps brachii is an important stabilizer of the humeral head. When the proximal end of the tendon is detached from the glenoid, it is rolled or knotted, sutured, and inserted through a keyhole shaped opening in the cortex of the humerus in the floor of the bicipital groove. This is performed through a longitudinal incision at the anterior aspect of the shoulder. Once proper fixation is obtained, the incision is closed and the arm is supported in a sling. Active elbow flexion and shoulder elevation are limited until proper fixation and healing are complete.

23450–23455

An anterior incision is made at the deltopectoral-pectoral interval. The coricoid process is identified and the tendon of the biceps (short head) is at times incised distal to coricoid for exposure. The anterior capsule is visualized through a small transverse incision of the subscapularis tendon which is tagged for identification and removed from its attachment on the capsule. The quality and laxity of the capsule are assessed and the joint is explored for damage to the labrum or glenoid. The joint is irrigated to remove any loose bodies. If there is no other abnormal laxity the capsule is advance superiorly and attached to the labrum with sutures. An appropriate amount of slack is taken up to provide stability within the joint. Once the capsule is reattached, the subscapularis tendon is reapproximated but not tightened and repaired. A subcutaneous drain is placed and the wound is closed. Report 23455 if Bankart type operation with or without stapling.

23460–23462

If there is significant damage to the glenoid where more than one third of the glenoid is deficient, a bone block procedure is performed to increase the surface area of the glenoid. The patient is placed in a lateral position or modified beach chair position. A horizontal or vertical incision is placed inferior to the scapular spine allowing a bone graft to be taken from the scapular spine if necessary. An additional incision is made at the lateral border of the acromion and carried posteriorly to the axillary crease. The deltoid is split to expose the infraspinatus and teres minor tendons. The capsule is exposed and incised with a T-shaped cut. The capsule is then reattached to the glenoid through drill holes or by means of suture anchors taking up slack on the inferior portion of the capsule. The capsular repair may be reinforced using the infraspinatus tendon if the local tissue is felt to be insufficient. The bone block is placed on the posterior inferior portion of the glenoid fossa and fixated wit a

screw. This bone fragment is usually obtained from the spine of the scapula through a posterior incision along the spine of the scapula. Report 23462 if performed with coracoid process transfer.

23465

The patient is placed in a lateral position or modified beach chair position. A horizontal or vertical incision is placed inferior to the scapular spine allowing a bone graft to be taken from the scapular spine if necessary. An additional incision is made at the lateral border of the acromion and carried posteriorly to the axillary crease. The deltoid is split to expose the infraspinatus and teres minor tendons. The capsule is exposed and incised with a T-shaped cut. The capsule is then reattached to the glenohumeral joint through drill holes or by means of suture anchors taking up slack on the inferior portion of the capsule. The capsular repair may be reinforced using the infraspinatus tendon if the local tissue is felt to be insufficient. When a bone block is used it is placed at the posterior inferior quadrant of the glenohumeral joint to increase the articulation surface of the glenoid. This technique is rarely used. Once the incision is closed the arm is placed in an Orthoplast splint with the arm in external rotation for the first 6 weeks. Motion is protected.

23466

The surgical approach may differ from patient to patient depending upon the patient's history. The incision is determined by the side of most significant instability. A separately reportable arthroscopic examination of the shoulder should be performed first to fully determine the extent of damage to the joint and the appropriate surgical approach. An anterior H-plasty is commonly used to tighten the capsule. In some cases, both medial and lateral capsular incisions may be required to provide sufficient capsular tension.

23470

A 14.0 cm curved incision is made from the superior aspect of the acromion along the deltopectoral interval to the deltoid insertion. The deltoid is retracted laterally and pectoralis medially. The fascia between the pectoral and the clavicle is divided and the subacromial space is freed with a gloved finger or periosteal elevator. The coricoacromial ligament is freed and often an acromioplasty is performed to allow for freedom of movement after surgery. The subscapularis tendon is tagged and removed from the capsule. The anterior joint capsule is divided and the glenohumeral joint is dislocated by further external rotation and extension of the arm. The joint is explored and all loose bodies are removed. The humeral head is removed with a reciprocating saw or osteotome. A trial prosthesis is placed along the proximal humerus as a guide for proper inclination of the osteotomy. A horizontal cut (osteotomy) is made as previously determined and a large curet is used to open the medullary canal for placement of the stem of the prosthesis. The canal is enlarged with a reamer to the appropriate size. The prosthesis is positioned in proper rotational alignment to articulate with the glenoid. Any remaining osteophytes (bone spurs) are removed. The joint is irrigated thoroughly. The prosthesis is reduced into the glenoid and the subscapularis tendon is sutured in place with multiple interrupted non-absorbable sutures with the shoulder is neutral position. The deltopectoral interval is closed loosely over drainage tubes. The arm is placed in a sling and swathe bandage.

23472

A 14.0 cm curved incision is made from the superior aspect of the acromion along the deltopectoral interval to the deltoid insertion. The deltoid is retracted laterally and pectoralis medially. The fascia between the pectoral and the clavicle is divided and the subacromial space is freed with a gloved finger or periosteal elevator. The coricoacromial ligament is freed and often an acromioplasty is performed to allow for freedom of movement after surgery. The subscapularis tendon is tagged and removed from the capsule. The anterior joint capsule is divided and the glenohumeral joint is dislocated by further external rotation and extension of the arm. The joint is explored and all loose bodies are removed. The humeral head is removed with a reciprocating saw or osteotome. In addition, a prosthetic device is placed proximally at the glenoid to articulate with the prosthetic humeral head. Prior to placement of the humeral prosthesis the joint is opened to fully expose the glenoid surface. The surface cartilage of the glenoid is removed. A power drill is used to cut a slot into the glenoid the exact size of the holding devise of the glenoid component. Small curets are used to remove cancellous bone from the base of the coricoid bone. With a bur, articular cartilage is removed from the surface of the glenoid. A trial glenoid component is used to properly prepare the bone and fit the prosthesis. Once the glenoid preparation is complete the glenoid vault is drilled and filled with polymethylmethacrylate (cement). The glenoid component is pushed into place and held until the cement is cured. Prior to final insertion of the humeral component, an anterior acromioplasty and acromioclavicular arthroplasty is performed if necessary. If large rotator cuff tears are found, they are repaired at this time. The joint is brought through full range of motion and fully irrigated. The subscapularis tendon is repaired to stabilize the joint, however, the joint capsule is not usually resutured. Drains are placed and the deltopectoral interval is sutured closed. The arm is placed in a sling and swathe.

23480

The physician performs an osteotomy (bone cut) of the clavicle. The physician makes an incision in the skin overlying the clavicle. Tissue is dissected down to the bone. Using a surgical saw or other sharp instrument, the physician cuts through the bone. Surgical screws, a metal plate, or wires may secure the

cut bone in the correct position. The wound is irrigated with antibiotic solution and the skin Is closed in layers.

23485

The physician performs an osteotomy (bone cut) of the clavicle that is not healing or has healed in an unacceptable position. The physician makes an incision in the skin overlying the clavicle. Tissue is dissected down to the bone. Using a surgical saw or other sharp instrument, the physician cuts through the bone. Surgical screws, a metal plate, or wires may secure the cut bone in the correct position. The physician harvests a bone graft from the patient through a separate incision. The physician then repairs the surgically created graft donor site. The graft is then placed in the clavicle. Surgical screws, plates, or other hardware secure the bone graft, osteotomy, and fracture. The incision is then closed in multiple layers.

23490–23491

In some cases the physician will choose to perform a preventative nailing or screwing of the clavicle to the coricoid process in order to gain better fixation and prevent further dislocation of the acromioclavicular joint. Access to the joint is obtained through a lateral incision over the acromion process. The skin and soft tissues are reflected back. The screw positioned and may be checked by separately reportable x-ray. The incision is closed with sutures and motion is protected for 4–6 weeks. The hardware is removed when ligament stability is determined. Report 23491 for treating the proximal humerus.

23500–23505

The physician treats a fracture of the clavicle bone without surgery or manipulation. Separately reportable x-rays confirm the stable position of the fractured pieces. No manipulation is required. The physician may apply a clavicle brace, tape, or splint until the fracture heals. In 23505, the fracture is displaced and manipulation is required. A local anesthetic may be applied. The physician then pushes or pulls on the bony pieces, or manipulates the shoulder in such a way to properly align the fracture. The physician may apply a clavicle brace, tape, or splint until the fracture heals.

23515

The physician treats a fracture of the clavicle with open surgery. The physician makes an incision overlying the fractured area of the clavicle. Tissue is dissected down to the bone and the fracture is identified. The physician debrides any nonviable tissues. Any tissue that has become lodged between the fracture pieces is removed. The physician applies screws, wires, or plates to secure the fracture. An external fixator may be applied on the outside of the skin. The wound is irrigated with antibiotic solution and the incision is closed. A splint or brace may also be applied on the outside of the clavicle or shoulder.

23520–23525

The physician treats a dislocation of the joint between the sternum and the clavicle (sternoclavicular) without making incisions and without any manipulation in 23520. The physician applies a splint or brace to hold the joint in place until it has healed. In 23525, manipulation is required. Anesthesia may be necessary. The physician pushes, pulls, or moves the arm and chest to restore the joint to correct position and alignment. After manipulation, the patient is placed in a brace or splint.

23530–23532

The physician treats a chronic or acute dislocation of the sternoclavicular joint. The physician makes an incision overlying the joint between the clavicle and sternum where the dislocation has occurred. The tissues are dissected down to the joint and the dislocation is visualized. The physician may debride the area. In 23532, the physician harvests a fascial graft from the patient through a separate incision. The physician then repairs the surgically created graft donor site. The fascial graft is then attached to the bones in the sternoclavicular joint, preventing recurrent dislocation. In both 23530 and 23532, the physician then reduces (realigns) the bones into the correct position. Fixation may be applied. The joint is irrigated with antibiotic solution. The incision is the closed in layers. A splint or brace may be applied to outside of the body.

23540–23545

The physician treats a dislocation of the acromioclavicular joint (between the acromion process of the scapula and the clavicle). In 23540 the physician places the affected shoulder and arm in a sling or other brace. In 23545 manipulation is necessary to correct the dislocation. Anesthesia may be necessary. The physician manipulates the joint by pushing or pulling on the shoulder and arm to align the bones. The physician then applies a sling or other brace.

23550

The physician treats an acute or chronic dislocation of the acromioclavicular joint (between the acromion process of the scapula and the clavicle). An incision is made overlying the shoulder at the articulation of the acromion of the scapula and the end of the clavicle. Dissection is carried through the tissues to the joint. Any nonviable tissue is removed. The bones are identified and the dislocation visualized. The physician then uses a heavy nonabsorbable suture, a wire, or screws to secure the two bones in their proper joint alignment. When the joint is restored, the wound is irrigated with antibiotic solution. The incision is closed in multiple layers. A sterile dressing

is applied. A sling or brace is applied to the shoulder and arm.

23552

The physician treats an acute or chronic dislocation of the acromioclavicular joint (between the acromion process of the scapula and the clavicle) with a fascial graft. An incision is made overlying the shoulder at the articulation of the acromion of the scapula and the end of the clavicle. Dissection is carried through the tissues to the joint. Any nonviable tissue is removed. The bones are identified and the dislocation visualized. The physician harvests a fascial graft from the patient through a separate incision. The physician repairs the surgically created graft donor site. The graft is a strong piece of connective tissue. The graft is then connected to the pieces of dislocated joint to restore alignment. The physician uses a heavy nonabsorbable suture, a wire, or screws to secure the two bones in their proper joint alignment. When the joint is restored, the wound is irrigated with antibiotic solution. The incision is closed in multiple layers. A sterile dressing is applied. A sling or brace is applied to the shoulder and arm.

23570

The physician treats a fracture of the scapula bone without surgery or any type of manipulation. Separately reportable x-rays confirm the stable position of the fractured pieces. The physician then places the shoulder in a sling or other brace until the fracture heals.

23575

The physician treats a fracture of the scapula bone without any incisions. Separately reportable x-rays confirm the nature of the fracture and the displacement of the pieces. With the patient under anesthesia, the physician manipulates (pushes, pulls, or moves) the scapula and arm to align the fractured pieces. Separately reportable serial x-rays may be necessary while the manipulation is performed to confirm alignment. The physician may apply traction devices to the body to maintain satisfactory fracture position. A brace, splint, or cast may be applied to hold the bones in the correct position until they are healed.

23585

The physician makes an incision overlying the area of the fractured scapula. The physician dissects the tissues down to the bone to visualize the fracture. Nonviable tissues or those between the fragments are debrided. The physician places the fragments back together in their correct anatomic position either manually or with instruments. Fixation devices may be applied to secure the fragments. The physician then applies screws, metal plates, sutures, or wire to hold the bones together. The wound is irrigated with antibiotic solution. The incisions are closed in layers with sutures.

CPT® Lay Descriptions

23600–23605

Separately reportable x-rays confirm a stable non-displaced fracture. No manipulation or open reduction is required. The arm is positioned in a sling and motion protected to allow adequate healing. Report 23605 if with manipulation, with or without skeletal traction.

23615–23616

An incision is made anteromedially extending posteriorly along the acromion to the lateral half of the spine of the scapula. The deltoid is detached from the exposed portion of the spine of the scapula. The deltoid is reflected down to expose the joint capsule and the humerus. The fractured portion of the proximal humerus (surgical or anatomical neck) is identified and the fracture is aligned. If the tuberosity is involved it is repaired. External or internal fixation may be used to stabilize the fracture site. Once the fracture is stabilized, the wound is irrigated. The deltoid is repositioned and sutured in place. The skin is sutured and the wound is covered with a soft dressing. The arm is positioned in a sling and motion is protected to allow for proper healing. Report 23616 when the fracture cannot be repaired and a prosthetic proximal humeral replacement is necessary.

23620–23625

Separately reportable x-rays determine a stable, non-displaced fracture. The arm is positioned in a sling and motion of the shoulder is protected to prevent pull of the muscles that attach to the bone of the upper arm (greater humeral tuberosity). Report 23625 if with manipulation.

23630

An anterior longitudinal incision is made and the underlying deltoid fibers are divided to expose the fracture site. Often this injury will include damage to the rotator cuff tendons requiring repair of the soft tissues in addition to the fracture site. The soft tissues are reflected to expose the bone and any loose bodies are removed. The fracture is stabilized by screw fixation and the soft tissues are reattached by suture. The skin incision is closed and a soft dressing is applied. The arm is placed in a sling and motion is protected to allow for adequate healing of the tissues.

23650–23655

The most common form of shoulder dislocation is the traumatic anterior inferior dislocation. A closed manipulation requires the patient to be positioned to allow the arm to hang forward. The physician applies gentle traction to distract the joint and manually relocates the glenohumeral joint back into position. Report 23655 if requiring anesthesia.

23660

A posterior dislocation would be more likely to require an open reduction procedure than an anterior dislocation. The shoulder is approached through a deltopectoral incision. The joint is inspected and the head of the humerus is reduced into its proper position. The subscapularis tendon is attached to the head of the humerus with sutures or screws. If there is significant posterior translation, the posterior capsule is tightened. The incision is closed and the arm is immobilized in 20 degrees of external rotation.

23665

The physician performs closed reduction of the shoulder with the patient positioned prone and the arm hanging toward the floor. Manual distraction is attempted. If not successful the physician may hang a 5 pound weight from the arm in attempt to reduce the shoulder into place. Once reduction is obtained the arm a neurovascular examination is performed. A repair to a humeral tuberosity fracture is addressed. The arm is immobilized for 3–6 weeks.

23670

The physician may choose to enter the shoulder anteriorly through a deltopectoral approach or superior through a deltoid splitting approach. The soft tissues are reflected back and the fracture observed. Once the joint is reduced into proper position the repair of the humeral tuberosity fracture is addressed. Larger fragments are stabilized with screws, wire sutures, staples, and heavy non-absorbable suture material. These fragments usually require the fixation device to be later removed to allow full motion of the shoulder. If the fragment is small it can be removed and the tendons of the rotator cuff are advanced and attached to the defect in the bone. Once the fracture is stable the incision is closed and the arm protected in a sling for 4–6 weeks.

23675

The patient may be given some form of anesthetic or analgesic and positioned prone to allow the arm to hang forward. Manipulation is performed to reduced the dislocation and the arm is positioned in a sling and protected for four to six weeks. Separately reportable x-rays and neurovascular examinations are performed pre- and postmanipulation.

23680

The dislocation may be reduced with closed manipulation but often the fracture is instable and requires internal fixation. Percutaneous pinning where pins are introduced through a small incision through the skin and placed into the bone at the fracture site. Intermedullary rod is placed through the shaft of the bone to stabilize the fracture as well as AO buttress plate and screws. All of these techniques require the hardware to be removed once bony fixation is stable to allow for full motion of the shoulder.

23700

Manipulation of the shoulder under anesthesia may be necessary to gain the loss of motion following surgical procedure or as in the case of frozen shoulder. The patient is positioned supine and given local or general anesthesia. Following full evaluation, the physician manipulates the shoulder to the appropriate range of motion. In the case of fracture, the appropriate fixation device will be positioned through open or closed procedure.

23800–23802

The shoulder is positioned in what is considered the most functional position, shoulder slightly abducted to the side with forward elevation. A dorsolateral semicircular incision is made across the glenohumeral joint. At the midpoint the incision is carried distally for 5.0 cm. The articular cartilage is removed from the head of the humerus (ball) and the glenoid cavity (socket). The head is split and a wedge of bone is removed. This wedge is where the acromion will rest when the arm is positioned in abduction. At this point bone grafting or plate fixation may be added to the procedure to stabilize the glenohumeral joint. If a plate is used a second procedure will be needed to remove the hardware. Cast application or external fixation may be used in a number of procedures. Report 23802 if with primary autogenous graft.

23900

The physician preforms a forequarter amputation (interthoracoscapular). The physician incises the skin overlying the shoulder and dissects the disease-free soft tissue away from the bone to create a skin flap to cover the wound. The clavicle is disarticulated from the sternum, and the chest wall is freed from muscular attachments to the arm. The quarter section is removed and the wound is closed in sutured layers. If enough disease-free tissue is not available for primary closure, the wound is packed closed with gauze.

23920–23921

The physician disarticulates the shoulder. The physician incises the skin overlying the shoulder. The rotator cuff is incised freeing the arm of ligamentous and muscular attachments. The arm is removed and the wound is closed in sutured layers. Report 23920 for the first amputation. Report 23921 for a secondary closure of the wound or scar revision.

23930

The physician makes an incision overlying the site of the abscess or hematoma of the upper arm or elbow area. Dissection is carried down through the subcutaneous tissues, into the deep muscles and below to expose the abscess or hematoma. The incision may be extended if the abscess or hematoma is larger than expected. The abscess is incised and drained and/or the hematoma is drained and removed. The physician then irrigates the area. The incision is repaired in multiple layers with sutures, staples, and/or Steri-strips.

23931

The physician incises and drains a bursa of the upper arm or elbow area (e.g., olecranon). A longitudinal incision is made along the posteromedial border of the elbow. The bursa is dissected out, incised, and drained. The wound is then irrigated with antibiotic solution. A drain tube is inserted. The physician repairs the incision in multiple layers. The elbow may be immobilized in a splint for one week.

23935

The physician makes an incision over the affected area of the humerus or elbow. Dissection is carried down to expose the bone. Drill holes are then made through the cortex and into the medullary canal in an outline of a window around the infected or abscessed bone. The area is drained and debrided of infected bony and soft tissue. The physician then irrigates the area with antibiotic solution. The wound is packed and left open, allowing the area to drain. Secondary closure is performed approximately three weeks later. Dressings are changed daily. A splint may be applied to limit elbow movement.

24000

The physician makes a longitudinal incision over the part of the elbow to be exposed (e.g., the anterior, posterior, medial, or lateral aspect). The soft tissues are dissected out to explore and identify infected tissues. Any necrotic tissue is removed. If a foreign body is present, (e.g., bullet, nail, gravel), it is exposed and removed. The wound is irrigated with antibiotic solution. The physician may leave the wound open for daily dressing changes, allowing secondary healing. If the incision is repaired, drain tubes are inserted and the incision repaired in multiple layers with sutures, staples, and/or Steri-strips. A splint may be applied to limit elbow motion.

24006

The physician makes an incision over the anterior part of the elbow. Dissection is carried down to expose the joint capsule of the elbow. The radial nerve is identified and protected. The anterior elbow joint capsule is incised and portions of it are removed. By excising the capsule, any scarring limiting elbow motion is minimal. If additional parts of the capsule are to be excised, an additional incision (e.g., medial elbow incision) may be made. The physician then repairs the incision in multiple layers with sutures, staples, and/or Steri-strips. The elbow is placed in a posterior splint.

24065–24066

The physician makes a small longitudinal incision over the site of the biopsy. The physician exposes the tumor or cyst in the subcutaneous tissue between the muscle and skin layers in 24065. In 24066, the tumor or cyst is deeper and within the muscle or below the muscle layer. A larger skin incision and more extensive dissection may be needed. The tumor is typically surrounded by a capsule. The physician then makes an incision through the capsule and removes a portion of the tumor for biopsy. The capsule around the tumor is closed with sutures. The physician repairs the incision is multiple layers with sutures, staples, and/or Steri-strips. A splint may be applied to limit elbow motion.

24075–24076

The physician makes an incision overlying the site of the tumor in either the upper arm or elbow. A subcutaneous tumor lies just below the skin layer in 24075. The tumor lies deeper in 24076, either between the fascia and muscle layer (subfascial), or within the muscle layer itself (intramuscular). The physician exposes the tumor by subcutaneous dissection. A deep tumor requires more extensive and deeper dissection for exposure. The tumor is then excised, including the capsule that surrounds it. The physician may extend the margin of resection to include some normal tissue from around the tumor to help ensure removal of tumor tissue. A drain tube is inserted in the wound. The physician repairs the incision in multiple layers with sutures, staples, and/or Steri-strips. A splint may be applied to limit elbow motion.

24077

The physician makes a long incision overlying the site of the tumor. The tumor is exposed through dissection. The physician identifies the tumor and its margins, then removes it. Because this type of tumor is spread across fascial planes, radical resection of surrounding normal tissue is also performed. Normal tissue of one or more compartments, from origin to insertion, may be removed with the tumor. The physician inserts one or two drains in the wound. The incision is repaired in multiple layers with sutures, staples, and/or Steri-strips. The arm may be placed in a posterior splint.

24100–24101

The physician makes a straight, 10.0 cm, lateral, longitudinal incision to access the elbow joint. The physician may also use a medial, anterior, or posterior approach. The synovium lies within the joint capsule. The elbow joint is exposed by freeing and reflecting the common origin of the extensor muscles. The physician incises the joint capsule to expose the synovium. A small portion of the synovium is excised for biopsy. In 24101, additional dissection is carried out to further explore the joint and soft tissues. Any loose or foreign bodies are then removed. The physician thoroughly irrigates the joint. A drain tube may be inserted. The capsule is closed with sutures. The physician repairs the incision in multiple layers with sutures, staples, and/or Steri-strips.

24102

The physician makes a straight, longitudinal, lateral incision beginning 5.0 cm above the lateral epicondyle, and extending 5.0 cm along the anterolateral surface of the forearm. The physician may also make a medial incision if significant ulnar nerve symptoms coexist. The elbow joint is exposed by freeing and reflecting the common origin of the extensor muscles. Inflamed and enlarged synovium is removed from all aspects of the joint. The physician inserts a drain, then repairs the incision in multiple layers with sutures, staples, and/or Steri-strips. A posterior, plaster, long arm splint is applied.

24105

The physician makes a longitudinal incision along the posteromedial border of the elbow. This bursa is located directly over the point of the elbow. The physician dissects down to expose the bursa. The bursa is then excised. The surrounding tissue is examined for any sign of infection. The wound is thoroughly irrigated with antibiotic solution. The physician then repairs the incision in multiple layers with sutures, staples, and/or Steri-strips.

24110–24116

The physician excises or curets a bones cyst or benign tumor of head or neck of radius or olecranon process in 24110. The physician makes an incision over the site of the cyst or tumor. Dissection is carried down to the bone. The cyst or tumor is removed by curettage with a high speed burr. If the amount of bone removed is small, a bone graft is not necessary and the incision is repaired in multiple layers with sutures, staples, and/or Steri-strips. If the amount of bone removed is significant, a bone graft is required. Report 24115 if an autograft is taken and inserted and 24116 if an allograft is inserted.

24120–24126

The physician makes a 10.0 cm longitudinal incision along the lateral aspect of the elbow. A posterior incision may also be made to access the olecranon process. To expose the radial head and/or neck, the common origin of the extensor muscles is reflected, and the joint capsule incised. The bone cyst or tumor is visualized on the affected bone. The physician removes bone surrounding the cyst or tumor by forming a cortical window sized larger than the cyst or tumor. The physician uses curets to remove all of the cyst or tumor. Bone in the cortical window is removed with power burs. If the strength of the bone is compromised, then an autograft or allograft is needed. In 24125, the physician harvests bone from the patient's iliac crest with an osteotome. In 24126 donor (allograft) bone from a bone bank is used. The cortical window cavity is then filled with the bone graft. Any surgically created graft donor site is closed with sutures and/or Steri-strips. If the capsule was incised, it is closed with sutures. The physician then repairs the incision in multiple layers with sutures, staples, and/or Steri-strips. The elbow may be placed in a long, posterior splint to limit motion.

24130

The physician makes a 5.0 cm to 6.0 cm longitudinal incision along the lateral aspect of the elbow. The elbow joint is exposed by freeing and reflecting the common origin of the extensor muscles. The joint capsule is incised and the radial head is exposed. The physician uses a bone cutting saw to excise the radial head. The capsule is closed with sutures and the incision is repaired in layers with sutures, staples, and/or Steri-strips.

24134

The physician performs a sequestrectomy of the shaft or distal humerus. The physician makes an incision along the shaft of the humerus over the involved area. To expose the affected portion of humerus, muscles are reflected, and the elbow joint capsule is incised. The infected area of bone or the bone abscess is exposed. Using an osteotome, the physician outlines a cortical window around the infected area, and the window is removed. Separated, dead bone (sequestra), purulent material, and scarred and necrotic tissue are removed. The physician may repair the incision loosely over drains, or the wound may be packed open with dressings.

24136–24138

The physician makes a 10.0 cm longitudinal incision along the lateral aspect of the elbow. To expose the radial head and/or neck, the common origin of the extensor muscles is reflected, and the joint capsule incised. In 24138, the physician makes a posterior incision on the elbow to access the olecranon process. The infected area of bone or the bone abscess is visualized. Using a drill, the physician outlines a cortical window around the infected area with an osteotome. The cortical window is removed. All sequestra (separated, dead bone), purulent material, and scarred and necrotic tissue is removed. The physician may repair the incision loosely over drains. If closure is not possible, the wound is packed open with dressings changed daily. The patient may be placed in a long posterior splint to limit elbow motion.

24140

The physician performs a partial excision to facilitate a craterization, saucerization, or diaphysectomy of bone in the humerus. The physician makes an incision along the shaft of the humerus over the involved area. To expose the affected portion of humerus, muscles are reflected, and the elbow joint capsule incised if necessary. The infected area of bone or the bone abscess is exposed. Using an osteotome, the physician outlines a cortical window around the infected area, and the window is removed. All necrotic bone, soft tissue, and purulent material removed. The infected bone is excised so that a crater-like, shallow depression is formed to facilitate drainage from the infected area of bone. The wound is packed open to allow drainage.

24145–24147

The physician makes a 10.0 cm longitudinal incision along the postero-lateral aspect of the elbow. To expose the radial head and/or neck, the common origin of the extensor muscles is reflected, and the joint capsule incised. The infected area of the bone is visualized. Using an osteotome, the physician outlines a cortical window around the infected area and removes the window. All necrotic bone and soft tissue and purulent material is removed. The infected bone is excised so that a crater-like, shallow depression is formed to facilitate drainage from the infected area of bone. The wound is packed open to allow drainage. In 24147, the physician makes a posterior elbow incision to access the olecranon process. A long posterior splint may be applied to limit elbow motion.

24149

The physician debrides undesirable tissue and releases a contracture of a muscle or tendon. With the patient under anesthesia, the physician makes a long longitudinal incision overlying the elbow. Depending on the extent of the excess bone to be removed or the severity of the contracture, additional incisions may be required. The incision is continued deep to the elbow joint capsule itself. Nerves, vessels, and tendons are retracted. The capsule is fully exposed. A thorough debridement is undertaken to excise unwanted soft tissue. The overgrown and excess bone is isolated and excised. The capsule is removed. The contracture of the elbow involving muscle, tendon, scar tissue, or soft tissue is identified and explored. The physician releases the offending tissue to allow full elbow range of motion. The wound or wounds are thoroughly irrigated and closed in layers. A dressing is applied.

24150–24151

The physician performs a radical resection of the shaft or distal humerus for a tumor. The physician makes an incision overlying the involved area of bone, dissecting down to expose the tumor site. The involved vessels and nerves are protected. Proximate muscles are detached extraperiosteally by sharp dissection, and the tumor is excised, including the immediately surrounding bone. Tissue is closed with layered sutures. Report 24151 if an autograft is performed during the repair.

24152–24153

The physician makes an anterolateral incision overlying the elbow or forearm. Dissection is carried down to expose the radial head or neck. The radial vessels and radial nerve are protected. The radial head is the most upper part of the radius and the neck extends just below the radial head. The tumor is then excised, including the radial head or neck. The physician selects the level of the radius to be divided. The physician then uses a bone saw to divide the bone at the appropriate level. Bone-holding forceps are used to elevate the bone from the wound, while

CPT® Lay Descriptions

the muscles are detached by sharp dissection. Radical resection may also include removal of surrounding soft tissues including, muscles, fascia, and vessels. In 24153, an autograft is necessary. The physician harvests the graft from the patient's iliac crest with an osteotome. The physician then closes the surgically created graft donor site. The bone is then placed in the area of the radial neck or head. The bone graft may need to be stabilized with either screws or wires. Suction drains are inserted into the wound. The physician then repairs the incision in multiple layers with sutures, staples, and/or Steri-strips. The elbow is placed in a posterior splint at 90 degrees for approximately two weeks.

24155

This procedure is a removal of the entire joint by resection of the distal humerus and the proximal radius and ulna. The physician makes a longitudinal incision along the lateral elbow. Dissection is carried down to expose the distal humerus and the proximal radius and ulna, which are then cut and removed from the elbow. The physician preserves the surrounding muscle attachments to maintain some support and function for moving the elbow. However, gross instability of the elbow is present. The incision is repaired in multiple layers using staples, sutures, and/or Steri-strips.

24160–24164

The physician makes an incision overlying the area of the implant of the elbow joint. The incision may be made on the medial, lateral, or posterior portion of the elbow. In 24164, the incision may be made along the lateral elbow to expose the radial head. Dissection is carried down to expose the implant (e.g., pin, wire, screw). The physician uses instruments to remove the implant from the bone. The incision is then repaired with sutures and/or Steri-strips.

24200–24201

The physician removes a foreign body of the upper arm or elbow area. If the foreign body is a result of trauma, an open wound may already exist. The physician may make a separate incision or access the foreign body through the open wound. Location of the foreign body may be determined prior to surgery by separately reportable x-rays. A subcutaneous foreign body is located between the skin and muscle layer in 24200. The foreign body is deep and may be within muscle in 24201. More extensive dissection and a larger incision may be necessary for a deep foreign body. Once the foreign body is visualized, it is removed. The physician may also debride any surrounding damaged soft tissue. The wound is thoroughly irrigated. Drains may be placed in the wound and the incision repaired in multiple layers with sutures, staples, and/or Steri-strips. A splint may be applied to limit elbow motion.

24220

Elbow arthrography provides information about the capsule size, the synovial lining, the articular surfaces of the joints, and detects loose bodies and capsular leaks. The patient is positioned either sitting or supine (lying face up) with the elbow flexed at 90 degrees. The physician prepares the elbow using sterile techniques. One of two injection sites may be used, either a lateral or posterior approach. The contrast medium is injected. A fluoroscope is then used to study the elbow. No incisions are made.

24300

Manipulation of the elbow under anesthesia may be necessary to regain the loss of motion following a surgical procedure or due to scar tissue. Following the induction of general anesthesia, the physician evaluates the elbow. The elbow is manipulated by stretching, rotation, and other maneuvers to gain the appropriate range of motion.

24301

The physician performs a muscle or tendon transfer of the upper arm or elbow. An example is transfer of the latissimus dorsi muscle. This transfer restores active elbow flexion by transferring the origin and belly of the latissimus dorsi to the arm and anchoring the origin near the radial head. The patient is placed sidelying with the affected side up. An incision is made starting at the loin and extending up to the axilla and then distally along the medial aspect of the arm to the anterior elbow. The physician then cuts free the origin of the latissimus dorsi. The muscle itself is cut free from the underlying abdominal muscles. The origin of the latissimus dorsi muscle is then sutured to the biceps tendon and the periosteal tissues about the radial tuberosity. The incision is repaired in multiple layers with sutures, staples, and/or Steri-strips.

24305

The physician lengthens a tendon of the upper arm or elbow. An anterior curvilinear incision is made, for example, over the anterior elbow to lengthen the biceps tendon. Dissection is carried down to expose the distal biceps tendon. The biceps tendon is divided by Z-plasty and then stretched into extension, causing it to stretch and release to a lengthened position. If the elbow joint capsule is thickened, the physician may elect to excise this part of the capsule and any fibrous bands or bone spurs in the anterior part of the elbow joint. A drain is inserted into the wound, and the incision is repaired in multiple layers using sutures, staples, and/or Steri-strips. The elbow is placed in a splint or cast in an extended position.

24310

For tenotomy of distal biceps tendon, an incision is made over the anterior elbow to expose the biceps tendon. The tendon is cut all the way through so as to release the flexion contracture. No repair of the tendon is made. The incision is repaired with sutures. The elbow may be placed in a splint to keep it in as much extension as possible.

24320

To perform a tenoplasty, the physician makes an incision from the deltopectoral groove to the midportion of the upper arm. The pectoralis major tendon is exposed through dissection and detached from its insertion on the humerus. The tendon of the long head of the biceps is then exposed and severed from its origin and withdrawn from the wound. An L-shaped incision is then made over the anterior aspect of the elbow. The distal portion of the long head of the biceps is divided and freed distally to its attachment on the radius. The biceps tendon and muscle is then withdrawn through the L-shaped incision. The tendon of the long head of the biceps is passed through two slits in the pectoralis major and looped on itself so that its proximal tendon is brought into the distal L-shaped incision. The end of the proximal tendon is then sutured through a slit in the distal tendon. The incisions are repaired in multiple layers using sutures, staples, and/or Steri-strips. A posterior plaster splint is applied with the elbow in flexion.

24330–24331

To perform flexor-plasty, the physician transfers the common origin of the biceps brachii and the brachialis so that it performs elbow flexion rather than forearm pronation. The physician makes a curved longitudinal incision over the medial side of the elbow. The ulnar nerve is identified and retracted for protection. The common origin of the pronator teres, flexor carpiradialis, palmaris longus, flexor digitorum sublimis, and flexor carpi ulnaris are detached as "one" from the medial epicondyle. A graft is then taken from the fascia lata. The physician obtains the graft by making an incision on the lateral thigh, exposing the fascia lata and harvesting a 4.0 cm to 5.0 cm graft. The physician then closes the surgically created graft donor site. One end of the graft is then sutured to the common origin, while the other end is attached 5.0 cm up the lateral side of the humerus. A cast is applied with the elbow in flexion. An anterior transfer of the triceps may be performed in conjunction with elbow flexor-plasty. For this procedure, a posterolateral incision is made over the lower upper arm. The triceps tendon is exposed and divided at its insertion. An anterolateral curvilinear incision is made on the anterior elbow so that the tuberosity on the radius can be exposed. Another 4.0 cm long fascia lata graft is harvested and attached to the triceps tendon. The other end of the fascia lata graft is attached to the tuberosity of the radius. This creates added elbow flexibility. A cast is applied with the elbow in flexion. Report 24331 if an extensor advancement is performed.

24332

Tenolysis involves transsection of adhesions that have formed between the tendon and its surrounding tissues. Beginning proximally along the supracondylar ridge and ending near the subcutaneous border of the ulna, the physician makes a deep dissection to the anterior aspect of the capsule. The triceps tendon is retracted posteriorly to expose the olecranon fossa and tenolysis of the triceps and posterior capsulectomy is performed. Tenolysis should be performed under a local anesthetic so that full release can be confirmed. If, however, general or regional anesthesia is used, the physician may check the adequacy of the capsulectomy with an incision proximal to the area of injury and manually by pulling the tendons.

24340

The physician treats a rupture of a distal biceps tendon by reattachment of the biceps tendon to the radius, direct reimplantation, or inserting a loop of fascia lata graft around the proximal radius. Reattachment of the biceps tendon to the radius is described. The patient is placed supine. The physician makes an anterior lateral incision on the lower upper arm and extending transversely across the antecubital fossa. The torn biceps tendon is identified and the tear is minimally debrided. Two Bunnell sutures are placed in the torn end. A second incision is made over the dorsal aspect of the proximal forearm to expose the radial tuberosity. The physician uses a high speed bur to evacuate a 5.0 mm to 7.0 mm defect in the radial tuberosity. Three holes are drilled through this window to the opposite side of the tuberosity. The physician places sutures through the holes and places the tendon into the window in the tuberosity. The sutures are pulled tight and secured. The incisions are repaired in multiple layers with drains inserted. The elbow is placed in a splint in 90 degrees of flexion and full supination.

24341

The physician repairs one of the muscles or tendons in the upper arm or elbow, not including those of the rotator cuff. With the patient soothed by general anesthesia, the physician makes an incision directly overlying the torn muscles or tendon. The incision is carried deep through the subcutaneous tissue. The extent of the tear is ascertained through debridement and exploration. The physician repairs the tissue using appropriate fixation devices such as suture, wire, or screw. The procedure can be performed primarily near the time of injury or afterward. Additional incisions are often required when a tendon is completely ruptured. When the repair is complete, the incision is closed in layers.

24342

The physician makes a posterior longitudinal incision, exposing the tendinous portion of the triceps. Drill holes are made in the olecranon. Sutures from the triceps tendon are then passed through the drill holes, pulled tight, and secured. The physician may harvest a fascia graft from the forearm. The proximal attachment of the fascia graft is left attached to the epicondyle. The distal part is detached, raised, and sutured to the distal triceps for reinforcement. The incision is then repaired in multiple layers with sutures, staples, and/or Steri-strips. The arm is immobilized in less than 90 degrees of flexion.

24343

The lateral collateral ligament (LCL) is the ligament of the elbow along the outer aspect that connects the distal end of the humerus to the proximal end of the ulna. It provides lateral stability to the joint and injury to the LCL can lead to elbow dislocation. Anterior-posterior and lateral x-rays of the elbow are taken and reported separately. The physician administers a local anesthetic block, makes an incision, and dissects the lateral ligament to the head and neck of the humerus to expose the anterior surface of the lateral epicondyle. Repair of a freshly torn collateral ligament usually requires the surgeon to make an incision through the skin over the area where the tear in the ligament has occurred. If the ligament has been pulled from its attachment on the bone, the ligament is reattached to the bone with either large sutures or a special metal bone staple. The ends of the ligament are sewed together to repair mid-ligament tears.

24344

The lateral collateral ligament (LCL) is the ligament of the elbow along the outer aspect that connects the distal end of the humerus to the proximal end of the ulna. It provides lateral stability to the joint and injury to the LCL can lead to elbow dislocation. Anterior-posterior and lateral x-rays of the elbow are taken and reported separately. The physician administers a local anesthetic block, makes an incision, and dissects the lateral ligament to the head and neck of the humerus to expose the anterior surface of the lateral epicondyle. The palmaris longus tendon is usually used for the graft repair. The physician makes a transverse wrist incision and spreads the areolar tissue to identify the tendon. A second transverse incision is made about eight centimeters above the first incision to again identify the tendon. The physician pulls on the tendon from both incisions to ensure that the same tendon has been isolated and makes a third transverse incision proximally. Alternatively, a tendon stripper can be used. The tendon is cut and reattached in a new position, either by stitching it to another tendon or through a hole drilled into the bone. The wound is closed and a dressing applied. The hand and wrist may be put in a plaster cast, splint, or bandage, depending on which tendons have been moved.

24345

The medial collateral ligament (MLC) is posterior to the axis of elbow flexion and primarily serves as the medial stabilizer of the flexed elbow joint. X-rays (reported separately) are taken to identify abnormally wide joint space on the medial side. An MRI (reported separately) may be taken to show focal discontinuity of the ligament and joint fluid extravasation. Repair of a freshly torn collateral ligament usually requires the surgeon to make an incision through the skin over the area where the tear in the ligament has occurred. If the ligament has been pulled from its attachment on the bone, the ligament is reattached to the bone with either large sutures or a special metal bone staple. The ends of the ligament are sewed together to repair mid-ligament tears. The procedure is normally performed under general anesthesia or with a local block.

24346

The medial collateral ligament (MLC) is posterior to the axis of elbow flexion and primarily serves as the medial stabilizer of the flexed elbow joint. X-rays (reported separately) are taken to identify abnormally wide joint space on the medial side. An MRI (reported separately) may be taken to show focal discontinuity of the ligament and joint fluid extravasation. The palmaris longus tendon is the most commonly used tendon graft for the elbow. The procedure is normally performed under general anesthesia. The physician makes a transverse wrist incision and spreads the areolar tissue to identify the tendon. A second transverse incision is made about eight centimeters above the first incision to again identify the tendon. The physician pulls on the tendon from both incisions to ensure that the same tendon has been isolated and makes a third transverse incision proximally. Alternatively, a tendon stripper can be used. The tendon is cut and reattached in a new position, either by stitching it to another tendon or through a hole drilled into the bone. The wound is closed and a dressing applied. The hand and wrist may be put in a plaster cast, splint, or bandage, depending on which tendons have been moved.

24350

The physician performs a lateral or medial fasciotomy. Fasciotomy may also be termed as a percutaneous release for tennis elbow. The more common problem is located on the lateral epicondyle. The physician makes a 1.5 cm to 2.5 cm incision anterior to the epicondyle. The common tendon origin of the extensors is exposed on the lateral elbow (or flexors on the medial side if this is where the incision was made). The physician uses a scalpel to free the tendinous origin of the common extensors or flexors from the epicondyle. The skin is closed with sutures and/or Steri-strips. The elbow is placed in a sling.

24351

The physician makes a 5.0 cm long incision overlying the lateral epicondyle. The origin of the common extensor tendon is exposed. The physician retracts the extensor longus tendon to expose the origin of the extensor brevis. Abnormal or unhealthy tissue, including the extensor brevis origin, is excised. The physician repairs the incision in multiple layers with sutures and Steri-strips. The arm is placed in a sling.

24352

The physician makes a 7.0 cm longitudinal incision over the lateral epicondyle of the humerus. The origin of the conjoined tendon is detached from the epicondyle and reflected distally from the underlying annular ligament. Care is taken not to enter the radio-humeral joint. The physician then uses a curved scalpel to incise the annular ligament circumferentially from the radial head to the ulna, and then detaches it. The distal portion of the annular ligament remains as a collar around the radial neck to preserve stability of the joint. A sharp osteotome is then used to remove the tip of the lateral epicondyle. The conjoined tendon is sutured back loosely to the epicondyle. The incision is repaired in multiple layers using sutures, staples, and/or Steri-strips. A sling may be applied.

24354–24356

The physician makes a 5.0 cm long curvilinear incision overlying the lateral epicondyle. The conjoined tendon of the extensor mechanism is exposed. This common extensor tendon is then excised from the bone and allowed to slide approximately 1.0 cm distally to a new resting length. Any abnormal surrounding tissue is excised as well. Using a 1/4 inch osteotome, the physician performs a partial ostectomy by removing a 2.0 mm thick fragment of the lateral epicondyle. The ostectomy enhances vascular supply to promote healing of the soft tissues. The incision is repaired in multiple layers with sutures, staples, and/or Steri-strips. The arm is placed in a sling. Report 24356 if the procedure is performed with a partial ostectomy.

24360

The physician makes a longitudinal incision over the lateral elbow. All soft tissue is dissected from the distal humerus. The elbow is then dislocated. Osteophytes and articular cartilage are removed from the distal humerus so that a smooth, rounded surface remains. Articular cartilage is left intact on the proximal ulna and radius. The physician uses a motorized dermatome to remove a thin split-thickness skin graft from the patient's lower abdomen. Small drill holes are made in the distal end of the humerus. The graft is then sutured into place over the distal end of the humerus with the dermal surface placed against the bone and the fat facing the new joint space. The elbow joint is reduced (realigned). The physician repairs the incision in multiple layers using sutures, staples, and/or Steri-strips. The elbow is placed in a posterior splint in 90 degrees of flexion.

24361

The physician makes a 10.0 cm longitudinal incision over the medial aspect of the elbow. The ulnar nerve is identified and retracted to protect it from injury. The joint capsule is excised, and the radius and ulna are separated from the humerus. A Kirschner wire is drilled into the trochlea (distal humerus) along the axis of the joint. Using an osteotome, high speed bur or saw, the physician trims and remodels the distal end of the humerus. A prosthesis is then fitted to the distal humerus and hammered into place. The ulna and radius are reduced to the prosthesis. If the radial head is severely deformed or arthritic, the physician may resect (remove) it. Other adjustments may be made, such as sculpturing the semilunar notch or olecranon. Sculpting allows better articulation with the prosthesis and better elbow motion. The flexor origins are reattached to the epicondyle. The physician repairs the incision in multiple layers with sutures, staples, and/or Steri-strips. A long arm cast or splint is applied with the elbow in 90 degrees of flexion.

24362

The physician makes a 10.0 cm longitudinal incision over the medial aspect of the elbow. The ulnar nerve is identified and retracted to protect it from injury. The joint capsule is excised, and the radius and ulna are separated from the humerus. A Kirschner wire is drilled into the trochlea (distal humerus) along the axis of the joint. Using an osteotome, high speed bur or saw, the physician trims and remodels the distal end of the humerus. A prosthesis is then fitted to the distal humerus and hammered into place. The ulna and radius are reduced to the prosthesis. If the radial head is severely deformed or arthritic, the physician may resect (remove) it. Other adjustments may be made, such as sculpturing the semilunar notch or olecranon. Sculpting allows better articulation with the prosthesis and better elbow motion. The flexor origins are reattached to the epicondyle. The physician repairs the incision in multiple layers with sutures, staples, and/or Steri-strips. For fascia lata ligament reconstruction, an additional incision may be necessary on the posterior aspect of the elbow and forearm. The radial head and olecranon are exposed. Through an incision on the lateral side of the thigh, a long rectangle of fascia lata is removed. The fascia is folded in half crosswise and the folded edge is anchored to the anterior part of the capsule with sutures. The distal half is then sutured in place over the trochlear notch. A fold of the same fascia is inserted between the radial head and ulna and fixed with sutures. The capsule is sutured closed. The incisions are repaired in multiple layers with sutures, staples, and /or Steri-strips. A long arm cast or splint immobilizes the elbow at 90 degrees of flexion.

24363

The patient is placed supine with the affected arm on the the chest and with a sandbag beneath the

CPT® Lay Descriptions

shoulder. Different types of prosthetic implants are available. Selection depends on capsuloligamentous structures, musculature integrity, and the amount of bone remaining at the elbow joint. A technique for a semiconstrained (two to three part prosthesis) hinged prosthesis is described. The physician makes a straight, midline, posterior incision. The ulnar nerve is identified and retracted for protection. The triceps mechanism is elevated from the olecranon. The collateral ligaments are preserved. A portion of the olecranon is cut and removed to allow implantation of the ulnar stem. The distal humerus is then prepared by removing cancellous bone with a curet. The physician then uses a rasp to open and contour the humeral and ulnar medullary canals for insertion of the prosthetic stems. Cement is inserted into the ulnar and humeral medullary canals with a cement gun or syringe. The elbow is flexed and the prosthesis is inserted into the humeral and ulnar medullary canals at the same time. The elbow joint is fully extended while the cement hardens. The triceps mechanism is sutured back to fascia. The ulnar nerve is positioned anterior to the elbow. The physician inserts drain tubes. The incision is repaired in multiple layers with sutures, staples, and/or Steri-strips. A posterior splint is applied to the elbow in 90 degrees of flexion.

24365

The physician makes a 5.0 cm to 6.0 cm longitudinal incision along the lateral aspect of the elbow. The elbow joint is exposed by freeing and reflecting the common origin of the extensor muscles. The joint capsule is incised and the radial head is exposed. The physician uses a bone cutting saw to excise the radial head. The capsule is closed with sutures and the incision is repaired in layers with sutures, staples, and/or Steri-strips.

24366

The patient is positioned supine (face up) or lateral (lying on one side) with the affected elbow up. The physician makes an incision beginning just above the lateral epicondyle and extending distally approximately 6.0 cm across the joint. Dissection is carried down to expose the capsule, that is then incised. The annular ligament is incised transversely so that the neck of the radius can be osteotomized. A bur or rasp is used to prepare the medullary canal of the radius to accept the implant. The implant is inserted into the medullary canal of the radius, and positioned into contact with the capitellum. The annular ligament is reattached. A suction drain is inserted. The physician then repairs the incision in multiple layers using sutures, staples, and/or Steri-strips. The arm may be placed in a posterior elbow splint at 90 degrees of flexion.

24400

The physician performs an osteotomy of the humerus with or without internal fixation. The physician makes a longitudinal incision overlying the involved

portion of the shaft of the humerus to expose the affected part of the bone. An osteotomy is made through the humerus, usually in a wedge shape. This allows the bone to be realigned. The physician may apply plates and screws to hold the bone together in the correct position (internal fixation). The incision is repaired in multiple layers with sutures, staples, and/or Steri-strips. The arm may be placed in a cast or splint for immobilization.

24410

The physician performs multiple osteotomies with realignment on the intramedullary rod, humeral shaft. The physician makes a longitudinal incision through skin, fascia, and muscle to expose the entire shaft of the bone subperiosteally, making an osteotomy through the proximal and distal metaphyses. Additional osteotomies, usually three or four, are performed to correct the alignment. Fragments are aligned, and a nail is inserted. Autografts grafts may be added if the cortex is thin. The periosteum is sutured over the bone and the wound is closed and dressed.

24420

The physician performs osteoplasty of the humerus for shortening or lengthening. An incision is made through skin, fascia, and muscle in the upper arm over the humeral shaft. Vessels and nerves are exposed and retracted. Dissection continues to expose the shaft of the humerus. An osteotomy is made at the determined point on the humerus. The physician removes a wedge of bone. To shorten the humeral shaft, a plate is attached to the distal segment with screws. Reduction forceps are used to hold and compress the osteotomy while the plate is attached to the proximal fragment with screws. To lengthen the bone, the segments are retracted, usually 2.0 mm to 3.0 mm, and fixed at that distance with plates and screws. X-rays (reported separately) are used to check rotational alignment of the segments. Drain tubes are inserted, the incision is repaired in multiple layers with sutures, staples, and/or Steri-strips, and the arm is immobilized.

24430

The physician repairs a nonunion or malunion of the humerus without using a graft. The physician exposes the nonunion or malunion of the humerus by making a 10.0 cm to 15.0 cm longitudinal incision through skin, fascia, and muscle over the fracture site. With a reciprocating saw, the bone is divided through the nonunion. The fragments are aligned. A compression plate is centered over the fracture and screws are inserted. The incision is repaired in multiple layers with sutures, staples, and/or Steri-strips. The limb is immobilized.

24435

The physician repairs a nonunion or malunion of the humerus with an iliac graft or autograft. The physician exposes the nonunion or malunion of the humerus by making a 10.0 cm to 15.0 cm longitudinal incision through skin, fascia, and muscle over the fracture site. With a reciprocating saw, the bone is divided through the nonunion. The fragments are aligned. A compression plate is centered over the fracture and screws are inserted. A bone graft is determined to be needed to help healing of the fracture due to loss of bone. Autogenous iliac bone is typically used, but proximal tibia may be used instead, either requiring an incision over the harvest site. The physician uses an osteotome to harvest strips of bone which are placed around the ends of the fracture in addition to the compression plate for internal fixation. Both incisions are repaired in multiple layers with sutures, staples, and/or Steri-strips. The limb is immobilized.

24470

The physician performs a hemiepiphyseal arrest. Angular deformities are typically a complication of fractures of the lateral condylar physis. The most common deformity is cubitus valgus. To treat cubitus valgus, the physician makes a longitudinal posterior incision along the distal humerus. The humerus is then exposed. If a nonunion exists from a previous condylar physeal fracture, it may be approached from the same incision. If a nonunion is present, the ends are denuded and a local bone graft is applied. The physician applies a cancellous screw to provide fixation and compression across the nonunion. An osteotomy is then performed across the distal humerus, correcting both the angulation and realigning the longitudinal axis of the humerus with that of the forearm. The osteotomy is secured with screws. The physician then repairs the incision in layers with sutures, staples, and/or Steri-strips. The elbow is immobilized in a splint or brace.

24495

The physician performs a decompression fasciotomy in the forearm with exploration of the brachial artery. The physician makes a longitudinal incision on the anterior forearm, from just lateral and proximal to the biceps tendon distal toward the radial styloid, excising the deep fascia, exposing brachioradialis laterally and biceps and brachialis medially, decompressing the compartment. The brachial artery is explored proximally to identify origin of decreased circulation. The fascial incision remains open; the skin incision may be left open or closed.

24498

The physician applies prophylactic treatment to prevent fracture. A longitudinal incision is made through skin, fascia, or muscle along the humerus to expose the affected part. Pins or a plate with screws are used to stabilize the bone. If defects in the bone do not allow for good internal fixation, methylmethacrylate cement may be used to fill in the gaps. Wiring may also be wrapped around the bone to

provide additional fixation. An intramedullary nail may also be inserted through the canal of the humerus to provide internal stabilization. The incisions are repaired in multiple layers with sutures, staples, and/or Steri-strips.

24500–24505

The physician treats a closed humeral shaft fracture without manipulation in 24500 or with manipulation in 24505. The segments are aligned and stable. Treatment involves immobilization, using one of several methods, of the elbow and possibly the glenohumeral joint for several weeks until union is established. Skeletal traction may be applied in 24505.

24515

The physician repair a humeral shaft fracture with a plate or screws, with or without cerclage. A lateral or anterolateral incision is made overlying a fracture site. The fracture is reduced by manipulation and bone reduction forceps. A compression plate with screws secures and compresses the fragments. Cerclage wiring might be used to facilitate fixation of the fracture. One or more wires may be placed around the humerus, over the fracture site. The incision is closed with sutures, staples, and/or Steri-strips.

24516

The physician repairs a humeral shaft fracture with insertion of an intramedullary implant, with or without cerclage and/or locking screws. A straight lateral incision is made through skin, fascia, and muscles to expose the fracture site. If there are multiple fragments or if there is a long spiral fracture, cerclage wires may be wrapped around the bone to hold the fragments in place. Using a guide rod to direct a reamer and rod, an intermedullary nail is placed within the humeral shaft. The nail may be locked in place proximally and distally with locking screws. The wound is irrigated, a drain may be inserted, and the wound is closed in layers.

24530–24535

Closed treatment of a supracondylar or transcondylar fracture is indicated when the fragments are not separated and appear stable. No manipulation is required in 24530. Supracondylar fractures in the adult are usually treated with a caption splint or hanging arm cast. In 24535, crossed screws or cross-threaded pins may be placed in medial and lateral pillars, engaging the posterior cortex of bone or lag screws may also be inserted through a small incision without opening the fracture. Transcondylar fractures may be treated conservatively with a hanging arm cast and elbow immobilization. The fracture may be reduced and fixed with percutaneous threaded Steinman pins inserted through the epicondyles.

24538

The physician performs a percutaneous skeletal fixation of a fracture in the supracondylar or transcondylar humerus. The elbow is prepared and draped.The physician makes an incision overlying the fracture. The fracture is reduced by applying longitudinal traction and manipulating the fracture into alignment. Pins are inserted through the condyles and metaphysis diagonally, avoiding the ulnar nerve. Pins are clipped and bent beneath the skin. An intercondyle extension may be performed. The incision is closed with layered sutures and the arm is immobilized.

24545–24546

The physician repairs a fracture in the humeral supracondylar or transcondylar with or without fixation or intercondylar extension. The physician makes a posterior incision from midline of the arm to just distal to the olecranon, exposing the olecranon, triceps tendon, and distal humerus. The ulnar nerve is isolated and retracted. Preserving as much soft tissue attachment as possible, the physician exposes and assembles the fragments, reducing the condyles and, if with internal fixation, fixing fragments with screws. Temporary wires may be used to hold fragments in place while inserting screws. Additional screws, pins or plates may be needed to fix the condyles to the metaphysis. The joint is irrigated, and the wounds are closed with drain placement if needed. Report 24546 if intercondylar extension is required.

24560–24565

The physician repairs a humeral epicondylar fracture without incision or manipulation. Closed treatment of a humeral epicondylar fracture is indicated when the fragments are not separated and appear stable. No manipulation is required. No incisions are made. The arm may be placed in a posterior elbow splint at 90 degrees of flexion. Report 24565 if manipulation is required.

24566

The physician fixates a humeral epicondylar fracture percutaneously. The physician uses separately reportable fluoroscopy to realign the fracture with manipulation. The fracture may involve the medial or lateral epicondyle. Once the bone is realigned, the physician fixates the pieces to the humeral shaft by driving a wire through the pieces and into the shaft.

24575

The physician treats a fracture of either the medial or lateral epicondyle of the humerus with or without fixation. The physician makes an incision in the skin overlying the fractured epicondyle. This is carried deep through the fascia to the bone. Fracture fragments are identified and manipulated into the appropriate anatomic position. The epicondyle is restored using fixation devices such as plates, screws, or wires if needed. An external device is utilized if needed. The wound is irrigated and closed in layers.

24576–24577

The physician repairs a fracture of the humeral condylar with closed treatment. Closed treatment of a humeral condylar fracture is indicated when the fragments are not separated and appear stable. No manipulation is required in 24576. The arm may be placed in a posterior elbow splint at 90 degrees of flexion. Report 24577 if manipulation is required to repair the fracture.

24579

The physician repairs the humeral condylar, medial or lateral, with or without fixation. The physician makes an incision exposing the posterior elbow. Skin and subcutaneous tissue are reflected to expose the olecranon and triceps tendon. The ulnar nerve is carefully retracted. The condyles are reduced and may be temporarily fixed with wires, while screws are placed across the major fragments. Small fragments may require excision. The incision is closed with sutures and the elbow is immobilized in a posterior elbow splint.

24582

The physician treats a fracture of the medial or lateral humeral condylar by manipulating the fracture in a closed fashion and inserting pins through the skin and bones to maintain appropriate position. Separately reportable anesthesia, either local or general, is first employed. Separately reportable x-rays, including fluoroscopic views, are obtained to ascertain the extent of the fracture. The physician manipulates the arm, elbow, and forearm in such a way to restore the fractured pieces to the acceptable position. The physician places pins through the skin and into the bones to maintain the reduction until healing is complete.

24586–24587

The physician treats a periarticular fracture and/or dislocation of the elbow. The physician may make more than one incision depending on the extent of the fractures and/or dislocation. If there is a dislocation, it is reduced (realigned) first. The fractures are then reduced and secured with plates, screws, pins, wires, or a combination of these. The physician may place a pin through the olecranon for skeletal traction in a patient with multiple injuries to temporarily stabilize the fracture and/or dislocation. In 24587, if joint surface congruity cannot be restored, the physician performs a total elbow arthroplasty. For elbow arthroplasty, the physician makes a straight, midline, posterior incision. The ulnar nerve is identified and retracted for protection. The triceps mechanism is elevated from the olecranon. The collateral ligaments are preserved. A portion of the olecranon is cut and removed to allow implantation of the ulnar stem. The distal humerus is then prepared by removing cancellous bone with a curet. The physician then uses a rasp to open and contour the humeral and ulnar medullary canals for insertion of the prosthetic stems. Cement is inserted into the ulnar and humeral medullary canals with a cement gun or syringe. The elbow is flexed and the prosthesis is inserted into the humeral and ulnar medullary canals at the same time. The elbow joint is fully extended while the cement hardens. The triceps mechanism is sutured back to fascia. The ulnar nerve is positioned anterior to the elbow. Arthroplasty may be performed in conjunction with some internal fixation for fracture reduction and stabilization.

24600–24605

The physician performs closed treatment of elbow dislocation when there are no fractures. The forearm typically dislocates posteriorly. The physician manually reduces (realigns) the dislocation with pressure to the area. The elbow is then placed in a posterior elbow splint or elbow brace at 90 degrees of flexion with the forearm supinated. The procedure is performed without anesthesia in 24600 or with anesthesia in 24605.

24615

To treat an acute or chronic elbow dislocation, the physician may use the Osborne-Cotterill technique of dislocation treatment. The physician makes a longitudinal incision over the lateral aspect of the elbow. The physician dissects open the elbow posterior to the lateral collateral ligament. Any bone fragments are removed. The physician then roughens the bone at the lateral epicondyle and lateral side of the capitellum. The physician uses an awl to make one or two transverse holes through the lateral condyle close to the articular surface of the humerus. Sutures are passed through these holes and through the posterolateral part of the capsule. The capsule is fixed to the bone as tightly as possible. The incision is repaired in multiple layers. A long arm cast or splint is applied with the elbow in 40 degrees of flexion for approximately four weeks.

24620

The physician treats a dislocation at the elbow. No incisions are made. The physician manually realigns the radial head back into position. If alignment of the ulnar fracture is not adequate, the physician may also manually align this fracture. Once satisfactory and stable reduction (realignment) is achieved, the elbow is placed in a posterior splint or cast. The elbow is immobilized at 120 degrees of flexion to prevent recurrent dislocation of the radial head.

24635

The physician makes a longitudinal incision along the lateral aspect of the elbow. Dissection is carried down to expose the radial head and proximal ulna. The physician then determines the status of the annular ligament. If the ligament is intact, the physician incises it so the radial head can be reduced. The ligament is then repaired with nonabsorbable sutures. More commonly the ligament is torn or avulsed,

requiring reconstruction. If so, a strip of fascia 1.3 cm wide and 11.0 cm long is dissected from the muscles of the forearm. If the ulnar fracture is stable, no internal fixation is required. If the fracture is unstable, internal fixation is typically applied rather than external fixation, unless there is a large, infected open wound. A compression plate or an intramedullary nail is used for internal fixation. The new annular ligament (fascial strip) is sutured about the radial neck. The incision is repaired in multiple layers with sutures, staples, and/or Steri-strips. The elbow is placed in a posterior splint or cast at 120 degrees of flexion, preventing redislocation of the radial head.

24640

To realign a subluxated (partially dislocated) radial head, the physician supinates the forearm (palm upward) while flexing the elbow. No incisions are made. If stability of the radial head is questionable, a cast or splint is applied with the elbow in 90 degrees of flexion.

24650–24655

The physician performs closed treatment without manipulation in 24650 for undisplaced fractures (e.g., Type I fracture). In 24655, the physician performs manual manipulation by applying pressure to realign the fractured bone. No incisions are made. The arm is placed in a posterior elbow splint or brace.

24665–24666

Types of fractures requiring open treatment have gross comminution of the head and neck, involve more than one-third of the articular surface, and/or interfere with forearm rotation (e.g., Type II and III radial head fractures). The physician makes an incision along the posterolateral aspect of the elbow. The common origin of the extensor muscles is reflected, and the joint capsule incised, exposing the radial head and neck. All loose particles of bone are removed and the elbow joint is thoroughly irrigated. For internal fixation, the fractured fragments are reduced. The physician then inserts AO screws or Herbert screws to stabilize the fracture. In 24666, the radial head is excised as well. The physician uses a bone cutting saw to excise the radial head. The physician repairs the capsule and the incision in multiple layers with sutures, staples, and/or Steri-strips. A posterior elbow splint is applied with the elbow at 90 degrees of flexion.

24670–24675

Closed treatment of an olecranon process fracture is indicated when the fragments are not separated and appear stable. No manipulation is required in 24670. When there is mild or slight separation of the fragments, manipulation is required. The physician manually manipulates the area, reducing the ulnar fracture in 24675. No incisions are made. The arm may be placed in a posterior elbow splint at 90 degrees of flexion.

24685

The physician treats a fracture of the olecranon process. The physician makes a 10.0 cm incision along the posterolateral border of the elbow. Dissection is carried down to expose the fracture. If the fracture is not comminuted, a figure-of-eight wire loop stabilizes the fracture. The physician drills a hole from side to side in the distal fragment. Wire is then passed through the drill hole in the distal fragment and through the triceps aponeurosis. This creates a figure-of-eight loop. The wire is pulled tight and twisted. If the fracture is more distal on the olecranon, a medullary pin or screw may be used as well. If medullary fixation is used, the pin or screw is inserted through the olecranon and into the medullary canal of the ulna. The physician then repairs the incision in multiple layers with sutures, staples, and/or Steri-strips.

24800–24802

The physician makes a posterior longitudinal or posterolateral incision. If the physician does not use a bone graft, then the triceps tendon is split and released from the olecranon. The radial head is excised and a posterior and anterior synovectomy is performed. The physician then trims the olecranon into a triangular shape with a saw. A triangular hole is created through the lower end of the humerus. The olecranon is inserted through the triangular hole in the lower humerus. The physician places a bone screw obliquely through the humerus and into the ulna. The triceps tendon is repaired with sutures. The physician repairs the incision in multiple layers and the elbow is immobilized in a long arm cast. If a bone graft is used, the physician prepares a bed for the graft in the posterior surface of the lower humerus. A cleft is the formed in the upper part of the tip of the olecranon. If local autograft bone is used, it is harvested from the surrounding healthy bone and no separate incision is required. The autograft is fitted into the olecranon cleft and humeral bed. If allograft (donor) bone is used, it is fitted in the same manner. In 24802, an autograft is harvested from the patient's upper tibia or iliac crest with an osteotome. The physician then repairs the surgically created graft donor site. One or two screws are then inserted through the graft and into the humerus to make it secure. Bone chips are packed into the the humeral-ulnar joint. The physician repairs the incision in multiple layers with sutures. A long arm cast is applied with the elbow in approximately 90 degrees of flexion.

24900

The physician amputates the arm through the humerus. The physician makes an incision distal to the intended level of bone section, and fashions anterior and posterior skin flaps. The brachial artery and vein are identified, double ligated, and divided just proximal to the level of bone section. Nerves are divided proximally to the site to ensure retraction proximal to the end of the stump. Muscles are sectioned slightly distal to stump. The humerus is divided and the end is smoothed. The triceps muscle is flapped over the end of the bone and sutured into the anterior fascia. The wound is closed over a drain tube with suction, and the fascia and skin flaps are closed.

24920

The physician amputates the arm through the humerus using an open, circular technique. The physician makes an incision distal to the intended level of bone section in a circular manner to the fascia, and fashions anterior and posterior skin flaps. The brachial artery and vein are identified, double ligated, and divided just proximal to the level of bone section. Nerves are divided proximally to the site to ensure retraction proximal to the end of the stump. Muscles are sectioned slightly distal to stump. The humerus is divided and the end is smoothed. The triceps muscle is flapped over the end of the bone and sutured into the anterior fascia. The wound is closed over a drain tube with suction, and the fascia and skin flaps are closed.

24925

The physician performs a secondary closure or scar revision of an existing amputation. The physician amputates the end of the stump through the humerus. The physician makes an incision distal to the intended level of bone section to the fascia, and fashions anterior and posterior skin flaps. The physician excises the granulation and scar tissues and remodels the soft tissues. Arteries and veins are identified, double ligated, and divided just proximal to the level of bone section. Nerves are divided proximally to the site. The humerus is divided and the end is smoothed. The wound is closed over a drain tube with suction, and the fascia and skin flaps are closed.

24930

The physician re-amputates the arm through the humerus. The physician makes an incision distal to the intended level of bone section, and fashions anterior and posterior skin flaps. The brachial artery and vein are identified, double ligated, and divided just proximal to the level of bone section. Nerves are divided proximally to the site to ensure retraction proximal to the end of the stump. Muscles are sectioned slightly distal to stump. The humerus is divided and the end is smoothed. The triceps muscle is flapped over the end of the bone and sutured into the anterior fascia. The wound is closed over a drain tube with suction, and the fascia and skin flaps are closed.

24931

The physician amputates the arm through the humerus bone and places a surgical implant in the arm. The physician makes an incision in a circular fashion around the entire arm distal to the level of the planned amputation of the humerus. The vessels and nerves are identified, divided, and ligated. The humerus bone is divided in two, completing the amputation. The physician spares the skin, soft tissue, and muscle needed to close the amputation incision. Any of a variety of implants, such as rods, are utilized to maintain the length of the arm or to replace a portion of the amputated humerus. Fixation devices are used. The entire incision is thoroughly irrigated. Retained muscle flaps are closed over exposed bone. The wound is closed in layers and a soft dressing is applied.

24935

The physician elongates a stump of an upper extremity. First, the physician obtains the bone graft. The physician incises the skin over the area where the bone graft is to be obtained (usually the iliac crest). The tissue is dissected away from the bone and the graft is harvested. The wound is closed in sutured layers. Next, the skin overlying the stump is incised to expose the bony stump. The graft is pinned or plated to the existing bone. The tissues are replaced around the bone and the wound is closed in sutured layers.

25000

The physician incises the extensor tendon sheath over the wrist. The physician incises the skin just proximal to the anatomic snuffbox. The tissues are dissected and the extensor retinaculum of the first extensor compartment is identified and incised. The incision is closed in sutured layers.

25001

The physician incises a flexor tendon sheath over the wrist. The physician makes a radial incision. The tissues are dissected to the tendon sheath. The compartment is identified and incised. When incising the flexor carpi radialis (FCR), the tendon sheath is opened proximal to distal. The fibro-osseous tunnel is released along the ulnar border of the trapezium. The incision is closed with layered suture.

25020

The physician performs a decompression fasciotomy of the forearm and/or wrist extensor or flexor compartment. The physician incises the skin and dissects to the deep muscular fascia. The fascia is incised and released. If possible, the skin is closed in sutured layers. Otherwise, it is packed open.

25023

The physician performs a decompression fasciotomy of the forearm and debrides any nonviable tissue, including muscles and nerves. The physician makes an incision over the flexor or extensor compartment of the forearm. This is carried deep to the fascia and the fascia itself is incised. The physician explores the compartment and debrides any nonviable tissue that may include muscle, nerve, or fascia. The wound is

irrigated and typically left open. Closure is accomplished during a later, separately reportable, procedure.

25024–25025

The physician begins the incision proximal to the antecubital fossa and extends the incision to the middle of the palm. The incision is carried no farther radially, mid-axis of ring finger to avoid injury to the superficial palmar branch of the median nerve. Alternatively, a lazy-S incision may be made extending from the proximal palmar ulnar forearm, curving across to radial palmar forearm, returning to the ulnar side, and extending into the mid palms just ulnar to the thenar crease. The incision frees the superficial and deep flexor wads and decompresses the median nerve by carpal tunnel release. Following a volar fasciotomy, which is made in the same line as the skin incision, the physician checks the compartment pressure to ascertain decompression of the deep flexor muscles. After volar decompression, the physician takes pressure measurements of the volar compartment, mobile wad, and dorsal compartments. A dorsal, linear, longitudinal forearm incision is made between the mobile extensor wad and the extensor digitorum communis muscle, and the two separate compartments are opened individually. If pressure in the mobile wad and dorsal compartments are greater than 15 mm Hg, the compartments are decompressed. Report 25025 for the debridement of individual superficial and deep muscles and/or nerves.

25028

The physician drains an abscess or hematoma from deep within the forearm or wrist. An incision is made overlying the abscess or hematoma. The physician carries dissection down through the tissue. The abscess or hematoma is exposed on all sides and removed. Antibiotic solution is applied to the area. The wound is closed in layers with sutures. If infection is present, the wound is left open to drain.

25031

The physician removes a bursa from the forearm or wrist. An incision is made overlying the bursa. Tissue is dissected down to the bursa. The physician then dissects around the bursa and removes it. The wound is then irrigated with antibiotic solution. The wound may be left open or surgical drains may be left in the wound.

25035

The physician makes a longitudinal incision overlying the forearm or a transverse or longitudinal incision overlying the wrist. Dissection is carried down through the subcutaneous, fascial, and muscle layers to expose the affected bone. Drill holes are made through the bone cortex in the outline of a window around the infected or abscessed bone. The area is drained and debrided of infected bony and soft tissue, then irrigated with antibiotic solution. The wound is

CPT® Lay Descriptions

packed and may be left open to allow drainage until secondary closure occurs in about three weeks. Dressings are changed daily. A splint may be applied to limit wrist motion.

25040

The physician makes an incision, opening the radiocarpal or midcarpal joint in the wrist to explore or drain the area or remove a foreign body. The physician dissects down to the bones of the wrist joint. The physician performs an arthrotomy of the affected joint by extending the incision into the joint space. If a mass or a foreign body is present, it is dissected free from surrounding tissue. The mass or foreign body is removed or drained as indicated. The incision may be closed or left open temporarily to drain.

25065–25066

The physician makes a small, longitudinal incision over the site of the biopsy of the forearm and/or wrist. The superficial tumor is located between the skin and muscle layers in 25065. The physician exposes the tumor by subcutaneous dissection. An incision is then made through the capsule that surrounds the tumor and removes a small portion of the tumor for biopsy. In 25066, the tumor or cyst is located deeper, either within muscle, or below the muscle layer. A larger skin incision may be needed and more extensive dissection may be required to visualize the tumor. The capsule around the tumor is closed with sutures. The incision is repaired in multiple layers with sutures, staples, and/or Steri-strips. If the wrist is involved, a splint may be applied to limit motion.

25075–25076

The physician makes an incision over the site of the tumor on the forearm and/or wrist. A subcutaneous tumor is located just underneath the skin layer. Soft tissue dissection is usually not very extensive. In 25076, the tumor lies deeper, either between the fascia and muscle layer, or within the muscle layer itself. This procedure may require a larger skin incision and more soft tissue dissection to expose and locate the tumor. Once the tumor is located and adequately exposed, it is excised, along with the capsule surrounding it. The physician may extend the margin of resection to include some of the normal tissue from around the tumor. The physician may insert a drain tube in the wound. The incision is then repaired in multiple layers using sutures, staples, and/or Steri-strips. If the wrist is involved, a splint may be applied to limit motion.

25077

The physician makes a longitudinal incision along the anterior or dorsal surface of the forearm. A longitudinal or transverse incision may be used for the wrist. Dissection is carried down to expose the tumor. The physician excises the tumor, including the capsule surrounding it. Due to the malignancy of the

tumor and its potential to spread, the physician extends the margin of resection to include significant amounts of surrounding soft tissue. This may include fascia, muscle layers, vessels and nerves, fatty tissue, and synovium. This procedure does not involve bone resection. Drain tubes may be inserted into the wound. The physician repairs the incision in multiple layers with sutures, staples, and/or Steri-strips. If the wrist is involved, a splint may be applied to limit motion.

25085

The physician performs a capsulotomy of the wrist. The physician makes an incision overlying the wrist joint. The tissues are dissected to the joint capsule. The physician makes an incision in the capsule, allowing better joint movement. The incision is then closed in multiple layers with sutures.

25100

The physician opens a joint in the wrist to take a biopsy of the bone or tissue within the joint. An incision is made overlying the wrist joint to be biopsied. The incision is extended by dissection down to the joint. The tissue or bone to be biopsied is excised. The incision is irrigated with antibiotic fluid then closed in multiple layers.

25101

The physician surgically opens the wrist joint to explore and remove any loose or foreign body. An incision is made overlying the wrist joint. The underlying tissues are divided down to the joint. The physician opens the joint through an arthrotomy incision. Using instruments, the physician explores the entire joint space. A loose or foreign body is removed. Biopsies are performed as needed. The physician then irrigates the joint and closes it in layers. The incision is then repaired in multiple layers with sutures.

25105

The physician opens the wrist joint to remove synovium of the joint. An incision is made overlying the wrist. The physician carries the incision down to the wrist joint. An arthrotomy cut is made to expose the joint. The physician then dissects the synovium from inside the joint away from the capsule and bones. The synovium is then removed. The joint is irrigated and closed. The physician irrigates the remainder of the incision and repairs it in multiple layers.

25107

The physician performs a distal radioulnar arthrotomy for repair of a triangular cartilage complex. The physician incises the skin over the wrist and locates the triangular cartilage complex. The defect is identified and either debrided or sutured to return to a correct anatomic state. The wound is closed in sutured layers.

25110

The physician makes an incision overlying the affected tendon in the anterior or posterior aspect (flexor or extensor tendons) of the forearm and/or wrist. Dissection is carried down to expose the affected tendon. The lesion is then excised or shelled out, leaving normal tissue intact. If incised, the tendon sheath is then closed. The incision is repaired in multiple layers with sutures, staples, and/or Steri-strips.

25111–25112

The physician removes a ganglion from the wrist in 25111 or a recurrent ganglion in 25112. An incision is made overlying the ganglion. The tissues are dissected around the ganglion, freeing the ganglion from surrounding tissue. (Scar tissue may be removed in 25112.) The physician may dissect deep within the wrist joint in order to excise all of the ganglion. The ganglion is then removed. The joint or muscle tissue may be repaired in 25112. The physician irrigates the wound with antibiotic solution then closes the wound in layers.

25115–25116

Radical excision is removal of all diseased and/or inflamed tissue and may include removal of a portion of surrounding normal tissue. The physician makes a longitudinal incision over the anterior aspect of the distal forearm and wrist. Dissection is carried down to expose the flexor tendons of the wrist in 25115 or the extensor tendons in 25116. The physician excises the bursa and any inflamed and hypertrophied tissues from around the tendons. The tendons are left intact, allowing them to glide better during wrist movement. The physician may perform a transposition of the dorsal retinaculum if enough tissue is removed from the wrist extensors. A transposition makes a smooth gliding surface no longer present between the extensor tendons and carpal bones of the wrist. The dorsal retinaculum is incised in the mid-line and tucked underneath the extensor tendons then closed with sutures. The incisions are repaired in multiple layers with sutures, staples, and/or Steri-strips. The wrist may be placed in a splint.

25118–25119

The physician performs a synovectomy of the extensor tendon sheath in the wrist. The physician makes a curved, longitudinal incision over the back of the wrist, radial to the ulna. A longitudinal incision is made through the deep fascia and the extensor retinaculum, entering the involved compartment. Hypertrophic synovium is removed from each extensor tendon sheath. If an area of a tendon appears frayed to the point of possible rupture, it may be sutured to an adjacent extensor tendon above and below the damaged area. After completing the tenosynovectomy, the physician evaluates the wrist. If synovitis is present, the joint is opened and a wrist synovectomy is performed. The dorsal retinaculum is

sutured back into place, deep to the exterior tendons. Closure is performed after a drain is placed. The wrist is held in a neutral position, the fingers in extension. Report 25119 if resection of the distal ulna is performed as part of the procedure.

25120–25126

The physician makes a longitudinal incision of the forearm overlying the shaft of the ulna or radius, depending on which bone is affected. Dissection is carried down through the fascia and muscles to expose the bone cyst or tumor. Once the cyst or tumor is visualized, bone is removed from around the cyst or tumor by forming a cortical window. The window is sized larger than the cyst or tumor. The physician uses a curet to remove all of the cyst or tumor. The surrounding bone within the cortical window is removed with a power bur. If the amount of bone removed from the cortical window is small and does not compromise the strength of the bone, no bone graft is needed. However, if the strength of the bone is compromised, autograft or allograft bone is used. In 25125, the physician uses autograft bone (bone from the patient). Using an osteotome, the physician harvests bone chips from the patient's iliac crest. The cortical window cavity is then filled with the bone graft. The physician then closes the surgically created graft donor site. In 25126, the physician uses allograft (donor) bone to fill the cortical window cavity. The physician then repairs the longitudinal incision in multiple layers with sutures, staples, and/or Steri-strips.

25130–25136

The physician excises or curets a bone cyst or benign tumor in the carpal bones. The physician identifies the bone cyst via roentgenograms (reported separately), exposing the region of the cyst through an appropriate approach. Dissection is carried down to the involved bone. The periosteum is reflected to expose the underlying bone cyst. The contents of the cavity are removed, including all portions of any soft tissue lining. Any sclerotic wall that surrounds the cyst is removed to expose normal bone. The wound is flushed with antibiotic and the soft tissue is closed in layers. Report 25135 if an autograft is employed during the procedure; report 25136 if allograft is employed during the procedure.

25145

Sequestrectomy is removal of a piece of dead bone that has separated from healthy bone. The physician makes an incision over the area of osteomyelitis or bone abscess. A longitudinal incision is typically used for the forearm and a curved or transverse incision for the wrist. Dissection is carried down to expose the infected part of the bone, which includes incising the capsule if the wrist joint is involved. Once the infected bone or abscess is exposed, the physician uses a drill to outline a cortical window around the area. The cortical window is then removed with an osteotome. All sequestra (separated dead piece of bone), purulent material, and scarred and necrotic tissue is removed. If possible, the skin is closed loosely over drains. If closure is not possible, the wound is left open and packed. The patient may be placed in either a posterior elbow splint or wrist splint to limit motion.

25150–25151

The physician makes a longitudinal incision along the lateral border of the forearm. A posterior or anterior incision may also be made to access different parts of the ulna. To access the radius in 25151, an incision is made along the postero-lateral or antero-lateral elbow or forearm. Dissection is carried down through soft tissues (depending on the approach, some muscle origins may be detached) to expose the infected part of the ulna. Using a drill, the physician outlines a cortical window around the infected area. This window is then removed with an osteotome. All necrotic bone, surrounding necrotic soft tissue, and purulent material is removed. The physician excises the infected bone so that a crater-like, shallow depression is formed to facilitate drainage from the infected area of bone. The wound is packed open and allowed to drain. A posterior elbow or wrist splint may be used to limit elbow and/or wrist motion.

25170

The physician makes a skin incision along the lateral, anterior, or dorsal aspect of the forearm, depending on the area of resection. Resection of the proximal ulna is described. The physician makes a longitudinal posterior incision. The triceps insertion is detached from the ulna. The physician then uses a bone saw to make an osteotomy cut in the ulna at the the appropriate level. While elevating the bone from the wound with bone-holding forceps, any remaining soft tissue is detached. The radius is then dislocated posteriorly so that the radial neck articulates with the trochlea. The triceps tendon is then sutured to the radial head. Drains are inserted into the wound, and the incision is repaired in multiple layers. A posterior splint is applied to the elbow at 90 degrees of flexion. No bone graft is used in this procedure.

25210

The physician removes one of the eight carpal bones of the wrist. An incision is made in the wrist overlying the carpal bone to be removed. The tissues are dissected down to the bone. The physician identifies the bone visually and dissects it free of the surrounding structures. Some ligaments may be reattached to other bones. The carpal bone is excised. The physician cleans the wound with antibiotic solution. The wound is repaired in multiple layers.

25215

The physician removes all four bones in the proximal row of the carpal bones of the wrist. An incision is made overlying the wrist. The physician carries the

incision down to the carpal bone. The physician identifies the two rows of carpal bones. The physician removes the bones one by one all four bones in the proximal row while preserving tendons, nerves, and blood vessels. Ligaments may need to be reattached to other bones. Each of the bones is dissected free and removed. The physician irrigates the wound with antibiotic solution. The wound is closed in multiple layers.

25230

The physician makes a bayonet-shaped incision along the radial aspect of the wrist. The radial artery and nerve are then exposed. The joint capsule is incised to expose the radial styloid. The physician uses a thin osteotome or thin oscillating saw blade to cut the radial styloid perpendicular to the long axis of the radius. The incision is repaired in multiple layers with sutures, staples, and/or Steri-strips. The wrist is placed in an anterior splint.

25240

The physician makes a medial longitudinal incision to expose the distal ulna. The ulna is located subcutaneously and does not require much dissection. The periosteum is incised and reflected to expose the distal ulna. Drill holes are made through the ulna 2.5 cm above the distal head. The physician uses bone-biting forceps to complete the division of the bone and remove the fragment. To stabilize the free end of the ulna, the physician reefs (overlaps) the periosteal envelope and ligament. The incision is repaired in layers with sutures, staples, and/or Steri-strips. Immobilization of the wrist is usually not necessary.

25246

The physician injects contrast material into the wrist joint for arthrography. The physician inserts a needle into the wrist and aspirates joint fluid for culture. Contrast material is injected into the wrist, and the wrist is manipulated to distribute the dye. As the dye fades, a second injection may be made.

25248

The physician removes a deeply implanted foreign body from the forearm or wrist. The physician incises the site and dissects to the foreign object. Separately reportable x-rays may be taken to locate the object. All parts of the object are removed. The wound is closed in sutured layers.

25250

The physician removes a prosthesis from the wrist. An incision is made overlying the wrist. The physician extends the incision deep to the wrist joint, opening the joint. The physician identifies the artificial joint piece that has failed. Using hand and powered instruments, the physician removes the prosthesis. The joint and incision both are irrigated with antibiotic solution and repaired in multiple layers. If infection is present, the incision is left open to drain temporarily.

25251

The physician removes all the parts of a wrist joint prosthesis from the wrist. An incision is made overlying the wrist. The physician may use the previous wrist surgery incision. The physician extends the incision down to the wrist joint by dividing and dissecting tissues. Some tissue may require debridement. The joint is entered through an arthrotomy cut. The physician identifies the pieces of artificial joint. Each piece is dissected free from the bone. Any loose pieces are removed. The entire joint is explored. The physician may smooth or debride the ends of the exposed bone. Any nonviable soft tissue and synovium is removed. The joint is irrigated with antibiotic solution. If infection is present, the joint and incision are left open for temporary drainage. Otherwise, the incisions are repaired in multiple layers.

25259

Manipulation of the wrist under anesthesia may be necessary to regain the loss of motion following a surgical procedure or due to scar tissue. Following the induction of general anesthesia, the physician evaluates the wrist. The wrist is manipulated by stretching, rotation, and other maneuvers to gain the appropriate range of motion.

25260–25263

The physician repairs a tendon or muscle, flexor, forearm and/or wrist. A "primary" repair is performed within the first few hours of post-injury. The physician identifies the proximal end of the tendon by extending the original laceration if needed for better exposure. Incisions to expose the injury vary in location and shape, but should never be straight, midline volar incisions that cross flexor creases. Before repairing the tendon, the volar plate is sutured if damaged. If the tendon laceration is more than 1.0 cm proximal to the insertion, end-to-end repair is done via suture (suture type is dependent on physician preference). If the tendon laceration is 1.0 cm or less from the insertion, advancement of the tendon and reinsertion into the distal phalanx is done via suture. To secure the tendon to the bone, a pullout wire is extended through the bone and fingernail. The wire is held in place by a button while healing of the tendon to bone occurs. Zone II and III tendon lacerations may involve the flexor digitorum profundus extending the original laceration if needed for better exposure. The two ends are repaired via the choice stitch of the surgeon. Sometimes identification of the proximal end involves making another incision over the wrist or forearm, depending on if the proximal end retracted proximally after the laceration. Zones IV and V tendon lacerations are rare and may involve a combination of nine flexor tendons. Repair is the same as for Zones II and III. After the tendon

repairs are completed at the involved level, skin closure is achieved via suture of the overlying layers. A post-operative splint and bulky dressing are applied. The splint should protect the repair by placing the flexor tendons on slack by holding the wrist and digits in flexion. In Zone I, II, and III injuries, usually a rubber band traction is utilized to flex the involved digits. Report 25263 if the repair is performed 10 days to three weeks post-injury.

25265

The physician repairs a tendon or muscle, flexor, forearm and/or wrist with a free graft. The physician first approaches the involved flexor muscle or tendon through a zig-zag incision on the palmar surface of the wrist or hand, depending on the area of tendon in need of the graft. Any pulleys that are in the area are preserved while the injured tendon is excised. A second incision is made, curvilinear, at the volar (palm side) distal forearm starting at the wrist crease and proceeding proximally. The musculotendinous junction of the involved muscles is identified and the tendon is pulled into this incision. The free graft is obtained. For retrieving the palmaris longus, the physician makes a transverse incision at the volar wrist. The palmaris longus is transected here and a silk-holding suture is placed in the distal end of the graft. The tendon is mobilized proximally and threaded through a circular tendon stripper. Holding tension on the graft at its distal end with a clamp, the stripper is firmly advanced into the proximal forearm. The muscle belly will fill the circular cutting blade and be divided, allowing the tendon to be withdrawn through one incision. The transverse skin incision is closed. The tendon graft is threaded through the forearm using a tendon passer. The distal juncture is secured using a Bunnell pullout wire technique. The distal incision is closed. The proximal juncture is made by interweaving the graft into the tendon of the involved muscle. This proximal wound is closed and wounds are dressed. A dorsal splint is applied maintaining wrist flexion to protect repair.

25270

The physician repairs a tendon or muscle, extensor, in the forearm and or wrist. The physician always debrides and cleanses the laceration first. In proximal forearm level injuries, the wound margins are debrided and extended by the physician as needed to evaluate the extent of the injury. Once both ends of the injured muscle are identified, they are approximated with multiple sutures of a synthetic, nonabsorbable material. Interrupted soft tissues are closed. The arm is supported in a separately reportable splint or cast that maintains a 45 degree extension of the wrist, and a 15–20 flexion of the metacarpophalangeal joints. The elbow is held in 90 degrees flexion if the involved muscles arise at or above the lateral epicondyle. In distal forearm level injuries, these injuries usually occur at the muscle tendon junction. The distal tendon usually accepts and hold sutures well, the proximal muscle belly does not. Multiple nonabsorbable sutures are placed in the fibrous tissue of the muscle belly proximal to where the tendon is identifiable as a distinct structure. The knots are buried between the tendon and the muscle. Small absorbable sutures may be used to repair the fascial margins of the muscle. After the opened soft tissues are closed, the same splinting method is used as described for proximal forearm injuries. In wrist level injuries, injuries to the extensor mechanism at the wrist level are associated with injuries to the retinaculum over the site should be excised. The tendon(s) is repaired using a standard suture of nonabsorbable material. If the abductor pollicis longus may have two to four slips, all portions of the tendon should be identified and repaired. If the level of injury is at or near the osseous insertion, the tendon(s) must be firmly reattached to the bone using nonabsorbable sutures. A pull-out wire technique may also be used. Repair of the abductor tendons must be protected by applying a splint (separately reportable) or cast holding the wrist in a 40 degree extension and radial deviation. The extensor pollicis are splinted in 45 degree wrist extension. Repair of finger extensors are splinted in 45 degree wrist extension and 15 degrees flexion of metacarpophalangeal joints.

25272

The physician repairs a tendon or muscle, extensor, secondary, with a tendon graft. A "secondary" repair is usually performed 10 days to three weeks post-injury. Proximal forearm level injuries — The physician makes a linear incision over the dorsal area of muscle interruption. If the tear occurred via severance of the involved muscle, the wound margins are debrided and extended proximally and distally to allow the physician to evaluate the extent of damage. Once both ends of the divided muscle are identified, multiple sutures of a synthetic nonabsorbable material are used to approximate the muscle ends. Interrupted soft tissues are closed. The extremity is supported in a plaster splint or cast that maintains the wrist in a 45 degree extended position, and the metacarpophalangeal joints in 15–20 degree flexion. The elbow is immobilized in 90 degrees of flexion if the involved muscles arise at or above the lateral epicondyle. Distal forearm level injures (musculotendinous). These injuries usually occur at the muscle tendon junction. Repair is achieved in the same fashion as already described, in addition to placement of small absorbable sutures in the fascial margins of the muscle. Wrist level injuries at this level involve damage to the extensor retinaculum. After the location of tendon injury is identified, the portion of the extensor retinaculum over the site should be excised. The tendons are repaired as already described. Lacerations on the radial side of the wrist may injure the short thumb extensor and the abductor pollicis longus tendons, as well as the radial wrist extensors. The abductor pollicis longus may have two to four slips or tendon segments — All portions of the tendon should be identified and

repaired. If the level of injury is at or near the osseous insertion, the tendon(s) must be firmly reattached to bone using nonabsorbable sutures. A pullout wire technique may also be used to reattach these tendons to their osseous insertions. Repair of the abductor tendon is protected by application of a splint or cast with the wrist in 40 degrees extension and slight radial deviation, and extension of the thumb metacarpal. Repair of the finger extensors is splinted in 45 degrees of wrist extension and 15 degrees of metacarpophalangeal joint flexion.

25274

The physician repairs a tendon or muscle, extensor, of the forearm and/or wrist, secondary with tendon graft. To approach the tendon or muscle needing repair, the physician makes an incision over the dorsal (back) of the proximal forearm at the site of the proximal tendon/muscle end. A second incision is made at the distal site of the involved tendon/muscle end. The desired free graft is obtained by making a transverse incision over the distal end of the muscle. The muscle is transected and a silk holding suture is placed in the distal end of the graft. The tendon is mobilized proximally under direct vision and threaded through a circular tendon stripper. Holding tension on the graft at its distal end with a clamp, the stripper is firmly advanced into the proximal forearm. The muscle belly fills the circular cutting blade and be divided, allowing the tendon to be withdrawn through one incision. The skin incision is closed. At the site of the tendon/muscle being repaired, the free graft is threaded through the dopal forearm between retracted ends of the involved extensor. The distal juncture is secured using a Bunnell pull-out wire technique. The distal incision is closed. The proximal juncture is made by interweaving the graft into the involved muscle. This wound is closed, and all wounds are dressed. Immobilization involves placing the proximal and distal interphalangeal joints in extension, the metacarpophalangeal joints in 60–70 degrees flexion, the thumb in the first projection, and the wrist in 10 degrees from the maximum extension.

25280

The physician lengthens or shortens the flexor or extensor tendon of the forearm and/or wrist. The physician makes a curved volar incision overlying the forearm. The muscle to be lengthened or shortened is identified and followed to the musculotendinous junction and further proximally until the muscle belly is identified. The physician makes transverse cuts in the aponeurosis, leaving none of the tendon intact with it. The wrist is placed in dorsiflexion for flexor procedure (palmarflexion for extensor procedure). The transverse cut in the aponeurosis will widen as the muscle lengthens, but the entire muscle-tendon unit will remain intact. The soft tissue is closed in layers and a bandage is applied.

25290

The physician repairs the flexor or extensor tendon, forearm and/or wrist. This procedure is indicated for mild Boutonniere deformity (extensor tenotomy) or for Swan-neck deformity (flexor tenotomy). The physician makes a dorsal transverse or oblique incision overlying the distal one-third of the middle phalanx and exposes the extensor tendon. This tendon is divided obliquely to enable it to lengthen and remain partially in apposition after the distal interphalangeal joint into flexion. The extensor tendon is not sutured. The wound is closed. No splinting is necessary if there is no mallet deformity.

25295

This tenolysis of the flexor or extensor tendon is indicated in the case of extrinsic extensor or flexor tendon tightness. In the case of flexor tightness, the physician approaches the involved flexor system through a zig-zag incision that is long enough to uncover the entire length of the flexor. The physician excises all limiting adhesions, whether the excess scarring is located proximally in the forearm and/or distally in the wrist. All involved tendons are released of motion-limiting adhesions. The retinacular pulley system is preserved. During the procedure, the patient's active motion is re-evaluated. To achieve this, a local anesthesia is supplemented by an intravenous analgesic-tranquilizer combination drug. After tissue closure, the physician applies a splint over the dressing. These must be applied in a manner that allows continued flexion to maintain tendon gliding through the lysed scars. The above techniques are the same for extrinsic extensors, except there is no critical annular pulley system to preserve, although the sagittal bands must be protected.

25300–25301

The physician performs a tenodesis at the wrist. In 25300, the physician exposes the flexor tendons at the wrist level. The terminal phalangeal flexors of the fingers to be tenodesed (usually all four) are identified in the depths of the wound. A window is made in the anterior surface of the distal radius proximal to the wrist. A similar second window is made more proximal. A criss-cross type of suture is passed through all four flexor digitonum profundi tendons side-by-side. The tendon is transected proximal to this suture. The tendons are drawn into the more distal window in the radius, through medullary canal, out the proximal window, and sutured back to themselves. The tension on the tenodesis is adjusted so that with the wrist in extension, the fingers naturally flex into the palm. With wrist flexion, the fingers can extend through the passive dorsal tenodesis of tension on the extrinsic extensors. All open soft tissues are sutured in layers. The wrist is immobilized in five to ten degrees of extension and with the metacarpophalangeal joints flexed and the interphalangeal joints extended. Report 25301 if the extensors of the fingers are repaired at the wrist.

25310–25312

The physician performs a flexor or extensor transplantation or transfer in the forearm and wrist. With the patient under anesthesia, the physician exposes the muscle to be transferred by making a longitudinal incision near its insertion. The insertion is released from near its bony attachment for transfer to the involved tendon. The entire tendon may not be released, but rather only the central portion. Through a separate incision, the physician exposes the involved tendon. A tunnel is prepared around or through the arm between the transferred and involved tendons. This tunnel must permit a straight line of pull between the two tendons. The transferred tendon is passed through the tunnel. A small, longitudinal hole is created in the involved tendon(s). The distal end of the transferred tendon is passed through the involved tendon(s) and sutured to that tendon. After these procedures are complete, all wounds are closed with sutures. Report 25312 if the procedure is performed with tendon grafts, each tendon.

25315–25316

The physician performs a flexor origin slide in the forearm or wrist for cerebral palsy. The physician makes a zig-zag incision from above the supracondylar region, distally through the middle and lower regions of the forearm. A periosteal elevator is inserted between the brachialis and the common flexor-pronator origin from the medial epicondyle. The elevator is brought out between the numeral and ulnar heads of the flexor carpi ulnaris on the anterior side of the elbow. The origin of the flexors is dissected using a scalpel to detach the muscle subperiosteally. The origins of the pronatorteres flexor carpi radialis, palmaris longus, and the numeral head of the flexor carpi ulnaris are released. The physician dissects the origins of the flexor digitonum superficialis. The ulnar head of the flexor carpi ulnaris is detached subperiosteally. The physician brings together the detached muscles from the proximal and ulnar sides at the interosseous space on the proximal side. Neurolysis of the median and ulnar nerves is performed. The muscles are slid distally the desired amount and are fixed in several places to periosteum and subcutaneous tissue. The ulnar nerve is transposed over the medial epicondyle. The wound is closed in layers. The elbow joint is maintained at 90 degrees, the wrist and fingers in extension, the forearm in supination. Report 25316 if this procedure is performed with a tendon transfer.

25320

The physician performs a capsulorrhaphy or reconstruction of the wrist using any method, including synovectomy, capsulotomy, and open reduction) to stem carpal instability. The wrist and finer extensors are retracted laterally and medially. The capsule is longitudinally cut over the involved carpus for exposure. If dislocation was present prior to surgery, this is reduced. The necessary fixation is carried out (i.e., Kirchner wires, screws). If the physician is performing a capsulodesis for scapholunate dissociation, a notch is made in the dorsum of the distal pole of the scaphoid proximal to the distal articular surface and distal to the mid-axis of rotation of the scaphoid. The dorsal capsuloligainentous flap is trimmed to attach into the distal pole of the scaphoid with a stainless steel pullout wire suture. This is passed through five drill holes to the volar tubercle of the scaphoid and the wire is tied at the level of the skin over felt and a button. The soft tissues are closed in layers.

25332

The physician performs an arthroplasty of the wrist. The physician makes a straight, dorsal, longitudinal incision centered over the wrist from the middle of the third metacarpal proximally. Skin and subcutaneous tissues are elevated off the fascia and retinaculum. The retinaculum over the fourth dorsal compartment is incised longitudinally and elevated medially and laterally. The extensor pollicis longus is freed, retracted radially, and left in the rerouted position at the end of the procedure. A longitudinal incision is made in the capsule. A capsular periosteal flap is elevated through the dorsal radioulnar ligaments. The distal radius is excised, as is the distal ulna if it is dislocated or severely involved. A cut is made through the hamate, capitate, trapezoid, and distal scapho-trapezoid area. The carpus is removed. The medullary canal of the radius is reamed. A fine awl is used to penetrate the base of the capitate and the shaft of the third metacarpal. The medullary canal of this bone is reamed. If using a double-stemmed component, an additional canal is prepared in the second metacarpal. Appropriate short canals are prepared in the carpal bones. With the wrist in 10 to 20 degree extension, the capsular-periosteal sleeves are repaired over the prosthesis. The extensor retinaculum may be used to reinforce the capsule, or may be repaired anatomically. The skin is closed over a deep and a superficial suction drain.

25335

The physician performs a centralization of the wrist on the ulna for conditions including radial club hand. The physician makes two incisions. A transverse incision is made over the end of the ulna to remove excess skin and fatty tissue and to expose the distal ulna. A Z-plasty incision may be needed on the radial surface of the distal forearm and wrist to give extra length to the tight skin on this side. The physician next incises the capsule, flexes the elbow, and reduces the carpus over the ulna. Insertions of the flexor carpi radialis and brachioradialis are cut. The distal end of the ulna is shaved to flatten its surface, and a Kirschner wire is drilled through the capitate and through the base of the third metacarpal. The second wire is removed and the ulnar wire is driven through the hole it created. The distal ulnacarpal capsule is pulled proximally over the ulna and sutured with nonabsorbable suture. The extensor carpiulnaris is

advanced distally over the fifth metacarpal tightly. The flexor carpi ulnaris is sutured with the extensor carpi ulnaris. The two incisions are closed. The wrist is placed in a neutral position, and a bulky dressing is applied.

25337

Restoring stability to a wrist with an unstable distal ulna or distal radioulnar joint may require just a few procedures, or it may dictate many procedures. In all cases, the physician must expose the distal radioulnar joint by making a curvilinear incision on the dopal wrist starting proximal to the ulna styloid and extending it dorsally, over the ulnar styloid to the carpus. The proximal and ulnar half of the extensor retinaculum is reflected radially. The extensor digiti minimi is retracted, revealing the styloid notch of the radius and the TFC. The capsule is sharply detached from the radius exposing the ulnar head. If a styloid fracture is found, two drill holes are made proximally from the fracture to exit facing the radius. A wire is passed either around or through the styloid using similar drill holes, and the two free ends of the wire are passed proximally through the fracture site into the previously drilled holes in the proximal shaft. The wire is twisted, compressing the styloid to the shaft. If the triangular fibrocartilaginous complex is avulsed from styloid, an intraosseous wiring as described above may be used to restore distal radioulnar stability. If the TFC is not avulsed, an intraosseous wire with a 24-gauge, or larger, should be used. The capsule is sutured closed, and the skin is closed in layers. Over the dressing, a longarm cast is applied with the elbow flexed, the forearm in zero degree extension, and the wrist in neutral.

25350–25355

The physician performs an osteotomy (bone cut) of the radius. An incision is made in the forearm overlying the distal third area of the radius in 25350 or the middle or proximal third in 25355. The physician performs dissection through the tissue layers and down to the bone. The periosteum is removed from the bone site where the osteotomy will be made. The physician then cuts through the radius. The physician then realigns the bone to the desired position. Metal plates and screws are typically applied to stabilize the bone. The wound is irrigated with antibiotic solution and then repaired in multiple layers. A cast or splint may be applied to further stabilize and support the bone.

25360–25365

The physician performs an osteotomy of the ulna in 25360 or of both the ulna and radius in 25365. The physician makes a longitudinal incision along the medial border of the forearm to expose the affected part of the ulna. Two separate incisions may be necessary in 25365. An osteotomy (bone cut) is made through the ulna, usually in a wedge shape. This allows the bone to be realigned. The physician applies plates and screws to hold the osteotomy together in the correct position. The incisions are then repaired in multiple layers with sutures, staples and/or Steri-strips. The arm may be placed in a splint for immobilization.

25370–25375

The physician treats the radius or ulna in 25370 or both in 25375. A longitudinal incision is made to expose the entire shaft of the bone. Two separate incisions may be necessary in 25375. The physician makes an osteotomy (bone cut) through the proximal and distal ends of the bone shaft. The bone shaft is then removed from the wound. The physician studies the bone shaft to determine how many times it must be osteotomized so that its segments can be threaded onto a medullary nail. The osteotomies are made, and each fragment placed end to end on the medullary nail. Because the cortex of the ulna and radius are very thin, a bone graft is usually added. This may be harvested from the surrounding area, or a separate incision may be needed. A separate incision would be made over the iliac crest, bone harvested, and the incision closed. The medullary nail is then inserted into place. The periosteum is sutured into place. The physician repairs the incision in multiple layers with sutures, staples, and/or Steri-strips. The arm is immobilized in a cast.

25390

The physician shortens the radius or ulna. An incision is made on the anterior aspect of the distal forearm. Any exposed arteries are carefully retracted. The physician continues dissection to expose the distal shaft of the radius or ulna. Based on preoperative x-rays, an osteotomy is made at the distal end of the radius or ulna. A more proximal osteotomy is then made which shortens the radius or ulna usually by 2.0 mm to 3.0 mm. The physician removes the bone fragment. A plate is then attached to the distal segment with screws. Reduction forceps hold and compress the osteotomy while the plate is attached to the proximal fragment with screws. Separately reportable x-rays are used to check radioulnar length. Drain tubes are inserted. The physician repairs the incision in multiple layers with sutures, staples, and/or Steri-strips. However, the forearm fascia is left open to minimize the chances of compartment syndrome. The forearm is placed in a splint.

25394

The physician shortens a carpal bone. The physician makes the incision over the area of the carpal bone. Dissection is carried down to the level of the carpal bone and an osteotomy is done. The bone is shortened. The amount of bone removed is dependent on the condition treated. The incision is closed with sutures.

25400–25405

The physician exposes a nonunion or malunion of the radius or ulna by making a 10.0 cm to 15.0 cm longitudinal incision over the fracture site. With a reciprocating saw, each bone is divided through the nonunion. The fragments are then aligned. A compression plate is centered over the fracture and screws are inserted. In 25405, a bone graft is needed to help heal the nonunion due to loss of bone. For example, if the nonunion is old, approximately 0.6 cm to 1.3 cm of bone is resected from the ends of the fragments. Autogenous iliac bone is typically used. Bone from the upper tibia may also be used. This requires an incision over the site of harvest. The physician uses an osteotome to harvest strips of bone. These strips are placed around the ends of the fracture along with the compression plate for internal fixation. The incision is repaired in multiple layers with sutures, staples, and/or Steri-strips. However, the deep fascial layer is not closed because of the potential to develop compartment syndrome. A long arm cast is applied with the elbow at 90 degrees of flexion.

25415–25420

The physician exposes the nonunions through two 10.0 cm to 15.0 cm longitudinal incisions One incision is made on the lateral aspect and one on the medial aspect of the forearm. With a reciprocating saw, the physician divides each bone through the nonunion. The fragments are then aligned. The physician centers a compression plate over the fracture and inserts screws. In 25420, a bone graft is needed to help bone healing of the nonunion due to loss of bone. For example, if the nonunion is old, approximately 0.6 cm to 1.3 cm of bone is resected from the ends of the fragments. Autogenous iliac bone graft is typically used. The physician makes an incision over the iliac crest. Once the bone is exposed, an osteotome is used to harvest strips of bone. These strips are placed around the ends of the fracture. Internal fixation with a compression plate is the same as for 25415. The incision are repaired in multiple layers with sutures, staples, and/or Steri-strips. However, the deep fascial layer is not closed because of the potential to develop compartment syndrome. A long arm cast is applied with the elbow in 90 degrees of flexion.

25425–25426

The physician repairs a defect of the radius or ulna in 25425 or of both the radius and ulna in 25426. The physician makes a longitudinal incision along the forearm. An anterior approach is made for the radius, medial for the ulna, or two incision for both. The defect is exposed through dissection. To harvest the bone graft, the physician makes a separate incision over the iliac crest. Bone from the upper tibia may also be used. The bone is exposed, and the physician uses an osteotome to harvest strips of bone. These bone strips are used to fill the defect. A screw or wire wrapped around the defect holds the bone graft in place. The incision is repaired in multiple layers with sutures, staples, and/or Steri-strips. However, the deep fascial layer is not closed because of the potential to develop compartment syndrome. The arm may be placed in a long arm cast with the elbow at 90 degrees of flexion.

25430

The physician makes an incision away from the iliac crest through the external oblique muscle. The internal oblique muscle is incised and isolated from the underlying transversalis muscle. The ascending branch is followed to its junction with the deep circumflex iliac vein, and the dissection proceeds to the isolation of the flap vessels to their origin at the external iliac crest vessels. The physician divides the transversalis muscle, identifies the iliacus muscle, and divides the iliacus at the site of the planned bone cut. The fascia and muscles are released from the lateral surface of the ilium to the level of the planned bone cut. The bone cuts are made with an oscillating saw. The direction and extent depend on the recipient bed defect. Following ligation of the pedicle and transfer, the bone portion of the flap is countered to meet the dimensions of the bone defect. The bone is secured to the plate and the soft tissue inset is completed prior to microvascular anastomosis. Free cancellous bone is packed into the opening osteotomies.

25431

Nonunion of the carpal bone refers to fractures that still allow free movement of bone ends more than six months after the injury and the start of treatment. In the case of a complex nonunion, the physician may take a graft from the medial aspect of the ulna and reinsert it into the prepared carpal site. Intravenous anesthesia is administered. An autogenous iliac bone graft is typically used for repair, which is obtained through an incision over the iliac crest. Once the bone is exposed, an osteotome is used to harvest strips of bone. These strips are placed between the carpal bones of the fracture through a 2.0 centimeter incision made at the base of the involved metacarpus. The physician centers a compression plate over the fracture and inserts screws. Lunate fractures require a short-arm spica cast or splint with thumb immobilization. Fractures of the pisiform can be immobilized with a volar splint. Injuries to the triquetrum are best treated with a sugar tong splint. Treatment of a hamate fracture involves a short-arm cast with the fourth and fifth metacarpophalangeal joints held in flexion.

25440

The physician performs this procedure when a scaphoid fracture has not healed and particularly if nonunion is accompanied by displacement of the fracture. The physician makes a 4.0 cm to 5.0 cm longitudinal incision along the radial border of the flexor carpi radialis tendon to expose the fracture site. The capsule is divided longitudinally, and the

underlying ligaments are retracted. An egg-shaped cavity is created in the fracture fragments. A cancellous bone graft is obtained and the graft is jammed between the fragments as they are distracted. The physician uses internal fixation such as a Kirschner wires to affix the bones if instability exists. If a radial styloidectomy is performed, the physician makes an incision on the radial wrist at the base of the thumb. Radial styloid bone is removed. The physician closes the incision(s) with sutures.

25441

The physician performs an arthroplasty on the wrist to relieve function-limiting wrist pain. The physician makes a T-shaped incision overlying the dorsal wrist. The capsule and synovium are incised and elevated. The distal end of the radius and the proximal carpal row are excised to accommodate the implant. The medullary canal of the third metacarpal is exposed and an awl is placed into the canal for reaming. The awl is removed, then the prosthetic awl is impacted into the base of the carpus and third metacarpal shaft. The medullary canal of the radius is then reamed and implanted with the prosthesis. Cement is injected into the medullary canal of the third metacarpal after previously inserting a small cancellous bone plug. The distal component is impacted home first. The proximal component is generally not cemented and is impacted only. The capsule is repaired over the prosthesis with strong sutures. A suction drain is placed beneath the capsule. The retinaculum is repaired over all of the extensor tendons. The skin is sutured closed, and the wrist is immobilized.

25442

The physician performs this arthroplasty to decrease ulnar bone overgrowth following resection of the distal ulna. The physician makes a dorsal ulnar longitudinal incision overlying the ulnar head. The extensor retinaculum is incised. The neck of the ulna is subperiosteally exposed and the ulnar head is resected at the neck. The cut edge of the ulna is smoothed and medullary canal reamed to accept the stem of the implant. The appropriately sized implant is tested and two drill holes are made 2.0 cm from the resected bone. The physician stabilizes the distal ulna by attaching the base of the sixth dorsal compartment retinaculum to the interosseous membrane with sutures. The distal end of the ulna is pressed volarly and is sutured tightly into the soft tissue on the radial side with the radial itself. The wound is closed with sutures over a drain. A conforming dressing is applied.

25443

The physician performs an arthroplasty with prosthetic replacement of the scaphoid. The physician makes a straight, longitudinal, or curvilinear incision over the anatomic snuff-box (superficial to the scaphoid), the "V" between your thumb and index finger. The capsule is incised longitudinally. The scaphoid is removed maintaining ligament stability. If a defect is found in the distal capsule, this is closed with a nonabsorbable suture. A hole is made in the proximal joint surface of the trapezium for insertion of the prosthetic stem. An implant is inserted. The implant is stabilized with sutures through drill holes in the lunate and radial styloid. The implant is also stabilized with a K-wire passed through the implant into an adjacent carpal bone or the radius. The capsule is closed, followed by skin closure. A compression dressing is applied.

25444

The physician performs an arthroplasty with prosthetic replacement of the lunate. The physician makes a straight, longitudinal or transverse incision over the dorsum of the wrist ulnar to Lister's tubercle of the radius. The fourth dorsal compartment is opened and the radiocarpal joint capsule is transversely cut. The scapholunate and lunate-triquetral interosseous ligaments are cut. The lunate is removed. If a defect in the volar ligamentous capsule is found, it is repaired. A hole is made in the middle of the triquetrum to accept the prosthetic stem. The implant is fixed to the carpus and radius with a K-wire. An absorbable suture may be placed through the scaphoid and prosthesis to increase stability. The distal capsule flap is sutured to the radius with nonabsorbable sutures. The wounds are closed and a bulky compression dressing is applied.

25445

The physician performs an arthroplasty with prosthetic replacement of the trapezium. The physician makes a straight, longitudinal cut from the middle of the thumb metacarpal to the radial styloid. The capsule is split longitudinally from the metacarpal to the scaphoid. The capsule and periosteum are elevated off the trapezium. The radial portion of the trapezoid is removed. The base of the first metacarpal is squared off. A triangular hole is made in the base of the metacarpal, and the canal is made to accept the implant stem. The size of the implant should be slightly smaller than a tight fit. The capsule is repaired and reinforced by suturing slips of the abductor pollicis and flexor carpi radialis muscles to the capsule. A K-wire is placed through the implant and into the trapezoid or capitate to stabilize the position for six weeks. The skin is closed, leaving the wire protruding through incision, and a bulky dressing is applied to keep the thumb abducted.

25446

The physician performs a total wrist arthroplasty. The physician makes a straight, dorsal, longitudinal incision centered over the wrist from the middle of the third metacarpal proximally. The skin and subcutaneous tissues are elevated off the underlying fascia and retinaculum. The retinaculum over the fourth dorsal compartment is incised longitudinally and elevated. The extensor pollicis longus is freed and

retracted radically. A longitudinal incision is made in the capsule overlying the distal radius. Ulnarly, a capsular periosteal flap is elevated through the dorsal radioulnar ligaments. Radially, the subperiosteal dissection continues to the radial styloid beneath the first dorsal compartment. The distal radius is excised, as is the distal ulna if it is dislocated or severely involved. A cut, made to match the shape of the prosthesis of choice, is made through the hamate, capitate, trapezoid, and distal scaphotrapezial area. The carpus is removed. The medullary canal of the radius is reamed. A fine awl is used to penetrate the base of the capitate and the shaft of the third metacarpal. The medullary canal of this bone is reamed. If using a double-stemmed component, an additional canal is prepared in the second metacarpal. The component is inserted into the canals. Appropriate short canals are prepared in the carpal bases. The metallic components are inserted. The prosthetic polyethylene ball is placed on the trunnion and motion is tested. When desired motion is achieved, cement is mixed and injected into the medullary canals. The capsular-periosteal tissues are repaired over the prosthesis. The extensor retinaculum may be used to reinforce the capsule. The skin is closed over a deep and a superficial suction drain.

25447

The physician performs an interposition arthroplasty of the intercarpal or carpometacarpal joints. The physician makes a zig-zag incision over the proximal one third of the first metacarpal and extends it along the first wrist extensor compartment. The metacarpal joint is vertically incised to release the capsule from the base of the metacarpal. The joint is completely dislocated to expose the metacarpal end. The physician resects the metacarpal based perpendicular to its long axis. The base is shaped to allow the insertion of a Swanson great toe prosthesis. The medullary canal of the metacarpal is reamed to accept the prosthetic stem. The stem is inserted and the base of the prosthesis is seated on the flat surface of the trapezium bone. A Kirschner wire is inserted through the first metacarpal and into the carpus to ensure alignment. The capsule and the wounds are sutured closed.

25449

The physician revises an arthroplasty, including removal of an implant in the wrist joint. The physician makes an incision over the wrist, reduces the joint if it is not already dislocated, and removes the device from the radius and the one or two metacarpals in which it was implanted. If necessary, a new device is placed into the wrist. The skin is closed in layers and a bulky dressing is applied.

25450–25455

The physician makes an incision overlying the distal forearm and along the medial (ulna) or lateral (radius) aspect in 25450 or both in 25455. The distal epiphyseal plate is located here. Dissection is carried down to expose the epiphyseal plate. The physician may elect to use a curet to scrape out the epiphysis (growth plate). A staple may be placed through the epiphyseal plate instead. Either procedure arrests further growth of that particular bone. The physician then repairs the incision in multiple layers with sutures, staples, and/or Steri-strips.

25490–25492

The physician applies prophylactic treatment. The physician treats the radius in 25490. A longitudinal incision is made along the forearm. Dissection is carried down to expose the affected part of the radius. In 25491, the ulna is treated. A longitudinal incision is required along the medial aspect of the ulna. In 25492, both the radius and ulna are treated, which may require two separate incisions. Pins or a plate with screws are used to stabilize the bone. If there are defects in the bone, such that the internal fixation does not provide good purchase with the bone, methylmethacrylate (cement) is used to fill in the gaps. Wiring (cerclage) may also wrapped around the bone to provide additional fixation. The physician may also insert an intramedullary nail through the canal of the radius to provide internal stabilization. This is usually inserted through the distal end of the radius. The incisions are repaired in multiple layers with sutures, staples, and/or Steri-strips.

25500–25505

The physician treats a radial shaft fracture without manipulation in 25500 or with manipulation in 25505. No incisions are made. If manipulation is required (25505), anesthesia may be necessary to relax the muscles. With the elbow at 90 degrees of flexion, the physician uses a combination of traction and countertraction while the radius is reduced. The patient may be placed in a long arm cast. The cast is removed after approximately 18 days and a functional brace is applied, allowing wrist and elbow movement, but limited pronation and supination.

25515

The physician treats a radial shaft fracture. For internal fixation, the physician may use either plate and screw fixation or a medullary nail. A plate and screw fixation is described. If the fracture is in the lower half of the radius, an anterior forearm incision is made. If the fracture is in the upper half of the radius, a posterior forearm incision is made. Dissection is carried down to expose the fractured fragments. The physician uses bone-holding forceps to reduce the fracture. A plate of appropriate length is selected and centered over the fracture. Plates with five or six holes are usually required. The screws are then inserted. The incision is repaired in multiple layers. The deep fascia is not closed because of the potential of developing compartment syndrome. Depending on the rigidity of the fixation, a cast or

splint may be applied. If there is a severe open wound with skin and soft tissue loss (e.g., gunshot wound), infection, bone loss, or comminution, the physician may apply external fixation (e.g., Hoffman device).

25520

The physician treats a radial shaft fracture and a dislocation of the distal radio-ulnar joint. No incisions are made. The physician may reduce the fracture and dislocation by manipulation with traction force. A long arm cast is applied to immobilize the elbow and wrist.

25525

The physician makes a 5 in to 6 in longitudinal incision over the anterior aspect of the forearm and centered over the fracture. Dissection is carried down to expose the pronator quadratus muscle, that is then freed from the radius. The physician reduces the fracture with bone-holding forceps. A plate of appropriate length is selected and centered over the fracture. The screws are then inserted. The pronator quadratus muscle is reattached. The incision is repaired in multiple layers with sutures, staples, and or Steri-strips. The deep fascia is not closed. The physician then places the arm in a cast. The physician may use an external fixation device for traumatic fractures (e.g., open wound). The physician may also apply percutaneous skeletal fixation. Kirschner wires are inserted through small stab incisions through the radius and into the ulna to stabilize the radius.

25526

The physician treats a radial shaft fracture, using fixation and open treatment. This procedure includes repair of the triangular fibrocartilage complex. After the affected hand is suspended in finger traps, the physician reduces the fracture and confirms the reduction radiographically. Under separately reportable radiographic guidance, a Kirschner wire is inserted from the tip of the radial styloid obliquely across the fracture site. A second pin is inserted in a slightly more longitudinal direction. Finger traps are removed and the pins are cut off approximately 2.0 cm above the skin and bent at right angles. If tears are present in the fibrocartilage complex, they are repaired with sutures. Skin incisions may be made to prevent skin tethering. A dressing and splint is applied.

25530–25535

The physician treats an ulnar shaft fracture without manipulation in 25530 or with manipulation in 25535. No incisions are made. If manipulation is required, the physician uses a combination of traction and countertraction with manual manipulation of the fracture. The patient is placed in a long arm cast with the elbow at 90 degrees of flexion. A functional splint or brace is then applied.

25545

The physician makes an incision along the subcutaneous border of the ulna, exposing the shaft fracture. The physician then reduces the fracture with bone-holding forceps. A plate of appropriate length is selected and centered over the fracture. The screws are then inserted. Only the subcutaneous tissue is closed. The skin incision is repaired with sutures, staples, and/or Steri-strips. Depending on the rigidity of the fixation, a cast or splint may be applied. If there is a severe open wound with skin and soft tissue loss (e.g., gunshot wound), the physician may apply an external fixator (e.g., Hoffman device).

25560–25565

For undisplaced and stable fractures, the physician immobilizes the elbow and wrist with a long arm cast. Separately reportable x-rays are taken to confirm that displacement does not occur. In 25565, the fractures are displaced and manual reduction is required. Analgesia or a certain degree of sedation may be necessary. The physician uses a combination of traction and manual manipulation to reduce the fractures. A long arm cast immobilizes the elbow and wrist.

25574–25575

When both the radius and ulna are fractured, the physician exposes and reduces both fractures prior to fixation. Separate incisions along the forearm may be needed to expose the fracture. In 25574, only one fracture is stabilized, requiring only one incision. The other fracture is stable and does not require fixation. In 25575, both radial and ulnar fractures require fixation, usually requiring separate incisions. Once the fracture site is exposed and reduced, internal fixation is applied. A plate of appropriate length is selected and centered over the fracture. The physician then inserts the screws. The incisions are repaired in multiple layers with sutures, staples, and/or Steri-strips. The deep fascia is not closed, preventing the development of compartment syndrome. Depending upon the rigidity of the fixation, a cast or splint may or may not be applied. If there is a severe open wound with skin and soft tissue loss (e.g., gunshot wound), infection, or a need to maintain length due to bone loss or comminution, the physician may choose to apply external fixation (e.g., Hoffman device).

25600–25605

The physician treats a distal radial fracture. A Colles fracture is a fracture of the distal radius with dorsal displacement. A Smith fracture is palmar displacement of the distal radius. The ulnar styloid is usually fractured. If good alignment and correct angulation of the distal radial articular surface is present, the physician immobilizes the wrist and forearm in a cast or splint until the fracture or epiphyseal separation is stable. In 25605, manipulation is required to reduce an unstable and/or displaced fracture or epiphyseal separation. Analgesia or sedation may be necessary to

achieve reduction. The physician uses a combination of longitudinal distraction of the fracture and manipulation of the distal fragment to achieve reduction. The wrist and forearm are placed in a cast or splint until the fracture or epiphyseal separation is stable.

25611

The physician treats a fracture of the distal radius. The physician first manipulates the area to reduce the fracture. The physician applies a combination of traction on the wrist and manipulation of the distal radius to reduce the fracture. An assistant maintains the reduction. Using a drill, the physician inserts two Kirschner wires percutaneously (directly through the skin) through the radial styloid, across the fracture, and into the opposite metaphyseal cortex of the ulna. The Kirschner wires are cut off just beneath the skin. The arm is immobilized in a cast. The wires are removed in six weeks. If there is a severely comminuted fracture of the distal radius that is not suitable for percutaneous Kirschner wire stabilization alone, the physician apply either a traction cast or an Ace-Colles external fixator. For application of a traction cast, the fracture or separation is first reduced, then a Steinman pin is inserted transversely through the proximal elbow. A second pin is inserted transversely through the bases of the second and third metacarpals. A plaster cast is applied above and below the elbow and incorporates the two pins. The pins and cast are left in place for approximately eight weeks. With an external fixator, the fracture or separation is first reduced by manipulation and traction. The external fixator is then applied to the forearm and wrist to stabilize the fracture or separation.

25620

The physician makes a 7.5 cm longitudinal incision along the antero-lateral aspect of the distal forearm. The physician exposes the fracture by dissecting between the planes of muscles and tendons of the lateral wrist area while protecting the median nerve. The pronator quadratus muscle is severed from the radius. The physician then reduces the fracture or separation. A small T-plate is fixed to the proximal fragment with one or two screws. Usually no screw is inserted through the distal part of the plate since it acts as a buttress and helps hold the fracture in reduction. Direct visualization and separately reportable x-rays are used to confirm correct reduction and restoration of the joint surface. The pronator quadratus is replaced at its origin on the radius. The incision is repaired in multiple layers using sutures, staples, and/or Steri-strips. The arm is then immobilized in a cast. If the fracture of the distal radius is severely comminuted and is not suitable for internal fixation, then the physician may apply an external fixator device (e.g., Ace-Colles fixator). The external fixator is applied to the forearm and wrist to stabilize the fracture or separation after open reduction.

25622–25624

The physician treats a scaphoid fracture of the wrist without open surgery or manual manipulation in 25622. Separately reportable x-rays confirm the position and alignment of the bone. In 25624, manipulation of the bone is required. The patient may require anesthesia. The physician manipulates the area by pushing on the wrist bones, particularly the scaphoid. The physician also pulls on the fingers and forearm, moving the fractured area back into position. Separately reportable x-rays confirm alignment. In both 25662 and 25624, a cast is then placed on the wrist and forearm with a thumb spica to hold the fracture in position.

25628

The physician treats a fracture of the wrist scaphoid bone. An incision is made over the scaphoid bone. The physician extends the incision down to the bone and the fracture is identified. Soft tissue is debrided as necessary. The physician places the bone fragments in their correct anatomical position. Typically, screws are applied to hold the pieces together. An external fixation device may be applied. The physician then irrigates the wound and closes it in multiple layers. A cast or splint is applied to provide additional support of the area.

25630–25635

The physician performs closed treatment of a fracture of the carpal bone, each bone. Triquetrum fractures are usually nondisplaced and respond well to casting or splinting for six weeks. Capitate fractures are generally treated by conservative casting, immobilizing the wrist and thumb. Hamate fractures are accompanied by fractures at the base of the ulnar metacarpal, and become asymptomatic after a four to six week-period of immobilization. Lunate fractures are similarly treated by immobilization. Report 25630 if no manipulation is performed; report 25635 if manipulation is performed, each bone.

25645

The physician performs open treatment of a fracture of the carpal bone. Only some carpal bones are treated with open procedures. For hook of the hamate fractures, the physician makes an incision over the ulnar aspect of the wrist. The fracture is reduced and fixed with Kirschner wires, or the hook is excised. The tissue is closed in layers and a compression dressing is applied. Trapezium fractures are often treated with open surgery and may require secondary surgery to treat symptoms of pain. Capitate fractures — especially if associated with scaphoid fractures — are often treated with reduction and internal fixation via Kirschner wires. In cases in which Lunate fractures do not respond well to immobilization, the physician may elect open treatment. An incision is

made over the lunate to excise avulsed fragments. The soft tissue is closed in layers and a compression dressing is applied.

25650

The physician treats an ulnar styloid fracture with a cast or splint. No manual manipulation and no incisions are required.

25651

The physician performs percutaneous skeletal fixation of an ulnar styloid fracture. Following fixation of the ulnar styloid fragment, the remaining depressed articular fragments are elevated and reduced with traction, direct pressure, or with use of a small incision and application of pointed reduction clamps.

25652

If closed reduction of the ulnar styloid fracture is not possible, the physician extends an incision down to the bone and identifies the fracture. Soft tissue is debrided as necessary. The physician places the bone fragments in their correct anatomical position. The wound is irrigated and closed in multiple layers. A cast or splint is applied to provide additional support.

25660

The physician repairs the dislocation of radiocarpal or intercarpal bones with manipulation. Sustained traction is held while the physician applies force to reduce the dislocated bone(s) into the proper anatomical position. Immobilization post-reduction depends on the physician's preference.

25670

The physician performs an open treatment of radiocarpal or intercarpal dislocation, one or more bones. The physician makes a dorsal incision overlying the wrist, and the dislocation is reduced. If involved ligaments are torn, they are repaired to stabilize the reduction. The physician may use the overlying capsule to reinforce the stabilization. The soft tissue is closed in layers and a compression dressing is applied.

25671

Percutaneous pinning is commonly performed at 10 days from injury. The physician may use fluoroscopic guidance to perform an initial closed reduction and to insert pins from the radial styloid to the ulnar cortex of the radius for percutaneous fixation.

25675

The physician performs a closed treatment of distal radioulnar dislocation with manipulation. The physician reduces the dislocation by pronation (if the ulna is involved) and supination (if the ulna is dorsal). The arm is immobilized.

25676

The physician performs an open treatment a distal radioulnar dislocation, acute or chronic. For a locked dislocation or incongruous reduction, the physician opens the joint for reduction, and repairs the triangular fibrocartilage (TFC)/ulnar collateral ligament complex (UCLC), stabilizing the repair with Kirschner wires. The physician incises the dorsum of the wrist on the ulnar side. The proximal and ulnar half of the extensor retinaculum is raised radially. The extensor digiti minimi is retracted to reveal the TFC. The capsule is detached from the radius and reflected ulnar. After the dislocated joint is reduced, the TFC lesion may be repaired or reconstructed using a local or grafted tissue from the retinaculum, extensor carpi ulnaris, or flexor carpiulnaris. Kirschner wires may be used to stabilize the repair, after which the overlying soft tissue is sutured closed and a bulky dressing is applied.

25680

The physician performs closed treatment of a trans-scaphoperilunar type of fracture dislocation using manipulation. After being placed in continual traction for five to 10 minutes, the patient's hand is dorsiflexed while maintaining traction. While stabilizing the lunate volar, gradual palmar flexion reduces the capitate. The wrist is immobilized in a dorsal plaster thumb spica splint at 30 degrees volar flexion. Usually, if the scaphoid is properly reduced (visualized via separately reportable radiographs), the midcarpal joint is adequately reduced as well.

25685

The physician performs open treatment of trans-scaphoperilunar type of fracture dislocation. The physician makes a longitudinal, volar incision overlying the wrist, radial to the flexor carpi radialis tendon. This muscle is retracted toward the ulnar side, and the wrist joint is opened exposing the scaphoid fracture. After the fracture is reduced, Kirschner wires are drilled into the scaphoid to hold the reduction. If fixation of the scaphoid adequately stabilizes the midcarpal joint, no further fixation is required. If separately reportable radiographs visualize even the slightest tendency of volar subluxation, or rotary instability of the lunate, the volar incision must be extended and occasionally, a dorsal incision must be made. In such cases, additional Kirschner wires should be introduced to stabilize the capitate-lunate joint. If this operation is performed within two to three weeks of injury, bone grafting is not used. If open reduction is delayed for more than three weeks post-surgery, bone grafting (reported separately) may be used. Capsular and skin closure is performed.

25690

The physician treats a lunate dislocation with manipulation. During sustained traction, the physician applies force to reduce the dislocated lunate. Immobilization post reduction depends on the physician's preference.

25695

The physician performs an open lunate dislocation. The physician makes both dorsal and volar incisions over the wrist. Through the dorsal longitudinal incision, the extensor tendons are retracted. The proximal pole of the scaphoid is retracted to expose the capitate. Through the volar longitudinal incision, the flexor tendons and median nerve are retracted to the radial side exposing a tear in the volar capsule and ligaments. The dislocated lunate is reduced through the volar approach by manually pushing it back between the capitate and radius while an assistant applies axial traction through the hand. The physician repairs the capsular-ligamentous complex tear with nonabsorbable sutures. On the dorsal side, the physician reduces the proximal pole of the capitate into the distal concavity of the lunate. The proximal pole of the scaphoid is reduced. Kirschner wires are drilled into the scaphoid, lunate, and capitate for stabilization. The physician repairs the dorsal ligamentous complex. The skin is closed.

25800–25810

The physician performs fusion of the wrist joint, including the radiocarpal, intercarpal and/or carpometacarpal joints. The physician exposes the wrist through a dorsal, longitudinal incision. A dorsal tenosynovectomy is performed, and the wrist capsule is elevated exposing the radiocarpal joint. The physician excises the distal ulna and performs a synovectomy of the radiocarpal joint. The radial collateral ligament is released from the radial styloid. The cartilage and sclerotic bond is removed from the distal radius and proximal carpal row. Using an awl, the physician makes a channel in the medullary canal of the radius, through which a Steinman pin is used for internal fixation. The pin is drilled through the carpus to exit between the second and third, or between the third and fourth metacarpal, depending on alignment between the carpus and the radius. One or two small staples, or an obliquely-placed Kirschner, may be used to provide additional fixation on the radiocarpal joint. The position of the wrist can be varied only five to 10 degrees by adjusting the direction of the pin as it is driven into the radius. A drain is placed in the subcutaneous and prior to skin closure. A milky compression dressing is applied, and the wrist is splinted in the desired position of fusion. Report 25800 if performed without bone graft. Report 25805 if performed with sliding graft. Report 25810 if performed with iliac or other autograft.

25820–25825

The physician performs intercarpal or radiocarpal fusion. The physician makes a curved dorsal incision from the bases of the second and third metacarpal to the tubercle. The wrist joint capsule is opened via a longitudinal incision centered over the capitate-lunate joint. The dorsal three-quarters of the capitate, lunate, and scaphoid bones are removed. Approximately 25 degrees of wrist dorsiflexion will lock the graft in place. If the graft needs further stabilization, crossed Kirschner wires may be used for fixation. The skin is closed in layers. A separately reportable long-arm cast is placed for six weeks. This is followed by a short-arm gauntlet for an additional six weeks. Report 25820 if a graft is not used. Report 25825 if a fitted circular or rectangular corticocanulous graft from iliac crest is removed and precisely shaped to fit the recipient. This graft is fit into the proximal row carpal area that has been removed.

25830

The physician performs fusion of the distal radioulnar joint and resection of the ulna, sometimes using a bone graft. The physician makes a dorsal, curvilinear incision over the distal radioulnar joint. The extensor retinaculum is reflected, uncovering the extensor carpi ulnaris and extensor digiti minimi tendons. The capsule is cut and reflected, exposing the ulnar head. A small lamina spreader may be used to view the sigmoid notch of the radius. The periosteum is stripped from the ulna just proximal to the articular surface. The dorsal radioulnar ligaments are stripped sharply. If the distal ulna has been removed, or part of the distal ulna is missing, the remaining portion is decorticated. The radius is prepared by making a notch in the ulnar aspect where the distal ulna can be slotted. The ulna is manually compressed into the notch, holding the forearm in 10–15 degree pronation. The physician drives a Kirschner wire from the ulna into the radius and two compression screws from the outer aspect of the ulna through both cortices of the radius. The extensor retinaculum is reconstructed and the skin is closed.

25900

In elective below-elbow amputations, the physician cuts the soft tissue flaps distal to the intended level of bone amputation. The physician dissects the superficial veins and cuts them at the level of the amputation. Cutaneous nerves are cut proximal to the level of the amputation. The dorsal and volar antebrachial fascia is cut, and, depending on the level of amputation, either the tendons or muscle bellies are divided after the radial and ulnar vessels are severed. Muscle bellies are incised just distal to the planned level of bony resection. Nerves are cut through a separate incision, and brought under the muscle. The anterior and posterior interosseous vessels should be ligated or coagulated with electrocautery. An incision in the periosteum is carried out sharply and circumferentially. The bone is transected at the desired level at this time and the specimen is removed. The bone ends are smoothed with a rasp. Closure is accomplished after hemostasis is obtained following tourniquet release. The skin flaps can be fashioned, and subcutaneous tissue and skin are closed in separate layers. A drain is sometimes placed. The stump is dressed and wrapped with an elastic bandage applied more firmly distally than proximally.

25905

The physician performs a guillotine amputation. Just distal to the level of intended bone section, the physician incises the skin in a circular manner down to the deep fascia and allows it to retract. The muscles at the edge of the retracted skin are divided. All vessels encountered are ligated and divided. All major nerves are divided at a proximal level so that they retract proximal to the end of the stump. The physician sections the bone at the ends of the retracted muscles. The bone end is covered by the distal muscle bulk, and the skin is stretched over the stump and sutured closed. The stump is covered with a compressive dressing to control post-surgical edema.

25907

The physician performs secondary closure or scar revision after the stump has granulated or healed by a scar. In this procedure, no additional bone is sectioned. The physician resects the scar and granulation tissue from the end of the stump. Skin flaps are fashioned as close as possible to the thick scar surrounding the granulating wound. The dense layer of scar tissue is excised from over the end of the bone. Additional muscle may be removed as well. The skin flaps are pulled over the end of the stump and connected with nonabsorbable sutures. A temporary drain or suction tubes may also be used.

25909

The physician performs a reamputation. A reamputation may be necessary at a proximal level to reach healthy tissue. The physician cuts the soft tissue flaps distal to the intended level of bone amputation. The physician dissects the superficial veins and cuts them at the level of the amputation. Cutaneous nerves are cut proximal to the level of the amputation. The dorsal and volar antebrachial fascia is cut, and, depending on the level of amputation, either the tendons or muscle bellies are divided after the radial and ulnar vessels are severed. Muscle bellies are incised just distal to the planned level of bony resection. Nerves are cut through a separate incision, and brought under the muscle. The anterior and posterior interosseous vessels should be ligated or coagulated with electrocautery. An incision in the periosteum is carried out sharply and circumferentially. The bone is transected at the desired level at this time and the specimen is removed. The bone ends are smoothed with a rasp. Closure is accomplished after hemostasis is obtained following tourniquet release. The skin flaps can be fashioned and subcutaneous tissue and skin are closed.

25915

The physician performs the Krukenberg procedure, a forearm amputation. The physician longitudinally splits the stump into radial and ulnar rays by making a dorsal, longitudinal incision toward the ulnar aspect of the forearm. Also, a volar, longitudinal incision is made toward the radial aspect of the forearm. The muscles left or transferred to the radial side of the forearm are the radial wrist extensors and flexors, the flexors of the index and long fingers, the index and long finger extensors, the pronator tercs, the palmaris longus, and the brachioradialis. The remaining muscles are left or inserted on the ulnar side of the forearm. On occasion, some muscles need resection to reduce bulk, but the pronator tercs must be preserved. The interosseous membrane is freed along its ulnar border. Skin closure is performed, ensuring the tactile skin is placed over the contact surfaces between the radius and ulna.

25920–25924

The physician disarticulates (amputates) the hand from the forearm through the wrist. The physician makes a long, palmar flap and a short, dorsal flap at a level distal to the radioulnar joint. These flaps are pulled back proximally and all veins are ligated. The physician cuts the superficial branch of the radial nerve and the dorsal sensory branch of the ulnar nerve. The lateral and medial antebrachial cutaneous nerves are cut. The radial and ulnar blood vessels are severed proximate to the wrist. The median nerve is cut while traction is applied. The flexor and extensor tendons are pulled distally and cut. The physician makes a transverse, dorsal incision of the dorsal radiocarpal ligament to view the radiocarpal joint. Circumferential dissection of the radiocarpal capsular and ligamentous attachments are carried out. The amputated specimen is removed. The styloid processes are rounded off, and the skin flaps are closed in two layers of subcutaneous tissue and skin. A soft dressing is applied distal to proximal. Report 25920 if an amputation through the wrist is performed. Report 25922 if a secondary closure or scar revision is performed on the stump. Report 25924 if a re-amputation is performed. All use a similar technique.

25927–25931

The physician amputates the fingers. The physician makes circumferential incisions around each digit excluding the thumb. These incisions are carried out at the mid-proximophalangeal level. The extensor digitonum communis of each digit (also the extensor indicis proprius of the index and the extensor digiti minimi of the little) are transected at the metacarpal bases. Individually, each metacarpal bone is transected and elevated from its soft tissue bed. The lumbar cals and dorsal interossei are sectioned. Identified blood vessels are ligated. Nerves are ligated and transected. The flexor tendons are transected and allowed to retract in the palm. The volar plate, ligaments, and palmar fascia at this level are all cut and amputated digits are removed. The open periosteal tubes are closed. The soft tissue flaps are drawn over the end of the stump, and interrupted sutures are used. A soft dressing is applied. Report 25927 if an amputation is performed. Report 25929 if a secondary closure or scar revision is performed. Report 25931 if a re-amputation is performed. All use a similar technique.

26010–26011

The physician drains an abscess located in a finger. In 26010, the physician lances an abscess located in the cutaneous tissue of a finger. In 26011, the abscess just reaches deep subcutaneous tissue and requires debridement and irrigation. The wound may be left open to drain.

26020

The physician drains fluid located in a tendon sheath located in a finger or in the palm. The physician incises the skin above the affected sheath and dissects to the tendon sheath. The sheath is lanced and drained. An irrigation catheter may be placed and the wound is irrigated for up to 48 hours. The operative incision is closed in sutured layers.

26025–26030

The physician drains a palmar bursa or multiple bursas located on the ulnar or radial side of the palm. The physician incises the skin over the bursa and dissects to the bursa. The bursa is lanced and irrigated with a catheter. The catheter is removed and the operative incision is closed in sutured layers. Report 26025 for a single bursa, report 26030 for multiple and/or complicated bursas.

26034

The physician opens the bone cortex to remove diseased bone. The physician incises the overlying skin and dissects to the bone. The periosteum is incised and lifted to expose the defect. The diseased bone is cureted and removed. The periosteum is closed and the operative incision is closed in sutured layers.

26035

The physician decompresses fingers and/or a hand damaged due to an injection injury. The physician incises the skin overlying the entry point of the injection injury. The tissue is dissected to the fascial or periosteal layers and injected material is removed. If the injected material has followed the periosteum or fascia proximally, the incision length is increased until all the injected material is removed. The wound is irrigated and closed in sutured layers.

26037

The physician decompresses the hand fascia. The physician incises the skin overlying the affected fascia. The fascia is incised and the underlying tissues are irrigated. The operative incision is closed in sutured layers.

CPT® Lay Descriptions

26040–26045

The physician incises the palmar fascia to release a Dupuytren's contracture. A Dupuytren's contracture is a shortening of the palmar fascia resulting in flexion deformity of a finger. In 26040, the physician makes a stab wound through the subcutaneous to the palmar fascia, which is incised. In 26045, the subcutaneous tissue is incised and retracted to expose the palmar fascia. The palmar fascia is incised to relieve tension and allow the hand to extend correctly. The operative wound is closed in sutured layers.

26055

The physician makes an incision in a tendon sheath to release tension in the tendon. (For example, this procedure would be performed to relieve trigger finger.) The physician incises the skin overlying the tendon and dissects to the tendon sheath The sheath is incised lengthwise. The operative incision is closed in sutured layers.

26060

The physician incises a tendon at the subcutaneous level. The physician incises the overlying skin. The tendon is severed through the subcutaneous tissue. The operative incision is closed in sutured layers. Report each digit separately.

26070–26080

The physician incises an infected joint and drains excess fluid or removes a loose or foreign body. The physician incises the overlying skin and dissects to the joint. The infected joint and surrounding tissue are explored. If excess fluid exists, the fluid is drained and a tube may be placed for drainage and/or irrigation. If a loose or foreign body is located, it is removed. The operative incision is closed in sutured layers. Report 26070 for the carpometacarpal joint, 26075 for the metacarpophalangeal joint, or 26080 for each interphalangeal joint.

26100–26110

The physician incises a joint to retrieve synovial fluid or tissue for biopsy. The physician incises the overlying skin and dissects to the joint. A syringe is injected through the synovial membrane and a small sample of synovial fluid or tissue is obtained. The operative incision is closed in sutured layers. Report 26100 for the carpometacarpal joint, 26105 for each metacarpophalangeal joint, or 26110 for each interphalangeal joint.

26115–26116

The physician excises a tumor or vascular malformation in a hand or finger. The physician incises the overlying skin and dissects to the tumor or vascular malformation. The blood vessels are ligated and the defective tissue or tumor is excised. The operative incision is closed in sutured layers. In 26115, the defect is located under the subcutaneous

tissue. In 26116, the defect is in deep, subfascial, intramuscular tissue.

26117

The physician performs a radical resection to remove a tumor from the soft tissue of a hand or finger. The skin overlying the tumor is incised and the surrounding tissue is dissected. The margins are sent to pathology and the wound is extended until margins are cleared. The skin is reapproximated over the remaining tissue and sutured closed.

26121–26125

The physician removes the palmar fascia. The physician incises the overlying skin and subcutaneous tissue. The palmar fascia is exposed and resected. Tendon sheaths are freed. The operative is closed in sutured layers if possible. Z-plasties are performed or skin grafts are obtained to close the wound if necessary. In 26121, the entire palmar fascia is removed. In 26123, part of the palmar fascia is removed and flexor tendons at proximal interphalangeal joints are released. Use 26125 to report additional digits.

26130

The physician removes the synovial membrane from the carpometacarpal joint. The physician incises the skin overlying the affected joint and the tissues are dissected. The joint capsule is incised and the synovium is removed. The operative incision is closed in sutured layers.

26135

The physician removes the synovial membrane from the metacarpophalangeal joint and reconstructs the intrinsic release and extensor hood. The physician incises the skin overlying the affected joint and the tissues are dissected. The joint capsule is incised and the synovium is removed. Ulnar deviation is corrected by intrinsic release (the tightening of the radial tendons). The hood of the joint is reconstructed. The operative incision is closed in sutured layers. Report each finger separately.

26140

The physician removes the synovial membrane from the proximal interphalangeal joint and reconstructs the extensor articulation. The physician incises the skin overlying the affected joint and the tissues are dissected. The joint capsule is incised and the synovium is removed. The extensor tendons are reattached to the joint. The operative incision is closed in sutured layers. Report each finger separately.

26145

The physician removes the synovial membrane from a flexor tendon sheath at the palm or finger. The physician incises the skin overlying the affected tendon. The tissue is dissected to the tendon sheath and the synovium is excised. The tendon is freed from surrounding tissue and the operative incision is closed in sutured layers. Report each tendon separately.

26160

The physician excises a lesion of the tendon sheath or joint capsule, such as a cyst or ganglion. The physician incises the overlying skin and dissects to locate the affected area. The lesion, cyst, or ganglion is identified and excised from the tendon sheath or joint capsule. The operative incision is closed in sutured layers.

26170–26180

The physician excises a flexor tendon in the palm or finger. The physician incises the overlying skin and dissects to the flexor tendon. The tendon is freed and resected. The operative incision is closed in sutured layers. Report 26170 for each palm flexor tendon, report 26180 for each finger flexor tendon.

26185

This procedure is rarely performed, but may be necessary in cases of sesamoid fracture or when performing a metacarpal-sesamoid synostosis. The physician makes a midlateral incision over the metacarpophalangeal joint of the thumb on the radial side. The radial side of the extensor apparatus is opened, and the radial carpal ligament is dissected. The opponens pollicis muscle is separated from its attachment to the metacarpal neck. The metacarpophalangeal joint is opened through incision. In the case of a fracture, the fractured bone is exposed and removed. In a synostosis, the lateral sesamoid bone is exposed, its cartilage is removed along with the cortex of the first metacarpal neck. Drill holes are placed in the metacarpal neck and a wire suture is passed around the sesamoid bone. The capsule and overlying tissue are sutured closed.

26200–26215

The physician removes a bone cyst or benign tumor in the metacarpal or proximal, middle, or distal phalanx of a finger. The physician incises the skin overlying the cyst or tumor and dissects to locate the bony defect. The tumor is excised or cureted from the bone. If a graft is needed for reconstruction, it is obtained from the distal radius or iliac crest. In 26200 the defect is located in a metacarpal bone; report 26205 if an autograft is obtained. In 26210 the defect is located in the proximal, middle, or distal phalanx of a finger; report 26215 if an autograft is obtained and used.

26230–26236

The physician excises part of a bone. The physician incises the skin overlying the affected bone. The bone defect is identified and removed creating a saucer or crater-like hole in the bone. The skin is reapproximated and sutured closed. Report 26230 for a metacarpal excision, 26235 for a proximal or middle

phalanx of finger, or 26236 for a distal phalanx of a finger.

26250–26262

The physician radically resects a bone for, e.g., a tumor. The physician incises the overlying skin and dissects to determine the extent of invasion. The bone and surrounding tissues are resected. If a graft is needed for reconstruction, it is obtained from the distal radius or iliac crest. Skin is approximated over the remaining digit and sutured in layers. In 26250, the metacarpal bone is excised; report 26255 if an autograft is obtained and used. In 26260, the proximal or middle phalanx of finger is excised; report 26261 if an autograft is obtained and used. In 26262 the distal phalanx of a finger is excised (no graft is possible as the entire finger is excised).

26320

The physician removes a previously placed implant from a finger or hand. The physician incises the overlying skin and dissects to the implant. The implant is removed and the operative incision is closed in sutured layers.

26340

Manipulation of the finger joint under anesthesia may be necessary to regain the loss of motion following a surgical procedure or due to scar tissue. Following the induction of general anesthesia, the physician evaluates the finger. The finger is manipulated by stretching, rotation, and other maneuvers to gain the appropriate range of motion.

26350–26352

The physician repairs or advances a single tendon not located in "no man's land." "No man's land" is located between the A1 pulley and the insertion of the superficialis tendon. The physician incises the skin overlying the proximal or distal phalanx and dissects to the tendon. The tendon is repaired with sutures or advanced to improve joint function. Primary repair is done immediately after injury. Secondary repair is done sometime after the incident of injury. If a graft is needed for secondary repair, it is obtained from the palmaris longus tendon or from the foot. The operative incision is closed in sutured layers. Report 26350 for each primary or secondary tendon repair without autograft. Report 26352 for each secondary tendon repair with autograft.

26356–26358

The physician repairs or advances a single tendon located in "no man's land." "No man's land" is located between the A1 pulley and the insertion of the superficialis tendon. The physician incises the skin overlying the medial phalanx and dissects to the tendon. The tendon is repaired with sutures or advanced to improve joint function. Primary repair is done immediately after injury. Secondary repair is done sometime after the incident of injury. If a graft is needed for secondary repair, it is obtained from the palmaris longus tendon or from the foot. The operative incision is closed in sutured layers. Report 26356 for each primary tendon repair without autograft. Report 26357 for each secondary tendon repair without autograft. Report 26358 for each secondary tendon repair with autograft.

26370–26373
The physician repairs or advances the profundus flexor tendon; the superficialis tendon is intact. The physician incises the skin overlying the damaged tendon. The tendon is repaired with sutures or advanced to improve joint function. Primary repair is done immediately after injury. Secondary repair is done sometime after the incident of injury. If a graft is needed for secondary repair, it is obtained from the palmaris longus tendon or from the foot. The operative incision is closed in sutured layers. Report 26370 for each primary tendon repair without graft. Report 26372 for each secondary tendon repair with free graft. Report 26373 for each secondary tendon repair without free graft.

26390
The physician excises a flexor tendon in a finger or hand and implants a synthetic rod for delayed tendon graft. The physician incises the overlying skin and dissects to the tendon. The tendon is freed. The proximal and distal ends are severed and the tendon is removed. The physician implants a synthetic rod so the surrounding tissue will form a natural tube for a tendon graft. The operative incision is closed. This code is reported once for each rod that is implanted.

26392
The physician removes a synthetic rod used to create a natural location for a tube graft and inserts a flexor tendon graft. The physician incises the overlying skin and dissects to the rod. The rod is removed. A graft is obtained from the palmaris longus tendon or from the foot and inserted in the new position. The proximal and distal ends are sutured into place and the operative incision is closed in sutured layers. This code is reported once for each rod that is removed and replaced by a tendon graft.

26410–26412
The physician repairs or advances a single extensor tendon located in the hand. The physician incises the skin overlying the tendon. The tendon is repaired with sutures or advanced to improve joint function. Primary repair is done immediately after injury. Secondary repair is done sometime after the incident of injury. If a graft is needed for secondary repair, it is obtained from the palmaris longus tendon or from the foot. The operative incision is closed in sutured layers. Report 26410 for each primary or secondary tendon repair without free graft. Report 26412 for each secondary tendon repair with free graft.

26415
The physician excises an extensor tendon in a finger or hand and implants a synthetic rod for delayed tendon graft. The physician incises the overlying skin and dissects to the tendon. The tendon is freed. The proximal and distal ends are severed and the tendon is removed. The physician implants a synthetic rod so the surrounding tissue will form a natural tube for a tendon graft. The operative incision is closed. This code is reported once for each rod that is implanted.

26416
The physician removes a synthetic rod used to create a natural location for a tube graft and inserts an extensor tendon graft. The physician incises the overlying skin and dissects to the rod. The rod is removed. A graft is obtained from the palmaris longus tendon or from the foot and inserted in the new position. The proximal and distal ends are sutured into place and the operative incision is closed in sutured layers. This code is reported once for each rod that is removed and replaced by a tendon graft.

26418–26420
The physician repairs or advances a single extensor tendon located in the finger. The physician incises the skin overlying the tendon. The tendon is repaired with sutures or advanced to improve joint function. Primary repair is done immediately after injury. Secondary repair is done sometime after the incident of injury. If a graft is needed for secondary repair, it is obtained from the palmaris longus tendon or from the foot. The operative incision is closed in sutured layers. Report 26418 for each primary or secondary tendon repair without free graft. Report 26420 for each secondary tendon repair with free graft.

26426–26428
The physician repairs or advances the central slip extensor tendon sometime after the injury. The physician incises the skin overlying the tendon. The tendon is repaired with sutures or advanced to improve joint function. If a graft is needed for secondary repair, it is obtained from the lateral bands or from the foot. The operative incision is closed in sutured layers. Report 26426 for each finger repair with local tissues. Report 26248 for each finger repair with a free graft.

26432
The physician repairs the distal insertion extensor tendon without incising the skin. The physician uses a splint to pin the finger in an extended position. If extensive damage occurred during injury, pins may be used to stabilize the joint.

26433–26434
The physician repairs the distal insertion extensor tendon, using a graft if necessary. The physician incises the overlying skin and dissects to the damaged tendon. The tendon is repaired with sutures to

improve joint function. If a graft is needed for secondary repair, it is obtained from the palmaris longus tendon or from the foot. The operative incision is closed in sutured layers. Report 26433 for primary or secondary repair without a graft, report 26434 for primary or secondary repair requiring a graft.

26437

The physician realigns an extensor tendon in the hand. The physician incises the overlying skin and dissects to the damaged tendon. The tendon is realigned to correct finger position. The operative incision is closed in sutured layers. Report each tendon separately.

26440–26442

The physician removes scar tissue to release a flexor tendon in a finger or palm. The physician incises the overlying tissue and dissects to the affected tendon. The scar tissue is debrided and removed, freeing the tendon. The operative incision is closed in sutured layers. In 26440 repair is limited to the palm or finger. In 26442, repair extends to the hand and finger. Report each tendon separately.

26445–26449

The physician removes scar tissue to release an extensor tendon in a finger or the dorsum of hand. The physician incises the overlying tissue and dissects to the affected tendon. The scar tissue is debrided and removed, freeing the tendon. The operative incision is closed in sutured layers. In 26445 repair is limited to the hand or finger. In 26449, repair extends to the finger, including forearm. Report each tendon separately.

26450–26455

The physician incises a flexor tendon. The physician incises the overlying skin and dissects to the flexor tendon. The tendon is incised. The operative incision is closed in sutured layers. In 26450, the tendon is located in the palm. In 26455, the tendon is located in a finger. Report each tendon separately.

26460

The physician incises an extensor tendon in a hand or finger. The physician incises the overlying skin and dissects to the extensor tendon. The tendon is incised. The operative incision is closed in sutured layers. Report each tendon separately.

26471–26474

The physician sutures the tendon to the proximal or distal interphalangeal joint for stabilization. The physician incises the overlying skin and dissects to the joint. The tendon is incised and sutured over the joint space, providing joint stabilization. The operative incision is closed in sutured layers. In 26471, the proximal joint is stabilized. In 26474, the

distal joint is stabilized. Report each tendon separately.

26476

The physician lengthens an extensor tendon in a hand or a finger. The physician incises the overlying skin and dissects to the tendon. The physician performs step cuts to lengthen the tendon. The operative incision is closed in sutured layers. Report each tendon separately.

26477

The physician shortens an extensor tendon in a hand or a finger. The physician incises the overlying skin and dissects to the tendon. The physician removes a section of the tendon and sutures the ends back together, shortening the tendon. The operative incision is closed in sutured layers. Report each tendon separately.

26478

The physician lengthens a flexor tendon in a hand or a finger. The physician incises the overlying skin and dissects to the tendon. The physician performs step cuts to lengthen the tendon. The operative incision is closed in sutured layers. Report each tendon separately.

26479

The physician shortens a flexor tendon in the hand or finger. The physician incises the overlying skin and dissects to the tendon. The physician removes a section of the tendon and sutures the ends back together, shortening the tendon. The operative incision is closed in sutured layers. Report each tendon separately.

26480–26489

The physician transfers or transplants a tendon; a free tendon graft may be used if necessary. The physician incises the overlying skin and dissects to the tendon to be moved. The tendon is freed, transferred and sutured into place. If a free tendon graft is used, it is obtained from the palmaris longus tendon or from the foot. The operative incision is closed in sutured layers. For transfer or transplant of a carpometacarpal or dorsum of hand tendon without a free graft report 26480 for each tendon; report 26483 if a free graft is used. For transfer or transplant of a palmar tendon without a free graft, report 26485 for each tendon; report 26489 if a free tendon graft is used.

26490–26494

The physician transfers the superficialis tendon to restore palmar abduction to the thumb. The physician incises the overlying skin and dissects to the superficialis tendon. The tendon is freed and transferred to restore function. If a graft is used, the graft is obtained from the palmaris longus or the abductor digiti minimi. The graft is approximated and sutured into place. The operative incision is closed in sutured layers. Report 26490 if no graft is used. Report 26492 if a graft is used. Report each tendon separately. In 26494 the hypothenar muscle is transferred. The muscle tendon is resected from its distal attachment, transferred to the site and sutured into place.

26496

The physician performs this procedure when opposition of the thumb is lost because of median nerve paralysis. Methods described using this code include (1) attaching the extensor pollicis brevis to the extensor carpi ulnaris around the ulnar border of the wrist; (2) attaching the extensor carpi radialis longus to the extensor pollicis longus around the ulnar border of the wrist; (3) attaching the extensor indicis proprius tendon, with a small portion of the extensor hood, to the flexor pollicis longus tendon just distal to the metacarpophalangeal (MP) joint; (4) attachment of the extensor digiti minimi around the ulnar border of the wrist to the thumb MP joint; (5) attachment of the extensor indicis proprius with a small portion of the extensor hood around the ulnar border of the wrist to the thumb MP joint; (6) transfer of the adductor pollicis to the tendon of the superficial head of the flexor pollicis brevis; (7) attachment of the flexor pollicis longus around the ulnar aspect of the flexor carpi ulnaris into the abductor pollicis brevis pularthrodesis of the interphalangeal joint.

26497–26498

The physician transfers a tendon to restore intrinsic function to the fingers. The physician incises the overlying skin and dissects to the affected tendon. The tendon is freed, transferred and sutured into place to restore function to the of the flexor digitorum profundus. The operative incision is closed in sutured layers. In 26497, intrinsic function is restored to the ring and small finger. In 26498, intrinsic function is restored to all four fingers.

26499

The physician corrects a claw finger. The superficialis technique involves splitting the flexor digitonum superficialis of the long finger into four slips. One slip is passed through the lumbrical canal of each finger to be inserted into the radial lateral band of the dorsal apparatus. This slip is sutured with the wrist in 30 degrees palmar flexion, the MP joints in 80 to 90 degree flexion, and the interphalangeal joints in full extension. In the dorsal approach, the tendon slips of the extensor carpi radialis brevis are passed superficial to the dorsal carpal ligament, through the intermetacarpal spaces, through the lumbrical canal volar to the deep transverse metacarpal ligament. The tendon is attached to the radial lateral bands of the long, ring and little fingers, and the ulnar lateral band of the index finger. A modification of the latter procedure involves detaching the extensor carpi radialis longus at its insertion and passing it deep to

the brachioradialis to the volar sides of the forearm proximate to the wrist. The grafts of the plantaris or palmaris tendons are used. The lateral bands are identified through dorsoradial incisions over the proximal phalanx (except the index finger, which has the ulnar lateral band exposed). The tendon slips are directed through the carpal tunnel volar to the deep transverse metacarpal ligament and into the lateral bands. The tendons are sutured with the wrist dorsiflexed 45 degrees, the MP joints are flexed 70 degrees, and the interphalangeal joints are fixed at zero degrees. Incisions are closed.

26500–26504

The physician reconstructs a tendon pulley. The physician incises the overlying skin and dissects to the damaged pulley located in the A1 position or the distal interphalangeal joint position. In 26500, the tendon pulley is reconstructed using neighboring tissue. In 26502, the physician obtains a fascial graft for reconstruction. In 26504, a tendon prosthesis is used for reconstruction.

26508

The physician incises the thenar muscle to release, for example, thumb contracture. The physician incises the overlying skin and dissects to the thenar muscle. The scarred muscle tissue is incised to release contracture. The operative incision is closed in sutured layers.

26510

The physician performs a cross intrinsic transfer to restore anatomic position and intrinsic function to the fingers. The physician incises the overlying skin and dissects to the affected tendons. The ulnar tendon is resected and transferred to the radial side of the joint, where it is sutured into place. The operative incision is closed in sutured layers.

26516–26518

The physician performs a capsulodesis to stabilize the metacarpophalangeal joint. The physician incises the overlying the skin and dissects to the M-P joint. The capsule of the joint is sutured to the proximal and distal bones to stabilize the joint. The operative incision is closed in sutured layers. In 26516 one digit is repaired. In 26517 two digits are repaired. In 26518 three or four digits are repaired.

26520–26525

The physician removes or incises the joint capsule to release contracture and restore function. The physician incises the overlying the skin and dissects to the metacarpophalangeal joint. The capsule of the joint is incised or resected and removed. The operative incision is closed in sutured layers. In 26520, the capsulectomy or capsulotomy is performed on the metacarpophalangeal joint. In 26525 the capsulectomy or capsulotomy is performed on the interphalangeal joint. Report each joint separately.

26530–26531

The physician performs an arthroplasty on the metacarpophalangeal joint. The physician incises the overlying the skin and dissects to the M-P joint. In 26530 the joint is reconstructed using neighboring tissue. In 26531, a prosthetic joint is used to replace the diseased joint. Report each joint separately. Report each tendon separately.

26535–26536

The physician performs an arthroplasty on the interphalangeal joint. The physician incises the overlying the skin and dissects to the I-P joint. In 26535 the joint is reconstructed using neighboring tissue. In 26536, a prosthetic joint is used to replace the diseased joint. Report each joint separately.

26540–26542

The physician performs a primary repair on a collateral ligament of a metacarpophalangeal joint, possibly using a graft or advancement. The physician incises the overlying the skin and dissects to the M-P joint. In 26540, the ligament is repaired with sutures. In 26541, a palmaris longus tendon or fascial graft is obtained. The graft is sutured into place. In 26542, an adductor tendon is advanced and sutured into place to stabilize the joint. The operative incision is closed in sutured layers.

26545

The physician uses a graft to repair a collateral ligament of an interphalangeal joint. The physician incises the overlying the skin and dissects to the I-P joint. A palmaris longus tendon or fascial graft is obtained and sutured into place. to stabilize the joint. The operative incision is closed in sutured layers. Report each joint separately.

26546

The physician performs this procedure to promote healing of a fractured phalanx or metacarpal that fails to heal. The physician makes an incision overlying the dorsal aspect of the fracture of the digit. The extensor mechanism is retracted and the fracture is exposed. Surgical resection of the nonunion itself may be performed. If this resection takes place, fibrous tissue must be removed until there are freshened fracture ends. If a resultant gap produces unacceptable shortening. Fixation such as Kirschner wires or pins, or AO plates is applied. The physician closes the incision with sutures.

26548

The physician repairs a volar plate of an interphalangeal joint. The physician incises the overlying the skin and dissects to the I-P joint. The plate of the joint is sutured to the proximal and distal bones to stabilize the joint. The operative incision is closed in sutured layers.

26550

The physician replaces all or part of a thumb with the index finger. The extent of an index finger used is determined by the size of the defect. The physician harvests the index finger with its tendons, blood vessels, and nerves intact and transfers the digit to the thenar eminence. If the thenar eminence must be created, the physician will transfer the index metacarpal along with the digit. If the index metacarpal is not needed, it is removed to provide space for function. The tendons are sutured to the new digit to provide abduction function. The skin is reapproximated and closed in sutured layers.

26551

The physician performs this procedure to provide functional thumb reconstruction in cases of traumatic thumb amputation and congenital absence of the thumb. Two surgical teams are employed, one at the hand and the other at the foot. One physician makes a linear incision over the dorsal aspect of the foot, traveling from proximal to distal, aiming toward the great toe. This incision stops at the base of the toe and a circular incision is made around the toe. The medial and lateral dorsal foot flaps are raised. The first dorsal metatarsal artery (FDMA) and deep peroneal nerve (DPN) are identified and exposed proximally to the dorsalis pedis artery (DPA). The portion of the DPA that passes to the plantar side of the foot is ligated. On the plantar surface, the flexor hallicis longus (FHL) is identified along with the plantar digital nerves and arteries on either side. The physician dissects into the web space between the great and second toes where the first plantar metatarsal artery (FPMA) is divided, as are vessels to the second toe. The DPN is split and the fibers to the great toe are divided. On the plantar surface, the digital nerves are divided. The FHL is divided through a separate incision in the midfoot, and is pulled into the distal wound. The tourniquet is released and adequate circulation is confirmed. The great toe is perfused for 20 minutes prior to completion of the dissection and transfer to the hand. The second surgical team begins preparing the hand soon after toe dissection begins. The physician on this team make a radially based palmar thumb skin flap. The dorsal incision extends into the wrist area where the cephalic vein, superficial radial nerve, dorsal dominant branch of the radial artery, and extensor tendons are identified. A transverse incision is made over the volar wrist to allow identification of the flexor pollicis longus (FPL). The thumb metacarpal or phalanx is cut squarely at a right angle to two vertically placed interosseous compression wires and longitudinally placed K-wire, which helps hold the digit in extension. Extensor tendon and flexor tendon repairs are performed. The abductor and adductor tendons are repaired to the extensor mechanism. The vascular repairs are completed using standard microvascular techniques. The superficial radial nerve and DPN are joined dorsally, and the digital nerve repairs are completed volarly. The skin is closed with drains. If a skin graft is necessary, it is placed dorsally over the area of the dorsal veins. The donor site is closed by removal of the metatarsal condyles and suturing of the volar plate and sesamoids to the distal metatarsal.

26553–26554

The physician sometimes uses this procedure in cases of traumatic thumb amputation or congenital absence. Two surgical teams are used to complete the transfer. The first team makes a linear incision over the dorsal aspect of the foot, lateral to the dorsalis pedis artery (DPA), traveling from proximal to distal, aiming toward the second toe. Depending on the joint used, the physician may save skin for a graft. The physician harvests two veins in the foot, the dorsalis pedis and metatarsal arteries, the deep peroneal nerve branch, and the extensor tendon to the second toe, and performs an osteotomy at the joint needed. Digital nerves are harvested from the plantar surface. The second team prepares for the toe by making an incision over the wrists where the cephalic vein, superficial radial nerve, dorsal dominant branch of the radial artery, and the flexor pollicis longus (FPL). The thumb metacarpal or phalanx is cut squarely at a right angle to its long axis after appropriate measurement. If the toe is being transferred to a different finger position, the vein, superficial nerve, digital artery, and extensor tendon are all dissected. To attach the toes to the needed position, the physician affixes the bones by crossed Kirschner wires. The flexor muscles are attached to those of the toe. The digital nerves are repaired, and the palmar wounds are closed. The extensor tendons are attached, followed by the approximation of the dorsal sensory nerves, followed by vascular anastomoses. Incisions are closed using sutures. Report 26554 if more than one toe must be transferred because of finger/thumb deficit.

26555

The physician removes a digit, including the metacarpal bone, to improve hand function following trauma or disease. The physician incises the skin overlying the damaged bone. The bone, tendons, nerves, and muscles are removed. The remaining fingers are reapproximated and sutured to provide correct positioning. The skin is reapproximated and closed in sutured layers.

26556

The physician performs this procedure if finger joint function is absent, disturbed, or destroyed because of congenital malformation, trauma, or disease. The graft may be an autograft or allograft. Techniques include (1) toe proximal interphalangeal joint (PIPJ) transfer for finger metacarpophalangeal joint (MPJ) and PIPJ reconstruction; (2) metatarsophalangeal (MTPJ) transfer for MPJ or trapeziometacarpal (TMJ) reconstruction; (3) PIPJ or digital interphalangeal joint (DIPJ) "finger bank" transfer. If performing the toe PIPJ transfer for finger PIPJ reconstruction, the physician will engage two teams to prepare the donor

and recipient sites simultaneously. One physician makes a longitudinal dorsal incision overlying the toe. The dorsalis pedis and first dorsal metatarsal arteries are dissected, as are dorsal veins. The tibial-side digital artery is divided distally at the level of the DIPJ. The fibular side artery is ligated. The extensor mechanism is cut proximally and distally and the joint is isolated by distal disarticulation through the DIPJ and proximal osteotomy through the first phalanx. The second team prepares the hand by excising the involved PIPJ and dissecting a suitable artery. The toe joint is transferred and stabilized with an intraosseous wire and longitudinal Kirschner wire. The extensor mechanism from the toe is attached to that of the finger. The artery from the toe is attached to that of the finger. At least two veins from the foot are sutured to veins of the hand. The foot wound is closed. The hand wound is also sutured closed. If performing the toe MTPJ transfer for MPJ reconstruction, the physician makes a curved incision to expose the finger joint. The ulnar side of the extensor hood is incised and retracted, and the joint is resected. The radial artery and the cephalic vein are identified through a separate incision. A small branch of the superficial radial nerve is dissected at the wrist level to be sutured to the nerve of the transplanted joint. The donor site is prepared by dissection of the great saphenous vein and first dorsal metatarsal artery. The terminal branch of the deep peroneal nerve is dissected. The toe graft is turned 180 degrees around its longitudinal axis, from dorsal to volar, and attached to the finger. The physician uses a Kirschner wire and anastomoses the vessels. The extensor mechanism is sutured and the skin is closed. The donor site is filled either with the finger joint or by bone graft.

26560–26562

The physician repairs a syndactyly (web finger) using skin flaps and grafts. The physician incises the skin of the web for digital release and the underlying tissues are freed. In 26560, the repair is accomplished with skin flaps from the incision area. In 26561, the physician obtains grafts to provide skin coverage. In 26562, the syndactyly is complex and involves the phalangeal bones and fingernails. When possible, the bones are separated. Bone grafts are obtained when necessary for reconstruction. When reconstruction is complete, the skin is reapproximated and closed in sutured layers.

26565–26567

The physician performs an osteotomy to correct the metacarpal or phalanx. The physician incises the skin and dissects to the bone. The bone is incised and removed. The operative incision is closed in sutured layers. In 26565 a metacarpal is corrected, in 26567, a phalanx of the finger is corrected.

26568

The physician performs an osteoplasty to lengthen a metacarpal or phalanx. The physician incises the skin and dissects to the defective bone. The periosteum is incised and pulled away from the bone. The bone is cut and the proximal and distal ends are distanced. The periosteum is laid over the bone, and the operative incision is closed in sutured layers. The hand is splinted in anatomic position until bone callous is formed.

26580

The physician repairs a cleft hand. A cleft hand is a malformation where the division between the fingers extends into the metacarpus. The middle digits may be absent and remaining digits are abnormally large. The physician incises the overlying skin and dissects to the deformity. The tissues are brought together with sutures, and the tendons are approximated to produce tensor and extensor function. Following correction of the metacarpus, the skin is reapproximated, reduced, and closed in sutured layers.

26587

The physician reconstructs the hand by removing a polydactylous (extra) digit where the digit contains both soft tissue and bone. The physician incises the skin at the base of the polydactylous digit. The bone is cut and the digit is resected. The skin is reapproximated, reduced, and closed in sutured layers.

26590

The physician corrects macrodactylia, which is an abnormal largeness of the fingers. The physician incises and retracts the skin to expose the underlying tissue. Reduction is accomplished by removing excess connective tissue and bone if necessary. The tissues are reanastomosed and secured with sutures. The operative incisions are closed in sutured layers.

26591

The physician repairs the intrinsic muscles of the hand to restore intrinsic function. The physician incises the overlying skin and dissects to the damaged muscle. The integrity of the tendons and muscles are tested. Defects are corrected to restore function. The operative incision is closed in sutured layers. When reporting this procedure, indicate which intrinsic muscle was repaired (interossei or lumbricales). Report each muscle separately.

26593

The physician releases the intrinsic muscles of the hand to restore intrinsic function. The physician incises the overlying skin and dissects to the contracted muscle. The intrinsic muscle is incised to release contracture. The operative incision is closed in sutured layers. When reporting this procedure, indicate which intrinsic muscle was released

(interossei or lumbricals). If microsurgery is used, report using modifier -20 or 09920. Report each muscle separately.

26596

The physician excises a constricting ring of finger using multiple Z-plasties. The physician cuts the restricted skin in z shaped incisions. The Z flaps are reapproximated, increasing skin surface area without using grafts. The flaps are sutured closed.

26600–26605

The physician treats a metacarpal fracture with or without manipulation. The physician uses an x-ray to determine the location and severity of the fracture. In 26600, the fracture does not require realignment. In 26605, the proximal and distal ends of the fracture are not in correct anatomical position, and the physician reduces the fracture to correct alignment. The bones are splinted in anatomic position. Report each bone separately.

26607

The physician treats a metacarpal fracture with manipulation and external fixation. The physician uses a separately reportable x-ray to determine the location and severity of the fracture. The physician reduces the fracture to correct alignment of the proximal and distal ends of the bone. External fixation is placed to stabilize the fracture. The bones are splinted in anatomic position. Report each bone separately.

26608

The physician fixates a metacarpal fracture using a percutaneously placed wire. The physician uses an x-ray to determine the location and severity of the fracture. The physician reduces the fracture to correct alignment of the proximal and distal ends of the bone. The physician drills a wire through the metacarpophalangeal joint, through the fracture, and into the proximal bone. The drill entry point dressed and the hand is splinted.

26615

The physician performs an open correction of a metacarpal fracture, internal or external fixation may be used. The physician uses an x-ray to determine the location and severity of the fracture. The physician incises the overlying skin to expose the fracture. A wire or plate may be placed for internal fixation. The operative incision is closed in sutured layers and the hand is splinted. Report each bone separately.

26641–26645

The physician manipulates a carpometacarpal dislocation or fracture dislocation of the thumb to restore anatomical position. The physician determines the dislocated position of the bone. The bone is relocated to correct anatomical position using external manipulation, and the hand is splinted. Report 26641 for dislocation without fracture, report 26645 for dislocation including fracture (Bennett fracture).

26650

The physician manipulates a carpometacarpal fracture dislocation of the thumb to restore anatomical position and secures the bone with a wire. The physician determines the dislocated position of the bone. The bone is relocated to correct anatomical position using external manipulation. The physician drills a wire through the metacarpophalangeal joint, through the fracture, and into the proximal bone. The drill entry point dressed and the hand is splinted.

26665

The physician performs an open reduction of a carpometacarpal fracture dislocation of the thumb. The physician uses an x-ray to determine the position and severity of the defect. The physician incises the overlying skin to expose the fracture, and the bones are reapproximated. A wire or plate may be placed for internal fixation. The operative incision is closed in sutured layers and the hand is splinted.

26670–26675

The physician treats a carpometacarpal (other than the thumb) dislocation using manipulation; anesthesia may be used if necessary. The physician determines the dislocated position of the bone. The physician uses external manipulation to relocate the bone. In 26670, dislocation is minor and no anesthesia is needed. In 26675, dislocation is major and anesthesia is required.

26676

The physician manipulates a carpometacarpal dislocation (other than the thumb) to restore anatomical position and secures the bone with a wire. The physician determines the dislocated position of the bone. The bone is relocated to the correct anatomical position using external manipulation. The physician drills a wire through the carpometacarpal joint. The drill entry point is dressed and the hand is splinted.

26685–26686

The physician performs an open reduction of a carpometacarpal dislocation on a joint other than the thumb. The physician uses a separately reportable x-ray to determine the position and severity of the defect. The physician incises the overlying skin to expose the dislocation. A wire or plates may be placed for internal fixation and external fixation may be used to further stabilize the dislocation. The operative incision is closed in sutured layers and the hand is splinted. Report 26685 for each joint that is repaired simply. Report 26686 for complex or multiple dislocations, or when delayed treatment of the dislocation is performed.

26700–26705

The physician treats a metacarpophalangeal dislocation using manipulation; anesthesia may be used if necessary. The physician determines the dislocated position of the bone. The physician uses external manipulation to relocate the bone. In 26700, dislocation is minor and no anesthesia is needed. In 26705, dislocation is major and anesthesia is required.

26706

The physician manipulates a metacarpophalangeal dislocation to restore anatomical position and secures the bone with a wire. The physician determines the dislocated position of the bone. The bone is relocated to correct anatomical position using external manipulation. The physician drills a wire into the metacarpophalangeal joint, through the fracture, and into the proximal bone. The drill entry point dressed and the hand is splinted.

26715

The physician performs an open reduction of a metacarpophalangeal fracture dislocation. The physician uses an x-ray to determine the position and severity of the defect. The physician incises the overlying skin to expose the fracture, and the bones are reapproximated. A wire or plate may be placed for internal fixation. The operative incision is closed in sutured layers and the hand is splinted.

26720–26725

The physician treats a phalangeal shaft fracture of the proximal or middle phalanx, finger, or thumb with or without manipulation. In 26720, no manipulation is necessary. In 26725, the physician manipulates the bones to restore anatomical position. The hand is splinted for stabilization.

26727

The physician treats a phalangeal shaft fracture of the proximal or middle phalanx, finger, or thumb with manipulation and secures it with a wire. The physician drills a wire into the tip of the finger bone, through the fracture, and into the proximal bone. The drill entry point dressed and the hand is splinted.

26735

The physician performs an open correction of a phalangeal shaft fracture. The physician uses an x-ray to determine the position and severity of the defect. The physician incises the overlying skin to expose the fracture, and the bones are reapproximated. A wire or plate may be placed for internal fixation. The operative incision is closed in sutured layers and the hand is splinted.

26740–26742

The physician treats an articular fracture involving a metacarpophalangeal or interphalangeal joint with or without manipulation. In 26740, no manipulation is necessary. In 26742, the physician manipulates the bones to restore anatomical position. The hand is splinted for stabilization.

26746

The physician performs an open reduction of an articular fracture involving a metacarpophalangeal or interphalangeal joint. The physician uses an x-ray to determine the position and severity of the defect. The physician incises the overlying skin to expose the fracture, and the bones are reapproximated. A wire or plate may be placed for internal fixation. The operative incision is closed in sutured layers and the hand is splinted.

26750–26755

The physician treats distal phalangeal fracture of the finger or thumb with or without manipulation. In 26750, no manipulation is necessary. In 26755, the physician manipulates the bones to restore anatomical position. The hand is splinted for stabilization.

26756

The physician treats a distal phalangeal fracture of the finger or thumb with manipulation and secures it with a wire. The physician drills a wire into the tip of the finger bone, through the fracture, and into the proximal bone. The drill entry point dressed and the hand is splinted.

26765

The physician performs an open reduction of a distal phalangeal fracture of the finger or thumb. The physician uses an x-ray to determine the position and severity of the defect. The physician incises the overlying skin to expose the fracture, and the bones are reapproximated. A wire or plate may be placed for internal fixation. The operative incision is closed in sutured layers and the hand is splinted.

26770–26775

The physician treats an interphalangeal joint dislocation using manipulation; anesthesia may be used if necessary. The physician determines the dislocated position of the bone and uses external manipulation to relocate the bone. In 26770, dislocation is minor and no anesthesia is needed. In 26775, dislocation is major and anesthesia is required.

26776

The physician manipulates an interphalangeal joint dislocation to restore anatomical position and secures the bone with a wire. The physician determines the dislocated position of the bone. The bone is relocated to correct anatomical position using external manipulation. The physician drills a wire through the interphalangeal joint for stabilization and the hand is splinted.

26785

The physician performs an open correction of an interphalangeal joint dislocation. The physician uses

an x-ray to determine the position and severity of the defect. The physician incises the overlying skin to expose the dislocated joint, and the bones are reapproximated. A wire may be placed for internal fixation. The operative incision is closed in sutured layers and the hand is splinted.

26820

The physician fuses the thumb in opposition. The physician incises the overlying skin and dissects to the metacarpalphalangeal joint. A bone graft is obtained from the distal radius or iliac crest and placed to secure the joint. A wire is placed through the joint until fusion is complete. The operative incision is closed in sutured layers and the thumb is splinted for stabilization.

26841–26844

The physician fuses the carpometacarpal joint of a finger or the thumb. Internal or external fixation may be used. The physician incises the overlying skin and dissects to the carpometacarpal joint. The joint is fixated with a wire, screws, or plates. The operative incision is closed in sutured layers and the hand is splinted. If a graft is obtained, the physician harvests bone from the distal radius or iliac crest. The graft is interposed between the two bones to prevent movement and a wire is placed through the joint until fusion is complete. In 26841, the thumb is treated; report 26842 if an autograft is obtained and used. In 26843, a finger joint is treated; report 26844 if an autograft is obtained and used. The operative incision is closed in sutured layers and the hand is splinted.

26850–26852

The physician fuses a metacarpophalangeal joint. Internal or external fixation may be used. The physician incises the overlying skin and dissects to the metacarpophalangeal joint. The physician may use a wire to stabilize the joint until fusion is complete. Report 26852 if an autograft is obtained and used. Bone is harvested from the distal radius or iliac crest and interposed between the two bones to prevent movement. The operative incision is closed in sutured layers and the hand is splinted.

26860–26863

The physician fuses an interphalangeal joint. Internal or external fixation may be used. The physician incises the overlying skin and dissects to the interphalangeal joint. The physician may use a wire to stabilize the joint until fusion is complete. Report 26861 for each additional interphalangeal joint. Report 26862 if an autograft is obtained and used. A graft is harvested from the distal radius or iliac crest and interposed between the bones to prevent movement. Report 26863 for autografts on each additional interphalangeal joints. The operative incision is closed in sutured layers and the hand is splinted.

26910

The physician amputates a metacarpal bone including a finger or the thumb. An interosseous transfer may be performed. The physician incises the overlying skin and dissects to the defective metacarpal bone. The bone is freed of all muscular and vascular attachments and removed, using a saw if necessary. Tissues that are no longer necessary for anatomical function are removed. Interossei muscles may be transferred to adjacent metacarpals to retain intrinsic muscle function. Soft tissue structures are returned to anatomic position; the skin is reapproximated, reduced and closed in sutured layers.

26951–26952

The physician amputates a finger or thumb, primary or secondary to injury. Neurectomies are performed. The overlying skin is incised and the tissues are dissected to the bone. The bone is removed, using a saw if necessary. The vessels and nerves are ligated using microsurgical techniques. Primary amputation is removal of the digit following an acute injury or infection. Secondary amputation is removal of the digit after conservative methods to preserve the digit have failed. In 26951, the wound is skin is approximated, reduced, and closed in sutured layers. In 26952, local advancement flaps are necessary for closure.

26990

The physician drains a deep abscess or hematoma of the pelvis or hip joint area. The physician makes an incision and carries dissection down through the soft tissues. Once the abscess or hematoma is visualized, all purulent matter (pus) or clotted blood is evacuated. The wound is irrigated with a catheter. For an infectious abscess, such as with tuberculosis, the wound is packed with gauze. For two to three weeks, the wound is irrigated several times each day with antibiotic solution. The packing is changed daily until the wound has closed by granulation tissue from within the area. If the area is infection free, the wound is repaired in multiple layers with sutures, staples, and/or Steri-strips.

26991

The physician makes an incision overlying the site of the infected bursa of the pelvis or hip joint area. Dissection is carried down to expose the bursa. The bursa is incised and drained. Any necrotic (dead) bursal tissue and surrounding soft tissue is removed. The wound is irrigated with antibiotic solution. The wound is typically left open to drain. The wound may also be irrigated and packed with gauze and antibiotic solution. The wound may be left open to heal by granulation tissue or may be repaired in layers once the area is free of infection.

26992

The physician makes an incision overlying the affected area of the pelvis and/or hip joint. Dissection is carried down to the bone. The physician reflects the muscles, while protecting the nerves and vessels. The periosteum (bone lining) is incised over the infection or abscess. A window of several holes is drilled through the bone cortex. All necrotic and desiccated bone (dying and dry) is removed and the area is debrided. The physician then evacuates any purulent matter. The wound is then irrigated with antibiotic solution. The physician may leave the wound open for drainage and repeated packing. The wound is repaired in multiple layers once the tissue is healthy and infection free.

27000

The physician makes a small incision approximately 0.5 inches long over the origin of the adductor muscles. Dissection is carried down to the adductor tendon. The physician uses a small blade to release (free by incision) the tendon. The incision is then repaired in layers with sutures and Steri-strips. A spica cast is applied for three to four weeks to keep the hip in abduction.

27001–27003

The physician performs a tenotomy of the adductor of the hip. An incision is made starting at the pubis and extending approximately 5 cm along the inner thigh, in line with the V adductor longus muscle. The tendinous origins of the adductor muscles are identified and then separated to allow lengthening. In 27003, the adductor muscles are separated from each other and the obturator nerve is located. The anterior and posterior branches of the nerve are then resected (excised). To perform a tenotomy, the tendinous origins of the adductor muscles are then divided. The physician repairs the incision in multiple layers. A cast may be applied for three to six weeks to hold the hip in abduction.

27005

The physician makes a 10.0 cm to 15.0 cm incision overlying the anterior iliofemoral area. The iliacus muscle and femoral nerve are identified and then separated. The iliacus muscle and psoas tendon are separated. The psoas tendon is transferred superiorly and sutured to the anterior capsule of the hip joint. The iliacus muscle is also sutured to the capsule. The incision is repaired in multiple layers.

27006

The patient is placed in a lateral position. A transverse incision is made starting just below the anterosuperior iliac spine and extending to just above the greater trochanter. The gluteus medius and minimus are tenotomized. To perform a tenotomy, the tendinous origins of the abductor muscles are separated. The incision is repaired in multiple layers over a suction drain.

27025

The physician performs a fasciotomy, treating a swollen area of the hip or thigh. The swelling applies pressure to the neurovascular tissues and muscles and may result in tissue death and loss of limb. One or more incisions are made over the affected area. The incisions may extend the length of the hip or thigh. The fascial planes are dissected out and separated to release pressure caused from swelling. Any necrotic tissue is removed as well. The wounds are left open for approximately 72 hours and repaired in multiple layers with sutures and/or staples.

27030

The physician may make an incision with a posterolateral approach. A previous hip surgery incision may be used if the infection is superficial. The wound is dissected to deep fascia. The structures are examined to determine whether the infection extends deeper and into the hip joint. If the infection is deeper, the joint is excised. The wound and hip joint are irrigated with an antibiotic solution. If the skin is not necrotic (dead) and skin edges can be approximated without tension, the wound may be closed. Suction tubes may be inserted for drainage. If the wound is left open, the area is irrigated and packed. The wound is allowed to heal by granulation tissue from within. Secondary closure is often not necessary.

27033

The physician explores the hip joint and may remove a loose or foreign body. The physician may use an anterior iliofemoral approach. The origin of the rectus femoris muscle is released (freed by incision) to expose the hip joint. The capsule surrounding the hip joint is incised to gain access to the joint. The physician explores all areas of the hip joint for a loose or foreign body (e.g., loose cartilage, bone fragment, bullet, etc.) The loose or foreign body will most likely be removed by the physician to prevent further irritation and damage to the hip joint. The capsule is repaired with sutures. The origin of the rectus femoris is reattached. The incision is repaired in multiple layers with sutures, staples, and/or Steri-strips.

27035

The physician makes an incision overlying a nerve of the hip joint. The physician uses either a posterior approach to the sciatic or an anterior approach to its branches (the femoral or obturator nerves). The physician dissects the tissue to locate and isolate the nerve. The nerve is then cut and the incision repaired in multiple layers.

27036

The physician performs surgery on the hip joint capsule. An incision is made over the hip. Sharp and blunt dissection is utilized to continue deep through the fascia to the hip capsule. The capsule itself is incised. The physician removes all or part of the capsule. Excess bone in and around the capsule is identified, exposed, and removed. To accomplish this, the physician releases some or all of the hip flexor muscle. After the capsule and the excess bone have been removed, the muscles are repaired as warranted. The wound is closed in layers. A drain may be left in the hip joint and later removed.

27040–27041

The physician performs a biopsy to evaluate soft tissue. The area for biopsy is in the subcutaneous tissue between the muscle and skin layers in 27040. The suspect area is deeper and may be within muscle in 27041. An incision is made to expose the area. A tumor is typically surrounded by a capsule. The physician makes an incision through the capsule, removing a portion of the tumor for biopsy. The incision is repaired in multiple layers using sutures, staples, and/or Steri-strips.

27047–27048

In 27047, the area of tumor is contained in the subcutaneous tissue between the muscle and skin layers. The physician makes an incision overlying the tumor of the pelvis or hip area. In 27048, the muscle surrounding the tumor is exposed. The physician makes an incision through the muscle, identifying the tumor. The physician then removes the tumor, as well as the capsule surrounding it. The incision is repaired in multiple layers with sutures, staples, and/or Steri-strips.

27049

The physician makes a skin incision overlying a soft tissue tumor of the pelvis and hip area. Dissection is carried down to where the tumor can be visualized. The tumor may extend for long distances along fascial planes, or may not be contained in a compartment. Radical resection includes removal of the tumor as well as surrounding soft tissues such as muscle, fascia, and neurovascular structures. The incision is repaired in multiple layers using sutures, staples, and/or Steri-strips.

27050

The patient is placed in a lateral decubitus (lying on the side) or prone (lying face downward) position. The physician makes an incision overlying the sacrum. Soft tissue dissection is carried down to expose the sacroiliac joint. Muscle and ligaments are also incised to access the joint. The physician takes a tissue sample. Muscles and ligaments are then reattached. The incision is repaired in multiple layers with sutures, staples, and/or Steri-strips.

27052

The physician uses a standard hip approach to access the hip joint. The capsule surrounding the hip joint is incised to expose the hip joint and to obtain the desired tissue for biopsy. The capsule is then sutured.

The incision is repaired in multiple layers with sutures, staples, and/or Steri-strips.

27054
The physician removes inflamed synovium of the hip joint. The physician incises the capsule to gain access into the hip joint. The diseased synovium is removed. The physician then sutures the capsule. The incision is repaired in multiple layers with sutures, staples, and/or Steri-strips.

27060–27062
The physician makes an incision overlying the ischial tuberosity at the base of the buttock. Dissection is carried down to expose the ischial bursa in 27060. For excision of a trochanteric bursa in 27062, an incision is made over the lateral aspect of the hip. The infected or calcified bursa is dissected out from the surrounding tissue and removed. The incision is repaired in multiple layers using sutures, staples, and/or Steri-strips.

27065
The physician makes an incision overlying the area to expose the superficial bone cyst or benign tumor. Dissection is carried down to the cyst or tumor. The lining of the bone (periosteum) is also incised to further expose the cyst or tumor. The physician may make a few cuts above and below the lesion for removal or may remove it with a curet, depending on the position and location. If the cyst or tumor is large enough to weaken the integrity of the bone, then a bone autograft may be necessary. Bone chips are harvested from the surrounding cancellous (spongy) bone. These bone chips replace the excised cyst or tumor. The incision is then repaired in multiple layers using sutures, staples, and/or Steri-strips.

27066–27067
The physician makes an incision overlying the area, exposing the deep bone cyst or benign tumor. Further soft tissue dissection is required. The lining of the bone (periosteum) is also incised to further expose the cyst or tumor. The physician may either make a few cuts above and below the area for removal or may remove it with a curet, depending on the position and location. If the cyst or tumor was large enough to weaken the integrity of the bone, then a bone autograft may be necessary. Bone chips are harvested from the surrounding cancellous (spongy) bone. These bone chips replace the excised cyst or tumor. In 27067, a separate incision is required to harvest bone from the patient's iliac crest. An oblique incision is made over the iliac crest. Dissection is carried down to the periosteum. The periosteum is incised, exposing the bone. The physician performs an osteotomy to obtain both cortical and cancellous bone and then closes the surgically created graft donor site. The incision is repaired in multiple layers using sutures, staples, and/or Steri-strips.

27070–27071
The physician makes an incision in the skin extending the length of the infected area. In 27071, the infected bone may be deeper and require more extensive tissue dissection. The periosteum is incised and any soft tissue is stripped away from the affected bone. The physician drains the abscess and excises all necrotic (dying) bone. The wound is then irrigated. Based on the location of the abscess, the physician may either close the wound or leave it open for drainage. After drainage the wound is repaired in multiple layers with sutures, staples, and/or Steri-strips.

27075
The patient is positioned for a lithotomy with the buttock elevated. For resection (excision) of the pubis and/or ischium, an incision is made from the pubic tubercle to the ischial tuberosity. The adductor and obturator muscles are detached from the pubis and ischium. Additional dissection is carried down to better expose the pubis and ischium. The remaining muscles and ligaments are released (freed by incision) while the pudendal and genital nerves and vessels are protected. The bone(s) is then separated and cut with bone-cutting forceps and an osteotome or saw. The bone segments are then removed. A separate incision is made to resect the ilium. As above, the portion of the ilium needing resection is dissected out by releasing muscles, tendons, and ligaments. The incisions are repaired in multiple layers.

27076
The patient is placed in a lateral decubitus (lying on the side) position. The physician makes an incision from the posterior crest of the ilium to the symphysis pubis. A vertical extension of this incision is made, extending into the proximal thigh. The physician carries dissection down, while protecting the femoral artery, vein, and nerve. The physician uses a saw to divide (separate) the ilium and the pubic bone. Any remaining soft tissue is released (freed by incision) from the segment of bone to be removed. The inguinal ligament is reattached to the iliopsoas tendon to prevent a hernia. The incision is repaired in multiple layers over a suction drain.

27077
The patient is placed in a supine position with the involved side elevated. The physician makes an incision extending from the posterosuperior iliac spine, along the iliac crest, to the symphysis pubis. A vertical incision is then made extending down into the upper thigh. The abdominal muscles are detached. All muscles that attach to the innominate bone are divided and detached. Vessels and nerves are also separated and/or ligated. The hip joint capsule is incised. The sacroiliac joint is exposed and divided with an osteotome. The innominate bone is then removed. The incision is repaired in layers.

27078–27079

The patient is positioned prone to access the ischial tuberosity and a lateral decubitus position to access the greater trochanter. The physician makes an incision overlying the involved bone and dissects through the deep layers. The ischial tuberosity or greater trochanter is exposed, then resected. The wound is closed in multiple layers with sutures. Formation of skin flaps is required for closure in 27079.

27080

The physician makes a 15 cm vertical incision over the coccyx. The coccyx is freed from surrounding soft tissue and then disarticulated from the sacrum (separated from the joint). The incision is repaired in multiple layers using sutures, staples, and/or steri-strips. If infection is present, the physician may pack the wound with gauze, allowing the wound to heal by granulation tissue from within.

27086–27087

The physician makes an incision overlying the site of the foreign body in the pelvis or hip. The foreign body is then removed from the subcutaneous tissue in 27086. Deeper dissection is required in 27087 and more attention may be given to possibly damaged vessels and/or nerves. The physician then irrigates the wound. The incision is repaired with sutures, staples, and/or Steri-strips.

27090

The patient is placed in a lateral decubitus position (lying on the side). The physician may access the prosthesis through the previous hip surgery incision. The physician exposes and incises the hip joint capsule. The hip is then manually dislocated. Any scar tissue is resected (excised). The physician disimpacts the femoral prosthesis, removing cement as needed. The physician then repairs the incision in multiple layers with sutures.

27091

The patient is placed in a lateral decubitus position (lying on the side). The physician may access the prosthesis through the previous hip surgery incision. Any scar tissue is resected. The physician exposes and incises the hip joint capsule. The hip is then manually dislocated. Methylmethacrylate (cement) is removed from the upper portion of the stem. The physician removes the stem with forceful blows. The physician removes any cement. The physician may make a bone window in the femoral cortex to remove additional cement. If there is bony ingrowth, flexible osteotomes may be used to remove the bone, allowing further stem retraction. The physician removes cement from the border of the implant with chisels and gouges. The physician then removes the acetabular components with instruments. Any remaining loose cement is removed with a large curet or other instrument. A spacer of methylmethacrylate formed into a cube shape may be inserted into the space between the femur and tibia. The spacer prevents the soft tissues from compressing the joint space. The spacer is secured until another prosthesis is inserted. Drains may be placed. The wound may be left open for healing or the incision is repaired in multiple layers.

27093–27095

The physician may apply skin traction to increase the space between the femoral head and acetabulum. Using a fluoroscope, the physician places a metallic marker over the femoral neck. The point is marked on the skin with ink. The femoral artery is palpated and marked on the skin as well, avoiding inadvertent puncture. Under sterile conditions, the physician inserts a needle (1 1/2" for children, 3 1/2" for adults) and passes it into the capsule (located by fluoroscope). The synovial fluid is aspirated for a culture check. After aspiration, a contrast agent is injected into the hip joint and the needle is removed. X-rays are then taken with the hip in neutral, external, and internal rotation for children and adults. The frog leg position is also taken for children. A second set of x-rays may be taken following the hip movements. The procedure is performed without anesthesia in 27093 and with anesthesia in 27095.

27096

The physician injects the sacroiliac joint, the articulation between the sacrum and ilium in the pelvis. The physician draws contrast, an anesthetic and/or steroid into a syringe. Through a posterior approach a needle (syringe attached) is inserted into the sacroiliac joint. The physician pushes on the syringe to deliver its content into the joint. The needle is withdrawn. CT or fluoroscopic guidance may be used to guide the sacroiliac injection.

27097

The hamstring tendon is a fibrous connective tissue extension that attaches the (hamstrings) muscles to bone. The hamstrings include the semitendinous, semimembranous, and biceps femoris; they flex and extend the thigh. The hamstrings origins are in the ischium or femur and the insertions are in the tibia and fibula. The physician makes an incision overlying the hamstring origin. Muscle and fascia is exposed. The physician makes multiple cuts in muscle fascia. The incision is then repaired in multiple layers.

27098

The patient is placed in the lithotomy position with the buttocks at the end of the operating table, and the legs in pelvic stirrups. The physician makes an incision starting just superior to the adductor longus tendon, and extending posteriorly in a straight line to the ischial tuberosity. The adductor longus tendon is then severed from its origin on the pubic ramus. Next, the physician releases by incision the origins of the pubic adductor brevis, gracilis, and adductor magnus tendons. The physician grasps the freed ends of the tendons with a clamp, holding them along the side of the ischial tuberosity. The ends of the tendons are then sutured to the tuberosity with nonabsorbable sutures. The incision is repaired in multiple layers. A spica cast may also be applied for three weeks.

27100

The physician performs a muscle transfer, substituting the external oblique muscle for a paralyzed abductor of the hip. An incision is made starting at the pubic tubercle and extending along the crest of the ilium to its mid-point. Two incisions are made in the aponeurosis of the external oblique, freeing it from its medial and lateral origins. An aponeurosis connects a muscle with the parts it moves. The cut edges of the external oblique are then folded under and sutured together to form a cone-shaped structure. The physician then makes a 6.0 cm lateral incision over the greater trochanter. Two holes are drilled through the greater trochanter, 1.0 cm in diameter. A subcutaneous tunnel is then made extending proximally across the ilium. The cone-shaped external oblique muscle is passed distally through the tunnel. While the hip is held in wide abduction, the end of the muscle (which serves as a tendon) is passed through the holes in the trochanter, and sutured firmly to itself. When desired, a strong tensor fascia latae tendon may be transferred posteriorly on the iliac crest as well. The incision is repaired in multiple layers. A spica cast is applied for four weeks.

27105

The physician makes an incision overlying the paraspinal muscle. The muscle is detached from its insertion point. The muscle is then transferred and reattached to the hip. The incision is repaired in multiple layers with sutures.

27110

The physician performs a transfer of the iliopsoas for weakened or paralyzed gluteus minimus and medius muscles. An incision is made along the anterior two-thirds of the iliac crest and extending distally along the inner border of the sartorius muscle to the middle of the thigh. Dissection is carried down to the deep fascia. The iliac crest is exposed. If there is a hip flexion contracture, the physician may release both of these at the same time by incision. Next, the femoral nerve is identified and moved from the surgical area. The abdominal muscles are then detached from the anterior two-thirds of the iliac crest. The lesser trochanter is identified and detached from the femur along with the insertion portion of the iliopsoas tendon. Using blunt and sharp dissection, the iliacus muscle is detached from the pelvis. The physician then makes an oval hole through the iliac wing and passes the iliopsoas tendon and the entire iliacus muscle through the hole. The greater trochanter is exposed through dissection. Using an awl and burr, a hole is made through the greater trochanter, through which the iliopsoas tendon is passed. Several strong sutures are used to anchor the tendon securely to the greater trochanter. The iliacus muscle is sutured to the ilium, and the abdominal muscles to the iliac crest. The incision is repaired in multiple layers. A spica cast is applied for three to four weeks, holding the hip in full abduction, extension, and neutral rotation.

27111

The physician makes an incision beginning lateral and posterior to the anterosuperior iliac spine. The incision then extends anteriorly and distally, crossing the tensor fascia latae. The periosteum along the crest of the ilium is then incised, reflecting the tensor fascia latae and gluteal muscles. The physician also reflects the attachment of the abdominal muscles until the iliacus is exposed. The anterosuperior iliac spine is resected along with the origin of the sartorius muscle. This muscle is reflected distally. The physician identifies the femoral nerve and vessels. The nerve and vessels are then retracted to identify the apex of the lesser trochanter. The physician uses an osteotome to divide or separate the trochanter. The tensor fascia latae is divided halfway between its origin and insertion, so that a trough can be cut in the wing of the ilium. The physician will then lay the iliopsoas in the trough. The iliopsoas is transferred laterally, determining its position on the femur. The thigh is held in full abduction during the transfer so that the iliopsoas has powerful tension. A small window is cut on the femur at this site, and the lesser trochanter is anchored to it. The vastus lateralis is sutured to the edge of the iliopsoas tendon and the iliacus muscle to the psoas. The tensor fascia latae is then repaired and the anterosuperior spine is anchored back to the ilium. The incision is repaired in multiple layers. A spica cast is applied with the hip in internal rotation, slight flexion, and full abduction for four weeks.

27120

Acetabuloplasty redirects the inclination of the acetabular roof by an osteotomy of the ilium. The Pemberton acetabuloplasty is described as follows. The patient is placed in a supine (face up) position. Using an anterior iliofemoral approach, the physician carries dissection down to expose the hip joint capsule and sciatic notch. The capsule is incised. Using a curved osteotome, a bone cut is made through the lateral cortex of the ilium. Another cut is made through the medial cortex of the ilium. After completing the osteotomy, a wide, curved osteotome is inserted into the front part of the osteotomy and used to lever the distal fragment distally, until the front edges are 2.5 cm to 3.0 cm apart. A wedge of bone is then resected (excised) from the iliac crest and placed in the initial osteotomy made earlier in the ilium. The wedge is driven firmly into place. If necessary, the graft may be secured with two pins. The hip is then reduced (repositioned) and the capsule is tightened with sutures. The incision is repaired in multiple layers. A spica cast is applied from the nipple line to the toes on the affected side and to above the knee on the opposite side. The cast is worn for approximately three months.

27122

The physician uses a standard approach to the hip. The hip joint capsule is then incised to expose the femoral head, neck, and acetabular rim. These components are resected (excised). The physician uses a curet to remove any remaining necrotic or infected bone. The physician then drains any intrapelvic abscesses. Two to three drains are inserted. The incision is repaired in layers with sutures, staples, and/or Steri-strips. The hip is immobilized in a cast or with traction.

27125

The physician makes a posterolateral incision over the hip with the patient in a lateral decubitus position (lying on the side). The fascia lata is incised and the muscles around the hip joint are retracted to visualize the capsule. The physician then incises the capsule, exposing the femoral neck. The femoral neck is resected (excised) with a reciprocating saw. The excised femoral head is measured with a caliper to determine the appropriate size for replacement. The physician prepares the femoral shaft by enlarging the canal with a rasp. The physician then selects the type of stem to be used. The stem is secured into the femoral shaft. The stem is inserted and pounded into place with an impactor. The physician then reduces (repositions) the femoral stem prosthesis. Hip motion and stability are evaluated. The capsule is then closed and the incision repaired in multiple layers.

27130

The physician makes an incision along the posterior aspect of the hip with the patient in a lateral decubitus (lying on the side) position. The short external rotator muscles are released by incision from their insertion on the femur, exposing the joint capsule. The physician incises the capsule. The hip is then dislocated posteriorly. The physician resects (excises) the femoral head with a reciprocating saw. The physician removes any osteophytes around the rim of the acetabulum with an osteotome. The acetabulum is then reamed out with a power reamer, exposing both subchondral and cancellous bone. The acetabular component is inserted. The femoral canal is then prepared using either a hand or power reamer. The excised femoral head is measured with a caliper to determine the appropriate size for replacement. The physician prepares the femoral shaft by enlarging the canal with a rasp. The physician then selects the type of stem to be used. The stem is secured into the femoral shaft. The stem is inserted and pounded into place with an impactor. The physician then reduces (repositions) the femoral stem prosthesis. The physician may augment the area with an autograft or allograft. The graft may be harvested from the resected (excised) femoral head. Donor bone

(allograft) may be used instead. The physician places the bone graft into the canal and/or acetabulum. The hip is reduced (repositioned). The external rotator muscles are reattached. The incision is repaired in multiple layers with suction drains.

27132

The physician performs a conversion of a previous hip surgery to total hip replacement. Total hip replacement is replacement of both the femoral head and acetabulum. The physician may access the area through the previous hip surgery incision, extending it to allow adequate exposure of the hip joint. Muscles are reflected as well. The physician removes any hardware (internal fixation). The physician incises the capsule. The hip is then dislocated. The physician resects (excises) the femoral head with a reciprocating saw. Next, the acetabulum is prepared. The physician removes any osteophytes around the rim of the acetabulum with an osteotome. The acetabulum is then reamed out with a power reamer, exposing both subchondral and cancellous bone. The acetabular component is inserted. The femoral canal is then prepared using either a hand or power reamer. The excised femoral head is measured with a caliper to determine the appropriate size for replacement. The physician prepares the femoral shaft by enlarging the canal with a rasp. The physician then selects the type of stem to be used. The stem is secured into the femoral shaft. The stem is inserted and pounded into place with an impactor. The physician then reduces (repositions) the femoral stem prosthesis. The physician may augment the area with an autograft or allograft. The graft may be harvested from the resected femoral head (autograft). Donor bone (allograft) may be used instead. The hip is reduced (repositioned). Any reflected muscles are reattached. The incision is then repaired in multiple layers with suction drains.

27134

The physician performs a revision of a total hip arthroplasty. With the patient in a lateral decubitus (lying on the side) position, the physician may access the hip through the previous hip surgery incision. Muscles are reflected. A trochanteric osteotomy may be performed with an oscillating saw. The physician incises the hip joint capsule. Any scar tissue is freed and removed. The physician then manually dislocates the hip. Cement is removed from the upper portion of the femoral stem with a motorized or hand instrument. The stem may then be removed. If the stem has fractured, the physician may drill a hole in the femoral shaft so that an instrument may remove the broken portion. Any remaining cement in the femoral shaft is then removed. The physician removes scar tissue and cement from around the acetabular component with chisels and gouges. The acetabular component is removed from its bed. The physician then reconstructs the acetabulum with either cement or screws and bone graft. The new femoral stem is inserted into the femoral shaft with or without cement. The physician may augment the area with an autograft or allograft. The physician harvests bone from the patient's iliac crest, repairing the surgically created graft donor site. An allograft (donor bone) may be used when additional bone is needed. The physician reduces (repositions) the hip and closes the capsule. The greater trochanter is wired into place. Suction drains may be placed in the wound. The incision is repaired in multiple layers with sutures, staples, and/or Steri-strips.

27137

The physician performs a revision of a total hip arthroplasty. With the patient in a lateral decubitus (lying on the side) position, the physician accesses the acetabular component through a previous hip surgery incision. Muscles are reflected. The physician may perform an osteotomy of the greater trochanter with an oscillating saw. The capsule is incised and the hip manually dislocated. Any scar tissue is removed from around the acetabulum. The physician removes cement from around the acetabular component with chisels and gouges. The acetabulum is then levered out from its bed. The acetabulum may need to be reamed out in preparation for the new component. The physician then reconstructs the acetabulum with or without cement. If the acetabulum is reconstructed without cement, the component is usually inserted and fixed with screws. Prior to the acetabulum placement, the physician may harvest a bone graft from the patient's iliac crest and close the surgically created graft donor site. Donor bone (allograft) may be used instead. If cement is used, it secures the new component in the acetabular bed. Once the cement has dried, the hip is reduced (repositioned) and the capsule closed. The physician may place suction drains in the wound. The incision is repaired in multiple layers with sutures, staples, and/or Steri-strips.

27138

With the patient in a lateral decubitus position (lying on the side), the physician may access the femoral component through the previous hip surgery incision. Muscles are reflected. The physician may perform an osteotomy of the greater trochanter. The hip joint capsule is exposed and incised. The physician then dislocates the hip joint. If cement was used on the previous arthroplasty, the physician uses a motorized or hand instrument to remove it from around the upper portion of the femoral stem. If loose enough, the stem is removed with forceful blows. If the stem cannot be removed, additional cement may need to be removed from the femoral shaft, so the stem can be extracted. The physician may then place cement in the femoral shaft and insert the new femoral component. If the revision is cementless, then donor bone (allograft) may be inserted as needed into the femoral shaft between the cortex and femoral component. The hip is reduced (repositioned). The physician reattaches the greater trochanter with wires.

The incision is repaired in multiple layers with sutures, staples, and/or Steri-strips.

27140

The physician makes a longitudinal incision over the greater trochanter with the patient in a lateral decubitus position (lying on the side). The physician then detaches the greater trochanter with a Gigli saw or osteotome. The physician may reposition the trochanter more lateral, or more distal and lateral. Repositioning increases the abductor lever arm and/or tightens the abductor musculature. The physician then drills holes to secure the trochanter to the femur with wire. If fixation is rigid, the patient may be allowed weight bearing. If not, the patient may be placed in skeletal traction for three weeks with the hip abducted. The incision is repaired in multiple layers.

27146

For a Salter innominate osteotomy, the patient is placed supine (face up). The adductor muscles are released by a subcutaneous tenotomy. The physician makes a small incision approximately 0.5 inch long over the origin of the adductor muscles. Dissection is carried down to the adductor tendon. The physician uses a small blade to release (free by incision) the tendon. The physician makes an incision from the middle of the iliac crest to the inguinal area. The rectus femoris is released from its attachment by incision. The physician then carries dissection down to expose and incise the joint capsule. If the ligamentous teres is hypertrophied, it is excised. If the femoral head remains unstable, an osteotomy of the innominate bone is performed. The hip is allowed to dislocate. The physician makes an osteotomy cut on the innominate bone using a Gigli saw. The osteotomy extends from the sciatic notch to the anteroinferior spine. The physician may then harvest a separately reportable full thickness bone graft from the anterior part of the iliac crest and close the surgically created graft donor site. The graft is trimmed to the shape of the wedge and inserted into the osteotomy. A Kirschner wire is drilled through the ilium, bone graft, and into the lower fragment. Another wire is placed parallel to the first. Joint stability is reevaluated. Any released muscles are reattached. The capsule is closed with sutures, giving added stability to the reduction. The incision is repaired in multiple layers. A single spica cast is applied for eight to 10 weeks.

27147

For a Salter innominate osteotomy, the patient is placed supine (face up). The adductor muscles are released by a subcutaneous tenotomy (incision). The physician makes a small incision approximately 0.5 inch long over the origin of the adductor muscles. Dissection is carried down to the adductor tendon. The physician uses a small blade to release (free by incision) the tendon. The physician then makes an incision from the middle of the iliac crest to the inguinal area. The rectus femoris is released from its attachment by incision. The physician then carries dissection down to expose and incise the joint capsule. If the ligamentous teres is hypertrophied, it is excised. Next, the physician reduces (repositions) the femoral head into the acetabulum. If the femoral head remains unstable, an osteotomy of the innominate bone is performed. The hip is allowed to dislocate. The physician makes an osteotomy cut on the innominate bone using a Gigli saw. The osteotomy extends from the sciatic notch to the anteroinferior spine. The physician may then harvest a separately reportable full thickness bone graft from the anterior part of the iliac crest and close the surgically created graft donor site. The graft is trimmed to the shape of the wedge and inserted into the osteotomy. A Kirschner wire is drilled through the ilium, bone graft, and into the lower fragment. Another wire is placed parallel to the first. The femoral head is reduced again into the acetabulum. Any released muscles are reattached. The capsule is closed with sutures, giving added stability to the reduction. The incision is repaired in multiple layers. A single spica cast is applied for eight to 10 weeks.

27151–27156

The patient is placed in a supine (face up) position. The physician makes an incision from the middle of the iliac crest to the inguinal area. The rectus femoris is released from its attachment by incision. The physician then carries dissection down to expose and incise the joint capsule. If the ligamentous teres is hypertrophied, it is excised. Next, the physician reduces (repositions) the femoral head into the acetabulum. If the femoral head remains unstable, an osteotomy of the innominate bone is performed. The hip is allowed to dislocate. The physician makes an osteotomy cut on the innominate bone using a Gigli saw. The osteotomy extends from the sciatic notch to the anteroinferior spine. The physician then harvests a separately reportable full thickness bone graft from the anterior part of the iliac crest and closes the surgically created graft donor site. The graft is trimmed to the shape of the wedge and inserted into the osteotomy. A Kirschner wire is drilled through the ilium, bone graft, and into the lower fragment. Another wire is placed parallel to the first. For femoral osteotomy, a lateral incision is made from the greater trochanter, extending down the leg 8.0 cm to 12.0 cm. Dissection is carried down to expose the lateral femur. Transverse and longitudinal orientation lines are made on the femoral cortex with an osteotome. The physician makes an osteotomy cut at the transverse line in a transverse or oblique direction. Another cut is made at an angle so that a wedge of bone can be removed to complete the correction. The rectus femoris is then reattached to its insertion point. In 27156, the hip is reduced as well. A side plate is secured to the femur with bone screws. The incision is repaired in multiple layers. A one and one-half spica cast is applied for eight to 12 weeks.

27158

The patient is placed in a supine position. The physician releases the adductor muscles by subcutaneous tenotomy (incision). The physician makes a small incision approximately 0.5" long over the origin of the adductor muscles. Dissection is carried down to the adductor tendon. The physician uses a small blade to release (free by incision) the tendon. The physician makes an incision from the middle of the iliac crest to the middle of the inguinal ligament. The head of the rectus femoris muscle is released. Dissection is carried down to expose the hip joint capsule, which is incised in a T-shaped fashion. The periosteum is stripped from the medial surface of the ilium, down to the sciatic notch. The ilium is then divided or cut with a Gigli saw in a straight line from the sciatic notch to the anteroinferior spine. A full-thickness bone graft is then removed from the iliac crest and trimmed to the shape of a wedge. The physician then closes the surgically created graft donor site. This allows the entire acetabulum together with the pubis and ischium to be rotated as a unit. The bone graft is then inserted into the osteotomy. Two Kirschner wires are drilled parallel to each other through the ilium and bone graft for fixation. The femoral head is reduced (repositioned) into the acetabulum. The capsule is repaired and tightened with sutures to add stability to the joint. The incision is repaired in multiple layers. The same procedure is then performed on the other side. Both hips are placed in spica casts for eight to twelve weeks, at which time the Kirschner wires may be removed under general or local anesthesia.

27161

With the patient in a lateral (on the side) position, the physician makes an incision extending from the anterosuperior iliac spine, over and to a point 10.0 cm below the greater trochanter. The fascia lata and gluteal muscles are divided or separated. Dissection is carried down to expose the hip joint. The physician incises the capsule. The physician makes two osteotomy cuts in the femoral neck without disturbing the blood supply to the capsule. The size of the osteotomies (bone cuts) is determined by facility adn radiologist. A Steinman pin may be drilled into the femoral neck before the osteotomy is completed to control the position of the proximal femur. The cut wedge of bone is then removed. The physician inserts several 5.0 mm Steinman pins through the femoral neck and across the osteotomy site and epiphyseal plate to prevent further slipping. The capsule is then closed. The incision is repaired in multiple layers. Steinman pins are removed after the epiphyseal plate has fused.

27165

The physician exposes the lateral aspect of the proximal femur by making a lateral longitudinal incision. The femur is divided or separated with an osteotome at a level slightly above the lesser trochanter. The physician then places the extremity in the corrected position. A rigid internal fixation device, such as a plate and screws, may stabilize the area. External fixation may be applied instead. The incision is repaired in layers with sutures, staples, and/or Steri-strips. A spica cast is applied for eight to 12 weeks.

27170

The physician makes an incision over the affected area. The physician harvests bone from the patient's iliac crest and closes the surgically created graft donor site. Bone chips are then packed around the non-union fracture site. An allograft (donor bone) may be used instead. The nonunion site may be stabilized with internal fixation. The incisions are repaired in multiple layers with sutures, staples, and/or Steri-strips.

27175–27176

Separately reportable x-rays are taken to determine the position of the slipped femoral epiphysis. The physician may then apply skin traction in 27175 with the limb in internal rotation for three to four days. Gradual improvement is accomplished without reduction. In 27176, the physician makes a small stab incision. Use of a fluoroscope determines the correct site for inserting pins through the lateral femoral cortex, femoral neck, and into the epiphysis to stabilize the slip. The small stab incision is closed with sutures. The patient is placed on crutches for four to six weeks.

27177

The physician makes an anterior iliofemoral incision with the patient in a supine (face up) position. Dissection is carried down to expose the capsule of the hip. The physician incises the capsule, retracting it to expose the femoral neck and epiphysis. A square window is made in the anterior surface of the femoral neck. Under separately reportable x-ray, the physician inserts a hollow mill through the window and drills across the epiphyseal plate and into the epiphysis. The tunnel is then enlarged with a curet. The physician makes a separate incision over the ilium and removes sections of bone from the outer surface of the ilium. The bone sections are sandwiched together, placed in the tunnel, and driven across the epiphyseal plate into the epiphysis. If the physician uses single or multiple pinning rather than a bone graft, an incision is made overlying the greater trochanter and upper femur. The physician then exposes the intertrochanteric area. Under separately reportable x-ray, the physician inserts a guide pin through the femur, femoral neck, and into the femoral head. One or two pins are inserted parallel to the guide pin. The guide pin is removed and the incision repaired in multiple layers. The physician may place the limb in skin traction.

27178

The physician treats a slipped femoral epiphysis by manipulating the area. Following manipulation by the physician, the reduction is confirmed with separately reportable x-ray. The epiphysis is then secured with Knowles pins or cannulated hip screws. An incision is made overlying the greater trochanter and upper femur. The physician then exposes the intertrochanteric area. Under separately reportable x-ray, the physician inserts a guide pin through the femur, femoral neck, and into the femoral head. One or two 3/16 inch Knowles pins are then inserted parallel to the guide pin. The guide pin is removed and the incision repaired in multiple layers. The physician may place the limb in skin traction.

27179

With the patient in a supine (face up) position, the physician makes an anterior iliofemoral incision. Dissection is carried down to expose the capsule, which is incised and retracted. Retraction of the capsule exposes the femoral neck and the slipped epiphysis. To correct the deformity, the physician resects a wedge of bone from the anteriosuperior aspect of the femoral neck with an osteotome. A single Knowles pin is drilled into the epiphysis. The physician uses the pin to rotate the epiphysis into its normal position and to hold it into place as well. The edges of the osteotomy are then brought together. The physician makes a short, lateral skin incision just below the greater trochanter. Under separately reportable x-ray, the physician inserts three Knowles pins through the incision, the trochanter, and into the neck and epiphysis. The single Knowles pin is removed from the epiphysis and the incision repaired in multiple layers. If fixation is secure, the limb may be placed in balanced suspension. Otherwise, a cast is applied from the nipple line to the toes on the affected side.

27181

With the patient in a supine (face up) position, the physician makes an anterior iliofemoral incision. Dissection is carried down to the hip joint capsule. The capsule is incised and retracted, exposing the femoral neck and epiphysis. A single Knowles pin is drilled into the epiphysis to control its position later. The physician resects a wedge of bone (osteotomy) from the anterosuperior part of the femoral neck. The physician then fractures the posterior cortex of the femoral neck. The Knowles pin is used to rotate the epiphysis into its normal position in the acetabulum. The physician rotates the thigh internally to oppose the osteotomy surfaces. A short, lateral skin incision is made just below the greater trochanter. Under separately reportable x-ray, the physician inserts three Knowles pins through the incision, the trochanter, and into the femoral neck and epiphysis. The single Knowles pin is then removed and the incision repaired in multiple layers. Depending on how secure the fixation is, the physician may either place the extremity in a balanced suspension, or apply a cast from the nipple line to the toes on the affected side.

27185

Epiphyseal arrest is performed to arrest or stop growth of the greater trochanter growth plate. The patient is placed in a sidelying position. The physician makes a straight incision over the greater trochanter. Dissection is carried down to expose the area. The physician uses a curet to scrape out the growth plate. Screw(s) or staples are then placed through the greater trochanter, across the growth plate, and into the femur. The incision is repaired in multiple layers.

27187

The patient is placed supine (face up) or in a sidelying position, depending on the area for treatment. The physician may make tiny incisions to insert pins under roentgenographic control. The physician may need to perform an open procedure. In an open procedure an incision is made and dissection carried down to the femoral neck or proximal femur. The internal fixation (nailing, plating with screws, or cerclage with wires wrapped around the femur) is applied. The physician may use cement (methylmethacrylate) as needed to secure the fixation or strengthen the bone. The incision is then repaired in multiple layers.

27193

The physician treats a pelvic ring fracture or dislocation. The displacement or dislocation is less than 1.0 cm. No manipulation is required. Treatment typically is bed rest and crutches.

27194

The physician performs manual manipulation to reduce (reposition) the fracture, dislocation, or subluxation of the pelvic ring. Vigorous manipulation may be necessary. The patient may require greater sedation. Anesthesia is required for placement of skeletal traction through the distal femur or proximal tibia. Separately reportable x-rays may be used to verify position of the reduced fracture, dislocation, or subluxation.

27200

For closed treatment of a coccygeal fracture, the physician will prescribe bed rest to alleviate symptoms. Sitting on a rubber ring may also lessen symptoms. Closed manual manipulation may be performed as well.

27202

The patient is positioned prone. The physician makes a vertical incision in the gluteal fold. Dissection is carried down to the coccyx. The fractured portion is removed or internal fixation is applied. The incision is then repaired in multiple layers.

27215

The physician makes an incision overlying the site of injury. Dissection is carried down to expose the avulsion and/or fracture. For an avulsion, a screw(s) is drilled through the bone fragment, reattaching the tendon and bone fragment to their original positions. The physician stabilizes an iliac wing fracture with a plate and screws across the fracture. The incision is repaired in multiple layers. Suction drains may be applied.

27216

With the patient in a supine (face up) position, the physician inserts two to three pins through the skin and into the iliac crest on both right and left sides. The pins are directed at specific angles. The physician attaches pin holders to each ring and curved ring segments to pin holders. The physician uses the rings to gently reduce (reposition) an unstable pelvic fracture or dislocation, if needed. Frame clamps are then attached to the rings and tightened down to secure fixation. The frame is left in place for approximately eight to 12 weeks.

27217

With the patient in a supine (face up) position, the physician makes a curvilinear, transverse incision above the superior pubic ramus. Dissection is carried down to expose the pubic symphysis and/or rami. The separation (fracture and/or dislocation) may be reduced (repositioned) by the physician by applying manual ilium-to-ilium compression. For internal fixation, a plate is applied with screws directed into the bone. The incision is then repaired in multiple layers with suction drains.

27218

With the patient in a supine (face up) position, the physician makes an incision along the anterior iliac crest. The iliacus muscle is dissected and reflected medially with the abdominal contents to expose the sacroiliac joint. If needed, the physician manipulates the pelvis and leg to reduce (reposition) the fracture or dislocation. Compression plates and screws achieve internal fixation. In other approaches reconstruction plates, transiliar rod fixators, or screws alone may be used for internal fixation of the ilium, sacroiliac joint, and/or sacrum. The incision is repaired in multiple layers with suction drains.

27220–27222

Closed treatment of an acetabulum fracture may be indicated when a fracture is non-displaced, bone is osteoporotic, or when only a minor portion of the acetabulum is involved. The patient may be placed in skin (Bucks) traction for eight to 12 weeks. The physician performs closed reduction (repositioning) with manipulation in 27222. General anesthesia is usually required. The physician may apply skeletal traction, placing a Kirschner wire or Steinman pin through the tibia by the tibial tuberosity. Weight is attached to provide a traction force. While traction force is applied along the axis of the leg, a lateral traction force is applied to the proximal thigh. The physician then manipulates the leg through abduction and internal rotation, and then adduction. Typically, skeletal traction is continued for eight to 12 weeks.

27226

For a posterior wall fracture, the patient is placed in a lateral position. The incision extends from the greater trochanter to within 6.0 cm of the posterosuperior iliac spine. For an anterior wall fracture, the physician approaches the fracture through the ilioinguinal area. The patient is positioned supine (face up). The physician makes an incision just above the symphysis pubis and extends it laterally to the iliac crest. For an anterior wall fracture, skeletal traction may be applied during the procedure. In both cases, extensive dissection of muscles and fascia is required to expose the fracture site. The joint is debrided of any free fragments. The fractured fragments are then reduced (repositioned). For a posterior wall fracture, internal fixation is achieved by using screws and a plate across the posterior wall to buttress the fragments. For an anterior wall fracture, internal fixation is usually achieved with the use of a two screw technique. The incision is then repaired in multiple layers using sutures, staples, and/or Steri-strips. Closed suction drainage is used.

27227

A transverse fracture involves both the anterior column and posterior column of the acetabulum. For transverse fractures, an approach as for a posterior wall fracture (see 27226) can often be used. If the fracture is more complex, different approaches may be used, providing exposure to both the anterior and posterior columns without making two separate incisions. Internal fixation is accomplished using screws and plate(s) techniques (see 27226). The incision is repaired in multiple layers using sutures, staples, and/or Steri-strips. Closed suction drainage is used.

27228

The patient is placed supine (face up). The physician makes an incision beginning at the upper portion of the symphysis pubis, extending upwards along the iliac crest, and ending at its most superior aspect. The origins of the abdominal muscles and iliacus are elevated from the iliac crest. Dissection is carried down through the inguinal canal, protecting vessels and nerves. The physician treats the anterior column fracture first by reducing the fragments and securing fixation with lag screws. The physician uses pointed reduction forceps to reduce (reposition) the fracture. The fracture is stabilized with a combination of lag screw and plate fixation. There may be an associated T-fracture which has a transverse pattern with a vertical split extending through the obturator ring. For a T-fracture, the physician makes a posterior

incision with the patient in a prone (face down) position. At times, the two column fracture and T-fracture can be treated from a posterior approach. An anterior approach may be necessary, in which the patient is turned from prone to supine. All incisions are repaired in multiple layers. Postoperative immobilization or traction is only necessary if satisfactory reduction and fixation are not achieved.

27230–27232

The physician treats a non-displaced, stable fracture of the femur. No manual manipulation is necessary in 27230. Manipulation is required in 27232 to treat a displaced fracture. The physician manually flexes the hip while applying manual traction force and internally rotating and abducting the hip. The patient may be placed in a supine (face up) position and Buck's (skin) traction applied. A splint may be applied to stabilize the fracture for three to six weeks. Skeletal traction may be necessary as well. A Steinman pin or Kirschner wire is inserted through the tibia near the tibial tuberosity. A weight is then attached. Traction may be continued for approximately six weeks.

27235

The physician makes a small stab incision (1.0 cm to 2.0 cm) overlying the lateral aspect of the thigh and just below the greater trochanter. A pin is then drilled at approximately a 45 degree angle through the cortex and neck and into the femoral head. Two to five additional pins are then inserted parallel to the first pin. Final x-rays are taken to confirm positions. The physician may then close the stab incision made for each pin with a single suture.

27236

The physician directly exposes the femoral fracture for treatment. The patient is placed in a supine (face up) position or slightly rolled up onto the other side. A 15.0 cm incision is made over the lateral hip. The fascia lata is split and the vastus lateralis muscle is detached from the femur. The physician then exposes the femoral neck and head. A small periosteal elevator or Kirschner wire is used to reduce (reposition) the fracture. The physician places guide pins through the bone and across the fracture. The guide pins help determine correct screw length. The physician may use cannulated screws or compression hip screws and a plate to achieve internal fixation. In some cases due to the risk of subsequent non-union or avascular necrosis, the physician may replace the femoral head with a femoral prosthesis. The femoral canal is reamed out. A prosthesis of the proper size and length is then selected and inserted into the femoral canal. The physician then reduces the prosthesis into the acetabulum. The incision is repaired in multiple layers with sutures, staples, and/or Steri-strips.

27238–27240

For a non-displaced, stable fracture in 27238, the physician applies a spica cast or brace. Manual manipulation is necessary to align fragments in 27240. The physician applies skeletal traction using a tibial pin. A Steinman pin is inserted transversely across the upper tibia. With the thigh supported in slings, weight is applied to create the traction force. Traction remains in place for approximately 12 weeks, after which a spica cast may be applied. If skeletal traction is not necessary, a form of Russell's skin traction is placed on the lower leg. This type of traction is a foam boot with an attached weight providing the traction force.

27244

The physician makes an incision over the upper lateral thigh, exposing the fracture area through tissue dissection. The patient is in a lateral decubitus (lying on the side) position or may be placed in traction on a table. The fracture is reduced (repositioned). Placement of an interfragmentary screw may achieve initial stability. A plate is inserted and screws stabilize the fragments. If additional fixation is needed, the physician may apply cerclage wiring, placing a wire around the fractured bones. The incision is repaired in multiple layers with sutures, staples, and/or Steri-strips.

27245

The patient is placed in a supine (face up) position, or slightly rolled up onto the opposite side. The physician makes an incision over the posterolateral aspect of the hip. The fascia lata is divided or separated. The vastus lateralis muscle is detached from its origin site. The physician will place the intramedullary nail into the canal medial to the tip of the greater trochanter. Both the proximal and distal canals are reamed in preparation for placement of the intramedullary nail. The physician reduces (repositions) the fracture with bone-holding forceps or cerclage wires (wires wrapped around the fragments), or both. The intramedullary nail, is then placed through the proximal fragment, into the canal, and driven into the shaft of the femur. The physician inserts a nail or screw into the femoral head by drilling a tunnel from the lateral cortex, passing through a hole in the intramedullary nail, and into the femoral head. The triflange nail is then driven through the tunnel, through the hole in the intramedullary nail and into the femoral head. The physician may elect to place cerclage wires for added stability. The vastus lateralis muscle is reattached and the fascia lata repaired as well. The incision is then repaired in multiple layers with sutures, staples, and/or Steri-strips.

27246–27248

The physician treats a greater trochanteric fracture without manipulation. The fracture is not displaced and may be treated with skin traction while in wide abduction. Other treatments include a spica cast applied for six weeks or protected weight bearing with crutches for four to six weeks. In 27248, the fracture

is displaced, requiring fixation. The physician makes a straight, lateral skin incision overlying the greater trochanter. Dissection is carried to visualize the fragment(s). The physician then applies bone screws, pegs, or wire loops to secure the fragment(s). External fixation may be applied. The incision is repaired in multiple layers with sutures, staples, and/or Steri-strips. Toe touch weight bearing with crutches is allowed for three to four weeks, followed by partial weight bearing for another three to four weeks.

27250–27252

The physician treats a hip dislocation without anesthesia in 27250 or with anesthesia in 27252. Two types of closed reduction techniques are used depending on the type of dislocation: the Stimson maneuver and the Allis maneuver. General or spinal anesthesia is applied. The Stimson maneuver is a procedure for posterior dislocations. The patient is positioned prone (face down) with the lower limbs hanging from the end of the table. Stabilizing pressure is placed on the sacrum. The physician holds the knee and ankle flexed to ninety degrees and applies gentle downward pressure to the leg, just below the knee. The Allis maneuver is a procedure for anterior dislocations. The patient is positioned supine (face up). The pelvis is stabilized and lateral traction force is applied to the inside of the thigh. The physician applies longitudinal traction in line with the axis of the femur, and then gently abducts and internally rotates the femur to achieve reduction. Other techniques similar to those described above may also be used. After reduction, light skin traction may be applied.

27253

The physician performs open treatment of a hip dislocation. The physician makes an incision along the posterior aspect of the hip. The gluteus maximus muscle is then split. The physician exposes the hip joint, allowing manual reduction of the dislocated hip. Reduction is accomplished without traumatizing the articular cartilage. The incision is repaired in multiple layers with sutures, staples, and/or Steri-strips.

27254

The physician treats a traumatic hip dislocation. The physician makes an incision along the posterior aspect of the hip. The gluteus maximus muscle is split and the hip joint exposed. Fractures of the acetabulum and femoral head are visualized. If the fractures remain stable and the joint surface congruent when reduced (repositioned), no internal fixation is required. If the fractures are not stable after reduction of the dislocation, then internal fixation is applied. Cancellous bone screws or Kirschner wires may stabilize the fractures. The incision is repaired in multiple layers with sutures, staples, and/or Steri-strips. The limb may be placed in skeletal or skin traction following the reduction. External fixation is applied if there is significant soft tissue trauma around the hip.

27256–27257

The physician treats a spontaneous hip dislocation. For an infant patient (age birth to six months) a Pavlik harness is applied. The harness is a dynamic flexion abduction orthosis. The harness consists of a chest strap, two shoulder straps, and two stirrups. The physician applies the harness with the child in a supine (face up) position. The harness holds the hip in 90 to 110 degrees of flexion, and moderate abduction. Skin traction may also be applied to infants of six to 18 months of age. A mechanical pulley is attached to the patient's leg with ace wraps securing the material to the skin. Weight is then attached to the other end of the pulley to apply the traction force to the hip, allowing a gentle reduction of the hip dislocation. The hip is maintained in approximately 30 to 40 degrees of flexion. Traction time varies from two to six weeks. A splint or hip spica cast is applied to hold the hips in abduction. In an older patient, reduction may be possible by applying skin traction to the affected lower extremity. The procedure is performed without anesthesia in 27256 or with anesthesia in 27257.

27258

The physician performs an open treatment of a spontaneous hip dislocation. The physician first performs an adductor tenotomy. The physician makes a small incision approximately 0.5" long over the origin of the adductor muscles. Dissection is carried down to the adductor tendon. The physician uses a small blade to release (free by incision) the tendon. The physician makes an incision from the middle of the iliac crest to a point midway between the anterosuperior iliac spine and the midline of the pelvis. Dissection is carried down to expose the capsule. The iliac epiphysis is detached from the ilium. The sartorius and rectus femoris tendons are divided or separated. The physician makes a T-shaped incision in the capsule. The entrance to the acetabulum is enlarged with sequential incisions in the labrum which surrounds the acetabulum. This allows the femoral head to then be reduced (repositioned). Once the reduction is concentric and stable, the capsule is tightened and closed with sutures, stabilizing the hip joint. The rectus femoris and sartorius tendons are sutured to their origins. The iliac epiphysis is also reattached. The incision is repaired in multiple layers. A double hip spica cast is applied with the hip in 90 degrees of flexion and 40 to 55 degrees of abduction.

27259

The physician first performs an adductor tenotomy (see 27000). The physician makes an incision from the middle of the iliac crest to a point midway between the anterosuperior iliac spine and the midline of the pelvis. Dissection is carried down to

expose the capsule. The iliac epiphysis is detached from the ilium. The sartorius and rectus femoris tendons are separated. The physician makes a T-shaped incision in the capsule. The entrance to the acetabulum is enlarged with sequential incisions in the labrum which surrounds the acetabulum. This allows the femoral head to then be reduced (repositioned). Once the reduction is concentric and stable, the capsule is tightened and closed with sutures, stabilizing the hip joint. The rectus femoris and sartorius tendons are sutured to their origins. The iliac epiphysis is also reattached. Femoral shaft shortening is performed as well. The physician makes both an anterior ilioinguinal and a straight lateral incision from the tip of the greater trochanter to the distal third of the femoral shaft. Open reduction is performed through the ilioinguinal incision. The femoral shaft is exposed through the lateral incision. A lag screw is inserted into the femoral neck. Once the bone cut is made at the appropriate distance below the first cut and angled to allow varus and derotation of the femur, the cut segment is removed. A side plate with screws secures the two segments. The incisions are repaired in multiple layers. A spica cast is applied with the extremity in neutral rotation and slight flexion and abduction.

27265–27266

The physician treats a post hip arthroplasty dislocation with manual manipulation. Distal manipulative traction is applied to the leg, reducing the dislocation. No anesthesia is necessary in 27265. Regional or general anesthesia is required in 27266.

27275

The patient is administered general anesthesia. If manipulation is performed to increase motion, the physician applies gradual pressure in the desired direction. The gradual pressure releases adhesions or scar tissue, increasing motion. Manipulation of the hip joint is a closed procedure, requiring no incision.

27280

The physician makes an incision along the posterior two-thirds of the iliac crest, continuing curved around the posterosuperior spine. The soft tissues are reflected to expose the ilium. A rectangular bone window is cut and removed from the ilium. The physician then removes cartilage from the sacral surface of the joint as well as from the joint surface of the block of bone. The physician then replaces the block of bone and countersinks it so that its cancellous surface contacts the cancellous bone of the sacrum. The edges of the bone window are osteotomized and the fragments turned inward to secure the block and promote bone formation. The incision is repaired in multiple layers using sutures. The physician may place the patient in a trunk and pelvic cast or brace.

27282

The physician makes an incision overlying the symphysis pubis. Dissection is carried down to the joint. Soft tissue between bone is excised. The physician may harvest a bone graft from the patient through a separate incision or from surrounding bone. The physician then closes the surgically created graft donor site. Internal fixation is applied to the fusion with screws and/or plates. The incision is repaired in multiple layers.

27284

To perform an intraarticular arthrodesis, the physician makes an anterior iliofemoral incision. The sartorius and rectus femoris muscles are then detached from their origins. The iliopsoas is reflected from the front of the hip joint. The physician dislocates the hip anteriorly. Cartilage is removed from the femoral head and acetabulum down to bleeding cancellous bone. The physician then packs the space between the surfaces of the femoral head and acetabulum with cancellous autogenous bone grafts. An example of the position in which the hip may be fused is: 30 degrees of flexion, 0 to 5 degrees of adduction, and 10 degrees of external rotation. The physician may use compression screws to increase the stability of the fusion. The sartorius and rectus femoris muscles are reattached. The screws are placed through the femoral head and into the supraacetabular area of the ilium. The incision is repaired in multiple layers with suction drains. The limb may be placed in a single spica cast or in balanced suspension.

27286

To perform an intraarticular arthrodesis, the physician makes an anterior iliofemoral incision. The sartorius and rectus femoris muscles are then detached from their origins. The iliopsoas is reflected from the front of the hip joint. The physician dislocates the hip anteriorly. Cartilage is removed from the femoral head and acetabulum down to bleeding cancellous bone. The physician packs the space between the surfaces of the femoral head and acetabulum with cancellous autogenous bone grafts. The physician then harvests a bone graft from the patient's iliac wing and crest and closes the surgically created graft donor site. The graft is positioned so it spans the anterior aspect of the hip from the pubic ramus to the femoral neck. The graft is secured with cancellous lag screws. The arthrodesis is performed so that the hip is in 10 degrees of external rotation, 0 to 5 degrees of adduction, and 30 degrees of flexion. A subtrochanteric osteotomy (bone cut) is made just below the lesser trochanter. The sartorius and rectus femoris muscles are reattached and the iliopsoas muscle is repositioned. The incision is repaired in multiple layers with suction drains. A one and one-half spica cast is applied.

27290

The patient is placed in a lateral (on the side) position with the operative side up. There are three parts to

this procedure including, anterior, perineal, and posterior. Each part requires a separate incision for exposure, dissection, and development of skin flaps. The physician separates the nerves and ligates the vessels. Vessels are ligated anteriorly and posteriorly; the sciatic nerve is cut high and tied. The pelvic ring, extending from the symphysis pubis to the attachment of the ilium to the sacrum, is sectioned and removed. Some muscle is retained, such as the gluteus maximus part of the skin flaps. The flaps are then closed with interrupted sutures over drains. The drains are removed in 48 to 72 hours.

27295

The physician makes an anterior racquet-shaped incision beginning at the anterosuperior iliac spine and curving distally and medially. The incision extends to a point on the medial aspect of the thigh, 5.0 cm below the origin of the adductor muscles. The femoral artery and vein are ligated. The femoral nerve is divided. The physician continues the incision around the posterior aspect of the thigh to 5.0 cm below the ischial tuberosity and then laterally to the base of the greater trochanter. All muscles around the hip are detached. The physician then detaches the gluteal muscles, reflecting the muscle mass proximally for later use as a flap. The sciatic nerve is ligated and separated. The physician incises the hip joint capsule and ligamentum teres to complete the disarticulation. The gluteal flap is then brought around the wound and sutured. The physician places a drain in the inferior part of the incision. The edges of skin are closed with nonabsorbable sutures.

27301

The physician makes an incision overlying the abscess, hematoma, or bursa of the thigh or knee. The area is exposed and aspirated or dissected. The physician may also explore the surrounding tissue requiring debridement and irrigation. If an infection is present, the incision may be left open for one to three weeks. If an abscess or hematoma is present, a temporary drain is placed in the wound and the incision may be closed in multiple layers.

27303

The physician makes an incision overlying a bone abscess of the femur or knee. Dissection is carried down to the bone. The bone may appear soft or pitted, needing debridement. In order to remove the infected bone and promote healing, the physician may make a "cortical window." This is accomplished by drilling several holes in the shape of an elongated window. The physician removes the cortical window to expose the abscess. The physician then debrides and irrigates the area. Gauze may be placed and the wound left open. The wound may be packed and a few sutures placed. The incision may be repaired in multiple layers.

27305

For release of the iliotibial band, the patient is placed in a lateral decubitus position (lying down on the side). The physician exposes the iliotibial tract through a 4.0 cm lateral, longitudinal incision just above the femoral condyle. The physician then incises the iliotibial tract, fascia lata, and intramuscular septum transversely 2.5 cm above the patella. In severe contractures, the physician may remove a segment of the iliotibial tract and septum. The incision is closed in multiple layers with sutures, staples, and/or Steri-strips.

27306–27307

The physician performs a percutaneous tenotomy (cut) of the adductor or hamstring muscle. The physician palpates the tendon to be released. A small incision is made to access the tendon. The physician's thumb presses down on the tendon to create tension. The physician then uses an 11-blade to make a cut through the tendon, releasing it. More than one tendon is released in 27307. The incision is closed with sutures.

27310

The physician makes an anterior or anteromedial incision to expose the knee joint. The incision extends above and below the patella. Dissection is carried down to the knee joint with the patella moved laterally to provide better exposure. Each compartment of the knee is then thoroughly examined and any foreign bodies are removed. If infection is present, any purulent exudate (pus secretion) is irrigated and debrided. The physician uses an antibiotic solution to irrigate the joint. With the presence of infection, the incision may be left open temporarily to allow drainage. If no infection is present, the incision is repaired in multiple layers.

27315

The physician performs an incisional resection of a segment of a nerve. The physician makes a transverse incision over the hamstring muscle. The fascia is divided to expose the nerves which supply the muscle. The appropriate nerve branch is identified by stimulating it with an electrical current, or gently pressing it with forceps. Once this is accomplished, the nerve is divided and removed from the muscle, resolving the clonus or spasm. The incision is repaired in multiple layers.

27320

The physician performs an incisional resection of a segment of a nerve. The physician makes a transverse incision over the distal portion of the popliteal (back of the knee) fossa. The fascia is divided to expose the tibial nerve. The appropriate nerve branch is identified by stimulating it with an electrical current, or gently pressing it with forceps. Once this is accomplished, the nerve is divided and removed from the muscle, resolving the clonus or spasm. The incision is repaired in multiple layers.

27323–27324

The physician locates the tumor or cyst in the subcutaneous tissue between the muscle and skin layers. An incision is made overlying the site and the tumor is exposed. The tumor is typically surrounded by a capsule. The physician makes an incision through the capsule and removes a portion of the tumor for biopsy. For 27324, the tumor is deeper and may be located within muscle. The capsule may be closed with sutures in 27323. The incision is repaired in multiple layers using sutures, staples, and/or Steri-strips in 27324.

27327–27328

The physician makes a 3.0 cm to 5.0 cm elliptical incision encompassing the tumor mass. The physician's hand retracts the tumor while excising the superficial fascia surrounding the mass. A few centimeters of underlying muscle may be resected as well with electrocautery. For 27328, the physician makes a deeper incision into the deep fascia within the muscle. The tumor is removed with additional muscle. Due to the elliptical incision, a separately reportable skin graft may be harvested and applied for wound closure. A temporary drain may be placed. The wound may be closed with single or multiple layers of sutures.

27329

The physician performs a radical resection of a tumor. Extensive removal of surrounding tissue, including a significant amount of muscle, is performed. For tumor of the quadriceps (thigh) muscle, an elliptical incision is made along the anterior thigh. Medial and lateral skin flaps are developed as part of the incision. All major vessels and nerves are identified from the tissue to be removed and are then dissected and mobilized. The muscles of the thigh are next dissected. Some muscles will be excised with the tumor, according to its location. In order to compensate for the loss of thigh muscles, the physician may perform a separately reportable transfer of remaining muscles to aid in knee function. Irrigation of the wound is completed. The incision is repaired in multiple layers with sutures, staples, and/or Steri-strips. One or two large, temporary drains may be used.

27330–27331

The physician usually makes an anteromedial incision to gain adequate exposure of the knee joint. The patella is shifted to the side to examine the area. Each compartment of the knee joint is visually examined. The physician may need to make an additional incision to further explore other areas of the knee joint. If there is suspicion that synovium may be diseased, a tissue biopsy is taken. Any loose bodies or foreign bodies are removed in 27331. Incisions are closed with sutures, staples, and/or Steri-strips. A temporary drain may be placed.

27332–27333
The physician makes an incision along the anteromedial or anterolateral aspect of the knee, depending on which cartilage is torn (medial or lateral in 27332 or both in 27333). Dissection is carried down to the cartilage. The patella is shifted to either side and the knee joint exposed. The torn cartilage is removed and the roughened edges are smoothed. A partial synovectomy and release or excision (partial or total) of plica may be performed. Plica is a fold, pleat, band, or shelf of synovial tissue (e.g., transverse suprapatellar, medial suprapatellar, mediopatellar and infrapatellar). Debridement of the chondral surface of the patella may be performed as well. A temporary drain may be applied. The incision is repaired in layers with sutures, staples, and/or Steri-strips.

27334–27335
The physician makes an anteromedial incision for anterior synovectomy. Once the knee joint is accessed, proliferative, diseased synovium is removed. If posterior synovectomy is required, the physician will position the patient prone and make an "s" shaped incision along the popliteal (back of the knee) area. Both anterior and posterior synovectomy is performed in 27335. Dissection is carried down to expose the knee joint. Diseased synovium is removed. Incisions are closed with sutures, staples, and/or Steri-strips. A temporary drain may be applied.

27340
The physician makes a small incision over the upper portion of the patella. The bursal sac is located in fat in front of the patella. Dissection is carried down to the area of infection or inflammation. The bursa is then removed. The incision is repaired in layers with sutures and Steri-strips.

27345
A Bakers cyst is located in the popliteal space (back of the knee). The physician makes a popliteal incision, carrying dissection down to expose the semimembranosis tendon. The cyst is typically located around this tendon. The cyst is then excised from the tendon. The incision is repaired in multiple layers with sutures.

27347
The physician excises a lesion of the meniscus or capsule of the knee. Types of lesions treated include a cyst or ganglion (fluid-filled sac). Lesions may be located in the meniscus — the cartilage between the knee joint — (following an injury), or on the capsule, the fibrous covering over the joint space. Through an incision over the knee the physician dissects the tissues to the level of the cyst or ganglion. The lesion

is excised, and the wound is closed with layered sutures.

27350
Patellectomy is removal of the patella. A hemipatellectomy or partial patellectomy is removal of cartilage from the patella or removal of a portion of the bone. A transverse "u" shaped incision is made over the anterior aspect of the knee joint just below the patella. The patella is then excised from the tissue surrounding it (capsule, quadriceps, and patellar tendons). The physician then takes the upper part of the capsule and quadriceps tendon medially and distally so that they overlap the lower part of the capsule. The physician sutures the capsule and tendon in place. Incisions are repaired with sutures, staples, and/or Steri-strips.

27355–27356
The physician makes an incision over the site of the cyst or tumor. Dissection is carried down to the bone. The cyst or tumor is removed by curettage with a high speed bur. If the amount of bone removed is small and does not compromise the load capacity, no bone graft is necessary and the incision is repaired in multiple layers. In 27356, an allograft (donor bone) is shaped then packed into the bone wound. The soft tissues are closed in layers. The incision is repaired with sutures, staples, and/or Steri-strips.

27357–27358
The physician makes an incision over the site of the bone cyst or tumor of the femur. Dissection is carried down through the muscle layers to expose the bone. The cyst or tumor is removed with a scalpel or by curettage with a high speed bur. A bone graft may be necessary to strengthen the weakened bone in 27357. The physician typically harvests bone from the patient's hip, making an incision over the iliac crest. The physician then closes the surgically created graft donor site. The bone graft is fashioned by the physician and packed into the site where the tumor or bone cyst was removed. Internal fixation is required in 27358 for more stability. Bone screws, compression plates, or an intramedullary nail may be used. The incision is repaired in multiple layers with sutures, staples, and/or Steri-strips. A temporary drain may be placed.

27360
The physician makes an incision over the affected bone to remove osteomyelitis (bone infection). Dissection is carried down to expose the infected bone. Only the necrotic (dying) bone is removed so as not to create large bony defects. Dying and infected soft tissue is removed as well. The physician may remove the bone by craterization (creation of a circular depression with an elevated area of the periphery). The physician may remove the bone with a saucerization technique, creating a saucerlike depression in the bone. The wound is irrigated with

antibiotic solution. The physician may repair the incision in multiple layers or may leave the wound open temporarily.

27365

The physician makes an incision overlying a tumor of the femur or knee. Adequate exposure is accomplished. Resection is performed including, adjacent periosteum and muscle, a cuff of normal bone both proximal and distal to the lesion, and skin and soft tissues as necessary. For a malignant neoplasm of the femur or knee, additional bone and/or soft tissue may need to be removed, thus compromising the stability or integrity of the femur or knee joint. Separately reportable procedures, such as reconstruction of ligaments and/or tendons, reattachment of muscles, placement of donor bone graft, and use of an external fixator may be necessary as well. The incision is then repaired in multiple layers.

27370

The patient is placed supine (lying on the back) on an x-ray table with the knee flexed over a small pillow. The knee is cleansed with Betadine and covered with a sterile drape. A skin anesthetic may be applied. The physician then passes a 20-gauge needle into the femoropatellar space. Air, and either a single or double contrast agent is then injected into the space. After the injection is complete, the patient is asked to move the knee to produce an even coating of the joint structures. Multiple roentgenographic views are then taken of the knee.

27372

The physician removes a foreign body (i.e., nail, piece of wood) in the thigh or knee. For a foreign body in the thigh, an incision is made overlying the object. Tissue is dissected around the object. The physician may need to suture damaged muscle or other soft tissues. The wound is irrigated with antibiotic solution. The incision will typically be closed, unless an infection is present, in which case it will be left open temporarily to drain.

27380–27381

An incision is made from the upper portion of the patella and extending to a point just medial to the lower part of the tibial tuberosity. The patellar tendon is exposed, and all scar tissue removed. The ruptured ends of the tendon are then debrided. Sutures are passed through the ruptured ends to bring them together. A fascia lata graft may be used for reinforcement of the suture line by being incorporated in both ends of the ruptures in a figure "8" fashion. Another technique for reinforcement is to sever the semitendinosus tendon, and then make transverse drill holes through the distal third of the patella and transversely through the tibial tuberosity. The semitendinosus tendon is then looped through the drill holes and sewn back onto itself at the tibial

tubercle. In 27381, the repair is augmented with tissues (tendon or fascia) from surrounding areas or allograft tissue. The incision is closed with sutures and staples or Steri-strips.

27385–27386

The physician makes an incision over the site of injury. Dissection is carried down to the ruptured muscle. The torn ends are debrided so that healthy muscle tissue can be accurately opposed. Nonabsorbable sutures are placed close together around the circumference of the muscle. In 27386, the repair may be reinforced by using strips of fascia lata tissue. The physician makes an incision over the fascia lata in order to obtain the needed tissue. The fascia lata strips are then interwoven with sutures around the ruptured muscle. Incisions are repaired with sutures and staples or Steri-strips.

27390–27392

The patient is positioned prone (lying face down). The physician then makes a 7.0 cm to 10.0 cm, longitudinal incision beginning just above the popliteal crease and extending upward. Dissection is carried down to expose the hamstring tendons. The tendon sheath is divided and the tendon is incised transversely at two levels, 3.0 cm apart. The physician flexes the hip while the knee remains extended, causing the tendon to lengthen. The tendon sheath is then closed. For 27391, two or three tendons are lengthened on the same leg. For 27392, the same technique is performed on both legs. The incision is then repaired in multiple layers.

27393–27395

The patient is positioned prone (lying face down). The physician then makes a 7.0 cm to 10.0 cm, longitudinal incision beginning just above the popliteal crease and extending upward. Dissection is carried down to expose the hamstring tendons. The tendon sheath is divided and the tendon is then incised transversely at two levels, 3 cm apart. The physician then flexes the hip while the knee remains extended, causing the tendon to lengthen. The tendon sheath is then closed. For 27394, two or three tendons are lengthened on the same leg. For 27395, the same technique is performed on both legs. The incision is then repaired in multiple layers.

27396–27397

The physician makes an incision to expose the hamstring muscle and the knee. Dissection is carried down to the hamstring. The muscles causing flexion may then be sutured to the quadriceps tendon or patella. This provides motor for active extension of the knee. Multiple transplants are performed in 27397. The incisions are closed in multiple layers.

27400

The physician makes a curvilinear incision over the biceps femoris tendon, extending just above the fibular head. The peroneal nerve is retracted so that the biceps tendon is exposed. This tendon is then divided and repositioned on the lateral femoral condyle where it is anchored firmly. A similar incision is then made on the medial side of the knee to expose the semimembranosus, semitendinosus, and gracilis tendons. The tendons are each divided and then anchored firmly to the medial femoral condyle. The incisions are then repaired in multiple layers.

27403
With the knee in 60 degrees of flexion, the physician makes a vertical incision on either the medial or lateral joint line area, depending on which meniscus needs repair. The meniscus is exposed and the edges of the tear are debrided with a small curet or scalpel. A rasp abrades the debrided edges of the tear, creating an increased inflammatory healing response. Sutures are then placed through the tear in the meniscus every 3.0 mm to 4.0 mm. The incision is repaired with sutures and Steri-strips.

27405–27409
For a primary collateral repair (27405), the physician makes an incision on either the lateral or medial aspect of the knee, depending on which ligament is torn (medial collateral or lateral collateral). Sutures may be used to tie the torn ends together. If the attachment of the ligament to the bone is torn away, a screw may be used for fixation. For a cruciate ligament primary repair (27407), an incision is made to gain access into the knee joint (the physician may use the arthroscope for part of the procedure). Screws and/or sutures are used to reattach the torn end to the bone. Both collateral and cruciate ligaments are repaired in 27409. Incisions are closed with sutures, staples, and/or Steri-strips. A temporary drain may be applied.

27418
A lateral parapatellar incision is made extending from the top of the patella to the tibial tubercle. Small osteotomes or an oscillating saw is used to free a 6.0 cm to 8.0 cm block of bone, which includes the tibial tubercle near its upper end. A small bony platform is made on the medial side of the long bone block. The block is elevated anteriorly and its upper end is swung up onto the platform, while the lower end pivots. Cancellous bone is removed from the lower end of the block in order to improve the cosmetic appearance. Two bone screws secure the block. Incisions are closed with sutures, staples, or Steri-strips. By elevating the tibial tubercle, forces are decreased on the underneath surface of the patella.

27420
An incision is made on the anteromedial aspect of the knee beginning above the patella and ending 1.3 cm below the tibial tuberosity. The area where the patellar tendon inserts into the tibial tuberosity is then resected, including a thin piece of bone 1.3 cm

square. The patellar tendon is then pulled medially and distally on the tibia and a site is selected for reattachment. At the site, an "I" shaped incision is made and the patellar tendon is secured here temporarily with sutures. Next, the insertion of the vastus medialis muscle is transformed laterally and distally and sutured in place. After the alignment of the patella has been checked, the patellar tendon is then anchored into the tibia with a staple. The incision is closed with sutures, staples, or Steri-strips.

27422
An anteromedial incision is made parallel to the quadriceps tendon and the patella. Dissection is carried down to the vastus medialis muscle/tendon to the site where it attaches to the patella. An incision is made along the vastus medialis tendon parallel to the patella. The tendon is then overlapped and sutured, pulling the patella more medially and allowing for improved patellar alignment. Tissue layers are closed with sutures. The incision is closed with sutures and Steri-strips.

27424
Patellectomy is removal of the patella. A transverse U-shaped incision is made over the anterior aspect of the knee just below the patella. The skin edges are retracted, and the incision is carried down through the quadriceps expansion at the level of the distal third of the patella. The patella is then excised from the capsule, quadriceps, and patellar tendons. The proximal part of the capsule and quadriceps tendon are taken medially and distally so that they overlap the distal part of the capsule by 1.3 cm and then sutured in place. The insertion of the vastus medialis is then freed and transferred distally and laterally. Incisions are closed in multiple layers with sutures.

27425
This procedure is typically performed arthroscopically. One cm long incisions are made on either side of the patellar tendon for arthroscopic access into the knee joint. An additional portal incision may be made just overlying and lateral to the upper part of the patella. Scissors or electrocautery release the lateral retinaculum holding the patella more laterally than it should be. A temporary drain may be applied, and incisions are closed with sutures and Steri-strips. The procedure may also be performed through open incisions or percutaneously.

27427–27429
The physician performs an extra-articular and/or intra-articular ligamentous reconstruction procedure of the knee. To perform a lateral extra-articular augmentation in 27427, the physician makes an incision over the distal iliotibial band. The band is then incised, elevated, and secured to the distal femur with a cancellous screw and washer. In 27428, the physician makes an anteromedial incision to access the knee joint. The torn ligament (collateral or

cruciate) is identified. The ligament is then reattached at its torn end. If reattachment is not possible, the physician will obtain a graft (such as a tendon) either harvested from the patient or a donor graft, and attach it to the original location of the ligament. In 27429, both extra- and intra-articular ligamentous reconstruction are performed. A temporary drain is applied and incisions are repaired in multiple layers with sutures, staples, and/or Steri-strips.

27430

The physician corrects a shortened or fibrotic quadriceps muscle. An anterior longitudinal incision is made from the upper one third of the thigh to the lower part of the patella. Deep fascia is divided and the rectus femoris muscle is separated from the vastus medialis and lateralis muscles. The vastus intermedius muscle is excised because it is usually scarred and is binding the posterior surface of the rectus femoris and patella to the femur. If the vastus medialis and lateralis muscles are badly scarred, then subcutaneous tissue and fat are interposed between them and the rectus. If these muscles are relatively normal, then they are sutured to the rectus at the lower one third of the thigh. Layers and incisions are closed with sutures and staples or Steri-strips.

27435

The physician corrects severe flexion contractures of the knee that cannot be corrected by more conservative means. The patient is positioned prone and a curvilinear incision (approximately 15.0 cm long) is made over the popliteal (back of the knee) space. The medial and lateral aspects of the joint capsule are exposed by dissecting through subcutaneous tissue and deep fascia. The common peroneal nerve and popliteal vessels and nerves are retracted. The medial and lateral portions of the capsule are divided, allowing the knee to be completely extended. The subcutaneous tissue and skin incisions are repaired in multiple layers.

27437–27438

The physician makes a medial patellar incision, exposing the underneath surface (subchondral bone) of the patella. Abrasion arthroplasty or a smoothing down of the bone surface is performed to encourage growth of new cartilage. If cancellous bone is exposed and abrasion arthroplasty would not be effective, the physician may place a prosthesis (also called hemiarthroplasty) on the back side of the patella in 27438. The underneath side of the patella is smoothed down to make room for the prosthesis. The physician then secures the prosthesis with screws or glue. The prosthesis sits in the trochlear groove in the position where the patella slides up and down when the knee bends and straightens. The incision is repaired in multiple layers with sutures, staples, and/or Steri-strips.

27440

The physician replaces the damaged or degenerated tibial portion of the knee joint. The physician makes a medial incision along the patella. Dissection is carried down to expose the knee joint and tibial plateau. The menisci and anterior cruciate ligament are removed. The physician may also need to release other soft tissues around the knee to correct contractures and restore range of motion. The physician makes a bone cut through the tibial plateau using a cutting-alignment jig. Peg holes are made on the remaining tibial plateau and the tibial component is placed into position. Screws and/or glue secure the component. The incision is repaired in multiple layers with sutures, staples, and/or Steri-strips.

27441

The physician replaces the damaged or degenerated cartilage of the tibial component of the knee joint. The physician makes a medial incision along the patella. Dissection is carried down to expose the knee joint and tibial plateau. The menisci and anterior cruciate ligament are removed. The physician may also need to release other soft tissues around the knee to correct contractures and restore range of motion. If the synovium around the knee joint is diseased, the physician may remove it as well. Any osteophytes (bony outgrowths) interfering with motion may be removed. The physician makes a bone cut through the tibial plateau using a cutting-alignment jig to achieve correct alignment. Peg holes are made on the remaining tibial plateau and the tibial component is placed into position. Screws and/or glue secure the tibial component. The incision is repaired in multiple layers with sutures, staples, and/or Steri-strips.

27442–27443

The physician replaces the damaged or degenerated cartilage of the femoral condyles or tibial plateau. The physician makes a medial incision along the patella and carries dissection down to expose the knee joint. If the femoral condyles are replaced, the physician uses a cutting-alignment jig to determine proper alignment of the bone cut and then resects or cuts the distal femur. Additional smaller cuts may be made on the femur for rotational alignment. The physician may need to release soft tissues around the knee to correct contractures and restore range of motion. If the tibial plateau is replaced, the physician first removes the menisci and other soft tissue as needed. A cutting alignment jig is used to determine proper alignment of the tibial bone cut. Once the bone cuts are made, peg holes are also made into the bone. The prosthesis is then placed into position and secured with screws and/or glue. In 27443, debridement and synovectomy are also performed. Any osteophytes interfering with range of motion are debrided and removed. The physician will also remove any diseased synovium present around the knee joint. The incision is repaired in multiple layers with sutures, staples, and/or Steri-strips.

27445

The physician exposes the knee joint by making a straight longitudinal incision directly over the knee. Bone cuts are made to resect the anterior and posterior femoral condyles. A tibial cutting guide is then used to remove a minimal amount of bone from the proximal tibia. A template is then placed on the cut tibial surface and an osteotome is used to remove a square of bone from the tibial surface as outlined by the hole in the tibial template. The stem of the tibial component is placed into the hole and the femoral component is placed on the distal femur. Two polyethylene bushings are inserted into the femoral component and then joined to the tibial component with the metal axle. The patellar component is applied by making a cut along the articular surface, making a peg hole, and then inserting the component. If the patella does not track properly, a separately reportable lateral retinacular release is performed. All components are then cemented into place. The joint is thoroughly irrigated. The incision is closed in multiple layers and placement of temporary suction drainage tubes.

27446

The physician replaces one diseased or damaged compartment of the knee, including the femoral condyle and tibial plateau on the same side. A medial incision is made along the patella and dissection is carried down to expose the knee joint. The physician prepares the selected compartment for arthroplasty by removing the meniscus. Other soft tissue around the compartment may also need to be released. Using a cutting-alignment jig, the physician makes bone cuts on the femoral condyle and tibial plateau of the compartment being replaced. The other compartment is left intact. Peg holes are then made into the bone and the femoral and tibial components are placed into position. The components are secured with screws and/or glue. The incision is repaired in multiple layers with sutures, staples, and/or Steri-strips.

27447

The physician replaces severely damaged or worn cartilage of the knee joint. A midline incision is made over the knee. Dissection is carried down to expose the knee joint. The physician may release soft tissues and/or ligaments in order to correct deformities and improve range of motion. The physician uses a cutting-alignment jig placed on the upper tibia to remove the tibial joint surface (both medial and lateral compartments) by making a bone cut. A cutting-alignment jig is also used on the femoral condyles to make the appropriate bone cut. Depending on the integrity of the joint surface of the patella, the physician may also make a bone cut to remove damaged cartilage. If the joint surface is healthy, it is left intact. Peg holes are usually made, and the components of the prosthesis are placed into position on the tibia, femur, and, if needed, the patella. The components are secured with glue and/or

bone screws. The incision is repaired in multiple layers with sutures, staples, and/or Steri-strips.

27448–27450

The physician performs an osteotomy of the femur. A medial or lateral incision is made to approach the femur. After the femur is exposed, a Kirschner wire is placed where a blade-plate is to be inserted. The physician then inserts the blade of the plate at the determined angle an osteotomy (bone cut) that is performed transversely. The physician may use a nail plate and screws for internal fixation in 27450. Alignment of the knee now allows weight bearing to occur on the healthier compartment of the knee joint. The incision is repaired in multiple layers with sutures, staples, and/or Steri-strips.

27454

The physician exposes the entire shaft of the femur with a long, longitudinal, lateral incision. An osteotomy (bone cut) is made through the proximal and distal ends of the femur. The femoral shaft is then removed. Osteotomies are made (three or four) on the shaft, and the fragments are threaded end-to-end and aligned on a nail. If the cortex of the bone is very thin, the physician may need to add a separately reportable bone graft. The nail is then inserted into the proximal and distal ends of the femur. The periosteum (bone lining) is sutured over the bone and the incision is repaired in multiple layers.

27455

The physician removes a wedge of bone from the upper tibia below the growth plate. To correct the tibial varum (Bowles) in an eight year old child, for example, a 3.0 cm to 4.0 cm lateral incision is made over the fibula. An oblique osteotomy of the fibula is then performed. An anterolateral incision is then made to gain access to the upper tibia. A Steinman pin is inserted through the midshaft of the tibia, parallel to the ankle joint, and another pin is inserted through the upper tibia parallel to the knee joint. The pins are used as guides to make a bony wedge cut (osteotomy) using a bone saw and chisel. The bone ends are then approximated, correcting the deformity. The physician may use an AO five-hole compression plate or staples for internal fixation. The excised bone wedge may be used as a bone graft to fill in any defects. The incisions are closed, and the leg placed in a cast with the knee in 30 to 45 degrees of flexion.

27457

The physician performs an osteotomy of the proximal tibia to remove loading forces from damaged cartilage and bone. The load is transferred to normal cartilage and bone of the opposite knee compartment. For a valgus osteotomy (bone cut), the physician makes an incision over the lateral proximal tibia. For a varus osteotomy, the incision is made medially. Dissection is carried down to the bone. For a valgus osteotomy, the fibular head is removed with an oscillating saw. The osteotomy is made approximately 2.0 cm below the joint line. The degree of correction has been calculated before surgery with x-ray films. The physician then uses an oscillating saw to cut a wedge of bone at the determined angle, three-quarters of the width through the tibia. The cut wedge is removed and an osteotome completes the bone cut. The cut edges of the osteotomy are brought together and secured with a staple. The incision is repaired in multiple layers with sutures, staples, and/or Steri-strips.

27465–27468

Femoral shortening or lengthening techniques equalize leg lengths or treat malunions of the femur. The physician shortens the femur in 27465. An incision is made to expose the tip of the greater trochanter. The femoral canal is reamed and prepared for the insertion of an intramedullary nail. Next the femur is exposed through a lateral longitudinal incision at the middle third of the thigh. Two bone cuts are made to remove a length of bone. After the cut segment is removed, the bone ends are approximated, and the intramedullary nail is inserted into the femoral canal. Plates and screws may be used for fixation if the intramedullary nail is contraindicated, as in osteomyelitis or a deformity that precludes the use of a nail. The leg is placed in a Thomas splint. For femoral lengthening in 27466, two puncture wounds are made laterally in the distal and proximal femur. Two holes at each end are drilled in the bone, and a screw is inserted in each drill hole. The physician makes a lateral longitudinal incision 6.0 cm to 8.0 cm long to expose the femur. At the osteotomy site, an oscillating saw cuts through the femur. The Wagner distraction apparatus is then attached to the two sets of screws, so that the apparatus is 1.0 cm to 2.0 cm lateral to the thigh. The incision is repaired in multiple layers. The device is then distracted up to 5 mm to 6.0 mm immediately. The apparatus is operated by a knob. Lengthening is about 1.5 mm or 1.0 cm per week. Both lengthening and shortening are performed in 27468. When the appearance of the femur is normal and the medullary has been reestablished, the plate and screws are removed.

27470–27472

The physician repairs a nonunion or malunion of the femur. The physician makes a lateral incision to expose the femur. If there is no distortion of the intramedullary canal, intramedullary nailing is performed for fixation of the nonunion. If failed internal fixation is present, the physician removes the plates and screws. If there is malalignment of the medullary canal, a compression plate and screws are used for repair. In 27472, there is a loss of bone. The physician harvests bone with an osteotome from the iliac crest or from the femur itself and closes the surgically created donor site. Copious amounts of bone are placed around the nonunion site. The

incision is repaired in multiple layers and a temporary drain is applied.

27475–27479

The physician performs epiphysiodesis to achieve complete arrest of the longitudinal growth at the physis (growth plate) of the longer limb. A 5.0 cm to 7.0 cm longitudinal incision is made along the lower femur, beginning just above the joint line. The distal femur physis is exposed. Osteotomes excise a rectangular piece of bone from the epiphyseal plate. The growth plate is then drilled in anterior, posterior, and distal directions. A curet is used to remove the growth plate. The physician harvests bone from the patient's hip or femur and closes the surgically created graft donor site. The separately reportable cancellous bone graft is then packed into the defect created by the removal of the growth plate. The rectangular piece of bone is reinserted into its original bed and securely seated with a mallet. The arrest procedure is the same whether performed on the medial or lateral side. The periosteum and incision are repaired in multiple layers. For 27477, the same procedure is performed for the proximal tibial and fibular epiphyseal growth plates. For 27479, a combination of distal femur and proximal tibia and fibula epiphyseal arrest is performed.

27485

The physician performs hemiepiphyseal arrest on the distal femur or proximal tibia or fibula. For genu valgus, arrest of the medial femoral physis and/or proximal tibia is performed to realign the knee joint. A 5.0 cm to 7.0 cm, longitudinal incision is made along the lower femur, beginning just above the joint line. The distal femur physis is exposed. Osteotomes excise a rectangular piece of bone from the epiphyseal plate. The growth plate is then drilled in anterior, posterior, and distal directions. A curet is used to remove the growth plate. The physician harvests bone from the patient's hip or femur and closes the surgically created graft donor site. The separately reportable cancellous bone graft is then packed into the defect created by the removal of the growth plate. The rectangular piece of bone is reinserted into its original bed and securely seated with a mallet. The periosteum and incision are repaired in multiple layers.

27486–27487

The physician performs a revision of a total knee arthroplasty. Typically, previous skin incisions are incorporated to expose the knee. One or both (femoral and tibial) components are removed as determined by the physician. In order to remove the components, an osteotome or saw may be used to loosen the cement or bone so that the prosthesis can be topped out with a mallet. If any cement is present, it is removed in order to protect and preserve as much bone as possible. Bone cuts are made to accommodate the new prosthesis. If significant bone defects are present on either the femur, tibia or both, a bone graft may be needed. An allograft (donor bone) may be packed into the defect. The components of the new prosthesis are placed into position and may be cemented for fixation. The femoral and entire tibial component are revised in 27487. The incision is repaired with sutures, staples, and/or Steri-strips.

27488

The physician inserts a temporary spacer into the knee joint. To remove the knee prosthesis, the physician makes an incision directly over the original incision line. The prosthesis is exposed. An osteotome or saw may loosen the cement or bone around the components, so that they may be tapped out with a mallet. The cement is removed a piece at a time to protect and preserve as much bone as possible. Once the prosthesis is removed, there is an open space where the knee prosthesis was between the femur and tibia. A spacer of methylmethacrylate formed into a cube shape may be inserted into the space between the femur and tibia. The spacer prevents the soft tissues from compressing the joint space. The spacer is secured until another prosthesis is inserted. The incision is repaired in multiple layers.

27495

The physician applies a prophylactic treatment to the femur. Methylmethacrylate may be applied to an area of resection because of malignancy. Fixation (nailing, pinning, plating, or wiring) and a prophylactic treatment may be an alternative to bone grafting.

27496–27497

The physician performs a decompression fasciotomy on one compartment of the thigh and/or knee. A longitudinal incision is made over the affected compartment. Dissection is carried down through the fascial layers to the muscle compartments. An incision may also be made through the intramuscular septum to release pressure. If any necrotic tissue is present, it is debrided. Debridement of nonviable muscle and/or nerve is performed in addition in 27497. The incision may be left open for two to five days and then repaired in multiple layers with sutures.

27498

The physician performs a decompression fasciotomy on multiple compartments of the thigh and/or knee. One incision may be used to gain access to one or two compartments of the thigh. If not, a longitudinal incision is made over each compartment. Once the incision is made, dissection is carried through the fascial layers to the muscle compartments. An incision may also be made through the intramuscular septum to release pressure. The incision may be left open for two to five days and then repaired in multiple layers with sutures.

27499

The physician performs a decompression fasciotomy of multiple compartments of the thigh and/or knee, and debrides any nonviable tissue. The physician makes one or more extensive longitudinal incisions over the involved compartments. The incisions are carried deep to the fascia of each compartment. These fascia are incised to expose the compartments and relieve the pressures. A thorough exploration is undertaken and the physician debrides any nonviable tissue. This would typically be muscle, but it may also include other tissues within the compartment. The incisions are normally left open for several days before secondary closure is accomplished.

27500

The physician treats a femoral shaft fracture without manipulation. The fractured segments are aligned and stable. Treatment may be with a molded long leg cast, cast brace, or spica cast for several weeks until union is established.

27501

The physician treats a supracondylar or transcondylar femoral fracture without manipulation. The fractured segments are aligned and stable and no manipulation is required. If there is an intercondylar extension of the fracture such as a "T" or "Y" fracture extending into the joint, the intra-articular relationships of the knee must be reestablished. Treatment may be with a molded long leg cast, cast brace, or spica cast for several weeks until union is established.

27502

Closed reduction of the fracture is required either by manual reduction by the physician or in conjunction with skin or skeletal traction. If skin traction is used, the leg is placed in full extension and bandages and straps are encircled around the leg starting at the foot and extending to the thigh. Weight is added to provide the traction force. The best application of skin traction is to temporarily provide comfort and support to the fractured limb until a definitive form of therapy is available. For skeletal traction, a pin is placed transversely through the proximal tibia with the knee in slight flexion. Traction weight is 15 to 20 pounds, and thereafter may be reduced gradually. If the physician is concerned about accurate reduction, a second pin may be placed through the distal femur, permitting early movement of the knee. Traction can maintain position until bone healing is well established. If traction is not needed, the extremity is placed in a spica cast or cast brace.

27503

The physician may reduce a displaced fracture manually without the use of skin or skeletal traction. If the intra-articular relationships of the knee cannot be reestablished manually, traction is generally not as effective as skeletal traction, but can be used by wrapping circular wraps around the lower extremity and attaching weight. Skeletal traction is more commonly used by placing a pin through the proximal tibia with the thigh, knee, and leg supported in suspension with some knee flexion. Traction weight of 15 to 20 pounds is applied and thereafter reduced gradually. The physician may need to perform manipulative reduction while in traction if accurate reduction cannot be obtained by traction alone. Traction is used to maintain position until bone healing is well established, or a cast or cast brace may be applied after the fracture becomes stable.

27506

With the patient in a lateral or supine (lying on the back) position, the physician makes a straight lateral incision to expose the fracture site. If there are large butterfly-type fragments or there is a long spiral fracture, cerclage wires may be wrapped around the bone to hold the fragments in place. The intramedullary nail is then put into place by making a 4.0 cm to 6.0 cm incision over the tip of the greater trochanter. The trochanteric fossa is exposed. A drill hole is made into the center of the femoral canal. A reaming guide is then used to ream out the intramedullary canal to the desired length, making room for the implant or nail. A nail-driving guide is inserted, and the nail is driven into place with a hammer. If it is a comminuted fracture, the physician may use interlocking screws to provide better fixation. One or two screws are placed proximally and/or distally through the femur and intramedullary implant. This technique helps secure rotatory stability. The interlocking screws may be removed after six to eight weeks.

27507

With the patient in a supine (lying on the back) or lateral decubitus (lying on the side) position, the physician makes a lateral or anterolateral incision. The fracture is reduced by manipulation and bone reduction forceps. A compression plate with screws and/or leg screws secure and compress the fragments. The physician may elect to use cerclage wiring in conjunction with plates or screws in order to facilitate fixation of the fracture. The wire is placed around the femur, over the fracture site. One or more wires may be used. The incision is closed with sutures, staples, and/or Steri-strips.

27508

Closed treatment of a femoral fracture of the distal end of the medial or lateral condyle is indicated if the intra-articular relationships of the knee are intact and stable, as found upon x-ray. If the fracture does not need reduction, then skeletal traction is not required. A spica cast brace is used until bony union is secure.

27509

Percutaneous skeletal fixation can be used for internal fixation in nonunions, malunions, and either open or closed fractures of the distal femur area. Fixation pins

are introduced through stab wounds (small incision over the bone). A small hole is drilled and a pin placed across the fracture line to hold it in place. Two, three, or more pins may be used. The ends of the pins are cut off beneath the skin, and the small incision closed with suture or Steri-strips. The pins are left in place approximately three to six weeks, and then removed.

27510

Closed treatment of femoral fracture of the distal end of the medial or lateral condyle is indicated if the intra-articular relationships of the knee are intact and stable upon x-ray. If reduction of the fracture is required, skeletal traction is most commonly used. A pin is placed through the proximal tibia and the leg is supported in suspension with some knee flexion. Traction weight is 15 to 20 pounds initially, and thereafter may be reduced gradually. If reduction cannot be obtained by traction alone, the physician may manually reduce the fracture under anesthesia. The physician may use a second pin through the distal femur to aid in accurate reduction and permit early movement in the knee. Traction can be used to maintain position until bone healing is well established.

27511

For open reduction, an incision is made along the medial or lateral femoral condyle area to expose the fracture site. The fragments are manually reduced and internal fixation is typically accomplished using a buttress blade plate or screw-plate with screws. The incision is then closed. When skin or other soft tissue damage is considerable, the physician may use external fixation which allows for proper wound care management in hopes of preventing infection.

27513

At times, this type of fracture may be treated closed initially with a trial period of traction. However, if reduction is not acceptable, open treatment may be required. Since this type of fracture includes a fracture line extending into the joint, it is important to secure accurate articular surface restoration and to retain the reduction. An incision is made over the medial or lateral femoral condyle to expose the fracture site. The fracture is reduced. Cancellous bone screws or bolts may be used to secure the condyle fracture, and a blade-plate with screws for the supracondylar fracture. The physician may repair only the condyles, leaving the patient in skeletal traction for treatment of the supracondylar portion of the fracture. If there is significant soft tissue or skin damage, external fixation may be used to allow for proper wound care management.

27514

A curvilinear incision is made along the lateral or medial distal end of the femur, exposing the fracture site. The physician reduces the fracture, ensuring restoration of the articular surface of the knee joint and of the patellofemoral groove. After reduction, if the fracture is stable, no internal fixation is used. However, with this type of fracture internal fixation is typically used. A dynamic condylar screw system or an angled blade-plate with screws may achieve internal fixation of the fracture. Under certain conditions such as extensive soft tissue damage or infection, the physician may use an external fixation device. However, its application to the distal femur fracture is quite limited. The incision is closed with sutures, staples, and/or Steri-strips, or left open for secondary closure.

27516–27517

An abduction type separation is caused by a blow to the lateral side of the distal femur. There may typically be a fracture in conjunction with the epiphyseal separation. If alignment and stability are adequate, a single hip spica cast is used with the knee immobilized in extension. For 27517, closed reduction is attempted first in a more problematic fracture or separation such as in a hyperextension injury. If this is unsuccessful, the physician may choose to insert a Steinman pin in the femur above the fracture or separation, and another pin in the proximal third of the tibia. Gentle skeletal traction is applied to disengage the fragments while the physician reduces the displacement. A hip spica cast is applied with the knee in 45 to 60 degrees of flexion. In three to four weeks, the cast and pins are removed and an above-knee cast is applied.

27519

The physician makes an anteromedial or anterolateral, longitudinal incision to expose the epiphysis on the distal femoral condyle area. The articular surface of the epiphysis is examined. The physician may use a Knowles pin placed into the displaced epiphyseal fragment, and use it as a handle to guide the displaced fragment back into position. Additional threaded pins or screws are then directed transversely across the epiphysis or across the metaphysis as needed to complete fixation. The incision is closed with sutures and placed in a splint or long leg brace. If there is an open wound associated with the injury, the wound is thoroughly irrigated and debrided. The physician may choose to use an external fixator to facilitate dressing changes and skin grafting procedures if needed.

27520

Closed treatment of a patellar fracture is indicated when there is 2.0 mm or less displacement, separation, or step off. X-ray determines any displacement. The leg is placed in either a long leg cast or splint to keep the knee immobilized for three to six weeks.

27524

A vertical midline incision is made beginning 5.0 cm above the patella and ending at the midportion of the patellar tendon. The patellar fracture is identified and the knee joint is irrigated and inspected for any loose fragments. Clotted blood is removed from the fracture surfaces. The physician may use two types of treatment, depending on the type of fracture. The physician may place tension band wiring through drill holes made in the fragments to hold them together. Other fractures require screw fixation placed perpendicular to the fractured surfaces. If the patellar fracture is so severely fragmented that internal fixation or tension band wiring cannot be used, then partial or complete removal of the patella is performed by the physician. If only a partial patellectomy is performed, then the patellar tendon is reattached to the remaining patella with sutures and wire. Dissection and/or soft tissue repair of surrounding tissues may be necessary. Incisions are closed with sutures, staples, and/or Steri-strips.

27530–27532

Closed treatment of a tibial plateau fracture is indicated when the fractured segments are stable, in good alignment, and the tibial joint surface is congruent. The physician may need to perform a manual reduction in 27532 to realign the fractured segments. The physician may also use skeletal traction such as Kirschner wire. A wire is placed through the tibia and a traction bow is applied, reducing or realigning the fractured segments.

27535–27536

The physician makes a vertical incision on the side of the patella overlying either the medial or lateral tibial plateau to correct a unicondylar (27535) fracture. A bicondylar fracture (27536) is treated by making both a medial and a lateral parapatellar incision. The incision extends downward to the upper portion of the tibia. If reduction is needed to realign the joint surfaces, the physician may use an AO distracter. This is an external device anchored with a screw in the tibia and one in the medial femoral condyle to distract the fractured fragments, allowing them to realign. Instead of a distracter, the physician may use a bone punch to raise fragments. Kirschner wires may be applied to provide provisional fixation of the fragments. A plate, such as a "T" or "L" plate, is then fitted to the contour of the bone. Screws are inserted to secure fixation and to compress the fragments so that healing may occur. The incision is closed with sutures, staples, and/or Steri-strips. The physician may treat the open fracture of the tibial plateau with an external fixation device.

27538

There are three types of fractures of the intercondylar spine and tibial tuberosity. Types I and II of the intercondylar spine and Type I of the tibial tuberosity are typically treated closed. If the fragment appears stable and is not displaced, no manipulation for reduction is needed. If the fragment is displaced, reduction may be achieved by extending the knee.

CPT® Lay Descriptions

The knee may also need to be aspirated. A splint or a locked, long-leg knee brace may be used for four to six weeks.

27540

If adequate closed reduction of the fragment cannot be achieved, an open procedure is needed to ensure normal knee range of motion and function. Open treatment is typically performed for Type III intercondylar spine fracture and Types II and III tibial tuberosity fracture. An anteromedial incision is made to expose the knee, and the fragments are identified. For the intercondylar spine fracture, the fragment is reduced by placing the knee in full extension. Two holes are drilled through the tibial epiphysis. A wire or nonabsorbable suture is passed through the lowest portion of the anterior cruciate ligament and through the drill holes and tied together. The knee is flexed and extended so the reduction is stable. For tibial tuberosity fracture, the fragment is reduced by extending the knee. Two small pins or a bone screw are placed through the fragment to hold it in place. The incision is closed. A splint or brace is applied with the knee in full extension for four to six weeks, after which the physician may remove the pins.

27550–27552

A positive diagnosis of a knee dislocation typically warrants immediate reduction. Radiographic evaluation is performed to help determine the direction of dislocation. Minor instabilities can be reduced without anesthesia by applying manual longitudinal traction (27550). If secondary restraints (ligaments) were damaged, anesthesia may be required in order to reduce the dislocation (27552). The knee is usually aspirated, and placed in a posterior splint for support. The physician may choose to do further tests to evaluate ligamentous, capsular, meniscal, and vascular integrity. The knee is usually placed in a splint or immobilizer.

27556–27557

In an open knee dislocation there is considerable soft tissue trauma. The physician may debride the injury and explore the popliteal space for arterial evaluation and/or repair. If the joint is unstable after the dislocation is reduced, the physician may decide to use internal or external fixation for a period of time. Two transfixion pins drilled across the joint can provide good stability against recurrent dislocation, or an external fixator can be used to immobilize the joint. The wound may be left open to allow for drainage and treatment of infection. For 27557, primary ligamentous repair is performed at the same time, or at a later date after certification of popliteal artery flow, or after artery repair. The torn ligaments are reattached with screws, staples, and/or sutures. The incision or wound is closed or left open temporarily depending on the size of the wound, or if an infection is present.

27558

In an open knee dislocation, there will be considerable soft tissue trauma. The physician may need to debride the injury and explore the popliteal space for arterial evaluation and/or repair. If the joint is unstable after the dislocation is reduced, the physician may apply internal or external fixation for a period of time. Two transfixion pins drilled across the joint can provide good stability against recurrent dislocation, or an external fixator can be used to immobilize the joint. Those ligaments not able to be repaired directly may need augmentation or reconstruction. Typically the posterior cruciate ligament and sometimes the anterior cruciate ligament will be reconstructed by drilling bone tunnels in the tibia and femur, and passing donor ligament grafts through the tunnels and into the knee joint to take the place of the torn ligaments. If there is a severely injured knee, then extra-articular repairs for the cruciate ligaments may be favored over multiple joint drill holes (see 27427, 27428, 27429). The incision or wound is closed or left open temporarily depending on the size of the wound, or if an infection is present.

27560–27562

When the patella dislocates, it typically moves to the lateral side of the knee and off of the femoral condyles. Frequently the physician is able to gently extend the knee, causing the patella to move back into its normal position without administering anesthesia (27560). If the patient is in pain and guarding excessively, the physician may use anesthesia (27562) to relax the patient so the patella can be realigned. An x-ray may be taken to check the position of the patella. A splint or brace may be applied to give the patella additional support.

27566

If there is significant damage to the patella, such as an osteochondral fracture, or severe cartilage breakdown associated with a patellar dislocation, then a partial or total patellectomy may need to be performed with this procedure. A medial longitudinal patellar incision is made to expose the patella and medial retinaculum. If the patella is still dislocated, it is reduced at this time. If significant damage has occurred to the patella as noted above, the physician may choose to remove a portion or all of it. This is done by incising the tendon that encases the patella and using a saw and osteotome to resect the damaged portion of the patella. The tendon sheath is closed with sutures. To repair the patellar dislocation, the physician places the sutures in the medial retinaculum to tighten it down, which in turn keeps the patella or the tendon sheath from moving out from the trochlear groove. The incision is closed with sutures, staples, and/or Steri-strips.

27570

The physician increases range of knee motion limited by adhesions or scar tissue. After general anesthesia is administered, the physician bends the knee and applies gradual pressure until the desired range of motion for the knee is achieved. Traction or other fixation devices may be applied.

27580

The physician makes a long incision along the inside of the patella. The patella is reflected laterally to expose the knee joint. Bone cuts are made to flatten out the joint surfaces of the femur and tibia. A U-shaped groove is made on the underneath side of the patella and a corresponding one on the femur. The patella is placed into the femoral groove and secured with screws. The physician makes an incision overlying the iliac crest, harvests a graft, and closes the surgically created graft donor site. The bone graft is placed between the joint surfaces. An external fixator compresses the joint surfaces. The knee is typically fused in 10 to 15 degrees of flexion. The incision is closed with sutures, staples, and/or Steri-strips.

27590–27591

The physician makes incisions so that equal anterior and posterior flaps are fashioned. Dissection is carried down to the femur. Arteries and veins are doubly ligated and transected. The sciatic nerve is divided. A Gigli saw is then used to section the femur and bevel the cut ends. The anterior and posterior myofascial flaps are sutured together and secured to the lower end of the femur through drill holes. Incisions are closed in layers and a temporary drain is applied. For fitting (27591) an immediate postoperative prosthesis (IPOP), a rigid dressing is applied at the time of amputation. A sterile, closed-end stump sock is placed over the dressings. Felt pads are used over bony prominences to evenly distribute the pressure. An elastic, plaster cast is applied over the amputation site. A belt suspension apparatus may be incorporated into the cast. If immediate weight bearing is planned, an end-plate is wrapped into the lower portion of the cast to allow attachment of a temporary prosthesis.

27592

An open amputation is one in which the skin is not closed over the end of the stump, but is rather followed by a secondary closure (reamputation, scar revision) at a later date. The purpose of this type of amputation is to prevent or eliminate infection so that final closure of the stump may be carried out without breakdown of the wound. This procedure is usually used in severe traumatic wounds with extensive destruction of tissue. Just below the intended bone section, the physician makes a circular incision down to the deep fascia. Muscles and nerves are divided and all vessels ligated. The bone is then sectioned, and the wound is dressed. Skin traction is applied by covering the stump with a stockinette which is glued to the skin. The free end of the stockinette is split into 4 tails and tied together over the stump. A rope is attached to the stockinette and traction of 3 to 5

pounds is applied in order to gradually stretch the skin over the stump, while the stump is healed by a scar. This may take two to three weeks or more. The stump is dressed at intervals while continuing the traction.

27594

The physician performs secondary closure or scar revision after the stump has granulated or healed by a scar. In this procedure, no additional bone is sectioned. The physician resects the scar and granulation tissue from the end of the stump. Skin flaps are fashioned as close as possible to the thick scar surrounding the granulating wound. The dense layer of scar tissue is excised from over the end of bone. Additional muscle may be removed as well. The skin flaps are pulled over the end of the stump and connected with nonabsorbable sutures. A temporary drain or suction tubes may also be used.

27596

After the stump has granulated or healed by scar, the physician performs secondary closure or scar revision. This procedure will usually be performed 2 to 3 weeks or more after the initial open amputation was completed. Additional bone is sectioned, usually at a more proximal or higher level. Skin flaps are fashioned and pulled down over the stump and closed with nonabsorbable sutures. A temporary drain or suction tubes are used as well.

27598

The physician performs disarticulation at the knee, which is a disjoining but not removal of bone above the knee. Equal anterior and posterior incisions are made around the knee. The patellar tendon is sectioned close to where it attaches to the tibial tubercle. The tendons surrounding the knee are divided from their insertions on the tibia. The same is done with the cruciate ligaments. Arteries and veins are ligated and nerves are divided. The patella is removed. A saw is used to remove the femoral condyles 1.5 cm above the level of the knee joint. The patellar tendon is pulled into the intercondylar notch and sutured to the remaining portions of the cruciate ligaments. The hamstring tendons are then sutured to the patellar tendon. A temporary drain is placed in the knee joint and the incision is closed in multiple layers.

27600–27602

The physician performs a decompression fasciotomy on the compartments of the leg to reduce high pressure within those compartments. The physician treats the anterior or lateral compartments of the leg in 27600, the posterior compartments in 27601, or the anterior and/or lateral and posterior compartments in 27602. The physician makes incisions overlying the compartments measured at dangerous levels. The incisions are carried deep to the respective fascia. The physician makes long incisions in the fascia to relieve the pressure. The fascial and skin incisions are left open. Any nonviable tissue is removed.

27603–27604

The physician drains an abscess or hematoma in 27603 or an infected bursa in 27604 from deep within the leg or ankle. An incision is made over the mass. The overlying tissues are dissected down to the area of the abscess, hematoma, or bursa. The mass is dissected free on all sides and removed. The physician then irrigates the area with antibiotic solution. In 27604, any nonviable or infected tissue is debrided. If infection is present, the wound is left open to drain. Otherwise, the incision is closed in multiple layers with sutures.

27605–27606

The physician performs a percutaneous tenotomy of the Achilles tendon. The physician infiltrates the skin and Achilles tendon with a local anesthetic about 1.0 cm above the insertion into the calcaneus. A knife blade or tenotome held vertically is inserted through the skin and subcutaneous tissue into the Achilles tendon. The blade is turned medially and laterally and swept back forth, creating a nick in the tendon, until the foot can be dorsiflexed at the ankle. Pressure is applied over the incision for about five minutes. A dressing and long leg cast is applied with the ankle in ten degree dorsiflexion and the knee in maximal extension. Report 27605 if performed with local anesthesia; report 27606 if general anesthesia is required.

27607

The physician makes an incision in the leg or ankle for osteomyelitis or bone abscess. The physician makes a longitudinal incision over the involved portion of the bone. The physician dissects through the overlying muscles and outlines a cortical window using a drill. The window is removed with an osteotome. The medullary canal is entered. Necrotic and infected matter is removed. The wound is closed loosely over drains.

27610

The physician opens the ankle for exploration of the joint or to drain an infection or remove a foreign body. The physician makes an incision overlying the ankle joint and exposes the joint. The physician explores the joint and drains any infection and/or removes a foreign body. A drain is placed and the wound is closed in sutured layers.

27612

The physician makes an incision along the Achilles tendon and retracts the muscles to expose the posterior ankle capsule. The capsule is incised to increase dorsiflexion. If the Achilles tendon is lengthened, the physician notches the tendon at the

medial and lateral aspects to release contracture. The wound is closed in sutured layers.

27613–27614

The physician biopsies a lesion in the soft tissue of the leg or ankle. The physician incises the skin over the lesion dissects to the lesion. The tissue sample is obtained and the incision is closed in sutured layers. In 27613, the lesion is superficial. In 27614, the lesion is located in deep tissue.

27615

The physician removes a malignant tumor from the soft tissue of a leg or ankle. A radical resection includes removal of involved tissues and compartment from origin to insertion. The physician makes an incision through the skin of the leg or ankle. The soft tissues are cleaned off the underlying bone. All of the muscles and fascia in the compartment are removed. Adjacent neurovascular structures are also removed. The remaining skin is reapproximated and closed in sutured layers.

27618–27619

The physician excises a subcutaneous tumor in the leg or ankle. The physician incises the skin and dissects to the tumor. The tumor is removed and the wound is closed in sutured layers. Report 27618 if the excision is subcutaneous. Report 27619 if the excision is deep, subfascial, or intramuscular.

27620

The physician makes an incision over the ankle joint and exposes the joint. The physician explores the joint and takes a biopsy if necessary and may remove a foreign body if one is present. The ankle capsule is closed and the tissues are sutured into place.

27625

The physician performs an arthrotomy (surgically opens the ankle joint) and removes the synovium. An incision is made overlying the ankle joint. The physician dissects the tissue down to the capsule of the joint. An incision is then made through the capsule and into the joint. The physician then removes the synovium through this arthrotomy. The joint is and the skin incision are both irrigated with antibiotic solution then repaired in multiple layers.

27626

To correct thickening of the synovium, the physician makes an incision over the tendon and exposes the tendon sheath. The synovium is the lining that bathes the joint in fluid. The physician removes the affected sheath from the tendon and the joint space is opened and the synovium is removed. The wound is irrigated and closed with sutures.

27630

The physician makes an incision over the site of the lesion on the tendon sheath or capsule. Dissection is

carried down to expose the tendon or capsule. The
tissues are then dissected around the lesion, freeing it
from surrounding tissue and the lesion is excised. The
operative site is irrigated with antibiotic solution and
the wound closed with layered sutures.

27635–27638

The physician makes an incision overlying the lesion.
Soft tissues are separated and the bone is exposed. A
cortical window with rounded edges is cut into the
bone so that the entire growth can be seen. The
physician scrapes the growth from the bone with a
curet and reams the site with a burr. The physician
may treat the growth with cryotherapy, cement or
cauterization. An autograft is necessary in 27637. An
allograft (donor bone) is inserted into the area in
27638. The wound is irrigated, closed, and dressed.

27640–27641

The physician makes a longitudinal incision, retracts
the tissue, and exposes the tibia. The periosteum is
divided from the bone. A portion bone is removed
creating a shallow crater-like or saucer-like depression
to facilitate drainage from infected areas of bone. A
drain is placed at the operative site and soft tissues are
sutured around the drain. The leg is immobilized. In
27640, the site of the infection is in the tibia; in
27641, the site is the fibula.

27645–27647

The physician removes a tumor with radical resection.
The physician incises the overlying skin and dissects
to the bone, freeing the involved bone from muscular
attachments and the tissue bed. The area affected by
tumor is removed, and the wound is closed in sutured
layers. Report 27645 if the tumor is located in the
tibia. Report 27646 if the tumor is located in the
fibula. Report 27647 if the tumor is located on the
talus or calcaneus.

27648

The physician injects radiopaque fluid into the ankle
for arthrography. The physician inserts a needle into
the ankle joint and aspirates if necessary. Opaque
contrast solution is injected into the ankle, and the
needle is removed. A separately reportable arthrogram
is taken of the ankle.

27650–27652

The physician repairs a ruptured Achilles tendon. An
incision is made overlying the tendon. The physician
extends the incision through the tissues to the
tendon. The physician identifies the tear and debrides
any rough edges. In 27652, the physician harvests a
fascial graft from the patient through a separate
incision. The physician then repairs the surgically
created graft donor site. The graft is then incorporated
into the repair of the tendon and secured to the area
with fixation (e.g., screw). The tendon is then
repaired, typically with a heavy nonabsorbable suture.
The wound is irrigated with antibiotic solution, then

closed in multiple layers. A cast, splint, or brace may
be applied.

27654

The physician repairs a secondarily torn Achilles
tendon. An incision is made overlying the tendon.
The physician extends the incision deep to the
tendon. The tear or rupture is identified. Because the
repair is secondary, significant scar tissue may be
debrided. Any nonviable tissue is also removed. A
graft may be harvested from the patient through a
separate incision. The physician then repairs the
surgically created graft donor site and the tendon
either with a suture or with both the graft and suture.
The graft may be secured to the area of repair with a
screw. The physician irrigates the wound with
antibiotic solution. The wound is closed in multiple
layers. A cast or splint may be applied.

27656

The physician repairs a fascial defect of the leg. The
physician incises the skin overlying the defect. If
underlying muscles are herniated through the fascial
defect, they are pulled to their correct anatomical
position and secured with sutures. The wound is
closed in sutured layers.

27658–27659

An incision is made overlying the flexor tendon in the
leg. The physician extends the incision deep to the
tendon. The tear or rupture is identified. If the repair
is secondary, significant scar tissue may be debrided.
Any nonviable tissue is also removed. The physician
then repairs the tendon either just with a suture or
with both the graft and suture. The graft may be
secured to the area of repair with a screw. The
physician irrigates the wound with antibiotic solution.
The wound is closed in multiple layers. A cast or
splint may be applied. Report 27658 for a primary
repair; report 27659 for a secondary repair.

27664–27665

The physician makes a midline longitudinal incision
to expose the extensor tendon. The surgical site is
irrigated and the ends of the torn tendon are realigned
to make for better attachment. The ends of the tendon
are brought together and sutured. The tendon is
attached to the retinaculum around the knee. Report
27664 for a primary repair. Report 27665 if the injury
is old and requires an inverted V incision in the
tendon to facilitate repair. In a secondary repair,
significant scar tissue may be debrided. Any nonviable
tissue is also removed. The physician then repairs the
tendon either just with a suture or with both the graft
and suture. The graft may be secured to the area of
repair with a screw. The wound is closed and the leg
is placed in a cast.

27675

The physician makes a longiitudinal curved incision
that extends from the distal end of the fibula, over the

lateral border of the foot to the cuboid bone. A possterior sin flap is elevated at the laterall malleolus, using the deep facia with its base attached to the tip of the lateral malleolus. The peroneal tendons and sheaths are identified and place in their appropriate anatomic position. The are secured in place with sutures or drill holes and suture anchors. The incision is closed in sutured layers.

27676

A longitudinal lateral ankle incision is made and a groove created in the posterior aspect of the fibular malleolus (fibular osteotomy). The peroneal tendons are placed in the groove and held in place either with a thick osteoperiosteal flap from the surface of the maleolus that is swung posteriorly over the tendons or with a wedge of bone cut from the lateral malleolus that is displaced posteriorly over the tendons. The wound is then irrigated and closed in sutured layers. A short leg case is usually applied and modified to walking cast once the stitches are removed.

27680–27681

The physician corrects a tightened or adhesed tendon sheath in the leg or ankle by making a longitudinal incision over the restricted tendon. Skin is retracted and scar tissue is removed. The physician dissects the tendon with a sharp instrument to free it from the bone. The wound is sutured and dressed with compression bandages. Report 27680 if the procedure is performed on a single tendon. Report 27681 if multiple tendons, requiring separate incisions, are freed from tightened or adhesed tendon sheaths.

27685–27686

The physician makes three incisions on the lateral side of the foot centered over the sinus tarsi. The physician exposes the extensor digitorum brevis tendon, and reflects it distally to expose the anterior part of the talocalcaneal joint. The calcaneocuboid joint is identified and all tight surrounding structures are released. A second incision is made on the medial side of the foot centered over the prominent head of the talus. The physician releases all tight structures on the medial and dorsal aspects of the head of the talus and the navicular. The anterior part of the talus is freed from its attachments to the navicular and calcaneus. If the peroneal, and extensor hallucis longus and extensor digitorum longus tendons remain contracted the physician lengthens them by Z-plasty. A third incision is made on the medial side of the Achilles tendon, lengthened by Z-plasty. The physician inserts a Steinmann pin through the navicular and into the neck of the talus to maintain the reduction. The wound is closed in layers and a long-leg cast with the knee flexed and the foot in proper position. The Steinmann pins are removed in eight weeks.

27687

The physician performs a gastrocnemius recession. To lengthen the gastrocnemius muscle using the Strayer procedure, the physician makes a posterior longitudinal incision 10.0 cm to 15.0 cm long overlying the middle of the calf. The medial sural nerve is retracted and the incision is deepened to the fascia to expose the gastrocnemius. This muscle is dissected bluntly from the underlying soleus muscle to their common tendon at the calcaneus. A probe or clamp is inserted deep to the gastrocnemius and its tendon is severed. The physician dorsaflexes the foot until there is a 2.0 cm to 2.5 cm gap between the two tendon segments. The two muscle bellies are dissected from their fascial attachments proximally to the popliteal fossa. The physician passes a finger from side-to-side beneath the muscle to completely separate the gastronemus from the soleus. The proximal part of the tendon is sutured to the soleus with fine interrupted silk sutures. The wound is closed.

27690–27692

Because this procedure iiinvolves transfer or transplant of a single tendon from a number of different sites on the foot, the exact procedure will differ depending on the specific tendon involved. When transfer of the anterior tibial tendon is perffformed, an anterior lower-leg incisionis made and the tendon extracted and passed posteriorly through the interosseous membrane to the calcaneus. A posterior heel incision is made and the tendon end is fixed to the calcaneous and/or Achellies tendon. The wound is closed in layers over a drain with a subcutaneous layer closed so that the skin can be brought together under minimal tension. The patient is placed into a dressing incorporating plaster splints.

27695–27696

The collateral ligament is two-part ligament that stabilizes the medial side of the ankle. The physician makes a curved incision across the inside of the ankle. The skin is reflected to expose the torn ligament. Holes are drilled diagonally across the talus and two non-absorbable sutures are placed through these holes and the ligament. Report 27696 if a similar procedure is performed to attach the ligament to the medial malleolus, which requires the placement of a screw through the fibula to the tibia. The wound is closed and dressed. The leg is immobilized in a long leg cast with the knee flexed to 30–45 degrees for four weeks followed by a walking cast for four weeks.

27698

This procedure reports a secondary repair of the collateral ligament of the ankle. There are several techniques, inclluding Watson-Jones, Evan and Chrisman-Snook. In a Watson-Jones repair, an ankle incision is made and the peroneus brevis tendon divided and mobilized. It is then passed through drill holes in the talus and fibular malleolus to reconstruct both the calcaneofibular and anterior talofibular ligaments (lateral collateral ligament). An Evans procedure involves mobilizing the peronoeus brevis tendon and passing it through a drill hole in the lateral fibular malleolus to reconstruct the collateral ligament. A Chrisman-Snook procedure involves dividing the peroneus brevis tendon and using it in the repair of the collateral ligament.

27700–27703

The physician performs arthroplasty to correct joint problems caused by arthritis. Three portal incisions are made at the front and sides of the ankle. Joint surfaces are smoothed and scar tissues are removed from the joint. If excessive damage is noted, the physician replaces damaged parts of the ankle with a prosthesis and reports 27702. Report 27703 if a loose component must be revised.

27704

The physician removes an implant. The preexisting skin incision is opened and the tibial and talus components are removed with accompanying cement. Bone grafts are placed in the resulting defect and the ankle is secured with either compression or screws. The wound is sutured and a cast is applied for up to 12 weeks.

27705–27709

The physician performs an osteotomy (bone cut) of the tibia in 27705, of the fibula in 27707, or of both in 27709. An incision is made in the skin overlying the osteotomy site. Separate incisions may be necessary to access both tibia and fibula in 27709. The physician dissects the tissues down to the bone. The bone is exposed. The physician makes a cut through the tibia, fibula, or both in the desired location and plane. The bone is then aligned to the proper position. Fixation, such as screws or plates may be applied to maintain position. The physician irrigates the area with antibiotic solution and then closes it in multiple layers. A splint, cast, or brace may be applied.

27712

The physician makes an incision along the shaft of the limb, exposing the bone. Another incision is made through the periosteum to expose the entire shaft. The physician cuts through the proximal and distal ends of the bone, temporarily removes the shaft, and makes three or four cuts through the shaft. These segments are threaded onto a medullary nail and shifted as necessary to alignment. Bone grafts are added if the cortex is extremely thin. The shaft is placed back into position with the medullary nail extending into the bone at either end. The periosteum is sutured over the bone and the wound is closed with sutures. The extremity is immobilized by cast until healed.

27715

The patient is placed prone and an incision is made over the distal lateral fibula. The physician places two screws 1.5 cm apart through fibula to the tibia, securing the fibula during the procedure. The fibula is cut above the screws. Incisions are made at the top and bottom of the tibia, and Schanz screws are placed parallel to the plane of the knee outside the leg. Another incision is made at the front of the tibia, making a transverse cut through the bone. The Achilles tendon may be lengthened. An external distraction device is attached to the screws and the distance increased by 1.5 cm per day or 10.0 cm per week. After the desired length is achieved either a shortened or lengthened a metal plate and screws are attached, with possible bone grafting. The wound is closed.

27720–27722

To correct nonunion of the tibia in 27720, the physician makes an incision on the medial aspect of the tibia through the periosteum. The bone is divided by transverse cuts and the pieces are manually rotated into position and stabilized with a metal plate and screws. In 27722, the physician makes an anteromedial incision and fibrous tissue is removed from the site. The ends of the fragments are roughened and the distal segment is hollowed out. A rectangular window is cut into the bone just above the site, cancellous bone is removed, and placed around the fixation site. The wound is closed, dressed and a cast is applied.

27724

The physician repairs a tibia fracture that has not healed or has healed in malalignment. An incision is made in the skin overlying the tibial fracture site. The incision is extended down to the bone. The physician identifies the fracture or malunion. Any scar tissue is debrided from around and between the fracture pieces so that the clean edges of bone can be approximated. A bone graft is harvested through a separate incision from the patient's ilium or from another bone. The physician then repairs the surgically created graft donor site. The graft is placed at the fracture site and the fracture is manipulated into the desired position and alignment. The physician then applies fixation, such as screws, plates, wires, or rods to stabilize the fracture. The wound is then irrigated with antibiotic solution and closed in multiple layers. A splint, brace, or cast may be applied.

27725

The physician repairs a fracture of the tibia that has not healed or has healed in malalignment. An incision is made in the skin overlying the fracture site. The physician extends the incision deep to the bone. The fracture or malunion is identified. Any scar tissue is debrided from around and between the fracture pieces. An osteotomy of the bone is performed if needed to correct the malalignment. Using the adjacent fibula as a strut, the fibula is attached to the tibia with fixation, such as plates, screws, or wires. This attachment allows the fibula to heal to the tibia in a synostosis. The physician irrigates the wound with antibiotic solution and closes it in multiple layers. A brace, cast, or splint may be applied.

27727

Congenital Anterolateral Bowing of the Tibia is a rare condition that is present in 1 in 250,000 live births. The affected leg is bowed forwards, and usually shortened. By age 2, the bowed tibia fractures spontaneously, and does not heal. However, before the fracture occurs, the physician may place the affected leg in a thermoplastic brace to protect it. Once the fracture occurs, it does not heal, and forms a pseudarthrosis (non-union). Surgical repair using fibula graft or using the Ilizarov technique of repair is often used.

27730–27742

The physician makes a 2.0 cm incision over the physis on the deformed side of the bone to correct epiphyseal. A 1.0 square cm bone block is removed from the physeal line. A curet is used to roughen the remaining walls of the block site. The block is then rotated and replaced in its original space. The wound is closed with sutures. Report 27730 if performed on the distal lateral bone (lower leg toward the ankle); report 27732 if performed on the distal fibula; report 27734 if performed on both the distal tibia and fibula (two bones of the lower leg); report 27740 if performed on both ends of the bones; and report 27742 if performed on the distal femur.

27745

Preventative nailing of a bone may be performed if a surgeon feels that a bone is not stable on its own despite the lack of a true fracture site. An incision is made to reflect the soft tissues and the periosteum is divided to expose the bone. The bone is plated or pinned as necessary. the soft tissues are repositioned and skin is closed with sutures. Often weight bearing is progressed as with normal fractures or internal fixation procedures.

27750

The physician treats a fracture of the tibial shaft without open surgery or any manipulation of the bones. Separately reportable x-rays confirm a fracture of the tibial shaft with or without a simultaneous fibular fracture. The position and alignment of the fracture fragments are stable. The physician applies a cast or brace to maintain the stability of the fragments.

27752

The physician treats a tibial shaft fracture without surgery but with manipulation of the bones. Separately reportable x-rays confirm a fracture of the tibial shaft with or without a simultaneous fibular

fracture. Using anesthesia, and with the use of skeletal traction as required, the physician manipulates the fracture. Manipulation is accomplished by pushing, pulling, rotating, or otherwise maneuvering the bones so they are properly aligned. Separately reportable x-rays confirm proper alignment. Skeletal traction may not be removed and a cast or brace may be applied to the leg to maintain stability of the bone.

27756

The physician treats a fracture of the tibia shaft by placing pins or screws through the skin and into the bone. Separately reportable x-rays confirm that the fracture, with or without an associated fibular fracture, can be treated without any long incisions or exposure of the bone. The physician makes small stab wounds in the skin overlying the fracture. Using separately reportable fluoroscopic x-ray as needed, the physician inserts the pins or screws through the small incisions and then through the fractured pieces. The pins or screws hold the fractured pieces together. The wounds are irrigated with antibiotic solution and the skin is closed. A sterile dressing is applied. The leg is placed in a cast, splint, or brace.

27758

The physician repairs a fracture of the shaft of the tibia using internal fixation devices. An incision is made overlying the fracture area of the tibia. The physician extends the incision deep to the bone, identifying and exposing the fracture. Tissue is debrided as needed. The physician manipulates the pieces of bone together under direct visualization. Fixation devices, such as plates and screws or cerclage wires, are applied to hold the fracture in the desired position. The wound is irrigated with antibiotic solution. The physician may close the wound in layers or the wound may be left open to drain.

27759

The physician makes an incision over the proximal tibia. The tissue is dissected. The physician carries the incision down to the bone. Separately reportable fluoroscopic x-ray may be used throughout the rest of the procedure to confirm stabilization of the fracture. The physician drills a hole in the proximal tibia and places a long guidewire into the marrow canal of the bone. This guide wire is threaded distally in the canal and across the fracture site to the distal tibia. Bone reamers are sequentially placed over the guide wire in even larger sizes to ream the inside of the bone. Reaming is continued until the desired size is reached. The physician then chooses the correct size rod to be implanted in the canal. The physician then inserts the rod into the proximal tibia over the guide wire and drives it down the intramedullary canal to the distal tibia. The guide wire is removed. The incision is irrigated with antibiotic solution and the skin is closed in layers. A splint or brace may be applied to the leg.

27760

The physician treats a fracture of the medial malleolus of the ankle without surgery or any manipulation of the bones. Separately reportable x-rays confirm the fracture is in an acceptable position. A cast or brace is placed on the leg to hold the fragments in place.

27762

The physician treats a fractured medial malleolus without open surgery but with manipulation of the fracture. Separately reportable x-rays confirm the fracture is in an unacceptable position. Using anesthesia as needed, the physician manipulates the fracture by pushing, pulling, or maneuvering the fracture into the desired position. Traction may be used to aid in the manipulation or for stabilization. A cast or brace is applied to the leg.

27766

The physician makes an incision overlying the medial malleolus near the ankle. The incision is extended through the tissue and deep to the bone. The fractured medial malleolus is identified. The physician places the fractured pieces of bone into proper position and alignment. The physician applies bone fixation devices, such as screws or pins, to secure the fractured pieces. The wound is irrigated with antibiotic solution and closed in multiple layers. A splint, cast, or brace is applied to the leg.

27780–27781

The physician treats a fracture of the fibula without open surgery or any manipulation of the bony fragments in 27780. Separately reportable x-rays are obtained that confirm a stable fracture of the proximal fibula or shaft. The physician applies a cast or brace to the leg to secure the fracture while it heals. In 27781, separately reportable x-rays confirm a fracture that is unstable and requires manipulation. Using anesthesia as needed, the physician pushes, pulls, or maneuvers the leg until the fracture is in the proper position and alignment. A cast or brace is then placed on the leg to hold the fracture in place while it heals.

27784

The physician makes an incision in the skin of the leg overlying the fractured area of the fibula. The tissues are dissected deep to the bone and the fracture is identified. Any nonviable tissue is debrided. The physician then places the bony fragments into their correct position and alignment. Fixation devices, such as plates, screws, or wires may be applied to maintain the fracture reduction. With the fracture stabilized, the physician irrigates the wound with antibiotic solution. The wound is closed in multiple layers. A cast, splint, or brace may be applied to the leg.

27786–27788

The physician treats a fracture of the distal fibula (also known as the lateral malleolus) without open surgery or any manipulation of the bones in 27786.

Separately reportable x-rays confirm the fracture of the distal fibula with the bony fragments in stable position. The physician applies a cast or brace to hold the fracture in place until it heals. In 27788, separately reportable x-rays confirm a fracture that is unstable and requires manipulation. Using anesthesia as needed, the physician pushes, pulls, or maneuvers the leg until the fracture is in the proper position and alignment. A cast or brace is then placed on the leg to hold the fracture in place while it heals.

27792

The physician makes an incision in the skin of the leg overlying the fractured area of the distal fibula. The tissues are dissected deep to the bone and the fracture is identified. Any nonviable tissue is debrided. The physician then places the bony fragments into their correct position and alignment. Fixation devices, such as plates, screws, or wires may be applied to maintain the fracture reduction. With the fracture stabilized, the physician irrigates the wound with antibiotic solution. The wound is closed in multiple layers. A cast, splint, or brace may be applied to the leg.

27808–27810

The physician treats a fracture of the ankle involving both the medial and lateral malleoli without open surgery or any manipulation of the fractured pieces in 27808. Separately reportable x-rays confirm the fracture of the medial and lateral malleoli of the ankle with the bony fragments in stable position. The physician applies a cast or brace to hold the fracture in place until it heals. In 27810, separately reportable x-rays confirm fractures of the medial and lateral malleoli that are unstable and require manipulation. Using anesthesia as needed, the physician pushes, pulls, or maneuvers the foot, ankle, and leg until the fracture is in the proper position and alignment. A cast or brace is then placed on the leg to hold the fracture in place while it heals.

27814

The physician makes incisions on each side of the ankle overlying fractures of the medial and lateral malleoli respectively. Each incision is carried deep through the soft tissues and down to the bone. The fractures are identified by exposing the fragments. Nonviable tissue and any intervening tissue between the ends of the fractured pieces are debrided. Each malleolus fracture is placed into its correct position one at a time. Bony fixation devices, such as metal plates, screws, wires, or pins are applied to stabilize the fractures. Fixation may be applied either internally to the bones or on the outside of the skin incision. When the fractures are appropriately stabilized, the skin incisions are thoroughly irrigated with antibiotic solution and closed in layers. A cast or brace may be applied to the leg.

27816–27818

The physician treats a fracture of the ankle involving all three of the malleoli (medial, lateral, and posterior) without open surgery or any manipulation of the fractured pieces in 27816. Separately reportable x-rays confirm the fracture of the malleolus of the ankle with the bony fragments in stable position. The physician applies a cast or brace to hold the fracture in place until it heals. In 27818, separately reportable x-rays confirm trimalleolar ankle fracture that is unstable and requires manipulation. Using anesthesia as needed, the physician pushes, pulls, or maneuvers the foot, ankle, and leg until the fracture is in the proper position and alignment. A cast or brace is then placed on the leg to hold the fracture in place while it heals.

27822–27823

The physician makes at least two separate incisions in the skin overlying the trimalleolar fracture. This fracture involves all three malleoli: medial, lateral, and posterior. The incisions are carried deep to the bones and the extent of each fracture is identified. Any nonviable or intervening tissue is dissected and debrided as needed. One at a time, the physician restores the fractured pieces to their correct positions. Using bony fixation devices, such as pins, plates, or screws, the physician repairs the fractures of the lateral and medial malleolus. The posterior malleolus (lip) fracture is left in position without applying fixation devices in 27822. In 27823, the posterior malleolus (lip) fracture is also repositioned to its correct position and secured similarly. Another incision may be required to obtain adequate fixation of all three fractures. The wounds are irrigated with antibiotic solution and closed in layers. A cast or brace is applied to the foot and leg.

27824–27825

The physician treats a fracture of the distal tibia extending into the ankle joint without open surgery or any manipulation of the fractured pieces. Separately reportable x-rays confirm the fracture of the distal tibia extending into the ankle joint (e.g., pilon or tibial plafond) with the bony fragments in stable position. Using anesthesia as needed, the physician applies a cast or brace to the foot and leg to hold the fracture in place until it heals. In 27825, separately reportable x-rays confirm a distal tibia fracture (e.g., pilon or tibial plafond) that is unstable and requires manipulation. Using anesthesia as needed, the physician pushes, pulls, or maneuvers the foot, ankle, and leg until the fracture is in the proper position and alignment. Traction may be applied. A cast or brace is applied to the foot and leg.

27826–27828

The physician treats a fracture of the distal tibia with fixation of the fibula only in 27826, the tibia only in 27827, or both in 27828. The physician makes an incision overlying the ankle to treat a fracture of the distal tibia, extending into the ankle joint (pilon or tibial plafond fracture). The incision is carried down to the bone. Often, two or more incisions are necessary in 27828. Any nonviable tissues are dissected and debrided as needed. The fracture pieces are placed in appropriate position. Using the fibula bone as a strut or splint, the physician applies fixation devices such as screws or plates to stabilize the fracture. No fixation devices are applied to the tibia in 27826. In 27827, the physician applies fixation to the tibia to stabilize the fractured pieces. In 27828, fixation is applied to both the tibia and fibula. The wound is thoroughly irrigated with antibiotic solution and closed in multiple layers. A cast, brace, or splint is applied.

27829

The physician makes an incision in the skin overlying the ankle. The tissues are dissected down to the distal joint between the tibia and fibula. Nonviable tissues are debrided as needed. The physician places the tibia and fibula in the correct position to reduce or realign the disruption. Fixation devices, such as screws are applied as needed to hold the joint (also know as a syndesmosis) in the correct position. The wound is thoroughly irrigated and then closed in multiple layers. A cast or brace may be applied to the leg.

27830–27831

The physician treats a dislocation of the proximal joint (near the knee) between the tibia and fibula without the use of anesthesia in 27830 or with anesthesia in 27831. Separately reportable x-rays are obtained that confirm the dislocation. No open surgery or extensive manipulation is necessary in 27830. Anesthesia is necessary in 27831 to perform manipulation of the leg and correctly aligning the bones. The physician applies a brace or splint to the leg and knee to hold the bones in appropriate position while healing takes place.

27832

The physician makes an incision overlying the joint between the tibia and fibula and near the knee to reposition a dislocation of these two bones. Tissue is dissected down to the joint and the joint is exposed. The physician identifies the dislocation and treats it one of several ways. The area may be treated by holding the joint together with fixation devices such as screws, pins, or wires. An external fixation device may be applied. The physician may excise or remove a piece of the proximal fibula. The physician then thoroughly irrigates the wound and closes it in multiple layers. A brace or splint may be applied to protect the joint and maintain its position until it heals.

27840–27842

The physician treats a dislocation of the ankle joint without anesthesia in 27840. Separately reportable x-rays confirm that the ankle joint requires no manipulation or open surgery. A cast or brace is applied to stabilize the dislocation. In 27842, anesthesia is required to perform manipulation of the dislocated ankle joint. Percutaneous skeletal fixation, such as pins, may be applied. The physician makes small incisions in the skin and inserts the pins through the skin and into the bones of the ankle joint. No open incisions are necessary. When the ankle joint is stabilized, the physician applies a cast or brace.

27846–27848

The physician treats a dislocation of the ankle joint with open surgery. An incision is made overlying the ankle joint and is extended deep to the joint. More than one incision may be necessary in 27848. Tissues are dissected around the joint. The joint may need to be surgically opened to restore it in the appropriate position. Percutaneous skeletal fixation may be applied to stabilize the dislocation. If applied, the physician makes small incisions in the skin, then inserts the pins through the skin and into the bones. No repair or internal fixation is necessary in 27846. In 27848, bony fixation devices, such as screws, plates, or wires are necessary. External fixation devices may also be applied on the outside of the ankle to maintain joint position. The physician then irrigates the joint and wound and closes the wound in multiple layers. A brace, splint, or cast is applied to maintain the relocated joint.

27860

The physician performs manipulation of the ankle with the patient under general anesthesia. The physician pushes, pulls, and maneuvers the foot, ankle, and leg to treat a stiff ankle. The physician may apply traction devices to the ankle to help perform the manipulations. Traction is then removed.

27870

The physician performs surgery on the ankle to fuse the ankle joint. The physician makes two or more incisions overlying the ankle joint, exposing the joint. The incisions are individually extended deep to the joint. The physician opens the joint through an arthrotomy incision. Tissue is dissected and debrided as necessary. The surfaces of the joint are then prepared so that they can be fused together. Preparation includes debriding and smoothing so that an intimate fit can be accomplished. Numerous methods can be used to fuse the joint, including screws, plates, or external fixation devices. The physician thoroughly irrigates the joint and closes the arthrotomy. The incisions are the irrigated and closed in layers. A cast or brace is applied to hold the newly fused joint in place until the bones heal together.

27871

The periosteum is stripped from the anteroposterior fibula, the lateral talus, and the calcaneus. The distal portion of the fibula is removed about 1.5 centimeters above the level of the distal tibia and the dissection is carried over the anterior distal tibia to the medial malleolus. The physician makes an incision along the tibia and the periosteum is stripped distally to the level of the calcaneus. Using a saw, the physician cuts through the neck of talus to mobilize and remove the talus either as one large fragment or morselize fragments. With the talus gone, the calcaneus can be seen. The distal end of the tibia is removed perpendicular to the long axis of the tibia. The physician uses a saw to remove the dorsal calcaneus and to create a flat surface for the arthrodesis. The two flat surfaces of the distal tibia and dorsal calcaneus are brought together to establish a varus/valgus and dorsiflexion/ plantar flexion alignment. A cut is made along the anterior tibia parallel to the cut made in the neck of the talus which creates a flat surface for apposing the neck of the talus. The bone surfaces are deeply scaled to prepare for internal fixation. Kirschner wires are used to place the tibia and calcaneus in apposition. Using an anterior cruciate guide, a pin is guided form the calcaneus across the fusion site to the anterior cortex of the tibia. Once satisfactory fixation has been achieved, cannulated screws are placed through the neck of the talus into the tibia. The wound is closed over a drain and a dressing incorporating plaster splints is applied. Marcaine is instilled through the drain tube into the wound.

27880

The physician performs an amputation of the leg below the knee. The physician makes an incision in the skin of the leg at the level where the amputation is to take place. The incision is carried completely around the leg. The tissue is dissected down to the bones. The large arteries, veins, and nerves are identified and tied off prior to being cut. Tissue is further debrided as needed. The tibia and fibula are identified. The physician surgically cuts the bones, completing the amputation. The wound is thoroughly irrigated and then closed in layers, including the skin. A soft dressing is placed over the stump.

27881

The physician performs an amputation of the leg below the knee and the fitting technique for an artificial leg. The physician makes an incision in the skin of the leg at the level where the amputation will be performed. The incision is extended completely around the leg. The tissue is dissected down to the bones. The large arteries, veins, and nerves are identified and tied off prior to being cut. Tissue is further debrided as needed. The physician surgically cuts the tibia and fibula individually to complete the amputation. The wound is thoroughly irrigated with antibiotic solution. The wound and skin are closed in multiple layers. The remaining stump is then fitted with a cast to prepare it for eventual placement of an artificial leg.

CPT® Lay Descriptions

27882

The physician places a pneumatic tourniquet on the thigh. The limb is measured for optimal stump length and marks are made to facilitate skin flap preparation. Progressive incisions are made through soft tissues, and nerves and vessels are ligated. The tibia and fibula are bisected with a circular saw, rounded, and smoothed. The calf muscles are brought forward over the ends of the tibia and fibula and attached to the connective tissue on the front of the stump. The tourniquet is released and bleeding points are electrocoagulated. A drainage tube is placed deep in the muscle flap and the skin flaps are closed and sutured. A soft dressing is applied, followed by a rigid dressing in preparation for prosthetic devices fabrication.

27884

The physician performs an amputation of the leg below the knee as part of a secondary closure of a wound or to revise a scar. The physician makes the necessary incisions on the leg where the amputation is to be performed. Open wounds are debrided as necessary. Scars are then excised. The physician dissects the tissue around the tibia and fibula. The tibia and fibula are then surgically cut to complete the amputation. The wounds are thoroughly irrigated with antibiotic solution and closed in layers. Any previous wounds left open are also irrigated and closed. Any scars that may cause problems with the use of an artificial leg are excised and revised. The stump may be placed in a soft dressing.

27886

The physician performs an amputation on the leg below the knee in a patient who has already undergone amputation. The physician identifies the additional area of the remaining stump requiring amputation. An incision is made in the skin at the appropriate site and extended laterally and medially around the leg. The tissue is dissected down to the bones. The large arteries, veins, and nerves are identified and tied off prior to being cut. Tissue is further debrided as needed. The physician surgically cuts the tibia and fibula individually to complete the reamputation. The wound is thoroughly irrigated with antibiotic solution. The wound and skin may be closed in multiple layers. If infection is present, the incision may be temporarily left open to drain.

27888

The physician performs an amputation of the foot near the ankle while leaving much of the soft tissue of the heel intact. The physician makes a long incision in the skin overlying the ankle at about the level of the medial and lateral malleoli. The incision is carried deep to the ankle joint. The talus bone is removed from the joint and the incision is carried to the heel bone (calcaneus). The soft tissues of the bottom of the heel are kept with the leg. The skin on the bottom of the foot is cut to complete the amputation of the foot.

The major arteries, veins, and nerves are identified and ligated. The wound is thoroughly irrigated with antibiotic solution and may be closed in layers. If infection of the foot is present, this operation is performed in two stages. The amputation is performed and then later the soft tissues and skin are repaired and closed. A soft dressing is applied.

27889

The physician performs an amputation of the ankle directly through the joint with removal of the foot. An incision is made overlying the ankle joint. The incision is carried around the ankle and deep to the joint. The tissues are dissected and the major arteries, veins, and nerves are identified then individually ligated. The ankle joint is opened through an arthrotomy incision and the foot is dislocated from the ankle joint and removed. Tissue is debrided as necessary. Muscles and tendons are attached to the remaining tibia and fibula bones as appropriate. The wound is thoroughly irrigated with antibiotic solution and may be closed in layers. If infection is present, the incision is temporarily left open to drain. A soft dressing, cast, or splint may be applied.

27892

The physician performs surgery on the anterior and/or lateral compartments of the leg reducing high pressure within the compartments. The physician makes incisions in the skin overlying the respective compartments. Multiple incisions may be required. The incisions are extended deep to the muscle fascia. Long incisions are made in the fascia to relieve the pressure. The muscles are carefully examined and any nonviable muscle or nerve tissue is debrided and removed. The physician may also debride and remove nonviable muscle tissue from within the compartments. The incisions in the fascia and skin are left open.

27893

The physician performs surgery on the posterior compartments of the leg to reduce high pressure within the compartments. The physician also removes muscle tissue from within the compartments that has become nonviable because of the high pressures. The physician makes incisions in the skin overlying the posterior compartments of the leg. Several incisions may be required. These are extended deep to the muscle fascia. Long incisions are made in the fascia the full length of the compartments. The underlying muscles are carefully examined. Any and all nonviable muscle and nerve tissue is debrided and removed. The fascia and skin incisions are left open.

27894

The physician performs surgery on all the compartments of the leg to reduce high pressures within the compartments. Muscle and nerve tissue that has become nonviable because of the high pressures is debrided. The physician makes multiple incisions in the skin overlying the respective compartments of the leg. These incisions are carried deep to the muscle fascia. Long incisions are then made in the fascia the full length of the muscles. The muscles in each compartment are carefully examined. Any nonviable muscle or nerve tissue is debrided. The incisions in the skin and the fascia are left open.

28001

The physician performs this procedure to correct bursa, fluid-filled sacks that reduce friction. The physician makes an incision over the bursa. Soft tissues are retracted and an incision is made in the bursa to drain fluid. An antibiotic is often injected to clear the infection. The incision is sutured and dressed.

28002–28003

An incision is made through skin and fascia to expose the infection. The infected tissue is removed, and the bursal sac may be removed or simply incised and drained. If the wound is large, the physician may leave the incision open after irrigating the area, treating it with antibiotic, and packing it with petroleum gauze. The wound heals from inside. Report 28003 if more than one incision is necessary.

28005

This procedure is performed for osteomyelitis of the calcaneus (heel) or other bones of the foot. The patient is placed prone. If the calcaneus is the involved bone, a longitudinal incision is made in the midline of the heel extending 2.5 cm to 4.0 cm from the attachment of the fifth metatarsal toward the back of the foot. The deeper tissues are divided. The heel bone is divided into two parts with an osteotome so that the infected portion can be removed. The wound is loosely closed over drain. A short leg cast, with a wind over the heel bone is applied. If the infection is in a bone other than the calcaneus, a similiar procedure would be performed at that site.

28008

There are two common techniques used in faciotomies of the foot and/or toes. Ffor flexion contracture of the toe, a plantar incision is made. A transverse division of the fibrotic and contractaed cord of planter fascia in the foot and/or toe is performed through one or more incisions. A percutaneous procedure may be performed instead which involves making a stab incision over the center of the plantar fascia where it attaches to the calcaneus. The plantar fascia is then transversely divided.

28010–28011

This procedure is performed to correct mallet or hammer toe. The physician makes a small incision at the crease of the toe where the tendon is restricted. The tendon is released from the bone and the toe is straightened. The incision is sutured and dressing

applied. Report 28011 if more than one toe is being straightened.

28020–28024

Arthrotomy is performed on joints of the foot to explore the joint, drain a fluid collection or abscess, or remove a foreign body. The physician makes a longitudinal incision over the affected joint. The soft tissue is reflected and the joint capsule is incised. The joint is explored. If fluid collection or infection is present it is drained. Any foreign bodies are removed. Report 28020 if the procedure is performed on the intertarsal or tarsometatarsal joint; report 28022 if the procedure is performed on the metatarsophalangeal joint; and report 28024 if the procedure is performed on the interphalangeal joint.

28030

The patient lies in the supine position and is placed under general anesthesia. A physician using loupe magnification marks the dorsal side of the affected web space, including both metatarsal heads and metatarsophalangeal joints. The physician makes a straight dorsal skin incision midline in the intermetatarsal space beginning at the metatarsal heads and extending to the terminal skin fold of the web space. A blade is used to deepen the incision through subcutaneous tissue to the level of the interosseous fascia. The layer is slit in to expose the transverse metatarsal ligament that is, also, divided. The physician uses a laminar spreader to spread the metatarsal heads and the nerve is dissected out in the web space to its bifurcation. The inflamed bursal tissue is removed, though the plantar fat pad generally is left intact. The physician dissects the nerve 3 centimeters and cleanly divided at its proximal point. The wound is irrigated with sterile saline solution. The subcutaneous tissue and skin are sutured and a sterile compression dressing is used to protect the wound.

28035

The physician releases the tarsal tunnel, decompressing the posterior tibial nerve. The tarsal tunnel is located on the inside of the ankle. A curved incision is made along the inner ankle, behind the medial malleolus. Dissection is carried down to expose the flexor retinaculum. The retinaculum is carefully released along the tunnel. The posterior tibial nerve is identified by blunt dissection and traced as it courses down through the tarsal tunnel. Three branches of the posterior tibial nerve are also traced at the point. Once the posterior tibial nerve and its terminal branches are released, the nerve is inspected to see if any other constrictions are present. The incision is closed layers without closing the retinaculum.

28043–28046

The physician removes a tumor of the foot under the skin. An incision is made over the tumor and it is determined to either be benign or malignant. If benign, it is dissected and removed. If malignant, it is dissected and the surrounding skin is removed. The wound is sutured and dressed. Report 28045 if the tumor is deeper in the foot; report 28046 if the entire muscle group must be removed.

28050–28054

Arthrotomy is performed to determine the type and extent of a growth. The physician makes the incision at the joint line and opens the skin to remove a part of the growth. The incision is often left open to allow for pathology confirmation of the growth's composition and allow for synovectomy if malignant. Once complete, the wound is sutured closed. Report 28050 for an intertarsal or tarsometatarsal joint; report 28052 for metatarsophalangeal joint; and report 28054 for an interphalangeal joint.

28060–28062

Heel pain originates deep within the foot, directly on the heel bone or within the foot's connective tissues, called the fascia. Pain can result when these tissues become irritated or inflamed, or when small spurs grow on the heel bone. Prior to surgery a tourniquet is applied to the ankle. The surgeon makes a longitudinal incision inside the heel and the fat that has filled the wound is separated with a key elevator. The medial third of the plantar fascia is identified using right angle retractors under direct vision. Report 28062 when the medial third of the plantar fascia is incised and a 1-centimeter segment is removed. The tourniquet is released and the skin closed with nonabsorbable sutures. A dressing and a removable walking boot are applied. The sutures are removed in about three weeks and weightbearing is increased; though the radical procedure increases postoperative recovery period.

28070–28072

The physician makes an incision on the top of the foot over the small bones of the foot in front of the ankle. The skin is reflected back to expose the tendons. They are divided and the soft tissue reflected back to expose the bones. The synovium is the lining between the bones that becomes thickened and inflamed with some disease processes. The synovium is removed by careful dissection. The bones are allowed back into their original position and the skin is closed with sutures. Report 28072 if the area of incision is further toward the toes, between the long bones of the foot and the phalanges (toes).

28080

Surgery for Morton's neuroma involves removal of the fibrous nerve growth from between the toes. The physician places a tourniquet at the ankle and a small incision is made on the top of the foot between the third and fourth metatarsal bones. The soft tissue is reflected in the web space and the bones are separated. Pressure is applied to the bottom of the

foot under the web space causing the neuroma to protrude upward. The neuroma is removed and the nerve trunk is cut to prevent regrowth. The tourniquet is removed and the incision is closed with sutures.

28086–28088

A synovectomy is performed to relieve pain in the active stages of disease before joint destruction. For this procedure description the flexor hallucis longus (FHL) tendon was used as the example. The patient is placed in a supine position with a tourniquet placed around the ankle. The physician makes a 5-centimeter incision behind the medial malleolus and toward the navicular. The neurovascular bundle is retracted, revealing the FHL in its fibroosseous sheath. The reticulum is released to the level of the sustentaculum tali and the tendon is inspected. A tenosynovectomy is performed and the tenosynovial tissue is debrided. Any nodules are excised and longitudinal tears are repaired. The FHL is released until the retinaculum no longer prohibits its motion. The distal soft tissue is approximated and the skin is sutured closed. A below-knee splint or cast is applied. This procedure will vary depending upon which tendon is affected. Use 28088 when affected tendon is the extensor tendon.

28090–28092

The physician makes an incision through the skin on the foot to expose a portion of the tendon requiring removal and suturing ends together, or a portion of the joint capsule or lining of the joint may be removed from the foot. The lesion, usually a cyst or benign ganglion growth, is excised or removed from the tissue surrounding the tendon. Every effort is made not to disrupt the tendon itself. The incision is closed and a soft dressing is applied. Report 28092 if the lesion is located in the toes. Report each toe separately.

28100–28108

The physician makes an incision along the lateral aspect of the heel bone and reflects back the skin and fat pad on the bottom of the bone. The periosteum or lining of the bone is divided and reflected. A window is cut into the bone completely surrounding the benign growth. The growth is scraped from the bone completely removing any evidence of abnormal tissue from the bone. The soft tissues are repositioned and the wound is closed with sutures and soft dressing. The patient is kept non-weight bearing for a period of time to allow for healing. Report 28102 if an iliac or other autograft is used; report 28103 if an allograft is used; report 28104 if bone cyst benign tumor, tarsa or metatarsal bones are excised or cureted; report 28106 if an iliac or other autograft is used; report 28107 if an allograft is used; report 28108 if excision or curettage of bone cyst or tumor is performed on the phalanges of the foot.

28110

The physician makes a lateral incision over the distal third of the fifth metatarsal bone to expose the metatarsal head. An osteotome is used to remove the lateral extension of the bone (bunionette). The cut is made along the shaft of the bone. The wound is irrigated and the soft tissues are sutured. Soft dressing is applied and weight bearing is allowed as tolerated.

28111–28114

The patient is placed under regional anesthesia and an ankle tourniquet is applied. The physician incises the first metatarsophalangeal joint and inserts a Weitlaner into the wound to remove the joint capsule as well as any proliferative synovial tissue. The physician detaches the adductor hallucis tendon from the base of the phalanx and cuts the metatarsal head and base with an osteotome. A longitudinal incision is made in the second and fourth dorsal web spaces, which exposes the base of the phalanx for excision with a bone cutter. The same is done for all the lesser toes. The physician uses blunt dissection to strip the plantar structures that are around the metatarsal head and places them on the plantar aspect of the foot. The fat pad is returned to its position under the metatarsal heads. If an arthrodesis is performed, the physician drives Steinmann pins through the tip of the toe and back across to the site of the arthrodesis. The skin is sutured closed and a dressing applied. Report 28111 for a complete excision of the first metatarsal head. Report 28112 for the excision of the second, third, or fourth metatarsal heads and 28113 for the fifth metatarsal head. Report 28114 when using a Clayton type procedure in the approach to the metatarsal heads. The physician makes an incision over the metatarsal heads that curves to overlie the first metatarsophalangeal joint. The exposed extensor tendons are retracted or, if contracted, cut in the line of the incision. The physician opens the incision by depressing the toes and the bases of the proximal phalanges, thus, delivering the heads into the wound. The metatarsal heads are dissected free with partial excision of the proximal phalanges, excluding the first metatarsal. Only the subcutaneous tissue and skin are sutured. If the extensor tendon has been cut, it is resutured.

28116

A tarsal coalition is an abnormal fusion of the tarsal bones or small bones of the foot near the ankle. A common procedure is for the physician to reproduce the division of the calcaneus and the navicular. An incision is made on the dorsal aspect of the foot. The soft tissues and tendons are reflected back to expose the bones. An osteotome is used to divide the calcaneus and the navicular. The ends of the bones are smoothed for better articulation or movement of the joint. The wound is irrigated and sutured closed.

28118

A mid-thigh tourniquet is placed on the leg to control bleeding. The physician makes a longitudinal incision on the lateral side of the ankle behind the ankle bone. The peroneal tendons are protected and the plantar fascia is reflected back to expose the calcaneus. A crescent shaped cut is made into the bone with a motor saw using a curved blade. The bottom of the heel bone is shifted backward to correct the deformity. The bone fragments are secured in place with a staple or wire. A short leg case is applied for six weeks. At that time the staple or wire is removed and full weight bearing is allowed.

28119

The physician applies a tourniquet to the ankle. The medial third of the plantar fascia is incised and, through the incision, the abductor hallucis muscle is elevated and a portion of the deep fascia of the abductor hallucis released, if required. To excise the spur, a key elevator is placed forward and back of the spur and the spur is transected with an osteotome. The cut spur is removed using a rongeur and the bone edges smoothed. Thrombin or bone wax can be packed at the cut edge of the bone. In some cases, part of the flexor digitorum brevis must be removed for a calcaneal spur that is deeply embedded. Once the spur is removed, the margins are smoothed with a bone rasp. The wound is irrigated and a dressing is applied.

28120–28124

The patient is placed prone with the ankle supported. A longitudinal incision is made along the midline of the heel from the bottom of the mid foot to the insertion of the Achilles tendon. The soft tissues are reflected back exposing the periosteum. The bone is split in two with an osteotome and divided to expose the interior of the bone. All infected material is removed, but the bone cortex is kept intact if possible. The wound is closed loosely over drains. A short leg cast is applied with the foot in neutral position and the ankle at 90 degrees. A window is cut over the calcaneus to permit dressing changes. Report 28122 if the incision is made dorsally over the tarsal bones. Report 28124 if the procedure is performed on the distal segment of the toe.

28126

This procedure is often performed in conjunction with others in an effort to correct alignment of the toes. A dorsal longitudinal incision is made on top of the foot where the toe joins the foot. The soft tissues are reflected back to expose the bone. A wedge of bone is cut out of and removed from the proximal phalanx. The remaining portions of the bone are then approximated to realign the toe. The bones are held in this position by a Kirschner wire that is drilled and placed through the end of the bone. The wound is sutured and the foot is elevated for 72 hours. After

CPT® Lay Descriptions

that time the patient is allowed to bear weight as tolerated in a wood soled shoe.

28130

The physician performs surgery on the astragalus, the bone that articulates with the fibula and tibia to form the ankle joint. The physician makes a curved incision overlying the lateral part of the ankle. The incision is carried down to the joint capsule of the subtalar and talonavicular joints. The capsule is excised and the surrounding ligaments are divided. The entire talus is removed. If further correction is needed, the physician may elect to excise the navicular bone in a procedure to be reported separately. The calcaneus is usually placed in the ankle mortise and held in place by inserting a Kirschner wire up through the heel into the tibia. The incision is closed in layers.

28140

The physician makes an incision on the dorsal aspect of the foot over the affected metatarsal. With the patient under anesthesia, the physician dissects to the metatarsal bone. The affected part of the metatarsal is cut with a bone saw on either end and removed. The incision is closed in layers with sutures, staples, and Steri-strips.

28150

The physician removes a single phalanx of a toe. An incision is made over the involved toe. This is carried deep through the fascia to the bone. The specific phalanx is identified. Using blunt and sharp dissection, the phalanx is isolated and exposed. The physician removes the bone as indicated. The wound is irrigated and the tissues are closed in layers to include the skin. Code for each phalanx removed.

28153

The physician makes an incision is over the first lesser metatarsophalangeal (MTP) joint along the border of the extensor hallucis longus tendon. Z-plasty or lengthening of the tendon may be necessary to expose the MTP joint. A complete synovectomy excises thickened synovium. If an excisional arthroplasty is performed, two Kirschner wires are introduced at the MTP joint and driven distally through the tip of the toe. The physician drives the Kirschner wires into the first metatarsal head to stabilize the hallux. The pins are bent at the tip of the toe to prevent migration. The Kirschner wires are cut off level with the surface of the skin. The soft tissue and the skin are closed with suture.

28160

The physician removes a part of the phalanges or interphalangeal joint for problems including trauma, infection, tumors, and gangrene resulting from diabetes. The physician makes an oblique incision over the toe and dissection is carried down to expose the affected bone. Using a small bone cutter, the

physician excises the involved bone that may include the interphalangeal joint. Any angular areas of bone are rounded to relieve internal and external pressure. Sutures are used to close the incision and skin flaps without tension.

28171–28175

Radical removal of a tumor involves complete removal of the affected tarsal bone, including the navicular, cuboid, or any of the three cuneiform bones, and the soft tissues that surround it. This is performed in order to prevent spreading of the tumor to adjacent tissues. If it is determined that the foot is going to be spared from amputation, then the affected bone and soft tissues would be removed through a dorsal incision at the front of the ankle. The skin and tendons are carefully reflected back and the bone is identified. The capsule is released and the bone is removed in one piece. Tissue samples are taken to determine the extent of tumor growth and need of soft tissue removal. Once complete, the wound is closed with sutures and dressing and cast are applied. Report 28173 if the resection is performed on the metarsal bone(s) in which case an incision is made longitudinally over the affected metatarsal bone(s). Report 28175 if the resection involves the phalanges (proximal, middle, or distal).

28190–28193

Subcutaneous refers to something under the skin. An incision is made through the skin and it is reflected to expose the foreign body. It is removed and the wound is irrigated and the wound is closed. A dressing is applied and aftercare may include antibiotic injection into the wound and orally. Weight bearing is allowed as the wound heals. Report 28192 if the foreign body lies deeper in the foot. Report 28193 if repair of torn tendon, nerves, and blood supply is required.

28200–28202

If the tendon has ruptured, surgery may be required to either repair the ruptured tendon - or to replace it with a tendon graft. Usually, another tendon in the foot, such as the tendon that bends the four lesser toes is used as a tendon graft to replace the function of the posterior tibial tendon. In cases of a fixed flatfoot, the physician may perform a fusion (or arthrodesis) of the foot that requires the removal of a joint between two bones and the two bones on either side of the joint are allowed to grow together. This type of operation is used to stop pain from joints or to realign the bones. Several joints must be fused to control the flatfoot after a posterior tibial tendon rupture. Report 28022 if a free graft is used for the repair. The patient may be placed in a cast for six to eight weeks.

28208–28210

A dorsal incision is made on top of the foot over the injured extensor tendon. The skin is reflected back and the ends of the tendon are exposed. They are cleaned up for easier attachment. The ends are brought together and sutured. The wound is closed and a soft dressing and cast are applied for 3 weeks. Report 28210 if secondary with free graft, each tendon.

28220–28222

The patient is in a supine position and general anesthesia is administered. A tourniquet is placed on the thigh to create a bloodless field desirable for the procedure. An incision is made over the flexor hallucis longus (FHL); a procedure often used to alleviate the pain associated with "Dancer's tendinitis." The deep fascia is divided and the surgeon retracts the neurovascular bundle. The fascia is opened and the surgeon frees the tendon from the any surrounding adhesions. The tendon is retracted and inspected for tears that should be debrided or repaired. The wound is irrigated and closed in layers with catgut A plaster cast or splint is applied. Report 28222 when the procedure is performed on multiple tendons.

28225–28226

The patient is in a supine position and general anesthesia is administered. A tourniquet is placed on the thigh to create a bloodless field desirable for the procedure. The foot and great toe is placed in a dosiflex position to simplify finding of the proximal and distal ends of the extensor hallucis longus. An incision is made over the dorsal aspect of the first metatarsal. The fascia is opened and the physician frees the tendon from the any surrounding adhesions. The tendon is retracted and inspected for tears that should be debrided or repaired. The wound is irrigated and closed in layers with catgut A short-leg compression dressing incorporating plaster splints is applied. Report 28226 when the procedure is performed on multiple tendons.

28230

A small incision is made on the back of the ankle and a sharp blade knife is inserted into the achillies tendon and rotated medially and laterally. The foot is forced into dorsiflexion to stretch the tendon to the appropriate length. Direct pressure is applied to control bleeding. A suture is made in the incision and a dressing is applied.

28232–28234

This procedure is often done for repair of hammer toe. A small incision is made on the crease of the toe on the bottom of the foot. The skin is reflected back and the tendon is exposed. The tendon is released from its attachment site allowing the toe to extend. This is usually is accompanied by other procedures. The incision is closed with sutures and a soft dressing is applied. Report 28234 if the incision is made on the dorsal toe and the extensor tendon is released.

28238

The physician advances the posterior tibial tendon with excision of the accessory navicular bone. The physician makes a longitudinal skin incision on the medial side of the foot from the tip of the medial malleolus to the medial cuneiform. Dissection is carried down to expose the posterior tibialis tendon. The accessory navicular is identified and removed with sharp dissection. The physician detaches the distal portion of the posterior tibialis tendon and drills a hole through the navicular. The tendon is passed through the drill hole and sutured back to itself or to surrounding periosteal tissue. Wounds are sutured closed.

28240

A dorsal incision is made over the first metatarsal bone extending to the middle of the big toe. The skin is reflected back to expose the underlying soft tissues. The abductor hallucis muscle is identified and its distal insertion is removed from the bone of the big toe. This allows the toe to move back out into proper alignment. The incision is closed with sutures and a soft dressing is applied. The patient can bear weight while using a wood soled shoe.

28250

A longitudinal incision is made on the medial side of the heel and is carried distally to the other side of the heel in order to expose the underlying soft tissues. The superficial and deep layers of the plantar fascia are separated from the muscle and fat by blunt dissection. This allows for freedom of movement of the fascia and releases the scar tissue. Once sufficient movement is obtained, the incision is sutured and a soft dressing is applied. Weight bearing is allowed as the wound heals.

28260–28262

This procedure is often performed in an effort to correct club foot deformity. A medial incision is made on the inner ankle to expose the underlying tissues. The skin and tendons are reflected back to expose the joint capsule of the talonavicular joint. The joint capsule is cut by sharp dissection to release the deformity of the mid foot. Several releases can be made from this approach. A particular order is followed in order to obtain the appropriate amount of release. The incision is closed with sutures and a cast is applied. Report 28261 if tendon lengthening is also performed. Report 28262 when posterior, medial, and subtalar soft tissue contractures are released to correct severe clubfoot deformity. The patient is placed supine and a posteromedial skin incision is made. The tibialis posterior, flexor digitorum longus, and flexor hallucis longus are identified and mobilized. The contracted tendons are lengthened. The talonavicular and talotibial joint capsules are incised. The joint capsules are cut by sharp dissection to release the deformity. Bones are then placed in correct alignment and secured with a single Kirschner wire

CPT® Lay Descriptions

28264–28272

Two straight incisions are made, one between the first and second metatarsals and the second in line with the fourth metatarsal. The tendons and nerve bundles are reflected back to expose the intermetatarsal space. The ligament there is divided by careful dissection. The dorsal capsule of the first tarsometatarsal joint is divided. The second tarsometatarsal joint is identified and divided. Similar incisions are made at the bases of other metatarsals. When sufficient motion is gained the bleeding is controlled and the incisions are closed with sutures. A series of short leg casts are applied for 8–12 weeks. Report 28270 if the joint capsule released is that between the tarsal and the toe. Report 28272 if the joint capsule released is that between the small bones of the toe.

28280

This procedure is performed when there is a deformity of the foot where toes are missing and a large gap exists between the toes present. A dorsal incision is made along the web space extending to the ends of both toes. The skin is reflected and the alignment of the bones are corrected with osteotomies of the base of the proximal phalanx. The toes are approximated and the incisions closed bringing the toes together and eliminating the gap between them. This produces an artificial syndactylism or webbing of the toes. A soft dressing is applied and weight bearing is allowed in two to three weeks.

28285

Hammertoe describes an abnormal flexion posture of the proximal interphalangeal joint of one of the lesser toes. Conservative treatment is usually unsuccessful. The physician makes an elliptical incision over the proximal interphalangeal joint 5.0 mm to 6.0 mm wide. A portion of the extensor tendon and joint capsule under the skin is removed. The collateral ligaments are cut to allow the toe to be flexed to 90 degrees. The head and neck of the proximal phalanx are removed with a small power blade saw and the ends of the bones are smoothed. The toe is checked for ROM and the extensor tendon is reattached and the incision is closed with sutures.

28286

An elliptical shaped incision is made in the skin under the fifth toe. The soft tissues are reflected back to expose the underlying structures. The proximal phalanx is removed leaving a space between the base of the metatarsal and the distal phalanx. The deep tissues and skin incisions are closed with sutures.

28288

The physician surgically removes a portion of a metatarsal head of the foot. A separate incision is made for each involved bone in the dorsal aspect of the foot. The tendons are retracted and preserved. The incision is carried deep to the particular metatarsal head. The bony spurs or prominences are excised

from the head using appropriate surgical instruments. The physician debrides and smooths the remaining bone. The wound is irrigated and closed in layers. Code for each metatarsal head removed.

28289

The physician corrects a hallux rigidus deformity and performs a cheilectomy. Hallux rigidus is a condition caused by degenerative (DJD) arthritic changes at the first metatarsophalangeal joint; the condition causes pain, limited range of motion, and dorsiflexion. In the context of this procedure a cheilectomy refers to excision of part of the lip of the first metatarsophalangeal joint. The podiatrist makes a dorsal incision over the first metatarsophalangeal joint. The extensor hallucis longus tendon is retracted, and the joint capsule is entered. Osteophytes and part of the metatarsal head are excised. Bony irregularities may be removed using a chisel, and edges smoothed with a rasp. When adequate dorsiflexion (60-80 degrees) is obtained the capsule is closed, the tendon is returned to its correct anatomical position, and the skin is closed with sutures.

28290

The physician surgically corrects a bunion of the foot using a Silver-type procedure. The physician makes an incision over the top of the foot between the first and second toes. The incision is carried deep to the head of the first metatarsal bone. The physician releases (frees) the structure of the lateral joint realigning the toe. A second incision is made over the medial aspect (inside) of the big toe and carried deep to the bone. The offending bony spur, known as a bunion, is then removed from the head of the first metatarsal bone. The sesamoid bones, which lie underneath this bone, are examined removed as needed. The incisions are irrigated and closed in layers.

28292

The physician surgically corrects a bunion of the foot using a Keller, McBride, or Mayo type procedure. The physician makes an incision along the medial aspect (inside) of the big toe. The incision is carried deep to the metatarsophalangeal joint. In a Keller procedure, the median eminence and one-third of the base of the proximal phalanx are resected. This is followed by repaaair of the plantar plate and stabilization with a longitudinal K-wire. In a McBride procedure, the adductor tendon and transverse metatarsal ligament are relased through an incision made between the first and second toe. Following the release of the contractured lateral structures, the subleuxated first MP joint is reduced and the median eminence excised. The medial cappsule of the first MP joint is imbricated through a medial arthrotomy incision. In a Mayo procedure, the first metatarsal head and its aarticular cartilage are removed and the remaining bone is restructured. Excision of a medial exostosis is performed. The external joint capsule is then configured so that it can be used ass cartilage between the metatarsal bone and the base of the first proximal phalanz. Fixation devises may hold the bone fragments in position. The wound is then closed in layers after thorough irritation.

28293

The physician treats a bunion of the foot by removing the joint of the big toe and replacing it with an artificial implant. The physician makes an incision over the big toe where it joins the foot. The incision is carried deep to the joint (first metatarsal phalanges joint). An incision is made in the joint capsule and it is exposed. The physician removes (resects) the surfaces of the bones in the joint. The sesamoid bones of the foot are examined and removed as necessary. The bones are placed in proper alignment and debrided further as needed. An artificial implant is placed in the joint and fixed to the bones. The incision is irrigated thoroughly and closed in layers.

28294

The physician treats a bunion of the foot with tendon transplants. The physician makes an incision over the top of the foot between the first and second toes. The incision is carried deep to the metatarsophalangeal joint. The extensor tendon of the big toe is identified and cut to restore the toe to its correct alignment. The extensor tendon is then reattached (transplanted) to the head of the metatarsal bone. Other tendons may also be cut and reattached until correct anatomical alignment is achieved. Any contracted structures are released as needed. The sesamoid bones are examined and removed as necessary. A second incision is typically made over the inside of the big toe. This incision is carried deep to the bony eminence, or bunion, which is surgically removed. The proximal phalanx and metatarsal bone are fused. The incisions are thoroughly irrigated and closed in layers.

28296

The physician treats a bunion of the foot with an osteotomy, a cut in the first metatarsal bone. The physician makes an incision in the skin over the top of the foot at the base of the big toe. Depending on the particular osteotomy to be performed, the incision may be made over the medial (inside) of the foot; or two separate incisions may be made. The incision is carried deep to the bone. Tissue is dissected and debrided as needed. The bony eminence, or bunion, is removed from the first metatarsal head. The physician then cuts through the bone, performing the desired osteotomy. The pieces of bone are realigned to their correct position. Fixation devices may hold the bone fragments in position. The wound is then closed in layers after thorough irrigation.

28297

The physician treats a bunion of the foot using a Lapidus-type procedure in which the joint between the first metatarsal bone and first cuneiform bone is fused. The physician makes an incision in the skin between the first and second toes on the top of the foot. The incision is extended deep to the first metatarsophalangeal joint. The physician releases the contracted structures of the lateral joint. A second incision is then made in the top of the foot over the first metatarsocuneiform joint. The joint capsule is exposed and opened. The articular cartilage of the joint is removed. The ends of the bones are fashioned so they fit intimately together. The joint and bones of the big toe are then manipulated into alignment. Fixation devices are needed to fuse the metatarsal and cuneiform bones. Prior to closing the incisions, the sesamoid bones are examined and removed as needed. The wounds are irrigated and closed in layers.

28298

The physician treats a bunion of the foot using a phalanx osteotomy (Akin procedure). This procedure consists of a removal of a bony wedge from the base for the proximal phalanx. A medial based wedge (0.3-0.4 mm) is cut allowing reorientation of bone while leaving the lateral cortex intact. The medial eminence then is excised. Fixation is accomplished by crossed K-wires. The wound is then closed is then closed in layers after through irrigation.

28299

The physician treats a severe hallux valgus (bunion) deformity of the foot by double osteotomy. The physician makes an incision over the first metatarsal. Various methods of double osteotomy may be performed. In a distal Austin double osteotomy, the soft tissue is corrected and a V-osteotomy made through the metatarsal head and neck that is displaced laterally to replace the metatarsal head over sesamoids. K wire fixation is used and a cast is applied.

28300–28302

The physician performs an osteotomy of the calcaneus with or without internal fixation in 28300. An incision is made on the lateral aspect of the foot. The sural nerve is exposed and retracted. The calcaneus is exposed by stripping off the peroneal sheath from the calcaneus. A saw blade is used to make an oblique cut in the calcaneus. Another cut is made to free a 4.0 mm to 8.0 mm wedge of bone. The physician gently manipulates and closes the osteotomy site, stabilizing the site with a screw, staple, or Steinman pin, if necessary. The incision is closed in layers and a plaster splint (reported separately) is applied. Report 28302 if this procedure is performed on the talus.

28304–28305

The physician makes an incision over the base of the first metatarsal, and over the second and third metatarsals depending on the extent and type of plantar flexion deformity. The physician retracts the tendons and incises the periosteum to expose the metatarsal. A sagittal saw is used to remove a wedge of bone. Samples screws, or Kirschner wires are used for fixation. After the immediate postoperative dressing, a short leg case is applied and worn for six to eight weeks. Report 28305 when a bone graft is necessary due to the segmental bone loss. For this procedure, the physician debrides the metatarsal joint and a bone graft from the iliac crest graft is shaped and placed between the prepared surfaces of the proximal phalanx and the first metatarsal. Steinmann pins are centered on the phalangeal articular surface and driven distally, crossing the interphalangeal joint and exiting at the tip of the toe. The physician uses a lamina spreader to place the bone graft and drives Steinmann pins across the bone graft into the metatarsal metaphysis until they penetrate the metatarsal cortex. The pins are severed at their tips of the tie, leaving a short extension to aid in later pin removal. The tissue and skin are sutured closed.

28306–28308

A dorsomedial incision is made over the big toe and the skin and soft tissues are reflected back. In many cases this procedure is performed in an effort to correct the poor alignment of the big toe. In addition to removal of the medial eminence, a cut is made through the metatarsal shaft and a portion of the bone is removed in order to correct the alignment of the bone. Wires are used to reattach the bone in its corrected alignment. Sutures are used to close the incision. Weight bearing is protected for several weeks. Report 28307 if a bone graft is used to correct the alignment of the first metatarsal shaft and attached with wire or screws. Report 28308 if the procedure is performed on other metatarsal bones.

28309

The physician treats a patient with a high arch (pes cavus) by performing osteotomies (bone cuts) on the metatarsal bones of the foot. Two or more incisions are made on the dorsal surface (top) of the foot over the metatarsal bones. The incisions are carried deep to the bones. Tissue is dissected and debrided as needed. The physician makes cuts through the metatarsal bones one at a time. The bones are each manipulated in such a way that the angles are changed. The manipulation allows the high arch to be shifted to an appropriate position. Multiple fixation devices such as screws, plates, or pins are applied to hold the bones in their new positions. The incisions are thoroughly irrigated and closed in layers.

28310–28312

A medial incision is made on the proximal phalanx or first digit of the big toe. The periosteum is divided from the bone and a wedge section of bone is removed. The toe is properly aligned and a screw is place through the bone to maintain alignment. The incision is closed with sutures. Weight bearing is allowed in six weeks at that time the screw is commonly removed. Report 28312 when procedure is performed on any other phalanges of any toe

28313

In this procedure the correction of the toe deformity is made by releasing soft tissues and possibly involving tendon transfers. It does not include cutting or realigning the shafts of the bones. An incision is made on top of the toe to be operated on. The involved tendons are identified and released and reattached at another portion of the bone and the joint capsule may be released to decrease the abnormal pull on the joint. Once proper alignment is obtained, the incisions are closed and a soft dressing is applied. Weight bearing is protected and gradually progressed.

28315

The sesamoid bone is a small bone that lies under the metatarsal heads of each toe. This procedure involves the removal of that bone. A dorsal incision is made between the first and second metatarsal bones proximal to the web space. The soft tissues are reflected in order to separate the two metatarsal heads. The inter-sesamoid ligament is released and the sesamoid bone is removed with small Kocher clamp or forceps. The soft tissues are replaced and the incision is closed with sutures. Weight bearing is permitted as the wound heals.

28320

Nonunion or malunion of the talus may result from trauma. Fractures are rare but may unite in malposition. The treatment of choice depends upon the portion of bone involved. If the top if the talus (articular surface) is involved, the treatment of choice is to fuse the talus to the tibia with bone grafting and casting. The same can be done for malunion of the calcaneus. In this case the calcaneus may be fused to the talus.

28322

An incision is made on the dorsum of the foot parallel with the shaft of the affected bones. The old fracture is exposed and divided with an osteotome. A small portion of the bone must be removed to produce a nonunion or division between the bone surfaces. The bones alignment is corrected and stabilized with a medullary pin. The incision is closed with sutures and a cast is applied. At three weeks the medullary pin is removed and a walking boot is applied. A felt pad is placed under the metatarsal region to maintain proper alignment.

28340–28341

Macrodactyly is the overgrowth of one or several adjacent digits of a hand or foot. The physician generally stages the surgery to control blood supply. In the first stage, reported using 28340, the physician removes the distal half of the middle phalanx and the tip of the remaining shaft is shaped to a pencil point. The articular surface of the distal phalanx is reamed to create a receptacle, which is fitted over the end of the middle phalanx. Kirschner wires are used to hold the position. An incision is made across the digit at the mid phalanx level and carried down to the midsagittal line. The soft tissue (up to 20 percent) is excised over the dorsum. A hump is created with the plantar tissue. In the second stage, reported using 28341, the physician performs the underlying bony work following the excision of soft tissue over the dorsum. Kirschner wire is used to stabilize the digit and the extensor tendon is shortened while the flexor tendon is left alone. Epiphysiodesis of the bones is performed during growth.

28344

This is a congenital anomaly where an extra toe is present. Correction is obtained by surgical removal of the accessory digit. An oval shaped incision is made at the base of the toe to be removed. The underlying tendons are drawn distally and divided. The joint capsule of the metatarsophalangeal joint is incised and the joint is disarticulated and the toe is removed. If x-rays reveal any development of an extra metatarsal bone, the incision is continued proximally and the bone is also removed. The incision is closed and a soft dressing is applied.

28345

The physician surgically corrects the congenital deformity of webbed skin between the toes of the foot. Separately reportable x-rays are obtained of the foot and toes to ensure that no extra bones are present. The physician operates on one web space at a time. The skin is incised between each toe and the excess tissue is removed. A thorough debridement is performed, including the removal of any extraneous subcutaneous or nonviable tissues. Skin grafts may be required depending on the extent of the webbing removed and the debridement performed. The incisions are individually closed in layers to ensure proper skin coverage of the toes. A soft dressing is typically applied.

28360

Cleft foot (lobster foot) is an anomaly in which a single cleft or division extends proximally into the foot, sometimes even as far as the midfoot. Generally one or more toes are missing and often their metatarsals are absent. The goal is to improve function of the foot. A V-shaped incision is made at the cleft and the skin of the opposing surfaces within the cleft is removed, but the dorsal and plantar skin flaps are left to close the cleft when sutured together. Any bone or joint deformity is corrected at the time of surgery. This may include capsulotomies and osteotomies of any retained metatarsals and phalanges. If pin fixation is required the pins and short leg cast are removed at six weeks.

28400

The physician treats a fracture of the calcaneus bone without open surgery or manipulation of the bone. Separately reportable x-rays confirm a fracture of the calcaneus bone with the fracture fragments in acceptable position. The physician places the foot and leg in a cast, brace, or splint to provide protection while the bone heels.

28405

The physician treats a fracture of the calcaneus without open surgery but with manipulation of the fracture pieces. Separately reportable x-rays confirm a fractured calcaneus with the fracture pieces in an unacceptable position. The physician pushes and otherwise maneuvers the fracture fragments into the proper position. No incisions are required.

28406

The physician treats a fracture of the calcaneus without open surgery but with the use of manipulation and pins placed through the skin and into the bone. With the patient under anesthesia, the physician pushes and otherwise maneuvers the fracture fragments into the proper position. Through small holes in the skin, the physician places pins that are driven into the pieces of the bone in appropriate places to hold the fracture in position for healing. X-rays (separately reported) are used to help guide the pins correctly. With the fracture reduced, the physician places the foot and leg in a cast, splint, or brace.

28415

The physician performs surgery on a fracture of the calcaneus bone. An incision is made in the skin overlying the fractured area of the calcaneus. The incision is extended deep to the bone. Tissues are dissected and debrided as required. The fracture fragments are identified. The physician places the bony pieces in their correct position. Fixation devices are applied either on the inside adjacent to the bone or various types of external fixation to hold the fracture together. These may include wires, screws, or pins. The incision is thoroughly irrigated and then closed in layers.

28420

The physician treats a fracture of the calcaneus with open surgery and the use of bone graft. The physician makes an incision in the skin overlying the fractured calcaneus. Tissues are dissected and debrided as needed as the incision is carried down to the bone. The fracture is identified and exposed. Through a separate incision, the physician obtains a bone graft from the patient's ilium and closes the surgically created graft donor site. The fractured pieces are placed in appropriate position and the bone graft is placed in and around the fracture site. Fixation devices are applied to hold the fracture and graft in the correct position. An external fixation device may be applied. The wound is irrigated thoroughly and closed in layers.

28430

The physician treats a fracture of the talus bone in the ankle without performing open surgery or any manipulation of the fracture. X rays (reported separately) confirm a fracture of the talus bone with the fractured pieces in an acceptable position. The physician applies a cast, brace, or splint to protect the ankle and keep the fracture positioned correctly. No incisions are required.

28435

The physician treats a fracture of the talus bone of the ankle without performing open surgery but with manipulation of the fracture. X rays (separately reported) confirm a fracture of the talus bone with the fractured pieces in an unacceptable position. With the patient under anesthesia (separately reported), the physician pushes, pulls, or otherwise maneuvers the foot, ankle, and leg to restore the fracture to a satisfactory position.

28436

The physician treats a fracture of the talus bone of the ankle without open surgery but with the use of manipulation and pins placed through small holes in the skin and then into the bone. With the patient under anesthesia, the physician pushes, pulls, or otherwise maneuvers the foot, ankle, and leg to restore the fracture to a satisfactory position. Surgical pins are placed through the skin and guided into the talus bone. The pins help manipulate the fracture pieces and hold them in the proper place. Screws may also be applied. X-rays (separately reported) are obtained to confirm the correct placement of the fixation and the fracture.

28445

The physician treat a fracture of the talus bone of the ankle with open surgery. An incision is made in the skin overlying the fractured talus. This is extended deep to the talus bone. Tissues are dissected and debrided as needed. The fracture is identified and exposed. Any intervening tissue between the fractured pieces is removed. The physician then reduces (realigns) the fracture, placing the pieces back into satisfactory position. Fixation devices are applied as needed to hold the fragments in place either internally or using an external device. The wound is thoroughly irrigated and closed.

28450

The physician treats a fracture of one of the tarsal bones, other than the calcaneus or the talus without performing open surgery or any manipulation. X-rays (separately reported) confirm a fracture of the navicular, cuboid, or one of the three cuneiforms, with the fragments in acceptable position. The physician applies a cast, brace, or splint to the foot and leg to protect the fracture and hold it in the appropriate position.

28455

The physician treats a fracture of one of the tarsal bones other than the talus or calcaneus without performing open surgery but with manipulation of the fracture. Separately reportable x-rays confirm a fracture of the navicular, cuboid, or one of the cuneiform bones with the fracture fragments in an unacceptable position. With the patient under anesthesia as needed, the physician pushes, pulls, or otherwise maneuvers the foot, ankle, or leg to restore the bony pieces to a satisfactory position.

28456

The physician treats a fracture of one of the tarsal bones other than the talus or calcaneus without open surgery but with the aid of manipulation and pins placed through skin and into the bone. The physician pushes, pulls, or otherwise maneuvers the foot, ankle, or leg to restore the fracture of the navicular, cuboid, or one of the cuneiforms to a satisfactory position. Pins or screws are placed through small holes in the skin and then guided into the bone. X-rays (separately reported) are used to help manipulate the fracture as needed. A cast, brace or splint is applied.

28465

The physician treats a fracture of one of the tarsal bones, other than the talus or calcaneus, with open surgery. The physician makes an incision in the skin of the foot overlying the particular fracture of the navicular, cuboid, or one of the three cuneiform bones. Tissue is dissected and debrided deep to the bone. The fracture is identified and exposed. The physician places the fracture fragments in their correct position. Any intervening or nonviable tissue is removed. Fixation devices such as screws, plates, pins, or wires are applied as needed to hold the fracture properly. External fixation devices may be applied. The incision is irrigated thoroughly and closed in layers.

28470

The physician treats a fracture of one of the five metatarsal bones without open surgery or any manipulation of the fracture. X-rays (separately reported) confirm a fracture of a metatarsal bone of the foot with the fracture fragments in acceptable position and alignment. The physician places the foot, ankle, and leg in a cast, splint, or brace as needed.

28475

The physician treats a fracture of one of the five metatarsal bones in the foot without performing open surgery but with manipulation of the fracture. X-rays (separately reported) confirm a fracture of the metatarsal bone with the bony pieces in an unacceptable position. The physician pushes, pulls, or other maneuvers the foot to restore the fracture fragments to a satisfactory position and alignment. X-rays (separately reportable) confirm desired results. The foot and leg are placed in a cast or brace.

28476

The physician treats a fracture of one of the five metatarsal bones without performing open surgery but with the use of manipulation and fixation pins that are placed through skin and into the bone. The physician pushes, pulls, or otherwise maneuvers the foot, toes, or ankle to restore the fractured bone to its proper position. Fixation pins, wires, or screw are inserted through small holes in the skin and then guided into the fracture pieces. X-rays (separately reported) are often used to aid in the proper placement of the fixation and to ensure that the fracture is in satisfactory position.

28485

The physician treats a fracture of one of the five metatarsals with open surgery. An incision is made overlying the particular metatarsal fracture. The tissues are dissected and debrided as needed. The fracture is identified and exposed. Any tissue between the fracture pieces is removed. The fracture fragments are reduced (realigned) to their correct position. Fixation devices are applied as needed to hold the fracture in place. External fixators may also be applied. The wound is thoroughly irrigated and closed in layers.

28490

The physician treat as a fracture of the big toe involving one or both of the bones without any open surgery or manipulation of the bones. X-rays (separately reported) confirm a fracture or fractures of the bones in the big toe with the fragments in an acceptable position for healing. The physician places a cast, sling, or brace on the toe and foot as needed.

28495

The physician treats a fracture of the big toe involving one or both of the bones without open surgery, but with manipulation of the fracture. X-rays (reported separately) of the big toe confirm a fracture or fracture of the bones in the big toe in an unacceptable position. With the patient under anesthesia as required, the physician pulls or pushes on the toe and foot to restore the bony pieces to their proper place. X-rays (separately reported) are taken to ensure that the fracture is aligned correctly. A cast, splint, or brace is placed on the toe and foot.

28496

The physician treats a fracture of the big toe involving one or both of the bones without open surgery but with pin fixation through the skin and manipulation of the fractures. The physician pushes, pulls, or otherwise maneuvers the toe and foot to place the fracture pieces in their appropriate position. Fixation devices such as pins or wires are inserted through small holds in the skin and guided into the bone. The fixation is used to manipulate the fracture further into proper position and to hold bones in the right place.

X-rays (separately reported) are used to confirm the desired placement and fracture alignment.

28505

The physician treats a fracture of the big toe involving one or both of the bones with open surgery. An incision is made in the skin overlying the big toe. The tissues are carefully dissected and debrided down to the bones. The fracture or fractures are identified and exposed. The physician places the fracture fragments into their proper position removing any intervening tissue. Fixation devices such as pins screws, wires, or plates are then applied to hold the bony pieces together as required. The wound is thoroughly irrigated and closed in layers. A cast, splint, or brace may be applied to the toe and foot.

28510

The physician treats a fracture of one of the four toes other than the big toe. No open surgery or manipulation of the toe or foot is required. X-rays (reported separately) of the toe confirm a fracture or fractures of the bones where the fragments are in an acceptable position. The physician applies a splint, brace, or cast to the toe and foot.

28515

The physician treats a fracture of one of the four toes other than the big toes involving one or more of the bones in the toe without performing open surgery but with manipulation of the toe and foot. X-rays (reported separately) confirm a fracture or fractures of the toe with the bony pieces in unacceptable positions for correct healing. The physician pulls or pushes on the toe or foot in such a way as to restore the bones to their correct alignment. X-rays (reported separately) are taken to confirm the desired result. A splint, cast or brace may be applied.

28525

The physician treats a fracture of one of the four toes, other than the big toe with open surgery and fixation devices as needed. An incision is made in the skin overlying the fractured toe. The tissues are dissected so that the fracture or fractures are identified and exposed. The physician places the fracture fragments into their correct position. Fixation devices are applied as needed to hold the bony pieces together. This may include pins, wires, or screws. The wound is thoroughly irrigated and closed in layers.

28530

The physician treats a fracture of a sesamoid bone in the foot without performing any open surgery. X-rays (separately reported) confirm a fracture of the sesamoid bone. The physician places the foot and ankle in a splint, brace, or cast to protect the bone while it heals.

CPT ® Lay Descriptions

28531

The physician treats a fracture of a sesamoid bone in the foot by open surgery. An incision is made in the foot over the fractured sesamoid bone. The incision is carried deep to the bone, tissue is dissected, and tissue is debrided to expose the fracture. The physician may apply a fixation device to hold the fracture together. The bone may be excised if it is nonviable. The wound is irrigated thoroughly and closed in layers.

28540

The physician reduces a tarsal bone dislocation, other than talotarsal, without requiring anesthesia. Separately reportable x-rays are obtained of the foot to demonstrate a tarsal bone dislocation in such a position that the physician can return it to the correct position without the need for anesthesia. The physician manipulates the involved bones to restore normal anatomy and function. Separately reportable x-rays are again obtained to note the desired outcome. A cast or brace is applied as indicated.

28545

The physician reduces a tarsal bone dislocation, other than talotarsal, with the use of anesthesia. Separately reportable x-rays are obtained of the foot to demonstrate a tarsal bone dislocation which will require anesthesia to reduce. Either general or regional anesthesia is employed. Without any surgical incision, the physician manipulates the involved bones so as to return them to the appropriate anatomic position. Separately reportable x-rays are obtained to confirm the adequacy of the reduction. A cast or brace is applied.

28546

The physician treats dislocation of a bone in the foot, other than talotarsal, with manipulation and percutaneous skeletal fixation. The physician performs this procedure on the joints of the mid-foot with the patient soothed by general anesthesia or a nerve block. The physician manually reduces the dislocation between the tarsal bones. Radiographs or fluoroscopy (reported separately) are typically used to confirm proper alignment and position. To stabilize the dislocation, small stab incisions are made, and holes are drilled through the bone. Pins are inserted through the drillholes and cross the affected joint(s) to maintain the reduction. The pins are cut just below the surface of the skin.

28555

The physician performs open treatment of dislocation of the tarsal bone, sometimes using internal or external fixation. With the patient under anesthesia, the physician makes an incision and dissects down to the dislocated tarsal bones that are located in the mid-foot. The physician reduces the dislocation. To stabilize the dislocation, the physician may elect either Kirschner wires placed through drill holes in the adjacent bone or bone screws. The incision is closed in layers with sutures and Steri-Strips. A cast may be applied. External fixation may be considered in cases in which there is severe soft tissue damage with open wounds or degloving of skin. The incisions are closed with sutures.

28570–28575

The physician treats talotarsal joint dislocation without surgery. The physician may use separately reportable x-rays to identify dislocation and congruency of joint surfaces. The physician manipulates the bones back into position. A short leg cast is applied with the foot in a plantar flexed position. Report 28570 if the manipulation is performed without anesthesia. Report 28575 if anesthesia is required to perform the procedure.

28576

The physician repairs the dislocation of a joint of the foot with percutaneous skeletal fixation, with manipulation. The physician performs this procedure with the patient soothed by general anesthesia or a spinal block. The physician manually reduces the dislocation between the talus and tarsal bones and uses separately reportable x-ray or fluoroscopy to confirm alignment and position. To stabilize the dislocation, small stab incisions are made and holes are drilled through the bones. Pins are inserted through the drill holes that cross the affected joint(s) and maintain the reduction. The pins are cut just below the surface of the skin.

28585

The physician treats a talotarsal joint dislocation, sometimes using internal or external fixation. This dislocation involves the talo-navicular joint. Open treatment is required in cases where closed reduction was unsuccessful, or where the dislocation is unstable. An incision is made over the dorsal part of the foot and dissection is carried down to expose the talo-navicular joint dislocation. The physician reduces the dislocation. The physician may elect to use Kirschner wires or screws that are placed through drilled holes in the talus and navicular to hold them in place. The incision is closed in layers with sutures and Steri-strips.

28600–28605

The patient is positioned supine on the table. The physician manually manipulates the foot in an effort to reposition the tarsal and metatarsal bones into proper alignment. Report 28600, if no anesthesia is required; however, pain medication may be given orally if needed. Report 28605 if performed with patient under general or regional anesthesia.

28606

With the patient under anesthesia, the foot is manually manipulated to correct the dislocation of the tarsometatarsal joint. A small stab incision is made over the tarsal bone and a small pin or screw is inserted to stabilize the affected tarsal and metatarsal bones. The incision is closed with one to two sutures and a cast is applied.

28615

A dorsal incision is made over the dislocated bones. The soft tissues are reflected back to expose the joint. The joint is properly aligned and stabilized with screw, plate or wire fixation. The incision is closed with sutures and a cast is applied. Weight bearing is allowed at six weeks. At that time the physician may or may not remove the metal fixation.

28630–28635

The patient is placed supine on the table. The physician manually manipulates the foot in order to reduce the dislocation of the metatarsophalangeal joint (joint between the long bone of the foot and the toe). Report 28630, if this is performed without anesthesia. Report 28635 if performed under general anesthesia.

28636

With the patient under anesthesia, the foot is manually manipulated to correct the dislocation of the long bone of the foot and the toe. A small stab incision is made over the metatarsal bone and a small pin or screw is inserted to stabilize the two bones. The incision is closed with one to two sutures and a cast is applied.

28645

A dorsal incision is made over the dislocated bones. The soft tissues are reflected back to expose the joint. The joint is properly aligned and stabilized with screw, plate or wire fixation. The incision is closed with sutures and a cast is applied. Weight bearing is allowed at six weeks. At that time the physician may or may not remove the metal fixation.

28660

The physician reduces a dislocation of an interphalangeal joint of a toe without the need of anesthesia. Separately reportable x-rays are obtained which identify the specific dislocation. The physician manipulates the toe without performing surgery to reduce the dislocation. Post reduction x-rays are obtained.

28665

The physician reduces a dislocation of an interphalangeal joint of a toe with the use of anesthesia. Separately reportable x-rays are obtained to identify the specific dislocation. A local or regional anesthetic is employed. The physician manipulates the toe to reduce the dislocation. Separately reportable x-rays are obtained to confirm that appropriate position has been accomplished.

28666

The physician reduces the dislocation of an interphalangeal joint of a toe with the use of percutaneous fixation. Separately reportable x-rays are obtained to demonstrate the dislocated joint. Anesthesia is typically employed. The physician inserts metal pins or wires directly through the sterilized skin of the toe and into the affected phalanges. The toe is manipulated with the help of these fixation devices to reduce the dislocation. Separately reportable x-rays are obtained to ensure that the joint is again anatomically correct. The pins or wires may be removed or retained for later removal.

28675

The physician reduces the dislocation of the interphalangeal joint of a toe by surgically opening the joint. Separately reportable x-rays are obtained to determine the extent of the dislocation. The patient is taken to the operating room and anesthesia is utilized. The physician makes a longitudinal incision over the dislocated bones. The incision is continued deep to the joint. The capsule is identified and opened. The physician identifies the dislocation and reduces it. This may require the use of internal or external fixation devices to complete the reduction and/or hold it in place. The wound is irrigated and closed in layers. A dressing is applied.

28705

The physician fuses several joints in and around the ankle. It can be performed in one operation or in two separate surgeries. In either case, the physician makes at least one incision around the ankle. Incisions are continued deep to the ankle mortise itself and to the following joints: the talocalcaneal, the talonavicular, and the calcaneocuboid. The capsule of each joint is opened, explored, and debrided. Osteotomies are performed so that viable bone is available on each side of the joints. The physician utilizes a variety of internal fixation devices such as pins, wires, plates, or screws to connect the bones together across each joint. This allows the bones to fuse together as they heal. Because of the extensive nature of the surgery, and the time required for healing, the surgery is frequently performed in two stages. Incisions are irrigated and closed as usual. A cast is applied until the fusion is solidly healed.

28715

The physician fuses the talonavicular, the calcaneocuboid, and the subtalar (talocalcaneal) joints. The physician makes incisions on each side of the foot. These are carried deep to the joints. Tendons are reflected and protected. Each joint is identified. Soft tissues are debrided. The capsules are opened and the joints visualized. Surgical curets are used to remove the articular cartilage of the joints one at a time so that viable bone is exposed. The physician uses any of a variety of surgical fixation devices including screws, plates, or wires to connect the bones of each individual joint together. The incisions are irrigated and closed in layers. A cast is applied and continued until all three joints are solidly fused.

28725

The physician fuses the subtalar (talocalcaneal) joint. An incision is made over the lateral ankle and foot. The physician extends this incision deep to the subtalar joint. Tendons and nerves are retracted and protected. Soft tissues are debrided. The joint capsule is incised and the joint is debrided as necessary. Surgical instruments including curets are utilized to remove the articular cartilage of the joint. Fixation devices such as screws, pins, or wires are employed to maintain fixation of the talus . The incision is closed in layers. A cast is typically applied.

28730

The physician performs surgery on the foot in which more than one of the midtarsal or tarsometatarsal joints are fused. The physician makes one or more incisions over the dorsal aspect of the foot in the skin overlying the affected joints. The incisions are continued deep through the subcutaneous tissue. Nerves and tendons are retracted. The physician identifies the specific problem joints of the tarsals and metatarsals, performing capsulotomies. The joints are entered, explored, and debrided. The physician utilizes any of a variety of friction devices to hold each joint in its fused position. The wounds are irrigated and closed in layers.

28735

The physician performs surgery on the foot in which more than one of the midtarsal or tarsometatarsal joints are fused. The metatarsals are also osteotomized to correct for a flat foot deformity. The physician makes one or more incisions in the dorsal skin of the foot overlying the affected joints and metatarsals. The incisions are continued deep to the particular joints. Nerves and tendons are retracted. The shafts of the metatarsals that will undergo osteotomy are isolated and debrided. The physician performs capsulotomy on each joint to be fused. The metatarsals are cut and realigned in a plantar flexion position to correct flatfoot deformity. The joints, debrided of their articular cartilage, are fashioned for a close fit. The physician utilizes any of a variety of fixation devices such as wires, plates, pins, or screws to hold the metatarsal and the joints in alignment. The incisions are irrigated and closed in layers.

28737

The physician fuses the navicular and cuneiform bones of the foot and advances distally with the posterior tibial tendon the calcaneonavicular, navicular cuneiform and cuneiform metatarsal ligaments. An incision is made over the medial aspect of the foot. This is carried to the tendon and ligaments. The physician creates an osteoperiosteal

flap incorporating the tibial tendon and the ligaments. The navicular-cuneiform and metatarsal-cuneiform joints are opened. The surfaces of the joints are denuded of their articular cartilage. The physician utilizes fixation devices such as screws, pins, wires, or plates to hold the joints in position. The flap of ligaments and tendon together is passed forward beneath the anterior tibia and transplanted to the first cuneiform bone and the base of the first metatarsal bone. Friction devices are employed to hold the flap. The incision is irrigated and closed in layers.

28740

The physician fuses one of the midtarsal or tarsometatarsal joints of the foot. Separately reportable x-rays are used to determine the particular joint to be fused. The physician makes an incision in the skin directly overlying the joint. Tendons and nerves are retracted and a capsulotomy is performed. The physician removes the articular cartilage of the bones on both sides of the joint. The bony surfaces are fashioned for a close fit. Any of a variety of fixation devices are used to hold the bones in proper alignment. The wound is irrigated and debrided. The incision is closed in layers.

28750

The physician fuses the joint between the great toe and the first metatarsal bone. A longitudinal incision is made on the dorsal surface of the first toe. It is deepened through the subcutaneous tissue and fascia to the first metatarsophalangeal joint. The nerves and tendons are retracted. A capsulotomy is performed. The physician makes parallel cuts of the metatarsal with a saw or osteotome. The two cuts are placed together in the desired alignment and position. Fixation devices hold the bones in position. The wound is irrigated and closed in layers.

28755

The physician fuses the interphalangeal joint on the great toe. An incision is made over the dorsal aspect of the toe directly overlying the joint. The incision is continued deep to the joint. A capsulotomy is performed. Parallel cuts are made on the two phalanges that constitute the joint. The physician then places the cut bones together. Pins or screws hold the bones in the correct alignment. The wound is irrigated and closed.

28760

The physician performs a Jones type procedure. The physician fuses the interphalangeal joint of the great toe and transfers the extensor hallucis longus tendon from its insertion on the phalanges to the first metatarsal bone. An incision is on the dorsal aspect of the great toe and distal first metatarsal. It is continued deep to the extensor hallucis longus tendon. The physician fuses the interphalangeal joint. Fixation devices hold the fusion in place for healing. The neck of the first metatarsal bone is identified dorsally. The extensor hallucis longus tendon is identified dorsally. The extensor hallucis longus tendon is attached to the metatarsal using any of a variety of fixation devices. The incision is irrigated and closed in layers.

28800

The physician amputates the foot across the midtarsal region. The physician makes the incision so that skin flaps are made dorsally and plantarly. The skin is refracted and the dissection is carried down through the soft tissue. The tendons are severed and allowed to retract. The dorsal and plantar ligaments of the calcaneocuboid and talonavicular joints are released so that the foot can be removed. The physician may also perform a percutaneous achilles tenotomy (reported separately) to prevent flexion contracture. Skin flaps are closed and a soft compression dressing is applied.

28805

The physician amputates the foot across the transmetatarsal region. The physician makes the incision so that skin flaps are made dorsally and plantarly. The skin is refracted and the dissection is carried down through the soft tissue. The tendons are severed and allowed to retract. The dorsal and plantar ligaments are released so that the foot can be removed. The physician may also perform a percutaneous achilles tenotomy (reported separately) to prevent flexion contracture. Skin flaps are closed and a soft compression dressing is applied.

28810

The physician performs an amputation of a metatarsal bone and its attached toe. An incision is made dorsally over the involved metatarsal and toe. This is carried deep to the tarsometatarsal joint. The joint and capsule are identified. A capsulotomy is performed and the metatarsal is disarticulated from the other toes. The incision is continued around the toe itself. Tendons are retracted or removed as indicated. The metatarsal bone and the toe are completely dissected free from the foot and removed. The wound is irrigated and debrided. It is closed in layers. A dressing and a cast or a brace are applied.

28820

The physician performs an amputation of a toe at the metatarsophalangeal joint. An incision is made over and around the affected toe where the toe joins the foot. The physician continues the incision deep to the metatarsophalangeal joint. The capsule is identified and a capsulotomy is performed. The proximal phalanx bone is disarticulated from the metatarsal bone. The joint is debrided. The tendon and soft tissues are excised for closure and skin coverage. The toe is excised free from the foot. The wound is irrigated and closed in layers. A dressing and firm-soled shoe are applied.

28825

The physician performs an amputation of a portion of a toe at the level of an interphalangeal joint. An incision is made over the involved toe. It is carried deep to the planned interphalangeal joint amputation site. Skin is preserved around the toe for closure. The physician extends the incision deep to the joint capsule. A capsulotomy is performed and the joint is disarticulated. Debridement is performed. The soft tissues are excised and prepared for the amputation. The desired portion of toe to include the disarticulated bone is excised free. The wound is irrigated and closed in layers. A dressing and post-operative shoe are applied.

29000

The physician constructs this body cast to provide a foundation for a halo in which the cervical spine must be stabilized. This involves use of a torso body cast to which the halo is attached. Casting material is applied tightly, beginning at the pelvis and extending up the torso to the upper chest. Extenders from the halo (which is already inserted around the head) can be attached to the body cast. This holds the halo very securely. An alternative is to use a prefabricated torso/chest brace that is placed on the upper torso. The previously applied halo is attached.

29010–29015

The physician applies a Risser jacket, a method of correction for a scoliotic curve. The physician places the patient face up on a canvas strap tied to a rectangular frame. A stockinette is stretched over the patient from the head to the knees. A metallic half-circle carrying a moveable jack with a metal plate to be directed toward the apex of the angulation of the ribs is suspended beneath the frame. The rib angulation area is protected by a heave piece of felt covered with a contoured square piece of plaster that rests on the plate. The jack is turned so that it presses the plate in a direction on the rib angulation that corrects the scoliotic curvature. A second jack may be applied to correct a double primary curve or a secondary lumbar curve. The cast is applied in sections while traction is applied to the head with a hatter and the pelvis with a pelvic belt attached to the plaster girdle. The casting begins with a well-molded neck and shoulder section and finishes with incorporating the entire trunk. Separately reportable spinal instrumentation largely eliminates the use of the Risser jacket. Report 29015 if this jacket includes the head.

29020–29025

The physician applies a turnbuckle jacket to treat scoliotic curves. The physician places the patient face up on a horizontal canvas strap attached to a rectangular frame. Traction is applied by pulling distally on the pelvis on the convex side of the scoliotic curve and the head is pulled toward the concave side. All bony prominences are padded well and two or three layers of felt are placed under the proposed location of the anterior hinge. A body cast is applied extending from the neck to above the knee on the convex side of the curve. Metal hinges are placed in the front and back of the cast toward the convex side of the curve. The cast is allowed to dry for three to five days, cut at the level of the hinges on the concave side forward and back to the hinges. Turnbuckle lugs are inserted into these cuts. A turnbuckle is attached to these edges. From the opposite side of the cast, the physician removes a large elliptical window between the hinges. The turnbuckle is turned each morning. When x-rays (reported separately) indicate the hinges are on the convex side of the curve, no further correction may be obtained by traction. The sides of the cast are reinforced with plaster and wood strips. The turnbuckle and lugs are removed. A large window is cut in the cast over the area of fusion. Report 29020 for application of the jacket. Report 29025 if the head is included in the jacket.

29035–29046

The physician applies a body cast, shoulder to hips. The physician applies two layers of stockinette to the patient's torso (armpits to hips), adding cotton and felt padding over bony prominences. Fiberglass or plaster cast is applied over the stockinette to create a rigid cast. Report 29035 for application of the cast. Report 29040 if the cast includes the head, Minerva type. Report 29044 if the cast includes one thigh. Report 29046 if the cast includes both thighs.

29049–29085

The physician applies a figure-of-eight cast to maintain shoulder retraction while a clavicle fracture heals. A cast method is seldom used; shoulder retraction is maintained with a figure-of-eight shoulder strap. Report 29049 for the cast itself. Report 29055 if the cast includes a shoulder spica. Report 29058 if the cast includes a plaster Velpeau. Report 29065 if the cast is constructed from shoulder to hand. Report 29075 if the cast is constructed from the elbow to finger. Report 29085 if the cast is constructed over the hand and lower forearm.

29086

The hand is placed in the functioning position, with the thumb opposed. The physician extends a synthetic stockinette from the proximal interphalangeal (PIP) joints of the hand to the wrist joint and cuts a hole for the thumb. The physician covers the gap at the thumb MCP joint by splitting the thumb tube to extend it proximal to the MCP joint. Synthetic cast padding is wrapped to cover the cast area two to three layers thick, with extra layers at the proximal wrist to protect the wrist joint during flexion and extension. The physician uses 1-inch or 2-inch casting tape to wrap the hand and thumb in a thumb spica. The wrapping starts with one full around the metacarpals and then wrapping the tape

around the thumb and hand in a figure-eight pattern, alternating the direction of the wrap around the thumb. The free ends of the stockinette are tucked under the second layer of wrap.

29105

The physician applies a splint from the shoulder to the hand. A long arm posterior splint is used to immobilize a number of injuries around the elbow and forearm. A cotton bandage is wrapped around the forearm from the midpalm region to midarm. Plaster strips or fiberglass splints are applied along the back of the arm and forearm, maintain the elbows and wrist in the desired position.

29125–29126

The physician applies a splint from the forearm to the hand. A short arm splint is used to immobilize the wrist. Cotton padding is applied from midforearm to the midpalm region. Plaster strips or fiberglass splint material are applied along the palm side of the hand, extending to midforearm, maintain the wrist in the desired position. An Ace wrap is applied by the physician to hold the splint material in position. Report 29125 if the splint is static, keeping the wrist totally immobilized. Report 29126 if the splint is dynamic, allowing some movement.

29130–29131

The physician applies a finger splint. This type of splint is applied to immobilize the digits. A twin layer of cotton padding is applied by the physician to the digit, covering the last to joints of that digit. Plaster casting or fiberglass splint material is applied to the finger from just beyond the knuckle to the tip of the finger. Usually the finger is immobilized in a straight position. Report 29130 if the splint applied is static for full immobilization. Report 29131 if the splint applied is dynamic for some movement.

29200–29280

The physician or a medical professional under the physician's direction performs strapping with tape on a patient of any age. In 29200, this technique was once more frequently used to compress the thorax offering some support and to limit deep inhalation following fracture. This support does not promote healing, but provides palliative relief. A thoracic elastic or canvas binder is more commonly used. Report 29220 if the strapping is performed on the low back; report 29240 if the strapping is applied to the shoulder; report 29260 if strapping is applied to the elbow or wrist; and report 29280 if strapping is applied to the hand or finger.

29305–29325

The physician applies a hip spica cast. The hip spica cast is ideal for patients of all ages who may have hip problems ranging from fractures to dislocations. The physician applies cast padding to the lower torso and hips and extends this down the affected leg in 29305.

It may extend below the knee depending on the physician's preference and the extent of hip immobilization desired. The hip is placed at the desired angle and casting material is placed over the padding material and allowed to dry. Report 29325 if the physician applies a one and one-half spica or a cast that envelopes both legs.

29345–29355

The physician applies a cast from the thigh to the toes. The physician places the ankle and knee at the desired angle. Cast padding is applied from the toes to the upper portion of the thigh. Casting material is moistened and applied in an overlapping pattern from the toes to the upper thigh and allowed to harden. Report 29355 if the cast is a walker or ambulatory type.

29358

The physician applies a long leg cast brace for a fracture. Code with caution: this cast is rarely applied, having been replaced by a pre-fabricated long leg brace. The physician places a metal or plastic support (with or without a hinge) on either side of the knee. Casting material is applied over the supports to hold them in place. The cast allows the knee to bend and straighten while stabilizing the knee during side-to-side movement.

29365

The physician applies a cylinder cast from thigh to ankle. This cast is used for fractures of the femur that extend into the knee joint. The knee is positioned at the desired angle. The cast and material are applied and allowed to dry.

29405–29425

The physician applies a cast below the knee to the toes. The physician positions the ankle at the desired angle. Cast padding is applied from the toes to just below the knees. Casting material is moistened and applied to the leg in an overlapping fashion and allowed to dry. Report 29425 if the cast is a walking or ambulatory type.

29435

The physician applies the patellor tendon bearing (PTB) cast for tibial shaft fractures. The cast is constructed to transfer weight to the upper tibia rather than the shaft of the tibia. The physician applies the casting material so that a shelf is formed under the tibial tuberosity/patellar tendon to bear the load of the cast. The foot is also included as part of the cast.

29440

The physician adds a walker to a previously applied cast. Lower extremity casts may be modified for walking with the addition of a walker. There are two types of walkers available: (1) those made of hard rubber and incorporated into the cast and (2) those

applied over the cast like a shoe or boot. If the rubber walker is used, it must be secured to the cast with additional plaster.

29445

The physician applies a rigid total contact leg cast. The rigid total contact leg cast is applied to feet and legs demonstrating venous stasis ulcers. Of primary importance in applying this cast is even distribution of contact of the cast over the foot, ankle, and lower leg. The method and cast material used varies with the applicator. Sometimes wound dressing must be applied over the ulcers prior to application of the cast. The cast begins at the foot and extends to just below the knee.

29450

The physician applies a clubfoot cast with molding or manipulation. The cast may be long or short. If applying a cast to the right foot, the physician uses the left hand to grasp the right heel of the patient, placing the thumb over the talar prominence. The physician's right hand grasps the forefoot. The thumb and index finger hold the metatarsophalangeal joint of the great toe and longitudinal traction is exerted on the forefoot. At the same time, gentle pressure is exerted over the head of the talus. After one to two minutes of traction, the foot elongates. It is held in this corrected position while a cast made of fast-setting plaster is applied by a second person over layers of sheet cotton. The cast may be applied only to the foot and connected to the leg in separate parts or the entire cast may be applied at one time. If applied to the left foot, the physician uses the right hand to grasp the heel.

29505

The physician applies a long leg splint from thigh to the ankle or toes. A long leg posterior splint is used to immobilize a number of injuries around the knee or ankle. The physician wraps cotton bandaging around the involved leg from the upper thigh to the ankle or toes. Plaster strips or fiberglass splint material are applied along the posterior aspect of the leg from the upper thigh to the ankle or toes. After the splint material dries, it is secured into place by an Ace wrap.

29515

The physician applies a short leg splint from calf to foot. A short leg splint is used to immobilize the ankle. The physician wraps cotton bandaging from just below the knee to the toes. Plaster strips or fiberglass splinting material are applied to the posterior of the calf, around the heel, and along the bottom of the foot to the toes. The splint material is allowed to dry. The splint is secured into place with an Ace wrap.

29520–29550

The physician or medical professional uses tape to strap a lower extremity. In 29520, taping of the hip

CPT® Lay Descriptions

for immobilization is rarely used because of the hip muscles' superior strength to that of the tape. A hip spica taping procedure may be used to hold analgesic packs in place and to offer mild support to injured hip adductor s or flexors. The patient stands with all weight on the unaffected leg. Six inch Ace wrap is usually used. The end of the wrap begins at the upper part of the thigh and immediately encircles the upper thigh and groin, crossing the starting point. When the starting end is reached the roll is taken completely around the waist and fixed firmly above the iliac crest. The wrap is carried around the thigh at groin level and up again around the waist. The end is secured with tape. Report 29520 if the site taped is the hip. Report 29530 if the site taped is the knee. Report 29540 if the site taped is the ankle. Report 29550 if the site taped is the toes.

29580

The physician applies an Unna boot to the leg of a patient. An Unna boot is typically used to treat or prevent venostasis dermatitis or ulcers of the lower leg. It is also used to control postoperative edema like that resulting from an amputation. The physician prepares this semirigid dressing by first making a paste of zinc oxide, gelatin, and glycerin. This is applied to the skin of the leg. A spiral or figure eight bandage is wrapped evenly over the leg. Paste is then reapplied and further bandages are applied in the same fashion until the desired rigidity is obtained. Elastic bandages are often added to the dressings for reinforcement. The dressing is typically replaced at least once a week or more often as needed.

29590

The physician applies Denis-Browne splint strapping to an infant to correct equinovarus deformity. It is performed on infants no later than two to three weeks after birth. The deformed foot is taped to foot plates attached to a crossbar that is no wider than the infant's pelvis. The foot is retaped weekly to maintain a snug fit. This method involves three phases. Phase One requires at least five to six weeks and consists of progressive external rotation and abduction of the foot. The foot is maintained in this for about five months. Phase Two consists of placing the foot in an open-toed shoe on the bar in the corrected position for an additional six months or until the infant begins walking. Phase Three consists of wearing the shoe and bar at night and a below-knee brace during the day. The day brace has a 90 degree plantar flexion stop and a spring dorsiflexion assist. This is continued for as long as necessary and usually for a minimum of 2 to 3 years.

29700–29715

The physician removes or bivalves a cast. These codes are used to remove a cast or to simply cut it in half for the purpose of either using one half the cast as a splint or for intermittent immobilization. A manual cast saw is used to make two cuts in the cast. One cut is extended along the medial edge of the cast. The second cut is extended along the lateral edge of the cast. These cuts are started proximally and are extended distally. Once the cuts are made, the cast may be removed. The front and back portion of the cast may be applied and secured using an Ace bandage intermittently for immobilization. Only one half may be Ace wrapped for splinting purposes. Report 29700 if the cast is a gauntlet, boot or body cast. Report 29705 if a full arm or full leg cast is removed. Report 29710 if a shoulder cast or hip spica, Minerva or Risser jacket is removed. Report 29715 if a turnbuckle jacket is removed.

29720

The physician repairs a spica, body cast, or jacket due to normal wear and tear, revision of the cast or jacket, or the cutting of a window to check the status of a wound, incision, or other area. Additional casting material is applied in the normal manner.

29730

The physician chooses this procedure to check the status of a wound that is underneath the cast or to visualize an area under the cast where infection may exist. A cast saw is used to cut an appropriately-sized section in the cast. This is removed to create a window. Once the status is determined, the physician may reinsert the section and hold it in place with casting material.

29740–29750

The physician wedges a cast. X-rays (reported separately) of a casted, fractured extremity may show slight malalignment. Wedging of the cast may correct this malalignment without having to remove the cast. The bony deformities identified by the physician and the necessary direction and amount of correction is decided. The necessary cut is made in the cast using a cast saw. A wedge of plastic or wood is wedged into the cast cut to redirect the pressure of the cast on the fracture site to correct the bony deformity. Report 29740 if the wedge is placed in a cast. Report 29750 if the cast wedge is placed in a cast that has been applied for correction of clubfoot deformity.

29800

The physician inserts an arthroscope into the temporomandibular joint to examine the joint space(s). The physician may lavage or wash the joint. The physician makes a 0.5 cm vertical incision anterior to the contour of the ear. The arthroscope is inserted into the joint through the incision. A needle is placed into the joint in front of the arthroscope to allow the saline from the arthroscope to flow out of the joint. An instrument may also be inserted through the arthroscope for biopsy of the synovium (lining of the joint). The arthroscope and outflow needle are then removed and the incision is closed with simple sutures.

29804

The physician inserts two arthroscopic cannulas into the temporomandibular joint. The physician introduces an arthroscope into one cannula to view the joint and operative field. Through the other arthroscopic cannula, small instruments are inserted and used to surgically repair the joint. The physician makes a 0.5 cm vertical incision anterior to the contour of the ear. The arthroscope is inserted through the incision into the joint. A second arthroscopic cannula is inserted into the joint through which instruments are inserted to repair the joint. A biopsy of the synovium (lining of the joint) may be performed. The arthroscopes are then removed and the incisions are closed with layered sutures.

29805

A general anesthetic is commonly administered for shoulder arthroscopic procedures. Two to four small poke hole incisions are made above the joint and sterile fluid is introduced into the joint space to provide a better view. A band is placed to restrict blood flow. A small incision is made on one side of the joint and the arthroscope is inserted. The inside of the joint may be viewed through the eyepiece or the image can be reproduced on a screen. A cannula may be introduced to take a synovial biopsy. Once the biopsy is completed, the physician irrigates the joint until it is clear of blood and loose particles. A long acting local anesthetic may be injected into the joint to help with post-operative pain. The joint is irrigated and suture or Steri-strip closes the incisions. The area is covered with a sterile dressing and a sling or shoulder immobilizer is applied.

29806

The patient is positioned side-lying with arm suspended using a weight and a pulley system. An anesthetic is administered. Two to four small poke hole incisions are made around the shoulder joint to allow access to all areas of the shoulder joint. A sterile solution is pumped through one of these incisions and into the joint to expand the joint for better visualization and to cleanse the joint. The arthroscope is inserted through a hole allowing the physician to perform a diagnostic arthroscopic exam by visualizing the shoulder joint. The coricoid process is identified and the tendon of the biceps (short head) is at times incised distal to coricoid for exposure. The anterior capsule is visualized through a small transverse incision of the subscapularis tendon which is tagged for identification and removed from its attachment on the capsule. The quality and laxity of the capsule are assessed and the joint is explored for damage to the labrum or glenoid. The joint is irrigated to remove any loose bodies. If there is no other abnormal laxity the capsule is advance superiorly and attached to the labrum with sutures. An appropriate amount of slack is taken up to provide stability within the joint. Once the capsule is reattached, the subscapularis tendon is reapproximated but not tightened and repaired. A

long acting local anesthetic may be injected into the joint to help with post-operative pain. The joint is irrigated and suture or Steri-strip closes the incisions. The area is covered with a sterile dressing and a sling or shoulder immobilizer is applied.

29807

SLAP lesions are injuries to the labrum that extend from anterior to the biceps tendon to posterior to the biceps tendon. For a SLAP lesion repair, the physician makes three incisions: one for the arthroscope, a second for the suture hook, and a third for a cannula. The surgeon prepares the bony bed with a small ball burr and drills or punches a hole at the cartilage bone junction of the superior labrum. A hook is passed through the anterior superior portal and the inside limb is grasped with a suture retrieval forceps. The physician sets an anchor into the drill hole by mounting the suture anchor on the inserter and sliding it down the suture. The physician closes the loop with a slipknot that is tied and tightened outside the cannula. A knot pusher secures the knot under arthroscopic control. A long acting local anesthetic may be injected into the joint to help with post-operative pain. The joint is irrigated and suture or Steri-strip closes the incisions. The area is covered with a sterile dressing and a sling or shoulder immobilizer is applied.

29819

To remove loose bodies, such as floating cartilage, the physician visualizes the foreign bodies and removes them with instruments passed through the portal holes. For a synovectomy, the physician makes several half-inch incisions to allow arthroscopic investigation of any problems associated with the synovium. Through the arthroscope, the physician removes the synovium from inside the shoulder joint using cutting tools and arthroscopic suction equipment. A long acting local anesthetic may be injected into the joint to help with post-operative pain. The joint is irrigated and suture or Steri-strip closes the incisions. The area is covered with a sterile dressing and a sling or shoulder immobilizer is applied.

29819–29826

The physician performs an arthroscopy to remove a loose or foreign body. The patient is positioned sidelying with arm suspended using a weight and a pulley system. Two to four small poke hole incisions are made around the shoulder joint to allow access to all areas of the shoulder joint. The arthroscope is inserted through a hole allowing the physician to visualize the shoulder joint. Loose bodies, such as floating pieces of cartilage, are seen and removed with instruments passed through the holes. Sutures and Steri-strips are used to close the poke holes. Report 29820 if performed with synovectomy, partial; report 29821 if performed with synovectomy, complete; report 29822 if performed with debridement, limited; report 29823 if performed with debridement, extensive; report 29825 if performed with lysis and resection of adhesions, with or without manipulation; and report 29826 if performed with decompression of subacromial space with partial acromioplasty, with or without coracoacromial release.

29820–29821

The patient is positioned side-lying with arm suspended using a weight and a pulley system. An anesthetic is administered. Two to four small poke hole (port) incisions are made around the shoulder joint to allow access to all areas of the shoulder joint. A sterile solution is pumped through one of these incisions and into the joint to expand the joint for better visualization and to cleanse the joint. The arthroscope is inserted through a hole allowing the physician to perform a diagnostic arthroscopic exam by visualizing the shoulder joint. The synovium is removed with a motorized synovial resector inserted through a port. The instruments are then removed and a long acting local anesthetic may be injected into the joint to help with post-operative pain. The joint is irrigated and suture or Steri-strip closes the incisions. The area is covered with a sterile dressing and a sling or shoulder immobilizer is applied. Report 29820 for a partial synovectomy and 29821 for a complete synovectomy.

29822–29823

The patient is positioned side-lying with arm suspended using a weight and a pulley system. An anesthetic is administered. Two to four small poke hole (port) incisions are made around the shoulder joint to allow access to all areas of the shoulder joint. A sterile solution is pumped through one of these incisions and into the joint to expand the joint for better visualization and to cleanse the joint. The arthroscope is inserted through a hole allowing the physician to perform a diagnostic arthroscopic exam by visualizing the shoulder joint. A long acting local anesthetic may be injected into the joint to help with post-operative pain. The joint is irrigated and suture or Steri-strip closes the incisions. The area is covered with a sterile dressing and a sling or shoulder immobilizer is applied. Report 29822 if the arthroscopic surgery is performed with limited debridement and 29823 if the procedure includes extensive debridement.

29824

The physician makes two to four small poke hole incisions around the shoulder joint to allow access to all areas of the joint. A sterile solution is pumped through one of these incisions and into the joint to expand the joint for better visualization and to cleanse the joint. The arthroscope is inserted through a hole allowing the physician to perform a diagnostic arthroscopic exam by visualizing the shoulder joint. The physician may shell the entire bone out of its periosteal lining, including the distal articular surface, when using arthroscopic guidance. A long acting local

anesthetic may be injected into the joint to help with post-operative pain. The joint is irrigated and suture or Steri-strip closes the incisions. The area is covered with a sterile dressing and a sling or shoulder immobilizer is applied.

29825

The physician makes two to four small poke hole incisions around the shoulder joint to allow access to all areas of the joint. A sterile solution is pumped through one of these incisions and into the joint to expand the joint for better visualization and to cleanse the joint. The arthroscope is inserted through a hole allowing the physician to perform a diagnostic arthroscopic exam by visualizing the shoulder joint. The physician may shell the entire bone out of its periosteal lining, including the distal articular surface, when using arthroscopic guidance. The physician lyses and resects adhesions, with or without manipulation. A long acting local anesthetic may be injected into the joint to help with post-operative pain. The joint is irrigated and suture or Steri-strip closes the incisions. The area is covered with a sterile dressing and a sling or shoulder immobilizer is applied.

29826

The physician makes two to four small poke hole incisions around the shoulder joint to allow access to all areas of the joint. A sterile solution is pumped through one of these incisions and into the joint to expand the joint for better visualization and to cleanse the joint. The subacromial space is decompressed and a partial acromioplasty, with or without coracoacromial release, is performed. The patient is seated with the torso raised and a sheet placed on the medial border of the affected scapula. Anterior, lateral, and posterior arthroscopic portals are established and a cannula is inserted through the anterior and lateral portals to accommodate the inflow and instrumentation. The arthroscope is inserted into the posterior portal, where it is driven into the subacromial space for visualization of the subacromial joint. A limited bursectomy is performed using a full radius shaver and, if necessary, the physician clears the entire undersurface of the antero-lateral acromion of soft tissue using intra-articular cautery. The acromial ligament may be released. A long acting local anesthetic may be injected into the joint to help with post-operative pain. The joint is irrigated and suture or Steri-strip closes the incisions. The area is covered with a sterile dressing and a sling or shoulder immobilizer is applied.

29830–29838

The physician performs elbow arthroscopy with the patient in a supine position. General anesthesia is preferred. The physician makes 1.0 cm portal incisions to insert the arthroscope into the elbow joint space. The five most commonly used portals are the lateral, anterolateral, anteromedial, posterolateral, and straight positions. The physician then places the arthroscope into the elbow joint and examines the humeral-ulnar and radial-ulnar joints. The elbow is flexed and extended, and pronated and supinated to allow visualization and examination of all joint spaces and surfaces. If there is evidence of synovial proliferation or inflammation indicating disease, the physician uses an instrument to obtain a small piece of synovium for biopsy. In 29830, the physician performs a diagnostic arthroscopy. In 29834, the physician examines all parts of the elbow joint with the arthroscope. Any loose bodies (e.g., small pieces of cartilage from chondral injuries) or foreign bodies (e.g., bullet or nail) are removed by identifying them through the arthroscope and using another portal incision to remove the object. In 29835, the physician may also perform a partial synovectomy, where in 29836 the physician may perform a complete synovectomy. In 29837, the physician perform a limited debridement. In 29838, the physician uses the arthroscope to examine all parts of the elbow joint. Debridement is performed on proliferative cartilage, a degenerative joint, or roughened or frayed articular cartilage. The physician uses instruments through the arthroscope to cut and remove inflamed and proliferated synovium and to clean and smooth the articular joint surfaces of the elbow. Extensive debridement includes all joints of the elbow. The portal incisions are closed with sutures or Steri-strips.

29840–29845

The physician performs wrist arthroscopy. The joint is distended using finger traps on the index and long fingers that are attached to a 10 pound weight pulley. Counter traction is applied to the arm with a second 10 lb pulley. The joint is injected with lidocaine and epinephrine to distend the capsule. A sterile wrap is applied to the forearm to prevent extravasation of fluid. Portal incisions are made. The scope is inserted. The physician then inspects the wrist joint. The wrist is manipulated to allow visualization of all joint spaces and surfaces. In 29840, a diagnostic arthroscopy is performed A synovial biopsy may also be obtained. In 29843, an infection is treated using lavage and drainage. Irrigation fluid is directed into each compartment of the wrist joint using the arthroscope for visualization. Lavage is continued until the fluid is clear. A motorized suction cutter may be used to remove encrusted fluid (exudate) and any fibrinous clots. Drains are placed as needed. The portal incisions are closed with sutures or Steri-strips. In 29844, the synovial membrane lining the joint capsule is partially removed and in 29845 it is completely removed. This is accomplished by use of a motorized, suction cutting resector. The joint is irrigated and all instruments are removed. Drains are placed as needed. The portal incisions are closed with sutures or Steri-strips.

29846

The physician performs wrist arthroscopy. The joint is distended using finger traps on the index and long fingers that are attached to a 10 pound weight pulley. Counter traction is applied to the arm with a second 10 lb pulley. The joint is injected with lidocaine and epinephrine to distend the capsule. A sterile wrap is applied to the forearm to prevent extravasation of fluid. Portal incisions are made. The scope is inserted. The physician then inspects the wrist joint. The wrist is manipulated to allow visualization of all joint spaces and surfaces. The joint is debrided, which involves removing any inflamed or devitalized tissue. The articular surfaces are cleaned and smoothed. If tears are present in the triangular fibrocartilage, the physician uses instruments through the arthroscope to suture the tears. The joint is irrigated and all instruments are removed. The portal incisions are closed with sutures or Steri-strips.

29847

The physician performs wrist arthroscopy. The joint is distended using finger traps on the index and long fingers that are attached to a 10 pound weight pulley. Counter traction is applied to the arm with a second 10 lb pulley. The joint is injected with lidocaine and epinephrine to distend the capsule. A sterile wrap is applied to the forearm to prevent extravasation of fluid. Portal incisions are made. The scope is inserted. The physician then inspects the wrist joint. The wrist is manipulated to allow visualization of all joint spaces and surfaces. The site of the fracture or instability is identified. The physician uses instruments through the arthroscope to manipulate the fracture or unstable area into proper alignment. Internal fixation, consisting of wires, pins, and/or screws, is applied. The joint is irrigated and all instruments are removed. The portal incisions are closed with sutures or Steri-strips.

29848

The patient is placed supine with the arm positioned on a hand table. Endoscopic release may be accomplished by a one or two portal technique. In a single portal technique, a small, 1 1/2 cm, horizontal incision is made at the wrist. Using a two portal technique, two small incisions are made, one in the palm and one at the wrist. The palmar skin, underlying cushioning fat, protective fascia, and muscle are not cut. The endoscope is introduced underneath the transverse carpal ligament. The endoscope allows the physician to view the procedure on a monitor. A special blade attached to the arthroscope is then used to incise the transverse carpal ligament from the inside of the carpal tunnel. The instruments are removed and the portal(s) closed with sutures or Steri-strips. A splint may be applied.

29850–29851

The physician makes 1.0 cm long portal incisions on either side of the patellar tendon for arthroscopic access into the knee joint. The knee joint is examined with the arthroscope and the fracture site is identified. Any loose bodies are removed and the physician may debride the knee joint. If the fracture is not displaced (29850) and appears stable, no fixation is needed. If the fracture is not stable (29851), the physician may reduce the fracture by manipulating it into place and applying one or more screws for adequate fixation. An additional incision may be made for better access in applying fixation. Incisions are closed with sutures and staples and/or Steri-strips. A temporary drain may be applied. A post-op brace or splint may be used.

29855–29856

The physician treats a unicondylar (29855) or bicondylar (29856) tibial fracture. The physician makes 1.0 cm long incisions on either side of the patellar tendon to access the knee joint and insert the arthroscope. The knee may be irrigated free of blood. The knee joint is then examined with the arthroscope and if possible, the fracture fragments are identified. A calibrated hole probe can be used to palpate the bone fragments and to measure their size and displacement. An osteotome or probe can sometimes be used in conjunction with the arthroscope to reduce the fracture fragments. If not, an additional incision is made 3.0 cm to 4.0 cm below the joint line. An impactor is used to elevate the fragment. The fracture may be stabilized with cancellous screws. Incisions are closed with sutures and Steri-strips.

29860

The physician performs an arthroscopy for diagnostic purposes with the patient supine, or in a sidelying position. The hip is abducted and then distracted with enough force to allow adequate visualization through the arthroscope. Once joint distraction has been verified radiologically, a needle is inserted with fluoroscopic guidance into the joint to create a portal just superior to the greater trochanter. Using the Seldinger technique, a wire is introduced through the needle. A small skin incision is made, a trocar is placed over the wire, and it is advanced to the hip capsule where the sharpened end is used to break through the hip capsule and into the joint. An arthroscope is placed over the trocar into the joint. Using the same technique, a second (anterolateral) port is established to aid in the examination of the joint structures and to pass instruments. The joint is examined and a portion of synovium may be removed for biopsy. The instruments are removed. A temporary drain may be placed, and the incisions are closed with Steri-strips and/or sutures.

29861

The physician performs an arthroscopy for removal of a loose or foreign body with the patient in a supine, or lateral (sidelying) position. The hip is abducted and then distracted with enough force to allow adequate visualization through the arthorscope. Once joint distraction has been verified radiologically, the

hip is prepped and draped; a needle is inserted (avoiding neurovascular structures), by use of fluoroscopic guidance, into the joint to create a portal just superior to the greater trochanter. Using the Seldinger technique a wire is introduced through the needle. A small skin incision is made, a trocar is placed over the wire, and is advanced to the hip capsule where the sharpened end is used to break through the hip capsule and into the joint. A fiberoptic arthroscope especially designed for hip arthroscopy is then placed over the trocar into the joint. Using the same technique, a second (anterolateral) port is established to aid in the examination of the joint structures, and to pass instruments. The joint is examined. Small loose bodies can be suctioned or irrigated from the joint. Larger loose bodies are divided into smaller pieces, or shaved, and then grasped by a special clamp and removed. The instruments are removed. A temporary drain may be placed, and the incisions are closed with steri-strips and/or sutures.

29862

The physician performs an arthroscopy to remove a lesion of the articular cartilage, and/or to resect the labrum with the patient in a supine, or sidelying position. The hip is abducted and then distracted with enough force to allow adequate visualization through the arthroscope. Once joint distraction has been verified radiologically, a needle is inserted with fluoroscopic guidance into the joint to create a portal just superior to the greater trochanter. Using the Seldinger technique, a wire is introduced through the needle. A small skin incision is made, a trocar is placed over the wire, and it is advanced to the hip capsule where the sharpened end is used to break through the hip capsule and into the joint. A fiberoptic arthroscope is placed over the trocar into the joint. Using the same technique, a second (anterolateral) port is established to aid in the examination of the joint structures and to pass instruments. If a third port is necessary, it is usually placed close to the anterolateral port. The joint is examined. The articular cartilage is debrided/shaved, or an abrasion arthroplasty is performed using special instruments until bleeding bone is reached. The joint is irrigated. A resection of the labrum (acetabular lip) may be performed. The instruments are removed. A temporary drain may be placed, and the incisions are closed with Steri-strips and/or sutures.

29863

The physician performs an arthroscopy with a synovectomy with the patient in a supine, or sidelying position. The hip is abducted and then distracted with enough force to allow adequate visualization through the arthorscope. Once joint distraction has been verified radiologically, a needle is inserted with fluoroscopic guidance into the joint to create a portal just superior to the greater trochanter. Using the Seldinger technique, a wire is introduced through the needle. A small skin incision is made, a trocar is placed over the wire, and it is advanced to the hip capsule where the sharpened end is used to break through the hip capsule and into the joint. An arthroscope is then placed over the trocar into the joint. Using the same technique, a second (anterolateral) port is established to aid in the examination of the joint structures, and to pass instruments. If a third port is necessary, it is usually placed close to the anterolateral port. The joint is examined. Using a special instrument passed through the anterolateral port, perilabial, ligamentum teres, and inferior capsule synovium may be excised and removed. The instruments are removed. A temporary drain may be placed, and the incisions are closed with Steri-strips and/or sutures.

29870

The physician performs a diagnostic arthroscopy of the knee. Portal incisions of 1.0 cm in length are made on either side of the patellar tendon for arthroscopic access into the knee joint. With the use of the arthroscope and a probe, each compartment of the knee is thoroughly examined for pathology. This includes examination of the patellar-articular surface, medial and lateral meniscus, cruciate ligaments, and joint surfaces. Additional portal incisions may be made to better access some compartments. If there is suspicion of a primary disease of the synovium, then a biopsy is performed. A temporary drain may be applied. Incisions are closed with sutures and Steri-strips.

29871

The physician makes 1.0 cm long portal incisions on either side of the patellar tendon to arthroscopically access the knee joint. Lavage is accomplished with a minimum of 4 liters of a physiologic solution. The irrigation solution is directed into each compartment while visualizing through the arthroscope. Lavage is continued until the outflow is clear. A motorized suction cutter is used to remove encrusted fluid (exudate) and any fibrinous clots. Drains are placed as needed and incisions are closed with sutures and Steri-strips. The drains are removed after 48 to 78 hours.

29874

The physician makes 1.0 cm long portal incisions on either side of the patellar tendon for arthroscopic access into the knee joint. A thorough exam is made of each compartment in the knee. Additional portal incisions may be made to gain better access to the knee compartments. Any loose bodies (fragments of cartilage or bone) encountered are removed through the portal incisions. Small loose bodies can be suctioned or irrigated from the joint. Larger loose bodies are grasped by a clamp and removed. Very large loose bodies may require enlargement of a portal or division with an arthroscopic scissor before removal. A temporary drain may be applied and incisions are closed with sutures and Steri-strips.

29875–29876

The physician performs an arthroscopic synovectomy. The physician makes 1.0 cm long portal incisions on either side of the patellar tendon for arthroscopic access into the joint. Proliferative, diseased synovium is removed with a motorized, suction, cutting resector. If the plica located along the medial side of the patella is inflamed, it may require removal. Removal is accomplished by dividing and excising the plica. The synovectomy is limited in 29875. For a more extensive synovectomy (29876), up to six portal incisions may be made to access all of the involved compartments of the knee. A temporary drain may be applied and incisions are closed with sutures and Steri-strips.

29877

The physician makes 1.0 cm long portal incisions on either side of the patellar tendon for arthroscopic access into the knee joint. Lesions in the articular cartilage are identified by the arthroscope and the use of a probe. Additional portal incisions may be made to provide better access to the cartilage lesions. Debridement of the unstable hyaline cartilage or partially fragmented cartilage is accomplished with a motorized suction cutter. This smoothes the roughened or damaged cartilage. Any loose bodies are removed. After debridement, the joint is thoroughly flushed. A temporary drain may be applied, and incisions are closed with sutures and Steri-strips.

29879

The physician makes 1.0 cm long portal incisions on either side of the patellar tendon for arthroscopic access into the knee joint. Lesions of the articular cartilage are identified by the arthroscope and the use of a probe. Additional portal incisions may be made to provide better access to the lesions. Debridement of the unstable or fragmented cartilage is accomplished with a motorized suction cutter. The cartilage is smoothed down to the layer of subchondral bone which promotes bleeding and regeneration of cartilage. Any loose bodies are removed. The physician may also drill holes into the subchondral bone or create tiny fractures (microfractures) to further promote cartilage regeneration. The joint is thoroughly flushed. A temporary drain may be applied. Incisions are closed with sutures and Steri-strips.

29880–29881

The physician makes 1.0 cm long portal incisions on either side of the patellar tendon for arthroscopic access into the knee joint. Once the meniscal tear is identified, additional portal incisions may be made to provide easier access to the area. There may be a tear on both the medial and lateral meniscus (29880) or on only the medial or the lateral meniscus (29881). The procedure is the same for either medial or lateral meniscal tears. Angled scissors, a motorized cutter, or punch forceps remove torn fragments. The remaining

CPT® Lay Descriptions

intact meniscus is then trimmed and contoured. A temporary drain may be applied and the incisions closed with sutures and Steri-strips.

29882–29883

The physician makes 1.0 cm long portal incisions on either side of the patellar tendon for arthroscopic access into the knee joint. The meniscal tear(s) is identified through the arthroscope. There may be a tear on only the medial or the lateral meniscus (29882) or both may be torn (29883). Depending on the site of the tear, other portal incisions may be made to gain better access. Angled scissors, motorized cutters, and punch forceps are used to debride the tear margins and break the surface of the adjacent synovium in preparation for repair. A 3.0 cm to 4.0 cm incision is made along the medial or lateral joint line, depending on which meniscus is torn. A cannula passes sutures through the meniscal tear and then out through the joint line incision. A temporary drain may be applied. Subcutaneous layers are sutured and skin closure is with Steri-strips. Typically, a hinged knee brace is applied after surgery.

29884

The physician makes 1.0 cm long portal incisions for arthroscopic access into and around the knee joint. A blunt trocar, a knife, scissors, or a mechanical shaver may remove any adhesions limiting range of knee motion. If a manipulation is performed, the physician will remove the arthroscope and apply gradual, progressive pressure to bend or straighten the knee. Manipulation helps the knee regain range of motion. A drain may be applied. Incisions are closed with sutures and Steri-strips.

29885

The physician makes a 1.0 cm long portal incision on either side of the patellar tendon. The defect is visualized through the arthroscope. Any loose bodies are removed with grasping instruments. A motorized suction cutter is used to debride the disrupted hyaline cartilage. Drill holes 2.0 cm in depth are made into the lesion, penetrating the vascular bone at the base of the defect. This promotes bleeding and subsequent healing of the lesion. The donor harvests bone from the patient's hip, rib, or skull and closes the surgically created donor site. The bone is sized to fit the defect. The physician then determines if a screw is needed for internal fixation. If so, a screw is placed. A temporary drain may be applied. The incisions are closed with sutures and Steri-strips.

29886

The physician makes a 1.0 cm long portal incision on either side of the patellar tendon. The defect is visualized through the arthroscope. A motorized suction cutter is used to debride the disrupted hyaline cartilage. Drill holes 2.0 cm in depth are then made into the lesion in order to penetrate the vascular bone at the base of the defect. This promotes bleeding and

subsequent healing of the lesion. The incisions are closed with sutures and Steri-strips. A temporary drain may be applied.

29887

The physician makes a portal incision 1.0 cm long on either side of the patellar tendon. The defect is visualized through the arthroscope. A motorized suction cutter debrides the disrupted hyaline cartilage. Drill holes 2.0 cm in depth are made into the lesion in order to penetrate the vascular bone at the base of the defect. This promotes bleeding and subsequent healing of the lesion. Internal fixation is accomplished by placing a screw into the lesion. The incisions are closed with sutures and Steri-strips. A temporary drain may be applied.

29888–29889

The physician makes a portal incision 1.0 cm long on either side of the inferior patella for arthroscopic access into the knee joint. If the ligament is intact but torn away from its bony attachment, the physician may reattach the ligament with a screw. If the ligament is nonfunctional, it is removed with the arthroscope. For an anterior cruciate ligament reconstruction (29888), a 5.0 cm to 12.0 cm incision is made on the anterior lower patella and upper tibia. A tunnel is drilled through the tibia into the knee joint. A second tunnel is drilled from inside the knee joint, up and through the femur. With the aid of the arthroscope for visualization, a new ligament graft is placed in the tibial tunnel and positioned inside the knee joint. The bony ends of the ligament are placed in the tibial and femoral tunnels. The ligament is secured with interference screws in both tunnels. For a posterior cruciate ligament reconstruction (29889), an additional 3.0 cm to 5.0 cm incision is made along the medial aspect of the knee joint to allow for proper location of the femoral tunnel. Incisions are closed with staples or Steri-strips. A temporary drain may be inserted.

29891

The physician performs an arthroscopy to excise an osteochondral defect, including drilling of the talus and/or tibia. The patient is placed supine with the hip and upper part of the leg elevated, rotated slightly forward, and with the lower part of the leg, ankle and foot resting on a cushioned platform. The ankle joint is distended to allow access for the first port. Distraction is usually not performed. The skin is superficially anterolateral incised. The tissues and tendons are separated to the joint capsule by a clamp, and a blunt trocar is inserted into the joint. The arthroscope in placed over the trocar, and advanced into the joint. A second anteromedial portal is established for further examination and for instrument passage. The joint is examined and any loose bodies are removed. The osteochondral defect of the talus and/or tibia is excised and the sides of the crater are contoured. Multiple holes may be drilled in the bone to promote vascularization. The joint is irrigated, and the instruments are removed. A temporary drain may be placed, and the incisions are closed with Steri-strips and/or sutures.

29892
The physician performs an arthroscopy to aid in the repair of a large osteochondritis dissecans lesion, talar dome fracture, or tibial plafond fracture. The patient is placed supine with the hip and upper part of the leg elevated, rotated slightly forward, and with the lower part of the leg, ankle, and foot resting on a cushioned platform. The ankle joint is distended to allow access for the first port. The skin is superficially incised. The tissues and tendons are separated to the joint capsule by a clamp, and a blunt trocar is inserted into the joint. The arthroscope is placed over the trocar and advanced into the joint. A second anteromedial portal is established for further examination and for instrument passage. The joint is examined, and any loose bodies are removed. A large osteochondritis dissecans lesion is excised, and the sides of the crater are contoured; a talar dome or tibial plafond fracture is treated. Internal fixation may be applied at the fracture site. A temporary drain may be placed, and the incisions are closed with Steri-strips and/or sutures.

29893
The physician performs a plantar fasciotomy using an endoscope. The patient is placed prone. The physician uses small or blunt incisions to create a passage for the endoscope. Other incisions may be made as needed for additional instruments. The physician advances the endoscope and identifies the osteomyelitis. The heel bone is divided into two parts with an instrument so the infected portion can be removed. The instruments are removed and the wound closed.

29894
The physician performs arthroscopy on an ankle joint to remove a loose body or foreign body from the ankle. After induction of anesthesia in the operating room, the physician makes two to four 0.5 cm incisions around the ankle. Using arthroscopic instruments, the physician enters the ankle through these small incisions. The offending loose body or foreign body is identified. Instruments are introduced through the portal incisions and utilized to remove the foreign body. The joint is examined through the arthroscope and irrigated. The skin portals are closed and a dressing is applied.

29895
The physician performs arthroscopy on an ankle joint to remove the synovial lining of the joint. With the patient soothed by general anesthesia, the physician makes two to four 0.5 cm skin incisions around the ankle. The physician introduces the arthroscope into the ankle and conducts an exam. The offending

synovial tissue is identified. Additional instruments are placed through the incisions. Using the arthroscope, the physician uses these instruments to excise the synovium. The joint is irrigated and the skin portals are closed. A dressing is applied.

29897
The physician performs arthroscopy on the ankle joint to minimally debride the joint. With the patient under general anesthesia, the physician makes two to four 0.5 cm skin incisions around the ankle joint. The arthroscope is introduced into the ankle joint and an examination is performed. The physician identifies areas of the joint where debridement is required. Additional surgical instruments are placed through the skin portals and into the joint. These are used to debride frayed, nonviable, or extraneous tissue. The ankle is irrigated and the skin incisions are closed. A dressing is applied.

29898
The physician performs arthroscopy on the ankle joint to extensively debride the joint. With the patient under general anesthesia, the physician makes two to four 0.5 cm skin incisions around the ankle joint. The arthroscope is introduced into the joint and the physician conducts an examination. Frayed cartilage, redundant synovium, defects in the articular surfaces, or bony abnormalities are identified. Additional arthroscopic instruments are placed into the joint through the skin incisions. These are used to extensively debride, excise, smooth, and/or wash out the offending tissues. A thorough irrigation is undertaken. The skin incisions are closed and a dressing is applied.

29900
The metacarpophalangeal joints consist of the convex heads of the metacarpals articulating with the concave bases of the proximal phalanges. The metacarpophalangeal joint of interest is placed for easy access and an injection of local anesthetic is administered. Incisions for portals are made in the respective metacarpal to allow the arthroscope and surgical instruments to be introduced into the joint. The arthroscope is inserted through a portal into the joint, and the surgical equipment is passed through a second portal. A third portal may have been made for pumping fluid in to expand the joint space for clearer visualization. A needle is inserted through the trocar and twisted to cut out the tissue segment for biopsy. The biopsy needle, trocar, and arthroscope are removed. The site is cleansed and a pressure bandage is applied.

29901
The metacarpophalangeal joints consist of the convex heads of the metacarpals articulating with the concave bases of the proximal phalanges. The metacarpophalangeal joint of interest is placed for easy access and an injection of local anesthetic is

administered. Incisions for portals are made in the respective metacarpal to allow the arthroscope and surgical instruments to be introduced into the joint. The arthroscope is inserted through a portal into the joint, and the surgical equipment is passed through a second portal. A third portal may have been made for pumping fluid in to expand the joint space for clearer visualization. Arthroscopic debridement is carried out over the surface of the lesion. The physician must avoid debridement of the adjacent joint surface, so as to avoid possible ankylosis. Closure of the wound includes a re-approximation of the attachment of adductor tendon to the dorsal extensor hood.

29902

The physician makes an incision along the midlateral aspect of the thumb, curves the incision over the MP joint, and extends the incision to the EPL tendon. The Stener lesion can be seen as a mass of tissue proximal to the adductor aponeurosis. A Stener lesion occurs when a torn distal edge of ulnar collateral ligament displaces superficially and proximalyl to the adductor aponeurosis. The ruptured end of ligament is no longer in contact with its area of insertion of the phalanx. A longitudinal incision is made through the aponeurosis volar to the edge of the EPL, leaving a rim of tissue on the tendon to be used for later closure. The adductor tendon is retracted volarly and the dorsal capsule is reflected to permit a clear view of the joint and the inside portion of the collateral ligament. The physician assesses the injury (i.e., ligament rupture at the insertion into the phalanx). The ulnar collateral ligament flap is partially dissected and mobilized off the metacarpal and the volar edge of the proximal phalange is debrided of soft tissue. The physician drills two parallel holes distally and dorsally to exit on the far side of the cortex. Sutures are passed through the distal ligament and pulled through the drill holes and tied over a padded button. Closure of the wound includes a re-approximation of the attachment of adductor tendon to the dorsal extensor hood.

30000–30020

The physician makes an incision to decompress and drain a collection of pus or blood in the nasal mucosa for 30000 or septal mucosa for 30020. A hemostat bluntly penetrates the pockets and allows the fluid to evacuate. Once decompressed, a small latex drain may be placed into the incision site. This allows an escape for any fluids that may continue to enter the pocket. If a drain is used, it is removed within 48 hours. The nasal cavity may be packed with gauze and Telfa to provide pressure against the mucosa and assist decompression after drainage. The incision may be closed primarily or may be left to granulate without closure.

30100

The physician removes mucosa from inside the nose for biopsy. This biopsy is performed when the mucosa is suspicious for disease. Some normal tissue adjacent to the diseased mucosa is also removed during the biopsy. This allows the pathologist to compare diseased versus nondiseased tissues. The excision site may be closed primarily with sutures or may be allowed to granulate without closure.

30110

The physician removes a polyp from inside the nose. Nasal polyps may obstruct both the airway passages and sinus drainage ducts in the nose. The area is approached intranasally. Topical vasoconstrictive agents are applied to the nasal mucosa. Local anesthesia is injected underneath and around the polyp. A scalpel or biting forceps excise the polyp. Small polyps may leave mucosal defects that do not require closure. With larger defects, the mucosa is closed with sutures in a single layer. The physician may place Telfa to pack the nasal cavity during the first 24 hours.

30115

The physician removes complicated nasal polyps in a hospital setting. Nasal polyps may obstruct both the airway passages and sinus drainage ducts in the nose. The area is approached intranasally. Topical vasoconstrictive agents are applied to the nasal mucosa. Local anesthesia is injected underneath and around the polyp. Large polyps are removed with a wire snare stretching the polyp base; the snare or a scalpel can be used to detach the polyp from its mucosal base. A scalpel or biting forceps excise smaller polyps. Small polyps may leave mucosal defects that do not require closure. With larger defects, the mucosa is closed with sutures in a single layer. The physician may place Telfa to pack the nasal cavity during the first 24 hours.

30117–30118

The physician removes or destroys intranasal soft tissue lesions using techniques such as cryosurgery, chemical application, or laser surgery. The lesion is approached intranasally in 30117 or through skin incisions externally in the lateral ala in 30118. The physician performs a lateral rhinotomy by retracting the lateral ala to expose the internal nose. Cryosurgery will freeze and kill soft tissue lesions. Laser surgery will vaporize and emulsify the lesions. Chemical application of topical vasoconstrictive agents and local anesthesia cauterizes vessels and limits post-surgical hemorrhage. No post-operative wound closure or intranasal packing is necessary.

30120

The physician surgically removes diseased tissue caused by rhinophyma from the external nasal tip. Local anesthesia is injected into the nasal tip. The excess tissue is removed by carving and recontouring hyperplastic tissue from the area. Scalpels, dermabrasion (planing with fine sandpaper or wire brushes), and lasers are common methods of removing this excess tissue. A thin layer of epithelium is maintained over the nasal cartilages to ensure adequate healing. Separately reportable skin grafting may be necessary for very large lesions.

30124–30125

The physician removes a dermoid (developmental) cyst of the nose that may be associated with the soft tissue only in 30124 or may extend into bone and/or cartilage in 30125. If associated with the nasal bone, the usual location is at the bone-cartilage junction. Dependent on the size and location, the cyst may be removed using either skin or intranasal incisions. A fistula opening may be present and its tract would be excised. Commonly, an incision is made overlying the cyst in the nasal skin. The cyst is then removed from its cavity using curets. The defect size dictates pos-removal cavity packing and/or separately reportable reconstruction. Incisions may be closed in single and multiple layers.

30130

The physician removes a part or all of the nasal turbinate located on the lateral wall of the nose. The inferior nasal turbinate is most commonly resected. The physician places topical vasoconstrictive drugs on the turbinate to shrink the blood vessels. A mucosal incision is made around the base of the turbinate. The physician fractures the bony turbinate from the lateral nasal wall with a chisel or drill. The turbinate is then excised from the lateral nasal wall. Electrocautery may control bleeding. The nasal mucosa is sutured in single layers. The nasal cavity may be packed with gauze.

30140

The physician removes a part or all of the turbinate bone through a submucous incision. The physician places vasoconstrictive drugs on the turbinate to shrink the blood vessels. A full thickness incision is made over the anterior-inferior surface of the turbinate and continued deep to bone. The physician lifts the mucoperiosteum with an elevator to expose the bony turbinate. A chisel or forcep is used to remove portions of the bony turbinate. Electrocautery may control bleeding. The turbinate mucosa is then closed in a single layer.

30150–30160

The physician resects a portion of the nose in 30150 or the total nose in 30160, leaving a surgical defect. The extent of the resection is determined by the extent of the tumor or trauma. A full thickness incision is made through the external nose. All diseased or damaged soft tissue is excised to clear margins. Underlying bone or cartilage may be removed. Exposed bone or cartilage is covered with mucosal flaps or separately reportable skin grafts.

30200

The physician injects a pharmacologic agent (i.e., steroids, sclerosing agents) into the submucosal tissue overlying the nasal turbinate. The inferior nasal turbinate is most commonly involved. Enlarged turbinates obstruct airflow through the nasal cavity. Turbinates with allergic hypertrophy or hypertrophy compensating for septal deviation may benefit from therapy.

30210

The physician displaces mucopurulent secretions (pus and mucous) from sinuses by gravity replacement with a second liquid. This therapy is effective for the ethmoid and sphenoid sinuses. While lying supine, the patient's head is hyperextended. The nose is filled with isotonic saline solution. The physician closes one nostril and applies suction to the other nostril. The patient repeats vowels or words (phonates), elevating the soft palate and creating negative pressure. While the patient is phonating, the physician suctions the nostril. The saline solution enters the sinus, displacing the secretions of the sinuses. The secretions are then suctioned from the nostril.

30220

The physician uses an alloplastic button to obturate (close) a nasal septal opening. This procedure is performed as an option to surgical reconstruction of the septum such as grafting. The commercially available alloplastic button is made of silicone rubber. The physician inserts the button into the septal perforation securing it with transseptal sutures.

30300–30310

The physician removes a foreign body from the inside of the nasal cavity, either in the office for 30300 or under general anesthesia for 30310. Foreign bodies are defined as objects not normally found in the body. An object may be embedded in normal tissue as a result of some type of trauma. Topical vasoconstrictive agents and local anesthesia are applied to the nasal mucosa. A small incision may be necessary to access the foreign body. Blunt dissection and retrieval of the object is performed with hemostats or forceps. Sutures may close the mucosa in a single layer if the size of the dissection requires.

30320

The physician removes a foreign body from deep within the nasal cavity, accessing the area with a lateral rhinotomy surgical approach. This foreign body is located in an area of difficult access and requires complex surgery to remove it. Foreign bodies are defined as objects not normally found in the body. The object may be embedded in normal tissue as a result of some type of trauma. Topical vasoconstrictive agents and local anesthesia are applied to the nasal mucosa. A full-thickness skin incision is made from the nostril extending along the nasal alar rim and continuing superiorly. The incision can extend to the

CPT® Lay Descriptions

medial aspect of the eyebrow if necessary. The lateral aspect of the nose is retracted, exposing the bony structures beneath the soft tissue. Blunt dissection and retrieval of the object is performed with hemostats or forceps. The surgical wound is closed in multiple layers.

30400

The physician performs surgery to reshape the external nose. No surgery to the nasal septum is necessary. The physician may perform surgery open (external skin incisions) or closed (intranasal incisions). Topical vasoconstrictive agents are applied to shrink the blood vessels and local anesthesia is injected into the nasal mucosa. After incisions are made, dissections expose the external nasal cartilaginous and bony skeleton. The cartilages may be reshaped with files. Fat may be removed from the subcutaneous regions. Incisions are closed in single layers. Steri-strip tape is used to support cartilaginous surgery of the nasal tip.

30410

The physician performs surgery to reshape the external nose. No surgery to the nasal septum is necessary. This surgery can be performed open (external skin incisions) or closed (intranasal incisions). Topical vasoconstrictive agents are applied to shrink the blood vessels and local anesthesia is injected in the nasal mucosa. After incisions are made, dissections expose the external nasal cartilaginous and bony skeleton. The cartilages may be reshaped by trimming or may be augmented by grafting. Local grafts from adjacent nasal bones and cartilage are not reported separately. The physician may reshape the dorsum with files. The physician then fractures the lateral nasal bones with chisels. Fat may be removed from the subcutaneous regions. Incisions are closed in single layers. Steri-strip tape is used to support cartilaginous surgery of the nasal tip. An external splint or cast supports changes in bone position.

30420

The physician performs surgery to reshape the external and internal nose. The nasal septum internally supports the shape of the external nasal appearance. The physician reshapes a fractured or deformed septum. Rhinoplasties can be performed open (external skin incisions) or closed (intranasal incisions). Topical vasoconstrictive agents are applied to shrink the blood vessels and local anesthesia is injected into the nasal mucosa. After incisions are made, dissections expose the external nasal cartilaginous and bony skeleton. The cartilages may be reshaped by trimming or may be augmented by grafting. Local grafts from adjacent nasal bones and cartilage are not reported separately. The physician may reshape the dorsum with files. Fat may be removed from the subcutaneous regions. A vertical incision is made in the septal mucosa and the mucoperichondrium is elevated from the septal

cartilage. Septal cartilage may be removed or grafted. The physician fractures the lateral nasal bones with chisels and manually repositions them in the desired positions. Incisions are closed in single layers. Steri-strip tape is used to support cartilaginous surgery of the nasal tip. An external splint or cast supports changes in bone position.

30430

The physician performs a second surgery to reshape the external nose and correct unfavorable results from the initial rhinoplasty. Secondary rhinoplasties can be performed open (external skin incisions) or closed (intranasal incisions). Topical vasoconstrictive agents are applied to shrink the blood vessels and local anesthesia is injected in the nasal mucosa. After incisions are made, dissections expose the external nasal cartilaginous and bony skeleton. The cartilages and nasal tip may be reduced by trimming or may be augmented by grafting. The bony dorsum may receive grafts. Local grafts from adjacent nasal bones and cartilage are not reported separately. Incisions are closed in single layers. Steri-strip tape is used to support cartilaginous surgery of the nasal tip.

30435

The physician performs a second surgery to reshape the external nose and correct unfavorable results from the initial rhinoplasty. Secondary rhinoplasties can be performed open (external skin incisions) or closed (intranasal incisions). Topical vasoconstrictive agents are applied to shrink the blood vessels and local anesthesia is injected in the nasal mucosa. After incisions are made, dissections expose the external nasal cartilaginous and bony skeleton. The physician refractures the lateral nasal bones with chisels and manually repositions them in the desired positions. The bony dorsum may receive grafts. Local grafts from adjacent nasal bones and cartilage are not reported separately. Incisions are closed in single layers. Steri-strip tape is used to support cartilaginous surgery of the nasal tip. An external splint or cast supports changes in bone position.

30450

The physician performs a second surgery to reshape the external nose and correct unfavorable results from the initial rhinoplasty. Secondary rhinoplasties can be performed open (external skin incisions) or closed (intranasal incisions). Topical vasoconstrictive agents are applied to shrink the blood vessels and local anesthesia is injected in the nasal mucosa. After incisions are made, dissections expose the external nasal cartilaginous and bony skeleton. The cartilages and nasal tip may be reduced by trimming or augmented by grafting. The bony dorsum may receive grafts as well. Local grafts from adjacent nasal bones and cartilage are not reported separately. The physician refractures the lateral nasal bones with chisels and manually repositions them in the desired position. Incisions are closed in single layers. Steri-strip tape is used to support cartilaginous surgery of the nasal tip. An external splint or cast supports changes in bone position.

30460

The physician reshapes the external nose and corrects secondary developmental cleft lip and/or palate deformities. Rhinoplasties can be performed open (external skin incisions) or closed (intranasal incisions). Topical vasoconstrictive agents are applied to shrink the blood vessels and local anesthesia is injected in the nasal mucosa. After incisions are made, dissections expose the external nasal cartilaginous and bony skeleton. The cartilages and nasal tip may be reduced by trimming or may be augmented by grafting. Local grafts from adjacent nasal bones and cartilage are not reported separately. Incisions are closed in single layers. Steri-strip tape supports cartilaginous surgery of the nasal tip.

30462

The physician reshapes the external and internal nose and corrects developmental cleft lip and/or palate deformities. Deflection of the nasal septum can cause airway obstruction and affect both support and appearance of the external nasal cartilages. Rhinoplasties can be performed open (external skin incisions) or closed (intranasal incisions). Topical vasoconstrictive agents are applied to shrink the blood vessels and local anesthesia is injected in the nasal mucosa. After incisions are made, dissections expose the external nasal cartilaginous and bony skeleton. The cartilages and nasal tip may be reduced by trimming or may be augmented by grafting. The physician makes a vertical incision in the septal mucosa and elevates the mucoperichondrium from the septal cartilage. Septal cartilage may be removed or grafted. The nasal dorsum may be a graft recipient. Local grafts from adjacent nasal bones and cartilage are not reported separately. The physician fractures the lateral nasal bones with chisels and manipulates the bones into the desired positions. Incisions are closed in single layers. Steri-strip tape supports cartilaginous surgery of the nasal tip. An external splint or cast supports changes in bone position.

30465

The physician repairs a nasal vestibular stenosis using a variety of techniques. Separately reportable cartilage (e.g., auricular composite) graft may be used to support the cartilaginous skeleton and vestibular soft tissue scarring. In one external approach the physician makes an incision in the upper lateral cartilage, in another approach a "V" shaped cut may be made. In either case the incision is followed by an osteotomy of the medial aspect of the nasal bones. A spreader graft is placed to widen the nasal vestibule. The incision is closed or closed in a V-Y manner (lengthens the columella) with suture.

30520

The physician reshapes the nasal septum, correcting airway obstruction. Topical vasoconstrictive agents are applied to shrink the blood vessels and local anesthesia is injected in the nasal mucosa. The physician makes a vertical incision in the septal mucosa and elevates the mucoperichondrium from the septal cartilage. The deviated portion of the bony and cartilaginous septum is excised or augmented by grafting. Local grafts from adjacent nasal bones and cartilage are not reported separately. If the cartilaginous septum remains bowed, partial or full-thickness incisions are made in the cartilage to straighten the septum. Excess cartilage is excised from the bone-cartilage junction. Incisions are closed in single layers. Transseptal sutures are placed. Septal splints may support the septum during healing.

30540

The physician reconstructs the congenitally absent openings between the nasal cavity and the pharynx (throat). Topical vasoconstrictive agents are applied and local anesthesia is injected in the nasal mucosa. A mastoid curet or scalpel is placed in the nose and passed to the closure along the floor of the nose. The physician gently punctures the closure to create an opening in the nasopharynx. Sequential rubber tubes of increasing size are then placed through the new opening. Once the new opening is dilated to the desired diameter, the rubber tubes are sutured to the nasal columella. The tubes remain for a three- to eight-week healing period to ensure patency of the new posterior nares after removal.

30545

The physician reconstructs the congenitally absent openings between the nasal cavity and the pharynx (throat). Topical vasoconstrictive agents are applied to the nasal mucosa. Local anesthesia is injected in the nasal mucosa and maxilla. A midpalatal incision is made extending posterior to the nasopalatine foramen to the soft palate. The mucoperiosteum is elevated, exposing the hard palate. Using drills and chisels, the physician creates bony windows at the posterior hard palate, removing bony obstructions between the nasal floor and the pharynx. The physician then places rubber tubes along the nasal floor through the new openings into the nasopharynx. The rubber tubes are sutured to the nasal columella. The palatal incision is closed in a single layer. The rubber tubes remain for a three- to eight-week healing period to ensure patency of the new posterior nares after removal.

30560

The physician removes mucosal scarring which blocks the passage of air in the nose. Nasal synechiae are formed when two bleeding mucosal surfaces contact forming scar tissue and eventual fibrosis. These patients are unable to breath through the nose. The physician makes an intranasal approach to the synechia. Topical vasoconstrictive agents are applied

CPT® Lay Descriptions

and local anesthesia is injected in the nasal mucosa. An attempt to minimize intra- and postoperative mucosal bleeding is made. A scalpel is used to excise the mucosal tissue. Mucosal edges are sutured with resorbable sutures. Postoperative gauze packing or splints may be used to absorb hemorrhage until mucosal healing occurs. Long term splinting may be necessary to prevent reformation of the synechiae.

30580

The physician closes an opening between the mouth and the maxillary sinus. The communication is through the maxillary bone and this tract is lined with epithelium. Local anesthesia is injected into the mucosa. The physician uses a scalpel to excise the epithelized tract. An incision is made into the palatal mucosa and a local mucosal flap is developed. The flap is sutured in multiple layers, covering the oromaxillary tract. Careful postoperative instructions are given to limit sinus pressure by not allowing nose blowing which would reopen the tract and impair healing.

30600

The physician closes an opening between the mouth and nasal cavity. The communication is through the maxillary hard palate and the tract is lined with epithelium. Local anesthesia is injected into the mucosa. The physician uses a scalpel to excise the epithelized tract. An incision is made into the palatal mucosa and a local mucosal flap is developed. The flap is sutured in multiple layers, covering the oronasal tract.

30620

The physician removes diseased intranasal mucosa and replaces it with a separately reportable split thickness graft. The surgery is performed on one nasal side. A lateral rhinotomy is made to expose the intranasal mucosa. The diseased mucosal tissue is excised from the septum, nasal floor, and anterior aspect of the inferior turbinate. A split thickness graft is then sutured to the recipient bed, covering the exposed cartilage and submucosal surfaces. Gauze packing and splints are placed in the grafted nasal cavity.

30630

The physician repairs perforations in the nasal septum. Topical vasoconstrictive agents are applied and local anesthesia is injected into the nasal mucosa. The physician creates local mucoperichondrial flaps on either side of the perforation with a scalpel. Each flap is designed only exposing one side of the septal cartilage while retaining mucosal coverage of the septal cartilage on the opposite side. The flaps are then sutured in a single layer to cover the perforation. Larger defects may require the use of separately reportable autogenous grafts (i.e., muscle fascia) in addition to local flaps. Transseptal sutures and septal

stents support the septal mucosa and maintain the new position of the flaps.

30801–30802

The physician uses electrocautery to reduce inflammation or remove excessive mucosa from the nasal turbinates. Cauterization may be superficial in 30801 or may be placed deep into the mucosa in 30802. Topical vasoconstrictive agents are applied to the nasal mucosa. A portion of the mucosa may be excised. Postoperative bleeding is minimal and there is no need for intranasal packing.

30901–30903

To control a less serious nosebleed in 30901, the physician applies electrical or chemical coagulation or packing materials to the anterior (front) section of the nose. Only limited electrical or chemical coagulation is used. To control a less responsive nosebleed in 30903, the physician uses extensive electrical coagulation or extensive packing in the anterior (front) section of the nose.

30905–30906

To control bleeding that is coming from the posterior (back) of the nose (nasopharynx), the physician places extensive packing into the nasal cavity through the back of the throat. Extensive electrical coagulation may be required. The patient may return (e.g., 30906) if the bleeding recurs.

30915

When nasal packing fails to control nasal hemorrhage, the physician administers a local anesthetic and makes an incision along the side of the nose near the inner canthus of the eye to expose the ethmoid arteries. The periosteum (periorbitum) is elevated. The anterior ethmoid artery is identified in the suture line between the frontal and ethmoid bones. The posterior ethmoid artery is located entering the posterior medial wall near the orbital apex. A clip or suture completes the ligation. The incision is repaired with a layered closure.

30920

When nasal packing proves inadequate to stop nasal hemorrhage, the physician makes an incision in the mucous membrane under the upper lip. The incision above the canine tooth on the side of the hemorrhage is commonly referred to as a Caldwell-Luc approach. An opening is created through the bone into the normal maxillary sinus. Through an operating microscope, the physician locates and incises the posterior wall of the maxillary sinus. Through this incision, The maxillary artery is isolated and ligated with sutures or a clip. The posterior maxillary sinus wall is repaired. The incision is repaired with a layered closure.

30930

The physician fractures a portion of the turbinate bone to reposition the nasal turbinate. This procedure is usually performed on the hypertrophied (enlarged) inferior turbinate obstructing the nasal airway. With repositioning, the hypertrophied turbinate should shrink in size, allowing normal air flow. Topical vasoconstrictive drugs are placed on the turbinate to shrink the blood vessels. Commonly, the physician uses a blunt instrument to out-fracture the turbinate. This can be performed with or without incisions. If visualization is necessary, the physician makes a full thickness incision over the anterior-inferior surface of the turbinate and continues it deep to bone. An elevator lifts the mucoperiosteum, exposing the bony turbinate. The physician fractures the bony turbinate with a chisel. Electrocautery may control bleeding. The turbinate mucosa is then closed in a single layer.

31000–31002

The physician irrigates infected sinuses through cannulas. Topical vasoconstrictive agents are applied. The maxillary sinus is entered in 31000 through the natural ostium or opening in the middle meatus of the nasal cavity or through an antral puncture beneath the inferior nasal turbinate. The sphenoid sinus is entered in 31002 through the sphenoethmoidal recess in the superior nasal cavity. A flexible cannula is inserted into these openings and the sinuses are irrigated with saline solutions. These lavages will reduce inflammation and remove purulent (pus) discharge in the sinuses.

31020

The physician surgically creates an opening from the nasal cavity into the maxillary sinus to allow adequate sinus drainage. An antral "window" is made either in the inferior meatus or by enlargement of the natural ostium in the middle meatus. Topical vasoconstrictive agents are applied to the nasal mucosa. Local anesthesia is injected into the nasal mucosa. Then a trocar is used to create an opening into the desired antral window location. The opening is enlarged with biting forceps. The maxillary sinus can then be inspected and irrigated with direct visualization. A temporary irrigation catheter may be placed into the sinus and secured with sutures to the nose. The nasal cavity may be packed for 24 to 48 hours if excessive bleeding occurs during the procedure.

31030–31032

The physician creates several maxillary sinus openings to allow adequate sinus drainage for treatment of irreversible maxillary sinus disease. An intraoral incision is made in the labial mucosa, exposing the canine fossa. The canine fossa is perforated with a trocar and biting forceps increase the opening into the maxillary sinus. Sinus mucosa is removed with curets. A second opening is made from the nasal cavity into the inferior meatus. Topical vasoconstrictive agents are applied to the nasal

mucosa and local anesthesia is injected. Then a trocar perforates an opening into the inferior meatus. The opening is enlarged with biting forceps. An antrochoanal polyp is present in 31032 within both the maxillary sinus and nasal cavity. The mucosa adjacent to the natural ostium is removed with the polyps. The intraoral incision is repaired in a single layer.

31040

The physician opens the pterygopalatine space to access the nerves or blood vessels located within the fossa. An intraoral incision is made in the maxillary buccal vestibule. An opening is then made in the anterior maxillary wall with drills and chisels. Electrocautery of the sinus membrane of the posterior maxillary wall is performed to control bleeding. Chisels then create an opening in the posterior maxillary wall. This bone is carefully removed, providing an entrance into the pterygopalatine space. Fat is abundant and protects the fossa's vidian nerve, the sphenopalatine ganglion, and the branches of the internal maxillary artery. These structures are dissected free from fat and may be ligated and sectioned. The intraoral incision is closed in a single layer.

31050–31051

The physician enters the diseased sphenoid sinus. While open, biopsies may be taken of the sphenoidal masses. The sinus mucosa or mucosal polyps are removed in 31051. Due to its location deep within the skull, the sphenoid sinus surgery is accessed through structures overlying the sinus. Most commonly, an intraoral incision is made in the maxillary labial vestibule. The nasal septal cartilage is dissected from the nasal floor and is detached from the anterior nasal spine. The anterior cartilaginous septum is displaced and dissection continues to the bony nasal septum. The physician uses rongeurs to remove the bony septum, exposing the sphenoid region. The anterior wall of the sphenoid sinus is also removed with rongeurs. The physician then uses an operating microscope to remove sinus contents. The nasal midline is reestablished and the cartilage is reattached to the nasal spine. Transseptal sutures are placed. The intraoral incision is closed in a single layer. The nose is packed and external nasal dressings may be placed.

31070

The physician uses a trephine to access the frontal sinus in 31070. In 31071, frontal sinusotomy is accomplished with an intranasal approach accessed through the agger nasi bone cells for drainage. The frontal sinus opening is obstructed by sinus disease, not allowing the sinus to drain into the nose. A small skin incision is made beneath the unshaven medial eyebrow. The dissection is carried to the frontal bone overlying the frontal sinus. The physician uses a round bur to make an opening into the sinus cavity. Tissue for culture may be taken at this time. The sinus is then irrigated with saline solutions. Two irrigation catheters are placed into the sinus through the bony opening. The wound is closed in layers. The catheters are then sutured to the skin. The exposed catheters are used to irrigate the sinus and are removed once the sinus inflammation subsides and the irrigation fluid starts to exit through the nose.

31075

The physician makes an external skin incision in the medial orbit to access the frontal sinus. The curvilinear incision is made beneath the eyebrow along the medial orbit extending to the superior aspect of the orbit. The dissection continues to the bone. The physician uses a drill and forceps to create an opening into the frontal sinus and, if needed, the ethmoid sinus. Pathologic tissue and diseased tissue membrane is removed with curets. The inferior wall of the sinus can be removed, increasing the drainage from the sinus into the nose. The wound is closed in multiple layers.

31080–31081

The physician removes the frontal sinus mucosa and places material into the sinus cavity to prevent regrowth of the sinus mucosa. To access the frontal sinus through a brow incision in 31080, a full thickness incision is made from the superior aspect of one eyebrow, extending through the nasofrontal junction to the opposite eyebrow. A bicoronal flap may access the frontal sinus in 31081. After the physician exposes the sinus, the frontal bone overlying the frontal sinus is removed with drills, saws, and chisels. The contents of the exposed sinus are removed with curets and burs. The nasofrontal duct is obstructed with an alloplastic or autogenous material (bone). The sinus cavity is then obliterated with autologous fat harvested from the abdomen or buttocks. The removed frontal bone is returned and secured with wires, plates, and/or screws. Incisions are repaired in multiple layers.

31084–31085

The physician removes the frontal sinus mucosa and places material into the sinus cavity to prevent regrowth of the sinus mucosa. In the frontal sinus access, an osteoplastic flap is used. The periosteum of the excised frontal bone is preserved. When the frontal sinus is accessed by brow incision in 31084, an incision is made from the superior aspect of one eyebrow, extending through the nasofrontal junction to the opposite eyebrow. A bicoronal flap accesses the frontal sinus in 31085. Dissection is carried to the periosteal layer. A template is made from a radiograph outlining the frontal sinus. The template is placed over the frontal sinus and the periosteum is excised around the template. The physician removes the frontal bone, with attached periosteum overlying the frontal sinus, using drills, saws, and chisels. The contents of the exposed sinus are removed with curets and burs. The nasofrontal duct is obstructed with an

alloplastic (synthetic) or autogenous material (i.e, bone). The sinus cavity is then obliterated with autologous fat harvested from the abdomen or buttocks. The frontal bone flap is returned and secured with sutures, wires, plates, and/or screws. The incisions are repaired in multiple layers.

31086–31087

The physician enters the frontal sinus to remove pathologic lesions and diseased sinus mucosa. In the frontal sinus access, an osteoplastic flap is used in which the periosteum of the excised frontal bone is preserved. When the frontal sinus is accessed by brow incision in 31086, an incision is made from the superior aspect of one eyebrow, extending through the nasofrontal junction to the opposite eyebrow. A bicoronal flap accesses the frontal sinus in 31087. Dissection is carried to the periosteal layer. A template is made from a radiograph outlining the frontal sinus. The template is placed over the frontal sinus and the periosteum is excised around the template. The physician removes the frontal bone with attached periosteum overlying the frontal sinus using drills, saws, and chisels. The contents of the exposed sinus are removed with curets and burs. No obliteration of the sinus is necessary. The frontal bone flap is returned and secured with sutures, wires, plates, and/or screws. The incisions are repaired in multiple layers.

31090

The physician enters three or more sinuses to remove diseased sinus contents using multiple approaches. Sinus disease may involve any of the maxillary, ethmoid, sphenoid, and/or frontal sinuses. The physician uses multiple approaches to the sinus including, intraoral, intranasal, skin and/or bicoronal incisions. Once the sinus is accessed, the physician removes its contents with curets. Incisions are repaired in both single and multiple layers, depending on the access.

31200

The physician removes diseased tissue from the ethmoid sinuses. The physician accesses the ethmoid sinuses through the nose. Topical vasoconstrictive agents are placed on the nasal mucosa to shrink the blood vessels. Local anesthesia is then injected into the nasal mucosa. The physician retracts the middle turbinate anteriorly, exposing the sinus opening. A small curet may be advanced into the anterior ethmoid cells. The physician uses the curet to remove any diseased tissue of the anterior sinus, and allows the sinus to drain.

31201

The physician removes diseased tissue from the anterior and posterior ethmoid sinuses. The physician accesses the ethmoid sinuses through the nose. Topical vasoconstrictive drugs are placed on the nasal mucosa. Local anesthesia is then injected into the nasal mucosa. The physician retracts the middle turbinate anteriorly, exposing the sinus opening. A small curet is used to remove the uncinate process in the bone. The physician may advance the curet into the anterior ethmoid cells. The physician then uses blunt forceps to open posterior bony cells. Curets remove diseased tissue and allow postoperative drainage of both the anterior and posterior ethmoid sinuses.

31205

The physician removes diseased tissue of the ethmoid sinuses. A curvilinear incision is made between the nasal dorsum and the medial canthus of the eye. Dissection is carried to the medial orbital bone. A bony window is made through the lamina papyracea bone, exposing the lateral ethmoid sinus. The physician then removes all diseased tissue. The nasal cavity is penetrated through the medial ethmoid region. Nasal gauze packing is placed through the extranasal incision. The external skin incision is repaired with a layered closure.

31225

The physician removes a portion of or all of the diseased maxilla. Incisions may be intraoral or may include skin incisions such as the Weber-Ferguson approach. Dissection is continued to expose and isolate the planned bony excision. The physician uses drills, saws, and chisels to fracture the maxilla from the midface. The fractured maxilla and adjacent tissue is then loosened and removed to "free margins" as determined with intraoperative tissue specimens sent to the pathologist for immediate microscopic examination. All sinus mucosa is removed. Exposed bone may be covered with a separately reportable split thickness skin graft. A splint may be placed to obturate (block) the mouth from the surgical area. All skin incisions are repaired with a layered closure.

31230

The physician removes the maxilla, eye, and orbital soft tissue. Incisions may be intraoral or may include skin incisions such as a modified Weber-Ferguson incision that includes incision in the upper eyelid. Dissection is continued to expose and isolate the planned bony excision. The physician uses drills, saws, and chisels to fracture the maxilla from the midface. The fractured maxilla and adjacent tissue is then loosened and removed to "free margins" as determined with intraoperative tissue specimens sent to the pathologist for immediate microscopic examination. The upper eyelid incision is dissected to the periosteum of the superior orbit. The maxilla is retracted downward, so the physician can visualize the optic nerve and blood vessels. The optic nerve is severed and the vessels are ligated. The maxilla, adjacent soft tissue, and orbital contents are removed in one specimen. All sinus mucosa is removed. Exposed bone is covered with a separately reportable split thickness skin graft. A splint may be placed to

obturate (block) the mouth from the surgical area. All skin incisions are repaired with a layered closure.

31231

The physician uses an endoscope for a diagnostic evaluation of the nose. An endoscope has a rigid fiberoptic telescope that allows the physician both increased visualization and magnification of internal anatomy. Topical vasoconstrictive agents are applied to the nasal mucosa and nerve blocks with local anesthesia are performed. The endoscope is placed into the nose and a thorough inspection of internal nasal structures is accomplished. No surgical procedure is performed.

31233

The physician uses an endoscope for a diagnostic evaluation of the nose and the maxillary sinus. An endoscope has a rigid fiberoptic telescope that allows the physician both increased visualization and magnification of internal anatomy. Topical vasoconstrictive agents are applied to the nasal mucosa and nerve blocks with local anesthesia are performed. The endoscope is placed into the nose and a thorough inspection of the internal nasal structures is accomplished. Then a trocar puncture is made either directly into the inferior meatus area of the nose or after a mucosal incision into the canine fossa of the maxilla. The endoscope is then placed into the maxillary sinus for evaluation. The intraoral mucosa may be closed in a single layer. The nasal puncture wound does not require closure. No other procedure is performed on the sinus at this time.

31235

The physician uses an endoscope for a diagnostic evaluation of the nose and the sphenoid sinus. An endoscope has a rigid fiberoptic telescope that allows the physician both increased visualization and magnification of internal anatomy. Topical vasoconstrictive agents are applied to the nasal mucosa and nerve blocks with local anesthesia are performed. The endoscope is placed into the nose and a thorough inspection of the internal nasal structures is accomplished. Then access to the sphenoid sinus is accomplished by a trocar puncture made directly into the sphenoid sinus after negotiation through the ethmoids or by cannulation of the sphenoid drainage system that enters the sphenoethmoidal recess. The endoscope is then placed into the sphenoid sinus for evaluation. The sphenoidal puncture wound does not require closure. No other procedure is performed on the sinus at this time.

31237

The physician uses an endoscope for a diagnostic evaluation of the nose. An endoscope has a rigid fiberoptic telescope that allows the physician both increased visualization and magnification of internal anatomy. Topical vasoconstrictive agents are applied to the nasal mucosa and nerve blocks with local anesthesia are performed. The endoscope is placed into the nose and a thorough inspection of the internal nasal structures is accomplished. Any identified lesions can be removed by intranasal instruments placed parallel to the endoscope. Scalpels, forceps, snares, and other instruments are used to remove diseased mucosa or lesions from the internal nose. The nose may be packed if excessive bleeding occurs.

31238

The physician uses an endoscope for a diagnostic evaluation of the bleeding nose. An endoscope has a rigid fiberoptic telescope that allows the physician both increased visualization and magnification of internal anatomy. Topical vasoconstrictive agents are applied to the nasal mucosa and nerve blocks with local anesthesia are performed. The endoscope is placed into the nose and a thorough inspection of the internal nasal structures is accomplished. Any bleeding sources are identified. Electrocautery instruments or lasers are placed parallel to the endoscope and are used to stop internal nasal bleeding.

31239

The physician uses an endoscope to visually and surgically assist during a dacryocystorhinostomy. When the lacrimal system is obstructed and excessive tearing is a problem for the patient, a dacryocystorhinostomy is performed. In this procedure, the new lacrimal drainage system is surgically created from the lower eyelid into the nose. An endoscope allows the physician both increased visualization and magnification of the internal anatomy. Topical vasoconstrictive agents are applied to the nasal mucosa and nerve blocks with local anesthesia are performed. The endoscope is placed into the nose. The nasolacrimal duct and other lacrimal structures are visualized. Endoscopy may aid in location of structures or enhance intranasal procedures like osteotomies and internal splinting with Teflon tubes.

31240

The physician uses an endoscope for an intranasal evaluation and surgical resection of a concha bullosa, an intranasal cyst has caused distention (stretching or swelling) of the turbinate bone. This swelling is called a concha bullosa. An endoscope has a rigid fiberoptic telescope that allow the physician both increased visualization and magnification of internal anatomy. Topical vasoconstrictive agents are applied to the nasal mucosa and nerve blocks with local anesthesia are performed. The endoscope is placed into the nose and thorough inspection of internal nasal structures is accomplished. A scalpel or biting forceps are introduced parallel to the endoscope and are used to excise the concha bullosa. Electrocautery may be used for hemostasis. The nasal cavity may be packed with Telfa or gauze for 24 to 48 hours.

31254–31255

The physician uses an endoscope for surgical resection of the anterior or posterior ethmoidectomy. Disease of the anterior ethmoid sinus may block maxillary sinus drainage. An endoscope allows both increased visualization and magnification of internal anatomy. Topical vasoconstrictive agents are applied to the nasal mucosa and nerve blocks with local anesthesia are performed. The endoscope is placed into the nose and a thorough inspection of internal nasal structures is accomplished. A scalpel or biting forcep is introduced parallel to the endoscope and is used to remove diseased tissues. Polyps may be excised. Electrocautery may be used for hemostasis. The nasal cavity may be packed with Telfa or gauze for 24 to 48 hours. Report 31255 if a total ethmoidectomy is performed.

31256–31267

The physician uses an endoscope for surgical resection of the maxillary sinus. Topical vasoconstrictive agents are applied to the nasal mucosa and nerve blocks with local anesthesia are performed. The endoscope is placed into the nose and a thorough inspection of internal nasal structures is accomplished. A scalpel or biting forcep is introduced parallel to the endoscope and is used to remove diseased tissues. Polyps may be excised. An antrostomy is performed in 31256, creating an opening for drainage from the maxillary sinus. Additionally, in 31267, the maxillary sinus may be opened and the mucosa removed. In either case, electrocautery may be used for hemostasis. The nasal cavity may be packed with Telfa or gauze for 24 to 48 hours

31276

The physician uses an endoscope for surgical resection of the frontal sinus. Topical vasoconstrictive agents are applied to the nasal mucosa and nerve blocks with local anesthesia are performed. The endoscope is placed into the nose and a thorough inspection of the internal nasal structures is accomplished. A scalpel or biting forceps is introduced parallel to the endoscope and is used to remove diseased tissues from the frontal sinus. Polyps are removed. An antrostomy is sometimes performed, creating an opening for drainage from the maxillary sinus. Electrocautery may be used for hemostasis. The nasal cavity may be packed with Telfa or gauze for 24 to 48 hours.

31287–31288

The physician uses an endoscope for surgical access of the sphenoid sinus. The sphenoid can be explored with direct access or through the posterior ethmoid sinus. The isolated access to the sphenoid sinus is through dilation of the sphenoid ostium. The middle turbinate may be fractured or partially removed for access. The ostium is cannulated and dilated. The physician uses forceps or a sphenoid punch to open the sinus cavity. Additionally, diseased mucosa or tissue is removed in 31288. The nose may be packed if excessive bleeding occurs.

31290–31291

The physician uses an endoscope for surgical access and repair of cerebrospinal fluid leaks in ethmoid and sphenoid sinuses. Topical vasoconstrictive agents and local anesthesia are applied to the nasal mucosa. The endoscope is placed into the nose. The middle turbinate may be fractured to provide access. In 31290, the ethmoid sinus is entered through the ethmoid bulla. In 31291, the sphenoid sinus can be explored through the posterior ethmoid sinus or through direct access. If accessed through the ethmoid sinus, the sphenoid ostium is cannulated and dilated. The physician uses forceps or a sphenoid punch to open the sinus cavity. Once the sinus cavity is entered, the cerebrospinal fluid leak is isolated. Local mucosal or muscle flaps may be developed to plug the defect. Autologous fat, muscle or fascia lata may also be used to seal the leak.

31292–31293

The physician uses an endoscope for surgical access to decompress the orbit. Decompression may occur through one orbital wall in 31292 or through two orbital walls in 31293. The inferior orbital wall is approached through a canine fossa puncture into the maxillary sinus. The inferior orbital wall is the roof of the maxillary sinus. Forceps remove orbital bone while preserving the orbital periosteum. This allows orbital contents to herniate into the maxillary sinus. The medial orbital wall can be approached through the ethmoid sinuses. The ethmoids are may be opened through the maxillary sinus or by a separate intranasal ethmoid approach. The medial wall of the orbit is the lateral wall of the ethmoids. Bone is carefully removed from this region, also allowing orbital contents to herniate into the ethmoid regions. The nose may be packed if excessive bleeding occurs.

31294

The physician uses an endoscope for surgical access to decompress the optic nerve in the posterior orbit. The optic nerve sends transmissions that provide the sense of sight. This nerve enters the posterior cone through the optic foramen (orbital apex). The orbital apex may be approached through the sphenoid sinus. The sphenoid sinus may be explored through the posterior ethmoid sinus or directly. The middle turbinate may be fractured or partially removed to provide access. Isolated access to the sinus is through cannulation and dilation of the sphenoid ostium. The physician uses a forcep or a sphenoid punch to gain entry into the sinus cavity. Bone is carefully removed from the lateral portion of the sinus, decompressing the optic nerve. The nose may be packed if excessive bleeding occurs.

31300

A laryngocele is an air-filled dilation of the laryngeal ventricle that connects with the laryngeal cavity. The physician first performs a tracheostomy on the patient. Using a horizontal neck incision, the physician exposes the larynx and performs a thyrotomy and laryngofissure, opening the larynx at the midline of the thyroid cartilage. The laryngocele or tumor is isolated, dissected, and excised. A cordectomy, the excision of all or part of the vocal cord, may also be performed. The incision is repaired in sutured layers.

31320

The physician first performs a tracheostomy on the patient. Using a horizontal neck incision, the physician exposes the larynx and performs a thyrotomy and laryngofissure, opening the larynx at the midline of the thyroid cartilage. The larynx is explored, but no other procedure is performed. The incision is repaired in sutured layers.

31360–31365

The physician removes the larynx in 31360, and removes the larynx and surrounding tissues in 31365. First, a tracheostomy is performed. Then the physician makes a low collar or midline cervical incision for 31360 or a horizontal neck incision for 31365. The strap muscles of the neck and thyroid isthmus are cut. Part or all of the hyoid bone is removed. The trachea and inferior pharangeal constrictor muscles are transected. By cutting the hypopharyngeal walls, the larynx is freed and removed. Resected tissues may include part of the esophagus and base of the tongue for 31360. In 31365, an extensive dissection may include removal of the sternocleidomastoid muscle, the submandibular salivary gland, the internal jugular vein and the lymph nodes of the lateral neck, under the chin and mandible, and the supraclavicular nodes. Any reconstruction performed at this time is separately reported. When either excision is completed, the incision is closed in sutured layers.

31367–31368

The surgeon removes the larynx in 31367, and the larynx and surrounding tissues in 31368. First, a tracheostomy is performed. Then, the physician approaches the larynx through the thyroid cartilage for 31367 or a horizontal neck incision for 31368. The epiglottis, false vocal cords, mucosal lining of the ventricles, part or all of the hyoid bone, and superior part of the laryngeal cartilage are removed in 31367. In 31368, an extensive dissection may include removal of the sternocleidomastoid muscle, the submandibular salivary gland, the internal jugular vein and the lymph nodes of the lateral neck, under the chin and mandible, and the supraclavicular nodes. Any reconstruction performed at this time is separately reported. When either excision is completed, the operative incision is closed in sutured layers.

31370–31382

The physician removes a portion of the larynx. First, a tracheostomy is performed. The physician makes a low collar or midline cervical incision. The strap muscles of the neck are retracted and a midline incision of the perichrondrium is made, exposing the larynx. The laryngeal cartilage is incised. In 31370, a horizontal incision is made above or below the affected area, and the diseased tissue is excised. The airway is reconstructed above to the pharnyx or below to the trachea. In 31375, the vocal cord and adjacent cartilage is resected. In 31380, incision are a made into both halves of the thyroid cartilage, and the anterior part of the thyroid cartilage and the affected portions of both vocal cords are excised. In 31382, the area of resection also includes part or all of the arytenoid. In each instance, the pharnyx is closed by suturing the perichondrium and strap muscles. The operative incision is closed in sutured layers.

31390

The physician removes the larynx and pharynx. First, a tracheostomy is performed. Then, the physician approaches the pharynx and larynx through a horizontal neck incision. The epiglottis, false vocal cords, mucosal lining of the ventricles, part or all of the hyoid bone, pharynx, and superior part of the laryngeal cartilage are removed. Extensive dissection may include removal of the sternocleidomastoid muscle, the submandibular salivary gland, the internal jugular vein and the lymph nodes of the lateral neck, under the chin and mandible, and the supraclavicular nodes. When either excision is completed, the operative incision is closed in sutured layers.

31395

The physician removes the larynx and pharynx and performs reconstruction with available tissues. First, a tracheostomy is performed. Then the physician approaches the pharynx and larynx through a horizontal neck incision. The epiglottis, false vocal cords, mucosal lining of the ventricles, part or all of the hyoid bone, pharynx, and superior part of the laryngeal cartilage are removed. Extensive dissection may include removal of the sternocleidomastoid muscle, the submandibular salivary gland, the internal jugular vein and the lymph nodes of the lateral neck, under the chin and mandible, and the supraclavicular nodes. Reconstruction of the pharyngeal area can be achieved in a number of ways; one of the most common is the myocutaneous flap reconstruction using the pectoralis major muscle and its overlying skin. The flap is rotated and inserted through a previously created tunnel between the clavicle and overlying skin. The flap is then sutured into place to reconstruct the pharynx. The operative incision is closed in sutured layers.

31400

The physician secures the arytenoid process. First, a tracheostomy is performed. Then, the physician exposes and transects the inferior pharyngeal constrictor muscle and continues dissection to reach the arytenoid cartilage. In an arytenoidectomy, the arytenoid cartilage is tacked against the thyroid ala to lateralize the arytenoid. In an Arytenoidectomy, the arytenoid cartilage is resected and removed. The operative incision is closed with layered sutures.

31420

The physician excises all or part of the epiglottis, the cartilage that protects the entrance to the larynx. The physician uses an intra-oral approach to access and remove the entire epiglottis or lesions involving the tip of the epiglottis. If the affected area is minor, no sutures are needed. If the area involve most or all of the epiglottis, the remaining tissues are sutured together.

31500

The physician places an endotracheal tube to provide air passage in emergency situations. The patient is ventilated with a mask and bag and positioned by extending the neck anteriorly and the head posteriorly. The physician places the laryngoscope into the patient's mouth and advances the blade toward the epiglottis until the vocal cords are visible. An endotracheal tube is then inserted between the vocal cords and advanced to the proper position. The cuff of the endotracheal tube is inflated.

31502

The physician removes the indwelling tracheotomy tube and replaces it with a new one. The procedure is performed before healing sufficient to form a fistula tract has taken place; usually a few days within placement of the original tube.

31505

The physician administers a topical anesthetic to the oral cavity, pharynx, and larynx and inserts the laryngoscope into the patient's mouth. The interior of the larynx is examined. In 31535, a lesion is biopsied with a Sharp basket or cup forceps. Sometimes staining with toluidine blue is used to delineate the biopsy site. In 31536, the physician uses an operating microscope to isolate and biopsy the lesions. This is usually done for smaller lesions.

31510

After applying topical anesthesia to the oral cavity and pharynx, the physician uses a laryngeal mirror to examine the patient's larynx, hypopharynx, and tongue. Suspect tissue may be stained with toluidine blue to delineate the biopsy site. The physician uses a sharp basket or cup forceps to obtain the biopsy specimen. Usually, no closure is required.

31511–31512

The physician removes a foreign body or lesion from the larynx. After applying topical anesthesia to the oral cavity and pharynx, the physician uses a laryngeal mirror to examine the patient's larynx, hypopharynx, and tongue. In 31511, the foreign body is grasped with a laryngeal forceps and withdrawn. In 31512, the lesion is identified and excised. Closure is seldom required for either procedure.

31513

After applying topical anesthesia to the oral cavity and pharynx, the physician examines the interior of the patient's larynx using a laryngoscope. The physician injects the vocal cord with glycerin, sesame oil, Gelfoam, or Teflon paste using a retractable needle fed through the laryngoscope. No other procedure is performed.

31515

The physician uses an aspirator to remove excess saliva or semi-solid foreign material from the larynx. After applying topical anesthesia to the oral cavity and pharynx, the physician inserts the laryngoscope through the patient's mouth. An aspirator is fed through the laryngoscope and the larynx is cleared of saliva and semi-solid foreign material. If a tracheoscopy is performed, a bronchoscope is inserted through the laryngoscope for microscopic visualization of the trachea and bronchi. No other procedure is performed.

31520–31525

The physician places a rigid laryngoscope to examine the patient's larynx. The physician administers a topical anesthetic to the oral cavity, pharynx, and larynx and inserts the laryngoscope through the patient's mouth. The interior of the larynx of a newborn is examined in 31520 and of a patient other than a newborn in 31525. If a tracheoscopy is performed, a bronchoscope is inserted through the laryngoscope for visualization of the trachea and bronchi. No other procedure is performed at this time.

31526

The physician uses an operating microscope to examine the interior of the larynx. After administering a topical anesthetic to the oral cavity, pharynx, and larynx, the physician inserts the laryngoscope into the patient's mouth and examines the larynx. If a tracheoscopy is performed, a bronchoscope is inserted through the laryngoscope for microscopic visualization of the trachea and bronchi. No other procedure is performed at this time.

31527

The physician administers a topical anesthetic to the oral cavity, pharynx, and larynx and inserts the laryngoscope through the patient's mouth. The interior of the larynx is examined. An obturator is an object that is used to close an opening. A wire is threaded through a cannulated needle which has been placed into the larynx. The end of the wire is grasped with forceps and drawn out through the laryngoscope. The wire is then drawn through the obturator and threaded through another needle in the supraglottic space. The external ends of the wire are then knotted over a stent.

31528–31529

The physician dilates the tracheobronchial stenosis. The physician administers a topical or general anesthetic and inserts the laryngoscope into the patient's mouth. The interior of the larynx is examined. The physician manipulates the laryngocope to dilate areas of the tracheobronchial stenosis. Use 31529 to report subsequent dilations. If a tracheoscopy is performed, a bronchoscope is inserted through the laryngoscope for visualization of the trachea and bronchi.

31530–31531

The physician administers a topical anesthetic to the oral cavity, pharynx, and larynx and inserts the laryngoscope into the patient's mouth. The interior of the larynx is examined. In 31530, the foreign body is located, grasped with biopsy forceps and withdrawn. In 31531, the physician additionally uses a microscope to locate and remove the foreign body.

31535–31536

The physician administers a topical anesthetic to the oral cavity, pharynx, and larynx and inserts the laryngoscope into the patient's mouth. The interior of the larynx is examined. In 31535, a lesion is biopsied with a sharp basket or cup forceps. Sometimes staining with toluidine blue is used to delineate the biopsy site. In 31536, the physician uses an operating microscope to isolate and biopsy the lesions. This is usually done for smaller lesions.

31540–31541

The physician removes a tumor of the vocal cords or epiglottis. The physician administers a topical anesthetic to the oral cavity, pharynx, and larynx and inserts the laryngoscope into the patient's mouth. The interior of the larynx is examined and the laryngeal tumor is isolated and dissected. The tumor and a portion of the underlying vocal cord are removed using stripping forceps. The procedure is performed with a direct laryngoscope in 31540. Additionally, an operating microscope is used in 31541. An operating microscope is usually used for smaller lesions.

31560–31561

The physician removes the arytenoid cartilage. The arytenoid cartilage helps the vocal cords function. First, a tracheostomy is performed. The physician administers a topical anesthetic to the oral cavity, pharynx, and larynx and inserts the laryngoscope into the patient's mouth. The interior of the larynx is examined and the arytenoid cartilage is exposed by excising the overlying mucosa. The arytenoid is then dissected from its muscular attachments and removed. The procedure is performed with a direct laryngoscope in 31560. Additionally, an operating microscope is used in 31561.

31570–31571

The physician injects the vocal cords with therapeutic serum. The physician administers a topical anesthetic to the oral cavity, pharynx, and larynx and inserts the laryngoscope into the patient's mouth. The interior of the larynx is examined and the physician injects the vocal cord at one to three sites with glycerin, sesame oil, Gelfoam, or Teflon paste. No other procedure is performed. The procedure is performed with a direct laryngoscope in 31570. Additionally, an operating microscope is used in 31571.

31575–31576

The physician administers a topical anesthetic to the oral cavity, pharynx, and larynx and uses a nasal or oral approach to insert a flexible fiberoptic laryngoscope. The interior of the larynx is examined in 31575. Additionally, in 31576, a lesion is biopsied with a sharp basket or cup forceps. Sometimes staining with toluidine blue is used to delineate the biopsy site.

31577–31578

The physician removes a foreign body from the larynx. The physician administers a topical anesthetic to the oral cavity, pharynx, and larynx and uses a nasal or intraoral approach to insert a flexible fiberoptic laryngoscope. The interior of the larynx is examined in 31577, the foreign body is located, grasped with biopsy forceps and withdrawn. In 31578, the physician locates and excises the lesion.

31579

The physician examines the larynx and vocal cord function. The patient is prepared with a nasal spray containing topical decongestant and anesthetic. The physician passes a flexible laryngoscope through the patient's nose into the pharynx and larynx, which are examined. The stroboscope responds to the fundamental frequency of the vibrating vocal cords, allowing the physician to see vocal cord function. No other procedure is performed.

31580–31582

The physician excises a laryngeal web, a congenital malformation of the larynx. The physician first performs a tracheostomy on the patient. Using a horizontal neck incision, the physician exposes the laryngeal web. In 31580, the web lies between the vocal cords. The physician excises the web and inserts a laryngeal keel, or spacer, between the vocal cords. The laryngotomy incision is closed. During a separate operative session after the larynx has had time to heal, the physician reenters the operative site through the

same incision and removes the keel. The incision is repaired in sutured layers. In 31582, the stenosis, or web, involves the arytenoid cartilages. The physician excises the affected area in the posterior glottis. A rib graft is obtained and sewn to provide posterior stability to the larynx and adjacent trachea. The operative incision is closed in sutured layers.

31584

The physician reduces a fractured larynx to its anatomical position. The physician first performs a low tracheostomy on the patient to secure the airway and prevent extravasation of air into the surrounding tissues. Using a horizontal neck incision, the physician exposes the thyroid cartilage and repairs the mucosal defects. The thyroid cartilage is stabilized with wire stents. The incision is repaired in sutured layers.

31585–31586

The physician examines the fractured larynx with a operating laryngoscope. If no mucosal tears are identified, the physician palpates the exterior laryngeal area while directly visualizing the glottic area. The larynx may be protected with a rigid surface cast. The cast is secured with a circumferential dressing. In 31585, no manipulation is needed to correct laryngeal damage. In 31586, the physician externally manipulates the thyroid cartilage while internally visualizing the laryngeal mucosa.

31587–31588

The physician restores a cricoid split. (A cricoid split is a break in the circular cartilage of the larynx.) The physician first performs a low tracheostomy on the patient. Using a horizontal neck incision, the physician exposes the cricoid split and restores it to its normal anatomical position (reduction). The cartilage is affixed with wire. At stent may be placed to maintain cricotracheal continuity. The incision is repaired in sutured layers. Report 31588 for laryngoplasty, not otherwise specified.

31590

The physician restores innervation to the larynx using a neuromuscular pedicle (flap). The physician makes a horizontal neck incision and dissects the strap muscles of the anterior neck. The descending branch of the hypoglossal nerve is located. The nerve and the muscle are rotated to the larynx and secured with sutures. The incision is closed in sutured layers.

31595

The physician severs the laryngeal nerve. The recurrent laryngeal nerve controls the action of the vocal cords. The physician makes a vertical incision and retracts the strap muscles and dissects the tissue until the nerve is exposed and identified. The physician then severs the recurrent laryngeal nerve prior to its point of branching. The incision is repaired in sutured layers.

31600–31610

The physician creates a tracheostomy. The physician makes a horizontal neck incision and dissects the muscles to expose the trachea. The thyroid isthmus is cut if necessary. The trachea is incised and an airway is inserted. After bleeding is controlled, a stoma is created by suturing the skin to the tissue layers. In 31600, the tracheostomy is a planned procedure. In 31601 it is performed on patients aged under two years. In 31603, it is performed under emergency conditions, trantracheal. In 31605, it is performed under emergency conditions, cricothyroid membrane. In 31610, skin flaps are used to create a more permanent stoma.

31611

The physician constructs a tracheal esophageal fistula for vocalization. The physician makes a horizontal neck incision and dissects the tissues between the tracheostoma and the esophagus. The esophagus is incised and a laryngeal speech prosthesis is inserted between the esophagus and the trachea, creating a fistula. The prosthesis, called a voice button or a Blom-Singer prosthesis, is a one-way valve enabling the patient to phonate. The physician closes the incision around the prosthesis.

31612

The physician punctures the trachea with a needle to aspirate secretions or inject a therapeutic agent. The physician palpates the site and inserts a hollow point needle. Secretions are aspirated or a therapeutic agent is injected. The needle is removed.

31613–31614

The physician revises a tracheal stoma. The physician incises the stoma area and resects redundant scar tissue or a poorly healing wound. The skin is re-anastomosed and sewn to the stoma in sutured layers. Report 31613 for performance of a simple revision and 31614 if a complex procedure is performed with flap rotation.

31615

The physician views the airway using a bronchoscope placed through an existing tracheostomy. The physician examines the conducting airways. The bronchoscope is removed.

31622–31624

The physician views the airway using a fiberoptic or rigid bronchoscope that is introduced through the nasal or oral cavity. The airway is anesthetized. The bronchoscope is inserted and advanced through the nasal or oral cavity, past the larynx to the bronchus. In 31622, the bronchus is inspected and cell washings may be obtained. In 31623, the bronchoscope is inserted down into the lungs to sample lung tissue with brushings. In 31624, the bronchoscopy includes bronchial alveolar lavage to sample lung tissue by irrigating with saline followed by suctioning the fluid. The bronchoscope is removed.

31625–31629

The physician views the airway using a fiberoptic or rigid bronchoscope that is introduced through the nasal or oral cavity. The airway is anesthetized. The bronchoscope is inserted. It is advanced through the larynx to the bronchus. In 31625, a sample of tissue is removed (biopsy) for study. In 31628 and 31629 the physician uses the views obtained through the bronchoscope to identify abnormal structures in the lung to be biopsied. Fluoroscopy (x-ray) may be used to assist with navigation of the bronchoscope tip to the abnormal tissue. In 31628, the physician passes special closed biopsy forceps through a channel in the bronchoscope, through the bronchial wall to obtain a tissue sample. In 31629, a needle is passed through a channel in the bronchoscope, through the bronchial wall to obtain an aspiration biopsy. The physician leaves the bronchoscope wedged in the bronchus to asses for and limit bleeding. The bronchoscope is removed.

31630

The physician views the airway using a bronchoscope introduced through the nasal or oral cavity, using local anesthesia of the patient's airway. The physician uses the views obtained through the bronchoscope to identify any narrowing or fracture of the trachea or bronchus. The physician introduces a wire through the narrowed airway. The bronchoscope is removed. A series of dilators or stents are passed over the wire to open the airway until sufficient dilation and/or reduction of the fracture is accomplished. When the stent is left in place, see code 31631.

31631

The physician views the airway using a bronchoscope introduced through the nasal or oral cavity, using local anesthesia of the patient's airway. The physician uses the views obtained through the bronchoscope to identify any narrowing or fracture of the trachea. The physician introduces a wire into the narrowed trachea. The bronchoscope is removed. A series of dilators or stents are passed over the wire to open the airway until sufficient dilation and/or reduction of the fracture is accomplished. A stent is left in place to maintain patency.

31635

The physician views the airway using a bronchoscope introduced through the nasal or oral cavity, using local anesthesia of the patient's airway. The physician uses the views obtained through the bronchoscope to locate the foreign body within the airway. The physician passes a snare, basket, or biopsy forceps through a channel in the bronchoscope to grasp the foreign body. The bronchoscope and foreign body are removed.

CPT® Lay Descriptions

31640

The physician views the airway using a bronchoscope introduced through the nasal or oral cavity, using local anesthesia of the patient's airway. The physician uses the views obtained through the bronchoscope to identify the tumor from within the airway. The physician may use fluoroscopy (x-ray) to assist with navigation of the bronchoscope tip to the abnormal tissue. The physician passes special forceps through channels in the bronchoscope to grasp and excise the tumor. The bronchoscope is removed.

31641

The physician views the airway, using a bronchoscope introduced through the nasal or oral cavity, using local anesthesia of the patient's airway. The physician uses the views obtained through the bronchoscope to identify the tumor and/or area of stenosis from within the airway. The physician may use separately reportable fluoroscopy (x-ray) to assist with navigation of the bronchoscope tip to the abnormal tissue. The physician passes a laser or freezing (cryo) probe through a channel in the bronchoscope to destroy the tumor or any areas of stenosis. The bronchoscope is removed.

31643

The physician views the airway using a bronchoscope with a fiberoptic camera and operating device. The airway is anesthetized and the bronchoscope is introduced through the nasal or oral cavity and advanced through the bronchus. A catheter is inserted through the bronchoscope into a lung cavity and is placed at the site where, in a separately reportable procedure, intracavitary radioelements will be applied.

31645–31646

The physician views the airway using a bronchoscope introduced through the nasal or oral cavity, using local anesthesia of the patient's airway. The physician uses the views obtained through the bronchoscope to identify the closest approach to the fluid collection or abscess from within the airway. The physician may use fluoroscopy (x-ray) to assist with navigation of the bronchoscope tip to the fluid collection or abscess. The physician passes a special needle through a channel in the bronchoscope into the fluid collection and aspirates fluid through the needle. The bronchoscope is removed. Code 31645 should be used for initial treatment only. Code 31646 should be used for any subsequent aspiration procedure(s).

31656

The physician views the airway using a bronchoscope introduced through the nasal or oral cavity, using local anesthesia of the patient's airway. The physician uses the views obtained through the bronchoscope to identify the bronchial segment to be studied. The physician may use fluoroscopy (x-ray) to assist with navigation of the bronchoscope tip. The physician passes a needle or catheter through a channel in the

bronchoscope into the bronchial segment and injects the contrast material for bronchography. The bronchoscope is removed.

31700

The physician places a transglottic catheter. The physician inserts a needle through the patient's glottis to establish a passageway. The glottis is incised, the catheter is placed, and secured with sutures.

31708

The patient inhales radiopaque gas in preparation for separately reportable laryngography or bronchography. The physician provides the patient with an inhaler holding a mixture of air and radiopaque gas. The patient inhales the gas and retains breath. More inhalant is pumped in for each exposure.

31710

The physician places an oral or nasal catheter that is threaded to the larynx. The catheter may be used to instill contrast material for a separately reportable bronchography.

31715

The physician injects contrast material for a bronchography into the trachea, just below the voice box. The physician palpates the laryngeal structures and identifies the tracheal rings. The physician inserts a needle into the trachea. After verifying placement, the physician injects the contrast material for a bronchography (reported separately).

31717

The physician catheterizes the trachea to obtain a bronchial brush biopsy. The physician inserts a needle through the cricoid cartilage or the trachea. A catheter is passed over the needle and a brush is placed through the catheter to obtain bronchial tissue. A bronchoscope may be used to guide the brush. The brush is withdrawn through the catheter and both are removed. The incision may be closed with sutures.

31720–31725

The physician aspirates sputum from the lungs using a nasal tracheal catheter. The physician passes a suction catheter through the nose into the trachea. Saline may be used to liquify secretions. The secretions are removed with suction and the catheter is removed. Report 31725 if a tracheobronchial approach with fiberscope is used at bedside.

31730

The physician introduces a needle wire dilator/stent into the trachea to relieve a subglottic stenosis. The physician places a needle through the cricoid membrane or trachea. A wire is passed through the needle and the needle is removed. A series of dilators or stents are passed over the wire to open the trachea. When sufficient dilation is gained, a stent or indwelling tube for oxygen therapy is left in place to maintain patency.

31750

The physician performs an anterior cervical incision and dissects surrounding tissues and muscles to expose the trachea. An airway is inserted and the trachea is incised. Surgical repair of the trachea is undertaken. End-to-end anastomosis of the trachea may be performed. For satisfactory reconstruction, it may be necessary for the physician to surgically repair the trachea using splints constructed from rib or costal cartilage to patch the length of the trachea. Once repair is achieved, the airway is removed and the incisions are closed.

31755

The physician performs an anterior cervical incision and dissects surrounding tissues and muscles to expose the trachea and pharynx. An airway may be inserted and the trachea and pharynx are incised. The physician incises the trachea and pharynx in such a way as to create an opening from the trachea to the pharynx. The physician may implant a device like the Singer-Blom prosthesis between the trachea and pharynx. The purpose of the prosthesis is to produce speech in a previously laryngectomized patient. Once repair is achieved, the airway, if inserted, is removed and the incisions are closed.

31760

The physician makes an incision in the thorax and approaches the trachea by opening the rib cage. An airway is inserted and the trachea is incised. Surgical repair of the trachea is undertaken. End-to-end anastomosis of the trachea may be performed. For satisfactory reconstruction, it may be necessary for the physician to surgically repair the trachea using splints constructed from rib or costal cartilage to patch the length of the trachea. Once repair is achieved, the airway is removed and the incisions are closed.

31766

The physician reconstructs the carina. The carina is the junction of the trachea and the bronchi. The physician uses a midline sternotomy or a lateral thoracotomy approach to access the carina. The carina is located and repaired primarily if possible. More extensive damage may be repaired with a Silastic stent or an autograft. A chest tube is inserted, and the wound is closed in sutured layers.

31770–31775

The physician repairs a bronchus. The physician makes a lateral thoracotomy incision to access the bronchus. An autograft or silastic stent may be used to repair the bronchus in 31770. A chest tube is inserted and the wound is closed in sutured layers. Report 31775 if an excision stenosis and anastomosis are performed with this procedure.

31780

The physician excises a tracheal stenosis and re-anastomoses the trachea. The physician makes a horizontal neck incision to access the stenosis. The trachea is incised and the stenosis is resected. The proximal and distal portions of the trachea are brought together and closed with sutures. The wound is closed in sutured layers.

31781

The physician excises a tracheal stenosis and re-anastomoses the trachea. The physician makes a cervicothoracic incision to access the stenosis. The trachea is incised and the stenosis is resected. The proximal and distal portions of the trachea are brought together and closed with sutures. The wound is closed in sutured layers.

31785

The physician excises a tracheal tumor or carcinoma. The physician makes a horizontal neck incision to access the mass. The trachea is incised and the mass is resected. If necessary, the proximal and distal portions of the trachea are brought together and closed with sutures. The wound is closed in sutured layers.

31786

The physician excises a tracheal tumor or carcinoma. The physician makes a thoracic approach to access the mass. The trachea is incised and the mass is resected. If necessary, the proximal and distal portions of the trachea are brought together and closed with sutures. The wound is closed in sutured layers.

31800–31805

The physician closes a wound or injury of the cervical trachea in 31800 or the intrathoracic trachea in 31805. The physician debrides the wound and closes the trachea with sutures. The tissues are closed in sutured layers.

31820–31825

The physician closes a tracheostomy or fistula. The physician excises the scarred tissue forming the tracheostomy or fistula. If the trachea has healed, it is closed with sutures. The remaining tissues of the tracheostomy or fistula are pulled together and the wound is closed in sutured layers. Report 31820 if the tracheostomy or fistula is closed without plastic repair; report 31825 if the tracheostomy or fistula is closed with plastic repair of the skin made to hide the repair.

31830

The physician revises a tracheostomy scar. The physician incises the skin around the tracheostomy scar and removes the scarred tissues. The incision is closed in sutured layers, leaving a less noticeable scar.

32000

The physician removes fluid from the chest cavity by puncturing through the space between the ribs. Using an aspirating needle attached to a syringe, the physician carefully passes the needle over the top of a rib, punctures through the chest tissues, and enters the pleural cavity. With the end of the needle in the chest cavity, the physician withdraws the fluid from the chest cavity by pulling back on the plunger of the syringe.

32002

The physician removes fluid from the chest cavity by puncturing through the space between the ribs. To enter the chest cavity, the physician carefully passes a trocar (a long, thin, sharp pointed instrument within a plastic tube) over the top of a rib, punctures through the chest tissues between the ribs, and enters the pleural cavity. With the end of the trocar in the chest cavity, the physician advances the plastic tube (catheter) into the chest cavity. The sharp instrument is removed leaving one end of the plastic catheter in place within the chest cavity. A syringe is attached to the outside end of the catheter and fluid is removed from the chest cavity by pulling back on the plunger of the syringe. The outside end of the tube may be connected to a water seal system to prevent air from being sucked into the chest cavity and to allow continuous or intermittent removal of fluid.

32005

The physician instills fluid into the chest cavity by puncturing through the space between the ribs. To enter the chest cavity, the physician carefully passes a trocar (a long, thin, sharp, pointed instrument within a plastic tube) over the top of a rib, punctures through the chest tissues, and enters the pleural cavity. With the end of the trocar in the chest cavity, the physician advances the plastic tube (catheter) into the chest cavity. The sharp instrument is removed leaving one end of the plastic catheter in place within the chest cavity. A syringe is attached to the outside end of the catheter and fluid is injected into the chest cavity. The fluid selected is designed to cause the adhesion of the surface of the lung to the inside surface of the chest cavity.

32020

The physician removes fluid from the chest cavity by puncturing through the space between the ribs. To enter the chest cavity, the physician carefully passes a trocar(a long, sharp, pointed instrument within a plastic tube) over the top of a rib, punctures through the chest tissues between the ribs, and enters the pleural cavity. With the end of the trocar in the chest cavity, the physician advances the plastic tube (catheter) into the chest cavity. The sharp trocar is removed leaving one end of the plastic catheter in place within the chest cavity. A large syringe is attached to the outside end of the catheter and the fluid (blood or pus) is removed from the chest cavity by pulling back on the plunger of the syringe. The outside end of the tube may be connected to a water seal system to prevent air from being sucked into the chest cavity and to allow continuous or intermittent removal of fluid.

32035

The physician removes the purulent fluid of an empyema by creating a drainage wound in the chest. Using a scalpel, an incision is made through the skin of the chest and the incision is deepened to expose a portion of a rib. To enter the chest cavity, a short segment of the exposed rib is removed using rib cutters. The resulting defect in the chest wall allows for the continuous release of pus from the empyema (abscess in the chest cavity).

32036

The physician removes the purulent fluid of an empyema (abscess in the chest cavity) by creating a drainage wound in the chest. Using a scalpel, an incision is made through the skin of the chest and the incision is deepened to expose a portion of a rib. To create a drainage site, a short segment of the rib is removed using rib cutters. The resulting defect in the chest wall allows for the continuous release of pus from the empyema. To ensure that the drainage wound stays open, a flap is created in the skin and subcutaneous tissues.

32095

The physician removes a sample of tissue from the lung or the pleura (the tissue covering the inside surface of the chest cavity or the surface of the lung). Using a scalpel, the skin between two ribs is incised and the tissues separated to expose the inside of the chest cavity. A representative sample of tissue is removed using a biopsy needle or by cutting with a scalpel or scissors. The surgical wound created is then closed by suturing.

32100

The physician opens the chest cavity widely to directly visualize and assess the organs and structures in the chest and/or to obtain tissue for study and analysis. Using a scalpel the surgeon makes a long incision around the side of the chest between two of the ribs. The incision is carried through all the tissue layers into the chest cavity. Rib spreaders are inserted into the wound and the ribs are spread apart exposing the lung, the heart, and other structures. The area of the chest cavity is explored by pushing aside the deflated lung with a gloved hand and large gauze sponges. Tissue can be sampled by using a biopsy needle or by grasping tissue and cutting it with a scalpel or scissors. After the removal of the instruments and gauze sponges the incision is closed in layers of sutures. A chest tube(s) may be used to provide drainage for the chest cavity. Alternately, the chest cavity can be opened and the operation performed through a vertical incision in the center of the chest through the sternum. The skin incision is carried down to the sternum bone and then a saw is used to split the sternum. With the sternum split in half, the chest is entered by spreading the sternum apart with a set of rib spreaders. When the procedure is complete, the wound is closed by using wires to bring the two halves of the sternum together and the skin is closed over the sternum by suturing.

32110

The physician opens the chest cavity widely to directly visualize and assess the organs and structures in the chest and to control bleeding and/or repair injury to the lung. Using a scalpel, the surgeon makes a long incision around the side of the chest between two of the ribs. The incision is carried through all the tissue layers into the chest cavity. Rib spreaders are inserted into the wound and the ribs are spread apart exposing the lung, the heart and other structures. The area of the chest cavity is explored by pushing aside the deflated lung with a gloved hand and large gauze sponges. The site of the injury is identified and repaired. After the removal of the instruments and gauze sponges the incision is closed in layers of sutures. A chest tube(s) may be used to provide drainage for the chest cavity. Alternately, the chest cavity can be opened and the operation performed through a vertical incision in the center of the chest through the sternum. The skin incision is carried down to the sternum bone and a saw is used to split the sternum. With the sternum split in half the chest is entered by spreading the sternum apart with a set of rib spreaders. When the procedure is complete the wound is closed by using wires to bring the two halves of the sternum together and the skin closed over the sternum by suturing.

32120

The physician opens the chest cavity widely to directly visualize and assess the organs and structures in the chest after recent surgery in the chest. Using a scalpel, the surgeon makes a long incision around the side of the chest between two of the ribs. The incision is carried through all the tissue layers into the chest cavity. Rib spreaders are inserted into the wound and the ribs are spread apart exposing the lung, the heart, and other structures. The area of the chest cavity is explored by pushing aside the deflated lung with a gloved hand and large gauze sponges. Repairs can be made as indicated and discovered while exploring the chest cavity. After the removal of the instruments and gauze sponges, the incision is closed in layers of sutures. A chest tube(s) may be used to provide drainage for the chest cavity. Alternately, the chest cavity can be opened and the operation performed through a vertical incision in the center of the chest through the sternum. The skin incision is carried down to the sternum bone and then a saw is used to split the sternum. With the sternum split in half, the chest is entered by spreading the sternum apart with a set of rib spreaders. When the procedure is complete,

the wound is closed by using wires to bring the two halves of the sternum together and the skin is closed over the sternum by suturing.

32124

The physician opens the chest cavity widely to directly visualize and separate the surface of the lung which has become adherent to the inside surface of the chest cavity. Using a scalpel, the surgeon makes a long incision around the side of the chest between two of the ribs. The incision is carried through all the tissue layers into the chest cavity. Rib spreaders are inserted into the wound and the ribs are spread apart exposing the lung. Using a gloved hand and a large moist gauze sponge the surgeon manually divides the tissues attaching the lung to the wall of the chest cavity. After the procedure is completed, the instruments and gauze sponges are removed and the incision is closed in layers of sutures. A chest tube(s) may be used to provide drainage for the chest cavity. Alternately, the chest cavity can be opened and the operation performed through a vertical incision in the center of the chest through the sternum. The skin incision is carried down to the sternum bone and then a saw is used to split the sternum. With the sternum split in half, the chest is entered by spreading the sternum apart with a set of rib spreaders. When the procedure is complete, the wound is closed by using wires to bring the two halves of the sternum together and the skin is closed over the sternum by suturing.

32140

The physician opens the chest cavity widely to remove one or more lung cysts. Using a scalpel, the surgeon makes a long incision around the side of the chest between two of the ribs. The incision is carried through all the tissue layers into the chest cavity. Rib spreaders are inserted into the wound and the ribs are spread apart exposing the lung. Space is made in the chest by packing the uninvolved lung away from the operative field by using large moist gauze sponges. In order to perform the procedure the pleural surface may require an operative procedure such as pneumonolysis (separation of the surface of the lung which has become adherent to the inside surface of the chest cavity). The lung cyst is located and removed by sharp and blunt dissection of the tissues. After the procedure is completed, the instruments and gauze sponges are removed and the incision is closed in layers of sutures. A chest tube(s) may be used to provide drainage for the chest cavity. Alternately, the chest cavity can be opened and the operation performed through a vertical incision in the center of the chest through the sternum. The skin incision is carried down to the sternum bone and then a saw is used to split the sternum. With the sternum split in half, the chest is entered by spreading the sternum apart with a set of rib spreaders. When the procedure is complete, the wound is closed by using wires to bring the two halves of the sternum together and the skin is closed over the sternum by suturing.

CPT® Lay Descriptions

32141

The physician opens the chest cavity widely to remove one or more lung bullae (large non-functional air sacs). Using a scalpel, the surgeon makes a long incision around the side of the chest between two of the ribs. The incision is carried through all the tissue layers into the chest cavity. Rib spreaders are inserted into the wound and the ribs are spread apart exposing the lung. Space is made in the chest by packing the uninvolved lung away from the operative field by using large moist gauze sponges. In order to perform the procedure the pleural surface may require an operative procedure such as pneumonolysis (separation of the surface of the lung which has become adherent to the inside surface of the chest cavity). The lung bullae is located and removed by sharp and blunt dissection of the tissues and often by folding and suturing of the tissues (plication). After the procedure is completed, the instruments and gauze sponges are removed and the incision is closed in layers of sutures. A chest tube(s) may be used to provide drainage for the chest cavity. Alternately, the chest cavity can be opened and the operation performed through a vertical incision in the center of the chest through the sternum. The skin incision is carried down to the sternum bone and then a saw is used to split the sternum. With the sternum split in half, the chest is entered by spreading the sternum apart with a set of rib spreaders. When the procedure is complete, the wound is closed by using wires to bring the two halves of the sternum together and the skin is closed over the sternum by suturing.

32150

The physician opens the chest cavity widely to remove a foreign body or fibrin deposit (thick insoluble protein deposit formed after the clotting of blood) in the pleura (the membranous tissues investing the lungs and lining the thoracic cavity). Using a scalpel, the surgeon makes a long incision around the side of the chest between two of the ribs. The incision is carried through all the tissue layers into the chest cavity. Rib spreaders are inserted into the wound and the ribs are spread apart exposing the lung. Space is made in the chest by packing the uninvolved lung away from the operative field by using large moist gauze sponges. The foreign body or fibrin deposit is located and removed by sharp and blunt dissection. After the procedure is completed, the instruments and gauze sponges are removed and the incision is closed in layers of sutures. A chest tube(s) may be used to provide drainage for the chest cavity. Alternately, the chest cavity can be opened and the operation performed through a vertical incision in the center of the chest through the sternum. The skin incision is carried down to the sternum bone and then a saw is used to split the sternum. With the sternum split in half, the chest is entered by spreading the sternum apart with a set of rib spreaders. When the procedure is complete, the wound is closed by using wires to bring the two halves of the sternum together and the skin is closed over the sternum by suturing.

32151

The physician opens the chest cavity widely to remove a foreign body in the lung. Using a scalpel, the surgeon makes a long incision around the side of the chest between two of the ribs. The incision is carried through all the tissue layers into the chest cavity. Rib spreaders are inserted into the wound and the ribs are spread apart exposing the lung. Space is made in the chest by packing the uninvolved lung away from the operative field by using large moist gauze sponges. The foreign body is located and removed by sharp and blunt dissection. After the procedure is completed, the instruments and gauze sponges are removed and the incision is closed in layers of sutures. A chest tube(s) may be used to provide drainage for the chest cavity. Alternately, the chest cavity can be opened and the operation performed through a vertical incision in the center of the chest through the sternum. The skin incision is carried down to the sternum bone and then a saw is used to split the sternum. With the sternum split in half, the chest is entered by spreading the sternum apart with a set of rib spreaders. When the procedure is complete, the wound is closed by using wires to bring the two halves of the sternum together and the skin is closed over the sternum by suturing.

32160

The physician opens the chest cavity widely to perform direct manual cardiac massage in the treatment of a cardiac arrest. Using a scalpel, the surgeon makes a long incision around the side of the chest between two of the ribs. The incision is carried through all the tissue layers into the chest cavity. Rib spreaders are inserted into the wound and the ribs are spread apart exposing the lung. Space is made in the chest by packing the uninvolved lung away from the operative field by using large moist gauze sponges. The heart is exposed and squeezed rhythmically to mimic cardiac contractions thus pumping blood through the body. The heart may be directly contra-shocked to produce spontaneous heart beats. After procedure is completed, the instruments and gauze sponges are removed and the incision is closed in layers of sutures. A chest tube(s) may be used to provide drainage for the chest cavity. Alternately, the chest cavity can be opened and the operation performed through a vertical incision in the center of the chest through the sternum. The skin incision is carried down to the sternum bone and then a saw is used to split the sternum. With the sternum split in half, the chest is entered by spreading the sternum apart with a set of rib spreaders. When the procedure is complete, the wound is closed by using wires to bring the two halves of the sternum together and the skin is closed over the sternum by suturing.

32200

The physician treats an abscess or cyst in the lung by draining the pus or fluid directly through the chest wall. Using a scalpel, the skin between two ribs is incised and the tissues separated to expose the inside of the chest cavity. The lung is cut with either scissors or a scalpel down to the abscess or the cyst. The abscess or cyst is opened and the fluid is allowed to drain through the wound created in the lung and the chest wall. A rubber drainage tube may be left in place to maintain or facilitate drainage. The incision is not sutured closed. The outside incision is dressed with bulky gauze dressing to absorb the drainage.

32201

The physician performs a pneumonostomy with percutaneous drainage of an abscess or cyst. The physician may create a small incision in the skin between two ribs proximal to the abscess or cyst in order to ease placement of drainage instruments through the skin into the lung (percutaneous). The physician uses a CAT scan or ultrasound to guide the placement of a drainage needle or trocar into the abscess or cyst. The physician advances the drainage needle or trocar through the chest wall into the lung to gain access to the abscess or cyst. The fluid is allowed to drain. Once the abscess or cyst is drained, a drainage catheter may be placed (and later removed). Sutures may be placed to secure the drainage catheter in place. The operative site is cleaned and bandaged. For radiological supervision and interpretation, see 75989.

32215

The physician treats repeat pneumothorax by producing adhesions between the surface of the lung and the inside surface of the chest cavity. To create the adhesions, a chemical solution is injected into the chest cavity and allowed to circulate over the surface of the lung and the inside surface of the chest cavity. The physicians injects the solution by passing a tube into the chest cavity. The physician carefully passes a trocar (a long, thin, sharp pointed instrument within a plastic tube) over the top of a rib and punctures through the chest tissues between the ribs and enters the pleural cavity. With the end of the trocar in the chest cavity, the physician advances the plastic tube (catheter) into the chest cavity. The sharp instrument is removed leaving one end of the plastic catheter in place within the chest cavity. A syringe is attached to the outside end of the catheter and fluid is injected into the chest cavity. The fluid selected is design to cause the formation of adhesive scar tissue between the surface of the lung and the inside surface of the chest cavity. Once the lung is stuck to the chest wall it can no longer collapse and allow the formation of a pneumothorax.

32220–32225

The physician removes a constricting membrane or layer of tissue from the surface of the lung (decortication) in order to permit the lung to fully expand. The physician opens the chest cavity widely. Using a scalpel, the surgeon makes a long incision around the side of the chest between two of the ribs. The incision is carried through all the tissue layers into the chest cavity. Rib spreaders are inserted into the wound and the ribs are spread apart exposing the lung. The constricting membrane is then stripped off the entire surface of the lung. In 32225, only a portion of the lung surface is removed. The chest wall incision is then sutured closed in layers. A chest tube(s) may be used to provide drainage for the chest cavity. Alternately, the chest cavity can be opened by a vertical incision in the front of the chest through the sternum. The skin incision is carried down to the sternum bone and then a saw is used to split the sternum. With the sternum split in half, the chest is entered by spreading the sternum apart with a set of rib spreaders. When the procedure is complete, the wound is closed by using wires to bring the two halves of the sternum together and the skin is closed by suturing.

32310

The physician removes the membranous tissue lining the inside surface of the chest cavity (the parietal pleura). The physician opens the chest cavity widely to gain access to the inside surface of the chest. Using a scalpel, the surgeon makes a long incision around the side of the chest between two of the ribs. The incision is carried through all the tissue layers into the chest cavity. Rib spreaders are inserted into the wound and the ribs are spread apart exposing the lung. The parietal pleura is stripped from the inside surface of the chest. The chest wall incision is then sutured closed in layers. A chest tube(s) may be used to provide drainage for the chest cavity. Alternately, the chest cavity can be opened and the operation performed through a vertical incision in the center of the chest through the sternum. The skin incision is carried down to the sternum bone and then a saw is used to split the sternum. With the sternum split in half, the chest is entered by spreading the sternum apart with a set of rib spreaders. When the procedure is complete, the wound is closed by using wires to bring the two halves of the sternum together and the skin is closed over the sternum by suturing.

32320

The physician removes a constricting membrane or layer of tissue from a portion of the surface of the lung (decortication) in order to permit the lung to fully expand and also removes the membranous tissue lining the inside surface of the chest cavity (the parietal pleura). The physician opens the chest cavity widely. Using a scalpel, the surgeon makes a long incision around the side of the chest between two of the ribs. The incision is carried through all the tissue layers into the chest cavity. Rib spreaders are inserted into the wound and the ribs are spread apart exposing the lung. The constricting membrane is then stripped off the surface of the lung. The parietal pleura is stripped from the inside surface of the chest. The chest wall incision is then sutured closed in layers. A chest tube(s) may be used to provide drainage for the chest cavity. Alternately, the chest cavity can be opened and the operation performed through a vertical incision in the center of the chest through the sternum. The skin incision is carried down to the sternum bone and then a saw is used to split the sternum. With the sternum split in half, the chest is entered by spreading the sternum apart with a set of rib spreaders. When the procedure is complete, the wound is closed by using wires to bring the two halves of the sternum together and the skin is closed over the sternum by suturing.

32400

The physician obtains a sample of the lining of the lung and/or the lining of the inside of the chest cavity by needle biopsy. Using a special pleural biopsy needle, the physician carefully passes the needle over the top of a rib, punctures through the chest tissues between two ribs, enters the pleural cavity and slightly punctures the surface of the lung. With the end of the needle in the chest cavity, the physician withdraws a piece of tissue. The needle is then withdrawn and the puncture site covered with a bandage. The procedure is often done under radiological guidance to assure more precise placement of the needle.

32402

The physician removes a sample of tissue from the pleura (the tissue covering the inside surface of the chest cavity or the surface of the lung). A small opening is created in the chest. The skin between two ribs is incised and the tissues separated to create a small opening in the chest. Under direct vision through this opening, a representative sample of tissue is removed using a biopsy needle or by cutting the tissue with a scalpel or scissors. The surgical wound created is then closed by suturing.

32405

The physician obtains a sample of the lung or the mediastinum (the tissues in the center of the chest between the two lung cavities) by puncturing through the space between two of the ribs with a needle. The procedure is often done under radiological guidance to assure more precise placement of the needle. Using a biopsy needle, the physician carefully passes the needle over the top of a rib, punctures through the chest tissues, enters the pleural cavity, and punctures into the area of concern in the lung or the mediastinum. With the end of the needle in the chest cavity, the physician withdraws a piece of tissue. The needle is then withdrawn and the puncture site covered with a bandage.

32420

The physician removes a collection of fluid in a lung by puncturing through the space between the ribs and entering the lung. Using an aspirating needle attached to a syringe, the physician carefully passes the needle over the top of a rib, punctures through the chest tissues, enters the pleural cavity, and directs the

needle into the fluid area of the lung. With the end of the needle in the fluid cavity within the lung, the physician withdraws the fluid by pulling back on the plunger of the syringe.

32440

The physician removes one lung in its entirety. The physician opens the chest cavity widely to gain access to the lung to be removed. Using a scalpel, the surgeon makes a long incision around the side of the chest between two of the ribs. The incision is carried through all the tissue layers into the chest cavity. Rib spreaders are inserted into the wound and the ribs are spread apart exposing the lung, heart, and other structures. The root of the lung is found by pushing aside the deflated lung with a gloved hand and large moist gauze sponges. Within the root of the lung, the blood vessels and bronchial tubes are clamped, tied off, and cut. The lung is then removed through the wide chest incision. After the removal of the instruments and gauze sponges, the chest incision is sutured closed in layers. A chest tube(s) may be used to provide drainage for the chest cavity. Alternately, the chest cavity can be opened and the operation performed through a vertical incision in the center of the chest through the sternum. The skin incision is carried down to the sternum bone and then a saw is used to split the sternum. With the sternum split in half, the chest is entered by spreading the sternum apart with a set of rib spreaders. When the procedure is complete, the wound is closed by using wires to bring the two halves of the sternum together and the skin is closed over the sternum by suturing.

32442

The physician removes one lung in its entirety. The physician opens the chest cavity widely to gain access to the lung to be removed. Using a scalpel, the surgeon makes a long incision around the side of the chest between two of the ribs. The incision is carried through all the tissue layers into the chest cavity. Rib spreaders are inserted into the wound and the ribs are spread apart exposing the lung, heart, and other structures. The root of the lung is found by pushing aside the deflated lung with a gloved hand and large moist gauze sponges. Within the root of the lung, the blood vessels and bronchial tubes are clamped, tied off, and cut. The lung and a segment of the trachea are then removed through the wide chest incision. The trachea is sutured to the main bronchial tube of the remaining lung in the other half of the chest. After the removal of the instruments and gauze sponges, the chest incision is sutured closed in layers. A chest tube(s) may be used to provide drainage for the chest cavity. Alternately, the chest cavity can be opened and the operation performed through a vertical incision in the center of the chest through the sternum. The skin incision is carried down to the sternum bone and then a saw is used to split the sternum. With the sternum split in half, the chest is entered by spreading the sternum apart with a set of rib spreaders. When the procedure is complete, the wound is closed by using wires to bring the two halves of the sternum together and the skin is closed over the sternum by suturing.

32445

The physician removes one lung in its entirety and the pleural membranes covering the lung and the inside surface of the chest cavity (the parietal pleura). The physician opens the chest cavity widely to gain access to the lung to be removed. Using a scalpel, the surgeon makes a long incision around the side of the chest between two of the ribs. The incision is carried through all the tissue layers down to the membrane lining the chest cavity. Rib spreaders are inserted into the wound and the ribs are spread apart, taking care to preserve the integrity of the chest lining. Holding a gauze sponge, the surgeon strips away the entire lining inside the chest all the way around to the root of the lung. This creates a sac of the parietal pleura that contains the entire lung. Within the root of the lung, the blood vessels and bronchial tubes are clamped, tied off, and cut. The lung and the pleural tissues of the inside of the chest wall are then removed through the wide chest incision. After the removal of the instruments and gauze sponges, the chest incision is sutured closed in layers. A chest tube(s) may be used to provide drainage for the chest cavity.

32480–32482

The physician removes a single lobe of one lung in 32480 and two lobes of one lung in 32482. In 32480, the physician opens the chest cavity widely to gain access to the lung to be removed. Using a scalpel, the surgeon makes a long incision around the side of the chest between two of the ribs. The incision is carried through all the tissue layers into the chest cavity. Rib spreaders are inserted into the wound and the ribs are spread apart exposing the lung. The lobe(s) to be removed is identified and isolated in the operative field by pushing aside the deflated lung with a gloved hand and large moist gauze sponges. Within the lobe(s) of the lung, the main blood vessels and bronchial tubes are clamped, tied off, and cut. The lobe(s) is then removed through the wide chest incision. After the removal of the instruments and gauze sponges, the chest incision is sutured closed in layers. A chest tube(s) may be used to provide drainage for the chest cavity. Alternately, the chest cavity can be opened and the operation performed through a vertical incision in the center of the chest through the sternum. The skin incision is carried down to the sternum bone and then a saw is used to split the sternum. With the sternum split in half, the chest is entered by spreading the sternum apart with a set of rib spreaders. When the procedure is complete, the wound is closed by using wires to bring the two halves of the sternum together and the skin is closed over the sternum by suturing.

32484

The physician removes a segment of a lobe of one lung. The physician opens the chest cavity widely to gain access to the lung to be removed. Using a scalpel, the surgeon makes a long incision around the side of the chest between two of the ribs. The incision is carried through all the tissue layers into the chest cavity. Rib spreaders are inserted into the wound and the ribs are spread apart exposing the lung. The segment to be removed is identified and isolated in the operative field by pushing aside the deflated lung with a gloved hand and large moist gauze sponges. Within the segment of the lung, the main blood vessels and bronchial tubes are clamped, tied off, and cut. The segment is then removed through the wide chest incision. After the removal of the instruments and gauze sponges, the chest incision is sutured closed in layers. A chest tube(s) may be used to provide drainage for the chest cavity. Alternately, the chest cavity can be opened and the operation performed through a vertical incision in the center of the chest through the sternum. The skin incision is carried down to the sternum bone and then a saw is used to split the sternum. With the sternum split in half, the chest is entered by spreading the sternum apart with a set of rib spreaders. When the procedure is complete, the wound is closed by using wires to bring the two halves of the sternum together and the skin is closed over the sternum by suturing.

32486

The physician removes a portion (lobectomy, bilobectomy or segmentectomy) of one lung and repairs a bronchial tube that has been partially resected. The physician opens the chest cavity widely to gain access to the lung to be removed. Using a scalpel, the surgeon makes a long incision around the side of the chest between two of the ribs. The incision is carried through all the tissue layers into the chest cavity. Rib spreaders are inserted into the wound and the ribs are spread apart exposing the lung. The portion of lung to be removed is identified and isolated in the operative field by pushing aside the deflated lung with a gloved hand and large moist gauze sponges. Within the lung, main blood vessels and bronchial tubes are clamped, tied off, and cut. The resected part of the lung is then removed through the wide chest incision. The segment of diseased or damaged bronchial tube is removed. The healthy end of the smaller bronchial tube in the remaining lobe is sutured to the main bronchial tube in the root of the lung. After the removal of the instruments and gauze sponges, the chest incision is sutured closed in layers. A chest tube(s) may be used to provide drainage for the chest cavity. Alternately, the chest cavity can be opened and the operation performed through a vertical incision in the center of the chest through the sternum. The skin incision is carried down to the sternum bone and then a saw is used to split the sternum. With the sternum split in half, the chest is entered by spreading the sternum apart with a set of rib spreaders. When the procedure is complete, the wound is closed by using wires to bring the two halves of the sternum together and the skin is closed over the sternum by suturing.

32488

The physician removes the remaining portion(s) of a lung from a prior partial lung removal. The physician opens the chest cavity widely to gain access to the lung to be removed. Using a scalpel, the surgeon makes a long incision around the side of the chest between two of the ribs. The incision is carried through all the tissue layers into the chest cavity. Rib spreaders are inserted into the wound and the ribs are spread apart exposing the lung. The entire remaining portion of lung is isolated in the operative field by pushing aside the deflated lung with a gloved hand and large moist gauze sponges. Within the root of the lung, the blood vessels and bronchial tubes are clamped, tied off, and cut. The lung is removed through the wide chest incision. After the removal of the instruments and gauze sponges, the chest incision is sutured closed in layers. A chest tube(s) may be used to provide drainage for the chest cavity. Alternately, the chest cavity can be opened and the operation performed through a vertical incision in the center of the chest through the sternum. The skin incision is carried down to the sternum bone and then a saw is used to split the sternum. With the sternum split in half, the chest is entered by spreading the sternum apart with a set of rib spreaders. When the procedure is complete, the wound is closed by using wires to bring the two halves of the sternum together and the skin is closed over the sternum by suturing.

32491

The physician removes part of an emphysematous lung. The physician opens the chest cavity widely to gain access to the lung to be removed. The physician makes a long incision around the side of the chest between two of the ribs, or the physician may use an incision through the center of the sternum. The incision is carried through all the tissue layers into the chest cavity, and rib spreaders are used to expose the lung. The lung tissue to be removed is identified and isolated in the operative field by pushing aside the deflated lung with a gloved hand and large moist gauze sponges. The lung tissue may be further isolated using a row of staples. The tissue is excised and instruments and gauze sponges are removed. The chest incision is sutured closed in layers (sternal wires are used if the chest was entered through a midline sternal incision). A chest tube(s) may be used to provide drainage for the chest cavity.

32500

The physician removes a wedge-shaped portion(s) of a lobe(s) of one or both lungs. The physician opens the chest cavity widely to gain access to the lung to be removed. Using a scalpel, the surgeon makes a long incision around the side of the chest between two of the ribs. The incision is carried through all the tissue

layers into the chest cavity. Rib spreaders are inserted into the wound and the ribs are spread apart exposing the lung. The area to be removed is identified and isolated in the operative field by pushing aside the deflated lung with a gloved hand and large moist gauze sponges. The healthy portions of the lung surrounding the area(s) to be removed are clamped with special clamps and the portion is removed by cutting the lung tissue isolated by the clamps. Sutures or surgical clips are used to repair the cut portion of the remaining lung tissue. After the removal of the instruments and gauze sponges, the chest incision is sutured closed in layers. A chest tube(s) may be used to provide drainage for the chest cavity. In another technique, the chest cavity can by opened and the operation performed through a vertical incision in the center of the chest through the sternum. The skin incision is carried down to the sternum bone and then a saw is used to split the sternum. With the sternum split in half, the chest is entered by using a set of rib spreaders to separate the sternum. When the procedure is complete, wires are used to bring the halves of the sternum together. The skin is closed over the sternum by suturing.

32501

During lobectomy or segmentectomy, the physician repairs part of a bronchus. After removing the lobes or lobe segments (see codes 32480, 32482, 32484 for procedure description), the segment of diseased or damaged bronchial tube is repaired and sutured to the main bronchial tube in the root of the lung. The remaining instruments and gauze sponges are removed from the chest cavity. The chest incision is sutured closed in layers (sternal wires are used if the chest was entered through a midline sternal incision). A chest tube(s) may be used to provide drainage for the chest cavity. List this code separately in addition to the primary procedure.

32520

The physician removes part of one lung and a portion of the chest wall. The physician opens the chest cavity widely to gain access to the lung to be removed. Using a scalpel, the surgeon makes a long incision around the side of the chest between two of the ribs. The incision is carried through all the tissue layers into the chest cavity. Rib spreaders are inserted into the wound and the ribs are spread apart exposing the lung, heart, and other structures. The area of lung and chest wall to be removed is identified and isolated in the operative field by pushing aside the deflated lung with a gloved hand and large moist gauze sponges. Within the lung, the blood vessels and bronchial tubes that go to the area to be removed are clamped, tied off, and cut. The affected area of chest wall is resected. After the removal of the instruments and gauze sponges, the chest incision and created defect are sutured closed in layers. A chest tube(s) may be used to provide drainage for the chest cavity.

32522

The physician removes part of one lung and a portion of the chest wall and reconstructs the created chest wall defect. The physician opens the chest cavity widely to gain access to the lung to be removed. Using a scalpel, the surgeon makes a long incision around the side of the chest between two of the ribs. The incision is carried through all the tissue layers into the chest cavity. Rib spreaders are inserted into the wound and the ribs are spread apart exposing the lung, heart, and other structures. The area of lung and chest wall to be removed is identified and isolated in the operative field by pushing aside the deflated lung with a gloved hand and large moist gauze sponges. Within the lung, the blood vessels and bronchial tubes that go to the area to be removed are clamped, tied off, and cut. The affected area of chest wall is resected. After the removal of the instruments and gauze sponges, the chest incision and created defect are sutured closed by reconstructing the damaged area. This may require complete or partial resection of one or two ribs and the use of muscle and/or skin flaps. A chest tube(s) may be used to provide drainage for the chest cavity.

32525

The physician removes part of one lung and a portion of the chest wall followed by major reconstruction of the created chest wall defect with prosthesis. The physician opens the chest cavity widely to gain access to the lung to be removed. Using a scalpel, the surgeon makes a long incision around the side of the chest between two of the ribs. The incision is carried through all the tissue layers into the chest cavity. Rib spreaders are inserted into the wound and the ribs are spread apart exposing the lung. The area of lung and chest wall to be removed is identified and isolated in the operative field by pushing aside the deflated lung with a gloved hand and large moist gauze sponges. Within the lung, the blood vessels and bronchial tubes that go to the area to be removed are clamped, tied off, and cut. A large affected area of chest wall is resected. After the removal of the instruments and gauze sponges, the chest defect is reconstructed. This requires complete or partial resection of two or more ribs and the use of muscle flaps and ridged prosthetic segment(s) that help fill in the chest wall defect and give stability to the area. Closing the skin over the prosthesis may require the use of pedicle or free skin grafts. A chest tube(s) may be used to provide drainage for the chest cavity.

32540

The physician removes an empyema (an abscess in the chest cavity between the lung and the chest wall) in its entirety including the pleural membranes surrounding the abscess. The physician opens the chest cavity to gain access to the abscess. Using a scalpel, the surgeon makes an incision around the side of the chest between two of the ribs. The incision is carried through all the tissue layers down to the membrane lining the chest cavity. Rib spreaders are inserted into the wound and the ribs are spread apart exposing the tissues, taking care to preserve the integrity of the chest lining. Holding a gauze sponge, the surgeon strips away the lining adherent to the chest wall and the abscess and carries this all the way around the entire abscess. This creates a sac that contains the abscess. The intact mass is then shelled out through the chest incision. After the removal of the instruments and gauze sponges, the chest incision is either sutured closed in layers leaving a drainage tube or the wound partially closed to allow drainage.

32601

The physician examines the inside of the chest cavity through either a rigid or flexible fiberoptic endoscope. The procedure can be done under local or general anesthesia. The surgeon makes a small incision between two ribs and by blunt dissection and the use of a trocar enters the thoracic cavity. The endoscope is passed through the trocar and into the chest cavity. The lung is usually partially collapsed by instilling air into the chest through the trocar, or if general anesthesia is used, the lung may be collapsed through a special double lumen endotracheal tube inserted through the mouth into the trachea. The contents of the chest cavity are examined by direct visualization and/or the use of a video camera. Still photographs may be taken as part of the procedure. At the conclusion of the procedure, the endoscope and the trocar are removed. A chest tube for drainage and re-expansion of the lung is usually inserted through the wound used for the thoracoscopy.

32602

The physician examines the inside of the chest cavity through either a rigid or flexible fiberoptic endoscope and takes a sample(s) of tissue. The procedure can be done under local or general anesthesia. The surgeon makes a small incision between two ribs and by blunt dissection and the use of a trocar enters the thoracic cavity. The endoscope is passed through the trocar and into the chest cavity. The lung is usually partially collapsed by instilling air into the chest through the trocar or, if general anesthesia is used, the lung may be collapsed through a special double lumen endotracheal tube inserted through the mouth into the trachea. The contents of the chest cavity are examined by direct visualization and/or the use of a video camera. Still photographs may be taken as part of the procedure. The tissue selected for biopsy is identified and a biopsy taken using a device through the endoscope or the insertion of an instrument through a second incision in the chest. At the conclusion of the procedure, the endoscope and the trocar are removed. A chest tube for drainage and re-expansion of the lung is usually inserted through the wound used for the thoracoscopy.

32603–32604

The physician examines the inside of the pericardial sac through either a rigid or flexible fiberoptic endoscope. The procedure can be done under local or general anesthesia. The physician makes a small incision between two ribs and by blunt dissection and the use of a trocar enters the thoracic cavity. The endoscope is passed through the trocar and into the chest cavity. The lung is usually partially collapsed by instilling air into the chest through the trocar or, if general anesthesia is used, the lung may be collapsed through a special double lumen endotracheal tube inserted through the mouth into the trachea. The endoscope is advanced to and into the pericardial sac as the physician views the structures and the anatomy of the area through the scope. The contents of the pericardial sac are examined by direct visualization and/or the use of a video camera. Still photographs may be taken as part of the procedure. At the conclusion of the procedure the endoscope and the trocar are withdrawn. A chest tube for drainage and re-expansion of the lung is usually inserted through the wound used for the thoracoscopy. In 32604, the tissue selected for bipsy is identified and a biopsy taken using a device inserted through the endoscope.

32605–32606

The physician examines the inside of the mediastinal space, through either a rigid or flexible fiberoptic endoscope. The procedure can be done under local or general anesthesia. The physician makes a small incision between two ribs and by blunt dissection and the use of a trocar enters the thoracic cavity. The endoscope is passed through the trocar and into the chest cavity. The lung is usually partially collapsed by instilling air into the chest through the trocar or, if general anesthesia is used, the lung may be collapsed through a special double lumen endotracheal tube inserted through the mouth into the trachea. As the physician views the structures and the anatomy of the area through the endoscope, the endoscope is advanced into the mediastinum (area inside the center of the chest cavity between the lungs). The contents of the mediastinal space are examined by direct visualization and/or by the use of a video camera. Still photographs may be taken as part of the procedure. In 32606, the tissue selected for biopsy is identifed and a biopsy taken using a device inserted through the endoscope. At the conclusion of the procedure, the endoscope and the trocar are withdrawn. A chest tube for drainage and re-expansion of the lung is usually inserted through the wound used for the thoracoscopy.

32650

The physician examines the inside of the chest cavity through either a rigid or flexible fiberoptic endoscope and induces adhesion of the surface of the lung to the inside surface of the chest cavity. The procedure can be done under local or general anesthesia. The physician makes a small incision between two ribs and by blunt dissection and the use of a trocar enters the thoracic cavity. The endoscope is passed through the trocar and into the chest cavity. The lung is usually partially collapsed by instilling air into the chest through the trocar or, if general anesthesia is used, the lung may be collapsed through a special double lumen endotracheal tube inserted through the mouth into the trachea. The contents of the chest cavity are examined by direct visualization and/or by the use of a video camera. Still photographs may be taken as part of the procedure. A second trocar and instruments may be inserted into the chest cavity through a second wound in the chest. Adhesion may be induced in one of two ways: either by abrading the surfaces of the lung and the inside of the chest cavity or by the instillation of chemicals into the chest cavity that bath the surfaces of the lung and the inside of the chest cavity. Most commonly, a chemical solution is instilled into the chest through the endoscope or second puncture site. At the conclusion of the procedure, the endoscope and the trocar are removed. A chest tube for drainage and re-expansion of the lung is usually inserted through the wound used for the thoracoscopy.

32651–32652

The physician examines the inside of the chest cavity through either a rigid or flexible fiberoptic endoscope and removes a portion of the tissue covering the surface of the lung. The procedure can be done under local or general anesthesia. The physician makes a small incision between two ribs and by blunt dissection and the use of a trocar enters the thoracic cavity. The endoscope is passed through the trocar and into the chest cavity. The lung is usually partially collapsed by instilling air into the chest through the trocar or, if general anesthesia is used, the lung may be collapsed through a special double lumen endotracheal tube inserted through the mouth into the trachea. The contents of the chest cavity are examined by direct visualization and/or by the use of a video camera. Still photographs may be taken as part of the procedure. A second and/or third trocar and instruments may be inserted into the chest cavity through a second and/or third wound in the chest. Under direct visualization through the endoscope, the physician strips away the membranous tissues covering a portion of the lung (or all of the lung ins 32652) using instruments inserted into the chest through the secondary sites. Code 32652 includes intrapleural pneumonolysis in which the physician divides the tissues attaching the lung to the wall of the chest cavity. At the conclusion of the procedure, the endoscope and the trocar are removed. A chest tube for drainage and re-expansion of the lung is usually inserted through the wound used for the thoracoscopy.

32653

The physician examines the inside of the chest cavity through either a rigid or flexible fiberoptic endoscope and removes a foreign body or a fibrin deposit (the thick tissue much like remains of a blood clot). The procedure can be done under local or general anesthesia. The surgeon makes a small incision between two ribs and by blunt dissection and the use of a trocar enters the thoracic cavity. The endoscope is passed through the trocar and into the chest cavity. The lung is usually partially collapsed by instilling air into the chest through the trocar or, if general anesthesia is used, the lung may be collapsed through a special double lumen endotracheal tube inserted through the mouth into the trachea. The contents of the chest cavity are examined by direct visualization and/or by the use of a video camera. Still photographs may be taken as part of the procedure. A second and/or third trocar and instruments may be inserted into the chest cavity through a second and/or third wound in the chest. The foreign body or fibrin deposit is located and then removed using instruments through the scope or the secondary sites. At the conclusion of the procedure, the endoscope and the trocar are removed. A chest tube for drainage and re-expansion of the lung is usually inserted through the wound used for the thoracoscopy.

32654

The physician examines the inside of the chest cavity through either a rigid or flexible fiberoptic endoscope and controls bleeding from a wound to the chest. The procedure can be done under local or general anesthesia. The physician makes a small incision between two ribs and by blunt dissection and the use of a trocar enters the thoracic cavity. The endoscope is passed through the trocar and into the chest cavity. The lung is usually partially collapsed by instilling air into the chest through the trocar or, if general anesthesia is used, the lung may be collapsed through a special double lumen endotracheal tube inserted through the mouth into the trachea. The contents of the chest cavity are examined by direct visualization and/or by the use of a video camera. Still photographs may be taken as part of the procedure. A second and/or third trocar and instruments may be inserted into the chest cavity through a second and/or third wound in the chest. Under direct visualization through the endoscope, the physician manipulates the instruments inserted through the secondary sites and localizes the site of the bleeding. The hemorrhage is controlled by clipping or cauterizing the damaged blood vessel. At the conclusion of the procedure, the endoscope and the trocar(s) are removed. A chest tube for drainage and re-expansion of the lung is usually inserted through the wound used for the thoracoscopy.

32655

The physician examines the inside of the chest cavity through either a rigid or flexible fiberoptic endoscope and removes one or more lung bullae (large non-functional air sacs). The physician makes a small incision between two ribs and by blunt dissection and the use of a trocar enters the thoracic cavity. The endoscope is passed through the trocar and into the

chest cavity. The lung is usually partially collapsed by instilling air into the chest through the trocar or the lung may be collapsed through a special double lumen endotracheal tube inserted through the mouth into the trachea. The contents of the chest cavity are examined by direct visualization and/or by the use of a video camera. Still photographs may be taken as part of the procedure. A second and/or third trocar and instruments may be inserted into the chest cavity through a second and/or third wound in the chest. Under direct visualization through the endoscope, the physician manipulates the instruments inserted through the secondary sites and localizes the bullae. The bulla(e) is removed by sharp and blunt dissection of the tissues which often requires folding and suturing of the tissues (plication). In order to perform the procedure, the pleural surface may require an operative procedure such as pneumonolysis (separation of the surface of the lung which has become adherent to the inside surface of the chest cavity). At the conclusion of the procedure, the endoscope and the trocar(s) are removed. A chest tube for drainage and re-expansion of the lung is usually inserted through the wound used for the thoracoscopy.

32656

The physician examines the inside of the chest cavity through either a rigid or flexible fiberoptic endoscope and removes the inside lining of the chest cavity (the parietal pleura). The physician makes a small incision between two ribs and by blunt dissection and the use of a trocar enters the thoracic cavity. The endoscope is passed through the trocar and into the chest cavity. The lung is usually partially collapsed by instilling air into the chest through the trocar or the lung may be collapsed through a special double lumen endotracheal tube inserted through the mouth into the trachea. The contents of the chest cavity are examined by direct visualization and/or by the use of a video camera. Still photographs may be taken as part of the procedure. A second and/or third trocar and instruments may be inserted into the chest cavity through a second and/or third wound in the chest. Under direct visualization through the endoscope the physician manipulates the instruments inserted through the secondary sites and strips away the parietal pleura from the inside surface of the chest. At the conclusion of the procedure, the endoscope and the trocar(s) are removed. A chest tube for drainage and re-expansion of the lung is usually inserted through the wound used for the thoracoscopy.

32657

The physician removes a wedge-shaped portions of a lobe of one or both lungs through either a rigid or flexible fiberoptic endoscope. The physician makes a small incision between two ribs and by blunt dissection and the use of a trocar enters the thoracic cavity. The endoscope is passed through the trocar and into the chest cavity. The lung is usually partially collapsed by instilling air into the chest through the trocar or the lung may be collapsed through a special double lumen endotracheal tube inserted through the mouth into the trachea. The contents of the chest cavity are examined by direct visualization and/or by the use of a video camera. Still photographs may be taken as part of the procedure. A second and/or third trocar and instruments may be inserted into the chest cavity through a second and/or third incision in the chest. Under direct visualization through the endoscope, the physician manipulates the instruments inserted through the secondary sites; and clamps the healthy portions of the lung surrounding the area to be removed. With the special clamps in place, the portion of lung is removed by cutting the lung tissue isolated by the clamps. The cut portions of the remaining lung tissue are repaired by suturing or clipping with surgical clips. At the conclusion of the procedure, the endoscope and the trocar(s) are removed. A chest tube for drainage and re-expansion of the lung is usually inserted through the wound initially created for the thoracoscope insertion.

32658

The physician examines the inside of the pericardial sac through either a rigid or flexible fiberoptic endoscope and removes a blood clot or foreign body. The procedure can be done under local or general anesthesia. The physician makes a small incision between two ribs and by blunt dissection and the use of a trocar enters the thoracic cavity. The endoscope is passed through the trocar and into the chest cavity. The lung is usually partially collapsed by instilling air into the chest through the trocar or, if general anesthesia is used, the lung may be collapsed through a special double lumen endotracheal tube inserted through the mouth into the trachea. The endoscope is advanced to and into the pericardial sac as the physician views the structures and the anatomy of the area through the scope. The contents of the pericardial sac are examined by direct visualization and/or by the use of a video camera. Still photographs may be taken as part of the procedure. The clot and/or foreign body is identified and removed using a device through the endoscope or using a second instrument introduced into the area through a second insertion site in the chest. At the conclusion of the procedure, the endoscope and the trocar are withdrawn. A chest tube for drainage and re-expansion of the lung is usually inserted through the wound used for the thoracoscopy.

32659

The physician operates on the pericardial sac (the sac surrounding the heart) through either a rigid or flexible fiberoptic endoscope and creates a hole in the pericardial sac for drainage. The procedure can be done under local or general anesthesia. The physician makes a small incision between two ribs and by blunt dissection and the use of a trocar enters the thoracic cavity. The endoscope is passed through the trocar and into the chest cavity. The lung is usually partially

collapsed by instilling air into the chest through the trocar or, if general anesthesia is used, the lung may be collapsed through a special double lumen endotracheal tube inserted through the mouth into the trachea. The endoscope is advanced to and into the pericardial sac as the physician views the structures and the anatomy of the area through the scope. The contents of the pericardial sac are examined by direct visualization and/or by the use of a video camera. Still photographs may be taken as part of the procedure. Using an instrument introduced through the endoscope or through a second wound in the chest, the physician creates an opening in the pericardial sac to allow constant drainage from the sac. The drainage opening is made by either the creation of a window (a flap) in the pericardium or by resecting (cutting away) a portion of the pericardium. At the conclusion of the procedure, the endoscope and the trocar are withdrawn. A chest tube for drainage and re-expansion of the lung is usually inserted through the wound used for the thoracoscopy.

32660

The physician removes the pericardial sac through either a rigid or flexible fiberoptic endoscope. The physician makes a small incision between two ribs and by blunt dissection and the use of a trocar enters the thoracic cavity. The endoscope is passed through the trocar and into the chest cavity. The lung is usually partially collapsed by instilling air into the chest through the trocar or the lung may be collapsed through a special double lumen endotracheal tube inserted through the mouth into the trachea. The endoscope is advanced to and into the pericardial sac as the physician views the structures and the anatomy of the area through the scope. The contents of the pericardial sac are examined by direct visualization and/or by the use of a video camera. Still photographs may be taken as part of the procedure. Using instruments introduced through a second and/or third wound in the chest, and manipulated by direct vision through the endoscope, the physician removes the pericardial sac. At the conclusion of the procedure, the endoscope and the trocar are withdrawn. A chest tube for drainage and re-expansion of the lung is usually inserted through the wound used for the thoracoscopy.

32661

The physician examines the inside of the pericardial sac through either a rigid or flexible fiberoptic endoscope and removes a cyst, tumor, or mass lesion inside the pericardial sac. The procedure can be performed under local or general anesthesia. The physician makes a small incision between two ribs and by blunt dissection and the use of a trocar enters the thoracic cavity. The endoscope is passed through the trocar and into the chest cavity. The lung is usually partially collapsed by instilling air into the chest through the trocar or, if general anesthesia is used, the lung may be collapsed through a special double lumen endotracheal tube inserted through the mouth into the trachea. The endoscope is advanced to and into the pericardial sac as the physician views the structures and the anatomy of the area through the scope. The contents of the pericardial sac are examined by direct visualization and/or by the use of a video camera. Still photographs may be taken as part of the procedure. The cyst, tumor, or mass is identified and removed using instruments guided through the endoscope or by using instruments introduced into the area through a second and/or third insertion site in the chest. At the conclusion of the procedure, the endoscope and the trocar are withdrawn. A chest tube for drainage and re-expansion of the lung is usually inserted through the wound initially created for the thorascope insertion.

32662

The physician removes a cyst, tumor, or mass from the mediastinum through either a rigid or flexible fiberoptic endoscope. The procedure can be done under local or general anesthesia. The physician makes a small incision between two ribs and by blunt dissection and the use of a trocar enters the thoracic cavity. The endoscope is passed through the trocar and into the chest cavity. The lung is usually partially collapsed by instilling air into the chest through the trocar or, if general anesthesia is used, the lung may be collapsed through a special double lumen endotracheal tube inserted through the mouth into the trachea. As the physician views the structures and the anatomy of the area through the endoscope, the endoscope is advanced to and into the mediastinum (area inside the center of the chest cavity between the lungs). The contents of the mediastinal space are examined by direct visualization and/or by the use of a video camera. Still photographs may be taken as part of the procedure. The cyst, tumor, or mass is identified and removed using instruments guided through the endoscope or by using instruments introduced into the area through a second and/or third insertion site in the chest. At the conclusion of the procedure, the endoscope and the trocar are withdrawn. A chest tube for drainage and re-expansion of the lung is usually inserted through the wound used for the thoracoscopy.

32663

The physician removes all or a segmental portion of a lobe of one lung through either a rigid or flexible fiberoptic endoscope. The physician makes a small incision between two ribs and by blunt dissection and the use of a trocar enters the thoracic cavity. The endoscope is passed through the trocar and into the chest cavity. The lung is usually partially collapsed by instilling air into the chest through the trocar or the lung may be collapsed through a special double lumen endotracheal tube inserted through the mouth into the trachea. The contents of the chest cavity are examined by direct visualization and/or by the use of a video camera. Still photographs may be taken as

part of the procedure. Additional instruments may be inserted into the chest cavity through a second and/or third wound in the chest. Under direct visualization through the endoscope, the physician manipulates the instruments inserted through the secondary sites and clamps the blood vessels and bronchial tubes going to the area of lung to be removed. With the special clamps in place the portion of lung is removed by dividing the vessel and bronchial tubes isolated by the clamps. Any cut portions of the remaining lung tissue are repaired by suturing or clipping with surgical clips. At the conclusion of the procedure, the endoscope and the trocar(s) are removed. A chest tube for drainage and re-expansion of the lung is usually inserted through the wound used for the thoracoscopy.

32664

The physician performs a sympathectomy inside of the chest cavity through either a rigid or flexible fiberoptic endoscope. The procedure can be done under local or general anesthesia. The physician makes a small incision between two ribs and by blunt dissection and the use of a trocar enters the thoracic cavity. The endoscope is passed through the trocar and into the chest cavity. The lung is usually partially collapsed by instilling air into the chest through the trocar or, if general anesthesia is used, the lung may be collapsed through a special double lumen endotracheal tube inserted through the mouth into the trachea. The contents of the chest cavity are examined by direct visualization and/or by the use of a video camera. Still photographs may be taken as part of the procedure. A second and/or third trocar and instruments may be inserted into the chest cavity through a second and/or third wound in the chest. Under direct visualization through the endoscope, the physician manipulates the instruments inserted through the secondary sites and localizes and isolates a portion of the sympathetic nerves as they course deeply through the chest. The sympathectomy is accomplished by clipping and/or cutting the nerves. At the conclusion of the procedure, the endoscope and the trocar(s) are removed. A chest tube for drainage and re-expansion of the lung is usually inserted through the wound used for the thoracoscopy.

32665

The physician repairs a diseased and malfunctioning esophagus by operating through a series of several ports through the chest wall, guided under direct visualization through an endoscope introduced into the chest cavity. The physician makes a small incision between two ribs and by blunt dissection and the use of a trocar enters the thoracic cavity. The endoscope is passed through the trocar and into the chest cavity. The lung is usually partially collapsed by instilling air into the chest through the trocar or the lung may be collapsed through a special double lumen endotracheal tube inserted through the mouth into

CPT® Lay Descriptions

the trachea. The contents of the chest cavity are examined by direct visualization and/or by the use of a video camera. Still photographs may be taken as part of the procedure. Several other trocars and instruments are inserted into the chest cavity through a series of similar puncture wounds placed at various locations in the chest. A second fiberoptic endoscope is passed through the mouth and guided into the esophagus just above the stomach to assist in the procedure. Under direct visualization through the chest endoscope, the physician manipulates the instruments inserted through the secondary chest sites and operates on the esophagus just above its junction with the stomach. The esophagus is presented to the physician by flexing the tip of the scope inside the esophagus. The outer longitudinal muscle of the esophagus is identified, and cut in a longitudinal fashion and the incision is carried down through the circular muscle layer of the esophagus. The length of the incision is carried onto the surface of the stomach about one centimeter. The depth of the incision in the esophageal wall is down to but not through the mucosal tissues lining the inside of the esophagus. Care is taken not to enter the inside of the esophagus. The incision relaxes the esophagus just above the stomach and allows food to more easily enter the stomach in those patients who have difficulty swallowing due to disease in this area of the esophagus. At the conclusion of the procedure, the endoscope and the trocar(s) are removed. A chest tube for drainage and re-expansion of the lung is usually inserted through the wound used for the thoracoscopy.

32800

The physician repairs a hernia of the chest wall that allows the bulging of the lung through a defect in the chest wall. The physician makes an incision through the skin overlying the defect and carries the incision down to the inside lining of the chest cavity. The defect is repaired by the folding and suturing of tissues or the rotation of muscle and/or thick fibrous tissue flaps over the area and suturing of the flap over the defect. Alternately, the defect can be covered by a synthetic mesh material which is sutured in place. The incision is then closed in layers of sutures.

32810

The physician treats a draining empyema (accumulation of pus in the chest cavity) by resecting a rib, irrigating the empyema space with an antibiotic solution intermittently over an extended period of time, and then closing of the empyema space in six to eight weeks. This code reports the closure portion only.

32815

The physician repairs a major bronchial fistula (an abnormal passageway between the remaining end of a bronchial tube and the chest that occurs sometimes after the removal of a lung or portion of a lung). The

physician enters the chest cavity through a vertical incision made in the middle of the front of the chest. The incision is carried down to the sternum which is split in order to enter the chest cavity at the root of the lung near the center of the chest. The fistula exposure often requires the resection of one or two of the upper ribs. The end of the bronchial tube is located and the stump of the bronchial tube is reamputated and the inside lining of the bronchial tube is treated with silver nitrate to destroy the mucus forming cells lining the bronchus. The stump is then sutured or stapled. The chest defect created is repaired and the sternum closed using wire sutures and the skin closed in layers of sutures. A chest tube may be inserted into the chest cavity for drainage closed

32820

The physician repairs and reconstructs the chest wall following a major disfiguring injury to the chest (e.g. a shotgun blast). Using prosthetic materials, muscle and skin flaps and possibly skin grafts, the surgeon repairs a large defect(s) in the chest wall. This may require the use of one or more stages to finish the reconstruction.

32850

The physician removes one or both lungs from a donor who has sustained devastating brain injuries such that the donor has been declared "brain dead." Prior to the removal of the organs, the surgeon maintains treatment of the patient to assure adequate functioning of the heart, lungs and circulatory system while preparations are made for surgery. The physician makes a long, mid-line vertical incision through all the layers of the skin down to the sternum bone. The sternum is split and the chest cavity entered. During the removal of the lung(s) the patient is usually placed on a cardiopulmonary bypass machine to maintain circulation to the organs. One or both lungs are removed in one block by dividing the trachea and the major arteries and veins that carry blood to and from the heart. The lung(s) is then transported under refrigeration to the recipient patient who may be hundreds of miles away. The donor patient is taken off life support and pronounced dead.

32851

The physician performs a single lung transplantation of the recipient patient. The physician makes a long, mid-line vertical incision through all the layers of the skin down to the sternum bone. The sternum is split and the chest cavity entered. The patient's original lung is deflated and the root of the lung isolated and the major arteries and veins that carry blood to and from the heart are identified and divided. The main bronchial tube to that lung is severed and the lung removed. The donor lung is placed in the chest cavity and its bronchial tube and arteries and veins sutured to the patients where the former lung was attached. Circulation and functioning of the donor lung is assured and the chest is closed. The sternum is closed using wire sutures and the skin closed in layers of sutures. A chest tube(s) is inserted into the chest cavity for drainage. During the procedure the patient's oxygenation and circulation is maintained by the patient's own heart and other lung.

32852

The physician performs a single lung transplantation of the recipient patient. The physician makes a long, mid-line vertical incision through all the layers of the skin down to the sternum bone. The sternum is split and the chest cavity entered. During the transplantation of the lung, the patient is placed on a cardiopulmonary bypass machine to maintain circulation to the organs. The patient's original lung is deflated and the root of the lung isolated and the major arteries and veins that carry blood to and from the heart are identified and divided. The main bronchial tube to that lung is severed and the lung removed. The donor lung is placed in the chest cavity and its bronchial tube and arteries and veins sutured to the site where the former lung was attached. Circulation and functioning of the donor lung is assured and the chest is closed. The sternum is closed using wire sutures and the skin closed in layers of sutures. A chest tube(s) is inserted into the chest cavity for drainage.

32853

The physician performs a double lung transplantation of the recipient patient. The physician makes a long, midline vertical incision through all the layers of the skin down to the sternum bone. The sternum is split and the chest cavity entered. The patient's original lungs are deflated sequentially and the root of the lung isolated and the major arteries and veins that carry blood to and from the heart are identified and divided. The tracheal tube to the lungs is severed and the lungs removed. The donor lungs are placed in the chest cavity either as a single unit or one at at time. The tracheal tube and arteries and veins sutured to the site where the former lungs were attached. Circulation and functioning of the donor lungs are assured and the chest is closed. The sternum is closed using wire sutures and the skin closed in layers of sutures. Chest tubes are inserted into the chest cavities for drainage.

32854

The physician performs a double lung transplantation of the recipient patient. The surgeon makes a long, midline vertical incision through all the layers of the skin down to the sternum bone. The sternum is split and the chest cavity entered. During the transplantation of the lungs, the patient is placed on a cardiopulmonary bypass machine to maintain circulation to the organs. The patient's original lungs are deflated and the root of the lung isolated and the major arteries and veins that carry blood to and from the heart are identified and divided. The tracheal tube to the lungs is severed and the lungs removed. The

donor lungs are placed in the chest cavity either as a single unit or one at at time. The tracheal tube and arteries and veins sutured to the site where the former lungs were attached. Circulation and functioning of the donor lungs are assured and the chest is closed. The sternum is closed using wire sutures and the skin closed in layers of sutures. Chest tubes are inserted into the chest cavities for drainage.

32900

The physician resects a rib(s) without entering the chest cavity. The surgeon make an incision in the skin overlying the rib to be removed and carries that incision through the tissues down to the rib. The tissues are dissected away from the rib taking care not to puncture through the pleural membrane on the inside surface of the rib. This avoids the egress of air into the chest cavity. With the tissue removed from the surface of the rib, the rib is cut at two places and the intervening section removed. The resulting defect may be covered by the use of muscle flaps grafted to the area. The remaining tissues and skin are closed by suturing in layers.

32905

The physician performs a thoracoplasty which is the removal of the skeletal support of a portion of the chest to treat chronic thoracic empyema (accumulation of pus in the chest cavity) when there is insufficient lung tissue to fill the chest space. The procedure is carried out primarily on the upper chest. An incision is made through the skin down to the ribs. The Schede operation consists of the extensive unroofing of an empyema space by resecting the overlying ribs and portions of membrane lining the chest cavity (parietal pleural peel). The muscles in the area are partially closed over gauze packing and the skin partially closed by suturing in layers. As the packing is withdrawn in stages a few days later, it is hoped that freshly granulation tissue fills in the space formerly occupied by the empyema. The original Schede type operation is rarely performed but several modifications are currently done.

32906

The physician closes a bronchopleural fistula and performs a thoracoplasty which is the removal of the skeletal support of a portion of the chest to treat chronic thoracic empyema (accumulation of pus in the chest cavity) when there is insufficient lung tissue to fill the chest space. The procedure is carried out primarily on the upper chest. An incision is made through the skin down to the ribs. The Schede operation consists of the extensive unroofing of an empyema space by resecting the overlying ribs and portions of membrane lining the chest cavity (parietal pleural peel). The bronchopleural fistula (an abnormal passageway between the remaining end of a bronchial tube that occurs sometimes after the removal of a lung or portion of a lung) is identified and resected, then closed by suturing. Closure of the

CPT® Lay Descriptions

fistula sometime requires the use of muscle flap grafts taken from outside the chest cavity. After the repair of the fistula, the muscles in the area are partially closed over gauze packing and the skin partially closed by suturing in layers. As the packing is withdrawn in stages a few days later, it is hoped that freshly granulation tissue fills in the space formerly occupied by the empyema. The original Schede type operation is rarely performed but several modifications are currently done.

32940

The physician opens the chest cavity and separates the surface of the lung which has become adherent to the inside surface of the chest cavity. Using a scalpel, the surgeon makes an incision around the side of the chest between two of the ribs. The incision is carried through all the tissue layers down to the tissue lining the chest cavity. Rib spreaders are inserted into the wound and the ribs are spread apart exposing the membrane lining the chest cavity (the parietal pleura). The surgeon separates the tissue between the periosteal membrane adherent to the inside surface of the lung and the parietal pleural membrane. This allows the movement of the lung within the chest cavity. The area or space created is packed or filled and the incision is closed in layers of sutures.

32960

The physician partially collapses a lung by injecting air into the chest cavity by puncturing through the space between the ribs. Using a needle attached to a syringe the physician carefully passes the needle over the top of a rib and punctures through the chest tissues and enters the pleural cavity. With the end of the needle in the chest cavity, the physician injects air into the chest cavity to create a partial collapse of one lung, most commonly used to treat tuberculosis. A small plastic tube may be passed through the chest and left in place for repeated injections of air.

32997

The physician performs total lavage on one lung. The physician views the airway using a fiberoptic or rigid bronchoscopy. The airway is anesthetized and the bronchoscope is introduced through the nasal or oral cavity and advanced to the lungs. Saline is introduced through the bronchoscope and the lung tissue is washed or bathed. The saline is removed by suction and the solution containing the cells that has been obtained in the procedure may be sent to pathology to diagnosis certain diseases, such as cancer. The procedure also may be performed to treat specific diseases or injuries.

33010–33011

The physician drains fluid from the pericardial space. The physician may perform this procedure using anatomic landmarks or under fluoroscopic or echocardiographic (ultrasound) guidance (separately reported). The physician places a long needle below

the sternum and directs it into the pericardial space. When pericardial fluid is aspirated, the physician may advance a guidewire through the needle into the pericardial space and exchange the needle over the guidewire for a drainage catheter. The physician removes as much pericardial fluid as is required, removes the needle or catheter, and dresses the wound. Report 33011 for each subsequent pericardiocentesis.

33015

The physician drains fluid from the pericardial space. The physician may perform this procedure using anatomic landmarks or under fluoroscopic or echocardiographic (ultrasound) guidance (separately reported). The physician places a long needle below the sternum and directs it into the pericardial space. When pericardial fluid flows back through the needle, the physician passes a guidewire through the needle into the pericardial space. The physician then exchanges the needle over the wire for an indwelling drainage catheter. The physician then attaches the catheter to a sterile drainage bag, sutures the indwelling catheter into place on the chest wall, and dresses the wound.

33020

The physician removes a clot or foreign body from the pericardial space. The physician performs a midline sternotomy, incising skin, fascia, and the sternum. The pericardium is incised and the clot or foreign body is removed. The pericardium is repaired loosely, leaving gaps for blood and fluid to drain into the pleural space. The sternum is reanastomosed with sternal wires and the skin is closed in sutured layers.

33025

The physician gains access to the pericardium through an incision through the sternum (median sternotomy), the subxiphoid space or the chest wall (lateral thoracotomy). The physician then makes an incision in the pericardium and creates an opening in the pericardium large enough to allow drainage of pericardial fluid into the pleural space. The physician then closes the sternal or chest wall incision and dresses the wound. The physician may leave chest tubes and/or a mediastinal drainage tube in place following the procedure.

33030–33031

The physician gains access to the pericardium through an incision through the sternum (median sternotomy). The physician then cuts away most or all of the pericardial tissue while the heart is still beating (without cardiopulmonary bypass), taking care to leave the phrenic nerves intact. The physician then closes the sternal or chest wall incision and dresses the wound. The physician may leave chest tubes and/or a mediastinal drainage tube in place following the procedure. Report 33031 if the procedure is performed with a cardiopulmonary bypass.

33050

The physician gains access to the pericardium through an incision through the sternum (median sternotomy) or the chest wall (lateral thoracotomy). The physician places cardiopulmonary bypass catheters (usually through incisions in the right atrial appendage and aorta or femoral artery). The physician stops the heart by infusing cardioplegia solution into the coronary circulation. The physician cuts away the pericardial cyst or tumor while the heart is still. The physician takes the patient off cardiopulmonary bypass, closes the surgical incisions and dresses the sternal or chest wall wound. The physician may leave chest tubes and/or a mediastinal drainage tube in place following the procedure.

33120

Cardiopulmonary bypass is employed. Venous tubes are placed in both caval veins. The part of the heart which is opened depends on where the tumor is located. Every effort is made to avoid making an incision in any ventricular wall. After the heart is opened, the tumor is resected with a margin of normal heart tissue. Any problems created by this resection (damage to heart valves, holes in the walls between heart chambers or the outside of the heart, injury to coronary arteries) are then repaired. All holes in the heart are closed. Cardiopulmonary bypass is stopped when heart function returns.

33130

Cardiopulmonary bypass is only required if a significant portion of the heart or major vessel must be removed with the tumor to get a margin of normal tissue around the tumor. The tumor and surrounding normal tissue are removed. Defects created in the heart, coronary arteries or major vessels are repaired.

33140–33141

The physician performs transmyocardial laser revascularization to restore the flow of blood and oxygen to the heart. Varying approaches may be employed. The procedure is frequently performed on the beating heart, although cardiopulmonary bypass may be initiated. In the beating heart: Using a scalpel the physician makes a 10 centimeters to 15 centimeters incision on the left side of the chest between the ribs and exposes the surface of the heart. The area of ischemia (in still vital tissue) is identified. A laser is inserted through the chest opening and is fired (between heartbeats) through the filled left ventricle. Between 10 channels to 40 channels (small holes) are created to encourage new capillary growth in the area. As the channels are created pressure is applied to each to help close the openings. When the procedure is completed the laser is removed and the wound is closed with layered sutures. If cardiopulmonary bypass was initiated it is

discontinued, the patient is rewarmed, and the heartbeat is restored. Report 33140 if the transmyocardial laser revascularization is performed alone. Report 33141 when it is performed at the time of another open cardiac procedure.

33200–33201

The left or right chest cavity is opened, depending on where the electrodes are to be placed and on which part of the heart has been used before. After the heart is exposed, electrodes are affixed to the appropriate areas of heart muscle. A pocket for the pacemaker generator is made and a subcutaneous tunnel is created through which the pacemaker wires travel from the heart to the generator pocket. The wires are tested, guided through the tunnel, and connected to the generator. The generator is placed in its pocket. The incisions are closed. Report 33201 if exposure to the heart is gained through an upper midline abdominal incision around the xiphoid process of the sternum.

33206–33211

Access to the central caval veins is obtained through the subclavian vein or jugular vein. The vein is penetrated with a large needle and a wire is passed through it. A fluoroscope (separately reported) is used to guide the wire into the right atrium. A pocket for the pacemaker generator is created and the wire is tested. The wire is connected to the generator and the generator is closed in its pocket. Report 33207 if the guide and pacemaker wires are placed in the right ventricle; report 33208 if elements of 33206 and 33207 are combined; report 33210 or 33211 if the pacemaker generator is not implanted but temporarily placed outside the body and a single (33210) or dual (33211) transvenous electrode(s) placed.

33212–33214

This operation proceeds under the assumption that permanent pacing wires are already in place. The old pacemaker generator pocket is opened, the old generator removed and the pacer wires tested. If a pacer wire is defective it is replaced and retested. The wires are connected to a new generator. The generator is placed into the old pocket and the pocket is closed. Report 33213 if inserting or replacing a dual chamber pacemaker pulse generator; report 33214 when a single chamber system is converted to a dual chamber system and a second lead is placed.

33216–33217

The operation is done if interrogation of the single chamber pacemaker generator or single chamber cardioverter-defibrillator generator suggests that there is a problem with either the electrode wire itself or the position of the wire. The generator is removed and the wire is tested. If the wire is not defective, it is repositioned. It is then reattached to the generator and tested. If the wire is defective, it is replaced. The old generator is then reattached to the wire. The

CPT® Lay Descriptions

generator is then replaced in its pocket and the pocket is closed. Report 33217 if both electrodes on a dual chamber permanent pacemaker or pacing cardioverter-defibrillator are tested.

33218–33220

In 33218, the pacemaker or cardioverter/defibrillator pocket is opened and the generator is removed. The electrode wire is tested. Repairs are performed. The wire is retested and then reconnected to the generator. The generator is placed back in its pocket and the pocket is closed. Report repair code 33220 if the pacemaker or cardioverter-defibrillator is a dual chamber model with two electrodes.

33222–33223

This operation is done for patient comfort, impending exposure of the generator through the skin, or complications from the original generator placement (eg., infection, bleeding) The pocket is opened. The generator is removed and the pocket is assessed. If it can be reused, it is revised. If not, a new pocket is formed somewhere within the reach of the pacemaker wires. The wires are then brought through a new subcutaneous tunnel into the new pocket and connected to a new or the old generator. The old pocket is closed and the generator is placed in the new pocket which is then closed. If the old pocket is to be used, the generator is simply reinserted and the pocket closed. Report 33223 when a cardioverter-defibrillator pocket is revised.

33233

In 33233, only the pulse generator is removed. The pacemaker generator pocket is opened. The generator is disconnected from the wire(s) and removed. The wire(s) are left in place in the pocket and the pocket is closed or a new pacemaker generator is inserted. If a new pacemaker is inserted, it is reported separately.

33234–33235

In 33234 and 33235, only the transvenous electrode(s) are removed. For 33234, the generator pocket is opened and the wire is disconnected from the generator. The wire is dissected from the scar tissue which has formed around it. Once the wire is completely freed, it is twisted in a direction opposite to that used for insertion (counter clockwise). The wire is then withdrawn. Bleeding from the tracts leading to the vein is controlled with sutures. A new wire may be placed, but is reported separately. Report 33235 for a dual lead system (removal of two wires).

33236–33237

Code 33236 reports the removal of a single lead epicardial pacemaker system and electrodes. The old pacemaker pocket is opened and the generator is removed. The old wires are cut and the incision is closed. The old chest incision is opened. The wires are pulled into the chest and they are followed onto the heart surface. The electrodes are then detached

from the heart. The chest incision is closed. Report 33237 if a dual lead epicardial system is being removed.

33238

Code 33238 reports thoracotomy with removal of transvenous electrode(s) only. The right chest is opened and the superior caval vein is dissected out. Tourniquets are placed around the vein above and below the planned site of opening into the vein. The tourniquets are tightened and a hole is made in the prior to opening the chest, the pacemaker pocket was opened, the generator removed and the wires were cut. The cut ends of the wires are pulled out through the hole in the caval vein. The ends of the wires which are still in the heart are twisted counter clockwise until they are free and then are withdrawn through the caval vein. The hole in the caval veins are closed and the tourniquets are released. The chest is then closed.

33240

This operation is done only when defibrillator electrodes are already in place. The previous pocket is opened or a new pocket is created for the defibrillator generator. AICD pulse generators are implanted subcutaneously usually in an either an infraclavicular or abdominal pocket. The electrodes are tested. The electrodes are then connected to the defibrillator and it is placed in the pocket. The pocket is then closed.

33241

In 33241, only the AICD pulse generator is removed. The subcutaneous generator pocket is opened and the generator is removed. The electrodes are detached from the generator and the electrodes are placed in the pocket. The pocket is then closed or a new cardioverter-debrillator generator is inserted.

33243

In 33243, only the electrodes are removed. The generator pocket is opened and the electrode wires are disconnected. The old chest incision is opened and the electrodes are dissected out and removed. The chest incision is closed.

33244

Code 33244 reports removal of electrodes only by transvenous extraction which is currently the most common technique for removing AICD electrodes since most cardioverter-defibrillator electrodes are now placed transvenously. The generator pocket is opened and the wire is disconnected from the generator. The wire is dissected from the scar tissue which has formed around it. Once the wire is completely freed, it is twisted in a direction opposite to that use for insertion (counter clockwise). The wire is then withdrawn. Bleeding from the tracts leading to the vein is controlled with sutures. A new wire may be placed, but is reported separately.

33245–33249

An implantable cardioverter-defibrillator (ICD) is a device designed to administer an electric shock to control cardiac arrhythmias and restore a normal heart beat. In 33245, placement of epicardial electrodes (leads) is performed by chest incision (thoracotomy). The chest cavity is opened. After the heart is exposed, electrodes are affixed to the appropriate areas of heart muscle. The electrodes are tested and then tunneled either under the costal margin to the upper abdomen where the pulse generator is placed or to the infraclavicular area if the generator is in that area. The chest is then closed. Report 33245 for either initial implantation or subsequent replacement of epicardial electrodes only. In 33246, in addition to epicardial electrode placement, the ICD generator is inserted. A subcutaneous pocket is created for the generator. The electrode wires are then tested, tunneled, and connected to the pulse generator. The generator is then placed in the pocket. All incisions are closed. Report 33246 when both ICD epicardial electrodes and the pulse generator are placed during the same surgical session. Code 33249 reports insertion of a pulse generator with transvenous electrode placement. Transvenous placement is currently the most common technique for placing ICD electrodes. Local anesthesia is administered. An incision is made in the infraclavicular area. The subcutaneous tissue is opened and a pocket is created for the pulse generator. Transvenous electrode placement is performed under separately reportable fluoroscopic guidance. The electrode catheter is advanced through the superior vena cava into the heart and placed in the appropriate site in the right ventricle (single chamber system) or in the right ventricle and atrium (dual chamber system). Multiple leads may be required for both single and dual chamber systems. Once all leads are placed, they are tested and connected to the pulse generator which is then placed in the previously prepared pocket. All incisions are closed.

33250

Cardiopulmonary bypass is usually required. The heart is exposed through the sternum. A mapping grid of electrodes is placed over the surface of the beating heart. The location of the arrhythmia source is determined. The source is then destroyed using electrical current, freezing, or cutting. Any bleeding is controlled with sutures. The chest is closed.

33251

Cardiopulmonary bypass is required. The heart is exposed through the sternum. A mapping grid of electrodes is placed over the surface of the beating heart. The right atrium is opened and a long cut is made around the tricuspid valve until the cut on the outside of the heart is seen. Any other focuses of the arrhythmia are destroyed with electrical current or freezing. The right atrium is closed. Cardiopulmonary bypass is discontinued when heart function returns.

33253

Atrial fibrillation is rapid, randomized muscle contraction of the atrial myocardium causing an irregular, rapid heart rate. The physician creates multiple incision lines to obliterate aberrant conduction of the atria. The physician performs a midline sternotomy, incising the skin, fascia, muscles, and sternum. The pericardium is incised and lines are placed for cardiopulmonary bypass. When bypass is established, the left and right atria are incised through to the endocardium, disrupting extranodal pacers. The atria incision lines are reanastomosed. The pericardium is repaired loosely, leaving gaps for blood and fluid to drain into the pleural space. The sternum is reanastomosed with sternal wires and the skin is closed in sutured layers.

33261

Following initiation of cardiopulmonary bypass, the physician exposes the heart through the sternum. A mapping grid of electrodes is placed over the surface of the beating heart. The location of the arrhythmia source is determined. The source is destroyed using electrical current, freezing or cutting, though not in the tricuspid valve. Any bleeding is controlled with sutures. The chest is closed.

33282–33284

The physician implants or removes an electronic device that is capable of recording heart rates and rhythms for over one year. In 33282, the physician uses a scalpel to make an incision and dissects down to the level of subcutaneous tissue located over the left pectoral or mammary area. A cardiac event (loop) recorder is implanted into the subcutaneous tissue. Electrodes that sense heart activity are located on the surface of the event recorder, making it unnecessary to place transvenous leads. The recorder continuously monitors the heart's electrical activity in a "loop" with new ECG information replacing old information. If symptoms occur the patient uses an external hand-held device to freeze a record of the event. In 33284, the physician removes the event recorder when sufficient information regarding the heart's activities has been obtained or when the batteries run out by incising down to the level of the recorder and removing it. In either surgery the incision is closed with sutures. This type of recorder is capable of storing many separate events. When appropriate a special "programmer" is used by the physician to retrieve the information that can be displayed, stored or printed.

33300–33305

The heart can be exposed through the sternum or either chest cavity (usually the left chest.) The pericardial sac is opened. Sutures with little patches of Teflon felt to closed the hole(s). The entire heart is inspected for additional holes. The chest is closed. Report 33305 if blood pressure must be supported during the repair.

33310–33315

The physician exposes the heart via the sternum. The foreign body is located by carefully feeling the heart. If possible, the object is removed from the surface of the heart. If necessary, a hole is made in one of the ventricles to remove the object. The holes are closed with sutures and small reinforcing patches of Teflon felt. Report 33310 if cardiopulmonary bypass is not initiated; report 33315 if cardiopulmonary bypass is initiated.

33320–33322

The physician gains access to the mediastinum through an incision through the sternum (median sternotomy) or the chest wall (lateral thoracotomy). The physician repairs the aorta or great vessels while the heart is still beating. The physician closes the surgical incisions and dresses the sternal or chest wall wound. The physician may leave chest tubes and/or a mediastinal drainage tube in place following the procedure. Report 33321 if performed with a shunt bypass; report 33322 if performed with a cardiopulmonary bypass.

33330

The physician gains access to the mediastinum through an incision through the sternum (median sternotomy) or the chest wall (lateral thoracotomy). The physician then sews in the aortic or great vessel graft while the heart is still beating. The physician closes the surgical incisions and dresses the sternal or chest wall wound. The physician may leave chest tubes and/or a mediastinal drainage tube in place following the procedure.

33332

The physician gains access to the mediastinum through an incision through the sternum (median sternotomy) or the chest wall (lateral thoracotomy). The physician uses purse string incisions to place a shunt (bypass) catheter around the abnormal area of the vessel to be repaired. The physician sews in the aortic or great vessel graft while the heart is still beating. The physician removes the bypass catheter, closes the surgical incisions and dresses the sternal or chest wall wound. The physician may leave chest tubes and/or a mediastinal drainage tube in place following the procedure.

33335

The physician gains access to the mediastinum through an incision through the sternum (median sternotomy) or the chest wall (lateral thoracotomy). The physician places cardiopulmonary bypass catheters usually through incisions in the right atrial appendage and aorta or femoral artery. The physician stops the heart by infusing cardioplegia solution into the coronary circulation. The physician sews in the aortic or great vessel graft while the heart is still. The physician takes the patient off cardiopulmonary bypass, closes the surgical incisions and dresses the

sternal or chest wall wound. The physician may leave chest tubes and/or a mediastinal drainage tube in place following the procedure.

33400

Cardiopulmonary bypass is initiated. The aorta is clamped from above the heart and a cold preserving solution is pumped through the heart. The aorta is opened near the valve. The spaces where the heart valve leaflets meet have been fused by inflammation and scarring in diseases requiring this operation. The scars between the leaflets are cut with a knife. The aorta is closed and the clamp is removed. Cardiopulmonary bypass is discontinued when heart function returns.

33401

This operation is of historical interest only. The following vessels are clamped or occluded with tourniquets: the superior caval vein, the inferior caval vein, and the aorta. The aorta is then quickly opened above the heart and the scar tissue between the valve leaflets are cut with a knife. The aorta is quickly closed and the clamps removed. The entire operation (except for opening and closing) must be done in no more than five minutes to prevent brain damage.

33403

Cardiopulmonary bypass is initiated. A purse string is placed in the left ventricular apex. The purse string is reinforced with small patches of Teflon felt. An incision is made in the center of the purse string. Blunt dilators are passed through the hole and across the aortic valve. Progressively larger dilators are inserted until the valve is wide open. The dilators break the scar tissues which are cut in an open aortic valvoplasty. The valve leaflets are frequently damaged to the point that the valve must be replaced. After the valve is fully dilated, the purse string is tied off. Cardiopulmonary bypass is discontinued when heart function returns.

33404

Cardiopulmonary bypass is required. A hole is made in the tip of the left ventricle and another is made in the aorta above the coronary arteries. The conduit is oriented so that the valve in it will only let blood flow out of the heart, but not back in. One end of the conduit is sewn to the hole in the tip of the heart. The other end is sewn to the hole in the aorta. Air is carefully removed from the heart and from the conduit. Cardiopulmonary bypass is discontinued when heart function returns.

33405

Cardiopulmonary bypass is initiated. A clamp is placed on the aorta well above the heart. A cold preserving solution is pumped into the coronary arteries to stop the heart. The aorta is opened just above the aortic valve. The valve leaflets are cut out and the annulus of the valve (ring of tissue where the valve leaflets normally attach to the aorta) is cleaned of calcium. The valve annulus size is measured and an appropriate artificial valve is selected. The artificial valve is then sewn to the valve annulus. The aorta is closed and the clamp is taken off. Cardiopulmonary bypass is discontinued when heart function returns.

33406

Cardiopulmonary bypass is initiated. A clamp is placed on the aorta well above the heart. A cold preserving solution is pumped into the coronary arteries to stop the heart. The aorta is opened just above the aortic valve. The valve leaflets are cut out and the annulus of the valve (ring of tissue where the valve leaflets normally attach to the aorta) is cleaned of calcium. At this point an allograft is selected. The tissue valve is then trimmed so that it can be sewn to the valve annulus. The aorta above the graft valve is trimmed so that the valve cusps can be suspended when the graft is in place. By doing so, the coronary arteries are not obstructed by the graft. The new valve is then sewn in place. The valve annulus size is measured and an appropriate artificial valve is selected. The artificial valve is sewn to the valve annulus. The aorta is closed and the clamp is taken off. Cardiopulmonary bypass is discontinued when heart function returns.

33410

Cardiopulmonary bypass is initiated. A clamp is placed on the aorta and above the heart. A cold preserving solution is pumped into the coronary arteries to stop the heart. The aorta is opened just above the aortic valve. The valve leaflets are cut out and the annulus of the valve (ring of tissue where the valve leaflets normally attach to the aorta) is cleaned of calcium. The valve annulus size is measured and an appropriate stentless tissue valve is selected, (the stentless valve is unique because unlike other valves it has no rigid external frame or sewing ring) and sutured directly into the aortic wall. The aorta is closed and the clamp is taken off. Cardiopulmonary bypass is discontinued when heart function returns. The wound is closed with layered suture.

33411

Cardiopulmonary bypass is initiated. A clamp is placed on the aorta well above the heart. A cold preserving solution is pumped into the coronary arteries to stop the heart. The aorta is opened just above the aortic valve. The valve leaflets are cut out and the annulus of the valve (ring of tissue where the valve leaflets normally attach to the aorta) is cleaned of calcium. At this point a homograft or a xenograph is selected. The tissue valve is trimmed so that it can be sewn to the valve annulus. The aorta above the graft valve is trimmed so that the valve cusps can be suspended when the graft is in place and so the coronary arteries are not obstructed by the graft. When the valve is sized, it must be greater than or equal to 19.0 mm on a normal sized adult. If a smaller

valve is inserted, the heart will slowly fail. To enlarge the valve, the aorta is cut longitudinally toward the heart and through the commissure (connecting point where two valve leaflets meet on the aortic wall) between the non-coronary leaflet (no coronary is near this leaflet) and the left coronary leaflet (leaflet near the left coronary artery) and across the valve annulus for a variable distance. The cut may need to extend onto the roof of the left atrium and onto the anterior leaflet of the mitral valve. The end of the cut is determined by the point at which the aortic root will accommodate at least a 19.0 mm valve. The anterior mitral leaflet, left atrial roof and the aorta are repaired with patches. The new valve is then sewn in place. The aorta is closed and the clamp is taken off. Cardiopulmonary bypass is discontinued when heart function returns.

33412

Cardiopulmonary bypass is initiated. A clamp is placed on the aorta well above the heart. A cold preserving solution is pumped into the coronary arteries to stop the heart. The aorta is opened just above the aortic valve. The valve leaflets are cut out and the annulus of the valve (ring of tissue where the valve leaflets normally attach to the aorta) is cleaned of calcium. At this point a homograft or a xenograph is selected. The tissue valve is then trimmed so that it can be sewn to the valve annulus. The aorta above the graft valve is trimmed so that the valve cusps can be suspended when the graft is in place and so the coronary arteries are not obstructed by the graft. When the valve is sized, it must be greater than or equal to 19.0 mm on a normal sized adult. If a smaller valve is inserted, the heart will slowly fail. The aorta is incised longitudinally toward a point just to the left of the right coronary artery. The cut is carried across the annulus and for a variable distance onto the right ventricular infundibulum. A triangular patch of pericardium or Dacron (a gusset, for example) is used to close the incision in the right ventricle and aorta and to enlarge the aortic annulus. The new valve is then sewn in place. The aorta is closed and the clamp is taken off. Cardiopulmonary bypass is discontinued when heart function returns.

33413

Cardiopulmonary bypass is initiated. The aorta and pulmonary artery are separated and the main pulmonary trunk is completely cleaned off. After the heart is stopped, the pulmonary trunk is detached from the branching point of the left and right pulmonary arteries. It is taken off the heart with a small lip of heart muscle. Care is taken when the muscle of interventricular septum is cut. It is possible to damage a large branch of the left anterior descending coronary artery when this muscle is cut. The aorta is then opened above the valve. The coronary arteries are detached from the aorta with a surrounding "button" of aortic wall. Next, the aortic valve and its annulus are removed from the heart. A length of the ascending aorta is also removed. The pulmonary artery is sewn to the heart in the aortic position. The commissures and cusps of the pulmonary valve are lined up to be in the same positions as their aortic counterparts were before the aortic valve was removed. The open end of the pulmonary artery is then sewn to the ascending aorta. The coronary arteries are re-implanted on the pulmonary artery in positions similar to their positions on the aorta. The pulmonary valve and artery from an organ donor are then sewn into the pulmonary position.

33414

The physician enlarges the aortic outflow track using what known as a Konno procedure. The physician performs a midline sternotomy, incising the skin, fascia, muscles, and sternum. The pericardium is incised and lines are placed for cardiopulmonary bypass. When bypass is established, the right ventricle is incised and the aortic outflow track is enlarged by incising the septum. Two patches are applied; the first is placed from the septum to the aortic annulus, enlarging the track. The second patch is placed from the base of the first patch at the septum, closing the right ventricle. The pericardium is repaired loosely, leaving gaps for blood and fluid to drain into the pleural space. The sternum is reanastomosed with sternal wires and the skin is closed in sutured layers.

33415–33416

Cardiopulmonary bypass is initiated. The aorta is opened and the left ventricular outflow tract is assessed below the valve. There is usually a clearly definable ring or shelf below the valve. This is taken off with a tool designed for the purpose. Usually, the left ventricular septal muscle is thickened. A trough of muscle tissue is then cut out of the left ventricular septal muscle. The aorta is closed. Cardiopulmonary bypass is discontinued when heart function returns. Report 33416 if there is no ring of subvalvular tissue to remove.

33417

Cardiopulmonary bypass is required. A piece of pericardium or Dacron is prepared. The aorta is clamped beyond the area of narrowing. The heart is then stopped with a cold preserving solution. The aorta is opened longitudinally across the area of narrowing. The aorta is then closed with a patch sewn onto the incision of the aorta. The clamp is then released. Cardiopulmonary bypass is discontinued when heart function returns.

33420

The left chest is opened. The pericardium is opened. A gloved finger is used to invert the left atrial appendage into the left atrium. The finger is placed across the mitral valve. Blunt tearing is used to open the areas between the leaflets, which have been obliterated by scar tissue and inflammation. The finger is removed and the chest is closed.

33422

Cardiopulmonary bypass is initiated. The left atrium is opened from the right side. The mitral valve is exposed. The scar tissue between the lateral ends of the valve leaflets is divided sharply. The left atrium is closed. Cardiopulmonary bypass is discontinued when heart function returns.

33425–33427

This operation is done to improve the ability of the mitral valve to close completely when the ventricle contracts. It is done in patients whose mitral valve has lost the ability to close normally. In almost all cases, this is the result of a mitral valve prolapse in which the mitral leaflets and the cords that tether them on the ventricle have become elongated. Cardiopulmonary bypass is initiated. The left atrium is opened and the mitral valve is then exposed. Redundant leaflet tissue is excised and defects in the valve leaflets are closed with sutures. The cords are also shortened with sutures. Valve closure is assessed after the repair. The left atrium is closed and cardiopulmonary bypass is discontinued when heart function returns. Report 33425 if the mitral valve diameter is enlarged requiring placement of a prosthetic ring. Report 33247 if a more extensive repair, including transfer of cords from the posterior leaflet to the anterior leaflet, is performed. A prosthetic ring may or may not be required with extensive reconstruction.

33430

Cardiopulmonary bypass is initiated. The left atrium is opened and the mitral valve is exposed. All leaflet tissue and its attached cords are cut out. Sutures are placed in the mitral annulus. The annulus is then sized and an appropriate artificial valve is selected (either a totally mechanical valve or a valve with plastic supports and tissue leaflets). The sutures are then passed through the sewing ring of the annulus and the sutures are tied down so the sewing ring is rightly adherent to the annulus. The left atrium is then closed. Cardiopulmonary bypass is discontinued when heart function returns.

33460

Cardiopulmonary bypass is initiated. The right atrium is opened and the tricuspid valve is exposed. The valve tissue and its cords are completely excised. The right atrium is closed. Cardiopulmonary bypass is discontinued when heart function returns.

33463–33464

Cardiopulmonary bypass is initiated with venous uptake tubes in both of the caval veins. The right atrium is opened valvuloplasty of the tricuspid valve almost always requires nothing more than reducing the diameter of the tricuspid valve. A double purse string of sutures is place around the circumference of the valve and tightened to reduce the valve diameter. The right atrium is then closed. Report 33464 if a stiff ring is used to the reduce the valve's diameter rather than purse strings.

33465

Cardiopulmonary bypass is initiated with venous uptake tubes in both caval veins. The right atrium is opened and the tricuspid valve leaflets are excised. A valve of an appropriate diameter is selected (usually it is a tissue/plastic valve, although a metal valve can also be used). Sutures are placed around the tricuspid valve annulus circumference. They are then brought through the sewing ring of the valve. The valve is then seated so that the sewing ring is resting on the annulus. The sutures are then tied tightly. The right atrium is closed. Cardiopulmonary bypass is discontinued when heart function returns.

33468

In this anomaly, the tricuspid valve annulus is displaced onto the right ventricle, the right ventricle becomes atrophied and the valve leaflets become tethered to the wall of the ventricle. Cardiopulmonary bypass is initiated with venous uptake tubes in both caval veins. The right atrium is opened. The valve is detached from the ventricular wall around its circumference. The edge of the cut valve is then sewn circumferentially around the lone port by the true junction of the right atrium and right ventricle. The right atrium is closed. Cardiopulmonary bypass is discontinued when heart function returns.

33470–33471

Cardiopulmonary bypass is not required. The heart is exposed through the sternum. A U-stitch reinforced with small patches of Teflon felt is placed in the right ventricular outflow tract muscle. A hole is made in the center of this U-stitch. Dilators are passed through the hole and across the valve. Gradually larger dilators are passed until the valve opening is large enough. The last dilator is removed and the U-stitch is tied to stop any bleeding. The chest is closed. In this operation, the valve is dilated from below. Report 33471 if the U-stitch is placed in the pulmonary artery and the valve is dilated from above.

33472–33474

The heart is exposed through the sternum. Tourniquets are placed around the superior and inferior caval veins. These are then tightened. A hole is made in the pulmonary artery and the pulmonary valve is cut opened through this hole. The hole in the pulmonary artery is then closed and the tourniquets are released. Report 33474 if cardiopulmonary bypass with two venous uptake tubes is used.

33475

Cardiopulmonary bypass is initiated with venous uptake tubes in both caval veins. The pulmonary

artery is opened and the pulmonary valve leaflets are cut out. Stitches are then placed around the circumference of the pulmonary annulus and the valve is sized. An appropriate artificial valve is selected. The stitches are then passed through the sewing ring of the valve. The sewing ring is then seated against the valve annulus an the stitches are tied. The hole in the pulmonary artery is closed. Cardiopulmonary bypass is discontinued when heart function returns.

33476–33478

Cardiopulmonary bypass is initiated. The right ventricular infundibular muscle is opened and the obstructing muscle bands are cut out. The valve may also need to be opened. If so, the valve is cut open. The hole in the right ventricle is closed with a patch of pericardium. Cardiopulmonary bypass is discontinued when heart function returns. Report 33478 if the operation if performed with a gusset, with or without commissurotomy or infundibular resection.

33496

This procedure is typically performed to repair a normal artificial prosthetic valve that is malfunctioning due to leakage around the valve sewing ring or when a normal prosthetic valve is impeded by blood clot or growth of surrounding tissue (pannus) into the functioning part of the valve. The exposes the heart through the sternum. Cardiopulmonary bypass is initiated. The prosthetic valve is exposed (this is most likely a prosthetic valve in the aortic or mitral position) and the valve is repaired. Cardiopulmonary bypass is discontinued when heart function returns. The incision is closed: the bones with wires or sutures, the soft tissues with sutures.

33500–33501

Cardiopulmonary bypass is initiated. The site of the fistula has bee previously determined by cardiac catheterization. The venous end of the fistula (ae) is (are) ligated with sutures. Cardiopulmonary bypass is often discontinued. If the fistula is to a cardiac chamber, that chamber is opened and the chamber end of the fistula is closed with a stitch. Report 33501 if cardiopulmonary bypass is not used and fistulae to a cardiac chamber cannot usually be repaired.

33502

This operation is usually done for a coronary artery which arises from the pulmonary artery instead of the aorta. It has a very poor prognosis. The artery is cleaned off near where it leaves the pulmonary artery. A suture is placed around the artery and it is ligated.

33503–33504

Cardiopulmonary bypass is almost always required for this operation. The coronary artery arising from the pulmonary artery is detached. The hole in the pulmonary artery is closed with stitches. A hole is made in the side of the aorta and the open end of the coronary artery is sewn to this hole. Report 33504 if cardiopulmonary bypass is required.

33505

Cardiopulmonary bypass is required. The operation is done in cases where the anomalous coronary is far from the aorta on the left lateral side of the pulmonary artery. Holes are made in the aorta and pulmonary at the level of the anomalous coronary and where the vessels touch each other. The holes are sewn together to create a direct aortopulmonary opening. A flap of pulmonary artery wall is created with the anomalous coronary at one end. The flap is fashioned into a tunnel with the flap as one side of the tunnel, the back wall of the pulmonary artery as the other side of the tunnel, the hole between the aorta and pulmonary artery as one end and the anomalous coronary as the other end. In this way, blood from the aorta is diverted into the anomalous coronary. The hole in the pulmonary artery is closed. Cardiopulmonary bypass is discontinued when heart function returns.

33506

Cardiopulmonary bypass is almost always required for this operation. The coronary artery arising from the pulmonary artery is detached. The hole in the pulmonary artery is closed with stitches. A hole is made in the side of the aorta and the open end of the coronary artery is sewn to this hole.

33510–33516

Cardiopulmonary bypass is initiated with a single, two-stage venous uptake tube. Saphenous vein is harvested from either leg. Vein may also be taken from the arm, the back of the leg, or from a cadaver. A clamp is placed on the aorta above the heart. Cold preserving solution is pumped through the coronary arteries to stop the heart. A point is chosen on the diseased coronary (aries) beyond the area of disease and a longitudinal incision is cut in it. The proximal part (the part nearest the thigh) of the vein is trimmed to the same length as the cut in the coronary artery and is cleaned off. the end of the vein is then sewn to the side of the coronary artery. A 3.0 mm to 6.0 mm hole is then punched in the ascending aorta and the other end of the vein graft is sewn to this hole. The clamp on the aorta is released. Cardiopulmonary bypass is discontinued when heart function returns. Report 33511 if two coronary venous grafts are needed; report 33512 if three are needed; report 33513 if four are performed; report 33514 if five are performed; report 33516 if six or more are performed.

33517–33523

Cardiopulmonary bypass is initiated with a single, two-stage venous uptake tube. Saphenous vein is harvested from the legs. Other veins grafts may be obtained from the arms, backs of the legs, or cadavers (organ donors.) These sources are inferior to the Saphenous vein. Arterial grafts may be obtained from the internal mammary artery (along the lateral side of the breastbone), the gastroepiploic artery (from the abdomen), the inferior epigastric artery (from the abdominal wall), or the radial artery (from the non-dominant hand). The most commonly used vessel is the internal mammary artery. It is left connected at one end to the arm artery from which it arises. Report 33518 if two venous grafts are performed; report 33519 if three venous grafts are performed; report 33521 if four are performed; report 33522 if five venous grafts are performed; and report 33523 if six or more are performed.

33530

For descriptions of the actual therapeutic procedure to be performed, please see the description of that procedure. The breast bone must be split again. Because the heart is invariably tightly adherent to the underside of the sternum in a redo operation, a vibrating saw is used to cut through it. After the sternum is cut, its halves are gently retracted while the tissues stuck to its under surface are carefully cut down. Once the sternum can be opened, the heart is exposed by cutting any chest tissues which have stuck to it since the last operation. It is usually necessary to initiate cardiopulmonary bypass before the heart is completely cleaned off.

33533–33536

Cardiopulmonary bypass is initiated with a single, two-stage venous uptake tube. Arterial grafts may be obtained from the internal mammary artery (along the lateral side of the breastbone), the gastroepiploic artery (from the abdomen), the inferior epigastric artery (from the abdominal wall), or the radial artery (from the non-dominant hand). The most commonly used vessel is the internal mammary artery. It is left connected at one end to the arm artery from which it arises. Report 33534 if two arterial grafts are placed; report 33535 if three are placed; report 33536 if four or more are placed.

33542

This operation is almost always done in conjunction with coronary artery bypass grafting. Prior to placing the bypass grafts, the aneurysm is opened and any clot is removed from the ventricle. The aneurysm is then opened widely and excised or opened, but not excised. The hole created by opening the aneurysm is then closed either with sutures directly or with a patch of Gortex, for example, or Dacron sewn into the hole. All stitches are placed in healthy (not aneurysm) heart tissue and care is taken to avoid the coronary arteries.

33545

This operation is always done in conjunction with coronary artery bypass grafting. The heart muscle involved in the infarction extends from the septum onto the surface of the heart. The heart is opened through this dead muscle and all dead muscle on the surface of the heart is cut out as is all the dead muscle in the septum. The septum is reconstructed by sewing in a patch of Gortex, for example or Dacron. The surface of the heart is closed either directly with sutures or with a patch sewn over the hole.

33572

This operation is only done when a coronary artery is so full of disease along its length that a good site for sewing on the bypass graft cannot be found. Coronary artery bypass grafts are almost always done along with the end arterectomy. The coronary artery to be cleaned out is opened along its length for a distance greater than that usually opened for a bypass alone, sometimes along its entire length. The plaque within the artery is separated from the outer layer of the arterial wall with a tool designed for the purpose. The plaque is removed from as much of the artery as is possible. A bypass graft is usually sewn to part of the hole left in the coronary. The rest of the hole is either closed directly with suture or a patch of opened vein graft is laid over the open artery and sewn to the coronary artery wall to close the hole.

33600–33602

Cardiopulmonary bypass is initiated. The appropriate heart chamber (right atrium for the tricuspid valve; left atrium for the mitral valve) is opened and the valve is assessed. The hole in the leaflet is cleaned of any infection. If it can be closed directly without distorting the valve significantly, then suture alone is used. If the hole is large, it is closed with a patch made of pericardium. The open heart chamber is then closed and cardiopulmonary bypass is discontinued when heart function returns. Report 33602 if the pulmonary artery or aorta are opened to gain access to the valve.

33606

The heart is exposed by dividing the breastbone longitudinally. Mechanical, extra corporeal circulation is established and the heart is stopped (cardiopulmonary bypass). The pulmonary artery is cut just before it divides into right and left branches. The pulmonary artery end is then connected to the side of the ascending aorta. A piece of Dacron graft is used to construct this connection. This allows the single ventricle to pump blood to the body.

33608

Mechanical, extra corporeal circulation is established and the heart is stopped (cardiopulmonary bypass). A hole is made in the pulmonary artery. This last hole is enlarged to cross any areas of narrowing. A cadaver ascending aorta is trimmed to the right length. A tube of artery or Dacron is sewn to the valve end of the cadaver aorta. The cadaver artery is then connected to the hole in the pulmonary artery. The tube of aorta or

Dacron is then sewn to the hole in the ventricle to close the hole and allow blood to flow through the new valved tube which now connects the ventricle to the pulmonary artery.

33610

The heart is exposed by dividing the breastbone longitudinally. Mechanical, extra corporeal circulation is established and the heart is stopped (cardiopulmonary bypass). The heart is opened and the hole in the wall between the two ventricles is enlarged so that blood will flow freely across it. A baffle is placed to direct blood that flows across the enlarged ventricular septal defect out the aorta.

33611–33612

Cardiopulmonary bypass is initiated. A hole is made in the right ventricle free wall. This exposes the hole between the right and left ventricles. A patch of either pericardium or Dacron is then sewn in place to block the hole and directs blood ejected from the left ventricle (i.e. blood coming from the lungs) out the aorta. If the pulmonary artery is of adequate size then blood will flow from the right ventricle to the lungs. If it is inadequate or if the valve does not open, a conduit containing a valve (natural or artificial) is sewn to the hole in the right ventricle free wall. The far end of the conduit is attached to the pulmonary artery. This then will allow blood to be pumped from the right ventricle to the lungs. Report 33612 if the obstructing muscles bundles in the outflow part of the right ventricle are excised when the heart is open.

33615

The right pulmonary artery (or left in situs inverses) is exposed from the main pulmonary trunk to the hilum of the lung. The superior vena cava is then detached from the right atrium. The atrial hole is closed. A hole is then made in the top part of the pulmonary artery and the cut end of the superior vena cava is connected to the hole in the pulmonary artery. Pulmonary blood flow then comes directly from the venous system and bypasses the heart. Later the process is completed by performing a Fontan operation.

33617

This operation is usually considered to be the second stage of a Glen Repair. Cardiopulmonary bypass with or without circulatory arrest is required. In this operation blood flow is directed from the inferior caval vein, through a tunnel created inside the right atrium to the pulmonary artery. All systemic venous return is diverted away from the heart and directly into the pulmonary circulation. The right atrium is widely opened. A large patch of either pericardium or Dacron is used in for one wall of the "tunnel." The lateral wall of the right atrium forms the other half of the "tunnel." The tunnel leads from the inferior caval vein, where it joins the right atrium, to the undersurface of the pulmonary artery. The "mouth" of

CPT® Lay Descriptions

the tunnel is then connected to a hole on the undersurface of the pulmonary artery. Previously, or at the same time, the superior caval vein will already have been directly connected to the upper surface of the pulmonary artery.

33619

Cardiopulmonary bypass and circulatory arrest are required. After the bypass pump is turned off the small aorta is opened on the inner surface of its arch up to the point where the aortic diameter becomes "normal." The pulmonary artery is removed and its connection to the branched pulmonary artery is closed with a patch. A large, rectangular patch of pericardium is then used to enlarge the small aorta. The pulmonary valve becomes the systemic arterial valve of the heart and is encircled by the large patch which becomes shaped like a tube as it is sewn along either side of the small ascending aorta and arch which have been opened longitudinally. The coronary arteries are small and still originate in the root of the abnormal aorta.

33641

Cardiopulmonary bypass is necessary. Two venous tubes are placed for the bypass machine — one draining the superior caval vein and the one draining the inferior caval vein. The right atrium is isolated by the putting tourniquets around the superior vena cava and inferior vena cava and their corresponding tubes. The right atrium is opened and the size and location of the arterial septal defect are assessed. If it is small enough or if the atrial septal tissue is sufficiently redundant, the defect is closed primarily with suture. If not, a patch of pericardium or Dacron is sewn to the edge of the defect to close it.

33645

Cardiopulmonary bypass is required. The operation is performed exactly as for a regular arterial septal defect, except that a patch is always required. Care is taken to place the patch so that 1) all pulmonary veins system and 2) there is no obstruction of the superior vena cava, RVC, or pulmonary veins by the patch.

33647

Cardiopulmonary bypass is established with the venous uptake tubes in both the superior and inferior caval veins. A hole in the right atrium or, if needed, a hole in one of the ventricles is made. The hole in the ventricle is made in the area of scar (if the ventricular septal defect is due to ischemia) or in the anterior part of the right ventricle (if the ventricular septal defect is congenital). Care is taken to avoid coronary arteries in which sometimes follow an anomalous course over the anterior right ventricle. All dead heart muscles is cut out (in ischemic ventricular septal defect) and the ventricular septal defect is then closed with a patch of Dacron or pericardium. The hole in the atrium or ventricle is then closed.

Cardiopulmonary bypass is discontinued when heart function is restored.

33660

Cardiopulmonary bypass is established using venous uptake tubes in both the superior and inferior caval veins. The right atrium is opened. A radially oriented cleft or division in the anterior leaflet of the mitral value is closed with the interrupted sutures. Care is taken to assure that the value classes properly after it is repaired. There is a raphe or line of denser value tissue marking the anatomic line between the two AR values. The ventricular septal defect is obliterated by sewing this line to the top of the septal muscle. The arterial septal defect is then closed with a patch of Dacron or pericardium. The right atrium is closed and cardiopulmonary pulmonary bypass discontinued after heart function is restored.

33665

Cardiopulmonary bypass is established with the venous uptake tubes in both the superior and inferior caval veins. A hole in the right atrium or, if needed, a hole in one of the ventricles is made. The hole in the ventricle is made in the area of scar (if the ventricular septal defect is due to ischemia) or in the anterior part of the right ventricle (if the ventricular septal defect is congenital). The AV value anatomy can be highly variable, ranging from normal mitral and tricuspid anatomy with a sub valvular ventricular septal defect to grossly abnormal AV value leaflet number position, but with 2 separate "values" present separated by a line of tissue. The AV valves are repaired. Repair is all is all that is done if valvular competence can be restored to the left AV valve. If not, this value is replaced with either a mechanical value on a tissue value.

33670

Cardiopulmonary pulmonary bypass is established using venous uptake tubes in both the superior and inferior caval veins. The right atrium is opened. A radially oriented cleft or division in the anterior leaflet of the mitral value is closed with the interrupted sutures. Care is taken to assure that the value classes properly after it is repaired. There is a raphe or line of denser value tissue marking the anatomic line between the two AR values. The ventricular septal defect is obliterated by sewing this line to the top of the septal muscle. The arterial septal defect is then closed with a patch of Dacron or pericardium. The right atrium is closed and cardiopulmonary pulmonary bypass discontinued after heart function is restored. Only a opening in the right atrium is made. The competency of the single AV value is assessed as is the imaginary line where the plane extending upward from the ventricular septal defect intersects the AV valve. The AV valve leaflets are divided along this line. The ventricular septal defect patch is placed. The valve leaflets are then resuspended by sewing them to the ventricular septal defect patch. The competency of the valves is assessed. The arterial septal defect is then closed with a patch sewn to the top of the ventricular septal defect patch or an extension of the ventricular septal defect patch is used to close the arterial septal defect (single patch technique). The hole in the right atrium is closed. Cardiopulmonary bypass is discontinued when cardiac function has returned.

33681

Cardiopulmonary bypass is established with tubes in both the caval veins. The ventricular septal defect can almost always be repaired through a hole in the right atrium, except in the case of a supracristal ventricular septal defect which ventricle is higher in the outflow part of the right ventricle. This type of ventricular septal defect is repaired most often through the pulmonary artery. All types of ventricular septal defects can be repaired through an opening in the right ventricle muscle, but this causes more damage and is avoided if possible. The ventricular septal defect is almost always repaired with a patch of either Dacron or pericardium. A primary closure rarely can be performed with stitches. After the ventricular septal defect is closed, the hole which has been either created in the right atrium, or right ventricle or pulmonary artery is closed. Cardiopulmonary bypass is discontinued when heart function returns.

33684

Cardiopulmonary bypass is established with venous uptake tubes in both the caval veins. Prior to operating, it has been established by echocardiography, cardiac catheterization or both that the diameter of the tricuspid valve is large enough to permit a normal cardiac output. If not the operation is combined with a modified Blalock-Taussig shunt. The right ventricle or pulmonary artery is opened. Through either opening, the infundibular muscle blocking blood flow to the pulmonary artery can be cut out and cuts can be made in the pulmonary valve to reduce the restriction to blood flow that it presents. The ventricular septal defect is then closed through either of these incisions, if possible. If it is not possible to close the ventricular septal defect with the exposure thus provided, the right atrium is opened and the ventricular septal defect closed. A patch is almost always used. All holes in the heart are then closed. Cardiopulmonary bypass is discontinued when heart function is restored.

33688

The patient is prepared for cardiopulmonary bypass as for 33681, but it is not established yet. The previously placed PA band is dissected out and removed. Stenosis at the site of the PA band is assessed before and after band removal with a pressure transducer connected to a needle probe which measures any pressure drop across the area of narrowing. Cardiopulmonary bypass is then established and the ventricular septal defect is repaired. If PA pressures proximal to the band site remain high after band removal and ventricular septal defect closure or if the surgeon feels the residual stenosis is too tight, cardiopulmonary bypass is restarted and either segment of pulmonary artery containing the area is removed with a primary repair of the pulmonary artery or an incision is made in the PA across the area of narrowing. This defect is then closed with a pericardial patch and CPB is discontinued.

33690

Cardiopulmonary bypass is not required. The pulmonary artery is exposed through either a median sternotomy or left thoracotomy. A band of heavy Dacron suture or tape is place around the base of the pulmonary artery. Once the PA pressure distal to the band is less than half of the systemic pressure and the patients arterial saturation is greater than 70 percent, the band is tight enough, but not too tight. The incision is closed.

33692

Repair of this defect assumes that the pulmonary artery annulus and right ventricular outflow tract are of adequate size to permit normal pulmonary blood flow. Cardiopulmonary bypass is required.

33694

In this defect the pulmonary valve annulus and/or the right ventricular infundibulum are too small to allow normal pulmonary blood flow. The ventricular septal defect is closed. Cardiopulmonary bypass is required. A longitudinal incision is made in the PA and carried proximally across the pulmonary valve annulus and onto the muscles of the right ventricular outflow tract. Infundibular muscle is removed if necessary. The defect is closed with a patch of pericardium. Cardiopulmonary bypass is discontinued when heart function returns.

33697

Cardiopulmonary bypass is required. A hole is made in the right ventricle and any muscular obstruction in the outflow tract of the right ventricle is removed. The pulmonary artery or its branches are opened longitudinally until normal-sized vessels are encountered. The ventricular septal defect is closed. An aortic graft from an organ donor is then trimmed to form a patch over the opened pulmonary artery. Any excess artery from the donor graft or a patch of pericardium or Dacron is sewn to the graft bellow the valve to use as a secondary patch for closing the hole in the right ventricle. The graft valve becomes the new pulmonary valve. After the patches and graft are sewn in place, cardiopulmonary bypass is stopped when heart function returns.

33702–33710

Cardiopulmonary bypass is required. After the heart is stopped, the aorta is opened and the fistula is identified. It is closed with a patch of pericardium.

Any aorta valve incompetence is repaired by shortening the redundant valve leaflet diameter with stitches that reef in its free edge. The hole in the aorta is then closed. Report 33710 if the sinus of valsalva fistula is closed through the right atrium or through as incision in the aorta.

33720

Cardiopulmonary bypass is required. The aorta is opened after the heart has stopped. Thrombus (clot) in the aneurysm is removed. The neck of the aneurysm is closed with stitches. The aortic valve is usually incompetent. If the aortic annulus is sufficiently dilated by the aneurysm the aortic valve may need to be replaced with either a mechanical aortic valve, a bio-mechanical valve or a tissue valve from an organ donor. After the valve is repaired or replaced, the aorta is closed. Cardiopulmonary bypass is discontinued after heart function returns.

33722

The physician closes a previously formed aortic-left ventricular tunnel. The physician performs a midline sternotomy, incising the skin, fascia, muscles, and sternum. The pericardium is incised and lines are placed for cardiopulmonary bypass. When bypass is established, the tunnel is isolated and ligated. The cardiac incision is closed. The pericardium is repaired loosely, leaving gaps for blood and fluid to drain into the pleural space. The sternum is reanastomosed with sternal wires and the skin is closed in sutured layers.

33730

The goal of repair of all types of TAPVR is to return pulmonary vein blood to the left atrium where it can then be pumped to the body. Pulmonary vein blood is replete with oxygen. The means by which this is done varies with whether the common vein and sinus (abnormal structures present only in these patients) returns above the heart, below the diaphragm, or at the level of the heart. Cardiopulmonary bypass is required. Sometimes, one pulmonary vein does not drain into the common vein or sinus. Usually, this is the left upper lobe vein. Its blood is directed into the left atrium by creating a connection between it and the left atrial appendage.

33732

This lesion is frequently considered to be related to TAPVR, but it is distinctly different. In this anomaly, there is a wall subdividing the left atrium between the pulmonary veins and the mitral valve. This restricts blood flow to the left ventricle and therefore to the rest of the body. Cardiopulmonary bypass is readied. The left atrium is opened and the membrane is cut out. The left atrium is then closed. Cardiopulmonary bypass is discontinued when heart function returns.

33735

This procedure is of historical interest only. The procedure requires either a median sternal opening or

a right chest opening. A purse string is placed in the right atrial appendage and the appendage is opened in the middle of the purse string. A finger or a dilating tool is then passed through the hole in the atrium and the wall between the right and left atria is torn open. The dilating instrument is removed and the purse string is tied to stop the bleeding.

33736–33737

This procedure is largely of historical interest. In most pediatric cardiac surgery centers, it has been supplanted by balloon dilation of a naturally occurring hole in the wall between the atrial chambers. No incision is needed for balloon dilation. Operative septostomy/septectomy requires cardiopulmonary bypass with venous uptake tubes in both caval veins. The right atrium is opened and the thin part of the wall between the right and left atria is cut out or opened widely. The goal is to allow free mixing of the blood from the right and left atria. Cardiopulmonary bypass is discontinued when heart function returns. Report 33737 if tourniquets are placed around the caval veins and the patient is placed head down so no air entering the right atrium crosses the wall between the right and left atria.

33750

In its unmodified form, this operation involves dividing the left subclavian artery, tying off the end of the artery going to the arm, and then creating a connection between the end of this artery coming from the heart and the side of the pulmonary artery. The difficulty with this operation is making the connection to the pulmonary artery exactly the right size to supply adequate, but not excessive blood flow to the lungs. Instead, a modified version of the operation is usually performed. The artery to the arm is not divided. Instead, one end of a 3.0 mm to 5.0 mm diameter tube of Gortex is sewn to the side of the artery to the arm and the other end is sewn to the side of the pulmonary artery. The size of the tube then determines the amount of blood flow to the lungs. Cardiopulmonary bypass is not required. The ductus arteriosus (a connection between the aorta and pulmonary artery that has been supplying blood to the lungs, but usually closes at birth) is then tied off.

33755

This procedure requires cardiopulmonary bypass. It is designed to allow adequate blood flow to the lungs. After cardiopulmonary bypass is initiated, the aorta is occluded above the heart. Holes are made in parts of the aorta and pulmonary artery which are next to each other. The holes are then sewn together. It is difficult to accurately control the diameter of the resulting connection and the resulting flow of blood into the lungs. Cardiopulmonary bypass is discontinued when heart function returns. The ductus arteriosus (a connection between the aorta and pulmonary artery that has been supplying blood to the lungs, but usually closes at birth) is then tied off.

33762

The operation is performed through the left side of the chest. Cardiopulmonary bypass is not required. One end of a 3.0 mm to 5.0 mm diameter tube made of PTFE (e.g., Gortex) is sewn to the side of the descending aorta and the other end is sewn to some part of the pulmonary artery. The ductus arteriosus (a connection between the aorta and pulmonary artery that has been supplying blood to the lungs, but usually closes at birth) is then tied off.

33764

The operation is done ether through an incision in the middle of the breast bone or through an incision in the left chest. Cardiopulmonary bypass is usually not required. One end of a 3.0 mm to 5.0 mm diameter tube made of Gortex is sewn to the side of the ascending aorta and the other end is sewn to some part of the pulmonary artery. The ductus arteriosus (a connection between the aorta and pulmonary artery that has been supplying blood to the lungs, but usually closes at birth) is then tied off.

33766

This operation is performed when there is an irreparable obstruction to blood flow through the right side of the heart. It is usually done as a prelude to a bidirectional or bilateral Glen procedure which is usually itself a prelude to a Fontan procedure. Cardiopulmonary bypass is usually required. The right (or the persistent left) superior caval vein is occluded and its connection with the heart is divided. The heart end of the of the superior caval vein is then oversewn (i.e., closed). The free end of the superior caval vein is then sewn to the side of the corresponding pulmonary artery. It is assumed that the corresponding pulmonary artery is isolated from the opposite lung either congenitally or surgically. The goal is to permit blood to flow directly from the superior caval vein to one of the lungs, thereby bypassing the right side of the heart.

33767

For this procedure, it is assumed that all the pulmonary arteries from both lungs communicate freely. Cardiopulmonary bypass is required. Circulatory arrest and deep cooling of the body are usually employed. The main pulmonary artery is often tied off. The superior caval vein is detached from its connection to the right atrium. The hole left in the right atrium is closed with sutures. The free end of the superior caval vein is then sewn to a hole in the side of the pulmonary artery. In this way, blood can flow to the lungs without passing through the right side of the heart. This operation is usually done as a prelude to a Fontan procedure.

33770

The physician gains access to the mediastinum through an incision through the sternum (median sternotomy). The physician places cardiopulmonary

bypass catheters usually through incisions in the right atrial appendage and aorta or femoral artery. The physician stops the heart by infusing cardioplegia solution into the coronary circulation. The physician then applies a large Dacron patch to direct oxygenated blood from the left ventricle through the large ventricular septal defect into the aortic valve and ascending aorta. The physician then ligates the proximal main pulmonary artery or oversews the pulmonic valve. The physician then places a fabric conduit or a human cadaveric homograft to direct unoxygenated blood from the right ventricle to the branch pulmonary arteries. The physician may place a bioprosthetic valve in the pulmonary outflow conduit if the pulmonary vascular resistance is elevated. The physician closes the cardiac incisions, takes the patient off cardiopulmonary bypass, closes the remaining surgical incisions and dresses the sternal or chest wall wound. The physician may leave chest tubes and/or a mediastinal drainage tube in place following the procedure.

33771

The physician gains access to the mediastinum through an incision through the sternum (median sternotomy). The physician places cardiopulmonary bypass catheters usually through incisions in the right atrial appendage and aorta or femoral artery. The physician stops the heart by infusing cardioplegia solution into the coronary circulation. The physician enlarges the ventricular septal defect anteriorly to avoid damage to the conduction bundles. The physician then applies a large Dacron patch to form a tunnel from the left ventricle through the large ventricular septal defect into the aortic valve and ascending aorta. The physician ligates the proximal main pulmonary artery or oversews the pulmonic valve. The physician places a fabric conduit to direct right ventricular flow to the pulmonary artery. The physician may place a bioprosthetic valve in the pulmonary outflow conduit if the pulmonary vascular resistance is elevated. The physician then closes the cardiac incisions, takes the patient off cardiopulmonary bypass, closes the remaining surgical incisions and dresses the sternal or chest wall wound. The physician may leave chest tubes and/or a mediastinal drainage tube in place following the procedure.

33774

The physician gains access to the mediastinum through an incision through the sternum (median sternotomy). The physician places cardiopulmonary bypass catheters through incisions in the low inferior vena cava, the superior vena cava, and aorta or femoral artery. The physician stops the heart by infusing cardioplegia solution into the coronary circulation. The physician excises the interatrial septum. The physician sews baffle material (pericardium or Dacron) to direct blood from the pulmonary veins to the right ventricle and the systemic venous drainage to the left ventricle. The physician may enlarge the pulmonary venous chamber with a woven Dacron or pericardial patch. The physician closes the cardiac incisions, takes the patient off cardiopulmonary bypass, closes the remaining surgical incisions and dresses the sternal or chest wall wound. The physician may leave chest tubes and/or a mediastinal drainage tube in place following the procedure.

33775

The physician gains access to the mediastinum through an incision through the sternum (median sternotomy). The physician places cardiopulmonary bypass catheters through incisions in the low inferior vena cava, the superior vena cava, and aorta or femoral artery. The physician stops the heart by infusing cardioplegia solution into the coronary circulation. The physician removes the pulmonary artery band (placed during a previous surgery) and dilates the pulmonary artery to normal size. If this is not possible, the physician removes the pulmonary band and constricted area of pulmonary artery, and applies a woven Dacron patch over the hole. The physician excises the interatrial septum. The physician then sews baffle material (pericardium or Dacron) to direct blood from the pulmonary veins to the right ventricle and the systemic venous drainage to the left ventricle. The physician may enlarge the pulmonary venous chamber with a woven Dacron or pericardial patch. The physician then closes the cardiac incisions, takes the patient off cardiopulmonary bypass, closes the remaining surgical incisions and dresses the sternal or chest wall wound. The physician may leave chest tubes and/or a mediastinal drainage tube in place following the procedure.

33776

The physician gains access to the mediastinum through an incision through the sternum (median sternotomy). The physician places cardiopulmonary bypass catheters through incisions in the low inferior vena cava, the superior vena cava, and aorta or femoral artery. The physician stops the heart by infusing cardioplegia solution into the coronary circulation. The physician closes the ventricular septal defect, usually with a Dacron patch. The physician then excises the interatrial septum. The physician sews baffle material (pericardium or Dacron) to direct blood from the pulmonary veins to the right ventricle and the systemic venous drainage to the left ventricle. The physician may enlarge the pulmonary venous chamber with a woven Dacron or pericardial patch. The physician then closes the cardiac incisions, takes the patient off cardiopulmonary bypass, closes the remaining surgical incisions and dresses the sternal or chest wall wound. The physician may leave chest tubes and/or a mediastinal drainage tube in place following the procedure.

33777

The physician gains access to the mediastinum through an incision through the sternum (median sternotomy). The physician places cardiopulmonary bypass catheters (through incisions in the low inferior vena cava, the superior vena cava, and aorta or femoral artery). The physician stops the heart by infusing cardioplegia solution into the coronary circulation. The physician makes an incision in the right ventricular outflow tract, resects the fibrous muscular tissue causing the subpulmonic obstruction, and sews the ventriculotomy closed. The physician then excises the interatrial septum. The physician then sews baffle material (pericardium or Dacron) to direct blood from the pulmonary veins to the right ventricle and the systemic venous drainage to the left ventricle. The physician may enlarge the pulmonary venous chamber with a woven Dacron or pericardial patch. The physician then closes the cardiac incisions, takes the patient off cardiopulmonary bypass, closes the remaining surgical incisions and dresses the sternal or chest wall wound. The physician may leave chest tubes and/or a mediastinal drainage tube in place following the procedure.

33778

The physician gains access to the mediastinum through an incision through the sternum (median sternotomy). The physician places cardiopulmonary bypass catheters through incisions in the low inferior vena cava, the superior vena cava, and aorta or femoral artery. The physician stops the heart by infusing cardioplegia solution into the coronary circulation. The physician removes the coronary ostia from the aortic root and sews them into the root of the pulmonary trunk. The pulmonary trunk and aortic root are each transected and interchanged to direct blood from the pulmonary veins through the left ventricle to the aorta, and the systemic venous drainage to the pulmonary trunk via the right ventricle. The physician closes the cardiac incisions, takes the patient off cardiopulmonary bypass, closes the remaining surgical incisions and dresses the sternal or chest wall wound. The physician may leave chest tubes and/or a mediastinal drainage tube in place following the procedure.

33779

The physician gains access to the mediastinum through an incision through the sternum (median sternotomy). The physician places cardiopulmonary bypass catheters through incisions in the low inferior vena cava, the superior vena cava, and aorta or femoral artery. The physician stops the heart by infusing cardioplegia solution into the coronary circulation. The physician removes the pulmonary artery band placed during a previous surgery and dilates the pulmonary artery to normal size. If this is not possible, the physician removes the pulmonary band and constricted area of pulmonary artery, and applies a woven Dacron patch over the hole. The physician removes the coronary ostia from the aortic root and sews them into the root of the pulmonary trunk. The pulmonary trunk and aortic root are each transected and interchanged to direct blood from the pulmonary veins through the left ventricle to the aorta, and the systemic venous drainage to the pulmonary trunk via the right ventricle. The physician then closes the cardiac incisions, takes the patient off cardiopulmonary bypass, closes the remaining surgical incisions and dresses the sternal or chest wall wound. The physician may leave chest tubes and/or a mediastinal drainage tube in place following the procedure.

33780

The physician gains access to the mediastinum through an incision through the sternum (median sternotomy). The physician places cardiopulmonary bypass catheters through incisions in the low inferior vena cava, the superior vena cava, and aorta or femoral artery. The physician stops the heart by infusing cardioplegia solution into the coronary circulation. The physician removes the coronary ostia from the aortic root and sews them into the root of the pulmonary trunk. The pulmonary trunk and aortic root are each transected and interchanged to direct blood from the pulmonary veins through the left ventricle to the aorta, and the systemic venous drainage to the pulmonary trunk via the right ventricle. The physician closes the ventricular septal defect, usually with a Dacron patch. The physician closes the cardiac incisions, takes the patient off cardiopulmonary bypass, closes the remaining surgical incisions and dresses the sternal or chest wall wound. The physician may leave chest tubes and/or a mediastinal drainage tube in place following the procedure.

33781

The physician gains access to the mediastinum through an incision through the sternum (median sternotomy). The physician places cardiopulmonary bypass catheters through incisions in the low inferior vena cava, the superior vena cava, and aorta or femoral artery. The physician stops the heart by infusing cardioplegia solution into the coronary circulation. The physician removes the coronary ostia from the aortic root and sews them into the root of the pulmonary trunk. The pulmonary trunk and aortic root are each transected and interchanged to direct blood from the pulmonary veins through the left ventricle to the aorta, and the systemic venous drainage to the pulmonary trunk via the right ventricle. The physician makes an incision in the right ventricular outflow tract, resects the fibrous muscular tissue causing the subpulmonic obstruction, and sews the ventriculotomy closed. The physician closes the cardiac incisions, takes the patient off cardiopulmonary bypass, closes the remaining surgical incisions and dresses the sternal or chest wall wound. The physician may leave chest tubes and/or a

mediastinal drainage tube in place following the procedure.

33786

The physician gains access to the mediastinum through an incision through the sternum (median sternotomy). The physician places cardiopulmonary bypass catheters usually through incisions in the right atrial appendage and aorta or femoral artery. The physician stops the heart by infusing cardioplegia solution into the coronary circulation. The physician applies a large Dacron patch to direct oxygenated blood from the left ventricle through the large ventricular septal defect into the aortic valve and ascending aorta. The physician then ligates the proximal main pulmonary artery or oversews the pulmonic valve. The physician then places a fabric conduit or a human cadaveric homograft to direct unoxygenated blood from the right ventricle to the branch pulmonary arteries after removing them from their origin(s) at the truncal vessel. The physician sews a pericardial patch in place to close the defect(s) in the truncal vessel. The physician may place a bioprosthetic valve in the pulmonary outflow conduit if the pulmonary vascular resistance is elevated. The physician then closes the cardiac incisions, takes the patient off cardiopulmonary bypass, closes the remaining surgical incisions and dresses the sternal or chest wall wound. The physician may leave chest tubes and/or a mediastinal drainage tube in place following the procedure.

33788

The physician gains access to the mediastinum through an incision through the sternum (median sternotomy). The physician places cardiopulmonary bypass catheters usually through incisions in the right atrial appendage and aorta or femoral artery. The physician stops the heart by infusing cardioplegia solution into the coronary circulation. The physician then identifies the coronary artery anomaly and reattaches the unperfused pulmonary artery to the pulmonic outflow tract, either directly or using Dacron graft. The physician ligates the patent ductus arteriosus, if present. The physician closes the cardiac incisions, takes the patient off cardiopulmonary bypass, closes the remaining surgical incisions and dresses the sternal or chest wall wound. The physician may leave chest tubes and/or a mediastinal drainage tube in place following the procedure.

33800

The physician performs a right lateral thoracotomy or, sometimes, a midline sternotomy and identifies the ascending aorta. The physician isolates and removes the thymus to allow the ascending aorta to be mobilized and pulled forward. The physician sutures the adventitia of the ascending aorta and base of the innominate artery to the periosteum of the posterior aspect of the sternum or anterior rib. The physician may perform a similar operation on descending aorta, depending upon the site of tracheomalacia. The physician then closes the thoracotomy or sternotomy, leaving chest or mediastinal tubes in place.

33802–33803

The physician gains access to the mediastinum through an incision through the left chest (posterolateral thoracotomy). The physician identifies the two aortic arches and occludes the smaller left arch with vascular clamps. The physician divides the arch and oversews and possibly ligates the divided ends. The physician dissects away the stumps of the divided left arch and frees them from their mediastinal attachments. The physician attaches traction sutures to the ligated stumps and to the endothoracic fascia anteriorly and posteriorly to minimize obstruction to the esophagus and trachea. The physician closes the remaining surgical incisions and dresses the chest wall wound. The physician may leave a chest tube and/or a mediastinal drainage tube in place following the procedure. Report 33803 if the procedure includes reanastomosis.

33813

Cardiopulmonary bypass is almost always required if the defect is in the wall between the right and left ventricle. If the hole is above the aortic and pulmonary valves, it may be possible to avoid cardiopulmonary bypass if the connection can be isolated and controlled with side-biting clamps on both the aorta and pulmonary artery.

33814

The physician gains access to the mediastinum through an incision through the sternum (median sternotomy). The physician places cardiopulmonary bypass catheters through incisions in the low inferior vena cava, the superior vena cava, and high aorta or femoral artery. The physician stops the heart by infusing cardioplegia solution into the coronary circulation. The physician then cross-clamps the aorta, places sump suction in the left atrium to obtain a bloodless surgical field. The physician then exposes the aortopulmonary septal defect by cutting through the ascending aorta or main pulmonary artery. The physician closes the defect with a Dacron fabric patch, closes the aortic or pulmonary arterial incision, takes the patient off cardiopulmonary bypass, closes the remaining surgical incisions and dresses the sternal wound. The physician may leave chest tubes and/or a mediastinal drainage tube in place following the procedure.

33820

The physician gains access to the mediastinum through an incision through the posterolateral left chest wall (posterolateral thoracotomy). The physician dissects through the posterior chest wall musculature to expose the superior mediastinum. The physician dissects away the tissues surrounding the ductus and then passes several heavy ligatures around

the ductus and ties it off (ligation). The physician closes the surgical incisions and dresses the chest wall wound. The physician may leave chest tubes and/or a mediastinal drainage tube in place following the procedure.

33822–33824

The physician gains access to the mediastinum through an incision through the posterolateral left chest wall (posterolateral thoracotomy). The physician dissects through the posterior chest wall musculature to expose the superior mediastinum. The physician dissects away the tissues surrounding the ductus and passes several heavy ligatures around the ductus and ties it off (ligation) at each end. The physician occludes the ductus with vascular clamps and divides the ductus with scissors. The physician closes the aortic end with suture, then closes the pulmonary stump. The physician removes the vascular clamps, sutures the pleura closed, closes the remaining surgical incisions and dresses the chest wall wound. The physician may leave chest tubes and/or a mediastinal drainage tube in place following the procedure. Report 33824 if the patient is 18 years and older.

33840–33845

The physician gains access to the mediastinum through an incision through the posterolateral left chest wall (posterolateral thoracotomy). The physician dissects through the posterior chest wall musculature to expose the superior mediastinum, clamping and ligating large collateral vessels as they are encountered. The physician dissects away the tissues surrounding the aorta. The physician clamps the aorta on either side of the coarctation and ties off and divides the ligamentum arteriosum (or patent ductus arteriosus, if present). The physician excises the stricture sutures the two ends of the aorta to each other. The physician then closes the mediastinal pleura and chest and dresses the chest wall wound. The physician may leave chest tubes and/or a mediastinal drainage tube in place following the procedure. Report 33845 if a graft is placed.

33851

The physician gains access to the mediastinum through an incision through the posterolateral left chest wall (posterolateral thoracotomy). The physician dissects through the posterior chest wall musculature to expose the superior mediastinum, clamping and ligating large collateral vessels as they are encountered. The physician dissects away the tissues surrounding the aorta. The physician clamps the aorta on either side of the coarctation and ties off and divides the ligamentum arteriosum (or patent ductus arteriosus, if present). The physician opens the aorta with a longitudinal incision that extends along the subclavian artery above and for a distance distally. The physician excises any extra tissue at the stricture site and sews in the left subclavian artery or a Dacron patch graft to attach and enlarge the aorta at the longitudinal incision. The physician closes the mediastinal pleura and chest and dresses the chest wall wound. The physician may leave chest tubes and/or a mediastinal drainage tube in place following the procedure.

33852

The physician surgically attaches the ascending and descending parts of the aorta, where normal connection is either too small or interrupted entirely. The physician gains access to the mediastinum through an incision through the sternum (midline sternotomy). The physician clamps the aorta and left carotid artery to allow completion of the end-to-side attachment of a Dacron mesh graft to the ascending aorta. The physician cross-clamps the graft and releases the proximal clamp and the left carotid artery clamp. The physician uses end-to-side attachment to secure the distal graft to the descending aorta. The physician closes the mediastinal pleura and chest and dresses the chest wall wound. The physician may leave chest tubes and/or a mediastinal drainage tube in place following the procedure.

33853

The physician surgically attaches the ascending and descending parts of the aorta, where normal connection is either too small or interrupted entirely. The physician gains access to the mediastinum through an incision through the sternum (midline sternotomy). The physician places cardiopulmonary bypass catheters (through incisions in the low inferior vena cava, the superior vena cava, and high aorta or femoral artery). The physician stops the heart by infusing cardioplegia solution into the coronary circulation. The physician clamps the aorta and left carotid artery to allow completion of the end-to-side attachment of a Dacron mesh graft to the ascending aorta. The physician cross-clamps the graft and releases the proximal clamp and the left carotid artery clamp. The physician uses end-to-side attachment to secure the distal graft to the descending aorta. The physician takes the patient off cardiopulmonary bypass, closes the mediastinal pleura and chest and dresses the chest wall wound. The physician may leave chest tubes and/or a mediastinal drainage tube in place following the procedure.

33860–33863

Cardiopulmonary bypass is required. Deep cooling of the body and circulatory arrest are often required, especially if the transverse arch of the aorta must be replaced. After circulatory arrest or if a cross-clamp can be placed on the aorta before its first branch, the aneurysm is opened. The hole in the aneurysm is lengthened along the aorta until the end of the aneurysm is reached. The aorta is divided at this point. A double layer of felt strips is placed circumferentially around the inner and outer circumference of the normal aorta with the aortic wall

sandwiched in between. A Dacron tube graft is then sewn to this end of the aorta and its felt layers. The aortic root where the aorta emerges from the heart is then assessed. This area is where the aortic valve is located. If the valve closes normally, the aortic root size is reduced using reefing stitches which also sew a double layer of felt to the aorta as previously described. This can only be done if the coronary arteries (which arise in this area) are not involved in the aneurysm. The open end of the Dacron tube is then sewn to the prepared aortic root. If the valve does not close normally, then it is replaced or repaired with reefing stitches which reduce the length of its valve leaflets. The operation otherwise proceeds as it does when the valve closes normally. Report 33861 if coronary arteries must be cut out of the aneurysm; report 33863 if the end of the Dacron tube sewn to the aortic root contains an artificial valve and the patient's valve is removed.

33870

This operation requires cardiopulmonary bypass. The patient's body temperature is lowered to 18–21 degrees centigrade and the bypass pump is stopped. The aneurysm is then opened along its length and a patch of aortic wall containing the openings of the arteries to the head and arms is cut out. Each of these vessels will have been surrounded by tourniquets which were tightened before the bypass pump was stopped. The hole in the aneurysm is lengthened along the aorta until the end of the aneurysm is reached. The aorta is divided at this point. A double layer of felt strips is placed circumferentially around the inner and outer circumference of the normal aorta with the aortic wall sandwiched in between. A Dacron tube graft is then sewn to this end of the aorta and its felt layers. The aortic root where the aorta emerges from the heart is then assessed. This area is where the aortic valve is located. If the valve closes normally, the aortic root size is reduced using reefing stitches which also sew a double layer of felt to the aorta as previously described. This can only be done if the coronary arteries (which arise in this area) are not involved in the aneurysm. The patch of aorta containing the openings for the vessels to the head and arms is sewn to a hole made in the top of the graft where it arches over.

33875–33877

A segment of the intrathoracic descending aorta is replaced with a tube of Dacron. This is done through an incision in the left chest cavity. The great concern in performing this operation is possible damage to the spinal cord. Preserving the spinal cord can be accomplished using a cardiopulmonary bypass circuit from above the aneurysm to below it, using deep cooling of the body and stopping the bypass machine, using perfusion of one or more spinal artery branches with blood pumped through it or using the "clamp and go" method in which no effort, except a speedy operation, is used to preserve the spinal cord. No matter what spinal cord preservation method is chosen, clamps are placed across the aorta above and below the aneurysm. The aneurysm is then cut out and the ends of any small branches are closed with sutures. One end of a Dacron tube graft is sewn to the end of the aorta above the aneurysm and the other end of the graft is sewn to the aorta below the aneurysm. The clamps on the aorta are then released. Report 33877 if aorta is exposed through the left chest.

33910–33915

This operation is only done for patients who are in extremis following a pulmonary artery embolism (i.e., a blood clot originating in one of the large veins in the leg breaks loose and travels into the heart via the caval vein where it obstructs blood flow to the lungs). Survival is low. If cardiopulmonary bypass is used, the physician opens the right atrium widely. If cardiopulmonary bypass is not used, the right atrium is opened through a hole in the middle of a purse string. The clot is "milked" out of the pulmonary artery into the right atrium and out the hole. Report 33910 if cardiopulmonary bypass is required and the right atrium is opened widely. Report 33910 if cardiopulmonary bypass is initiated. Report 33915 if cardiopulmonary bypass is not initiated.

33916–33917

Cardiopulmonary bypass is required. Only the main and branch pulmonary arteries can be treated. The blocked arteries are opened along their lengths. The inner layer of the of each artery is removed. The outer layer of each artery is then closed either with suture directly or with a patch of pericardium, saphenous vein or Dacron. Report 33917 when a pulmonary stenosis is repaired by reconstruction with a patch or graft.

33918–33919

Anomalous pulmonary arteries are almost never present in pulmonary atresia, but are frequently present in pulmonary stenosis. In this operation, the anomalous pulmonary arteries are removed from their connections to the systemic arteries, sewn together (unifocalization) and then connected to some part of the main, true pulmonary artery. Report 33919 if cardiopulmonary bypass is employed.

33920

Cardiopulmonary bypass is required. A hole is made in the right ventricle and any muscular obstruction in the outflow tract of the right ventricle is removed. The pulmonary artery or its branches are opened longitudinally until normal-sized vessels are encountered. The ventricular septal defect is closed. An aortic graft from an organ donor is then trimmed to form a patch over the opened pulmonary artery. Any excess artery from the donor graft or a patch of pericardium or Dacron is sewn to the graft below the valve to use as a secondary patch for closing the hole

in the right ventricle. The graft valve becomes the new pulmonary valve. After the patches and graft are sewn in place, cardiopulmonary bypass is stopped when heart function returns.

33922

Cardiopulmonary bypass is required. After it is started, cuts are made all the way across the pulmonary artery just above and just below the part of the artery containing the disease. The pulmonary artery is then closed directly or is closed using either a piece of the pulmonary artery or a piece of the aorta from an organ donor which is placed as an interposition graft.

33924

During a separately reportable congenital heart procedure, the physician ligates and takes down a previously formed systemic-to-pulmonary artery shunt. The shunt is ligated and the systemic arteries are returned to their correct anatomic position.

33930

This is usually performed when other organs (liver, kidneys, intestines, pancreas) are taken from an organ donor. Cold preserving solutions are then infused into the aorta and pulmonary arteries. After enough of those solutions have been given, the heart and lungs are removed by transection, en bloc. This includes the aorta well above the heart, and the right atrium, the atrial septum, and the left atrium completely and as close to the patient's spine (or as posteriorly as possible). The heart/lung block is placed in a sealable plastic bag containing some of the ice-cold preserving solution for transport to the recipient or storage until the recipient is ready.

33935

The patient is placed on cardiopulmonary bypass and the heart and lungs are removed. The donor's organs are placed by sewing the left atrium of the donor to the left atrium of the recipient's first, and then sewing together their atrial septums and their right atrium. The donor aorta is then trimmed to an appropriate length and sewn to the ascending aorta of the recipient. Immunosuppressive drugs may be given to the patient before, during and after the operation. Cardiopulmonary bypass is discontinued when the donor's heart function returns.

33940

This is usually done when the heart is from an organ donor. Cold preserving solutions are then infused into the aorta and pulmonary arteries. After enough of those solutions have been given, the heart is removed moved by transection. The heart is placed in a sealable plastic bag containing some of the ice-cold preserving solution for transplant to the recipient or storage until the recipient is ready.

33945

The patient is placed on cardiopulmonary bypass. Cardiac transplantation may be performed by one of two techniques: total orthotopic heart replacement or heterotropic implantation. A total orthotopic heart replacement involves excising the ventricles, atrial appendages, and most of the coronary sinus from the donor heart. The recipient heart is then opened. The atria, aorta, and pulmonary artery of the recipient heart are anastomosed to the donor heart. The sinoatrial nodes of both the donor and recipient heart are left intact. In a heterotropic implantation, the donor's organs are placed by sewing the left atrium of the donor heart to the left atrium of the recipient, and then sewing together the atrial septums and the right atrium. The donor aorta is then trimmed to an appropriate length and sewn to the ascending aorta of the recipient. Immunosuppressive drugs may be given to the patient before, during, and after the operation. Cardiopulmonary bypass is discontinued when the donor heart begins functioning in the recipient.

33960

This operation is rarely done solely for pulmonary insufficiency (ECMD.) It can be done for either right of left ventricular failure or both. Cardiopulmonary bypass is required. For right ventricular failure, a pump uptake tube is placed in the right ventricular apex. A pump delivery tube is placed in the pulmonary artery. The pump is then turned on and the patient is weaned off of cardiopulmonary bypass. For left ventricular failure, the pump uptake tube is placed either in one of the pulmonary veins or in the left ventricle apex. The arterial delivery tube is placed in the aorta. The pump is then turned on and the patient is removed from cardiopulmonary bypass. Use 33960 for the initial 24 hours.

33961

This procedure involves maintaining the functioning of the external pumps, assessing the recovery of the patient's heart muscle, maintaining the patient's level of blood thinners, and assessing the need for either emergency placement of an implantable ventricular assist device, a total artificial heart or a donor heart transplant. Use 33961 for each additional 24-hour time period. Use 33961 in conjunction with 33960.

33967

An intra-aortic balloon catheter, usually with a 40 cc volume capacity, is inserted into the femoral artery and advanced under fluoroscopy to the distal portion of the aortic arch. After correct placement of the intra-aortic balloon assist device (IAB) in the descending aorta with its tip at the distal aortic arch, the balloon is connected to a drive console. The console consists of a pressurized gas reservoir, a monitor for ECG and pressure wave recording, adjustments for inflation/deflation timing, triggering selection switches and battery back-up power sources. Either

helium or carbon dioxide is used for inflation. Inflation and deflation are synchronized to the patients' cardiac cycle. Inflation at the onset of diastole results in proximal and distal displacement of blood volume in the aorta. Deflation occurs just prior to the onset of systole. Once the patient's cardiac performance improves, weaning from the intra-aortic balloon catheter pump (IABP) begins by gradually decreasing the balloon augmentation ratio under control of hemodynamic stability.

33968

The physician removes an intra-aortic balloon assist device (IABP). In a previous separately reportable procedure an IABP was inserted. When the patient is stabilized they are weaned off of the IAPB. The pump is turned off and the IABP catheter with the attached balloon is withdrawn from the femoral artery. Pressure is placed over the wound in the groin for a specified period of time. A light dressing is then applied. The patient may be placed at bed rest and observed for several hours to avoid problems that could arise from bleeding or a hematoma at the puncture site.

33970

This operation is done to help support the function of the left ventricle of the heart. The left or right femoral artery is exposed in the groin. After the vessel is occluded above and below the proposed insertion site, the artery is opened transversely. The end of a small tube of Gortex may then be sewn to the side of the artery, although this is only done sometimes. Tip of the balloon catheter is then inserted into the artery (or Gortex tube). The clamp occluding the artery upstream is released and the balloon catheter is advanced up the femoral artery an into the aorta above the level of the kidney arteries, but not beyond the left arm artery. It is then connected to a pump and the pump is turned on. The pump inflates and deflates the balloon during each heartbeat cycle.

33971

The previously placed balloon pump is withdrawn and the artery is occluded above and below the hole. If a Gortex sleeve has been used, it is simply tied off and no other repair is needed. If the balloon was directly introduced into the artery, the hole is sewn shut. If sewing the hole shut narrows the artery significantly, the hole can be patched with a piece of saphenous vein or Dacron. If the entire arterial diameter has been damaged, the segment of artery containing the hole can be removed and the artery replaced with an interposition graft of either Saphenous vein or Dacron tube.

33973

The procedure is done when 1) the femoral arteries cannot be readily exposed in the operating room because of patient positioning; 2) the arteries are occluded by atherosclerosis or trauma; 3) there will be a need to reopen the patient's chest soon. A balloon placed in this fashion must be removed in the operating room and his chest must be reopened. A purse string is placed in the aorta. A hole is made in the aorta in the middle of the purse string. The balloon is inserted through this hole until it lies beyond the left arm artery but above the kidney arteries. The purse string is then tightened with a tourniquet. The chest incision is not closed. The balloon is driven by a pump outside the patient.

33974

The physician removes an ascending aortic intra-aortic balloon assist device during performance of a primary procedure. If the sternum is open, the physician removes the aortic balloon while tightening purse-string sutures around the hole. When hemostasis is assured, the pericardium is repaired loosely with or without graft, leaving gaps for blood and fluid to drain into the plural space. The sternum is reanastomosed with sternal wires and the skin is closed in sutured layers. If the sternum is closed, a Dacron-tube graft (reported separately) is used as a vehicle for balloon removal. As the balloon is removed, the Dacron-tube graft tightens around the aortic incision to create aortic hemostasis.

33975–33976

Cardiopulmonary bypass is required. For right ventricular failure, a pump uptake tube is placed in the right ventricular apex. A pump delivery tube is placed in the pulmonary artery. The pump is then turned on and the patient is weaned off cardiopulmonary bypass. For left ventricular failure, the pump uptake tube is placed either in one of the pulmonary veins or in the left ventricle apex. The arterial delivery tube is placed in the aorta. The pump is then turned on and the patient is removed from cardiopulmonary bypass. The implanted pump is placed in a pocket formed in the upper abdominal wall, but outside the abdominal cavity. Tubes for the pump drive are brought out through separate incisions in the skin. The pump is then started and the patient is weaned off cardiopulmonary bypass. The device is removed when the patient's ventricle recovers, a total artificial heart is placed or the patient undergoes heart transplantation. Report 33976 if biventricular support is needed.

33977–33978

Cardiopulmonary bypass is required. The pump is stopped. All the tubes are removed and any holes in the heart or vessels are closed. The device is then removed from the patient's body. Cardiopulmonary bypass is discontinued when the patient's heart function returns. An intraaortic balloon pump is often required to allow discontinuation of bypass. All wounds are closed. Report 33978 if biventricular support is needed.

33979–33980

Physician makes a midline incision extending from the sternal notch to the umbilicus. Sternotomy is performed prior to creation of the pocket. The preperitoneal fat is dissected from the undersurface of the rectus sheath using low power cautery. Superiorly the dissection is carried to the undersurface of the diaphragm until the apex of the heart can be palpated just lateral to the inferior phrenic artery and vein and carried well back into the retroperitoneum. The preperitoneal space is opened to allow room for the device outflow valve and graft conduit. The muscular attachment of the right hemidiaphragm to the medial edge of the sternum is divided to allow room for the graft. A small incision is made and a tunneling device is passed subcutaneously inferiorly around the umbilicus, and into the pocket through the rectus sheath at its most inferior aspect. The tunneler is screwed onto the end of the driveline, which is then pulled back through the tunnel to the skin. The drive line is not attached to the skin. Cardiopulmonary bypass is instituted using standard aortic and dual stage venous cannulae. The apex of the left ventricle is elevated. The physician cores out a piece of ventricle and places the apical cuff sutures. An apical vent is passed into the left ventricle. Pledgeted 2-0 Ethibond sutures are placed circumferentially partial thickness into the myocardium then passed through the sewing ring of the apical cuff. Once the apical cuff is secure, a cruciate incision in the diaphragm opposite the ventricular apex is made just lateral to the inferior phrenic vessels, and the inflow cannula is brought into the chest. The inflow cannula is inserted through the apical cuff until the entire sintered titanium surface is within the cuff. The Dacron tie of the inflow cuff is secured and an additional plastic band and Dacron tie used to reinforce the connection and flatten out the silicone cuff. Blood is allowed to passively fill the device and exit via the outflow valve. A partial occluding clamp is placed on the right lateral aspect of the ascending aorta and a longitudinal aortotomy performed. The periaortic adventitia is left in place, and a strip of pericardium is incorporated into the anastomosis. The apex and heel of the anastomosis are reinforced with interrupted 4-0 prolene pledgeted horizontal mattress stitches. Inotropic support is started before separating from bypass and activating the LVAD. The device is switched to automatic mode after the cessation of cardiopulmonary bypass. Transesophageal echocardiography is used to ensure adequate ventricular decompression and a bubble study is performed to rule out a patent foramen ovale. A thermodilution cardiac output is performed and compared to the output from the LVAD. In the presence of severe coagulopathy the chest may need to be packed open. The device is removed (33980) when the patient's ventricle recovers, an artificial heart is placed, or the patient undergoes heart transplantation.

34001

To remove a blood clot in the carotid, subclavian, or innominate artery, the physician makes an incision in the skin of the neck usually in front of the sternocleidomastoid muscle over the site of the clot, or immediately above it. The artery is isolated and dissected from critical structures. The artery may be clamped above and below the clot, and then incised. The physician removes the blood clot and sutures the artery. The clamps are removed. If a catheter is required, it is threaded past the clot and a small balloon at its tip is inflated. The catheter is withdrawn, capturing and retrieving the clot. The physician may make several passes to remove all of the clot. The blood vessel is repaired with sutures and the skin incision is repaired with a layered closure.

34051

The physician exposes the innominate or subclavian artery by making an incision in the anterior chest (midline sternotomy or lateral thoracotomy). The physician identifies the embolus or thrombus and occludes the artery proximal to the clot. The physician then makes a small incision in the artery proximal to the clot. The physician withdraws the clot by passing a Fogarty balloon catheter beyond the clot, inflating, and withdrawing the balloon. The physician establishes proof of patency by injecting contrast in the artery under fluoroscope. The physician sutures the arteriotomy closed, removes the vascular clamp or tie, and closes the chest wall the embolus or thrombus and occludes the artery proximal to the clot. The physician makes a small incision in the artery proximal to the clot. The physician withdraws the clot using ring forceps, or by passing a Fogarty balloon catheter beyond the clot, inflating, and withdrawing the balloon. The physician establishes proof of patency by injecting contrast in the artery under fluoroscope. The physician then sutures the arteriotomy closed, removes the vascular clamp or tie, and closes the chest wall. The physician may then establish proof of patency by injecting contrast in the artery under fluoroscope. The physician then sutures the arteriotomy closed, removes the vascular clamp or tie, and closes the chest wall wound. The physician may leave chest tubes and/or a mediastinal drainage tube in place following the procedure.

34101

To remove a blood clot in the axillary, brachial, innominate, or subclavian artery, the physician makes an incision in the skin of the arm at the site of the blood clot or above it. The artery is isolated and dissected from critical structures. The artery may be clamped above and below the clot, and incised. The physician removes the blood clot and repairs the artery. The clamps are removed. If a catheter is required, it is threaded past the clot and a small balloon at its tip is inflated. The catheter is withdrawn, capturing and retrieving the clot. The physician may make several passes to remove all of

the clot. The blood vessel is repaired with sutures and the skin incision is repaired with a layered closure.

34111

To remove a blood clot in the radial or ulnar artery, the physician makes an incision in the skin of the arm, over the site of the clot or immediately above it. The artery is isolated and dissected from adjacent critical structures. The artery may be clamped above and below the clot, and incised. The physician removes the blood clot and repairs the artery. The clamps are removed. If a catheter is required, it is threaded past the clot and a small balloon at its tip is inflated. The catheter is withdrawn, capturing and retrieving the clot. The physician may make several passes to remove all of the clot. The blood vessel is repaired with sutures and the skin incision is repaired with a layered closure.

34151

To remove a blood clot in the renal, celiac, mesentery, aortoiliac artery, the physician makes an incision in the skin of the abdomen over the site of the clot or immediately above or below it. The vein is isolated and dissected from adjacent critical structures. The artery may be clamped above and below the clot, and then incised. The physician removes the blood clot. The clamps are removed. If a catheter is required, it is threaded past the clot and a small balloon at its tip is inflated. The catheter is withdrawn, capturing and retrieving the clot. The physician may make several passes to remove all of the clot. The blood vessel is repaired with sutures and the skin incision is repaired with a layered closure.

34201

To remove a blood clot in the femoropopliteal or aortoiliac artery, the physician makes an incision in the skin of the leg over the femoral artery. The artery is isolated and dissected from adjacent critical structures. The artery may be clamped above and below the clot and incised. The physician removes the blood clot and repairs the vessel. The clamps are removed. If a catheter is required, it is threaded past the clot and a small balloon at its tip is inflated. The catheter is withdrawn, capturing and retrieving the clot. The physician may make several passes to remove all of the clot. The blood vessel is repaired with sutures and the skin incision is repaired with a layered closure.

34203

To remove a blood clot in the popliteal-tibio-peroneal artery, the physician makes an incision in the skin of the leg over the femoral or popliteal artery. The artery is isolated and dissected from adjacent critical structures. The artery may be clamped above and below the clot, and then incised. The physician removes the blood clot. The clamps are removed. If a catheter is required, it is threaded past the clot and a small balloon at its tip is inflated. The catheter is withdrawn, capturing and retrieving the clot. The physician may make several passes to remove all of the clot. The blood vessel is repaired with sutures and the skin incision is repaired with a layered closure.

34401

The physician exposes the vena cava by making an abdominal incision. The physician identifies the thrombus by venogram and may perform a contralateral femoral venogram to rule out inferior vena caval involvement. The physician makes an incision in the vena cava. The physician withdraws the clot by passing a Fogarty balloon catheter beyond the clot, inflating, and withdrawing the balloon. The physician may attempt to reduce the risk of pulmonary embolism by increasing intrathoracic pressure in a ventilated patient. The physician may establish proof of patency by repeat venography. The physician then sutures the venotomy closed and closes the wound.

34421

To remove a blood clot in the vena cava, iliac, or femoropopliteal vein, the physician makes an incision in the skin of the upper leg over the site of the clot or immediately above or below it. The vein is isolated and dissected from adjacent critical structures. The vein may be clamped above and below the clot, and then incised. The physician removes the blood clot. The clamps are removed. If a catheter is required, it is threaded past the clot and a small balloon at its tip is inflated. The catheter is withdrawn, capturing and retrieving the clot. The physician may make several passes to remove all of the clot. The blood vessel is repaired with sutures and the skin incision is repaired with a layered closure.

34451

The physician exposes the common femoral, superficial femoral, and Saphenous veins by making an inguinal incision. The physician identifies the thrombus by venogram and may perform a contralateral femoral venogram to rule out inferior vena caval involvement. The physician makes an incision in the distal common femoral vein. The physician withdraws the proximal clot by passing a Fogarty balloon catheter beyond the clot, inflating, and withdrawing the balloon. The physician may attempt to reduce the risk of pulmonary embolism by increasing intrathoracic pressure in a ventilated patient or asking the patient to perform a Valsalva maneuver if the procedure is performed under local anesthesia. The physician cuts down and introduces a Fogarty catheter via the popliteal vein, advancing the catheter toward the femoral vein while extruding thrombus through the femoral venotomy. The physician may establish proof of patency by repeat venography. The physician sutures the venotomy closed and closes the inguinal wound.

34471

To remove a blood clot in the subclavian vein, the physician makes an incision in the skin of the neck over the site of the clot or immediately above or below it. The vein is isolated and dissected from adjacent critical structures. The vein may be clamped above and below the clot, and then incised. The physician removes the blood clot. The clamps are removed. If a catheter is required, it is threaded past the clot and a small balloon at its tip is inflated. The catheter is withdrawn, capturing and retrieving the clot. The physician may make several passes to remove all of the clot. The blood vessel is repaired with sutures and the skin incision is repaired with a layered closure.

34490

To remove a blood clot in the axillary and subclavian vein, the physician makes an incision in the skin of the arm over the site of the clot or immediately above or below it. The vein is isolated and dissected from adjacent critical structures. The vein may be clamped above and below the clot, and then incised. The physician removes the blood clot. The clamps are removed. If a catheter is required, it is threaded past the clot and a small balloon at its tip is inflated. The catheter is withdrawn, capturing and retrieving the clot. The physician may make several passes to remove all of the clot. The blood vessel is repaired with sutures and the skin incision is repaired with a layered closure.

34501

The physician makes an incision in the skin overlying the site of the incompetent valve. The femoral vein is isolated and dissected from adjacent critical structures. The physician affixes vessel clamps above and below the malfunctioning valve. The physician opens the vein and repairs the valve leaflets by suture plication (tacking the excess valve material). The vein is repaired with sutures. The clamps are removed and the skin incision is repaired with a layered closure.

34502

The physician exposes the inferior vena cava by making an incision in the anterior abdomen. The physician clamps the vena cava proximally and sutures any defects closed. The physician may replace or bypass abnormal vena caval tissue with synthetic graft material. The physician may inject intravenous contrast under fluoroscope to demonstrate appropriate flow. The physician unclamps the vena cava and closes the abdominal wall incision. The physician may leave a surgical drain in place.

34510

The physician makes an incision in the skin overlying the site of the malfunctioning valve. The vein is isolated and dissected from adjacent critical structures. The physician affixes vessel clamps above and below the vein and excises the section of vein containing the malfunctioning valve. A section of harvested vein containing functional valves is then sutured end-to-end to the vein. The clamps are removed and the skin incision is repaired with a layered closure.

34520

The physician makes an incision in the skin overlying the site of the incompetent valve. The incompetent vein is isolated and dissected from adjacent critical structures. The physician affixes vessel clamps above and below the vein. The divided section of incompetent vein is connected to a nearby vein with functioning valves, placing competent values above the incompetent vein. Both the vein and the skin incision are closed with sutures.

34530

The physician makes an incision in the skin overlying the site of the greater Saphenous vein just below the knee. The vein is isolated and dissected from adjacent critical structures. The physician affixes vessel clamps above and below the incision site. The dissected section of Saphenous vein is then connected to the popliteal vein in an end-to-side anastomosis. The other end of the Saphenous vein is closed with sutures. Once the Saphenous vein and the popliteal vein are connected, the clamps are removed and the skin incision is repaired with a layered closure.

34800–34804

Endovascular repair or dissection of an infrarenal aortic aneurysm requires the skills of both a vascular surgeon and a radiologist. In endovascular repair a small incision is made in the groin over one or both femoral artery(ies). Under separately reportable fluoroscopy, a synthetic stent graft, approximately 6 inches long and contained inside a long plastic holding capsule, is threaded through the arteries to the site of the infrarenal aneurysm. Once the stent is in place, the holding capsule is removed. The stent graft, activated by heat, expands like a spring and becomes anchored to the artery wall serving as a substitute channel to carry blood. If full expansion of the prosthesis does not occur automatically, a balloon catheter is then threaded to the graft site and inflated within the endovascular prosthesis until full expansion is achieved. The catheter is removed and the arteriotomy site is closed. The aneurysm, excluded from the blood flow, typically shrinks over time. Report 34800 when a tube or straight prosthetic graft is used; 34802 when a modular bifurcated prosthetic graft (one docking limb) is used; 34804 when a unibody bifurcated prosthetic graft is used.

34808

Endovascular placement of iliac artery occlusion device is performed during separately reportable endovascular placement of infrarenal aortic aneurysm graft. Before the aneurysm can be repaired, the iliac artery below the aneurysm must be temporarily

occluded. Under separately reportable fluoroscopy, an iliac artery occlusion device is threaded through the arteries and placed distal to the aneurysm. When the aneurysm repair is complete the endovascular occlusion device is removed.

34812

The physician creates a femoral cutdown incision to expose one of the femoral arteries. The physician punctures the femoral artery with a large needle and passes a guidewire via the needle into the femoral artery. The physician removes the needle while leaving the guidewire in place, enlarges the arterial opening slightly with a blade, then slides an introducer sheath over the guidewire into the arterial lumen. Exposure of the femoral artery is followed by endovascular repair of an abdominal aneurysm. Under separately reportable fluoroscopy, a synthetic stent graft, approximately 6 inches long and contained inside a long plastic holding capsule, is threaded through the arteries to the site of the abdominal aneurysm. Once the stent is in place, the holding capsule is removed. The stent graft, activated by heat, expands like a spring and becomes anchored to the artery wall serving as a substitute channel to carry blood. If full expansion of the prosthesis does not occur automatically, a balloon catheter is then threaded to the graft site and inflated within the endovascular prosthesis until full expansion is achieved. The catheter is removed and the arteriotomy site is closed. The aneurysm, excluded from the blood flow, typically shrinks over time.

34813

During separately reportable endovascular repair of an abdominal aortic aneurysm, a diseased or damaged femoral artery is repaired by femoral-femoral bypass. Through incisions in the skin of the upper thighs, the physician isolates and dissects a section of the femoral arteries. The physician creates a bypass using a harvested vein. Once vessel clamps have been affixed above and below the area of anastomosis, the femoral artery may be cut through below the diseased or damaged area and sutured to one end of a harvested vein. The vein is sutured to the femoral artery in the opposite leg, resulting in a bypass of the damaged or blocked area. When the clamps are removed, the section of vein forms a new path through which blood can easily bypass the blocked area. The blocked or damaged portion of the artery is not removed. After the graft is complete, the skin incisions are repaired with layered closures.

34820

The physician exposes the iliac artery to facilitate introduction of the endovascular prosthesis or to perform temporary iliac artery occlusion procedure during endovascular therapy using either an abdominal or retroperitoneal incision. If the artery has been exposed for the purpose of placing a temporary occlusion device, the clamp is placed. If the artery has been exposed to facilitate introduction of the endovascular prosthesis, the physician first punctures the artery with a large needle and then passes a guidewire via the needle into the iliac artery. The physician removes the needle while leaving the guidewire in place, enlarges the arterial opening slightly with a blade, then slides an introducer sheath over the guidewire into the arterial lumen. Under separately reportable fluoroscopy, a synthetic stent graft, approximately 6 inches long and contained inside a long plastic holding capsule, is threaded through the arteries to the site of the infrarenal aneurysm. Once the stent is in place, the holding capsule is removed. The stent graft, activated by heat, expands like a spring and becomes anchored to the artery wall serving as a substitute channel to carry blood. If full expansion of the prosthesis does not occur automatically, a balloon catheter is then threaded to the graft site and inflated within the endovascular prosthesis until full expansion is achieved. The catheter is removed and the arteriotomy site is closed.

34825–34826

Cases of incomplete exclusion, called endoleaks, can occur at the proximal or distal fixation sites, through the body of the graft or from patent lumbar arteries in the aneurysm sac. Endoleaks sometimes seal on their own but may also require additional endovascular procedures. Using separately reportable aortography the site of the leak is identified. The proper extension prosthesis is selected. Under separately reportable fluoroscopy, the extension prosthesis, contained inside a long plastic holding capsule, is threaded through the arteries to the site of the leak. Once the extension prosthesis is in place, the holding capsule is removed. The extension prosthesis, activated by heat, expands like a spring and becomes anchored to the artery wall at the site of the endoleak. If full expansion of the prosthesis does not occur automatically, a balloon catheter is then threaded to the graft site and inflated within the endovascular prosthesis until full expansion is achieved. The catheter is removed and the arteriotomy site is closed. Report 34825 for placement of an extension prosthesis in the initial vessel and 34826 for placement of an extension prosthesis in each additional vessel.

34830–34832

An attempted endovascular repair of an aortic aneurysm originating below the renal arteries (infrarenal) fails necessitating open repair of the aneurysm as well as repair of any trauma associated with the endovascular attempt. An incision is made in the abdomen from just below the diaphragm to the umbilicus. The aorta is exposed, the aneurysm identified, and the aorta and other arteries inspected for injury resulting from the failed endovascular procedure. Repair of the aneurysm is accomplished by temporarily clamping the aorta both above and below the aneurysm. It is usually possible to place the upper clamp just below the origins of the renal arteries so that the kidneys continue to receive blood flow throughout the operation. Blood flow to the legs is interrupted while the aorta is clamped. The aneurysm is opened lengthwise and any thrombi (blood clots) removed. The aneurysm wall is not removed. The aorta is cut above and below the aneurysm and a prosthetic graft made of synthetic material is sutured in place between the two ends. The aneurysm wall is then wrapped around the synthetic graft. The clamps are removed allowing blood to flow through the graft and into the vessels of the lower extremities. The surgical wound is then closed. Repair using a tube prosthesis is reported with 34830; repair with an aorto-bi-iliac prosthesis is reported with 34831; and repair with a aorto-bifemoral prothesis is reported with 34832.

35001–35002

The physician makes an incision in the neck in front of the sternocleidomastoid muscle. The section of the carotid or subclavian artery (35001) or the ruptured section (35002) is isolated and dissected from adjacent critical structures. Vessel clamps are affixed above and below the defect. The repair may be accomplished by removing the segment of artery containing the aneurysm and suturing the exposed ends of the vessel in an end-to-end fashion or the aneurysm may be bypassed with a venous or synthetic graft. If a large section is removed, a harvested or synthetic graft is inserted into the defect, or a patch may be sutured into place to open up the diameter of the vessel. The skin incision is repaired with a layered closure.

35005

The physician makes an incision in the skin overlying the neck. The enlarged or blocked section of the vertebral artery is isolated and dissected from muscles and adjacent critical structures. A portion of a cervical vertebra may be removed to access the defect. Vessel clamps are affixed above and below the defect, which may be repaired or removed. The repair may be accomplished by removing the segment of artery containing the aneurysm and suturing the exposed ends of the vessel in an end-to-end fashion or the aneurysm may be bypassed with a venous or synthetic graft. If a large section is removed, a harvested or synthetic graft is inserted into the defect. Instead of a complete graft, a patch may be sutured into place to open up the diameter of the vessel. Once the vessel is repaired, the clamps are removed. The skin incision is repaired with a layered closure.

35011–35013

The physician makes an incision in the skin of the arm or axilla. The enlarged or blocked section of the axillary or brachial artery (35011) or the ruptured section (35013) is isolated and dissected from adjacent critical structures. Vessel clamps are affixed above and below the defect, which may be repaired or removed. The repair may be accomplished by removing the segment of artery containing the aneurysm and suturing the exposed ends of the vessel in an end-to-end fashion or the aneurysm may be bypassed with a venous or synthetic graft. If a large section is removed, a harvested or synthetic graft is inserted into the defect. Instead of a complete graft, a patch may be sutured into place to open up the diameter of the vessel. Once the vessel is repaired, the clamps are removed. The skin incision is repaired with a layered closure.

35021

The physician exposes the innominate or subclavian artery by median sternotomy or lateral thoracotomy. The physician anticoagulates the patient with heparin, then clamps the aortic arch widely around the origin of the innominate artery, then clamps the right common carotid and right subclavian arteries. The physician excises the aneurysmal tissue. The physician may use a woven Dacron patch graft or harvested vein to repair the aneurysmal artery. The physician unclamps the aorta, as well as the right common carotid and right subclavian arteries. The physician closes the sternotomy or thoracotomy, leaving a chest tube in place.

35022

The physician exposes the innominate or subclavian artery by median sternotomy or lateral thoracotomy. The physician clamps the aortic arch widely around the origin of the innominate artery, then clamps the right common carotid and right subclavian arteries. The physician excises the ruptured aneurysmal tissue. The physician may use a woven Dacron patch graft or harvested vein to repair the aneurysmal artery. The physician unclamps the aorta, as well as the right common carotid and right subclavian arteries. The physician closes the sternotomy or thoracotomy, leaving a chest tube in place.

35045

The physician makes an incision in the skin overlying the arm. The enlarged or blocked section of the radial or ulnar artery is isolated and dissected from adjacent critical structures. Vessel clamps are affixed above and below the defect, which may be repaired or removed. The repair may be accomplished by removing the segment of artery containing the aneurysm and suturing the exposed ends of the vessel in an end-to-end fashion or the aneurysm may be bypassed with a venous or synthetic graft. If a large section is removed, a harvested or synthetic graft is inserted into the defect. Instead of a complete graft, a patch may be sutured into place to open up the diameter of the vessel. Once the vessel is repaired, the clamps are removed. The skin incision is repaired with a layered closure.

35081

The physician exposes the abdominal aorta using a transperitoneal approach, placing a long incision in the mid abdomen. The physician retracts the transverse colon and small bowel to allow dissection and exposure of the aorta. The physician places an umbilical tape or rubber catheter around the aorta proximal to the aneurysm. The physician exposes the iliac arteries and achieves control of blood flow with umbilical tape or rubber catheters. The physician anticoagulates the patient and cross-clamps the iliac arteries and proximal aorta. The physician opens and clears the aneurysm, controls collateral bleeding from the lumbar arteries with suture, then sutures a Y-shaped knitted Dacron graft to the proximal aorta. The physician sutures the distal ends of the graft to the iliac arteries. The physician may then anastomose the inferior mesenteric arteries and any aberrant or accessory renal arteries to the Dacron graft. The physician then sutures the remaining aneurysmal shell around the graft and closes the retroperitoneum. The physician closes the abdominal wound, leaving drains in place.

35082

The physician quickly exposes the abdominal aorta using a transperitoneal approach, placing a long incision in the mid abdomen. The physician retracts the transverse colon and small bowel to allow dissection and exposure of the aorta. The physician quickly achieves control of bleeding by pushing the liver aside and compressing the aorta manually against the spine. The physician resuscitates the patient with fluids and blood products if necessary, then cross-clamps the aorta proximal to the dissection. The physician exposes the iliac arteries and achieves control of blood flow with umbilical tape or rubber catheters. The physician then anticoagulates the patient (if bleeding is controlled) and cross-clamps the iliac arteries and proximal aorta. The physician opens and clears the aneurysm, controls collateral bleeding from the lumbar arteries with suture, then sutures a Y-shaped knitted Dacron graft to the proximal aorta. The physician then sutures the distal ends of the graft to the iliac arteries. The physician then sutures the remaining aneurysmal shell around the graft and closes the retroperitoneum. The physician closes the abdominal wound, leaving drains in place.

35091

The physician exposes the abdominal aorta using a transperitoneal approach, placing a long incision in the midabdomen. The physician retracts the transverse colon and small bowel to allow dissection and exposure of the aorta. The physician places an umbilical tape or rubber catheter around the aorta proximal to the aneurysm. The physician then exposes the iliac arteries and achieves control of blood flow with umbilical tape or rubber catheters. The physician then anticoagulates the patient and cross-clamps the iliac arteries and proximal aorta. The physician opens and clears the aneurysm, controls collateral bleeding from the lumbar arteries with suture, then sutures a Y-shaped knitted Dacron graft to the proximal aorta. The physician sutures the distal ends of the graft to the iliac arteries. The physician may then anastomose the inferior mesenteric arteries and any aberrant or accessory renal arteries to the Dacron graft. The physician then sutures the remaining aneurysmal shell around the graft and closes the retroperitoneum. The physician closes the abdominal wound, leaving drains in place.

35092

The physician quickly exposes the abdominal aorta using a transperitoneal approach, placing a long incision in the midabdomen. The physician retracts the transverse colon and small bowel to allow dissection and exposure of the aorta. The physician quickly achieves control of bleeding by pushing the liver aside and compressing the aorta manually against the spine. The physician resuscitates the patient with fluids and blood products if necessary, then cross-clamps the aorta proximal to the dissection. The physician then exposes the iliac arteries and achieves control of blood flow with umbilical tape or rubber catheters. The physician anticoagulates the patient (if bleeding is controlled) and cross-clamps the iliac arteries and proximal aorta. The physician opens and clears the aneurysm, controls collateral bleeding from the lumbar arteries with suture, then sutures a Y-shaped knitted Dacron graft to the proximal aorta. The physician then sutures the distal ends of the graft to the iliac arteries. The physician may then anastomose the celiac, inferior mesenteric, and/or renal arteries to the Dacron graft. The physician then sutures the remaining aneurysmal shell around the graft and closes the retroperitoneum. The physician closes the abdominal wound, leaving drains in place.

35102

The physician exposes the abdominal aorta using a transperitoneal approach, placing a long incision in the mid abdomen. The physician retracts the transverse colon and small bowel to allow dissection and exposure of the aorta. The physician places an umbilical tape or rubber catheter around the aorta proximal to the aneurysm. The physician exposes the iliac arteries and achieves control of blood flow with umbilical tape or rubber catheters. The physician then anticoagulates the patient and cross-clamps the iliac arteries and proximal aorta. The physician opens and clears the aneurysm, controls collateral bleeding from the lumbar arteries with suture, then sutures a Y-shaped knitted Dacron graft to the proximal aorta. The physician sutures the distal ends of the graft to the iliac arteries. The physician may anastomose grafts from other involved iliac vessels (common, hypogastric, external) to the Dacron graft. The physician then sutures the remaining aneurysmal shell around the graft and closes the retroperitoneum. The physician closes the abdominal wound, leaving drains in place.

35103

The physician quickly exposes the abdominal aorta using a transperitoneal approach, placing a long incision in the mid abdomen. The physician retracts the transverse colon and small bowel to allow dissection and exposure of the aorta. The physician quickly achieves control of bleeding by pushing the liver aside and compressing the aorta manually against the spine. The physician resuscitates the patient with fluids and blood products if necessary, then cross-clamps the aorta proximal to the dissection. The physician then exposes the iliac arteries and achieves control of blood flow with umbilical tape or rubber catheters. The physician then anticoagulates the patient (if bleeding is controlled) and cross-clamps the iliac arteries and proximal aorta. The physician opens and clears the aneurysm, controls collateral bleeding from the lumbar arteries with suture, then sutures a Y-shaped knitted Dacron graft to the proximal aorta. The physician then sutures the distal ends of the graft to the iliac arteries. The physician may then anastomose the celiac, inferior mesenteric, and/or renal arteries to the Dacron graft. The physician then sutures the remaining aneurysmal shell around the graft and closes the retroperitoneum. The physician closes the abdominal wound, leaving drains in place.

35111

The physician exposes the splenic artery using an abdominal incision. If the aneurysm involves the proximal or distal (hilar) splenic artery, the physician may either repair the aneurysm using harvested venous material or synthetic graft material or simply tie off the diseased artery and vein. If the aneurysm involves the middle splenic artery, which is surrounded by pancreatic tissue, the surgeon may tie off the artery to avoid dissection of the pancreas. The physician then closes the abdominal wound, leaving drains in place.

35112

The physician quickly exposes the splenic artery using an abdominal incision, and gains control of bleeding by clamping the proximal splenic artery. If the aneurysm involves the proximal or distal (hilar) splenic artery, the physician may either repair the aneurysm (using harvested venous material or synthetic graft material) or simply tie off the diseased artery and vein. If the aneurysm involves the middle splenic artery, which is surrounded by pancreatic tissue, the surgeon may tie off the artery to avoid dissection of the pancreas. The physician then closes the abdominal wound, leaving drains in place.

35121

The physician exposes the involved hepatic, celiac, renal, or mesenteric artery using an abdominal incision, retracting and dissecting past large and small bowel. If the aneurysm involves an artery whose vascular distribution has adequate collaterals (the common hepatic artery, for example), the physician may simply tie off the diseased artery. Otherwise, the physician repairs the aneurysm, often using harvested vein graft, harvested internal iliac artery graft, or synthetic graft material. The physician then closes the abdominal wound, leaving drains in place.

35122

The physician quickly exposes the involved hepatic, celiac, renal, or mesenteric artery using an abdominal incision, retracting and dissecting past large and small bowel. The physician controls bleeding by clamping or compressing the involved artery proximal to the rupture. If the aneurysm involves an artery whose vascular distribution has adequate collaterals (the common hepatic artery, for example), the physician may simply tie off the diseased artery. Otherwise, the physician repairs the aneurysm, often using harvested vein graft, harvested internal iliac artery graft, or synthetic graft material. The physician then closes the abdominal wound, leaving drains in place.

35131

The physician exposes the involved iliac arterial branch(es) using a low abdominal incision. The physician repairs the aneurysm, clamping off the affected artery proximally and distally, replacing the affected arterial segment with harvested venous material or synthetic graft material such as Dacron mesh. The physician confirms arterial patency with a Doppler probe or by angiography. The physician then closes the abdominal wound, leaving drains in place.

35132

The physician quickly exposes the involved iliac arterial branch(es) using a low abdominal incision. The physician gains control of bleeding by clamping or compressing the proximal segment of the affected artery. The physician repairs the aneurysm, clamping off the affected artery proximally and distally, replacing the affected arterial segment with harvested venous material or synthetic graft material such as Dacron mesh. The physician confirms arterial patency with a Doppler probe or by angiography. The physician then closes the abdominal wound, leaving drains in place.

35141–35142

The physician makes an incision in the skin of the leg. The enlarged or blocked section of the femoral artery (35141) or ruptured section (35142) is isolated and dissected from adjacent critical structures. Vessel clamps are affixed above and below the defect, which may be repaired or removed. The repair may be accomplished by removing the segment of artery containing the aneurysm and suturing the exposed ends of the vessel in an end-to-end fashion or the aneurysm may be bypassed with a venous or synthetic graft. If a large section is removed, a harvested or synthetic graft is inserted into the defect. Instead of a complete graft, a patch may be sutured into place to

open up the diameter of the vessel. Once the vessel is repaired, the clamps are removed. The skin incision is repaired with a layered closure.

35151–35152

The physician makes an incision in the skin over the leg. The enlarged or blocked section of the popliteal artery (35151) or the ruptured section (35152) is isolated and dissected from adjacent critical structures. Vessel clamps are affixed above and below the defect, which may be repaired or removed. The repair may be accomplished by removing the segment of artery containing the aneurysm and suturing the exposed ends of the vessel in an end-to-end fashion or the aneurysm may be bypassed with a venous or synthetic graft. If a large section is removed, a harvested or synthetic graft is inserted into the defect. Instead of a complete graft, a patch may be sutured into place to open up the diameter of the vessel. Once the vessel is repaired, the clamps are removed. The skin incision is repaired with a layered closure.

35161–35162

The physician makes an incision in the skin over the site of the enlarged or blocked section of artery (35161) or a ruptured section of artery (35162) and isolates and dissects it from adjacent critical structures. Vessel clamps are affixed above and below the defect, which may be repaired or removed. The repair may be accomplished by removing the segment of artery containing the aneurysm and suturing the exposed ends of the vessel in an end-to-end fashion or the aneurysm may be bypassed with a venous or synthetic graft. If a large section is removed, a harvested or synthetic graft is inserted into the defect. Instead of a complete graft, a patch may be sutured into place to open up the diameter of the vessel. Once the vessel is repaired, the clamps are removed. The skin incision is repaired with a layered closure.

35180

The physician makes an incision in the skin of the head or neck over the site of the unnatural opening, a congenital fistula, that exists between an artery and vein. The fistula is isolated and dissected from adjacent critical structures, and vessel clamps are applied to the vein and the artery. The walls of the artery and vein creating the fistula are each sutured closed. A graft or patch graft may be required to complete the repair. The fistula is tied off, or it may be excised. Once the fistula has been eliminated, the clamps are removed and the skin incision is repaired with a layered closure.

35182

The physician exposes the congenital arteriovenous fistula by choosing an incision appropriate to the fistula site. The physician examines the fistulous connection and repairs it by ligation (tying it off), if possible. The physician may repair the fistula by clamping the connection from both sides, dividing the

CPT® Lay Descriptions

connection with scissors, and closing each side with suture. The physician may sew in synthetic graft material or vein material harvested from the patient to enlarge the arterial or venous lumen. The physician may confirm vessel patency with Doppler probe or angiography prior to closing the wound. The physician may leave surgical drains in place.

35184

The physician makes an incision in the skin of an extremity over the site of the unnatural opening, a congenital fistula, that exists between an artery and vein. The fistula is isolated and dissected from adjacent critical structures, and vessel clamps are applied to the vein and the artery. The walls of the artery and vein creating the fistula are each sutured closed. A graft or patch graft may be required to complete the repair. The fistula is tied off, or it may be excised. Once the fistula has been eliminated, the clamps are removed and the skin incision is repaired with a layered closure.

35188–35189

The physician makes an incision in the skin of the head or neck over the site of the unnatural opening, a fistula, created through trauma. The fistula connects an artery to a vein. The fistula is isolated and dissected from adjacent critical structures, and vessel clamps are applied to the vein and the artery. The walls of the artery and vein creating the fistula are each repaired and closed. A graft or patch graft may be required to complete the repair. The fistula is tied off or excised. Once the fistula has been eliminated, the clamps are removed and the skin incision is repaired with a layered closure. Report 35189 if either fistula is in the thorax or abdomen.

35190

The physician makes an incision in the skin of an extremity at the site of the unnatural opening, a fistula, created through trauma. It connects an artery to a vein. The fistula is isolated and dissected from adjacent critical structures, and vessel clamps are applied to the vein and the artery. The walls of the artery and vein creating the fistula are each repaired and closed. A graft or patch graft may be required to complete the repair. The fistula is tied off or excised. Once the fistula has been eliminated, the clamps are removed and the skin incision is repaired with a layered closure.

35201

The physician makes an incision in the skin of the neck over the site of an injured blood vessel. The vessel is isolated and dissected from adjacent critical structures, and vessel clamps are applied. The edges of the injured vessel may be trimmed to ease repair. A patch graft may be sutured over the defect or the hole in the vessel may be repaired with sutures. The clamps are removed and the skin incision is repaired with a layered closure.

35206

The physician makes an incision in the skin of an upper extremity over the site of an injured blood vessel. The vessel is isolated and dissected from adjacent critical structures, and vessel clamps are applied. The edges of the injured vessel may be trimmed to ease repair. A patch graft may be sutured over the defect or the hole in the vessel may be repaired with sutures. The clamps are removed and the skin incision is repaired with a layered closure.

35207

The physician makes an incision in the skin of the hand or finger over the site of an injured blood vessel. The vessel is isolated and dissected from adjacent critical structures, and vessel clamps are applied. The edges of the injured vessel may be trimmed to ease repair. A patch graft may be sutured over the defect or the hole in the vessel may be repaired with sutures. The clamps are removed and the skin incision is repaired with a layered closure.

35211

The physician exposes the abnormal blood vessel (arterial or venous) by choosing a thoracic incision appropriate to the involved vessel. The physician places cardiopulmonary bypass catheters (through incisions in the low inferior vena cava, the superior vena cava, and high aorta or femoral artery). The physician stops the heart by infusing cardioplegia solution into the coronary circulation. The physician examines the abnormal vessel and repairs it by ligation (tying it off), if possible. The physician may repair the vessel by clamping it proximally and distally to the defect, and suturing the defect closed. The physician may choose to repair the vessel by sewing in synthetic graft material or vein material harvested from the patient in order to enlarge the lumen of the repaired vessel (patch graft). The physician then confirms vessel patency with Doppler probe or angiography prior to taking the patient off cardiopulmonary bypass and closing the wound. The physician leaves chest and, possibly, mediastinal drains in place.

35216

The physician exposes the abnormal blood vessel (arterial or venous) by choosing a thoracic incision appropriate to the involved vessel. The physician examines the abnormal vessel and repairs it by ligation if possible. The physician may repair the vessel by clamping it proximally and distally to the defect, and suturing the defect closed. The physician may choose to repair the vessel by sewing in synthetic graft material or vein material harvested from the patient in order to enlarge the lumen of the repaired vessel (patch graft). The physician confirms vessel patency with Doppler probe or angiography prior to closing the wound. The physician leaves chest and, possibly, mediastinal drains in place. If repair is accomplished with a venous bypass (rather than patch) graft, use 35246. If repair is accomplished with a synthetic bypass (rather than patch) graft, use 35276.

35221

The physician exposes the abnormal blood vessel (arterial or venous) by choosing an abdominal incision appropriate to the involved vessel. The physician examines the abnormal vessel and repairs it by ligation (tying it off), if possible. The physician may repair the vessel by clamping it proximally and distally to the defect, and suturing the defect closed. The physician confirms vessel patency with Doppler probe or angiography prior to closing the wound. The physician leaves surgical drains in place.

35226

The physician makes an incision in the skin of a lower extremity over the site of an injured blood vessel. The vessel is isolated and dissected from adjacent critical structures, and vessel clamps are applied. The edges of the injured vessel may be trimmed to ease repair. A patch graft may be sutured over the defect or the hole in the vessel may be repaired with sutures. The clamps are removed and the skin incision is repaired with a layered closure.

35231

The physician makes an incision in the skin in the neck over the site of an injured blood vessel. The vessel is isolated and dissected from adjacent critical structures, and vessel clamps are applied. The defect is too extensive to repair directly, so the physician removes a short length of vein. The physician repairs the injured vessel with a length of vein harvested from another site in the body or with cadaver vein. The vein is sutured end-to-end to the vessel, replacing the excised portion, or is used as a patch to repair a large hole in the side of the vessel. A patch graft may be sutured over any remaining the defect. The clamps are removed and the skin incision is repaired with a layered closure.

35236

The physician makes an incision in the skin of an upper extremity over the site of an injured blood vessel. The vessel is isolated and dissected from adjacent critical structures, and vessel clamps are applied. The defect is too extensive to repair directly, so the physician removes a short length of vein. The physician repairs the injured vessel with a length of vein harvested from another site in the body or with cadaver vein. The vein is sutured end-to-end to the vessel, replacing the excised portion, or is used as a patch to repair a large hole in the side of the vessel. A patch graft may be sutured over any remaining defect. The clamps are removed and the skin incision is repaired with a layered closure.

35241

The physician exposes the abnormal blood vessel (arterial or venous) by choosing a thoracic incision appropriate to the involved vessel. The physician places cardiopulmonary bypass catheters through incisions in the low inferior vena cava, the superior vena cava, and high aorta or femoral artery. The physician stops the heart by infusing cardioplegia solution into the coronary circulation. The physician examines the abnormal vessel and repairs it by clamping proximally and distally to the defect, and sewing in venous graft material harvested from the patient in order to bypass the abnormal area of the vessel (bypass graft). The physician confirms vessel patency with Doppler probe or angiography prior to taking the patient off cardiopulmonary bypass and closing the wound. The physician leaves chest and, possibly, mediastinal drains in place. If repair is accomplished with a venous patch (rather than bypass) graft, use 35211. If repair is accomplished with a synthetic bypass (rather than venous bypass) graft, use 35271.

35246

The physician exposes the abnormal blood vessel (arterial or venous) by choosing a thoracic incision appropriate to the involved vessel. The physician examines the abnormal vessel and repairs it by clamping proximally and distally to the defect, and sewing in vein material harvested from the patient in order to bypass the abnormal portion of the repaired vessel (bypass graft). The physician confirms vessel patency with Doppler probe or angiography prior to closing the wound. The physician leaves chest and, possibly, mediastinal drains in place. If repair is accomplished with a venous patch (rather than bypass) graft, use 35216. If repair is accomplished with a synthetic bypass (rather than venous bypass) graft, use 35276.

35251

The physician exposes the abnormal blood vessel (arterial or venous) by choosing an abdominal incision appropriate to the involved vessel. The physician examines the abnormal vessel and repairs it by clamping proximally and distally to the defect, and sewing in vein material harvested from the patient in order to bypass the abnormal area of the diseased vessel (bypass graft). The physician then confirms vessel patency with Doppler probe or angiography prior to closing the wound. The physician leaves surgical drains in place. If repair is accomplished with a venous patch (rather than bypass) graft, use 35221. If repair is accomplished with a synthetic bypass (rather than patch) graft, use 35281.

35256

The physician makes an incision in the skin of a lower extremity over the site of an injured blood vessel. The vessel is isolated and dissected from adjacent critical structures, and vessel clamps are applied. The defect is too extensive to repair directly, so the physician removes a short length of vein. The physician repairs the injured vessel with a length of vein harvested from another site in the body or with cadaver vein. The vein is sutured end-to-end to the vessel, replacing the excised portion, or is used as a patch to repair a large hole in the side of the vessel. A patch graft may be sutured over any remaining defect. The clamps are removed and the skin incision is repaired with a layered closure.

35261

The physician makes an incision in the skin of the neck over the site of an injured blood vessel. The vessel is isolated and dissected from adjacent critical structures, and vessel clamps are applied. The defect is too extensive to repair directly, so the physician removes a short length of vein. The physician repairs the injured vessel with a length of synthetic graft material. The synthetic vein is sutured end-to-end to the vessel, replacing the excised portion. A patch graft may be sutured over any remaining defect. The clamps are removed and the skin incision is repaired with a layered closure.

35266

The physician makes an incision in the skin of an upper extremity over the site of an injured blood vessel. The vessel is isolated and dissected from adjacent critical structures, and vessel clamps are applied. The defect is too extensive to repair directly, so the physician removes a short length of vein. The physician repairs the injured vessel with a length of synthetic graft material. The synthetic vein is sutured end-to-end to the vessel, replacing the excised portion. A patch graft may be sutured over any remaining defect. The clamps are removed and the skin incision is repaired with a layered closure.

35271

The physician exposes the abnormal blood vessel (arterial or venous) by choosing a thoracic incision appropriate to the involved vessel. The physician places cardiopulmonary bypass catheters (through incisions in the low inferior vena cava, the superior vena cava, and high aorta or femoral artery). The physician stops the heart by infusing cardioplegia solution into the coronary circulation. The physician examines the abnormal vessel and repairs it by clamping proximally and distally to the defect, and sewing in synthetic graft material in order to bypass the abnormal area of the vessel (bypass graft). The physician then confirms vessel patency with Doppler probe or angiography prior to taking the patient off cardiopulmonary bypass and closing the wound. The physician leaves chest and, possibly, mediastinal drains in place. If repair is accomplished with a venous patch (rather than bypass) graft, use 35211. If repair is accomplished with a venous bypass (rather than synthetic bypass) graft, use 35241.

35276

The physician exposes the abnormal blood vessel (arterial or venous) by choosing a thoracic incision appropriate to the involved vessel. The physician examines the abnormal vessel and repairs it by clamping proximally and distally to the defect, and sewing in synthetic graft material in order to bypass the abnormal portion of the repaired vessel (bypass graft). The physician then confirms vessel patency with Doppler probe or angiography prior to closing the wound. The physician leaves chest and, possibly, mediastinal drains in place. If repair is accomplished with a venous patch (rather than bypass) graft, use 35216. If repair is accomplished with a venous bypass (rather than synthetic bypass) graft, use 35246.

35281

The physician exposes the abnormal blood vessel (arterial or venous) by choosing an abdominal incision appropriate to the involved vessel. The physician examines the abnormal vessel and repairs it by clamping proximally and distally to the defect, and sewing in synthetic graft material in order to bypass the abnormal area of the diseased vessel (bypass graft). The physician then confirms vessel patency with Doppler probe or angiography prior to closing the wound. The physician leaves surgical drains in place. If repair is accomplished with a venous patch (rather than bypass) graft, use 35221. If repair is accomplished with a venous bypass (rather than synthetic bypass) graft, use 35251.

35286

The physician makes an incision in the skin of a lower extremity over the site of an injured blood vessel. The vessel is isolated and dissected from adjacent critical structures, and vessel clamps are applied. The defect is too extensive to repair directly, so the physician removes a short length of vein. The physician repairs the injured vessel with a length of synthetic graft material. The synthetic vein is sutured end-to-end to the vessel, replacing the excised portion. A patch graft may be sutured over any remaining defect. The clamps are removed and the skin incision is repaired with a layered closure.

35301

The physician makes an incision in the skin of the neck over the site of plaque or abnormal lining of the carotid, vertebral, or subclavian artery. The vessel is isolated and dissected from adjacent critical structures, and vessel clamps are applied. A temporary vascular shunt may be placed, bypassing the area and allowing blood supply to continue uninterrupted during the procedure. The vessel is incised. Using a blunt, spatula-like tool, the plaque and the vessel lining are separated from the artery and removed. The edge of the normal artery lining may be sutured to the artery wall to prevent separation when blood flow resumes. After the plaque and lining are removed, a patch graft taken from another portion of the patient's body, a cadaver, or a synthetic source may be applied and sutured to the vessel. This enlarges the diameter of the artery. The vessel clamps are removed and the skin incision is repaired with a layered closure.

35311

The physician exposes the innominate or subclavian artery by median sternotomy or lateral thoracotomy. The physician clamps the aortic arch widely around the origin of the diseased artery, then clamps the distal end(s) of the diseased artery. After making a longitudinal incision in the diseased artery, the physician uses a spatula to remove the atherosclerotic material. The physician may tack (suture) down the inner layer of the artery with a few 6-0 sutures before closing the artery with suture. A woven Dacron patch graft or harvested vein may be used to enlarge the arterial lumen (patch graft). The physician then unclamps the aorta, as well as the distal arterial clamp(s), then closes the sternotomy or thoracotomy, leaving a chest tube in place.

35321

The physician makes an incision in the skin of the axilla or arm over the site of a blood clot, plaque, or abnormal lining of the axillary or brachial artery. The vessel is isolated and dissected from adjacent critical structures, and vessel clamps are applied. The vessel is incised. Using a blunt, spatula-like tool, the plaque and the vessel lining are separated from the artery and removed. The edge of the normal artery lining may be sutured to the artery wall to prevent separation when blood flow resumes. After the plaque and lining are removed, a patch graft taken from another portion of the patient's body, a cadaver, or a synthetic source may be applied and sutured to the vessel. This enlarges the diameter of the artery. The vessel clamps are removed and the skin incision is repaired with a layered closure.

35331

The physician exposes the abdominal aorta using a transperitoneal approach, placing a long incision in the mid abdomen. The physician retracts the transverse colon and small bowel to allow dissection and exposure of the aorta. The physician then exposes the iliac arteries and achieves control of blood flow with umbilical tape or rubber catheters placed proximal to the diseased area. The physician then anticoagulates the patient and cross-clamps the iliac arteries and proximal aorta. A longitudinal incision down the affected portion of abdominal aorta allows the physician to use a spatula to remove the atherosclerotic material. The physician may tack (suture) down the inner layer of the aorta with small sutures. A woven Dacron patch graft or harvested vein may be used to enlarge the aortic lumen (patch graft). The physician then sutures the aorta closed, closes the retroperitoneum, and closes the abdominal wound, leaving drains in place.

35341

The physician exposes the involved mesenteric, celiac, or renal artery using an abdominal incision, retracting and dissecting past large and small bowel. The physician clamps the aorta to isolate the involved vessel, places a longitudinal incision down the affected vessel, and uses a spatula to remove the atherosclerotic material. If there is significant stenosis at the arterial takeoff, the physician may open the aorta and remove the atherosclerotic material from within the aorta before suturing the aorta and diseased artery closed. The physician may use harvested vein to enlarge the arterial lumen (patch graft). The physician may perform arteriography or use a Doppler probe to establish patency of the vessel, before closing the abdominal wound, leaving drains in place.

35351

The physician exposes the involved iliac artery using an abdominal incision, retracting and dissecting past large and small bowel. The physician clamps the aorta to isolate the involved vessel, places a longitudinal incision down the affected vessel, and uses a spatula to remove the atherosclerotic material. If there is significant stenosis at the arterial takeoff, the physician may open the aorta and remove the atherosclerotic material from within the aorta before suturing the aorta and diseased artery closed. The physician may use harvested vein to enlarge the arterial lumen (patch graft). The physician may perform arteriography or use a Doppler probe to establish patency of the vessel before closing the abdominal wound, leaving drains in place.

35355

The physician exposes the involved iliac artery using abdominal and femoral incisions, retracting and dissecting past large and small bowel. The physician exposes the femoral artery via the femoral incision. The physician clamps the aorta to isolate the involved vessel, places a longitudinal incision down the involved vessel, and uses a spatula to remove the atherosclerotic material. If there is significant stenosis at the arterial takeoff, the physician may open the aorta and remove the atherosclerotic material from within the aorta before suturing the aorta and diseased artery closed. The physician may use harvested vein to enlarge the arterial lumen (patch graft). The physician may perform arteriography or use a Doppler probe to establish patency of the vessel before closing the abdominal and femoral wounds, leaving drains in place.

35361

The physician exposes the involved iliac artery using an abdominal incision, retracting and dissecting past large and small bowel. The physician clamps the proximal aorta above the diseased area, places a longitudinal incision down the distal aorta and affected iliac artery, then uses a spatula to remove the

CPT® Lay Descriptions

atherosclerotic material before suturing the aorta and iliac artery closed. The physician may use harvested vein to enlarge the aortic or arterial lumen (patch graft). The physician may perform arteriography or use a Doppler probe to establish patency of the vessel before closing the abdominal wound, leaving drains in place.

35363

The physician exposes the involved abdominal aorta and iliac artery using an abdominal incision, retracting and dissecting past large and small bowel. The physician exposes the involved femoral artery via a femoral incision and dissection. The physician clamps the proximal aorta above the diseased area, places a longitudinal incision down the distal aorta and affected iliac artery, then uses a spatula to remove the atherosclerotic material before suturing the aorta and iliac artery closed. The physician places a longitudinal incision down the femoral artery and uses a spatula to remove any atherosclerotic material before sewing the femoral artery closed. The physician may use harvested vein to enlarge the aortic or arterial lumen (patch graft). The physician may perform arteriography or use a Doppler probe to establish patency of the vessel. The physician then closes the femoral and abdominal wounds, leaving drains in place.

35371–35372

The physician makes an incision in the skin over the leg at the site of a blood clot, plaque, or abnormal lining of the common femoral artery (35371) or the deep (profunda) femoral artery (35372). The vessel is isolated and dissected from adjacent critical structures, and vessel clamps are applied. The vessel is incised. Using a blunt, spatula-like tool, the plaque and the vessel lining are separated from the artery and removed. The edge of the normal artery lining may be sutured to the artery wall to prevent separation when blood flow resumes. After the plaque and lining are removed, a patch graft taken from another portion of the patient's body, a cadaver, or a synthetic source may be applied and sutured to the vessel. This enlarges the diameter of the artery. The vessel clamps are removed and the skin incision is repaired with a layered closure.

35381

The physician makes an incision in the skin of the leg over the site of a blood clot, plaque, or abnormal lining of the femoral, and/or popliteal, and/or tibioperoneal arteries. The vessels are isolated and dissected from adjacent critical structures, and vessel clamps are applied. The vessels are incised. Using a blunt, spatula-like tool, the plaque and the vessel lining are separated from the arteries and removed. The edge of the normal artery linings may be sutured to the artery walls to prevent separation when blood flow resumes. After the plaque and lining are removed, patch grafts taken from another portion of

the patient's body, a cadaver, or a synthetic source may be applied and sutured to the vessels. This enlarges the diameter of the arteries. The vessel clamps are removed and the skin incision is repaired with a layered closure.

35390

The physician makes an incision in the skin of the neck over the site of plaque or abnormal lining of the carotid, vertebral, or subclavian artery. The vessel is isolated and dissected from adjacent critical structures, and vessel clamps are applied. A temporary vascular shunt may be placed, bypassing the area and allowing blood supply to continue uninterrupted during the procedure. The vessel is incised. Using a blunt, spatula-like tool, the plaque and the vessel lining are separated from the artery and removed. The edge of the normal artery lining may be sutured to the artery wall to prevent separation when blood flow resumes. After the plaque and lining are removed, a patch graft taken from another portion of the patient's body, a cadaver, or a synthetic source may be applied and sutured to the vessel. This enlarges the diameter of the artery. The vessel clamps are removed and the skin incision is repaired with a layered closure. Use 35390 in conjunction with 35301.

35400

The purpose of this procedure is to use an endoscope to look inside a blood vessel. The physician places an introducer sheath in the vessel to be examined, using percutaneous puncture or a cutdown technique. The physician places a special angioscopy catheter through the introducer sheath into the vessel to be examined. The physician advances the angioscope through the vessel, clearing the view with injections of saline. Once the inside of the vessel has been examined, the angioscope and sheath are withdrawn. Vessel hemostasis is achieved using sutures or manual pressure.

35450–35460

The physician makes an incision in the skin overlying the femoral artery. The artery is dissected from adjacent critical structures, and vessel clamps are applied. The physician may nick the artery to create an opening into which a catheter with a balloon attached is inserted into the vessel and threaded. The catheter is fed into the narrowed portion of the aorta, where its balloon is inflated in the narrowed area. The blood vessel is stretched to a larger diameter, allowing a more normal outflow of blood through the area. Several inflations may be performed along the narrowed area. The catheter is slowly withdrawn after deflation. Occasionally, the opening in the artery is repaired with sutures. The skin incision is repaired with a layered closure. Report 35450 if performed on the renal or another visceral artery; report 35452 if performed on the aortic artery; report 35454 if performed on the iliac artery; report 35456 if performed on the femoral-popliteal artery; report

35458 if performed on the brachiocephalic trunk or branches; report 35459 if performed on the tibioperoneal trunk and branches; and report 35460 if venous.

35470–35476

The physician isolates the femoral artery or (on occasion) the popliteal artery and inserts a large needle through the skin and into the artery. A guidance wire is threaded through the needle into the artery. The needle is removed. A catheter with a balloon attached follows the wire into the artery. The wire is removed. The catheter is fed through the arterial system and into the narrowed portion of the tibioperoneal trunk and, if necessary, one of its branches. There, the balloon is inflated. The blood vessel is stretched to a larger diameter, allowing a more normal outflow of blood through the area. Several inflations may be performed along the narrowed area. The catheter is slowly withdrawn after deflation. Pressure is applied to the puncture site to stop the bleeding after the catheter is removed. Report 35470 if tibioperoneal trunk or branches are treated; report 35471 if renal or visceral; report 35472 if aortic; report 35473 if iliac; report 35474 if femoral popliteal; report 35475 if brachiocephalic trunk or branches; report 35476 if venous.

35480–35485

The physician creates a femoral cutdown incision to expose one of the femoral arteries. The physician punctures the femoral artery with a large needle and passes a guidewire via the needle into the femoral artery. The physician removes the needle while leaving the guidewire in place, enlarges the arterial opening slightly with a blade, then slides an introducer sheath over the guidewire into the arterial lumen. The physician then slides an appropriately sized guidewire through the atherectomy catheter or device, and inserts the guidewire/atherectomy catheter combination through the introducer sheath into the aorta. The physician fluoroscopically positions the atherectomy device at the aortic stenosis and activates the device to remove the stenotic tissue. The physician then rechecks the diameter of the lesion by angiography. The physician may perform several passes with the atherectomy device. The physician then removes the atherectomy catheter, guidewire, and introducer sheath, closing the femoral arteriotomy with suture. The physician then closes the femoral cutdown incision with suture. Report 35480 if the occlusion is in the renal or other visceral artery; report 35481 if it is located in the aortic artery; report 35482 if it is located in the iliac artery; report 35483 if it is located in the femoral-popliteal artery; report 35484 if it is located in the brachiocephalic trunk or branches; and report 35485 if located in the tibioperoneal trunk and branches.

35490–35495

The physician punctures the femoral artery with a large needle and passes a guidewire via the needle into the femoral artery. The physician removes the needle while leaving the guidewire in place, enlarges the arterial opening slightly with a blade, then slides an introducer sheath over the guidewire into the arterial lumen. The physician then slides an appropriately sized guidewire through the atherectomy catheter or device, and inserts the guidewire/atherectomy catheter combination through the introducer sheath up the aorta and out into the involved renal or other visceral artery. The physician fluoroscopically positions the atherectomy device at the arterial stenosis and activates the device to remove the stenotic tissue. The physician then rechecks the diameter of the lesion by angiography. The physician may perform several passes with the atherectomy device. The physician then removes the atherectomy catheter, guidewire, and introducer sheath, compressing the femoral artery manually until hemostasis is achieved. Report 35490 if performed in the renal or other visceral artery; report 35491 if performed in the aortic artery; report 35492 if performed in the iliac artery; report 35493 if performed in the femoral-poplital artery; report 35494 if performed in the brachiocephalic trunk or branches; report 35495 if performed in the tibioperoneal trunk and branches.

35500

The physician harvests a vein from an upper extremity (arm) to use for a planned bypass procedure on a lower extremity vessel (leg) or coronary artery. An incision is made over the site on the arm. Tissue is dissected to the vein. The portion of the vein to be removed is released from the surrounding structures, and is tied off above and below the portion of vein to be removed. The vein is removed. The wound is closed with layered sutures. The portion of vein removed is prepared for use in a separately reportable bypass graft procedure of a leg vessel or coronary artery.

35501

Through an incision in the skin of the neck in front of the sternocleidomastoid muscle, the physician isolates and dissects the carotid artery, separating it from adjacent critical structures. The physician creates a bypass around the section of carotid artery that is damaged or blocked, using a harvested vein graft and one of two methods of repair after vessel clamps have been affixed above and below the defect. In the first method of repair the carotid artery may be cut through below the damaged area and sutured to one end of the harvest vein (end-to-end), which is then sutured to the same carotid artery beyond the affected area. In the second method, the ends of the harvested vein are sutured into the side of the carotid arterial wall at two places (end-to-side). Either method results in a bypass of the damaged area. When the clamps are removed, the section of vein graft forms a new path through which blood can easily bypass the blocked area. The damaged or blocked carotid artery is not removed. After the graft is complete, the skin incision is repair with a layered closure.

35506

Through an incision in the skin at the side of the neck, the physician isolates and dissects the subclavian and carotid arteries, separating them from adjacent critical structures. To create a bypass around a section of subclavian artery that is damaged or blocked, the physician uses a harvested vein and one of two methods of repair. After vessel clamps have been affixed above and below the damaged area, the graft is sewn to the side of the carotid artery and either sewn to the side of the subclavian artery beyond the affected area (end-to-side) or sewn to the cut end of the subclavian artery after dividing it beyond the affected area (end-to-end). The damaged or blocked portion of the subclavian artery is not removed. When the clamps are removed in either case, the section of vein graft forms a new path through which blood can easily bypass the blocked area. After the graft is complete, the skin incision is repaired with a layered closure.

35507

Through an incision in the skin of the neck in front of the sternocleidomastoid muscle, the physician isolates and dissects the carotid and subclavian arteries, separating them from adjacent critical structures. The physician creates a bypass around a section of carotid artery that is damaged or blocked, using a harvested vein and one of two methods of repair. After vessel clamps have been affixed above and below the damaged area, the graft is sewn to the side of the subclavian artery and either sewn to the side of the carotid artery beyond the affected area (end-to-side) or sewn to the cut end of the carotid artery after dividing it beyond the affected area (end-to-end). The damaged or blocked portion of the carotid artery is not removed. When the clamps are removed in either case, the section of vein graft forms a new path through which blood can easily bypass the blocked area. After the graft is complete, the skin incision is repaired with a layered closure.

35508

Through an incision in the skin of the neck, the physician isolates and dissects the vertebral and carotid arteries, separating them from adjacent critical structures. The physician creates a bypass around a section of vertebral artery that is damaged or blocked, using a harvested vein and one of two methods of repair. After vessel clamps have been affixed above and below the damaged area, the graft is sewn to the side of the carotid artery and either sewn to the side of the vertebral artery beyond the affected area (end-to-side) or sewn over the cut end of the vertebral artery after dividing it beyond the affected area (end-

to-end). The damaged or blocked section of the vertebral artery is not removed. When the clamps are removed, the section of vein graft forms a new path through which blood can easily bypass the blocked area. After the graft is complete, the skin incision is repaired with a layered closure.

35509

Through incisions in the skin of the neck, the physician isolates and dissects the carotid arteries, separating them from adjacent critical structures. The physician creates a bypass around a section of carotid artery that is damaged or blocked, using a harvested vein and one of two methods of repair. After vessel clamps have been affixed above and below the damaged area, the ends of the vein graft are sutured into the side of the carotid arterial wall (end-to-side). In the second method, the carotid artery may be cut through above the damaged area and sutured to one end of a harvested vein, which is then sutured to the side of the carotid artery on the opposite side of the neck (end-to-end). In either case, the blocked or damaged section of artery is not removed. When the clamps are removed, the section of vein graft forms a new path through which blood can easily bypass the blocked or damaged area. After the graft is complete, the skin incisions are repaired with layered closures.

35511

Through incisions in the skin at the base of the neck, the physician isolates and dissects the subclavian arteries, separating them from adjacent critical structures. The physician creates a bypass around a section of subclavian artery that is damaged or blocked, using a harvested vein and one of two methods of repair after vessel clamps have been affixed above and below the defect. In the first method of repair the ends of the vein graft are sutured into the sides of the walls of the two subclavian arteries, resulting in a bypass of the damaged area. In the second method, the subclavian artery may be cut through beyond the damaged area and sutured to one end of a harvested vein, which is then sutured to the subclavian artery on the opposite side of the neck. In either case, the blocked or damaged portion of the artery is not removed. When the clamps are removed, the section of vein graft forms a new path through which blood can easily bypass the blocked area. After the graft is complete, the skin incisions are repaired with a layered closure.

35515

Through an incision in the skin of the neck, the physician isolates and dissects the vertebral and subclavian arteries, separating them from adjacent critical structures. The physician creates a bypass around a section of vertebral artery that is damaged or blocked, using a harvested vein and one of two methods of repair. Once vessel clamps are affixed above and below the defect, the ends of the harvested vein are sutured into the sides of the subclavian and vertebral arterial walls resulting in a bypass of the damaged area (end-to-side). In the second method, the vertebral artery can be cut through above the damaged area and sutured to one end of a harvested vein (end-to-end). The remaining end is then sutured to the subclavian artery. In either case, the blocked or damaged vertebral artery is not removed. When the clamps are removed, the section of vein graft forms a new path through which blood can easily bypass the blocked area. After the graft is complete, the skin incision is repaired with a layered closure.

35516

Through an incision in the skin at the base of the neck and axilla, the physician isolates and dissects the subclavian and axillary arteries, separating them from adjacent critical structures. The physician creates a bypass around a section of subclavian artery that is damaged or blocked, using a harvested vein and one of two methods of repair. Once vessel clamps have been affixed above and below the defect, the ends of the harvested vein are sutured into the sides of the subclavian and axillary arterial walls resulting in a bypass of the damaged area (end-to-side). In the second method, the subclavian artery may be cut through before the damaged area and sutured to one end of a harvested vein, which is then sutured to the axillary artery (end-to-end). The blocked or damaged portion of the subclavian artery is not removed. When the clamps are removed, the section of vein graft forms a new path through which blood can easily bypass the blocked area. After the graft is complete, the skin incisions are repaired with a layered closure.

35518

The physician makes an incision in the skin of both axillae. The physician creates a bypass around a section of axillary or subclavian artery that is damaged or blocked, using a harvested vein and one of two methods of repair. Once vessel clamps have been affixed above and below the defect, the ends of the harvested vein are sutured into the sides of the two axillary arterial walls, resulting in a bypass of the damaged area. In the second method, the axillary artery may be cut through beyond the damaged area and sutured to one end of a harvested vein, which is then passed across the front of the chest under the skin and sutured to the side of the opposite axillary artery. The blocked or damaged portion of the axillary or subclavian artery is not removed. When the clamps are removed, the section of vein graft forms a new path through which blood can easily bypass the blocked area. After the graft is complete, the skin incisions are repaired with layered closures.

35521

The physician makes incisions in the skin of the axilla and upper thigh. The axillary and femoral arteries are isolated and dissected from adjacent critical structures. The physician creates a bypass around a section of lower aorta or iliac artery that is damaged

or blocked using a harvested vein and one of two methods of repair. Once vessel clamps have been affixed above and below the areas of anastomosis, the harvested vein is sutured to an incision in the side of the axillary artery and passed through a subcutaneous tunnel on the side of the body and to the upper thigh. The harvested vein is then sutured to the femoral artery (common, deep, or superficial) in either an end-to-side or end-to-end fashion. The blocked or damaged portion of lower aorta or iliac artery is not removed. When the clamps are removed, the section of vein graft forms a new path through which blood can easily bypass the blocked area. After the graft is complete, the skin incisions are repaired with layered closures.

35526

The physician exposes the aorta by median sternotomy and exposes the carotid or subclavian artery extending this incision in the appropriate direction. The physician clamps the middle part of the right anterolateral aspect of the anterior ascending aorta with a J clamp. The physician then makes a 2.0 cm to 3.0 cm longitudinal incision in the clamped portion of the aorta and sews the venous graft to the aortic incision. The physician clamps the vein and releases the aortic clamp to assess the anastomosis for leaks. The physician clamps the distal end of the diseased artery (carotid or subclavian). The physician then makes a longitudinal incision in the diseased artery, distal to the blockage, and sews the venous graft to the arterial incision. The physician may also use harvested vein to enlarge the arterial lumen (patch graft). The physician removes the clamp from the vein graft. The physician may perform arteriography or use a Doppler probe to establish patency of the graft. The physician then closes the sternotomy or thoracotomy, leaving a chest tube in place.

35531

The physician exposes the involved mesenteric or celiac artery using an upper midline abdominal incision, retracting and dissecting past large and small bowel. The physician exposes the distal thoracic aorta, administers heparin for anti coagulation, and clamps the aorta both proximal and distal to the celiac axis origin. The physician then cuts out an elliptical disk of aortic wall from the anterior surface of the aorta. The physician exposes the involved vessel (mesenteric or celiac artery) and divides it proximal to the occlusion, closing off the proximal stump with suture. The physician sews a venous graft from the clamped aorta to the undiseased distal artery. The physician may use harvested vein to enlarge the arterial lumen (patch graft). The physician may perform arteriography or use a Doppler probe to establish patency of the graft. The physician then closes the abdominal wound, leaving drains in place.

35533

Through incisions in the skin of the axilla and both upper thighs, the physician creates a bypass using a harvested vein around a section of lower aorta that is damaged or blocked. Once vessel clamps have been affixed above and below the area of anastomosis, the harvested vein is sutured to the side of the axillary artery and passed through a subcutaneous tunnel to the upper thigh, where it is sutured end-to-end or end-to-side to the femoral artery. A second harvested vein is sutured end-to-side to the femoral artery or to the vein graft descending from the axilla where it joins the femoral artery, and is passed through another subcutaneous tunnel to the opposite thigh, where it is sutured end-to-end or end-to-side to the femoral artery. When the clamps are removed, the two grafted vein limbs form a new path through which blood can easily bypass the blocked area. The section of blocked or damaged lower aorta is not removed. After the graft is complete, the incisions are repaired with layered closures.

35536

The physician performs a bilateral subcostal incision from the right midrectus position extending into the left flank, and dissects past bowel and pancreas to expose the splenic vein. The physician exposes the splenic artery by careful dissection. The physician then exposes the left renal artery by dissecting through the posterior parietal peritoneum, partially clamps it, and excises an ellipse of renal artery at its upper border. The physician then performs end-to-side anastomosis of vein graft material from the splenic artery to the renal artery. The physician removes the clamps and assesses the anastomotic sites for leaks. The physician may perform Doppler studies or arteriography to establish patency of the graft. The physician then closes the abdominal wound, leaving drains in place.

35541

The physician exposes the involved abdominal aorta and iliac artery using an abdominal incision, retracting and dissecting past large and small bowel. The physician partially clamps the aorta above the diseased area and places a longitudinal incision down the clamped portion of the aorta. The physician sews in a (two) venous graft(s), clamps the graft(s) and removes the aortic clamp to assess the anastomosis(es) for leaks. The physician then clamps the iliac artery(ies) distal to the stenosis, incises and attaches the distal venous graft to the iliac artery(ies). The physician may also use harvested vein to enlarge the aortic or arterial lumen (patch graft). The physician may perform arteriography or use a Doppler probe to establish patency of the graft. The physician then closes the abdominal wound, leaving drains in place.

35546

The physician makes an incision in the skin of the abdomen over a section of damaged or blocked lower aorta. The artery is isolated and dissected. Through a separate skin incision in the upper thigh, the femoral artery is isolated and dissected from adjacent critical structures. The physician creates a bypass around the damaged or blocked lower aorta using a harvested vein. Once vessel clamps have been affixed above the defect, the lower aorta may be cut through or tied off with sutures above the damaged or blocked area and sutured to one end of the harvested vein in an end-to-end or side-to-side fashion. The graft to one femoral artery is passed through a tunnel on the inside of the upper thigh and sutured to the femoral artery. If a bifemoral bypass is accomplished, a second harvested vein is placed in a similar fashion to the second side. When the clamps are removed, the two grafted vein limbs form a new path through which blood can easily bypass the blocked area. The blocked or damaged portion of artery is not removed. After the graft is complete, the skin incisions are repaired with layered closures.

35548

The physician makes an incision in the skin of the abdomen over a section of damaged or blocked lower aorta. The artery is isolated and dissected from adjacent critical structures. Through a separate skin incision in the upper thigh, the femoral artery is isolated and dissected from adjacent critical structures. The physician creates a bypass around the damaged or blocked artery using a harvested vein. Once vessel clamps have been affixed above the defect, the lower aorta may be cut through or tied off with sutures above the damaged area and sutured to one end of the harvested vein. The vein graft is then sutured to the iliac artery. A second vein is sutured to the iliac artery and the other end is passed through a tunnel on the inside of the upper thigh and sutured to a point on the femoral artery. When clamps are removed, the grafted vein forms a new path through which blood can easily bypass the blocked area. After the graft is complete, the skin incisions are repaired with layered closures.

35549

The physician makes an incision in the skin of the abdomen over a section of damaged or blocked lower aorta. The artery is isolated and dissected from adjacent critical structures. Through a separate skin incision in the upper thigh, the femoral artery is isolated and dissected from adjacent critical structures. The physician creates a bypass around the damaged section using a harvested vein. Once vessel clamps are affixed above the defect, the lower aorta is cut through or tied off with sutures above the damaged or blocked area and sutured to one end of the harvested vein. The free end of the harvested vein is sutured to the iliac artery. A second vein is sutured in place to join the aorta to the opposite iliac artery. Another vein is sutured to the iliac artery and passed through tunnels into the upper thigh where it is sutured to the femoral artery in the upper thigh. When the clamps are removed, the two grafted vein limbs form a new path through which blood can easily bypass the blocked area. After the grafts are complete, the skin incisions are repaired with layered closures. This procedure is repeated on the other side.

35551

The physician makes an incision in the skin of the abdomen over a section of damaged or blocked lower aorta. The artery is isolated and dissected from adjacent critical structures. Through a separate skin incision in the upper thigh, the femoral artery is isolated and dissected, and through a third skin incision behind the knee, the popliteal artery is isolated and dissected. The physician creates a bypass around the damaged artery that supplies the femoral-popliteal artery, using a harvested vein. Once vessel clamps have been affixed above the defect, the lower aortic artery is cut through or tied off with sutures above the damaged area and sutured to one end of the harvested vein. The graft is passed through a tunnel on the inside of the upper thigh and sutured to a point on the femoral artery. A third vein graft is sutured to the femoral artery and passed through a tunnel, where it is joined to the popliteal artery. It is also sutured. When the clamps are removed, the grafted vein forms a new path through which blood can easily bypass the blocked area. After the graft is complete, the skin incisions are repaired with layered closures.

35556

Through incisions in the skin of the leg overlying the femoral and popliteal arteries, the physician isolates and dissects a section of artery that is damaged or blocked. The physician creates a bypass around the superficial femoral artery, using a harvested vein and one of two methods of repair. Once vessel clamps have been affixed above and below the defect, the superficial femoral artery may be cut through above the damaged or blocked area and sutured to one end of a harvested vein. The vein is then passed through a tunnel down the thigh muscles and behind the knee and sutured to the popliteal artery. In the second method, the ends of the harvested vein are sutured into the side of the femoral and popliteal arterial walls, resulting in a bypass of the damaged area. When the clamps are removed, the section of vein forms a new path through which blood can easily bypass the blocked area. The blocked or damaged portion of artery is not removed. After the graft is complete, the skin incisions are repaired with layered closures.

35558

Through incisions in the skin of the upper thighs, the physician isolates and dissects a section of the femoral arteries. The physician creates a bypass using a harvested vein. Once vessel clamps have been affixed

above and below the area of anastomosis, the femoral artery may be cut through below the damaged area and sutured to one end of a harvested vein, which is then sutured to the femoral artery in the opposite leg, resulting in a bypass of the damaged or blocked area. When the clamps are removed, the section of vein forms a new path through which blood can easily bypass the blocked area. The blocked or damaged portion of the artery is not removed. After the graft is complete, the skin incisions are repaired with layered closures.

35560

The physician exposes the involved abdominal aorta and renal artery using an abdominal incision, retracting and dissecting past large and small bowel. The physician partially clamps the aorta below the renal takeoff and places a small longitudinal incision down the clamped portion of the aorta. The physician sutures in a venous graft, clamps the graft and removes the aortic clamp to assess the anastomosis for leaks. The physician then clamps the renal artery distal to the stenosis, incises the renal artery and attaches the distal venous graft to the distal renal artery. The physician may also use harvested vein to enlarge the renal arterial lumen (patch graft). The physician may perform arteriography or use a Doppler probe to establish patency of the graft. The physician then closes the abdominal wound, leaving drains in place.

35563

The physician exposes the iliac arteries using an abdominal incision, retracting and dissecting past large and small bowel. The physician partially clamps the patent (non-diseased) iliac artery and places a longitudinal incision down the clamped portion of the aorta. The physician sews in a venous graft, clamps the graft and removes the iliac clamp to assess the anastomosis for leaks. The physician then clamps the diseased iliac artery distal to the stenosis, places a distal incision and attaches the distal venous graft to the diseased iliac artery. The physician may also use harvested vein to enlarge the aortic or arterial lumen (patch graft). The physician may perform arteriography or use a Doppler probe to establish patency of the graft. The physician then closes the abdominal wound, leaving drains in place.

35565

Through incisions in the skin of the lower abdomen overlying the iliac artery and in the skin of the upper thigh overlying the femoral artery, the physician isolates and dissects a section of common iliac artery. The physician creates a bypass around the iliac artery, using a harvested vein and one of two methods of repair. Once vessel clamps have been affixed above and below the defect, the iliac artery may be cut or tied off with sutures above the damaged area and sutured to one end of a harvested vein. The graft is passed through a tunnel on the inside of the upper thigh and is sutured to the side of the femoral artery. In the second method, the end of the harvested vein is sutured to the side of the iliac artery. Either method results in a bypass of the damaged area. When the clamps are removed, the section of vein forms a new path through which blood can easily bypass the blocked area. After the graft is complete, the skin incisions are repaired with layered closures.

35566

Through incisions in the skin of the leg overlying the superficial femoral artery, the physician isolates and dissects sections of the femoral and anterior tibial, posterior tibial, or peroneal arteries. The physician creates a bypass around the affected artery using a harvested vein. Once vessel clamps have been affixed above and below the defect, the superficial femoral artery may be cut through above the damaged area and sutured to one end of a harvested vein, which is then passed through an intramuscular tunnel and sutured to the anterior tibial, posterior tibial, peroneal, or other distal vessel. In the second method, the ends of the harvested vein are sutured to the side of the femoral artery and anterior tibial, posterior tibial, peroneal, or other distal vessel wall, resulting in a bypass of the damaged area. When the clamps are removed, the section of vein forms a new path through which blood can easily bypass the blocked area. The blocked or damaged portion of artery is left in place and not removed. After the graft is complete, the skin incisions are repaired with layered closures.

35571

Through incisions in the skin of the leg overlying the popliteal arteries, the physician isolates and dissects a section of arteries from adjacent critical structures. The physician creates a bypass around the artery, using a harvested vein and one of two methods of repair. Once vessel clamps have been affixed above and below the defect, the popliteal artery may be cut through above the damaged area and sutured to one end of a harvested vein, which is then sutured to the tibial, peroneal, or other distal artery. In the second method, the ends of the harvested vein are sutured into the side of the popliteal and the tibial or peroneal arterial wall resulting in a bypass of the damaged area. When the clamps are removed, the section of vein forms a new path through which blood can easily bypass the blocked area. After the graft is complete, the incisions are repaired with layered closures.

35582

Through an incision in the skin of the abdomen overlying the lower aorta, the physician isolates and dissects the lower aorta from adjacent critical structures. Vessel clamps are affixed above and below the anastomosis site. The physician sutures a synthetic graft into the aorta in either end-to-end or end-to-side fashion. Each limb of the graft is passed through a tunnel on each side of the upper thigh and is sutured to the side of the common femoral artery. A long skin incision exposes the greater Saphenous vein along its length and all side branches are tied off. The valves are destroyed so blood can flow backward toward the feet. The upper end of the Saphenous vein is divided and sutured into the superficial femoral artery, either end-to-end or end-to-side. The lower end is divided and sutured into the popliteal artery. The clamps are removed, and blood flows backward toward the feet, as if the vein were an artery. When the procedure is complete, the skin incisions are repaired with layered closures.

35583

Through an incision in the skin of the leg overlying the greater Saphenous vein, the physician isolates and dissects the greater Saphenous vein from adjacent critical structures from the upper thigh to the level of the knee. Vessel clamps are affixed above and below the site of the anastomosis to the femoral and popliteal arteries. All side branches of the Saphenous vein are tied off. The vessel's valves are destroyed. The upper end of the Saphenous vein is divided and sutured into the femoral artery either end-to-end or end-to-side. The lower end is divided and sutured into the popliteal artery either end-to-end or end-to-side. The clamps are removed, and blood flows backward toward the feet, as if the vein were an artery. When the procedure is complete, the skin incision is repaired with a layered closure.

35585

Through an incision in the skin of the leg overlying the greater Saphenous vein, the physician isolates and dissects the greater Saphenous vein from adjacent critical structures. Vessel clamps are affixed above and below the site of anastomosis in the femoral artery and the distal artery. All side branches of the Saphenous are tied off. The vessel's valves are destroyed. The upper end of the Saphenous vein is divided and sutured either end-to-end or end-to-side in the femoral artery above the blockage. The lower end is divided and sutured either end-to-end or end-to-side to the anterior tibial, posterior tibial, or peroneal artery below the blockage. The clamps are removed, and blood flows backward toward the feet, as if the vein were an artery. When the procedure is complete, the skin incision is repaired with a layered closure.

35587

Through an incision in the skin of the leg overlying the greater Saphenous vein from the knee to the ankle, the physician isolates and dissects the greater Saphenous vein from adjacent critical structures along its length. Vessel clamps are affixed above and below the site of anastomosis on the popliteal and distal arteries. All side branches of the Saphenous vein are tied off. The vessel's valves are destroyed. The upper end of the Saphenous vein is divided and sutured into the popliteal-tibial artery. The lower end is divided and sutured into the peroneal artery. The clamps are removed, and blood flows backward through the vein toward the feet, as if it were an artery. When the procedure is complete, the incision is repaired with a layered closure.

35600

The physician harvests an artery from an upper extremity (arm) to use for a planned bypass procedure on a coronary artery. An incision is made over the site on the arm. Tissue is dissected to the artery. The portion of the artery to be removed is released from the surrounding structures and is tied off above and below the portion of artery to be removed. The artery is removed. The wound is closed with layered sutures. The portion of artery removed is prepared for use in a separately reportable bypass graft procedure of a coronary artery.

35601

Through an incision in the skin of the neck in front of the sternocleidomastoid muscle, the physician isolates and dissects the carotid artery, separating it from adjacent critical structures. The physician creates a bypass around the section of carotid artery that is damaged or blocked, using a synthetic vein graft and one of two methods of repair. After vessel clamps have been affixed above and below the damaged area, the carotid artery may be cut through below the damaged area and sutured to one end of the synthetic vein (end-to-end), which is then sutured to the same carotid artery beyond the affected area. In the second method, the ends of the synthetic vein are sutured into the side of the carotid arterial wall at two places (end-to-side). Either method results in a bypass of the damaged area. When the clamps are removed, the section of synthetic graft forms a new path through which blood can easily bypass the blocked area. The damaged or blocked carotid artery is not removed. After the graft is complete, the skin incision is repaired with a layered closure.

35606

Through an incision in the skin at the side of the neck, the physician isolates and dissects the subclavian and carotid arteries, separating them from adjacent critical structures. To create a bypass around a section of subclavian artery that is damaged or blocked, the physician uses a synthetic vein and one of two methods of repair. After vessel clamps have been affixed above and below the damaged area, the graft is sewn to the side of the carotid artery and either sewn to the side of the subclavian artery beyond the affected area (end-to-side) or sewn to the cut end of the subclavian artery after dividing it beyond the affected area (end-to-end). The damaged or blocked portion of the subclavian artery is not removed. When the clamps are removed in either case, the section of synthetic graft vein forms a new path through which blood can easily bypass the blocked area. After the graft is complete, the skin incision is repaired with a layered closure.

35612

Through incisions in the skin at the base of the neck, the physician isolates and dissects the subclavian arteries, separating them from adjacent critical structures. The physician creates a bypass around a section of subclavian artery that is damaged or blocked, using a synthetic vein and one of two methods of repair. Once vessel clamps have been affixed above and below the defect, the ends of the synthetic vein graft are sutured into the sides of the walls of the two subclavian arteries, resulting in a bypass of the damaged area. In the second method, the subclavian artery may be cut through beyond the damaged area and sutured to one end of a synthetic vein, which is then sutured to the subclavian artery on the opposite side of the neck. In either case, the blocked or damaged portion of the artery is not removed. When the clamps are removed, the section of synthetic vein graft forms a new path through which blood can easily bypass the blocked area. After the graft is complete, the skin incisions are repaired with a layered closure.

35616

Through an incision in the skin at the base of the neck and axilla, the physician isolates and dissects the subclavian and axillary arteries, separating them from adjacent critical structures. The physician creates a bypass around a section of subclavian artery that is damaged or blocked, using a synthetic vein and one of two methods of repair. Once vessel clamps have been affixed above and below the defect, the ends of the synthetic vein are sutured into the sides of the subclavian and axillary arterial walls resulting in a bypass of the damaged area (end-to-side). In the second method, the subclavian artery may be cut through before the damaged area and sutured to one end of a synthetic vein, which is then sutured to the axillary artery (end-to-end). The blocked or damaged portion of the subclavian artery is not removed. When the clamps are removed, the section of synthetic vein graft forms a new path through which blood can easily bypass the blocked area. After the graft is complete, the skin incisions are repaired with a layered closure.

35621

The physician makes incisions in the skin of the axilla and upper thigh. The artery is isolated and dissected from adjacent critical structures. The physician creates a bypass around a section of lower aorta or iliac artery that is damaged or blocked using a synthetic vein and one of two methods of repair. Once vessel clamps have been affixed above and below the areas of anastomosis, the synthetic vein is sutured to an incision in the side of the axillary artery and passed through a subcutaneous tunnel on the side of the body and to the upper thigh. The synthetic vein is then sutured to the femoral artery (common, deep, or superficial) in either an end-to-side or end-to-end fashion. The blocked or damaged portion of lower aorta or iliac artery is not removed. When the clamps are removed, the section of synthetic vein graft forms a new path through which blood can easily bypass the blocked area. After the graft is complete, the skin incisions are repaired with layered closures.

35623

The physician makes incisions in the skin of the axilla and behind the knee or in the lower leg. The artery is isolated and dissected from adjacent critical structures. The physician creates a bypass around a section of lower aorta or iliac artery that is damaged or blocked using a synthetic vein and one of two methods of repair. Once vessel clamps have been affixed above and below the areas of anastomosis, the synthetic vein is sutured to an incision in the side of the axillary artery and passed through a subcutaneous tunnel on the side of the body and behind the knee or upper thigh. The synthetic vein is then sutured to the popliteal or tibial artery in either an end-to-side or end-to-end fashion. The blocked or damaged portion of lower aorta or iliac artery is not removed. When the clamps are removed, the section of synthetic vein graft forms a new path through which blood can easily bypass the blocked area. After the graft is complete, the skin incisions are repaired with layered closures.

35626

The physician exposes the aorta by median sternotomy and exposes the carotid or subclavian artery extending this incision in the appropriate direction. The physician clamps the middle part of the right anterolateral aspect of the anterior ascending aorta with a J clamp. The physician then makes a 2–3 centimeter longitudinal incision in the clamped portion of the aorta and sews the arterial or synthetic graft to the aortic incision. The physician clamps the graft and releases the aortic clamp to assess the anastomosis for leaks. The physician clamps the distal end of the diseased artery (carotid or subclavian). The physician then makes a longitudinal incision in the diseased artery, distal to the blockage, and sews the graft to the arterial incision. The physician may also use graft material to enlarge the arterial lumen (patch graft). The physician removes the clamp from the graft. The physician may perform arteriography or use a Doppler probe to establish patency of the graft. The physician then closes the sternotomy or thoracotomy, leaving a chest tube in place.

35631

The physician exposes the involved mesenteric or celiac artery using an upper midline abdominal incision, retracting and dissecting past large and small bowel. The physician exposes the distal thoracic aorta, administers heparin for anticoagulation, and clamps the aorta both proximal and distal to the celiac axis origin. The physician then cuts out an elliptical disk of aortic wall from the anterior surface of the aorta. The physician exposes the involved vessel

(mesenteric or celiac artery) and divides it proximal to the occlusion, closing off the proximal stump with suture. The physician sews a synthetic or arterial graft from the clamped aorta to the undiseased distal artery. The physician may use graft material to enlarge the arterial lumen (patch graft). The physician may perform arteriography or use a Doppler probe to establish patency of the graft. The physician then closes the abdominal wound, leaving drains in place.

35636–35641

The physician performs a bilateral subcostal incision from the right midrectus position extending into the left flank, and dissects past bowel and pancreas to expose the splenic vein. The physician exposes the splenic artery by careful dissection. The physician then exposes the left renal artery by dissecting through the posterior parietal peritoneum, partially clamps it, and excises an ellipse of renal artery at its upper border. The physician performs an end-to-side anastomosis of synthetic or arterial graft material from the splenic artery to the renal artery. The physician removes the clamps and assesses the anastomotic sites for leaks. The physician may perform Doppler studies or arteriography to establish patency of the graft. The physician then closes the abdominal wound, leaving drains in place. Report 35641 if performed in the aortoiliac or bi-iliac arteries.

35641

The physician makes an incision in the abdominal wall and separates the muscles to expose the internal organs, which are then checked for any undetected disease. The physician next locates the aorta and iliac arteries and isolates the obstruction by clamping the vessels. An artificial graft, commonly of polyester or polytetrafluoroethylene, is made ready. Synthetic grafts are preferred in aortoiliac or bifemoral bypasses since they more closely match the luminal dimensions of the replaced arteries. The graft is sewn into place, with one end anastomosed to the aorta and the other end to the iliac artery. The physician removes the clamps, blood then flows freely, and the physician assesses the anastomotic sites for leaks. The physician may perform Doppler studies or arteriography to establish patency of the graft. The abdominal wound is closed in layers.

35642

Through an incision in the skin of the neck, the physician isolates and dissects the vertebral and carotid arteries, separating them from adjacent critical structures. The physician creates a bypass around a section of vertebral artery that is damaged or blocked, using a synthetic vein and one of two methods of repair. After vessel clamps have been affixed above and below the damaged area, the synthetic graft is sewn to the side of the carotid artery and either sewn to the side of the vertebral artery beyond the affected area (end-to-side) or sewn to the cut end of the vertebral artery after dividing it beyond the affected area (end-to-end). The damaged or blocked section of the vertebral artery is not removed. When the clamps are removed, the section of synthetic vein graft forms a new path through which blood can easily bypass the blocked area. After the graft is complete, the skin incision is repaired with a layered closure.

35645

Through an incision in the skin of the neck, the physician isolates and dissects the vertebral and subclavian arteries, separating them from adjacent critical structures. The physician creates a bypass around a section of vertebral artery that is damaged or blocked, using a synthetic vein and one of two methods of repair. Once vessel clamps are affixed above and below the defect, the ends of the synthetic vein are sutured into the sides of the subclavian and vertebral arterial walls resulting in a bypass of the damaged area (end-to-side). In the second method, the vertebral artery can be cut through above the damaged area and sutured to one end of a synthetic vein (end-to-end). The remaining end is then sutured to the subclavian artery. In either case, the blocked or damaged vertebral artery is not removed. When the clamps are removed, the section of synthetic vein graft forms a new path through which blood can easily bypass the blocked area. After the graft is complete, the skin incision is repaired with a layered closure.

35646–35647

The physician makes an incision in the skin of the abdomen over a section of damaged or blocked lower aorta. The artery is isolated and dissected. Through a separate skin incision in the upper thigh, the femoral artery is isolated and dissected from adjacent critical structures. The physician creates a bypass around the damage or blocked lower aorta using a synthetic vein. Once vessel clamps have been affixed above the defect, the lower aorta may be cut through or tied off with sutures above the damaged or blocked area and sutured to one end of the synthetic vein in an end-to-end or side-to-side fashion. The graft to one femoral artery is passed through a tunnel on the inside of the upper thigh and sutured to the femoral artery. A second synthetic vein is placed in a similar fashion to the second side. When the clamps are removed, the two grafted synthetic vein limbs form a new path through which blood can easily bypass the blocked area. The blocked or damaged portion of artery is not removed. After the graft is complete, the skin incisions are repaired with layered closure.

35650

The physician makes an incision in the skin of both axillae. The physician creates a bypass around a section of axillary or subclavian artery that is damaged or blocked, using a synthetic vein and one of two methods of repair. Once vessel clamps have been affixed above and below the defect, the ends of the synthetic vein are sutured into the sides of the two

axillary arterial walls, resulting in a bypass of the damaged area. In the second method, the axillary artery may be cut through beyond the damaged area and sutured to one end of a synthetic vein, which is then passed across the front of the chest under the skin and sutured to the side of the opposite axillary artery. The blocked or damaged portion of the axillary or subclavian artery is not removed. When the clamps are removed, the section of synthetic vein graft forms a new path through which blood can easily bypass the blocked area. After the graft is complete, the skin incisions are repaired with layered closures.

35651

The physician makes an incision in the skin of the abdomen over a section of damaged or blocked lower aorta. The artery is isolated and dissected from adjacent critical structures. Through a separate skin incision in the upper thigh, the femoral artery is isolated and dissected and through a third skin incision behind the knee, the popliteal artery is isolated and dissected. The physician creates a bypass around the damaged artery that supplies the femoral-popliteal artery, using a synthetic vein. Once vessel clamps have been affixed above the defect, the lower aortic artery is cut through or tied off with sutures above the damaged area and sutured to one end of the synthetic vein. The graft is passed through a tunnel on the inside of the upper thigh and sutured to a point on the femoral artery. A third vein graft is sutured to the femoral artery and passed through a tunnel, where it is joined to the popliteal artery. It is also sutured. When the clamps are removed, the grafted synthetic vein forms a new path through which blood can easily bypass the blocked area. After the graft is complete, the skin incisions are repaired with layered closures.

35654

Through an incision in the skin of the axilla and both upper thighs, the physician creates a bypass around a section of lower aorta that is damaged or blocked, using a synthetic graft. Once vessel clamps have been affixed above and below the defect, the synthetic graft is sutured to the side of the axillary artery and passed through a subcutaneous tunnel to the upper thigh where it is sutured end-to-end or end-to-side to the femoral artery. A second synthetic graft is sutured end-to-side to the femoral artery and passed through another subcutaneous tunnel to the opposite thigh where it is sutured end-to-end or end-to-side to the femoral artery. The section of blocked artery is not removed. When the clamps are removed, the two synthetic grafted limbs form a new path through which blood can easily bypass the blocked area. After the graft is complete, the skin incisions are repaired with layered closures.

35656

Through incisions in the skin of the leg overlying the femoral and popliteal arteries, the physician isolates and dissects a section of artery that is damaged or blocked. The physician creates a bypass around the superficial femoral artery, using a synthetic vein and one of two methods of repair. Once vessel clamps have been affixed above and below the defect, the superficial femoral artery may be cut through above the damaged or blocked area and sutured to one end of a synthetic vein, which is then passed through a tunnel down the thigh muscles to behind the knee and sutured to the popliteal artery. In the second method, the ends of the synthetic vein are sutured into the side of the femoral and popliteal arterial walls, resulting in a bypass of the damaged area. When the clamps are removed, the section of synthetic vein forms a new path through which blood can easily bypass the blocked area. The blocked or damaged portion of artery is not removed. After the graft is complete, the skin incisions are repaired with layered closures.

35661

Through incisions in the skin of the upper thighs, the physician isolates and dissects a section of the femoral arteries. The physician creates a bypass using a synthetic vein. Once vessel clamps have been affixed above and below the area of anastomosis, the femoral artery may be cut through below the damaged area and sutured to one end of a synthetic vein, which is then sutured to the femoral artery in the opposite leg, resulting in a bypass of the damaged or blocked area. When the clamps are removed, the section of synthetic vein forms a new path through which blood can easily bypass the blocked area. The blocked or damaged portion of the artery is not removed. After the graft is complete, the skin incisions are repaired with layered closures.

35663

The physician exposes the iliac arteries using an abdominal incision, retracting and dissecting past large and small bowel. The physician partially clamps the patent (non-diseased) iliac artery and places a longitudinal incision down the clamped portion of the aorta. The physician sews in a synthetic or arterial graft, clamps the graft and removes the iliac clamp to assess patency of the anastomosis. The physician then clamps the diseased iliac artery distal to the stenosis, places a distal incision and attaches the distal graft to the diseased iliac artery. The physician may also use graft material to enlarge the aortic or arterial lumen (patch graft). The physician may perform arteriography or use a Doppler probe to establish patency of the graft. The physician then closes the abdominal wound, leaving drains in place.

35665

Through incisions in the skin of the lower abdomen overlying the iliac artery, and in the skin of the upper thigh overlying the femoral artery, the physician isolates and dissects a section of common iliac artery. The physician creates a bypass around the iliac artery,

using a synthetic vein and one of two methods of repair. Once vessel clamps have been affixed above and below the defect, the iliac artery may be cut or tied off with sutures above the damaged area and sutured to one end of a synthetic vein. The graft is passed through a tunnel on the inside of the upper thigh and is sutured to the side of the femoral artery. In the second method, the end of the synthetic vein is sutured to the side of the iliac artery. Either method results in a bypass of the damaged area. When the clamps are removed, the section of synthetic vein forms a new path through which blood can easily bypass the blocked area. After the graft is complete, the skin incisions are repaired with layered closures.

35666

Through incisions in the skin of the leg overlying the superficial femoral artery, the physician isolates and dissects sections of the femoral and anterior tibial, posterior tibial or peroneal arteries. The physician creates a bypass around the affected artery using a synthetic vein. Once vessel clamps have been affixed above and below the defect, the superficial femoral artery may be cut through above the damaged area and sutured to one end of a synthetic vein, which is then passed through an intramuscular tunnel and sutured to the anterior tibial, posterior tibial, peroneal, or other distal vessel. In the second method, the ends of the synthetic vein are sutured to the side of the femoral artery and anterior tibial, posterior tibial, peroneal, or other distal vessel wall, resulting in a bypass of the damaged area. When the clamps are removed, the section of synthetic vein forms a new path through which blood can easily bypass the blocked area. The blocked or damaged portion of artery is left in place and not removed. After the graft is complete, the skin incisions are repaired with layered closures.

35671

Through incisions in the skin of the leg overlying the popliteal arteries, the physician isolates and dissects a section of artery from adjacent critical structures. The physician creates a bypass around the artery, using a synthetic vein and one of two methods of repair. Once vessel clamps have been affixed above and below the defect, the popliteal artery may be cut through above the damaged area and sutured to one end of a synthetic vein, which is then sutured to the tibial, peroneal, or other distal artery. In the second method, the ends of the synthetic vein are sutured into the side of the popliteal and the tibial or peroneal arterial wall resulting in a bypass of the damaged area. When the clamps are removed, the section of synthetic vein forms a new path through which blood can easily bypass the blocked area. After the graft is complete, the incision is repaired with layered closures.

35681–35683

In 35681 the physician constructs a composite graft from donor and synthetic materials. One common composite would involve the reconfiguring of a harvested vein into a length of larger diameter graft material. The harvested vein would be split lengthwise and then wrapped in a spiral and sutured around a larger diameter mandrill. This length of composite graft would be used to complete the primary procedure. In 35682 a graft is constructed using tissue acquired from two veins at separate locations in the patient's body for the transplantation. In 35863 a graft is constructed using three or more segments of vein from two or more locations in the patient's body. In all three procedures veins are harvested by making an incision over the site where the vein will be removed. Tissues are dissected down to the vein and the vein is released from surrounding tissues. The vein is tied off above and below the area of vein that is to be removed. The vein is removed. The wound is closed with layered sutures. The portion of vein(s) removed is prepared for use in a separately reportable bypass graft procedure.

35685

The physician places a vein patch or cuff at a distal arterial anastomosis site during a bypass graft, synthetic conduit procedure of the lower extremity. The physician harvests the vein to be used for the vein patch from a previously chosen site. The vein patch is positioned and anastomosed between the distal portion of the synthetic vein graft and the native artery, end-to-end or side-to-end. The physician returns to the bypass graft surgery having performed this additional procedure.

35686

The physician creates a fistula between an artery and vein during a lower extremity bypass procedure. The physician harvests the vein to be used for creation of the fistula from a previously chosen site. The vein is anastomosed between the tibial or peroneal artery and a vein at or beyond the distal bypass anastomosis site. The physician returns to the bypass graft surgery having performed this adjuvant (additional) procedure.

35691

The physician performs a supraclavicular incision and exposes the vertebral and carotid arteries by careful dissection. The physician clears the adventitia of the chosen translocation site in the posterolateral wall of the common carotid artery. The physician anticoagulates the patient with heparin and divides the vertebral artery above the stenotic area. The physician ligates the proximal vertebral stump with suture and makes a small arteriotomy in the common carotid arterial wall with an aortic punch. The physician attaches the vertebral artery using an end-to-side anastomosis to the carotid artery. The physician may perform arteriography or use a Doppler probe to establish patency of the graft. The physician then closes the supraclavicular wound, leaving a drain in place.

35693

The physician performs a supraclavicular incision and exposes the vertebral and subclavian arteries by careful dissection. The physician clears the adventitia of the chosen translocation site in the subclavian artery lateral to the thyrocervical trunk. The physician anticoagulates the patient with heparin and divides the vertebral artery above the stenotic area. The physician ligates the proximal vertebral stump with suture and makes a small arteriotomy in the subclavian artery wall with an aortic punch. The physician attaches the vertebral artery using an end-to-side anastomosis to the subclavian artery. The physician may perform arteriography or use a Doppler probe to establish patency of the graft. The physician then closes the supraclavicular wound, leaving a drain in place.

35694

The physician performs a supraclavicular incision and exposes the carotid and subclavian arteries by careful dissection. The physician clears the adventitia of the chosen translocation site in the subclavian artery lateral to the thyrocervical trunk. The physician anticoagulates the patient's blood with heparin and divides the carotid artery above the stenotic area. The physician ligates the proximal carotid stump with suture and makes a small arteriotomy in the subclavian artery wall with an aortic punch. The physician attaches the carotid artery using an end-to-side anastomosis to the subclavian artery. The physician may perform arteriography or use a Doppler probe to establish patency of the graft. The physician then closes the supraclavicular wound, leaving a drain in place.

35695

The physician performs a supraclavicular incision and exposes the carotid and subclavian arteries by careful dissection. The physician clears the adventitia of the chosen translocation site in the posterolateral wall of the common carotid artery. The physician anticoagulates the patient's blood with heparin and divides the subclavian artery distal to the stenotic area. The physician ligates the proximal subclavian stump with suture and makes a small arteriotomy in the common carotid artery wall with an aortic punch. The physician attaches the subclavian artery using an end-to-side anastomosis to the carotid artery. The physician may perform arteriography or use a Doppler probe to establish patency of the graft. The physician then closes the supraclavicular wound, leaving a drain in place.

35700

This code is only used with other codes to identify the reoperation aspect of this procedure, which usually requires more effort when performed again. Through incisions in the skin of the leg, overlying the affected artery, the physician isolates the graft. The physician makes an incision in the proximal portion of the graft and passes a Fogarty balloon catheter through the graft to clear and straighten it. If an arteriograph indicates the graft must be replaced, the physician makes a second incision distal to the inguinal incision, releases the graft, and places vein clamps above and below the stricture. The physician replaces the graft by suturing the ends of a new graft to the side of the arteries to form a bypass of the damaged area. The clamps are removed. After the stricture is controlled or the graft is otherwise complete, the incisions are repaired with layered closures.

35701

Through an incision in the skin overlying the carotid artery and in front of the sternocleidomastoid muscle, the physician dissects out around the carotid artery, freeing it so it can be carefully examined. The artery is freed from any surrounding scar tissue that may be compressing it. Finding no perforations or other signs of injury, the physician repairs the skin incision with a layered closure.

35721

Through an incision in the skin overlying the femoral artery, the physician dissects around the sartorius and/or adductor longus muscles as necessary to access the femoral artery. The physician dissects out around the femoral artery, freeing it so it can be carefully examined. The artery is freed from any surrounding scar tissue that may be compressing it. Finding no perforations or other signs of injury, the physician repairs the skin incision with a layered closure.

35741

Through an incision in the skin overlying the popliteal artery, the physician dissects around the popliteal vein and other critical structures as necessary to access the popliteal artery. The physician dissects out around the popliteal artery, freeing it so it can be carefully examined. The artery is freed from any surrounding scar tissue that may be compressing it. Finding no perforations or other signs of injury, the physician repairs the skin incision with a layered closure.

35761

Through an incision in the skin overlying the vessel to be examined, the physician dissects around any muscle, vessels, and/or other structures as necessary to access the vessel. The physician dissects out around the vessel, freeing it so it can be carefully examined. The artery is freed from any surrounding scar tissue that may be compressing it. Finding no perforations or other signs of injury, the physician repairs the skin incision with a layered closure.

35800

Through an incision in the neck over the affected area, the physician isolates the vessel and explores it for postoperative complications such as hemorrhage, thrombosis, or infection. The physician dissects any

adjacent critical structures as necessary to access the vessel. The complication is identified and corrected. A hemorrhage is controlled by ligation or suture repair of the artery. Thrombosis requires opening of the artery and the removal of the clot. Any infection is drained, and sometimes a temporary tube is placed so the infection can continue to drain. The physician sutures the skin incision with a layered closure once the postsurgical complication has been treated.

35820

The physician reopens the original incision site and inspects the operative area for active bleeding, hematoma, thrombus, and exudate. The physician removes or debrides any observed hematoma, thrombus, and infected tissues. The physician looks for and corrects any active bleeding sites using electrocautery or ligation of bleeding vessels. The physician may leave an infected wound open, but generally closes the incision, leaving drains and chest tubes in place.

35840

The physician reopens the original incision site and inspects the operative area for active bleeding, hematoma, thrombus, and exudate. The physician removes or debrides any observed hematoma, thrombus, and infected tissues. The physician looks for and corrects any active bleeding sites using electrocautery or ligation of bleeding vessels. The physician may leave an infected wound open, but generally closes the incision, leaving drains in place.

35860

Through an incision in the extremity over the affected area, the physician isolates the vessel and explores it for postoperative complications such as hemorrhage, thrombosis, or infection. The physician dissects any adjacent critical structures as necessary to access the vessel. The complication is identified and corrected. A hemorrhage is controlled by ligation or suture repair of the artery. Thrombosis requires opening of the artery and the removal of the clot. Any infection is drained, and sometimes a temporary tube is placed so the infection can continue to drain. The physician sutures the skin incision with a layered closure once the postsurgical complication has been treated.

35870

The physician opens the abdomen under antibiotic cover and exposes the graft-enteric fistula site by careful dissection (most often aortic/Dacron anastomosis with a fistulous connection to the duodenum). The physician disconnects the fistula and repairs the enteric defect using two layers of suture. The physician examines the vascular prosthesis, removes the prosthesis and sews in appropriate new bypass grafts if there is obvious graft infection. If there is no obvious infection, the physician repairs the graft with local sutures. The physician then closes the wound, leaving drains in place.

35875–35876

Through an incision in the skin overlying the arterial or venous graft, the physician isolates the site of the thrombus. The physician dissects any muscle, overlying vessel, and/or adjacent critical structures to access the graft. To excise the thrombus from the graft, the blood vessel is clamped above and below the thrombus, an incision is made into the vessel or graft and the thrombus is removed. The graft or vessel is sutured at the site of the thrombectomy and the clamps are removed. To remove the thrombus with a catheter, the physician makes an incision in the vessel above or below the graft and threads the catheter past the thrombus. A balloon or tool at the tip of the catheter is inflated or extended. The physician withdraws the catheter, repeating as necessary, to capture and retrieve all of the thrombus. The blood vessel is repaired with sutures. After either procedure, the skin incision is repaired with a layered closure. In 35876, the thrombotic graft is removed, the graft site is repaired with sutures, and, avoiding the repair site, a new graft is sutured into place on the vessel. The skin incision is then repaired with a layered closure.

35879–35881

The physician revises a lower extremity arterial bypass with vein-patch angioplasty or segmental vein interposition. A previous lower-extremity arterial bypass graft(s) requires open revision due to graft-threatening stenosis. The physician makes an incision in a lower extremity over the site of a previous arterial bypass graft. Dissection is carried down to the graft. In 35879 angioplasty of the stenosed area is performed by excising the area of stenosis and using a patch of vein to close the created wound. In 35881 a segment of vein is excised from another area. The area of stenosis is excised and the vein segment is positioned between the two ends of the graft and anastomosed in an end to end fashion. In this procedure a thrombectomy is not performed. The wound is closed with layered sutures.

35901

Through an incision in the skin of the neck overlying the graft, the physician dissects around any muscle, vessels, or other structures to access the graft site. The physician dissects around the vessel, and applies vessel clamps above and below the graft. The physician excises above and below the existing infected graft. The blood vessel is repaired with sutures. A special catheter may be left in place to help drain infection. The skin is loosely closed. If the excised graft is replaced with a new graft, report the appropriate revascularization code.

35903

Through an incision in the skin of the extremity overlying the graft, the physician dissects around any muscle, vessels or other structures to access the graft site. The physician dissects around the vessel, and applies vessel clamps above and below the graft. The

physician excises above and below the existing infected graft. The blood vessel is repaired with sutures. A special catheter may be left in place to help drain infection. The skin is loosely closed. If the excised graft is replaced with a new graft, report the appropriate revascularization code.

35905

Through an incision in the skin of the thorax overlying the graft, the physician dissects around any muscle, vessels or other structures to access the graft site. The physician dissects around the vessel, and applies vessel clamps above and below the graft. The physician excises above and below the existing infected graft. The blood vessel is repaired with sutures. A special catheter may be left in place to help drain infection. The skin is loosely closed. If the excised graft is replaced with a new graft, report the appropriate revascularization code.

35907

Through an incision in the skin of the abdomen overlying the graft, the physician dissects around any muscle, vessels or other structures to access the graft site. The physician dissects around the vessel, and applies vessel clamps above and below the graft. The physician excises above and below the existing infected graft. The blood vessel is repaired with sutures. A special catheter may be left in place to help drain infection. The skin is loosely closed. If the excised graft is replaced with a new graft, report the appropriate revascularization code.

36000–36005

In 36000, the physician places a needle or a catheter through a puncture in the skin and into a peripheral vein. In 36002, the physician injects a pseudoaneurysm (a pulsatile hematoma with a fibrous capsule) and maintains persistent communication with the adjacent vessel. The vessel wall does not heal and blood flows back and forth between the vessel and hematoma during the cardiac cycle. Under ultrasound control, the physician advances a 22-gauge needle into the lumen of the pseudoaneurysm and injects Thrombin to cause thrombosis of the pseudoaneurysm. In 36005, an opaque substance is injected through the catheter for venography. Once the procedure is complete, the catheter is removed and pressure is applied to stop bleeding at the injection site.

36010

The physician punctures a distal vein (typically antecubital, internal jugular, subclavian, or femoral) with a large needle and passes a guidewire via the needle into the punctured vein. The physician removes the needle while leaving the guidewire in place, and enlarges the skin opening slightly with a blade. The physician may then slide an introducer sheath over the guidewire into the venous lumen, or may slide the catheter directly into the venous lumen

CPT® Lay Descriptions

without using an introducer sheath. If using an introducer sheath, the physician inserts the catheter into the vein through an O-ring in the introducer sheath (this prevents blood from leaking around the catheter) into the superior or inferior vena cava. The physician may check the catheter position with fluoroscope or with an x-ray.

36011–36012

Through a puncture through the skin, the physician passes a needle into the vein and threads a guidewire through the needle into the vein. The needle is removed and the wire is passed to the desired location in the venous system. A catheter then follows the wire into the selected point in the vein and the wire is removed. A first order branch from the vena cava (36011) is any initial vessel draining directly into the vena cava (e.g., renal vein or jugular vein). A second order branch of the vena cava (36012) is any vein draining into a first order branch (e.g., left adrenal, petrosal sinus). Contrast material for venography is injected into the catheter that has traveled to an area upstream of the site under investigation. Once the procedure is complete, the catheter is removed, and pressure applied to stop bleeding at the injection site.

36013

The physician punctures a distal vein (typically antecubital, internal jugular, subclavian, or femoral) with a large needle and passes a guidewire via the needle into the punctured vein. The physician removes the needle while leaving the guidewire in place, and enlarges the skin opening slightly with a blade. The physician then slides an introducer sheath over the guidewire into the venous lumen. The physician inserts the catheter into the vein through an O-ring in the introducer sheath (this prevents blood from leaking around the catheter) and advances the catheter into the right heart or main pulmonary artery, using fluoroscopic guidance or while measuring pressures through the catheter lumen to ensure that the catheter tip is in the desired place. The physician may then use the catheter to inject contrast material to perform venography or pulmonary arteriography.

36014

The physician punctures a distal vein (typically antecubital, internal jugular, subclavian, or femoral) with a large needle and passes a guidewire via the needle into the punctured vein. The physician removes the needle while leaving the guidewire in place, and enlarges the skin opening slightly with a blade. The physician then slides an introducer sheath over the guidewire into the venous lumen. The physician inserts the catheter into the vein through an O-ring in the introducer sheath (this prevents blood from leaking around the catheter) and advances the catheter into one of the main pulmonary arteries (right or left) using fluoroscopic guidance and possibly measuring pressures through the catheter lumen to ensure that the catheter tip is in the desired

place. The physician may then use the catheter to inject contrast material to perform venography or pulmonary arteriography.

36015

The physician punctures a distal vein (typically antecubital, internal jugular, subclavian, or femoral) with a large needle and passes a guidewire via the needle into the punctured vein. The physician removes the needle while leaving the guidewire in place, and enlarges the skin opening slightly with a blade. The physician then slides an introducer sheath over the guidewire into the venous lumen. The physician inserts the catheter into the vein through an O-ring in the introducer sheath (this prevents blood from leaking around the catheter) and advances the catheter into one of the segmental or subsegmental pulmonary arteries using fluoroscopic guidance and possibly measuring pressures through the catheter lumen to ensure that the catheter tip is in the desired place. The physician may then use the catheter to inject contrast material to perform venography or pulmonary arteriography.

36100–36120

Through the skin of the neck (for the carotid or vertebral artery in 36100) or through the skin of the arm (into the brachial artery and upstream to the aortic arch in 36120) the physician inserts a needle into the underlying artery. A guidewire is threaded through the needle into the artery, and the needle is removed. A catheter follows the wire into the artery. The wire is removed. Contrast material is injected through the catheter into the artery for arteriography. Once either procedure is complete, the catheter is removed, and pressure applied to the puncture site to stop bleeding.

36140

Through a puncture in the skin over an extremity artery, the physician injects a needle into that artery and threads a guidewire through it. The needle is removed. A catheter then follows the wire into the artery, and the wire is removed. Contrast material for arteriography is injected into the catheter placed upstream of the site under investigation. Once the procedure is complete, the catheter is removed, and pressure applied to stop bleeding at the injection site.

36145

Through a puncture in the skin overlying the artificial fistula, graft, or cannula of a dialysis patient, the physician inserts a catheter into the fistula or supplying artery or draining vein. The catheter is guided into the fistula and vessel to an area upstream of the site under investigation, and contrast material is injected into it. Once the procedure is complete, the catheter is removed from the shunt.

36160

The physician punctures the left lumbar area, typically just above a rib, to direct a large needle into the aorta. When pulsatile red blood is obtained through the needle, indicating successful aortic puncture, the physician passes a guidewire via the needle into the punctured aorta. The physician removes the needle while leaving the guidewire in place, and enlarges the skin opening slightly with a blade. The physician then slides a catheter over the guidewire into the aortic lumen and secures the catheter in place with suture.

36200

The physician punctures a distal artery (typically femoral, brachial, radial, or axillary) with a large needle and passes a guidewire via the needle into the punctured artery. The physician removes the needle while leaving the guidewire in place, and enlarges the skin opening slightly with a blade. The physician then slides an introducer sheath over the guidewire into the arterial lumen. The physician inserts a catheter into the artery through an O-ring in the introducer sheath (this prevents blood from leaking around the catheter) and advances the catheter into the aorta. The physician may then use the catheter to inject contrast material to perform aortography, measure aortic pressures, or to administer medication.

36215–36216

The physician passes a needle into the skin into an extremity artery, usually in the upper thigh. A guidewire is threaded through the needle into the vessel. The needle is removed. The wire is threaded into the aorta and up to the thoracic aorta where it is manipulated into a branch off the aortic arch. A catheter follows the wire into a first order thoracic or brachiocephalic artery. The wire is removed. The catheter may pass through the first order vessel into a second order thoracic or brachiocephalic artery. Contrast material for arteriography is injected into the catheter that has been guided to an area upstream of the site under investigation. In 36215, the catheter remains in a first order artery. In 36216, the catheter travels further to a second order artery. Upon completion, the catheter is removed, and pressure applied to stop bleeding at the puncture site.

36217–36218

The physician punctures the skin and underlying artery with a needle and threads a guidance wire through the needle into the artery. The needle is removed. The guidewire is manipulated into the specific artery. A catheter then follows the wire into a first order thoracic or brachiocephalic artery. The catheter passes through the first order vessel into the second order thoracic or brachiocephalic artery. The catheter continues to a third order vessel. Contrast material for arteriography is injected into the catheter that has been guided to the site under investigation. Once the procedure is complete, the catheter is

removed, and pressure applied to stop bleeding at the injection site. Use 36218 for an additional second order, third order, and beyond, thoracic or bachiocephalic branch, within a vascular family. Used 36218 in addition to 36216 or 36217.

36245–36246

The physician inserts a needle through the skin and into an underlying artery, usually a lower extremity artery, and threads a guidewire through the needle and into the artery. The needle is removed. The wire is then threaded into the specific vessel. A catheter then follows the wire into the artery branch. The wire is removed. Contrast material for arteriography is injected into the catheter that has been guided to the site under investigation. In 36245, the catheter remains in a first order artery. In 36246, the catheter travels farther, to a second order artery. Once the procedure is complete, the catheter is removed, and pressure applied to stop bleeding at the injection site.

36247–36248

The physician inserts a needle through the skin and into an underlying artery. A guidewire is threaded through the needle into the artery and the needle is removed. The guidewire is then manipulated into the specific artery. A catheter follows the wire into the third order abdominal, pelvic, or lower extremity artery branch. Contrast material for arteriography is injected into the catheter that has been guided to the site under investigation. Once the procedure is complete, the catheter is removed, and pressure applied at the injection site. Report 36247 for a placement in the initial third order or more selective abdominal, pelvic, or lower extremity artery branch, within a vascular family. Use 36248 of and additional second order, third order, and beyond, abdominal, pelvic, or lower extremity artery branch, within a vascular family. Use 36248 in addition to 36246 or 36247.

36260

The physician performs an upper abdominal incision and exposes the hepatic artery. The physician then punctures the hepatic artery with a large needle and passes a guidewire via the needle into the punctured artery. The physician removes the needle while leaving the guidewire in place. The physician then slides the infusion catheter over the guidewire into the arterial lumen. The physician secures the catheter with suture and closes the abdominal wound around the proximal end of the infusion catheter. The physician may then use the catheter to administer chemotherapeutic medication.

36261

The physician performs an upper abdominal incision and exposes the hepatic artery, locating the previously implanted infusion catheter. The physician may unkink the catheter or replace it over a wire. The physician secures the catheter with suture and closes the abdominal wound around the proximal end of the infusion catheter. The physician may then use the catheter to administer chemotherapeutic medication.

36262
The physician performs an upper abdominal incision and exposes the hepatic artery while carefully dissecting free the previously implanted infusion catheter. The physician then removes the catheter, and may repair the arteriotomy with suture. The physician closes the abdominal wound, and may leave a drain in place.

36400
A needle is inserted through the skin to puncture the femoral or jugular vein of a child younger than age 3. The vein is used for the withdrawal of blood or for the infusion of intravenous medication. A soft flexible catheter may be placed for prolonged therapy. Once the procedure is complete, the needle is withdrawn and pressure is applied over the puncture site to control bleeding.

36405–36406
A needle is inserted through the skin to puncture a vein of a child under age 3. In 36405, the scalp vein is used for the withdrawal of blood or for the infusion of intravenous medication. A catheter may be placed for prolonged therapy. In 36406, a vein other than femoral, jugular, sagittal sinus, or scalp is used. Once the procedure is complete, the needle is withdrawn, and pressure is applied over the puncture site to control bleeding.

36410
The physician inserts a needle into the skin to puncture any vein in a person 36 months old or older. This vein is used for the withdrawal of blood, or for the infusion of intravenous medication. A catheter may be placed for prolonged therapy. Once the procedure is complete, the needle is withdrawn and pressure is applied over the puncture site to control bleeding.

36415
A needle is inserted into the skin over a vessel to puncture and withdraw blood from a vein, or the physician may prick the finger, heel, or ear and collect in a pipette the blood that pools at the puncture site. In either case, the blood is used for diagnostic study and no catheter is placed.

36420–36425
The physician makes an incision in the skin directly over the vessel and dissects the area surrounding the vein. A needle is passed into the vein for the withdrawal of blood or for the infusion of intravenous medication of a patient under 12 months of age (in 36420) or over 12 months of age (in 36425). A catheter may be left behind. Once the procedure is

complete, the incision is repaired with a layered closure.

36430
The physician transfuses blood or blood components to a patient. The physician establishes venous access with a needle and catheter and transfuses the blood products.

36440
The physician performs a push transfusion on a child 2 years old and under. The physician calculates the amount of blood to be transfused and slowly injects it into the patient using a needle or existing catheter.

36450–36455
The physician performs an exchange transfusion on a newborn. The physician calculates the blood volume to be transfused. A needle is placed in an artery or in an existing arterial catheter. The patient's blood is removed and replaced simultaneously to maintain blood pressure. Report 36455 if the child is other than a newborn.

36460
The physician performs a blood transfusion to a fetus. The physician uses separately reportable ultrasound guidance to locate the umbilical vein. A needle is directed through the abdominal wall into the amniotic cavity. The umbilical vein is pierced and fetal blood is exchanged with transfused blood. The needle is withdrawn and the fetus is observed under separately reportable ultrasound.

36468
The physician inserts a tiny needle through the skin and directly into the tiny, distended veins in the arms, legs, or trunk. A solution (hypertonic saline and other solutions) is injected into these veins. The solution causes the walls of the veins to become inflamed, collapse, and then stick together so the veins close.

36469
The physician inserts a tiny needle through the skin and directly into the tiny, distended veins in the face. A solution (hypertonic saline and other solutions) is injected into these veins. The solution causes the walls of the veins to become inflamed, collapse, and then stick together so the veins close.

36470–36471
The physician inserts a tiny needle through the skin and directly into any single vein (in 36470) or multiple veins (in 36471). A solution (hypertonic saline and other solutions) is injected into these veins. The patient stands while the injection is given. The leg or legs are elevated thereafter, and wrapped in an elastic dressing. The solution causes the walls of the veins to become inflamed, collapse, and then stick together so the veins close.

36481

The physician numbs the right lateral abdominal wall with local anesthetic. The physician places a large needle through the skin into the liver, maneuvering the needle through the liver into the intrahepatic portal vein, injecting contrast under fluoroscope for localization. The physician then places a wire through the needle, retrograde into the portal vein. The physician removes the wire over the needle, and advances a catheter over the wire, through the skin and liver into the portal vein. The physician secures the catheter with suture. Alternative methods include placing a catheter via the internal jugular vein, or using a transsplenic approach.

36488–36489

A needle is inserted into the skin overlying the subclavian, jugular, or any other vein and into the vein itself. A wire may be inserted through the needle into the vein, and the needle is removed. The physician threads a catheter along the wire into the vessel and removes the wire. The catheter tip is advanced into the superior or inferior vena cava. The catheter may be passed through a subcutaneous tunnel and brought out through at a point distant from the entry into the vein. The catheter will be used in long-term monitoring or treatment of a patient age 2 years or less (in 36488) or over 2 years (in 36489). The catheter is used to supply necessary nutrients, for dialysis or chemotherapy treatments, or for venous pressure monitoring.

36490–36491

Through a skin incision over the vein, the physician isolates and dissects the vein for placement of a catheter for long-term treatment of a patient age 2 years or less (in 36490), or over 2 years (in 36491). The vein is nicked and the catheter is inserted and the tip advanced into the vena cava. The skin is sutured closed. The catheter is left in the vein until treatment is completed. The catheter is used to supply necessary nutrients, for dialysis or chemotherapy treatments, or for venous pressure monitoring.

36493

The physician repositions, through external manipulation, a catheter within a vein. This repositioning may be necessary because of poor venous blood flow through the existing catheter or improper placement within the vena cava. The repositioned catheter will remain in place and is used for extended treatment.

36500

The physician inserts a needle through the skin and into a peripheral vein. A guidewire is threaded through the needle into the vessel. The needle is removed. The wire is manipulated into the vein draining from the organ to be sampled. The catheter follows the guidewire into the vein. Once the catheter has been placed, the guidewire is removed and the

blood sample obtained. The catheter is removed and pressure is applied to the puncture site to stop the flow of blood.

36510

The physician catheterizes the umbilical vein for diagnostic or therapeutic purposes. The physician cleanses the umbilical cord stump and locates the umbilical vein. A catheter is inserted in the vein for reasons including blood sampling or administering medication.

36520

The physician draws and separates a patient's blood to eliminate destructive elements (plasma, leukocytes, platelets, etc.), and retransfuses the cleansed blood. The physician establishes venous access or attaches the machine to an existing central venous catheter line. The blood is removed and cycled through the pheresis machine and returned to the patient through a catheter and a needle inserted in the vein.

36521

A portion of the patient's blood is removed from a vein. In a special machine, certain cells and/or fluid (plasma) are removed using a technique called extracorporeal affinity column adsorption. The cells and/or plasma is/are re-infused back to the patient through a return catheter to a vein.

36522

The physician draws a patient's blood and exposes the blood to light to eliminate destructive elements. The physician establishes venous access or attaches the machine to an existing central venous catheter line. The blood is removed and cycled through the pheresis machine where it is exposed to therapeutic wavelengths of light. The conditioned blood is returned to the patient through a catheter and a needle inserted in the vein.

36530

The physician implants an intravenous infusion pump. The physician incises the skin over the internal jugular vein and pierces the vein to insert the venous access catheter. The catheter is threaded to the lower portion of the superior vena cava; placement is confirmed with separately reportable fluoroscopy. The physician incises the skin and creates a pouch for the pump. The venous access line is tunneled from the neck to the pouch incision. The pump is placed in the pocket and connected to the venous access line. The wounds are closed in sutured layers.

36531

The physician revises an intravenous pump. The physician incises the skin over the pump connection. The pump and the connection to the venous catheter are located and disconnected. First venous access is tested for patency. If the line is clotted, it is removed and replaced. The pump is purged and tested for patency. If defective, the pump is replaced. The venous access and pump are reconnected, and the incision is closed in sutured layers.

36532

The physician removes an intravenous infusion pump. The physician incises the skin over the pump. The pump and the connection to the venous catheter are isolated and disconnected. The venous access line is removed; pressure may be applied to the vein to control bleeding. The pump is dissected from the surrounding tissues and removed. Bleeding is controlled and the wound is closed in sutured layers.

36533

The physician implants a venous access device, with or without a subcutaneous reservoir. The physician incises the skin overlying the internal jugular vein and pierces the vein to insert the venous access catheter. The catheter is threaded to the lower portion of the superior vena cava; placement is confirmed with separately reportable fluoroscopy. The physician incises the skin and creates a pouch for the reservoir. The venous access line is tunneled from the neck to the pouch incision. The reservoir is placed in the pocket and connected to the venous access line. The wounds are closed in sutured layers.

36534

The physician revises a venous access device and/or subcutaneous reservoir. The physician incises the skin over the device connection. The device/subcutaneous reservoir and the connection to the venous catheter are located and disconnected. First, venous access is tested for patency. If the line is clotted, it is removed and replaced. Next, the device or reservoir is tested for patency. If defective, the device is replaced. The venous access and device are reconnected, and the incision is closed in sutured layers.

36535

The physician removes a venous access device and/or reservoir. The physician incises the skin over the device connection. The device/subcutaneous reservoir and the connection to the venous catheter are located and disconnected. The venous access line is removed; pressure may be applied to vein to control bleeding. The device or reservoir is dissected from the surrounding tissues and removed. Bleeding is controlled and the wound is closed in sutured layers.

36540

A blood specimen is obtained from a previously placed partially or completely implanted venous access device. Partially implanted venous access devices are catheters that have external access (Hickman, Broviac, Groshong, Quinton). Completely implanted devices are those that have access through a subcutaneous port (Port-A-Cath, Infusaport). If the specimen is to be obtained from a partially implantable venous access device, the rubber top is

cleaned with alcohol. A clean syringe with a needle or needleless adaptor is inserted and the heparin solution is withdrawn. A new syringe is placed in the rubber top and blood is collected in appropriate type of blood collection tube. Once the blood draw is complete, a previously prepared syringe containing heparin solution is used to flush the catheter. An implantable access device requires the use of a percutaneous noncoring needle to accomplish the blood draw. The skin is cleansed with alcohol or iodine solution. The needle is placed into the port. Heparin is withdrawn. A second needle is inserted and the blood specimen obtained. The port is then flushed with heparin solution.

36550

To remove a clot from an intravenous catheter, the physician injects a thrombolytic agent (e.g., Streptokinase) into the catheter that dissolves the clot. The patient is observed for any abnormal signs of bleeding.

36600

The physician inserts a needle through the skin and punctures the artery to withdraw blood for testing. No catheter is left in the artery. Pressure is applied to the puncture site to stop the flow of blood.

36620–36625

The physician accesses, in most cases, the ulnar or radial artery to insert a cannula, or tube-shaped portal. In 36620, the physician inserts a needle through the skin to puncture the artery, and then inserts a cannula. In 36625, the physician makes an incision in the skin overlying the artery and dissects the surrounding tissue to access it. The artery is sometimes nicked with a thin-bladed scalpel before the physician inserts the cannula. This cannula acts as a portal for sampling, monitoring or transfusion. Once the procedure is complete, the cannula is removed. In an open procedure, the opening in the artery may be sutured and the incision repaired with a layered closure. Pressure is applied to the puncture if a percutaneous approach is used.

36640

The physician accesses the artery supplying the area to be treated. To insert a cannula, or tube-shaped portal for prolonged infusion therapy, the physician makes an incision above the artery and dissects the surrounding tissue to access it. The artery is sometimes nicked with a thin-bladed scalpel before the physician inserts the catheter. The catheter may be advanced to a site immediately upstream of the site to be treated. This catheter acts as a portal for the infusion of chemotherapy drugs and will remain in place until chemotherapy is completed. The catheter is removed, the hole in the artery is repaired, and the incision is repaired with a layered closure

36660

The physician catheterizes an umbilical artery in a newborn for diagnostic or therapeutic purposes. The physician prepares the umbilical artery and passes a catheter sheath inside the lumen for arterial access. The catheter is attached to a pressure line which maintains patency of the arterial lumen. The access is used for diagnostic or therapeutic purposes, allowing the drawing of blood for separately reportable tests or instillation of medication for therapeutic purposes.

36680

The physician inserts a special needle through the skin and through the muscle tissue to puncture the bone marrow cavity, usually in the tibia or femur, of a patient whose vessels otherwise seem inaccessible. This needle is then used as a method of infusing fluids into the blood vessels in the bone marrow.

36800

The physician isolates two veins, usually in the nondominant forearm, and inserts a needle through the skin and into each vessel. A guidance wire may be threaded through the needle into each vessel. The needle is removed. An end of a single cannula is inserted into each puncture, and any guidance wire removed. The cannula remains external, and may be left in place for several days. (This hemodialysis cannula is used to remove blood from the vein, route it through the dialysis machine, then reinfuse it.)

36810

The physician isolates an artery and a vein, usually in the nondominant forearm, and inserts a needle through the skin and into each vessel. A guidewire may be threaded through the needle into each vessel. The needle is removed. An end of a single cannula is inserted into each puncture, and any guidance wire removed. The Scribner cannula remains external, and may be left in place for several days. (This hemodialysis cannula is used to remove blood from the vessel, route it through the dialysis machine, then reinfuse it.)

36815

The physician repositions an external cannula or removes it, followed by closure of the insertion site using sutures on the vessels or skin as necessary. The cannula forms a ready connection between the artery and vein, or vein and vein, for hemodialysis or another purpose.

36819

A vascular surgeon creates a connection between an artery or a vein. Performed in the operating room, the surgeon dissects down to the vein and artery and then creates a connection between the two using one of several methods. This code is for using the basilic vein in the upper arm inverted from end to end.

36820

The physician creates a connection between an artery or vein, using a forearm vein in the arm - inverted end to end. The physician dissects down to the vein and artery. The subfascial plane is identified and elevated laterally to the flexor carpi radialis (FCR) and medially to the brachioradialis (BR). The plane between the BR and FCR is dissected and the perforating vessels are identified and cauterized. The pedicle is followed to the antecubital fossa. The tourniquet is released, and the vessels are further cleaned of their adventitia under loupe visualization. Using microvascular techniques, a suture for the arterial anastomosis is performed and closure is completed. Suction drains are placed in the neck. If a Doppler is to be used for postoperative assessment, a suture is placed to mark the pedicle site. A splint is fabricated and secured to the arm with an elastic bandage.

36821

Through an incision, usually in the skin over an artery in the nondominant wrist or antecubital fossa, the physician isolates a desired section of artery and neighboring vein. Vessel clamps are placed on the vein and adjacent artery. The vein is dissected free, divided, and the downstream portion of the vein is sutured to an opening created in the adjacent artery, usually in an end-to-side fashion, allowing blood to flow both down the artery and into the vein. Large branches of the vein may be tied off to cause flow down a single vein. The skin incision is repaired with a layered closure. This arteriovenous anastomosis will allow an increased blood flow through the vein, usually for hemodialysis.

36822

Using one of two methods, the physician either punctures the skin or makes an incision in the skin, of the upper thigh, to position a tube (cannula) to form a ready connection to an artery and a vein. In one method, a needle is passed into the vessel and a flexible wire is passed through the needle into the same vessel. The needle is removed and a cannula is passed over the wire into the vessel. Once the cannula is positioned, the wire is withdrawn. In the second method, a small incision is made into the vessel. The cannula is placed directly into the vessel. Once the treatment is complete, the cannula is withdrawn and the skin incision is repaired with a layered closure.

36823

Using one of two methods, the physician either punctures the skin or makes an incision in the skin of an extremity to position a tube (cannula) to form a ready connection to an artery and a vein. In one method, a needle is passed into the vessel and a flexible wire is passed through the needle into the same vessel. The needle is removed and a cannula is passed over the wire into the vessel. Once the cannula is positioned, the wire is withdrawn. In the second method, a small incision is made into the vessel. The cannula is placed directly into the vessel. The procedure allows the blood to circulate outside of the body. This code includes hyperthermia and the insertion and removal of the cannula. It also includes chemotherapy perfusion supported by a membrane oxygenator/perfusion pump. The arteriotomy and venotomy sites are closed with layered suture.

36825–36830

The physician makes an incision in the skin over an artery and vein, and the vein and artery are dissected free. A vessel clamp is affixed to each. A length of harvested vein (in 36825) or synthetic vein (in 36830) is sutured to the incised artery and vein, usually in an end-to-side fashion. The graft is passed in a superficial subcutaneous tunnel that is created bluntly and connects the arterial and venous sites. The clamps are removed, allowing the blood to flow through the graft, creating an arteriovenous fistula. The skin incision is repaired with a layered closure.

36831

The physician removes a blood clot from a surgically created connection between an artery and a vein (arteriovenous fistula). The procedure involves making an incision over the site of an existing fistula. The fistula is isolated and dissected free. Vessel clamps are affixed above and below the fistula. The blood clot is removed, the clamps are taken off, and the incision is repaired by layered suture. The procedure may involve a vein acquired from the patient or the construction of a synthetic graft.

36832–36833

In 36832, the physician makes an incision at the site of an already existing artificial fistula between an artery and a vein. The fistula is dissected free. Vessel clamps are affixed above and below the fistula, which is then incised. Revisions are made to the fistula at its juncture to the vein and/or artery and may require creating an entirely new anastomosis with a graft obtained from a separate site or created with synthetic material. After the repair has been made, the fistula is sutured, the clamps removed, and the skin incision repaired with a layered closure. Report 36833 when the physician removes a blood clot at the fistula site in addition to revising the existing arteriovenous fistula.

36834

The physician makes an incision in the skin over the site of an already existing artificial fistula between an artery and a vein. The fistula is isolated and dissected free. Vessel clamps are affixed above and below the fistula, which is then incised. To reduce the size of an aneurysm, a portion of the fistula wall may be removed and the remaining tissue sutured together. Other revisions may be required. After the repair or revision has been made, the clamps are removed and the incision is repaired with a layered closure.

36835

Through an incision in the skin overlying a large vein or artery of a child, the physician dissects the vessel that will receive a synthetic shunt. The vessel may be clamped. The vessel is nicked, and a needle threads a guidance wire into the vein or artery. The shunt follows, and the wire is removed. The physician sutures the synthetic shunt either end-to-end, or end-to-side, to the vein or artery. The shunt is most often used for access in hemodialysis.

36860–36861

To remove a blood clot lodged in a previously placed cannula, the physician may inject a solution containing enzymes into the cannula to dissolve the clot (in 36860) or the physician may, after injecting a solution containing enzymes, insert a balloon catheter (in 36861) into the cannula to retrieve a clot there. The balloon is inserted and inflated beyond the clot. Then the catheter is slowly pulled out, capturing and retrieving the clot. Once the clot is dissolved or retrieved, the catheter is removed and the cannula is left in place.

36870

Under separately reportable radiologic guidance, a percutaneously placed catheter is advanced to the site of a thrombus or clot that has formed in a previously created connection between an artery and a vein, (arteriovenous fistula). The catheter is inserted into the clot and the clot is fragmented. Injection of urokinase may be required to dissolve the clot or percutaneous pharmacomechanical thrombolysis may be performed. Pharmacomechanical thrombolysis involves both injection of urokinase and mechanical fragmentation of the clot. Suction is applied and the clot fragments are removed through the catheter. The catheter is removed and pressure is applied at the insertion site.

37140

The physician places a long right thoracoabdominal incision and exposes the liver. The physician exposes the inferior vena cava and portal vein through careful dissection. The physician places a plastic sling around the portal vein and ties it closed, just proximal to its bifurcation. The physician then clamps and divides the portal vein. The physician applies a partial exclusion vascular clamp to the front of the vena cava and removes a small oval of tissue from the vena cava to allow end-to-side anastomosis of portal vein to the inferior vena cava. The physician removes the clamps and checks for appropriate flow without anastomotic leakage. The physician closes the incision, leaving a chest tube in place (but no abdominal drains, as this may lead to protein loss from postoperative drainage of ascites).

37145

The physician performs an abdominal incision and exposes the left renal vein and inferior vena cava. The physician transects the left renal vein and attaches it to the portal circulation by sewing the vena caval end to the portal vein, the superior mesenteric vein, or the splenic vein. Alternatively, the physician may divide the portal vein and attach its splanchnic end to the end of the transected renal vein. The physician assesses patency of the anastomosis and may measure venous pressures before closing the abdomen.

37160

The physician performs an upper midline vertical abdominal incision and retracts the transverse colon in a cephalad direction. The physician exposes the anterior surface of the inferior vena cava and frees the posterior surface of the superior mesenteric vein after careful dissection through the root of the transverse mesocolon. The physician isolates a long segment of the superior mesenteric vein with ties and partially occludes the inferior vena cava. The physician removes an ellipse of tissue from the inferior vena cava and performs and end-to-side anastomosis of Dacron graft to the inferior vena cava. The physician then occludes the superior mesenteric vein, cuts an ellipse from its anterior surface, and sews the end of the Dacron graft to the side of the superior mesenteric vein. The physician assesses patency of the anastomosis and may measure venous pressures before closing the abdomen.

37180

The physician performs a bilateral subcostal incision from the right midrectus position extending into the left flank, and dissects past bowel and pancreas to expose the splenic vein. The physician dissects the splenic vein free, ligating the splenic vein towards the left and using the central (right) end of the vein for the anastomosis. The physician then exposes the left renal vein by dissecting through the posterior parietal peritoneum. The physician exposes the left renal vein, partially clamps it, and excises an ellipse of renal vein at its upper border. The physician then performs and end-to-side anastomosis of the splenic vein to the renal vein, using harvested vein graft material if extension is required. The physician removes the clamps. The physician may measure superior mesenteric (portal), renal, and splenic venous pressures. The physician may perform venography to establish patency of the graft. The physician then closes the abdominal wound.

37181

The physician performs a bilateral subcostal incision from the right midrectus position extending into the left flank, and dissects past bowel and pancreas to expose the splenic vein. The physician dissects the splenic vein free, ligating or clipping any vessels in continuity to the vein. The physician then exposes the left renal vein by dissecting through the posterior parietal peritoneum. The physician exposes the left renal vein, partially clamps it, and excises an ellipse of renal vein at its upper border. The physician then

performs and end-to-side anastomosis of the splenic vein to the renal vein, using harvested vein graft material if extension is required. The physician removes the clamps and divides the coronary (right gastric) vein, left gastric vein, and gastroepiploic veins. The physician may measure superior mesenteric (portal), renal, and splenic venous pressures. The physician may perform venography to establish patency of the graft. The physician then closes the abdominal wound.

37195

The physician remedies a stroke-causing blood clot obstructing blood flow to the brain. The physician infuses a thrombolytic ("clot-busting") drug through an intravenous catheter to help dissolve the clot and restore normal blood flow to the brain.

37200

A needle is inserted through the skin and into a blood vessel, and a guidewire is threaded through the needle into the vessel. The needle is removed. A catheter is then threaded into the vessel, and the wire extracted. The catheter equipped with a biopsy instrument travels to the area to be sampled. The instrument extracts for biopsy tissue affixed to the vessel wall. Pressure is applied over the puncture site to stop bleeding after the catheter is removed. This procedure may also be performed through a skin incision with direct exposure of the access vessel.

37201–37202

A needle is inserted through the skin and into a blood vessel, and a guidewire is threaded through the needle into the vessel. The needle is removed. A catheter equipped with an infusion tip is then threaded into the vessel, and the wire extracted. In 37201, the catheter travels to the point of a blood clot and drugs are infused until the clot is dissolved. In 37202, the catheter travels to the point of vasospasms and drugs are infused to reduce the spasms. Pressure is applied over the puncture site to stop the bleeding after the catheter is removed. This procedure may also be performed through a skin incision with direct exposure of the access vessel.

37203

A needle is inserted through the skin and into a blood vessel, and a guidewire is threaded through the needle into the vessel. The needle is removed. A catheter is then threaded into the vessel, and the wire extracted. The catheter equipped with a grasping instrument travels to the site of the foreign body. The instrument grasps the foreign body, typically a fractured catheter, and retrieves it. Pressure is applied over the puncture site to stop bleeding after the catheter is removed. This procedure may also be performed through a skin incision with direct exposure of the access vessel.

37204

A needle is inserted through the skin and into a blood vessel, and a guidewire is threaded through the needle into the vessel. The needle is removed. A catheter is then threaded into the vessel, and the wire extracted. The catheter travels to the point of the malformation and beads or another vessel-blocking device are released. The beads or other devise block the vessel. The catheter is then removed and pressure is applied over the puncture site to stop bleeding.

37205–37206

A needle is inserted through the skin and into a blood vessel, and a guidewire is threaded through the needle into a noncoronary blood vessel. The needle is removed. A catheter with a stent-transporting tip is then threaded into the vessel, and the wire extracted. The catheter travels to the point where the vessel needs additional support, and the compressed stent(s) is passed from the catheter into the vessel, where it expands to support the vessel walls. The catheter is then removed and pressure is applied over the puncture site to stop bleeding. 37205 is used for one stent placed by the physician. Use 37206 for each additional stent placed.

37207–37208

The physician makes an incision in the skin overlying the vessel to be catheterized. The vessel is dissected, and nicked with a small blade. A catheter with a stent-transporting tip is then threaded into the vessel. The catheter travels to the point where the vessel needs additional support, and the compressed stent(s) is passed from the catheter into the vessel, where it expands to support the vessel walls. The catheter is then removed and the vessel may be repaired. The skin incision is repaired with a layered closure. This procedure may be done in one vessel (37207) or may be repeated in multiple vessels (37208). Use 37208 for each additional vessel.

37209

The physician sterilizes the exposed arterial catheter and surrounding skin, generally with iodine solution. The physician passes a wire through the catheter into the artery and removes the catheter over the wire while manually compressing the entry site to prevent bleeding. The physician then passes a new catheter over the wire, removes the wire and secures the catheter to the skin with suture.

37250–37251

Intravascular ultrasound may be used during diagnostic evaluation of the noncoronary artery or vein It may also be used both before and after a therapeutic intervention upon a noncoronary artery or vein to assess patency and integrity of the vessel. A needle is inserted through the skin and into a blood vessel. A guide wire is threaded through the needle into a noncoronary blood vessel. The needle is removed. An intravascular ultrasound catheter is

placed over the guide wire. The ultrasound catheter is used to obtain images from inside the vessel to assess area and extent of disease prior to interventional therapy as well as adequacy of therapy after interventional therapy. Code 37250 is reported for the initial vessel. In 37251, the physician advances the ultrasound catheter into additional vessels to assess patency and structure. The catheter and guide wire are removed, and pressure is applied over the puncture site to stop bleeding.

37565

Through an incision in the skin at side of neck in front of the sternocleidomastoid muscle, the physician isolates and dissects the internal jugular vein, separating it from critical structures. Using a vascular clip or ligature, the blood flow is reduced and the vein is ligated. Once the vein has been tied off, the skin incision is repaired with a layered closure.

37600

Through an incision in the skin at the side of neck in front of the sternocleidomastoid muscle, the physician isolates and dissects the external carotid artery, separating it from critical structures. Using a vascular clip or ligature, the blood flow is reduced and the artery is ligated. Once the artery has been tied off, the skin incision is repaired with a layered closure.

37605–37606

Through an incision in the skin at the side of neck, the physician isolates and dissects the internal or common carotid artery, separating it from critical structures. After vessel clamps have been affixed above and below the injured or affected artery, the physician sutures the artery to permanently stop the flow of blood through it (37605). The physician may apply a gradual occluding clamp (37606) to assess the effect of a ligation prior to complete occlusion (37605). Once the artery has been ligated or the occluding clamp has been placed, the vessel clamp is removed and the skin incision is repaired with a layered closure.

37607

The physician exposes the arteriovenous fistula by careful dissection. The physician then isolates the fistula with ties or clamps. The physician may then tie the arteriovenous fistula off completely (ligation) with suture, or the physician may partially obstruct (banding) the lumen of the fistula with a broader band in order to reduce flow. The physician then closes the skin incision.

37609

Through an incision in the skin in front of the ear, the physician isolates and dissects the temporal artery, separating it from critical structures. Using a vascular clip or ligature, the artery is ligated or tissue samples are taken for biopsy. Once the artery has been tied off, the skin incision is repaired with a layered closure.

37615

Through an incision in the skin in the side of neck, usually in front of the sternocleidomastoid muscle, the physician isolates and dissects the ruptured or otherwise traumatized vessel, separating it from critical structures. Using a vascular clip or ligature, the vessel is ligated with sutures. Once the vessel has been tied off, the skin incision is repaired with a layered closure.

37616

The physician performs an incision of the chest wall (thoracotomy or median sternotomy) to best expose the involved artery. The physician identifies the injured artery and quickly clamps it to reduce blood loss. The physician then ties off the artery completely (ligation), proximal and distal to the site of injury. The physician closes the chest, leaving chest tubes in place.

37617

The physician performs an abdominal incision to best expose the involved artery. The physician identifies the injured artery and quickly clamps it to reduce blood loss. The physician then ties off the artery completely (ligation), proximal and distal to the site of injury. The physician closes the abdomen, leaving drains in place.

37618

Through an incision the skin of an extremity, usually over the damaged or traumatized vessel, the physician isolates and dissects the vessel, separating it from critical structures. Using a vascular clip or ligature, the vessel is ligated with sutures or vascular clips. Once the vessel has been tied off, the skin incision is repaired with a layered closure.

37620

The physician performs an upper midline abdominal incision and dissects to expose the inferior vena cava. The physician interrupts vena caval flow by tying the cava off with suture, folding it (plication), or clipping it. The physician closes the abdomen, leaving drains in place. The physician may place an intravascular umbrella device using a percutaneous (venous) approach. The physician places a needle in the femoral (or internal jugular) vein, advances a guidewire through the needle, removes the needle over the wire, and advances an introducer sheath over the wire into the femoral vein. The physician then advances the umbrella device through the introducer sheath into the inferior vena cava under fluoroscopic guidance. The physician then removes the introducer sheath and compresses the femoral vein manually until hemostasis is achieved.

37650

Through a small incision in the skin of the upper leg overlying the femoral vein, the physician isolates and dissects the femoral vein from other critical structures. After affixing vessel clamps, the physician either ligates the vein or inserts a catheter into the femoral vein. A guidewire may be inserted prior to the catheter, then removed. Through the catheter, the physician places an occluding device (one that blocks blood flow) in the vein. The catheter is removed and the skin incision is repaired with a layered closure.

37660

The physician performs a lower midline abdominal incision and dissects to expose the common iliac vein. The physician interrupts common iliac venous flow by tying the common iliac vein off with suture. The physician closes the abdomen, leaving drains in place.

37700

Through multiple small incisions in the skin of the upper thigh and along the femoral vein or its branches lower in the thigh, the physician isolates and separates the Saphenous vein at the point it joins the femoral vein or at several points farther down the leg. The physician affixes vessel clamps and ligates sections of the Saphenous vein along the leg as necessary. Once the ligations are completed, each skin incision is repaired with a layered closure.

37720–37730

The physician makes a skin incision in the upper thigh or upper leg exposing the long or short Saphenous vein (in 37720) or the long and short Saphenous veins (in 37730). Additional skin incisions are made at the knee and the ankle and along the leg as necessary. A long wire is threaded through the length of the vein and brought out at the ankle. The vein is tied to the end of the wire and the wire is pulled out along with the vein. Pressure is held along the course of the vein to stop bleeding. Once the vein has been removed, the skin incisions are repaired with layered closures. The leg is wrapped with an elastic pressure dressing postoperatively.

37735

The physician makes a skin incision in the upper thigh and the upper leg exposing the long and short Saphenous veins. Additional skin incisions are made at the ankle and along the leg as necessary. A long wire is passed through the length of the vein and brought out at the ankle. Each vein is tied to the end of the wire and the vein is pulled out along with the wire. The physician uses a scalpel to remove the skin ulcer from the leg. The ulcer site is then covered with a piece of skin which has been shaved from another part of the patient's body. Veins that connect superficial veins with deep veins may be tied off. The tough, fibrous envelope containing the muscle of the leg is split and removed at points where the superficial and deep veins connect. The skin incisions are repaired with layered closures. The leg is wrapped with an elastic pressure dressing postoperatively.

37760

Through incisions along the course of the Saphenous vein, the veins connecting the deep and superficial veins of the leg are isolated. They are then ligated, isolating the two systems along the course of the leg. The incisions may be sutured or covered with skin grafts shaved from another part of the patient's body.

37780

The physician makes an incision in the skin overlying the short Saphenous vein at its junction with the saphenopopliteal vein at the knee. The vessels are dissected and ties are placed around the short Saphenous vein which is cut apart between the ties. Once the ties are in place and the vein has been divided, the skin incision is repaired with a layered closure.

37785

The physician makes small incisions in the skin over localized areas of superficial varicose veins along the leg. These veins are then isolated and dissected free of neighboring tissue, and tied with sutures or stripped out bluntly. Pressure is applied over the site to stop bleeding. All incisions are repaired with a layered closure. The legs are wrapped in an elastic pressure dressing postoperatively.

37788–37790

Through an incision in the skin near the base of the penis, the physician isolates the penile artery and separates it from critical structures. In 37788, a neighboring artery in the groin or lower abdomen is also isolated and dissected and a vessel clamp applied. The end of the neighboring artery is sewn into the penile artery in an end-to-side fashion, or a piece of harvested vein may be used to connect the two arteries to establish an adequate blood flow to the penis. The clamps are removed and incision is repaired with a layered closure. In 37790, through an inguinoscrotal incision, lateral to the root of the penis, and along the spermatic cord, the physician exposes the suspensory ligaments and detaches them from the pubic bone, The physician incises the superficial layer of Buck's fascia, exposing and suture-ligating each leaking vein. A segment of deep dorsal vein is dissected, ligated at both ends, and resected. The physician reattaches the suspensory ligaments and when the procedure is complete, closes the skin incision with a layered closure.

38100–38102

The physician makes a midline incision and dissects tissue around the spleen. The short stomach vessels are doubly ligated and cut. The splenic recess is dissected and the splenic artery and vein are divided and cut individually. The physician removes the spleen. A drain may be placed and the wound is irrigated. The incision is closed with sutures or staples and a dry sterile dressing is applied. Report 38101 if performing a partial splenectomy; report 38102 if performing a total splenectomy in conjunction with another procedure.

38115

The physician makes an upper midline incision and dissects around the spleen until it is exposed. Lacerations are sutured. The damaged segment of the spleen is resected and removed and the edges are sutured. The wound is irrigated and the incision is closed using sutures or staples and a dry sterile dressing.

38120

The physician performs a laparoscopic splenectomy. The patient is placed in a right lateral decubitus position, left arm over the head. With the patient under anesthesia, the physician makes a small incision in the abdominal wall and inserts a trocar just below or above the umbilicus. The physician insufflates the abdominal cavity and places the laparoscope through the umbilical incision. Additional small incisions are performed and trocars are placed into the peritoneal space to be used as ports for instruments, video camera (the camera allows the physician to operate both by viewing through the laparoscope and on a video monitor), and/or an additional light source. Dissection is carried down to the level of the spleen with care taken to identify tail of the pancreas. Electrocautery is used to divide ligaments and the spleen is mobilized. Short gastric vessels may be transected to gain additional exposure. The splenic vessels are transected and the spleen is excised using special instruments to insure hemostasis. The freed spleen is isolated and pouched. Pieces of the spleen are then suctioned from the pouch through a trocar. The laparoscope and trocars are removed. The incisions are closed with sutures.

38200

The physician makes an incision in the left lower axilla. An 18 or 20 gauge sheath catheter is inserted into the middle of the soft sponge-like tissue of the spleen. The splenic vein is visualized and the catheter is placed. Around 2.0 cc to 3.0 cc of dye are injected per second totaling 15.0 cc to 20.0 cc of radiopaque dye. X-rays are taken every second for 12 seconds. The catheter is removed and the incision is covered with a dressing.

38220

Bone marrow samples are usually taken from the pelvic bone or sternum. The skin over the bone is first cleaned with an antiseptic solution. A local anesthetic is injected and the physician inserts a needle, known as a University of Illinois needle, beneath the skin and rotates it until the needle penetrates the cortex. At least half a teaspoon of marrow is sucked out of the bone by a syringe attached to the needle. If more marrow is needed, the needle is repositioned slightly, a new syringe is attached, and a second sample is taken. The samples are transferred from the syringes to slides and sent to a laboratory for analysis.

38221

Bone marrow samples are usually taken from the pelvic bone or sternum. The skin over the bone is first cleaned with an antiseptic solution. A local anesthetic is injected and the needle is inserted, rotated to the right, then to the left, withdrawn, and reinserted at a different angle. This procedure is repeated until a small chip is separated from the bone marrow. The needle is again removed, and a piece of fine wire threaded through its tip transfers the specimen onto sterile gauze. Samples contain bone marrow of which the structure has not been disturbed or destroyed. The bone must be decalcified overnight before it can be properly stained and examined.

38230

This procedure is for the removal of donor bone marrow. The physician places a large bore needle into the marrow cavity of the sternum, iliac crest, or ribs. The bone marrow is aspirated with a large syringe and placed in a sterile container. The puncture wound is covered with a sterile dressing.

38231

The physician collects peripheral stem cells from the blood system through venipuncture for transplantation. A needle is inserted in the vein and blood taken through a catheter. The blood is passed through a series of filters in which the large stem cells are collected. The remaining blood is stored or returned to the donor. This code is reported per collection.

38240–38241

This procedure is for the implantation of donor bone marrow. The recipient's immune system is first suppressed using radiation or chemotherapy. The harvested bone marrow is injected into the recipient by intravenous drip therapy in a sterile environment. Report 38241 if transplant is autologous.

38300–38305

The physician performs this procedure to drain inflamed lymph nodes. The physician makes an incision over the affected lymph node and the abscess or infection is drained. The wound is irrigated and closed with sutures or Steri-strips. Report 38305 if the procedure is extensive.

38308

This procedure is performed to correct lymphangiomas, which are primarily found in the neck. The physician makes an incision over the site of the tumor. The tissue, muscles, nerves, and blood vessels are dissected away from the tumor. The tumor is removed. The incision is closed with sutures, wound drains are placed, and a sterile dressing is applied.

38380–38382

This procedure is performed to suture or tie the thoracic duct to correct chylothorax, the presence of lymphatic fluid with the pleural or lung space. The physician makes an incision at the base of the neck, dissects the tissue, and visualizes the origin of the duct near C2 vertebra. The duct is tied or tied and cut. The incision is sutured. Report 38381 if using a thoracic approach; report 38382 if using an abdominal approach.

38500–38530

The physician performs a biopsy on or removes one or more superficial lymph nodes. The physician makes a small incision through the skin overlying the lymph node. The tissue is dissected to the node. A small piece of the node and surrounding tissue is removed, or the entire node may be removed. The incision is then repaired with a layered closure. Report 38505 if a needle is used; report 38510 if deep cervical nodes are biopsied; report 38520 if deep cervical nodes with excision scalene fat pads are checked; report 38525 if deep axillary nodes are biopsied; and report 38530 if internal mammary nodes are biopsied.

38542

The physician makes an incision over one of three jugular groups and retracts tissue. The nodes are isolated and excised. The incision is closed by sutures.

38550

The physician removes a rapidly growing sac containing fluid from the lymph system. The physician makes an incision in the axilla or neck over the sac. The surrounding tissue is cut away and the sac is exposed. The sac is removed, the skin is sutured, and a dry sterile dressing is applied.

38555

The physician makes incisions in the axilla or neck over the sac. The surrounding tissue is cut away and separated, and the sac is exposed. The sac is removed and the surrounding tissue is sutured with drains inserted. Skin flaps are sutured together over the wound.

38562–38564

The physician makes a midline abdominal incision just below the navel. The surrounding tissue, nerves, and blood vessels are dissected away, and the pelvic and/or para-aortic lymph nodes are visualized. The nodes are removed. The wound is closed with sutures or staples. Report 38564 if retroperitonial lymphadenectomy is performed.

38570

The physician performs laparoscopic retroperitoneal lymph node biopsies. The physician places a trocar at the umbilicus into the abdominal or retroperitoneal space and unsufflates the peritoneal or retroperitoneal space. The laparoscope is placed through the umbilical trocar and additional trocars are placed into the peritoneal or retroperineal space. The lymph nodes are identified, dissected free of surrounding structures and sampled for further separately reported analysis. The trocars are removed and the incisions are closed.

38571

The surgeon performs laparoscopic bilateral pelvic lymphadenectomy. The surgeon places a trocar at the umbilicus into the abdominal or retroperitoneal space and insufflates the peritoneal or retroperitoneal space. The laparoscope is placed through the umbilical trocar and additional trocars are placed into the abdominal or retroperitoneal space. The iliac vessels are identified and the lymph nodes are dissected from the surrounding structures and removed. The trocars are removed and the incisions are closed.

38572

The physician performs laparoscopic bilateral pelvic lymphadenectomy and pari-aortic lymph node sampling. The physician places a trocar at the umbilicus and insufflates the abdominal or retroperitoneal cavity. The laparoscope is placed through the umbilical port and additional trocars are placed into the peritoneal or retroperitoneal space. The iliac vessels are identified and the lymph nodes are dissected from the vessels and surrounded structures and removed. Dissection is continued up onto the aorta and para-aortic nodes are sampled. The trocars are removed and the incisions are closed.

38700

The physician makes a curved incision beginning below the ear curving down to the top of the hyoid bone and continuing toward the chin. The tissues are dissected and the targeted structures are exposed. The submental and submandibular lymph nodes are removed along with the submandibular gland and surrounding tissues. The incision is sutured with drain if necessary.

38720

The physician makes a large curved incision starting at the ear, going down the neck, and continuing to the chin. Incision may also be made starting at the original incision and continuing down the neck. The skin flaps are folded back and held in place with retractors. The tissue, lymph tissue, blood vessels, nerves, and muscles targeted for removal are dissected away and removed. The incision is closed with sutures.

38724

This lymph-removal procedure is performed to preserve the spinal accessory nerve, jugular vein, and the sternocleidomastoid muscles. The physician makes a large curved incision starting at the ear, going down the neck, and continuing to the chin. Other

incisions may be made down the neck from the original incision. Skin and tissue are retracted and the physician removes the lymph nodes The incision is closed with sutures, including wound drains connected to suction. A tracheotomy may be performed.

38740–38745

The physician makes a diagonal incision across the lower axilla, exposing the axillary vein. The fatty tissue, lymph nodes, and vessels beneath the vein are dissected free. A drain is placed and connected to suction. The tissue and skin is closed with sutures. Report 38745 if a complete procedure is performed.

38746

The physician makes a large vertical chest incision over the sternum. The tissues are dissected away the sternum is exposed. The chest cavity is entered through the sternum, which is split and retracted. Lymph nodes near the lungs, around the heart, and behind the trachea are removed. The area is irrigated, the retractors are removed, and the incision is closed with sutures or staples.

38747

The physician makes a midline abdominal incision. The abdominal contents are exposed, allowing the physician to locate the lymph nodes. Each lymph node grouping, with or without para-aortic and vena caval nodes, is dissected away from the surrounding tissue, nerves, and blood vessels, and removed. The incision is closed with sutures or staples.

38760–38765

The physician makes an incision across the groin area. The surrounding tissue, nerves, and blood vessels are dissected away, and the inguinal and femoral lymph nodes are visualized. The nodes are removed by group. The wound is closed with sutures or staples. Report 38765 if performing pelvic lymphadenectomy concurrently.

38770

The physician makes a low abdominal vertical incision. The surrounding tissue, nerves, and blood vessels are dissected away, and the pelvic lymph nodes are visualized. The nodes are removed by group. The wound is closed with sutures or staples.

38780

The physician makes a large midline abdominal incision. The surrounding tissue, nerves, and blood vessels are dissected away, and the lymph nodes are visualized. The nodes are then removed by group. Some surrounding tissues may also be removed. The wound is closed with sutures or staples.

38790

Vital blue dye is injected into the subcutaneous tissues for outlining of skin lymphatics. As soon as the lymphatic vessels are visualized by their blue color, the radiologist makes a small longitudinal incision over the area. Exposure of the lymph vessel is accomplished, the vessel is made taut, and it is cannulated with a 27 or 30 gauge needle with a fine catheter attached. A small amount of dye is injected to ensure correct placement, and the needle is advanced 2.0 to 3.0 mm into the vessel. The needle and catheter are secured. Dye is injected with a 10.0 cc syringe. X-rays are made and repeated 24 hours later. The physician removes the needle and closes the incision with sutures.

38792

The physician injects dye or contrast material into the patient to identify the sentinel lymph node. As soon as the node is visualized, the radiologist makes a small longitudinal incision over the area. The node is exposed and cannulated with a 27 or 30 gauge needle attached to a find catheter. A small amount of dye is injected to ensure correct placement, and the needle is advanced 2–3 mm into the node. The needle and catheter are secured. Dye is injected with a 10 cc syringe. X-rays are taken and repeated 24 hours later. The physician removes the needle and closes the incision by suture.

38794

Exposure of the lymph vessel is accomplished, the vessel is made taut, and it is cannulated with a 27 or 30 gauge needle with a find catheter attached. The needle and catheter are secured. Medication is injected. The physician removes the needle and closes the incision with sutures.

39000–39010

The physician makes an incision low in the front of the neck, pulling back the sternomastoid muscles and the cranial vessels to the side and drawing the trachea and thyroid to the center. The space behind the esophagus is exposed. The foreign body is removed, biopsy of any abnormal mass performed, and Penrose drains are placed. The incision is closed with sutures or staples. Report 39010 if using a transthoracic approach.

39200

The physician makes an incision from in front of the axilla just below the nipple line. The incision extends below the tip of the shoulder blade and ascends to halfway between the spinal column and the shoulder blade. The physician exposes the rib cage, retracting muscles. A rib spreader is used to ease access to the thoracic cavity. The cyst is located and removed. The rib spreader is removed, and the wound is closed with sutures or staples.

39220

The physician makes an incision from in front of the axilla just below the nipple line. The incision extends below the tip of the shoulder blade and ascends to

halfway between the spinal column and the shoulder blade. The physician exposes the rib cage by cutting through the muscles. The chest cavity is entered between the ribs by using a rib spreader. The tumor is located and dissected from the surrounding tissue. The wound is closed using sutures or staples.

39400

The physician makes a small incision in the notch above the sternum. The mediastinoscope is inserted and the explorations are carried out between the trachea and the major vessels. The mediastinal lymph nodes, thymus, and thyroid are visualized, and biopsy is performed through the mediastinoscope. The scope is removed, and the incision is closed with sutures or Steri-strips.

39501

The physician makes an abdominal or chest incision and exposes a tear in the diaphragm. The tear is repaired with nonabsorbable sutures. Occasionally the tear may be so extensive that an artificial patch is used to repair defects or reinforce sutures. The incision is closed with sutures or staples, and a dressing is applied.

39502

The physician makes an incision across the abdomen. The herniated stomach is returned to its appropriate position in the abdomen, and the hernia sac is cut away and removed. The enlarged opening in the diaphragm through which the esophagus passes is narrowed by placing sutures in the two pillars connecting the spinal column and diaphragm. Reforming the stomach, cutting the vagus nerve or altering the size of the stomach-intestinal opening may be performed as well. Drains are placed, and the wound is sutured closed.

39503

The physician makes an incision across the abdomen. The herniated stomach is returned to its appropriate position in the abdomen, and the hernia sac is cut away and removed. The enlarged opening in the diaphragm through which the esophagus passes is narrowed by placing sutures in the two pillars connecting the spinal column and diaphragm. Reforming the stomach, cutting the vagus nerve or altering the size of the stomach-intestinal opening may be performed as well. Drains are placed, and the wound is sutured closed.

39520–39531

The physician makes an incision across the chest. Tissues are dissected and the esophagus, diaphragm, and upper part of the stomach are exposed. The physician creates a segment of intrabdominal esophagus held in place by a support of folds or tucks in the stomach surrounds about 280 degrees of the distal esophagus. The incision is closed with sutures or staples. Report 39530 if thoracoabdominal; report 39531 if thoracoabdominal with dilation of stricture.

39540–39541

This procedure is performed to repair a massive injury in the diaphragm allowing organs to protrude into the chest cavity. The physician makes an incision in the chest or abdomen. The abdominal contents are drawn back into the abdomen, and the hole in the diaphragm is exposed. The opening is closed with sutures or by insertion of a patch. The tear is repaired with nonabsorbable sutures. The incision is closed with sutures or staples. Report 39541 if the hernia is chronic.

39545

The physician makes an incision across the chest or abdomen. The abdominal contents are drawn back into the abdomen, and the diaphragm is exposed. The connective tissue is used to stitch folds or tucks into the diaphragm to restore it to its original position. The incision is closed with sutures or staples.

39560

The surgeon removes all or part of the diaphragm, the large muscle separating the chest and abdominal cavities. The patient is taken to the operating room, the abdomen and/or chest are surgically opened, and the operation is preformed. This code involves a simple repair using sutures.

39561

The surgeon removes all or part of the diaphragm, the large muscle separating the chest and abdominal cavities. The patient is taken to the operating room, the abdomen and/or chest are surgically opened, and the operation is preformed. This code involves a complex repair using muscle or synthetic material for patching some of the area.

40490

The physician performs a biopsy of a lesion on the lip. An incision is made in the lip and a portion of the lesion as well as some normal tissue is removed. The surgical wound is then closed directly.

40500

The physician removes the diseased vermilion border of the lip. The mucosa from the skin to the labial mucosa is separated from the underlying muscle and removed. The remaining labial mucosa is advanced and sutured to the skin, covering the exposed muscle and forming a new vermilion.

40510

The physician removes a lesion on the lip using a transverse wedge technique. Incisions are made perpendicularly through the skin and mucosa. The lesion and surrounding tissue are removed. The physician extends the incisions 1.0 cm below the

surgical wound and advances the tissue flaps. The incisions are sutured primarily.

40520

The physician removes a lesion on the lip. A "V" incision is made around the lesion. The lesion and surrounding tissue are removed. The surgical wound is closed primarily.

40525

The physician removes a lesion on the lip. A "V" incision may be made around the lesion and through the full thickness of the lip. The lesion and surrounding tissues are removed. A local skin flap is incised and advanced to the site of the surgical wound and sutured into place with a layered closure.

40527

The physician removes a lesion on the lip. A "V" incision is made around the lesion and through the full thickness of the lip. The lesion and surrounding tissues are removed. A skin flap from the upper lip is incised and cross advanced to the surgical site of the lower lip. The flap is sutured with a layered closure.

40530

The physician performs a lip resection to remove a tumor. An incision may be made through the midline of the lip and extended vertically over the chin. The tumor and surrounding tissues are removed. The oral cavity is closed primarily, and the lip and chin are closed with layered sutures.

40650

The physician repairs a laceration of the full thickness of the lip. The tissues of the vermilion are closed with layered sutures.

40652–40654

The physician repairs a laceration extending through the full thickness of the lip. A laceration or surgically created wound of up to one-half (e.g., 40652) or over one-half (e.g., 40654) of the vertical height of the lip is closed with layered sutures.

40700

The physician surgically corrects a unilateral developmental cleft lip/nasal deformity. The cleft margins are incised to define the full-thickness anatomic layers of mucosa, muscle, and skin. Various incisions are designed to preserve lip length and symmetry while limiting the scar contracture (permanent shortening) which increases the probability of an unacceptable cosmetic result. The physician closes the prepared margins in anatomic layers from the intraoral mucosa through the muscle with final closure of the skin.

40701

The physician surgically corrects the bilateral developmental cleft lip/nasal deformity in one operation. The cleft margins of both sides are incised to define the full-thickness anatomic layers of mucosa, muscle, and skin. Various incisions are designed to preserve lip length and symmetry while limiting the scar contracture (permanent shortening) which increases the probability of an unacceptable cosmetic result. The physician closes the prepared margins in anatomic layers from the intraoral mucosa through the muscle with final closure of the skin.

40702

The physician performs two surgeries to correct a bilateral cleft lip/nasal deformity. This may be necessary because of the severity or the vascular compromise of the deformity. Typically, the cleft lip is repaired first and nasal deformities repaired in a second surgical session. In stage one, the cleft margins are incised to defined full-thickness anatomic layers of mucosa, muscle, and skin. Various incisions are designed to preserve lip length and symmetry while limiting the scar contracture (permanent shortening) which increases the probability of an unacceptable cosmetic result. The prepared margins are then closed in anatomic layers from the intraoral mucosa through muscle with final closure of the skin. The second surgery is performed after adequate healing of the first surgical site.

40720

The physician performs a second cleft lip/nasal repair after unfavorable results from a first surgical correction. This failure may be due to scar contracture (permanent shortening), wound dehiscence (splitting), or infection. The cleft margins are recreated to define the full-thickness anatomic layers of mucosa, muscle, and skin. The prepared margins are again closed in anatomic layers from the intraoral mucosa through muscle with final closure of the skin.

40761

The physician performs a complicated cleft lip/nasal repair using pedicled flaps from the lower lip. This is necessary because of inadequate quantity or quality of upper lip soft tissue. The cleft margins are incised to define the full-thickness anatomic layers of mucosa, muscle, and skin. A pedicle flap is designed from the lower lip based on blood supply. The flap is created with a full-thickness incision and rotated on its pedicle to the desired location. The flap is then sutured in multiple layers to the recipient tissue location. The prepared cleft margins are then closed in anatomic layers from the intraoral mucosa through muscle with final closure of the skin.

40800–40801

The physician drains an abscess, cyst, or hematoma within the vestibule of the mouth. The vestibule is part of the oral cavity outside the dentoalveolar structures. It includes the mucosal and submucosal tissue of the lips and cheeks. The physician makes an incision in the tissue overlying the abscess, cyst, or hematoma. Tissues are then dissected and the fluid drained. Multiple incisions or large lesions (e.g., 40801) may be treated. The physician may place a drain. If a drain is placed, it is later removed.

40804–40805

The physician removes a foreign body embedded in the vestibule of the mouth. The vestibule is part of the oral cavity outside the dentoalveolar structures. It includes the mucosal and submucosal tissue of the lips and cheeks. The physician may simply grasp the object with an instrument and remove it, or incisions may be made in the mucosa to free and remove the object. The foreign body may be large or more difficult to access (40805). Closure of the wound may be needed.

40806

The physician incises the labial frenum. This procedure is often performed to release tension on the frenum and surrounding tissues.

40808

The physician performs a biopsy on a lesion in the vestibule of the mouth. The vestibule is the part of the oral cavity outside the dentoalveolar structures; it includes the mucosal and submucosal tissue of the lips and cheeks. The physician makes an incision in the vestibule and removes a portion of the lesion and some surrounding tissue. The incision is closed simply.

40810–40812

The physician removes a lesion in the mucosa and submucosa of the vestibule of the mouth. The vestibule is the part of the oral cavity outside the dentoalveolar structures; it includes the mucosal and submucosal tissue of the lips and cheeks. The physician makes an incision around the lesion and through submucosal tissue, removing the entire lesion. No repair of wound (e.g., 40810) or simple repair of the wound (e.g., 40812), such as a sutured closure, is performed.

40814

The physician removes a lesion in the mucosa and submucosa of the vestibule of the mouth. The vestibule is the part of the oral cavity outside the dentoalveolar structures; it includes the mucosal and submucosal tissue of the lips and cheeks. An incision is made around the lesion and through submucosal tissue, removing the entire lesion. Complex repair of the surgical wound left after excision of the lesion is required. This may include advancement of tissue flaps, rearrangement of tissue, or complex suturing techniques.

40816

The physician removes a lesion in the mucosa and submucosa of the vestibule of the mouth. The vestibule is the part of the oral cavity outside the dentoalveolar structures; it includes the mucosal and submucosal tissue of the lips and cheeks. An incision is made around the lesion and through submucosal tissue removing the entire lesion. Underlying muscle is removed. Complex repair of the surgical wound left after excision of the lesion is required. This may include advancement of tissue flaps, rearrangement of tissue, or complex suturing techniques.

40818

The physician harvests mucosa from the vestibule and grafts it elsewhere in the mouth. The vestibule is the part of the oral cavity outside the dentoalveolar structures; it includes the mucosal and submucosal tissue of the lips and cheeks. A retractor is used to hold the mucosa to be grafted. The physician uses a scalpel to make an incision through the mucosa, usually in an elliptical shape. The physician grasps the mucosa with an instrument and the scalpel is used to cut just beneath the mucosa, freeing it from the underlying tissues. Any remaining fat or muscle attached to the mucosa is removed and the tissue is grafted to another part of the mouth. The surgical wound is then closed directly.

40819

The physician removes the frenum. Incisions are made around the frenum and through the mucosa and submucosa. The underlying muscle is removed (excised) as well. The excision may extend to the interincisal papilla. The mucosa is then closed simply, or the physician may rearrange the tissue as in a Z-plasty technique.

40820

The physician destroys a lesion in the vestibule of the mouth without excising it. Destruction may be accomplished by using a laser or electrocautery to burn the lesion, cryotherapy to freeze the lesion, or chemicals to destroy the lesion.

40830–40831

The physician sutures a laceration of the vestibule of the mouth measuring 2.5 cm or less in length. The physician performs a simple closure without submucosal sutures or tissue rearrangement (e.g., 40830). Extensive tissue damage or crushing, requiring submucosal sutures or closure of laceration of over 2.5 cm (e.g, 40831) may be necessary.

40840–40843

The physician deepens the vestibule of the mouth in edentulous (without teeth) patients, allowing a complete denture to be worn. This procedure may be performed in several ways. The physician may rearrange the patient's own tissue or the submucosal tissue may be dissected freeing it from bone. The mucosa is moved deeper into the vestibule. Skin or other tissues may also be grafted into the mouth. An anterior procedure (e.g., 40840) may be performed or a unilateral (e.g., 40842) or bilateral procedure (e.g.,

40843) may be performed on the posterior portion of the mouth.

40844

The physician deepens the vestibule of the mouth in edentulous (without teeth) patients, allowing a complete denture to be worn. This procedure is performed on the entire edentulous arch of the mouth and may be performed in several ways. The physician may rearrange the patient's own tissue or the submucosal tissue may be dissected freeing it from bone. The mucosa is moved deeper into the vestibule. Skin or other tissues may also be grafted into the mouth.

40845

The physician deepens the vestibule of the mouth in edentulous (without teeth) patients, allowing a complete denture to be worn. This procedure is performed for complex cases, such as those in which the physician must lower muscle attachments to provide enough space for deepening the vestibule. Skin grafting from other areas of the body into the mouth is often required.

41000

The physician makes a small incision through the mucosa in the floor of the mouth overlying the abscess or cyst. The abscess or cyst is opened with a surgical instrument and the fluid is drained.

41005

The physician makes a small incision in the sublingual space to drain a superficial abscess or cyst beneath the mucosa. The abscess or cyst is opened with a surgical instrument and the fluid is drained. An artificial drain may be placed.

41006

The physician makes a small incision in the sublingual space between the mucosa and the mylohyoid muscle. The abscess or cyst is opened with a surgical instrument and the fluid is drained. An artificial drain may be placed.

41007

The physician makes a small incision through the mucosa anteriorly in the floor of the mouth. The physician then dissects through the mylohyoid muscle and into the submental space. The abscess or cyst is opened with a surgical instrument and the fluid is drained. An artificial drain may be placed.

41008

The physician makes a small incision in the mucosa of the floor of the mouth to drain an abscess or a cyst within the submental space. Deeper dissection of tissue is required to reach the submandibular space. The abscess or cyst is opened with a surgical instrument and the fluid is drained. An artificial drain may be placed.

41009

The physician makes a small incision through the mucosa in the posterior floor of the mouth. The physician then dissects into the masticator space. The abscess or cyst is opened with a surgical instrument and the fluid is drained. An artificial drain may be placed.

41010

The physician makes an incision in the lingual frenum, freeing the tongue and allowing greater range of motion. Sutures may be placed. The frenum is simply incised and not removed.

41015

The physician drains an abscess, cyst or hematoma from the floor of the mouth in the sublingual space. The physician makes an extraoral incision in the skin below the inferior border of the mandible. The tissues are dissected through the submandibular or submental space and into the sublingual space. The fluid is then drained and an artificial drain may be placed. If placed, the drain is later removed.

41016

The physician drains an abscess, cyst or hematoma from the floor of the mouth in the submental space. The physician makes an extraoral incision in the skin below the inferior border of the mandible. The tissues are dissected to the submental space. The fluid is then drained and an artificial drain may be placed. If placed, the drain is later removed.

41017

The physician drains an abscess, cyst or hematoma from the floor of the mouth in the submandibular space. The physician makes an incision under the angle of the mandible, or between the angle and the chin, and below the inferior border of the mandible. Dissection is limited to the submandibular space. The fluid is then drained and an artificial drain may be placed. If placed, the drain is later removed.

41018

The physician drains an abscess, cyst or hematoma in the masticator space. The skin incision is made just beneath the angle of the mandible and dissection is limited to the masticator space. The fluid is then drained and an artificial drain may or may not be placed. If placed, the drain is later removed.

41100–41105

The physician performs an incisional biopsy on a lesion in the anterior two-thirds (e.g., 41100) or the posterior one-third (e.g., 41105) of the tongue. The physician makes an incision in the tissue, usually in an elliptical shape, which typically includes part diseased tissue and part normal tissue. Incisions are then made beneath the tissue and the specimen removed. The surgical wound is usually sutured simply.

41108

The physician performs an incisional biopsy on a lesion on the floor of the mouth. An incision is made in the tissue usually in an elliptical shape, which typically includes part diseased tissue and part normal tissue. Incisions are then made beneath the tissue and the specimen is removed. The surgical wound is usually sutured simply. The specimen is then sent to a pathologist.

41110

The physician removes a lesion in any area of the tongue. Incisions are made completely around and under a lesion, typically in an elliptical shape, removing the entire lesion. Due to the small size of the lesion, no suturing or closure of the surgical wound is necessary. A raised lesion (peduncle) may simply be cut off at the base.

41112–41113

The physician removes a lesion in the anterior two-thirds (e.g., 41112) or the posterior one-third (e.g., 41113) of the tongue. Incisions are made in the tissue completely around and under a lesion, typically in an elliptical shape, removing the entire lesion. The surgical wound is sutured.

41114

The physician removes a lesion in an area of the tongue. Incisions are made in the tissue completely around and under a lesion, removing the entire lesion. A flap of mucosa from another part of the tongue is incised, moved and sutured to repair the surgical wound. The donor site is closed with sutures.

41115

The physician removes (excises) a tight or short lingual frenum to free the tongue and allow greater range of motion. The physician makes incisions in the frenum both near the tongue and near the mandible which ultimately connect as they move posteriorly. The entire frenum is excised. The surgical wound may be sutured.

41116

The physician removes a lesion of the floor of the mouth. The physician makes incisions in the tissue completely around and under the lesion, usually in an elliptical shape. The lesion is removed, usually with some surrounding normal tissue as well. The surgical wound is typically sutured simply.

41120–41130

The physician removes less than one half (e.g., 41120) or one half (e.g., 41130) of the diseased (often malignant) tongue. The physician makes incisions around the portion of the tongue to be removed and extends the incisions through the entire thickness of the tongue. Scalpels, scissors, electrocautery or lasers may be used. The diseased portion is then removed. After obtaining good hemostasis (controlling bleeding) the tongue is sutured closed to repair the surgical wound. Tissue grafting to close the wound is rarely needed.

41135

The physician removes a part of the diseased (often malignant) tongue. The physician makes incisions in the tissue around the portion of the tongue to be removed and extends the incisions through the entire thickness of the tongue. Scalpels, scissors, electrocautery or lasers may be used. The diseased portion is then removed. After obtaining good hemostasis (controlling bleeding) the tongue is then sutured to repair the surgical wound. Tissue grafting to close the wound is rarely needed. In addition, a unilateral radical neck dissection is performed. This is a procedure where lymph nodes, muscles, blood vessels and other tissue are removed on one side of the neck.

41140

The physician removes the entire tongue. The physician makes incisions through the entire thickness of the tongue. Scalpels, scissors, electrocautery or lasers may be used. The tongue is then removed. A tracheostomy may be performed. A tracheostomy is a procedure where an incision is made in the front of the neck, below the larynx. The physician dissects the tissues down to the trachea. An incision is made through the tracheal wall and an artificial airway is inserted into the trachea, which extends out to the neck. The patient then breathes through this airway. No radical neck dissection is performed.

41145

The physician removes the entire tongue. The physician makes incisions through the entire thickness of the tongue. Scalpels, scissors, electrocautery or lasers may be used. The tongue is then removed. A tracheostomy may be performed. A tracheostomy is a procedure where an incision is made in the front of the neck, below the larynx. The physician dissects the tissues down to the trachea. An incision is made through the tracheal wall, and an artificial airway is inserted into the trachea, which extends out to the neck. The patient then breathes through this airway. In addition, a unilateral radical neck dissection is performed. This is a procedure where lymph nodes, muscles, blood vessels and other tissues are removed on one side of the neck.

41150

The physician removes part or all of the diseased or cancerous tongue, mandible, and the tissue of the floor of the mouth. The physician makes an incision both extraorally in the skin and intraorally through the mucosa. The physician makes incisions through the entire thickness of the tongue. Scalpels, scissors, electrocautery or lasers may be used. The tongue is then removed. The tissue of the mouth floor is

removed with a scalpel and the diseased portion of the mandible is removed. After removal of the diseased tissue, continuity of the mandible is reestablished. This is done either with metal plates initially and bone grafting at a later time, or with immediate bone grafting. Skin or mucosal grafting may be needed. The skin and mucosal incisions are repaired with layered sutures.

41153

The physician removes part or all of the diseased or cancerous tongue, and the tissue of the floor of the mouth. The physician makes an incision both extraorally in the skin and through the mucosa inside the mouth. The physician makes incisions through the entire thickness of the tongue. Scalpels, scissors, electrocautery or lasers may be used. The tongue is then removed. The tissue of the mouth floor is removed with a scalpel. The physician also removes lymph nodes and other soft tissue between the floor of the mouth and the hyoid bone. Skin or mucosal grafting may be needed. The skin and mucosal incisions are repaired with layered sutures.

41155

The physician removes part or all of the diseased or cancerous tongue, mandible, and the tissue of the floor of the mouth. The physician makes an incision both extraorally in the skin and through the mucosa inside the mouth. The physician makes incisions through the entire thickness of the tongue. The tongue is then removed. The tissue of the mouth floor is removed with a scalpel and the diseased mandible is removed. After removal of the diseased tissue, continuity of the mandible is reestablished. This is done either with metal plates initially and bone grafting at a later time, or with immediate bone grafting. In addition, a radical neck dissection is performed. This is a procedure where lymph nodes, muscles, blood vessels and other tissue are removed. Skin, mucosal grafting, or tissue flaps may be needed. The skin and mucosal incisions are repaired with layered sutures.

41250–41251

The physician sutures a laceration of the mouth floor and/or anterior two-thirds of the tongue (e.g., 41250) or the posterior one-third (e.g., 41251) measuring 2.5 cm or less. This is done simply without tissue rearrangement.

41252

The physician sutures a laceration of the mouth floor or portion of the tongue, measuring 2.6 cm or more. Complex closure techniques are used. These may include tissue rearrangement, extensive submucosal suturing, debridement of grossly contaminated lacerations, or repair of through-and-through lacerations.

41500

The physician applies K-wire (Kirschner wire) for temporary fixation of the tongue. The K-wire is threaded through one side of the mandible, through the tongue, and then through the opposite side of the mandible.

41510

The physician makes an incision in the commissure (corner) of the mouth. The tongue is sutured to the lip in the area previously incised to enlarge the mouth. The tongue is later sectioned from the mouth in a second surgical session.

41520

The physician alters the frenum by rearranging the tissue using a Z-plasty technique. An incision in the shape of a "Z" is made through the frenum, and the submucosal tissues are incised. The incision is then reapproximated in a different position and sutured.

41800

The physician drains an abscess, cyst, or hematoma from dentoalveolar structures. The physician may make gingival incisions to provide drainage. An artificial drain may be placed and removed at a later time. On occasion, drainage may be obtained by probing the gingival sulcus.

41805

The physician removes a foreign body embedded in the soft tissue of the dental alveolus (gingival or alveolar mucosa). The physician may simply grasp the object with an instrument and remove it. If the object is further embedded, incisions may be made in the mucosa near the object to remove it. Sutures may or may not be necessary.

41806

The physician removes a foreign body embedded in the bone of the dental alveolus (gingival or alveolar mucosa). The physician may simply grasp the object with an instrument and remove it. If the object is further embedded, mucosal incisions may be made and bone removed with drills or osteotomes. The incision is then sutured simply.

41820

The physician excises or trims hypertrophic (overgrown) gingiva to normal contours. The physician excises the overgrown gingiva using a scalpel, electrocautery, or a laser. Periodontal dressing or packing is often placed.

41821

The physician removes a small piece of gingiva from the back or top of a tooth. A scalpel, a laser, or electrocautery is used to excise the tissue and establish normal gingival contours around the tooth. A periodontal dressing may then be applied.

41822

The physician excises soft tissue overlying the tuberosities, reducing the size of the tuberosity. The physician makes wedged or elliptically shaped incisions through the soft tissue of the tuberosity. The tissue is then removed and the surgical wound is sutured directly.

41823

The physician removes the tuberosity producing more favorable bone contours. The physician makes an incision through the mucosa of the tuberosity, and exposes the underlying bone. Drills, osteotomes, or files are used to remove and contour the bone. The tissue is then sutured directly over the bone. Some soft tissue may be excised prior to closure for adaptation over the newly contoured bone.

41825–41826

The physician removes a lesion or tumor of the dentoalveolar structures. If the lesion is within the mucosa, the physician makes incisions around the lesion and dissects it away from adjacent structures. If the lesion is within the bone, the mucosa is incised and the underlying bone exposed. The lesion is then removed from the bone and the incision closed with layered sutures. No repair (e.g., 41825) or simple repair of the surgical wound (e.g., 41826) may be required.

41827

The physician removes a lesion or tumor of the dentoalveolar structures. If the lesion is within the mucosa, the physician makes incisions around the lesion and dissects it away from adjacent structures. If the lesion is within the bone, the mucosa is incised and the underlying bone exposed. The lesion is then removed from the bone. The resultant surgical wound is closed with sutures. Complex repair, such as tissue rearrangement (tissue flaps), tissue grafting, or complex suturing techniques may be required.

41828

The physician excises hyperplastic or excessive mucosa from the alveolus. Incisions are made in the hyperplastic tissue, separating it from the normal mucosa. The excessive tissue is then removed. The resultant defect may be directly sutured, or left to heal without suturing. With large amounts of excess tissue, more than one surgical session may be required or tissue grafting may be necessary to eliminate all of the tissue.

41830

The physician removes a portion of the alveolus. Incisions are made through the mucosa to expose the alveolar bone. Curets, drills, or osteotomes are used to remove the diseased alveolar bone or sequestrum. The mucosa may be sutured directly over the surgical wound, or it may be packed and allowed to heal secondarily.

CPT® Lay Descriptions

41850

The physician destroys a lesion of the dentoalveolar structures without excision. The physician may use different techniques of lesion destruction. Electrocautery may be used to burn the lesion, cryotherapy to freeze the lesion, or chemical injections to destroy the lesion. A laser which produces high-intensity light may be used to destroy the lesion. No suturing is required and the resultant surgical wound is left to heal secondarily.

41870

The physician takes mucosa from one area of the mouth and grafts it around the teeth to repair areas of gingival recession. The physician uses a scalpel to remove a small piece of mucosa, usually from the hard palate. After preparing the recipient site, the physician sutures the graft in the area of gingival recession.

41872

The physician alters the contours of the gingiva. Areas of gingiva may be excised or incisions may be made through the gingiva to create a gingival flap. The flap may then be sutured in a different position, trimmed, or both. Any incisions made are closed with sutures.

41874

The physician alters the contours of the alveolus by selectively removing sharp areas or undercuts of alveolar bone. The physician makes incisions in the mucosa overlying the alveolus, exposing the alveolar bone. Drills, osteotomes, or files are used to contour the bone. The mucosa is sutured in place over the contoured bone.

42000

The physician drains an abscess of the palate or uvula. The abscess is opened with a surgical instrument and the fluid is drained. The wound is allowed to heal without closure.

42100

The physician performs a biopsy on a lesion of the palate or uvula. An incision is made in the tissue, usually in an elliptical shape and typically including part diseased and part normal tissue. Incisions are then made beneath the tissue and the specimen is removed. The surgical wound is usually sutured simply.

42104–42107

The physician removes a lesion in any area of the the palate or uvula. Incisions are made completely around and under a lesion, typically in an elliptical shape, removing the entire lesion. Due to the small size of the lesion, no suturing or closure of the surgical wound is necessary in 42104. Removal of larger lesions may require simple closure (42106) or local flap closure (42107).

42120

The physician resects the palate or area of a lesion. The physician excises the lesion and any adjacent tissue where the lesion may have spread. The surgical wound is then repaired by intermediate or complex closure, adjacent tissue transfer, or graft.

42140

The physician removes the uvula with a full-thickness incision. Electrocautery may be used to control hemorrhage. Sutures may be used to close the mucosa in a single layer.

42145

The physician removes elongated and excessive tissues of the uvula, soft palate, and pharynx. Incisions are made in the soft palate mucosa and a wedge of mucosa is excised. Excessive submucosal tissue is then removed and the uvula is partially excised. The midline at the uvula is sutured first. The physician then closes the remaining mucosa in a single layer, reapproximating the soft palate and thus increasing the diameter of the oropharynx.

42160

The physician destroys a lesion of the palate or uvula. Destruction may be accomplished by using a laser or electrocautery to burn the lesion, cryotherapy to freeze the lesion, or chemicals to destroy the lesion.

42180–42182

The physician repairs a laceration of the palate measuring 2.0 cm or less in length. The physician performs a simple closure without submucosal sutures or tissue rearrangement (e.g., 42180). Extensive tissue damage or crushing, requiring submucosal sutures or tissue rearrangement of over 2 cm (e.g., 42182) may be necessary.

42200

The physician repairs the developmental cleft opening of the palate. The cleft size and location will dictate the type of repair to be performed. The physician closes the opening between the oral and nasal cavities with a partition of soft tissue. Typically, incisions are made in the palatal mucosa adjacent to the alveolar (tooth-bearing) bone. The mucosa is elevated and loosened from the bony palate. Then the margins of the cleft are incised and dissected to develop mucosal and muscular layers. These incised midline margins are closed in multiple layers, thus closing the communication between the oral and nasal cavities.

42205

The physician repairs the developmental cleft opening of the palate which extends through the alveolar ridge (tooth-bearing region of maxilla). The cleft size and location will dictate the type of repair performed. The physician closes the opening between the oral and nasal cavities with a partition of soft tissue. Closure of the alveolar ridge will benefit development of both the maxilla and the teeth. Typically, incisions are made in the palatal mucosa adjacent to the alveolar bone. The mucosa is elevated and loosened from the bony palate. Then the midline margins of the cleft are incised and dissected to develop mucosal and muscular layers. The physician closes the midline margins in multiple layers.

42210

The physician repairs the developmental cleft opening of the palate and reconstructs the alveolar ridge (tooth-bearing region) of maxilla. The cleft size and location will dictate the type of repair performed. The physician closes the opening between the oral and nasal cavities with a partition of soft tissue. Bony reconstruction of the alveolar ridge can stabilize maxillary segments, benefit development of the teeth, and aid dental rehabilitation of chewing functions. Typically, incisions are made in the palatal mucosa adjacent to the alveolar bone. The mucosa is elevated and loosened from the bony palate. Then the midline margins of the cleft mucosa and gingiva are incised and dissected to develop mucosal and muscular layers. Through a separate incision, the physician harvests bone from the hip or skull and closes the surgically created wound. The bone is placed in the alveolar cleft, reestablishing normal contours of the maxilla. The physician then closes all midline incisions in multiple layers and gingival incisions in a single layer.

42215

The physician revises previous repairs of the cleft palate. Wound dehiscence (splitting), infection, or scarring after initial surgeries could cause oral/nasal recommunication, developmental growth restrictions, or velopharyngeal incompetence. The defect will dictate the repair to be performed. Typically, incisions are made in the palatal mucosa adjacent to the alveolar (tooth-bearing) bone. The mucosa is elevated and loosened from the bony palate. Then the previous midline incisions are excised and dissected to develop mucosal and muscular layers. The physician resutures all midline incisions in multiple layers and gingival incisions are closed in a single layer.

42220

The physician revises the previous cleft palate incisions to lengthen the soft palate. Wound dehiscence (splitting), infection, or scarring after initial surgeries could cause developmental growth restrictions or velopharyngeal incompetence. The defect will dictate the repair performed. Typically, the soft palate lengthening is accomplished with the use of mucosal advancement flaps. Incisions are made in the palatal mucosa adjacent to the alveolar (tooth-bearing) bone. The mucosa is elevated and loosened from the bony palate. The pedicled flaps utilizing posterior palatine blood supply are developed and sutured to increase the anterior-posterior length of the

soft palate. The physician sutures all remaining midline incisions in multiple layers.

42225

The physician revises previous cleft palate incisions with pharyngeal flap techniques. Through the soft palate, a midline incision is made to expose the posterior pharyngeal wall. The physician incises a flap from the posterior pharyngeal wall through the mucosa, submucosa, and muscle. This flap is sutured to the soft palate. Revision of previous surgical incisions may be necessary. All remaining midline incisions are sutured in multiple layers.

42226

The physician uses both advancement flaps and pharyngeal flaps to lengthen the soft palate. Typically, the soft palate lengthening is accomplished with the use of mucosal advancement flaps. Correction of velopharyngeal incompetence is accomplished by pharyngeal flap techniques. A midline incision through the soft palate is made to expose the posterior pharyngeal wall. The physician incises a flap from the posterior pharyngeal wall through mucosa, submucosa, and muscle. This flap is sutured to the soft palate. Advancement flaps utilizing posterior palatine blood vessels are used to lengthen the soft palate by suturing techniques that increase the anterior-posterior length of the soft palate. All remaining midline incisions are sutured in multiple layers.

42227

The physician uses mucosal island flaps to lengthen the soft palate. Incisions are made in the palatal mucosa adjacent to the alveolar (tooth-bearing) bone. The mucosa is elevated and loosened from the bony palate. Advancement flaps utilizing posterior palatine blood vessels are used to lengthen the soft palate by suturing techniques that increase the anterior-posterior length of the soft palate. All remaining incisions are sutured in multiple layers.

42235

The physician repairs the hard palate by closing the communication between the oral and nasal cavities. A combination of mucosal and mucoperiosteal flaps are used to repair the defect. The margins of the defect are incised and dissected to develop mucosal, muscular, and mucoperiosteal layers. The mucoperiosteum of the vomer (nasal septum) is elevated and sutured to the mucoperiosteum of the hard palate. This closes the communication between the oral and nasal cavities. Incisions are then made in the palatal mucosa adjacent to the alveolar (tooth-bearing) bone. The mucosa is elevated and loosened from the bony palate. The palatal mucosa is closed in multiple layers.

42260

The physician repairs a fistula communication from the nasal or sinus regions to the nasolabial region of the midface. The repair is dependent on the size of the fistular tract. For small defects, an excision of the epithelized tract is made from source to skin surface. This wound is sutured in multiple layers. In larger defects, a nasolabial flap may be necessary after excision of the fistula. A nasolabial flap is designed, incised, and rotated to the defect region. The flap is sutured over the defect in multiple layers.

42280

The physician takes impressions of the maxilla. A palatal prosthesis is customized from the cast model of the impression.

42281

The physician inserts a palatal prosthesis prepared by an outside laboratory. The prosthesis is retained by pins and augments the palate.

42300–42305

The physician drains an abscess of the parotid gland. An incision is made intraorally through the tissue overlying the gland. The physician then dissects through the tissue overlying the abscess. The abscess is opened with a surgical instrument and the fluid is drained. Report 42305 if the excision is complicated.

42310

The physician drains an abscess of the submaxillary (submandibular) or sublingual gland. An incision is made intraorally through the tissue overlying the gland. The physician then dissects through the tissue overlying the abscess. The abscess is opened with a surgical instrument and the fluid is drained.

42320

The physician drains an abscess of the submaxillary (submandibular) salivary gland. An incision is made extraorally through the skin overlying the gland. The physician then dissects through the tissue overlying the abscess. The abscess is opened with a surgical instrument and the fluid is drained. A drain may be placed.

42325

The physician creates a fistula (or tube-like passage from a cavity to a free surface or to another cavity) in a sublingual salivary cyst for drainage purposes. These retention cysts may achieve a large size and burrow into the tissue planes of the neck.

42326

The physician creates a fistula (or tube-like passage from a cavity to a free surface or another cavity) in a sublingual salivary cyst for drainage purposes. These retention cysts may achieve a large size and burrow into the tissue planes of the neck. A prosthesis for

maintaining the patency of the fistula is inserted into the area.

42330

The physician makes an incision in the submandibular, sublingual or parotid ducts to remove a sialolith (a stone). An incision is made intraorally in the mucosa overlying the duct and tissue is dissected to the duct. The physician removes the stone. The incision is usually not closed.

42335

The physician makes an incision in the submandibular duct to remove a sialolith (a stone). An incision is made intraorally in the mucosa overlying the duct and tissue is dissected to the duct. A large stone and portion of surrounding tissue must be removed. The incision is usually not closed.

42340

The physician makes an incision in the parotid gland usually to remove a sialolith (a stone). An incision is made extraorally in the skin overlying the gland or the mucosa overlying the duct. Tissue is dissected to the gland. The physician removes the stone. The incision is closed with layered sutures.

42400–42405

The physician performs a needle or incisional biopsy of a salivary gland. For a needle biopsy (e.g., 42400), a needle is inserted through the skin overlying the salivary gland. The physician takes a tissue sample from the gland and withdraws the needle. For an incisional biopsy (e.g., 42405), an incision is made in the skin overlying the salivary gland. Tissues are dissected to the gland. An incision is made in the tissue of the gland, and a small piece of the gland is removed. The surgical wound is sutured.

42408

The physician removes a sublingual salivary cyst. An incision is made intraorally in the floor of the mouth overlying the cyst. The physician then removes the cyst.

42409

The physician incises and removes the mucosa overlying the cyst on the floor of the mouth. The roof of the cyst is removed and the remaining sides of the cyst wall are sutured to the mucosa, creating a pouch. The saliva drains through the pouch. The pouch shrinks in size to a small opening in the floor of the mouth. Saliva from the sublingual gland then flows through this opening.

42410–42426

The physician excises a portion or all of the parotid gland with or without facial nerve preservation and unilateral neck dissection. The physician makes a preauricular incision with a curved cervical extension to the midpoint of the mandible. The anterior and posterior skin flaps are retracted and the tissues are retracted to expose the parotid gland, leaving the fascia over the gland intact. In 42410, the main trunk of the facial nerve is visualized and the lateral (superficial) lobe of the parotid gland is freed and excised. In 42415, the facial nerve is identified and the lateral lobe is lifted off the branches of the nerve using dissection. A nerve stimulator may be used to test nerve integrity. In 42420, the facial nerve is identified and the entire the lateral lobe is lifted off the branches of the nerve using dissection. A nerve stimulator is used to test nerve integrity. The nerve is retracted so the deep parotid gland can be removed without damaging the facial nerve. The nerve stimulator is used often to ensure nerve integrity. In 42425, the physician removes the entire gland without capsule disruption, sacrificing the facial nerve. In 42426, the physician removes the entire gland without capsule disruption, sacrificing the facial nerve. The incision is then extended inferiorly to dissect the unilateral neck for lymph node excision.

42440

The physician removes a diseased, infected, blocked, or injured submandibular gland. The physician makes an incision in the skin of the neck below the inferior border of the mandible and near the angle of the mandible. The underlying tissues are then dissected to the submandibular gland. The gland is exposed, freed from surrounding tissue, and removed. The incision is then closed with sutures.

42450

The physician removes a diseased, infected, blocked, or injured sublingual gland. The physician makes an intraoral incision in the mucosa overlying the gland. Tissues are dissected down to the gland. The gland is exposed, freed from surrounding tissue, and removed. The incision is then closed with sutures.

42500–42505

The physician repairs a salivary duct by inserting a hollow plastic or silicone tube into the duct. The tube is threaded through the duct. The duct is allowed to heal and may be sutured around the tube. In 42505, repair of the duct is complex and may be delayed. The tube is later removed and patency is restored.

42507

The physician makes an intraoral incision overlying the parotid duct. The path of the duct is diverted into a new position and sutured to the mucosa so that the opening of the duct is in a different location. To bypass a blockage, the duct may be cut behind the blockage and repositioned so that saliva can flow freely into the mouth. This procedure is performed on both parotid ducts.

42508

The physician makes an intraoral incision overlying the parotid duct. The path of the duct is diverted into

a new position and sutured to the mucosa so that the opening of the duct is in a different location. To bypass a blockage, the duct may be cut behind the blockage and repositioned so that saliva can flow freely into the mouth. This procedure is performed on both parotid ducts. The physician also removes a submandibular gland. The physician makes an incision in the skin of the neck below the inferior border of the mandible. The underlying tissues are then dissected to the submandibular gland. The gland is exposed, freed from the surrounding tissue, and removed. The incision is then closed with sutures..

42509

The physician makes an intraoral incision overlying the parotid duct. The path of the duct is diverted into a new position and sutured to the mucosa so that the opening of the duct is in a different location. To bypass a blockage, the duct may be cut behind the blockage and repositioned so that saliva can flow freely into the mouth. This procedure is performed on both parotid ducts. The physician also removes both submandibular glands. The physician makes an incision in the skin of the neck below the inferior border of the mandible. The underlying tissues are then dissected to the submandibular gland. The gland is exposed, freed from the surrounding tissue, and removed. The incision is then closed with sutures. The mucosal incisions are closed directly.

42510

The physician makes an intraoral incision overlying the parotid duct. The path of the duct is diverted into a new position and sutured to the mucosa so that the opening of the duct is in a different location. To bypass a blockage, the duct may be cut behind the blockage and repositioned so that saliva can flow freely into the mouth. This procedure is performed on both parotid ducts. The physician then ligates both submandibular ducts. An incision may be made over the duct. Suture material is tied around the ducts to stop the flow of saliva. The mucosal incisions are closed directly.

42550

The physician inserts a small catheter into the duct of a salivary gland. A radiopaque dye (a dye which projects white on x-rays) is then injected into the duct. The duct is filled with the dye back to and including the gland, if possible. An x-ray is then taken. The x-ray shows the duct and gland filled with the dye, demonstrating the structure, blockages or disease affecting the structure.

42600

The physician closes a salivary fistula. The physician makes an incision around the fistula and excises the fistula down to the level of the duct. After excision of the fistula, the incision is closed directly.

CPT® Lay Descriptions

42650

The physician inserts a probe into the salivary duct to dilate a narrowed section. The physician repeats the procedure with progressively larger probes until the desired amount of dilation is achieved.

42660

The physician introduces a catheter and dilates or expands the salivary duct. A radiopaque dye may be injected into the duct to outline the structure of the duct and any disease process. The catheter is then removed.

42665

The physician makes an intraoral incision overlying a salivary duct and dissects to the layer of the duct. The duct is then ligated (tied) and the incision is closed.

42700

The physician drains an abscess near or on a tonsil. The patient is given a topical anesthetic or placed under general anesthesia. Using an intraoral approach with a mouth gag, the physician incises the mucus membrane of the abscess. The abscess cavity is opened with angulated closed forceps or hemostat. The wound is irrigated and left open.

42720

The physician drains an abscess located on or near the pharynx. Retropharyngeal indicates the abscess is located on the back of the pharynx; parapharyngeal indicates the abscess is near the pharynx. The patient is given a topical anesthetic or placed under general anesthesia. Though an intraoral approach, the physician locates the abscess using a diagnostic needle puncture and aspiration at the point of maximal fluctuation on the pharynx. The physician incises the mucus membrane to open the abscess. The pus is evacuated using suction and sponging.

42725

The physician drains an abscess located on or near the pharynx. The patient is placed under general anesthesia. The physician makes an incision beneath the angle of the jaw and carries out a blunt dissection to locate and isolate the abscess. The physician incises the mucus membrane of the abscess. The pus is evacuated; a gauze or rubber drain may be inserted into the abscess cavity. The incision is repaired in sutured layers.

42800–42802

The physician obtains a biopsy of the oropharynx or hypopharynx. After the airway is secured with an endotracheal tube, a mouth gag is placed. The physician obtains a tissue sample through an incisional or snare technique. Bleeding is controlled through electrocautery, the wound is not closed. In 42800, tissue in the oropharynx is biopsied. In 42802, tissue in the hypopharynx is biopsied. If the lesion is

deep in the hypopharynx, an operating laryngoscope is used to visualize the area.

42804–42806

The physician obtains a biopsy of the oropharynx or hypopharynx. After the airway is secured with an endotracheal tube, a mouth gag is placed. The physician obtains a tissue sample through an incisional or snare technique. Bleeding is controlled through electrocautery, the wound is not closed. In 42804, tissue with a visible in the nasopharynx is biopsied. In 42806, tissue in the nasopharynx is biopsied to survey for an unknown primary lesion. If the lesion is deep in the nasopharynx, an operating laryngoscope is used to visualize the area.

42808

The physician removes or destroys a lesion of the pharynx. The physician uses an intraoral approach to excise or destroy the lesion. Destruction may be accomplished using a laser, cryosurgery, or electrocoagulation to cause the tissue to coagulate. Methods of excision may include avulsion, or curettage.

42809

The physician removes a foreign body from the pharynx. After applying a topical anesthetic to the mouth and pharynx, the physician uses an intraoral approach with the aid of a tongue blade to visualize the foreign body. The foreign body is visualized, grasped with forceps and removed.

42810

The physician removes a branchial cleft cyst or vestige that is confined to the skin and subcutaneous tissues of the neck. A branchial cleft is an embryological remnant that resembles gills. Normally, the clefts involute before the fetal stage. The physician makes a horizontal neck incisions just below the jaw line to access and remove the cyst or vestige. The operative incision is repaired in sutured layers.

42815

The physician removes a branchial cleft cyst or vestige that has extended beyond the skin and subcutaneous tissue. A branchial cleft is an embryological remnant that resembles gills. Normally, the clefts involute before the fetal stage. The physician makes one or two horizontal neck incisions just below the jaw line. The cyst or vestige is dissected from the surrounding muscle and fascia. If a fistula is present, a surrounding elliptical skin excision is performed. Any ducts of the cyst are dissected and traced to a pharyngeal communication. The cyst, vestige, and ducts are removed. A tissue drain is placed and the wound is closed in sutured layers.

42820–42821

The physician removes the tonsils and adenoids. The patient is placed under general anesthesia. The physician uses an intraoral approach to access the tonsils and adenoids. First, the physician removes the tonsils by grasping the tonsil with a tonsil clamp and dissecting the capsule of the tonsil. The tonsil is removed. Bleeding vessels are clamped and tied. Bleeding may also be controlled using silver nitrate and gauze packing. Next the adenoids are are removed. Using a mirror or nasopharyngoscope for visualization, the physician uses an adenotome or a curet and basket punch to excise the adenoids. Alternate surgical techniques for a tonsillectomy and adenoidectomy include electrocautery, laser surgery, and cryogenic surgery. Report 42820 if the patient is under 12 years. For patients 12 years or older, report 42821.

42825–42826

The physician removes the tonsils. The tonsillectomy is the primary procedure, or can be performed as a secondary procedure. The patient is placed under general anesthesia. The physician uses an intraoral approach to access the tonsils. First, the physician removes the tonsils by grasping the tonsil with a tonsil clamp and dissecting the capsule of the tonsil. The tonsil is removed. Bleeding vessels are clamped and tied. Bleeding may also be controlled using silver nitrate and gauze packing. Alternate surgical techniques for a tonsillectomy include electrocautery, laser surgery, and cryogenic surgery. Report 42825 if the patient is under 12 years. For patients 12 years or older, report 42826.

42830–42836

The physician removes the adenoids. Using a mirror or nasopharyngoscope for visualization, the physician uses an adenotome or a curet and basket punch to excise the adenoids. Alternate surgical techniques for an adenoidectomy include electrocautery, laser surgery, and cryogenic surgery. For adenoidectomy performed as a primary procedure (the initial removal of the adenoid), report 42830 for patients under 12 years; report 42831 for patients 12 years and older. When performed as a secondary procedure (secondary procedure to remove portions of the adenoid missed during the primary procedure), report 42835 if the patient is under 12 years; report 42836 for patients 12 years and older.

42842–42845

The physician removes the tonsils, tonsillar pillars, and/or the retromolar trigone, along with any affected area of the maxilla or mandible involved in the tumor. First, the physician performs a tracheostomy. The involved tissue is resected. In addition to the above areas, radical resection may include a hemiglossectomy or a total glossectomy, as well as a full neck dissection. In 42842, the wound is so extensive that it is packed open and grafted at a later session. In 42844, the wound is less extensive and can be closed either primarily with sutured layers. In 42845 a flap is rotated up from the chest. If the wound included a resection of the mandible or maxilla, a fibular bone graft or a metal plate may be used to reconstruct the jaw.

42860

The physician removes portions of the tonsils not excised during primary resection or that have developed polyps. The physician uses a mouth gag to visualize the tonsillar pillars, and cauterizes and/or snares the affected tissue. No closure is required.

42870

The physician removes or destroys the lingual tonsils. Because the abscessed tonsil restricts the airway passage, the physician is present during intubation in case an emergency airway is needed. The physician uses an endotracheal tube or an operating laryngoscope with jet ventilation to ventilate the patient. Using an intraoral approach, the physician uses a laser to destroy the lingual tonsils.

42890

The physician removes the affected portion of the pharyngeal wall. The physician makes a vertical incision in the neck and retracts the strap muscles. The affected area of the pharynx is excised and the pharyngeal walls are reapproximated and closed with sutures. The incision is closed in sutured layers. Occasionally, the area removed includes part of the thyroid ala, hyoid bone, and wall of the pyriform fossa. Procedures include: anterior transhyoid pharyngotomy, lateral pharyngotomy, and median labiomandibular glossotomy. Reconstructive surgery is required for closure.

42892

The physician removes the affected portion of the pharyngeal wall or pyriform sinus. The physician makes a vertical incision and retracts the strap muscles. The mucosa of the upper pyriform sinus and the affected portion of the pharynx are excised. The lateral and posterior pharyngeal walls are reapproximated and closed with sutures. The operative incision is closed in sutured layers.

42894

The physician removes the affected portion of the pharyngeal wall or pyriform sinus. The physician makes a vertical incision and retracts the strap muscles. The mucosa of the upper pyriform sinus and the affected portion of the pharynx are excised. Myocutaneous flap reconstruction of the pharyngeal area is achieved using the pectoralis major muscle and its overlying skin. The flap is rotated and inserted through a previously created tunnel between the clavicle and overlying skin and sutured into place to reconstruct the pharynx. The operative incision is closed in sutured layers.

CPT ® Lay Descriptions

42900

The physician locates and sutures a wound or injury to the pharynx. The physician uses an intraoral or transhyoid approach, depending on the location and extent of the wound. For an intraoral approach, the physician uses a mirror for visualization. For a transhyoid approach, the physician makes a horizontal incision directly below the jaw line. The physician sutures the wound. If a transhyoid approach is used, the operative incision is closed in sutured layers.

42950

A variety of techniques may be used for pharyngeal reconstruction including skin grafts, tongue flaps, regional cutaneous flaps and microvascular free-tissue transfer. Skin grafts are commonly harvested from the forehead, deltopectoral, nape of the neck, and pectoralis major. Reconstruction is performed when direct wound closure or reapproximation is not possible.

42953

The physician repairs a tear at the pharyngeal esophageal junction. After the airway is secured, the physician makes a horizontal neck incision and retracts superficial tissues to expose the pharyngeal esophageal junction. The defect is identified, irrigated to reduce infection, and closed in sutured layers.

42955

The physician creates an opening to the pharnyx for long term feeding. The physician makes a horizontal incision below the jaw line to create a communication between the pharyngeal lumen and the exterior of the patient's neck. The incision is sutured to create an opening for placement of a feeding tube.

42960–42962

The physician controls bleeding of the oropharynx. Primary hemorrhaging occurs within 24 hours after surgery; secondary hemorrhaging occurs 24 hours to two weeks after surgery. In 42960 and 42961, hemorrhaging is controlled using methods such as clot evacuation and applying pressure with sponges, electrocautery, or application of vasoconstrictor solutions such as tannic acid, silver nitrate, and epinephrine. Cellulose sponges that expand when placed in the tonsillar cavity may be used. Report 42961 when extensive bleeding requires hospitalization. In 42962, surgery is required to control hemorrhaging. Surgical intervention methods include suture ligation of bleeding vessels. In cases of profuse bleeding, emergency ligation of the external carotid artery may be performed. The tonsillar pillars may be approximated with mattress sutures to control post-tonsillectomy bleeding.

42970–42972

The physician controls bleeding of the nasopharynx. Primary hemorrhaging occurs within 24 hours after

surgery; secondary hemorrhaging occurs 24 hours to two weeks after surgery. In 42970 and 42971 hemorrhaging is controlled using methods such as clot evacuation and application of vasoconstrictor solutions such as tannic acid, silver nitrate, and epinephrine; electrocautery; and posterior or anterior nasal packing. Report 42971 when extensive bleeding requires hospitalization. In 42972, surgery is required to control hemorrhaging. Surgical intervention methods include ligation of ethmoidal arteries using silver clips and/or electrocautery. The physician uses a nasal or intraoral approach for secondary surgery.

43020

The physician makes an incision in the esophagus to remove a foreign body. The physician makes a horizontal or oblique incision in the lateral neck. Then the physician makes an incision in the esophagus and uses forceps to grasp and extract the foreign body. The incision is closed with sutured layers.

43030

The physician incises the cricopharyngeal muscle. The physician makes a lateral neck incision to expose the cricopharyngeal muscle. The physician then makes a second lateral incision through the cricopharyngeal muscle. The operative incision is repaired with sutured layers.

43045

The physician makes an incision in the esophagus to remove a foreign body. For a thoracic approach, the physician incises and dissects the left posterior chest wall to access the esophagus. The physician incises the esophagus and uses forceps to grasp and remove the foreign body. The esophageal incision is closed with sutures. The left posterior chest wall is closed with sutured layers.

43100

The physician removes a lesion in the esophagus. The physician makes a horizontal or oblique incision of the lateral neck. Next, the physician makes an incision in the esophagus and excises the lesion. The remaining esophageal borders are sutured together. The operative incision is closed in sutured layers.

43101

The physician removes a lesion in the esophagus. For a thoracic approach, the physician incises and dissects the left posterior chest wall to access the esophagus. For an abdominal approach, the physician makes an upper midline abdominal incision to access the esophagus transhiatally. The physician then excises the lesion. The remaining esophageal borders are sutured together. The operative incision is closed with sutured layers.

43107

The physician removes most or all of the esophagus and attaches the stomach to the pharynx or cervical esophagus. The physician gains access to the esophagus through two incisions. The first is an oblique cervical incision. The second is a horizontal upper midline abdominal incision. The physician divides the esophagus either at the cervical level (for a esophagogastrostomy) or at its origin at the pharynx (for a pharyngogastrostomy). The esophagus is removed through the abdominal incision and divided from the stomach. The stomach is pulled up through the posterior mediastinum and anastomosed to the pharynx or the remaining cervical esophagus. If the stomach is used as the esophageal conduit, a pyloroplasty may be performed to open the pyloric sphincter. The operative incisions are repaired in sutured layers.

43108

The physician removes most or all of the esophagus and uses a bowel or colon graft for reconstruction. The physician gains access to the esophagus through two incisions. The first is an oblique cervical incision. The second is a horizontal upper midline abdominal incision. The physician divides the esophagus either at the cervical level (for a esophagogastrostomy) or at its origin at the pharynx (for a pharyngogastrostomy). The esophagus is removed through the abdominal incision and divided from the stomach. Next, a colon or bowel graft is obtained. A portion of the colon or small bowel is excised and freed of attachments, taking care to preserve its major vascular supply. Gastrointestinal continuity is reestablished by securing the distal and proximal bowel margins. Finally, the excised portion of the colon or bowel is attached to the pharynx or cervical esophagus and the stomach. This anastomosis (the attaching the two organs that are normally not attached) creates a usable esophagus. If the stomach is used as the esophageal conduit, a pyloroplasty may be performed to open the pyloric sphincter. The operative incisions are repaired in sutured layers.

43112

The physician removes the esophagus through abdominal, chest and neck incisions and replaces the esophagus with stomach. The physician makes a midline abdominal incision. Next the stomach is dissected free of surrounding structures and the esophagus is mobilized as it passes through the diaphragm to the stomach. Next, the physician makes an incision in the right chest between the ribs and exposes the esophagus. The esophagus is mobilized under direct vision in the chest from the diaphragm to the neck. Next, a longitudinal incision is made in the left or right neck and the esophagus is identified and mobilized in the neck. The esophagus is divided at its junction with the stomach and in the neck and the esophagus is removed. Next, the stomach is pulled up through the middle of the chest into the neck and the

stomach is connected to the stump of the esophagus in the neck. The incisions are closed.

43113

The physician removes the esophagus through abdominal, chest and neck incisions and replaces the esophagus with colon or small bowel. The physician makes a midline abdominal incision. Next, the stomach is dissected free of surrounding structures and the esophagus is mobilized as it passes through the diagram to the stomach. Next, the physician makes an incision in the right chest between the ribs and exposes the esophagus. The esophagus is mobilized under direct vision in the chest from the diaphragm to the neck. The esophagus is divided at its junction with the stomach and in the neck and the esophagus is removed. The physician selects an appropriate segment of colon or small bowel. The bowel is divided proximal and distal to this segment and the bowel ends are reapproximated. The selected segment of colon or small bowel is pulled up through the middle section of the chest and connected to the stump of the esophagus in the neck and to the stomach in the abdomen. The incisions are closed.

43116

The physician removes the affected portion of the esophagus and replaces it with a graft from the large or small intestine. The physician gains access to the esophagus through an oblique cervical incision. The physician resects the affected portion of the cervical esophagus. Next, the physician obtains a graft from the large or small intestine. To do this, the physician makes a midline abdominal incision and frees a portion of the large or small intestine of muscular and vascular attachments. The intestine is resected and interposed to reestablish gastrointestinal continuity in the cervical esophagus. Microsurgical techniques are used to create a new blood supply for the graft. The distal and proximal portions of the remaining intestine are reconnected (anastomosis).

43117

The physician removes the distal esophagus and possibly the proximal stomach through abdominal and chest incisions and replaces the esophagus with the remaining stomach. The physician makes a midline abdominal incision. The stomach is dissected free of surrounding structures and the esophagus is mobilized as it passes through the diaphragm to the stomach. The esophagus is divided at its connection to the stomach or the stomach may be divided near its middle portion. Next, a right chest incision is made between the ribs to expose the esophagus. The distal esophagus is mobilized under direct vision and divided above its diseased segment. The distal esophagus and attached proximal stomach are them removed. The remaining stomach is pulled up into the chest and connected to the stump of the proximal esophagus. Drains are placed into the chest near the new anastomosis and the incisions are closed.

43118

The physician removes the distal esophagus and possibly proximal stomach through abdominal and chest incisions and replaces the esophagus with colon or small bowel. The physician makes a midline abdominal incision. The stomach is dissected free of surrounding structures and the esophagus is mobilized as it passes through the diaphragm to the stomach. The esophagus is divided at its connection to the stomach or the stomach may be divided near its middle portion. Next, an appropriate segment of colon or small bowel is selected and the bowel is divided proximal and distal to this segment and the bowel ends re-approximated. One end of the selected bowel segment is connected to the remaining stomach and the other end is placed through the diaphragm into the chest. Next, a right chest incision is made between the ribs to expose the esophagus. The distal esophagus is mobilized under direct vision and divided above its diseased segment. The distal esophagus and attached proximal stomach are removed. The remaining end of the segment of colon or small bowel that has been attached to the stomach is pulled up into the chest and connected to the stump of the proximal esophagus. Drains are placed into the chest near the new anastomosis and the incisions are closed

43121

The physician removes the affected part of the esophagus and proximal stomach, then reattaches the remaining stomach to the esophageal stump. The physician accesses the esophagus through a right postero-lateral thoracotomy; no abdominal incision is made. The physician resects the affected portion of the distal esophagus and sometimes a portion of the proximal stomach. The resected area is removed. The stomach or gastric remnant is pulled up into the thorax and sutured to the esophageal stump. If the stomach is used as the esophageal conduit, a pyloroplasty may be performed to open the pyloric sphincter. The operative incision is closed in sutured layers.

43122

The physician removes the distal esophagus and possibly proximal stomach through a combined abdominal and chest incision and replaces the esophagus with the remaining stomach. The physician makes a midline abdominal incision that may extend onto the lower chest between the ribs. Next, the stomach is dissected free of surrounding structures and the esophagus is mobilized as it passes through the diaphragm to the stomach. The esophagus is divided proximally above the diseased area and distally at its junction with the stomach or the middle portion of the stomach may be divided. The distal esophagus and attached proximal stomach are removed. The remaining stomach is connected to the stump of the esophagus. The incision is closed.

43123

The physician removes the distal esophagus and possibly the proximal stomach through a combined abdominal and chest incision and replaces the esophagus with colon or small bowel. The physician makes a midline abdominal incision that may extend onto the chest between the ribs. Next, the stomach is dissected free of surrounding structures and the esophagus is mobilized as it passes through the diaphragm to the stomach. The esophagus is divided proximally above the diseased area and distally at its junction with the stomach or the middle portion of the stomach may be divided. The distal esophagus and attached stomach are removed. Next, an appropriate segment of colon or small bowel is selected. The bowel is divided proximal and distal to the segment and the bowel ends are re-approximated. The selected segment of bowel is connected proximally to the remaining esophageal stump and distally to the remaining stomach. The incision is closed.

43124

The physician removes the esophagus with no attempt to reconstruct the esophagus. The physician first creates a permanent tracheoplasty. The physician accesses the esophagus through an oblique cervical incision, a thoracotomy, and/or a midline abdominal incision and resects the affected portion of the esophagus. The esophageal stump is sutured to the cervical incision, creating a connection from the exterior of the neck to the esophageal lumen to provide drainage of saliva and mucus. The operative incisions are closed with sutured layers.

43130–43135

The physician removes a diverticulum from the hypopharynx or esophagus. A diverticulum is pouch that occurs normally or because of a defect in the muscular membrane. In 43130 (cervical approach), the physician makes a lateral incision in the neck. In 43135 (thoracic approach), the physician incises and dissects the left posterior chest wall. The physician may dissect the cricopharyngeous muscle to expose the diverticulum. If a myotomy is necessary, the physician makes a vertical incision through the cricopharyngeous muscle. The physician clamps the diverticulum and closes using sutures or staples. The operative incision is closed with sutured layers.

43200–43202

The physician uses an esophagoscope to view the entire esophagus. The physician passes either a rigid or flexible esophagoscope through the patient's mouth and into the esophagus. In 43200, specimens may be obtained by brushing or washing the esophageal lining with saline, followed by aspiration. In 43202 bite biopsy forceps are used to obtain samples of the esophageal mucosa that appear abnormal.

43204–43205

The physician uses an esophagoscope to view the entire esophagus and identify and treat varices. Varices are dilated, enlarged, and tortuous veins. The physician passes either a rigid or flexible esophagoscope through the patient's mouth and into the esophagus to identifies the varices. In 43204, the physician passes a sclerotherapy needle through the scope, and injects the varices with an agent that causes fibrosis (scarring). The result is obliteration of the varices. In 43205, the physician uses a suction tip to lift the varix and places a rubber band around the base of the varix, which will slough away within several days.

43215

The physician uses an esophagoscope to locate and remove a foreign body from the esophagus. The physician passes either a rigid or flexible esophagoscope through the patient's mouth and into the esophagus. The foreign body is located. It may be suctioned, or grasped with forceps and retracted through the scope. An alternative technique that may be used for objects too large to grasp is to pass a balloon beyond the foreign body. The balloon is inflated then simultaneously withdrawn with the scope and the foreign body.

43216–43217

The physician uses an esophagoscope to locate and remove a tumors, polyps, or lesions from the esophagus. The physician passes either a rigid or flexible esophagoscope through the patient's mouth and into the esophagus and locates the lesion. In 43216 the base of the lesion is electrocoagulated and severed using biopsy forceps or bipolar cautery. In 43217 a snare loop is placed around the base of the lesion and closed (the tissue is electrocoagulated and severed as the loop is closed). The severed tissue is withdrawn through the scope. If the lesion is removed using laser therapy, electrocoagulation, or injection of toxic agents, report 43228.

43219

The physician uses an esophagoscope to examine the esophagus and to place a plastic tube or stent. This procedure usually follows dilation for an obstruction. The physician passes either a rigid or flexible esophagoscope through the patient's mouth and into the esophagus. A guidewire is placed through the scope. (If the procedure follows dilation, the guidewire used for dilation is simply left in place.) The stent or plastic tube is advanced down the esophagus over the guidewire. The position of the stent is confirmed with the scope.

43220

The physician uses an esophagoscope to place a balloon and dilate the esophagus. The physician passes either a rigid or flexible esophagoscope through the patient's mouth and into the esophagus.

The balloon is advanced down the esophagus through the scope. A guidewire may used. After entering the obstructed region, the balloon is briefly inflated several times.

43226

The physician passes either a rigid or flexible esophagoscope through the patient's mouth and into the esophagus. A guidewire is placed through the scope and the scope is removed. A dilator is passed into the esophagus over the guidewire. This may be repeated several times using progressively larger dilators.

43227

The physician uses an esophagoscope to access and control bleeding of the esophagus. The physician passes either a rigid or flexible esophagoscope through the patient's mouth and into the esophagus. Control of bleeding may be achieved using several endoscopic methods including laser therapy, electrocoagulation, rubber band ligation, and injection of the bleeding vessel with sclerosants, ethanol, or adrenaline.

43228

The physician uses an esophagoscope to locate and remove a tumors, polyps, or lesions from the esophagus. The physician passes either a rigid or flexible esophagoscope through the patient's mouth and into the esophagus and locates the lesion. The lesion is destroyed using laser therapy, electrocoagulation, or injection of toxic agents. If the lesion is destroyed using hot biopsy forceps, bipolar cautery report 43216 instead. If destroyed using snare technique, report 43217 instead.

43231

The physician uses an esophagoscope to view the entire esophagus and performs an endoscopic ultrasound examination. The physician passes either a rigid or flexible esophagoscope through the patients' mouth and into the esophagus. The entire esophagus is examined and the area of interest is identified. Then either the esophagoscope is removed and replaced with an echoendoscope, or an ultrasound probe is passed through the already placed esophagoscope. The echoendoscope or ultrasound probe is fitted with a water-filled balloon near the tip; the tip contains a transducer that picks-up the ultrasound frequency and relays it to a processor, outside of the body. The water-filled tip is positioned in the esophagus, against the esophageal wall next to the area of interest. The area is scanned and an ultrasound image is projected through the processor to a monitor in real-time. When the ultrasound examination is complete the echoendoscope, or esophagoscope and ultrasound probe is removed.

43232

The physician uses an esophagoscope to view the entire esophagus and performs a transendoscopic ultrasound-guided intramural or transmural fine needle aspiration/biopsy. The physician passes either a rigid or flexible esophagoscope through the patients' mouth and into the esophagus. The entire esophagus is examined and the area of interest is identified. The esophagoscope may be removed. A radial scanning echoendoscope is inserted and ultrasound scanning is performed, or an ultrasound probe is passed through the already placed esophagoscope. The site for a fine needle aspiration biopsy is determined. If a radial scanning echoendoscope is used it is removed and is replaced with a curvilinear array echoendoscope. The echoendoscope or ultrasound probe is fitted with a water-filled balloon near the tip; the tip contains a transducer that picks-up the ultrasound frequency and relays it to a processor, outside of the body. The water-filled tip is positioned in the esophagus, against the esophageal wall next to the predetermined fine needle aspiration (FNA) biopsy site. The area is scanned and an ultrasound image is projected through the processor to a monitor in real-time. A FNA needle is passed through the scope to the biopsy site and the needle is inserted through the wall of the esophagus to the lesion, or other structure, such as a lymph node. The area is biopsied. When the FNA is complete the echoendoscope, or esophagoscope and ultrasound probe is removed.

43234

The physician uses an endoscope to examine the upper gastrointestinal tract. The physician passes an endoscope through the patient's mouth into the esophagus. The entire esophagus, stomach, duodenum and sometimes the jejunum are viewed.

43235–43239

The physician uses an endoscope to examine the upper gastrointestinal tract for diagnostic purposes. The physician passes an endoscope through the patient's mouth into the esophagus. The entire esophagus, stomach, duodenum and sometimes the jejunum are viewed to determine if bleeding, tumors, erosions, ulcers, or other abnormalities are present. In 43235, specimens may be obtained by brushing or washing the esophageal lining with saline, followed by aspiration. In 43239, single or multiple biopsy samples may be obtained for biopsy using bite biopsy forceps.

43240

The physician uses an endoscope to examine the upper gastrointestinal tract and performs transmural drainage of a pseudocyst. The physician passes an endoscope through the patient's mouth into the esophagus. The entire esophagus, stomach, duodenum and sometimes the jejunum are examined. The site for drainage of the pseudocyst is identified. A needle is passed through the scope to the site and the

needle is inserted through the small intestinal wall into the pancreatic pseudocyst. The pseudocyst is drained. The endoscope is removed.

43241

The physician uses an endoscope to examine the upper gastrointestinal tract and places an intraluminal (through the endoscope) tube or catheter. The physician passes an endoscope through the patient's mouth into the esophagus. The entire esophagus, stomach, duodenum, and, sometimes, the jejunum are viewed. The physician then places a tube or catheter through the endoscope. The endoscope is removed.

43242

The physician uses an endoscope to examine the upper gastrointestinal tract and performs a transendoscopic ultrasound-guided intramural or transmural fine needle aspiration/biopsy. The physician passes an endoscope through the patient's mouth into the esophagus. The entire esophagus, stomach, duodenum and sometimes the jejunum are viewed. The endoscope may be removed. A radial scanning echoendoscope is inserted and ultrasound scanning is performed, or an ultrasound probe is passed through the already placed endoscope. The site for a fine needle aspiration biopsy is determined. If a radial scanning echoendoscope is used, it is removed and is replaced with a curvilinear array echoendoscope. The echoendoscope or ultrasound probe is fitted with a water-filled balloon near the tip; the tip contains a transducer that picks-up the ultrasound frequency and relays it to a processor, outside of the body. The water-filled tip is positioned in the esophagus, stomach, or small intestine against the tissue wall next to the predetermined fine needle aspiration (FNA) biopsy site. The area is scanned and an ultrasound image is projected through the processor to a monitor in real-time. A FNA needle is passed through the scope to the biopsy site and a biopsy is taken of the tissue or the needle is inserted through the wall of the tissue into the lesion, or other structure, such as a lymph node. The area is biopsied. When the FNA is complete the echoendoscope, or endoscope and ultrasound probe is removed.

43243–43244

The physician uses an endoscope to examine the upper gastrointestinal tract to identify and treat esophageal and/or gastric varices. Varices are dilated, enlarged, and twisted (tortuous) veins. The physician passes an endoscope through the patient's mouth into the esophagus. The entire esophagus, stomach, duodenum and sometimes the jejunum are viewed. The physician identifies the varices. For 43243, the physician passes a sclerotherapy needle through the scope, and injects the varices with an agent that causes fibrosis (scarring). The result is obliteration of the varices. For 43244, the physician uses a suction tip to lift the varix. Next, the physician places a rubber band around the base of the varix, which will slough away within several days.

43245

The physician uses an endoscope to examine the upper gastrointestinal tract to locate an obstruction. The physician passes an endoscope through the patient's mouth into the esophagus. The entire esophagus, stomach, duodenum, and sometimes the jejunum are viewed. If the gastric outlet (pylorus) is obstructed, the physician dilates it using various methods, such as a balloon, guide wire, or bogie. If balloon dilation is performed, the balloon is inflated briefly several time to enlarge the gastric outlet. When the dilation is complete, the balloon and endoscope are removed.

43246

The physician uses an endoscope to examine the upper gastrointestinal tract to guide placement of a gastrostomy tube. The physician passes an endoscope through the patient's mouth into the esophagus. The entire esophagus, stomach, duodenum and sometimes the jejunum are viewed. The endoscope is used to guide the placement of a percutaneous gastrostomy tube. The tube is inserted through an incision of the abdomen. When in place, the tube connects the gastric lumen with the exterior abdominal wall.

43247

The physician uses an endoscope to examine the upper gastrointestinal tract to locate and remove a foreign body. The physician passes an endoscope through the patient's mouth into the esophagus. The entire esophagus, stomach, duodenum and sometimes the jejunum are viewed. The foreign body is located. It may be suctioned, or grasped with forceps and retracted through the endoscope.

43248

The physician uses an endoscope to examine and dilate a portion of the upper gastrointestinal tract. The physician passes an endoscope through the patient's mouth into the esophagus. The entire esophagus, stomach, duodenum and sometimes the jejunum are viewed. A guidewire is placed through the endoscope and the scope is removed. A dilator is passed into the esophagus over the guidewire. This may be repeated several times using progressively larger dilators.

43249

The physician visualizes the esophagus, stomach and proximal small bowel with an endoscope and dilates an esophageal stricture. The physician inserts the endoscope through the mouth into the esophagus. The endoscope is advanced under direct vision through the esophagus into the stomach. The stomach is visualized and the endoscope is advanced into and through the duodenum and into the proximal jejunum if possible. The endoscope is carefully withdrawn. If an esophageal stricture is present a balloon on a catheter is advanced through the endoscope and through the stricture. The balloon is inflated to correct volume, pressure, and duration according to the package insert. The endoscope is removed.

43250–43251

The physician uses an endoscope to examine the upper gastrointestinal tract and locate and remove tumors, polyps, or other lesions. The physician passes an endoscope through the patient's mouth into the esophagus. The entire esophagus, stomach, duodenum and sometimes the jejunum are viewed to locate the lesion. Report 43250, when the base of the lesion is electrocoagulated and severed using biopsy forceps or bipolar cautery. Report 43251 when a snare loop is placed around the base of the lesion and closed (the tissue is electrocoagulated and severed as the loop is closed). The severed tissue is withdrawn through the endoscope. The endoscope is removed.

43255

The physician uses an endoscope to access and control bleeding of the upper gastrointestinal tract. The physician passes an endoscope through the patient's mouth and into the esophagus. Control of bleeding may be achieved using several endoscopic methods including laser therapy, electrocoagulation, rubber band ligation, and injection of the bleeding vessel with sclerosants, ethanol, or adrenaline. The endoscope is removed.

43256

The physician uses an endoscope to examine the upper gastrointestinal tract and performs a transendoscopic stent placement. The physician passes an endoscope through the patient's mouth into the esophagus. The entire esophagus, stomach, duodenum and sometimes the jejunum are viewed. The endoscope is placed at the site of an obstruction or stricture, the necessary stent length is determined and predilation of the obstruction or stenosis may be performed. The stent (endoprosthesis) is introduced into the site of the obstruction. Using a commercial delivery system a plastic covering over the stent is removed and the stent self-deploys, shoring-up the walls at a specific site in the esophagus or proximal small intestine. When necessary, a balloon catheter is placed into the stent and gently inflated to more fully deploy the stent. The delivery system and endoscope are removed.

43258

The physician uses an endoscope to locate and remove tumors, polyps, or lesions from the upper gastrointestinal tract. The physician passes an endoscope through the patient's mouth into the esophagus. The entire esophagus, stomach, duodenum and sometimes the jejunum are viewed to locate the lesion. The lesion is destroyed using laser

CPT® Lay Descriptions

therapy, electrocoagulation, or injection of toxic agents. The endoscope is removed.

43259

The physician uses an endoscopic ultrasound transducer to examine the esophageal and gastric wall. The physician passes an endoscope equipped with an ultrasound transducer through the patient's mouth into the esophagus. The entire esophagus, stomach, duodenum and sometimes the jejunum are viewed through ultrasound to help determine the extent of cancerous tissue. The endoscope is removed.

43260–43272

The physician performs an endoscopic retrograde cholangiopancreatography (ERCP) for diagnostic or therapeutic reasons, depending on the code. The physician passes the endoscope through the patient's oropharynx, esophagus, stomach, and into the small intestine. The ampulla of Vater is cannulated and filled with contrast. The common bile duct and the whole biliary tract including the gallbladder are visualized. Report 43261 if performed with biopsy; report 43262 if performed a with sphincterotomy/papillotomy; report 43263 if performed with a pressure measurement of sphincter of Oddi; report 43264 if performed with an endoscopic retrograde removal of stones from biliary and/or pancreatic ducts; report 43265 if performed with an endoscopic retrograde destruction, lithotripsy of stones; report 43267 if performed with an endoscopic retrograde insertion of nasobiliary or nasopancreatic drainage tube; report 43268 if performed with an endoscopic retrograde insertion of tubor stent into bile or pancreatic duct; report 43269 if performed with an endoscopic retrograde removal of foreign body and/or change of tube or stent; report 43271 if performed with an endoscopic retrograde balloon dilation of ampulla, biliary and/or pancreatic ducts; and report 43272 if performed with an ablation of tumors, polyps or other lesions not amenable to removal by hot biopsy forceps, bipolar cautery or snare technique.

43280

The physician performs an esophagogastric fundoplasty using a laparoscope. With the patient under anesthesia, the physician places a trocar at the umbilicus into the abdomen and insufflates the abdominal cavity. The physician places a laparoscope through the umbilical incision and additional trocars are placed into the peritoneal or space. Additional instruments are introduced through the trocars. The physician identifies the fundus and the esophagus and resects them. The fundus is wrapped around the lower end of the esophagus, which is rejoined to the stomach with sutures. The trocars are removed and the incisions are closed with sutures.

43300–43305

The physician repairs a defect in the esophagus using plastic repair or reconstruction. The physician makes a lateral neck incision to access the esophagus. The defect is identified and repaired. For 43305, the physician also transects the tracheoesophageal fistula. The physician closes the the tracheal opening and repairs the esophagus. The operative incision is closed in sutured layers.

43310–43312

The physician repairs a defect in the esophagus using plastic repair or reconstruction. The physician makes a thoracic incision to access the esophagus. In 43310, the defect is identified and repaired. For 43312, the physician also transects the tracheoesophageal fistula. The physician closes the the tracheal opening and repairs the esophagus. The operative incision is closed in sutured layers.

43313–43314

The patient is placed in the supine position with the left shoulder elevated and the head extended. A cervical incision is made along the anterior margin of the left sternocleidomastoid muscle, which is retracted laterally. The sternothyroid and sternohyoid muscles are divided, as well as for the branches of the ansa hypoglossi. The inferior pole of the thyroid gland is mobilized and retracted anteriorly. A dissection plane between the trachea and esophagus at the inlet of the thorax can be approached, entered, and dissected. The tracheal and esophageal defects are closed primarily. If the defect is large, a pedicled muscle patch is required to replace the tracheal defect (43314). A denervated and vascularized muscle pedicle is sutured to loose areolar tissue adjacent to the trachea on the opposite side. The esophagus is closed in two layers. The trachea is closed in one layer, with sufficient sutures to make an airtight closure.

43320

The physician performs a plastic repair of the lower esophagus where it joins the upper area (cardia) of the stomach. The physician may also transect the vagus nerve and/or enlarge the pylorus, the distal portion of the stomach. The physician accesses the esophagus through an upper abdominal or lateral thoracic incision. The diseased portion of the esophagus is resected. An anastomosis between the esophageal stump and the cardiac portion of the stomach is created. If the lesion is secondary to acid reflux, a vagotomy may be performed. The anterior and posterior trunks of the vagus nerve are transected to decrease acid production. If the gastric outlet area is decreased, a pyloroplasty may be performed to enlarge the pyloris. The operative incision is repaired in sutured layers.

43324

The physician mobilizes the lower end of the esophagus and folds the fundus of the stomach around it. The physician accesses the lower esophagus through an upper abdominal incision. The fundus of the stomach is moved up and wrapped around the terminal 3.0 cm to 4.0 cm of the esophagus and sutured into place. The lower esophageal sphincter passes through a short tunnel of stomach muscle, which prevents reflux through the sphincter. When performed for hiatal hernia, this procedure may include a sutured tightening of the junction of the diaphragmatic crura behind the esophagus.

43325

The physician pulls up part of the gastric fundus to cover the affected distal esophagus. A bougie (dilating instrument) is placed in the distal esophagus to maintain the esophageal opening. The physician accesses the esophagus and stomach through a transverse abdominal incision. The physician picks up the stomach 1.0 cm below the gastroesophageal (GE) junction and attaches it 1.0 cm above the GE junction. This fundic patch is sutured to the esophagus. Next, a Nissen fundoplication is performed by wrapping the rest of the fundus around the esophagus and suturing it into place. The operative incision is closed in sutured layers.

43326

The distal portion of the esophagus is lengthened by constructing a tube made of the stomach wall. The physician accesses the esophagus and stomach through a lateral thoracotomy. A bougie (dilating instrument) is passed through the esophagus into the stomach so the bougie spans the gastroesophageal junction. The stomach is divided along the bougie with a GIA stapler, forming a gastric tube which effectively lengthens the esophagus. The fundus of the stomach is dissected, wrapped around the distal esophagus and gastric tube, and sutured into place. The operative incision is closed in sutured layers.

43330–43331

The esophagus is repaired using a fundic flap. The physician accesses the esophagus through an upper abdominal or a thoracic incision. For an abdominal approach, report 43330. For a thoracic approach, report 43331. The physician makes an incision into the muscular layers of the distal esophagus and cardia of the stomach (myotomy), leaving a gastric fundic flap. The flap is pulled up along the esophagus, and sutured onto the margins of the myotomy. Repair of a hiatal hernia is performed by restoring the herniated portion of the stomach back to the abdomen, then narrowing the hiatal opening of the diaphragm by suturing the left and right crura together. All operative incisions are closed in sutured layers.

43340–43341

The physician removes the affected esophagus and stomach, using the remaining stomach and jejunum to restore gastrointestinal continuity. The physician accesses the esophagus and stomach through an upper abdominal or a thoracic incision. For an abdominal approach, report 43340. For a thoracic approach, report 43341. The physician resects the affected part of the esophagus. The stomach is advanced through the hiatus and sutured to the esophageal remnant. The antral portion of the stomach is excised, and the proximal jejunum is sutured to the gastric remnant. The distal end of the duodenum is anastomosed to the jejunum; the proximal end of the duodenum is sutured closed to form a blind pouch. The operative incision is closed in sutured layers.

43350–43352

The physician connects the esophagus to the exterior of the body, creating a fistula for drainage. In 43350, the physician makes an upper midline abdominal incision to access the esophagus. In 43351, the physician uses a lateral thoracotomy to access the esophagus. In 43352, access is gained through a cervical incision. The physician makes an incision in the esophagus, or uses the esophageal stump as an opening. The proximal limb of the esophagus is exteriorized and sutured into place, creating a connection from the exterior of the body to the esophageal lumen for mucus drainage. The operative incision is closed in sutured layers.

43360–43361

The physician repairs the esophagus and other gastronomic structures for a number of reasons. The physician uses a thoracoabdominal approach either as a continuous incision or separate thoracic and abdominal incisions. The stomach is mobilized and repositioned in the chest in the original esophageal bed and sutured to the esophageal stump. The incision and esophageal stoma are closed. A jejunostomy tube is left in place. Report 43361 if performed with colon interposition or small bowel reconstruction, including bowel mobilization, preparation, and/or anastomosis.

43400

The physician accesses the esophagus through a midline abdominal or thoracic incision, and makes a longitudinal incision in the esophagus. The physician locates the varices (tortuous, dilated veins) and ligates them with sutures. The esophagotomy is closed with sutures. The operative incision is closed in sutured layers.

43401

The physician uses a stapler to transect and repair the esophagus to remove esophageal varices. Varices are twisted, tortuous veins. The physician accesses the esophagus and stomach through an abdominal or thoracic incision. A stapler, placed through an incision in the anterior wall of the stomach, is directed upward into the esophagus. The stapler is positioned to transect the area around the varices. When the stapler is fired, the esophagus is simultaneously transected and re-anastomosed. The stapler is removed, and the incision in the stomach is repaired. The operative incision is closed in sutured layers.

43405

The physician ligates or staples the esophagus to promote healing of a preexisting esophageal perforation. The physician makes a midline upper abdominal incision and retracts the soft tissues to expose the gastroesophageal junction. the physician staples or ligates the junction of the stomach and esophagus. A gastrostomy is created for feeding. The distal end of the esophagus may be exteriorized as a mucus fistula. The operative incision is closed in sutured layers.

43410–43415

The physician sutures a wound or injury to the esophagus. The physician accesses the esophagus through a lateral neck, midline abdominal, or thoracic incision. For a cervical approach, report 43410. For a thoracic or transabdominal approach, report 43415. The physician then exposes the affected segment of the esophagus, which is repaired by suturing. The operative incision is closed in sutured layers.

43420–43425

The physician closes an opening in the esophagus and returns it to its natural position. The physician accesses the defect through an oblique cervical incision along the border of the sternocleidomastoid muscle, a midline abdominal incision, or a thoracic incision. For a cervical approach, report 43420. For a thoracic or transabdominal approach, report 43425. The physician closes the opening with sutures and repositions the esophagus to its normal anatomical position. The operative incision is closed in sutured layers.

43450

The physician dilates the esophagus using an unguided dilator. The physician passes a dilator into the patient's throat down into the esophagus until the end of the dilator passes the stricture. A stricture is a decrease in the esophagus opening as a result of cicatricial (scar) contraction or a deposit of abnormal tissue. The dilator is withdrawn after it passes the stricture. This may be repeated several times to dilate the esophagus to an acceptable size.

43453

The physician dilates the esophagus by passing dilators over a guidewire. The physician uses a fluoroscope to place a guidewire into the patient's throat, down the esophagus, and into the stomach. A

series of olive-shaped metal dilators (Eder-Puestou) are passed over the guidewire and withdrawn. The process is repeated until the esophagus is dilated to an acceptable size.

43456

The physician dilates the esophagus using a dilator that passes from the stomach through the esophagus. The physician uses a fluoroscope to place a guidewire into the patient's throat, down the esophagus, and into the stomach. A dilator is inserted through a gastrostomy tube and attached to the guidewire. Tension on the oral end of the wire pulls the dilator into the distal esophagus. The process is repeated until the esophagus is dilated to an acceptable size.

43458

The physician uses a balloon to dilate the esophagus which is constricted due to achalasia. In achalasia, the smooth muscles of the gastrointestinal tract fail to relax in response to normal stimulus. The physician uses a fluoroscope to place the balloon at the gastroesophageal junction. The balloon is inflated and deflated several times until the esophagus is dilated to an acceptable size. It is possible to use a guidewire to place the balloon.

43460

The physician inserts a multilumen tube into the esophagus through which a balloon is passed for the tamponade of bleeding esophageal varices. The balloon is inflated to exert pressure on the varices to stop bleeding. The balloon is left inflated so coagulation can occur before the physician proceeds with definitive treatment.

43496

The physician makes an abdominal incision to gain access to the omentum. The greater omentum is reflected to reveal the underlying small intestine. The jejunum is identified and removed. The remaining jejunum is reattached and the omentum is replaced. The free section of jejunum is transferred to another site with anastomosis of its vessels to another structure. Most commonly, the free transfer of a short segment of jejunum occurs between the pharynx and esophagus with microvascular anastomosis of jejunal vessels to the external carotid artery branches and the jugular vein. Portions of the pharynx and/or esophagus have already been resected with removal of cervical esophageal and hypopharyngeal carcinoma. Operative sites are sutured closed.

43500–43510

The physician performs a gastrostomy and explores gastric area, removes a foreign body or corrects a mucosal defect. The physician makes a midline epigastric incision and retracts the skin and underlying tissues laterally. The stomach is incised and explored. In 43500, a foreign body is removed. In 43501, a bleeding ulcer is identified and bleeding is controlled with electrocautery or ligation of vessels, and the mucosa is drawn over the ulcer and sutured. In 43502, an esophagogastric laceration is identified and bleeding is controlled with electrocautery or ligation of vessels, and the mucosa is drawn over the defect and sutured. In 43510, the physician introduces dilators into the esophagus from the stomach to increase the diameter of the esophagus. When dilation is complete, a stent is placed and secured with sutures to maintain to patency. After exploration or repair, the stomach is closed in sutured layers, the soft tissues are returned to anatomical position, and the operative incision is closed in sutured layers.

43520

The physician incises the pyloric muscle. The physician makes a small subcostal incision over the pyloric olive. The peritoneum is incised, the tissues are retracted, and the pylorus is identified. The serosa is incised and the tension of the pyloric muscle is released with longitudinal incisions. The peritoneum is sutured closed and the operative site is closed in sutured layers.

43600

The physician obtains a biopsy of the stomach through an endoscope, capsule or tube. The physician anesthetizes the oropharynx and sedates the patient. An endoscope, capsule or tube is passed into the stomach and the stomach mucosa is biopsied. The physician uses a capsule or tube for biopsy of a random location. An endoscope is used for biopsy of a specific lesion.

43605

The physician makes a midline abdominal incision. The peritoneum is incised and tissues are retracted to identify the anterior surface of the stomach. An incision is made in the stomach and the physician explores the mucosa to obtain biopsies. Once biopsies are acquired, the stomach incision is closed with sutures or staples. The peritoneum is sutured closed and the abdominal incision is closed using layered sutures.

43610

The physician performs a local excision of a tumor of the stomach. The physician makes a midline abdominal incision. Next, the stomach is dissected free of surrounding structures and the area of the tumor identified. The tumor is excised with a normal margin of stomach around the tumor. The defect created in the stomach is closed with sutures or a stapling device. The incision is closed.

43611

The physician performs a local excision of a tumor of the stomach. The physician makes a midline abdominal incision. Next, the stomach is dissected free of surrounding structures and the area of the

tumor identified. The tumor is excised with a normal margin of stomach around the tumor. The defect created in the stomach is closed with sutures or a stapling device. The incision is closed.

43620

The physician removes the stomach and approximates a limb of small bowel to the esophagus (Roux-en-Y esophagojejunostomy). The physician makes a midline abdominal incision. Next, the stomach is dissected free of surrounding structures and its blood supply is divided. The stomach is divided at the gastroesophageal junction and at the gastroduodenal junction and removed. The proximal jejunum is divided and the distal end of bowel is connected to the esophagus. The divided proximal jejunum is connected to the limb of small bowel distal to the esophageal anastomosis to restore intestinal continuity. The incisions are closed.

43621

The physician removes the stomach and approximates a limb of small bowel to the esophagus (Roux-en-Y esophagojejunostomy). The physician makes a midline abdominal incision. Next, the stomach is dissected free of surrounding structures and its blood supply is divided. The stomach is divided at the gastroesophageal junction and at the gastroduodenal junction then removed. The proximal jejunum is divided and the distal end of bowel is connected to the esophagus. The divided proximal jejunum is connected to the limb of small bowel distal to the esophageal anastomosis to restore intestinal continuity. The incisions are closed.

43622

The physician removes the stomach and forms a pouch of small bowel and approximates this to the esophagus. The physician makes a midline abdominal incision. Next, the stomach is dissected free of surrounding structures and its blood supply divided. The stomach is divided at the gastroesophageal junction and the gastroduodenal junction then removed. The proximal jejunum is divided and the distal end of bowel is folded upon itself and approximated in such a way to form a pouch. The pouch is connected to the esophagus. The divided proximal jejunum is connected to the limb of small bowel distal to the esophageal anastomosis to restore intestinal continuity. The incisions are closed.

43631

The physician removes the distal stomach and approximates the proximal stomach to the duodenum. The physician makes a midline abdominal incision. The distal stomach (antrum) is dissected free from surrounding structures and the blood supply to the antrum is divided. Next, the gastroduodenal junction is divided and the stomach is divided in its middle portion removing the antrum. An anastomosis is made between the proximal stomach and the duodenum with either staples or sutures. The incision is closed.

43632

The physician removes the distal stomach and approximates the proximal stomach to the jejunum. The physician makes a midline abdominal incision. The distal stomach (antrum) is dissected free from surrounding structures and the blood supply to the antrum is divided. Next, the gastroduedenal junction is divided and the stomach is divided in its middle portion removing the antrum. An anastomosis is made between the proximal stomach and the jejunum with either staples or sutures. The incision is closed.

43633

The physician removes the distal stomach (antrum) and performs an anastomosis between the proximal stomach and a Roux-en-Y limb of jejunum. The physician makes a midline abdominal incision. Next, the distal stomach is dissected free of surrounding structures and the blood supply to the antrum is divided. The gastroduodenal junction and the middle portion of the stomach are divided and the antrum is removed. The vagus nerves, as they pass from the esophagus onto the stomach, are usually divided. The proximal jejunum is divided and the distal limb of jejunum is connected to the proximal stomach. The proximal jejunum is connected to the limb of jejunum distal to the gastrojejunostomy to restore intestinal continuity. The incisions are closed.

43634

The physician removes the distal stomach (antrum) and performs an anastomosis between the stomach and a pouch formed of jejunum. The physician makes a midline abdominal incision. The distal stomach is dissected free of surrounding structures and the blood supply to the antrum is divided. The gastroduodenal junction and the middle portion of the stomach are divided and the antrum is removed. The vagus nerves, as they pass from the esophagus onto the stomach, are usually divided. The proximal jejunum is divided and the distal end is folded upon itself and approximated in such a way to form a pouch. The pouch is then connected to the proximal stomach and the proximal end of the divided jejunum is connected to the jejunal limb distal to the pouch anastomosis to establish intestinal continuity. The incision is closed.

43635

The physician performs this with a separately reportable partial distal gastrectomy and repairs the stomach and severs vagus nerves. The physician uses a midline abdominal approach. The distal stomach (antrum) is dissected free and the blood supply to the antrum divided. The distal stomach is removed and the proximal stomach is sutured to the duodenum. Truncal vagotomy is performed by severing both right and left vagus nerves just below the diaphragm. This

subsidary code is listed separately in addition to primary procedures 43631, 43632, 43633, and 43634.

43638

The physician removes the proximal stomach through an abdominal or chest incision and performs an anastomosis between the esophagus and distal stomach. The physician makes a midline abdominal incision or a left chest incision. The stomach and distal esophagus are dissected free of surrounding structures. The gastroesophageal junction and the middle portion of the stomach are divided and the proximal stomach is removed. During this process the vagus nerves are divided. The physician performs an anastomosis between the esophagus and the remaining distal stomach. The incision is closed.

43639

The physician removes the proximal stomach through an abdominal or chest incision and performs an anastomosis between the esophagus and distal stomach. The physician makes a midline abdominal incision or a left chest incision. The stomach and distal esophagus are dissected free of surrounding structures. The gastroesophageal junction and the middle portion of the stomach are divided and the proximal stomach is removed. During this process the vagus nerves are divided. The physician performs an anastomosis between the esophagus and the remaining distal stomach. The incision is closed.

43640–43641

The physician severs the vagus nerves and widens the pyloric canal, with or without making an incision in the stomach. The physician uses a midline upper abdominal incision to expose the muscular band surrounding the distal opening of the stomach. A longitudinal incision is made in the pylorus. The incision is closed with a single full thickness suture layer. The two branches of the vagus nerve are exposed and a truncal vagotomy is performed by severing both right and left vagus nerves. A gastrostomy may be created by inserting a tube from the stomach to the external surface of the abdominal wall. Report 43641 if performed with a parietal cell procedure.

43651

The physician performs laparoscopic truncal vagotomy. The physician places a trocar through an incision above the umbilicus and insufflates the abdominal cavity. The laparoscope is placed through the supraumbilical port and additional troacars are placed into the abdominal cavity. The fascial anterior to the esophagus is incised and the distal esophagus is mobilized. The anterior and posterior vagal nerve trunks are identified and divided. The physician removes a small segment of each nerve. The trocars are removed and the incisions are closed.

43652

The physician performs laparoscopic selective or highly selective vagotomy. The physician places a trocar though an incision above the umbilicus and insufflates the abdominal cavity. The laparoscope is placed through the supraumbilical port and additional trocars are placed into the abdominal cavity. The distal esophagus is mobilized and the anterior and posterior vagal nerve trunks are identified. The main nerve trunks are followed down onto the stomach and the branches from the nerves to the proximal half of the stomach are divided. The trocars are removed and the incisions are closed.

43653

Using a laparoscope, the physician constructs a temporary or permanent gastrostomy for feeding. With the patient under anesthesia, the physician places a trocar at the umbilicus into the abdomen and insufflates the abdominal cavity. The physician places a laparoscope through the umbilical incision. An additional trocar is inserted through the abdominal wall into the intra-abdominal cavity at a previously determined site where the gastrostomy will reside. The gastrostomy tube is pulled through the trocar from outside the abdomen into the intra-abdominal cavity. The physician identifies the stomach and introduces instruments to open the organ and create a viable receptacle for the tube. The tip of the gastrostomy tube is inserted into the stomach, and the tube is clamped off on the outside of the body and sutured into place on the stomach. Additional sutures are placed in the abdominal wall to hold the gastrostomy tube in place and to secure the tube. The trocars are removed and the incisions are close with stapes or sutures.

43750

The physician places a gastrostomy tube into the stomach. A small incision is made through the skin and fascia. A large bore needle with a suture attached is passed through the incision into the lumen of the stomach. The needle is snared and the needle and suture are removed via the mouth. The gastrostomy tube is connected to the suture and passed through the mouth into the stomach and out the abdominal wall. The gastrostomy tube is sutured to the skin.

43752

The physician places a naso- or oro-gastric tube. In nasogastric tube placement the patient is placed in an upright position. The physician checks the nostrils for obstruction and selects the nostril for the tube insertion. The physician may swab the nostril and spray the oropharynx with medication to numb the nasal passage and suppress the gag reflex. Next, the physician lubricates the tube, the tip of the nose is elevated, and the nasogastric tube is introduced into the nostril. The tube is advanced and the position of the tube is checked to ensure it is aligned to enter the oropharynx. As the patient swallows the physician advances the tube through the pharynx, esophagus, and into the stomach. A separately reportable x-ray may be taken. Air is injected into the tube (at the nose) while the physician listens with a stethoscope positioned at the stomach for the air to come out of the tube. Gastric contents are aspirated. These precautions are performed to ensure the tube is positioned in the stomach. The nasogastric tube is taped to the nostril. If the tube is fitted with a balloon (at the end of the tube in the stomach), it is inflated to hold the tube in place.

43760

The physician changes a gastrostomy tube. If the old gastrostomy tube has been placed endoscopically, the physician must remove it by snaring it and pulling it out through the mouth. A new tube can be placed either percutaneously through the abdominal wall via the existing tract or endoscopically. A small incision is made through the skin and fascia. A large bore needle with suture attached is passed through the incision into the lumen of the stomach. The needle is snared and the needle and suture are removed via the mouth. The gastrostomy tube is connected to the suture and passed through the mouth into the stomach and out the abdominal wall. The gastrostomy tube is sutured to the skin.

43761

The physician repositions a gastric feeding tube through the duodenum for enteric nutrition. Under separately reportable fluoroscopic guidance, the physician passes the gastric feeding tube through the stomach into the distal duodenum.

43800

The physician repairs the pylorus. The physician makes an upper abdominal incision through skin, fascia, and muscles to expose the pylorus, a muscular band surrounding the distal opening of the stomach. A longitudinal incision is made in the pylorus. The incision is closed with a single full thickness suture layer.

43810

The physician performs a gastrodueodenostomy. The physician uses an upper midline epigastric incision through fascia and muscle. The distal end of the greater curvature of the stomach is removed. The duodenum is mobilized and connected to the greater curvature. The anastomosis is closed with interrupted stitches and the abdominal incision is closed.

43820–43825

The physician performs a gastrojejunostomy to create a direct passage between the stomach and jejunum. The physician makes an upper abdominal incision to expose the stomach and small intestine. The distal portion of the stomach is resected and the jejunum is anastomosed to the gastric stump. The duodenal stump is closed. The vagal nerves are preserved. Report 43825 if a vagotomy is also performed.

43830–43831

The physician constructs a temporary or permanent gastrostomy for instillation of nutrients. After making a midline incision in the upper abdomen, the physician chooses a gastrostomy site on the middle anterior surface of the stomach. Stay sutures are placed and a small stab wound is made between purse string sutures. A gastrostomy tube is inserted and the purse string sutures are tied. The gastrostomy tube is withdrawn through a stab wound in the abdominal wall and stay sutures are placed in the posterior fascia. The abdominal incision is closed. Report 43831 if performed to facilitate feeding a neonate.

43832

The physician constructs a permanent gastrostomy for instillation of nutrients. After a small midline upper abdominal incision, the physician creates a flap with its base at the greater curvature of the stomach. The flap is converted into a tube by closure of the stomach incision. The tube is brought through the skin surface via a stab wound or tunnel. The end of the tube is everted slightly and sutured to the skin. The abdominal incision is closed with sutures.

43840

The physician repairs an ulcer, wound, or injury to the stomach or duodenum. The ulcer or wound is exposed by the physician via a midline upper abdominal incision or a transverse supraumbilical incision through skin, fascia, and muscle. The perforation is sutured closed and the peritoneal cavity is irrigated and suctioned to remove contamination. The abdominal fascia and peritoneum are closed in one layer. The skin and subcutaneous layers are not closed unless the perforation is less than two hours old.

43842–43843

The physician alters the stomach's size to help stem morbid obesity. The physician exposes the lesser curvature of the stomach via a midline abdominal incision through skin, fascia, and muscles. In 43842, double row of staples is placed in the upper portion of the stomach to create a small stoma. A small strip of mesh or a Silastic ring is wrapped around the stoma and stapled to itself. Report 43843 if the technique used is other than the vertical-banded gastroplasty, and allows for staples restricting other parts of the stomach.

43846

The physician partitions the stomach and performs a small bowel anastomosis to the proximal stomach (Roux-en-Y gastrojejunostomy) in order to bypass the majority of the stomach. The physician makes a midline abdominal incision. Next, the stomach is mobilized and the proximal stomach is divided with a

stapling device leaving only a small proximal pouch in continuity with the esophagus. The proximal small bowel is divided and the distal limb of divided bowel is connected to the proximal gastric pouch. The proximal end of the divided bowel is connected to the bowel limb distal to the gastric anastomosis to restore intestinal continuity. The incision is closed.

43847

The physician partitions the stomach and performs a small intestine anastomosis to the proximal stomach (Roux-en-Y gastrojejunostomy) in order to bypass the majority of the stomach. The physician makes a midline abdominal incision. Next, the stomach is mobilized and the proximal stomach is divided with a stapling device leaving only a small proximal pouch in continuity with the esophagus. The small intestine is reconstructed so that it is partially bypassed to limit the amount of area available for absorption of nutrients. The incision is closed.

43848

The physician reapproximates a previously partitioned stomach in order to restore normal gastrointestinal continuity. The physician makes a midline abdominal incision. Next, the stomach and previous anastomoses are dissected free of surrounding structures. The gastrojejunostomy is taken down and the previously divided stomach is reapproximated. The limb of jejunum from the gastrojejunostomy is reapproximated to the small bowel to restore normal intestinal continuity. The incision is closed.

43850–43855

The physician revises and constructs an anastomoses between the stomach and the duodenum. The physician exposes the stomach and small intestine via a midline upper abdominal incision through skin, muscles, and fascia. The connection between the stomach and duodenum (gastroduodenostomy) is severed and the duodenal stump is closed. An 8.0 cm to 10.0 cm segment of the jejunum is reversed and anastomosed to the distal end of the stomach. The excised duodenum and segment of jejunum are connected to the jejunum. The abdominal incision is closed. Report 43855 if a vagotomy is performed in conjunction with this procedure.

43860–43865

The physician revises an anastomoses between the stomach and the jejunum. The physician exposes the stomach and small intestine via a midline upper abdominal incision through skin, muscles, and fascia. About 8.0 cm to 10.0 cm of the jejunum limb is divided, reversed and connected to the distal end of the stomach. The short reversed segment is connected to the jejunum and the remnant of jejunum and duodenum are anastomosed to the long segment of jejunum. A partial gastrectomy or intestine resection may be performed. The abdominal incision is closed.

Report 43865 if a vagotomy is performed in conjunction with this procedure.

43870

The physician closes a gastrostomy no longer needed. The physician enters through previous gastrostomy. The stomach is dissected free of the abdominal wall. The stomach gastrostomy site is closed with sutures. The abdominal incision is closed with layered sutures.

43880

The physician closes a gastrocolic fistula. The physician exposes stomach and colon via a midline abdominal incision through skin, fascia, and muscle. The fistula is excised and the bowel mobilized. The fistula is located and resected. The abdominal incision is closed.

44005

The physician frees intestinal adhesions. The physician enters the abdomen through a midline abdominal incision. The bowel is freed from its attachments to itself, the abdominal wall and/or other abdominal organs. The abdominal incision is closed.

44010

The physician opens the duodenum, explores the segment, collects tissue samples for biopsy, or removes a foreign body. The physician exposes the proximal duodenum via a midline upper abdominal incision through skin, fascia, and muscles. The duodenum is incised in a longitudinal fashion and the area of concern is exposed. The physician may choose during exploration to excise tissues, biopsy, or remove foreign bodies. The duodenum is closed with transverse interrupted sutures. The abdominal incision is closed.

44015

The physician places a tube in the jejunum for feeding during a separately reportable operation. The physician makes an abdominal incision. A section of proximal jejunum is selected and a tube is placed in the jejunum and brought out through the abdominal wall. This segment of jejunum is securely tacked to the inside of the abdominal wall. The incision is closed.

44020

The physician makes an incision in the small intestine (enterotomy) for biopsy, exploration or foreign body removal. The physician makes an abdominal incision. Next, the selected segment of small intestine is mobilized and incised to expose the area of interest. A biopsy is taken or a foreign body is removed. The enterotomy is closed with staples or sutures. The abdominal incision is closed.

44021

The physician places a tube in the small bowel for decompression. The physician makes an abdominal

incision. Next, the small bowel is dissected free of surrounding structures. The proximal small bowel is incised (enterotomy) and a tube is threaded through the small bowel. The proximal end of the tube is brought out through the abdominal wall. The bowel is tacked to the inside of the abdominal wall where the tube goes through. The abdominal incision is closed.

44025

The physician makes an incision in the colon (colotomy) through which the colon is explored for biopsy or foreign body removal. The physician makes an abdominal incision. Next, the selected segment of colon is mobilized and a colotomy is made in the area of interest. The colon is explored and biopsy performed or foreign body removed. The colotomy is closed with staples or sutures. The abdominal incision is closed.

44050–44055

The physician reduces a volvulus, intussusception or internal hernia through an abdominal incision. The physician makes an abdominal incision. Next, the abdomen is explored and the twisted segment of bowel (volvulus), telescoped segment of bowel (intussusception) or internal hernia is manually reduced. The bowel is inspected to insure viability. The incision is closed. Report 44055 if the problem is corrected by lysis of duodenal bands or reduction of midgut volvulus.

44100

The physician performs a peroral biopsy of the small intestine with a capsule. The physician places a biopsy capsule attached to a tube through the mouth and directs it into the small intestine usually with fluoroscopy. The capsule blade is fired by placing suction on the tube and a biopsy obtained. The tube and capsule are withdrawn.

44110

The physician removes one or more lesions in the small or large intestine through an incision in the colon (colotomy) or small intestine (enterotomy) without bowel resection. The physician makes an abdominal incision. Next, the segment of small intestine or colon containing the lesions is mobilized. An incision is made in the small intestine or colon and the lesions are removed. The enterotomy or colotomy is closed with staples or sutures. The abdominal incision is closed.

44111

The physician removes one or more lesions in the small or large intestine through multiple incisions in the colon (colotomy) or small intestine (enterotomy) without bowel resection. The physician makes an abdominal incision. Next, the segments of small intestine or colon containing lesions are mobilized. Incisions are made in the small intestine or colon and the lesions are removed. The enterotomies or

CPT® Lay Descriptions

colotomies are closed with staples or sutures. The abdominal incision is closed.

44120

The physician resects a segment of small intestine and performs an anastomosis between the remaining bowel ends. The physician makes an abdominal incision. Next, the selected segment of small bowel is isolated and divided proximally and distally to the remaining bowel and removed. The remaining bowel ends are reapproximated using either staples or sutures. The incision is closed.

44121

The physician resects one or more segments of small bowel and performs an anastomosis between the remaining bowel ends. The physician makes an abdominal incision. Next, the selected segments of small bowel are isolated and divided proximally and distally to the remaining bowel and removed. The remaining bowel ends are reapproximated using either staples or sutures. The incision is closed.

44125

The physician resects a segment of small bowel and brings the proximal end of bowel through the abdominal wall onto the skin as a stoma. The physician makes an abdominal incision. Next, the selected segment of small bowel is isolated and divided proximally and distally to the remaining bowel and removed. The proximal end of the remaining small bowel is brought through a separate incision in the abdominal wall onto the skin as a stoma. The initial incision is closed.

44126–44128

The physician resects a segment of small intestine and may perform tapering to fit the area of anastomosis. The physician makes an abdominal incision. The selected segment of small intestine is isolated and divided proximally and distally to the remaining bowel and removed. An end-to-end anastomosis of the proximal rectum to the distal and canal is performed. The remaining bowel ends are reapproximated using either staples or sutures. The incision is closed. Report 44126 for a single resection and anastomosis. Report 44127 when tapering (gradually narrowing toward one end) of the bowel is performed with the resection and anastomosis. Report 44128 for each additional resection and anastomosis beyond the first one.

44130

The physician performs a small bowel anastomosis and may bring one end of small bowel through the abdominal wall onto the skin as a stoma. The physician makes an abdominal incision. A segment of small bowel may be resected. Next, a small bowel anastomosis is performed with either staples or sutures. An end or loop of small bowel may be brought through a separate incision in the abdominal

wall onto the skin as a stoma. The initial incision is closed.

44132–44133

The physician performs a donor enterectomy. The cadaver or living donor is placed supine on the operating room table. After adequate preparation, the physician performs a midline abdominal incision, tissue is incised, and muscles are separated down to the level of the small intestine. In 44132 the small intestine is mobilized and excised. In 44133 a portion of the small intestine is excised and the bowel is anastomosed. Any bleeding is controlled, the area is irrigated, and the incision is closed with layered sutures. A sterile dressing is applied. In both procedures the intestinal allograft is placed in a prepared solution, where it is maintained until needed for a separately reportable intestinal allotransplantation.

44135–44136

The physician performs an intestinal allotransplantation. The patient is placed supine on the operating room table. After adequate preparation, the physician performs a midline abdominal incision, tissue is incised, and muscles are separated down to the level of the small intestine. The area of small intestine to be transplanted is located. An incision is made through the intestine, the area is examined, and the free intestinal edges are debrided or excised in order to accept the intestinal transplant. The previously excised small intestinal allograft, from a cadaver (44135) or partially excised small intestinal allograft, from a living donor (44136) are removed from the maintenance solution, and irrigated. The allograft is sized and is anastomosed first to one free end of the patient's small intestine and then the opposite end of the patient's small intestine. Any bleeding is controlled, the area is irrigated, and the small bowel is anatomically positioned in the abdominal cavity. The wound is closed with layered sutures over a drain. A sterile dressing is applied.

44139

The physician mobilizes the splenic flexure in conjunction with a partial colon resection. The physician makes an abdominal incision. The attachments between the splenic flexure of the colon and the lateral abdominal wall and spleen are dissected free and taken down to mobilize the colon. This is done to mobilize adequate length of colon in conjunction with a partial colon resection. At the completion of the procedure the abdominal incision is closed.

44140

The physician resects a segment of colon and performs an anastomosis between the remaining ends of colon. The physician makes an abdominal incision. Next, the selected segment of colon is isolated and divided proximally and distally to the remaining colon and removed. The remaining ends of colon are reapproximated with either staples or sutures. The incision is closed.

44141

The physician resects a segment of colon and brings the proximal end of colon through the abdominal wall onto the skin as a colostomy. The physician makes an abdominal incision. Next, the selected segment of colon is isolated and divided proximally and distally to the remaining colon and removed. The proximal end of colon is brought through a separate incision on the abdominal wall and onto the skin as a colostomy. Alternately, the remaining bowel ends may be reapproximated and a loop of colon proximal to the anastomosis brought through a separate incision on the abdominal wall onto the skin as a loop colostomy. The initial incision is closed.

44143

The physician resects a segment of colon and brings the proximal end of colon through the abdominal wall onto the skin as a colostomy. The physician makes an abdominal incision. Next, the selected segment of colon is isolated and divided proximally and distally to the remaining colon and removed. The proximal end of colon is brought through a separate incision on the abdominal wall onto the skin as a colostomy. The distal end of colon is closed with staples or sutures and left in the abdomen. The initial incision is closed.

44144

The physician resects a segment of colon. The proximal and distal ends of colon are brought through the abdominal wall onto the skin as a colostomy and mucus fistula. The physician makes an abdominal incision. Next, the selected segment of colon is isolated and divided proximally and distally to the remaining colon and removed. The proximal end of colon or terminal ileum and the distal end of colon are brought through separate incisions on the abdominal wall onto the skin as an ileostomy or colostomy and mucus fistula. The initial abdominal incision is closed.

44145

The physician resects a segment of distal colon or rectum and performs a low colorectal anastomosis in the pelvis. The physician makes an abdominal incision. Next, the distal colon and rectum are mobilized and the selected segment divided proximally and distally to the remaining colon. An anastomosis is created between the proximal colon and remaining rectum in the pelvis with either staples or sutures. The incision is closed.

44146

The physician resects a segment of distal colon or rectum and performs a low colorectal anastomosis in the pelvis and creates a proximal colostomy. The physician makes an abdominal incision. Next, the

distal colon and rectum are mobilized and the selected segment divided proximally and distally to the remaining colon. An anastomosis is created between the proximal colon and remaining rectum in the pelvis with either staples or sutures. A loop or end of colon proximal to the anastomosis is brought out through a separate incision in the abdominal wall onto the skin as a colostomy to divert the fecal stream. The initial incision is closed.

44147

The physician removes a segment of colon and rectum through a combined abdominal and perineal approach with a proximal colostomy or coloanal anastomosis. The physician makes an abdominal incision. The distal colon and rectum are mobilized. The colon is divided above the pelvic brim and the rectum is divided distally. The distal rectum and anus may be resected from a perineal approach and a proximal colostomy formed. The distal end of colon may be brought down and approximated to the anus with sutures or staples. The abdominal incision is closed.

44150

The physician removes the entire colon and performs an ileostomy or an anastomosis between the ileum and rectum. The physician makes an abdominal incision. Next, the entire colon is mobilized and the colorectal junction and terminal ileum is divided. The colon is removed. The terminal ileum is approximated to the rectum or brought out through a separate incision on the abdominal wall onto the skin as an ileostomy. The initial incision is closed.

44151

The physician removes the entire colon and creates a reservoir of distal ileum (Kock pouch). The reservoir is brought out through the abdominal wall as a continent stoma. The physician makes an abdominal incision. Next, the entire colon is mobilized. The colorectal junction and terminal ileum is divided and the colon removed. The distal ileum is folded upon itself and approximated to form a pouch and valve. The distal end of the pouch is brought through a separate incision on the abdominal wall onto the skin an a continent ileostomy. The initial incision is closed.

44152

The physician removes the entire colon and proximal rectum, strips the mucosa from the distal rectum and performs an anastomosis between the terminal ileum and anus. The physician makes an abdominal incision. Next, the entire colon and rectum are mobilized. The terminal ileum and proximal rectum are divided and the colon is removed. The mucosa of the distal rectum is stripped from a perineal approach. The terminal ileum is pulled through the remaining muscular cuff of the rectum and approximated to the anus with sutures. A loop of ileum may be brought out through the abdominal wall onto the skin as an ileostomy proximal to the anastomosis. The initial incision is closed.

44153

The physician removes the entire colon and proximal rectum, strips the mucosa from the distal rectum and performs an anastomosis between a created pouch of ileum and the anus. The physician makes an abdominal incision. Next, the entire colon and rectum are mobilized. The terminal ileum and proximal rectum are divided and the colon is removed. The mucosa of the distal rectum is stripped from a perineal approach. The terminal ileum is folded upon itself and approximated in order to form a pouch. The pouch is pulled through the remaining muscular tube of the rectum and approximated to the anus with sutures. A loop of ileum may be brought out through a separate incision on the abdominal wall onto the skin as an ileostomy proximal to the anastomosis. The initial incision is closed.

44155

The physician removes the entire colon and rectum and brings the terminal ileum out through the abdominal wall onto the skin as an ileostomy. The physician makes an abdominal incision. Next, the entire colon and rectum are mobilized, the proximal rectum and distal ileum are divided, and the colon and proximal rectum are removed. The distal rectum is mobilized and removed through a perineal approach. The terminal ileum is brought out through a separate incision on the abdominal wall onto the skin as an ileostomy. The abdominal and perineal incisions are closed.

44156

The physician removes the entire colon and rectum and creates a pouch from the terminal ileum (Kock pouch) that is brought out through the abdominal wall as a continent ileostomy. The physician makes an abdominal incision. Next, the entire colon and rectum are mobilized, the proximal rectum and distal ileum are divided, and the colon and proximal rectum are removed. The distal rectum is mobilized and removed through a perineal approach. The terminal ileum is folded upon itself and approximated to form a pouch with a valve. The end of the pouch is brought out through a separate abdominal incision onto the skin as a continent ileostomy. The abdominal and perineal incisions are closed.

44160

The physician makes an abdominal incision and removes a segment of the colon and terminal ileum and performs an anastomosis between the remaining ileum and colon. The physician makes an abdominal incision. Next, the selected segment of colon and terminal ileum are isolated and divided proximal and distal to the remaining bowel and removed. An anastomosis is created between the distal ileum and

remaining colon with staples or sutures. The incision is closed.

44200

The physician performs laparoscopic enterolysis to free intestinal adhesions. With the patient under anesthesia, the physician places a trocar at the umbilicus into the abdominal or retroperitoneal space and insufflates the abdominal cavity. The physician places a laparoscope through the umbilical incision and additional trocars are placed into the abdomen. Intestinal adhesions are identified and instruments are passed through to dissect and remove the adhesions. The trocars are removed and the incisions are closed with sutures.

44201

The physician constructs a jejunostomy using a laparoscope. With the patient under anesthesia, the physician places a trocar at the umbilicus into the abdomen and insufflates the abdominal cavity. The physician places a laparoscope through the umbilical incision and additional trocars are placed into the peritoneal or space. Additional instruments are introduced through the trocars. The physician identifies the jejunum and resects it, re-routing it to an opening created in the skin. An ostomy is created in the skin. The trocars are removed and the incisions are closed with sutures.

44202–44203

With the patient under general anesthesia, a urinary catheter is inserted and the patient is placed in a supine or Trendelenburg position on the operating table. A 15-mmHg carbon dioxide pneumoperitoneum is established with a laparoscopic port placed through the umbilicus using a direct open technique; the laparoscope is positioned in the abdominal cavity and a diagnostic laparoscopy is performed. The remaining laparoscopic ports are placed under direct vision. The transverse colon is located and maintained in upward traction. The ligament of Treitz is identified and the small intestine is run. The section of small intestine is marked and suspended with traction sutures through the mesentery. The peritoneum overlying the mesentery is scored and segment of bowel marked for resection is devascularized. The bowel is divided proximal and distal to the segment with a stapler. The segment is brought out through an enlarged trocar site. The divided bowel ends are anastomosed with staples and inspected. The mesentery is closed with interrupted sutures. The trocars and laparoscope are removed and the incisions are closed with sutures. Report 44203 for each additional small intestine resection and anastomosis beyond the first.

44204–44205

With the patient under general anesthesia, a urinary catheter is inserted and the patient is placed supine or in a Trendelenburg position on the operating table. A 15-mmHg carbon dioxide pneumoperitoneum is established with a laparoscopic port placed through the umbilicus using a direct open technique; the laparoscope is positioned in the abdominal cavity and a diagnostic laparoscopy is performed. The remaining laparoscopic ports are placed under direct vision. The physician incises peritoneum along both sides to mobilize the colon. The greater omentum and colon are separated by incision to mobilize the hepatic and splenic flexures. The colon is mobilized centrally onto its mesentery and the mesenteric vessels are divided intracorporeally using titanium clips. The colon is divided with an endoscopic stapler, and the specimen is removed through an enlarged trocar site. If the procedure is being performed for malignancy, a wound protector is used. In 44204, the divided bowel ends are anastomosed and inspected. In 44205, for the ileocolostomy with removal of terminal ileum, the abdomen is deflated and the laparoscope and trocar incisions are closed. The segment of terminal ileum and cecum is removed and an anastomosis is done between the remaining ileum and colon and brought out through the trocar site to an opening created in the skin. The abdomen is deflated and the laparoscope and trocar incisions are closed.

44300

The physician places a tube in the small bowel for feeding or the cecum for decompression. The physician makes an abdominal incision. Next, a segment of proximal small bowel or the cecum is isolated. A tube is placed into the small bowel or cecum and brought out through the abdominal wall. The incision is closed.

44310

The physician brings a loop or end of jejunum or ileum through the abdominal wall onto the skin as a stoma. The physician makes an abdominal incision. Next, the selected segment of jejunum or ileum is isolated. A loop or end of the selected segment of bowel is brought through a separate incision on the abdominal wall onto the skin as a stoma. The initial incision is closed.

44312

The physician revises an ileostomy through an incision around the stoma with release of scar tissue. The physician makes and incision around the ileostomy site. Next, the stoma is dissected free of the surrounding abdominal wall and constricting scar tissue is released. The stoma is reapproximated to the skin or the distal end of the stoma may be transected. Additional ileum may be pulled through the abdominal wall and approximated to the skin as a revised ileostomy.

44314

The physician revises an ileostomy by forming a new stoma site. The physician makes an abdominal incision. Next, the previous ileostomy is completely taken down. The distal ileum is brought through a new incision on the abdominal wall onto the skin as an ileostomy at a new site. The initial incision and former stoma site are closed.

44316

The physician forms a reservoir of distal ileum (Kock pouch) and brings it through the abdominal wall onto the skin as a continent ileostomy. The physician makes an abdominal incision. Next, the distal ileum is folded upon itself and approximated in such a way to form a pouch with a valve. The end of the pouch is brought through a separate incision on the abdominal wall onto the skin as a continent ileostomy. The initial incision is closed.

44320

The physician brings a loop, end of colon, or cecum through the abdominal wall onto the skin as a stoma. The physician makes an abdominal incision. Next, the selected segment of colon or cecum is isolated. A loop, end of colon, or cecum is brought through a separate incision on the abdominal wall onto the skin as a stoma (cecostomy or colostomy). The initial incision is closed.

44322

The physician performs multiple biopsies of the colon wall and brings a loop of colon or cecum through the abdominal wall onto the skin as a stoma. The physician makes an abdominal incision. Next, multiple biopsies are obtained along the length of the colon wall. A loop of colon or cecum is brought through a separate incision on the abdominal wall onto the skin as a stoma (colostomy or cecostomy). The initial incision is closed.

44340

The physician revises a colostomy through an incision around the stoma site with release of scar tissue. The physician makes an incision around the stoma site. Next, the stoma is dissected free of the surrounding abdominal wall and constricting scar tissue is released. The stoma is reapproximated to the skin or the distal stoma is transected and additional colon pulled through the abdominal wall and approximated to the skin as a revised colostomy.

44345

The physician revises a colostomy by forming a new stoma site. The physician makes an abdominal incision. Next, the previous colostomy is completely taken down. The distal end of colon is brought through a separate incision on the abdominal wall onto the skin at a new site as a revised colostomy The initial incision and previous stoma site are closed.

44346

The physician performs a colostomy revision and repairs a paracolostomy hernia. The physician makes an abdominal incision. Next, the previous colostomy site is taken down. The hernia at the former colostomy site is repaired. The end of colon is brought through a separate incision on the abdominal wall at a new site and onto the skin as a revised colostomy. The initial incision and previous stoma site are closed.

44360

The physician performs endoscopy of the proximal small bowel and may obtain brushings or washings. The physician places an endoscope through the mouth and advances it into the small intestine. An abdominal incision may be made to mobilize the small bowel and assist in running the bowel over the endoscope. The lumen of the small bowel is examined and brushings or washings may be obtained of suspicious areas. The endoscope is withdrawn at the completion of the procedure. If an incision was made, it is closed.

44361

The physician performs endoscopy of the proximal small bowel and obtains biopsies. The physician places an endoscope through the mouth and advances it into the small intestine. An abdominal incision may be made to mobilize the small bowel and assist in running the bowel over the endoscope. The lumen of the small bowel is examined and biopsies are obtained of suspicious areas. The endoscope is withdrawn at the completion of the procedure. If an incision was made, it is closed.

44363

The physician performs endoscopy of the proximal small bowel and removes a foreign body. The physician places an endoscope through the mouth and advances it into the small intestine, An abdominal incision may be made to mobilize the small bowel and assist in running the bowel over the endoscope. The bowel lumen is examined and the foreign body located. A snare or forceps is advanced through the endoscope and the foreign body grasped and removed. The endoscope is withdrawn at the completion of the procedure. If an incision was made, it is closed.

44364

The physician performs endoscopy of the proximal small bowel and removes a tumor or polyp by snare technique. The physician places an endoscope through the mouth and advances it into the small intestine. An abdominal incision may be made to mobilize the small bowel and assist in running the bowel over the endoscope. The bowel lumen is examined and the polyp or tumor is located and removed with a snare placed through the endoscope. The endoscope is withdrawn at the completion of the procedure. If an incision was made it is closed.

44365

The physician performs endoscopy of the proximal small bowel and removes a tumor or polyp with hot biopsy forceps or cautery. The physician places an endoscope through the mouth and advances it into the small intestine. An abdominal incision may be made to mobilize the small bowel and assist in running the bowel over the endoscope. The bowel lumen is examined and the polyp or tumor is located and removed with hot biopsy forceps or cautery placed through the endoscope. The endoscope is withdrawn at the completion of the procedure. If an incision was made, it is closed.

44366

The physician performs endoscopy of the proximal small bowel and controls an area of bleeding. The physician places an endoscope through the mouth and advances it into the small intestine. An abdominal incision may be made to mobilize the small bowel and assist in running the bowel over the endoscope. The bowel lumen is examined and the area of bleeding is identified and controlled. The endoscope is withdrawn at the completion of the procedure. If an incision was made, it is closed.

44369

The physician performs endoscopy of the proximal small bowel and ablates a tumor or polyp or other lesion. The physician places an endoscope through the mouth and advances it into the small intestine. An abdominal incision may be made to mobilize the small bowel and assist in running the bowel over the endoscope. The bowel lumen is examined and the tumor, polyp, or other lesion is identified and ablated. The endoscope is withdrawn at the completion of the procedure. If an incision was made it is closed.

44370

The physician uses an endoscope to examine the proximal small intestine and performs a transendoscopic placement of a stent in the small intestine. The physician places an endoscope through the mouth and advances it into the small intestine. The lumen of the entire small intestine is visualized. The endoscope is placed at the site of an obstruction or stricture, the necessary stent length is determined and predilation of the obstruction or stenosis may be performed. The stent (endoprosthesis) is introduced into the site of the obstruction. Using a commercial delivery system ,a plastic covering over the stent is removed and the stent self-deploys, shoring-up the walls at a specific site in the small intestine beyond the second portion of duodenum, not including the ileum. When necessary, a balloon catheter is placed into the stent and gently inflated to more fully deploy the stent. The delivery system and endoscope are removed.

44372

The physician performs endoscopy of the proximal small bowel and places a percutaneous jejunostomy tube. The physician places an endoscope through the mouth and advances it into the small intestine. The bowel lumen is visualized and transilluminated through the abdominal skin. A needle is placed through the skin into the lumen of the jejunum under visualization of the endoscope. A wire is threaded through the needle into the bowel lumen. The needle is removed. A jejunostomy tube is placed over the wire, through the skin, into the jejunum, and secured into place. The endoscope is withdrawn.

44373

The physician performs endoscopy of the proximal small bowel and converts a percutaneous gastrostomy tube to a percutaneous jejunostomy tube. The physician places an endoscope through the mouth and advances it into the stomach. A jejunostomy tube is advanced through the previously placed gastrostomy tube. The jejunostomy tube is grasped with a snare or forceps placed through the endoscope and advanced with the endoscope into the proximal jejunum. The endoscope is withdrawn.

44376

The physician performs endoscopy of the entire small bowel and may obtain brushings or washings. The physician places the endoscope through the mouth and advances it into the small intestine. An abdominal incision may be made to mobilize the small bowel and assist in running the bowel over the endoscope. The lumen of the entire small bowel is visualized and brushings or washings may be obtained. The endoscope is withdrawn at the completion of the procedure. If an incision was made, it is closed.

44377

The physician performs endoscopy of the entire small bowel and performs biopsies. The physician places the endoscope through the mouth and advances it into the small intestine. An abdominal incision may be made to mobilize the small bowel and assist in running the bowel over the endoscope. The lumen of the entire small bowel is visualized and biopsies are performed. The endoscope is withdrawn at the completion of the procedure. If an incision was made, it is closed.

44378

The physician performs endoscopy of the small intestine, which may include the ileum, and controls an area of bleeding. The physician places the endoscope into the mouth and advances it into the small intestine. The lumen of the small intestine is visualized and any area of bleeding is controlled using various methods, such as cautery, injection, or laser. In some cases, a separately reportable abdominal incision is made to mobilize the small bowel and assist in running the bowel over the endoscope. The endoscope is withdrawn at the completion of the procedure.

44379

The physician uses an endoscope to examine the entire small intestine and performs transendoscopic placement of a stent in the small intestine. The physician performs endoscopy of the entire small bowel and places a transendoscopic stent. The physician places an endoscope through the mouth and advances it into the small intestine. The lumen of the entire small intestine is visualized. The endoscope is placed at the site of an obstruction or stricture and the necessary stent length is determined. The stent (endoprosthesis) is introduced into the site of the obstruction. Using a commercial delivery system, a plastic covering over the stent is removed and the stent self-deploys, shoring-up the walls at a specific site in the small intestine beyond the second portion of the duodenum, including the ileum. When necessary, a balloon catheter is placed into the stent and gently inflated to more fully deploy the stent. The delivery system and endoscope are removed.

44380

The physician performs endoscopy through an ileostomy and may obtain brushings or washings. The physician places the endoscope through the ileostomy and advances the endoscope into the small intestine. The small bowel lumen is visualized and brushings or washings may be obtained. The endoscope is withdrawn at the completion of the procedure.

44382

The physician performs endoscopy through an ileostomy and obtains material for biopsies. The physician places the endoscope through the ileostomy and advances the endoscope into the small intestine. The small bowel lumen is visualized and biopsies are obtained. The endoscope is withdrawn at the completion of the procedure.

44383

The physician uses an endoscope through an ileostomy to view the ileum and places a transendoscopic stent. The physician places an endoscope through the mouth and advances it into the small intestine. The lumen of the entire ileum is visualized The endoscope is removed. The endoscope is placed at the site of an obstruction or stricture and the necessary stent length is determined. The stent (endoprosthesis) is introduced into the site of the obstruction. Using a commercial delivery system, a plastic covering over the stent is removed and the stent self-deploys, shoring-up the walls at a specific site in the ileum. When necessary, a balloon catheter is placed into the stent and gently inflated to more fully deploy the stent. The delivery system and endoscope are removed.

44385

The physician performs endoscopy of an intestinal pouch and may obtain brushings or washings. The physician places the endoscope into the pouch,

CPT® Lay Descriptions

through the anus, or abdominal wall stoma. The lumen of the pouch is visualized and brushings or washings may be obtained. The endoscope is removed at the completion of the procedure.

44386

The physician performs endoscopy of an intestinal pouch and obtains biopsies. The physician places the endoscope into the pouch through the anus or abdominal wall stoma. The lumen of the pouch is visualized and biopsies are obtained. The endoscope is removed at the completion of the procedure.

44388

The physician performs colonoscopy through an abdominal wall colostomy and may obtain brushings or washings. The physician places the endoscope through the colostomy and advances the endoscope through the colon. The lumen of the colon is visualized and brushings or washings may be obtained. The endoscope is withdrawn at the completion of the procedure.

44389

The physician performs colonoscopy through an abdominal wall colostomy and obtains biopsies. The physician places the endoscope through the colostomy and advances the endoscope through the colon. The lumen of the colon is visualized and biopsies are obtained. The endoscope is withdrawn at the completion of the procedure.

44390

The physician performs colonoscopy through an abdominal wall colostomy and removes a foreign body. The physician places the endoscope through the colostomy and advances the endoscope through the colon. The lumen of the colon is visualized. The foreign body is isolated and grasped with a snare or forceps (placed through the endoscope) and removed. The endoscope in withdrawn at the completion of the procedure.

44391

The physician performs colonoscopy through an abdominal wall colostomy and controls an area of bleeding. The physician places the endoscope through the colostomy and advances the endoscope through the colon. The lumen of the colon is visualized and the area of bleeding is identified and controlled. The endoscope is withdrawn at the completion of the procedure.

44392

The physician performs colonoscopy through an abdominal wall colostomy and removes a tumor, polyp, or other lesion with hot biopsy forceps or cautery. The physician places the endoscope through the colostomy and advances the endoscope through the colon. The lumen of the colon is visualized and the tumor, polyp, or lesion is identified and removed with hot biopsy forceps or cautery. The endoscope is withdrawn at the completion of the procedure.

44393

The physician performs colonoscopy through an abdominal wall colostomy and performs ablation of a tumor, polyp, or other lesion. The physician places the endoscope through the colostomy and advances the endoscope through the colon. The lumen of the colon is visualized and the tumor, polyp, or other lesion is identified and ablated. The endoscope is withdrawn at the completion of the procedure.

44394

The physician performs colonoscopy through an abdominal wall colostomy and removes a tumor, polyp or other lesion with a snare. The physician places the endoscope through the colostomy and advances the endoscope through the colon. The lumen of the colon is visualized and the tumor, polyp or other lesion is identified and removed with a snare placed through the endoscope. The endoscope is withdrawn at the completion of the procedure.

44397

The physician uses a colonoscope to examine the colon through an abdominal wall colostomy and places a transendoscopic stent. The physician places the endoscope through the colostomy and advances the endoscope through the colon. The lumen of the colon is visualized. The endoscope is placed at the site of an obstruction or stricture and the necessary stent length is determined. The stent (endoprosthesis) is introduced into the site of the obstruction. Using a commercial delivery system, a plastic covering over the stent is removed and the stent self-deploys, shoring-up the walls at a specific site in the large intestine. When necessary, a balloon catheter is placed into the stent and gently inflated to more fully deploy the stent. The delivery system and colonoscope are removed.

44500

A long, Miller-Abbott style gastrointestinal tube with a mercury-filled balloon at the bottom is introduced, usually nasally, and used to clear gastrointestinal strictures. The patient is seated lower than the person performing the procedure and the dilator is placed in the posterior pharynx. The patient swallows and the tube and balloon are carried into the small intestine. The balloon is then inflated and withdrawn until resistance is encountered. The balloon is then partially deflated, withdrawn a little more, and re-inflated. This process is repeated several times to achieve dilation of the stricture. This procedure may be done without fluoroscopy or with fluoroscopy by instilling a diluted contrast into the balloon.

44602

The physician performs suture closure of a single small bowel perforation. The physician makes an abdominal incision. Next, the abdomen is explored and the small bowel perforation is identified and repaired with sutures. The incision is closed.

44603

The physician performs suture closure of multiple small bowel perforations. The physician makes an abdominal incision. Next, the abdomen is explored and the small bowel perforations are identified and repaired with sutures. The incision is closed.

44604

The physician performs suture closure of a colon perforation. The physician makes an abdominal incision. Next, the abdomen is explored and the colon perforation is identified and repaired with sutures. The incision is closed.

44605

The physician performs suture closure of a colon perforation and forms a colostomy proximal to the repair. The physician makes an abdominal incision. Next, the abdomen is explored and the colon perforation identified and repaired with sutures. A loop or end of colon proximal to the repair is brought out through a separate incision on the abdominal wall onto the skin as a colostomy. The initial incision is closed.

44615

The physician performs an abdominal incision to gain access to the site of an intestinal narrowing (stricture). Once identified, the intestinal stricture is incised (enterotomy) in a longitudinal manner. The physician may find it necessary or prudent to dilate the stenotic intestine to complete proper repair. The intestine is repaired or sutured. The two divided portions of the incised intestine may be reapproximated after one segment is drawn into the other (invagination) end to end (enterorrhaphy). The abdominal incision is sutured or stapled closed.

44620

The physician takes down and closes an enterostomy (stoma) of the small intestine or colon. The physician makes an incision around the stoma or a separate abdominal incision may be made. Next, the stoma is mobilized and taken down from the abdominal wall and the stoma is closed. The abdominal incisions are closed.

44625

The physician takes down an enterostomy (stoma) of small intestine or colon, other than colorectal. The stoma is resected and an anastomosis between the bowel ends is completed. The physician makes an incision around the stoma or a separate abdominal incision may be made. Next, the stoma is mobilized and taken down from the abdominal wall. The stoma is resected and the bowel ends are reapproximated with staples or sutures. The abdominal incisions are

closed. Report 44625 if with resection and anastomosis other than colorectal.

44626

A surgeon closes a previously-existing enterostomy, or a surgically created opening, in the large or small intestine. This code includes both resection of the intestine and a colorectal anastomosis, or a reconnection of the colon and rectum.

44640

The physician takes down and closes an intestinal cutaneous fistula. The physician makes an abdominal incision. Next, the bowel is mobilized and the fistula is identified and taken down from the abdominal wall and skin. The segment of bowel containing the fistula is resected and the bowel ends reapproximated with staples or sutures. The abdominal wall incisions are closed.

44650

The physician closes a connection (fistula) between loops of small bowel or between the small bowel and colon. The physician makes an abdominal incision. Next, the enteroenteric or enterocolic fistula is identified and divided. The ends of the fistula may be closed with sutures or the segments of bowel involved with the fistula may be resected and the bowel ends reapproximated in order to completely remove the involved areas. The incision is closed.

44660

The physician closes a connection between the small bowel and bladder (enterovesical fistula). The physician makes an abdominal incision. Next, the enterovesical fistula is identified and divided. The ends of the fistula are closed with sutures. The incision is closed.

44661

The physician closes a connection between the small or large intestine and bladder (enterovesical fistula) by resecting a portion of the intestine or bladder. The physician makes an abdominal incision. Next, the enterovesical fistula is identified and divided. The connection of the fistula to the bladder is resected and the bladder is closed with sutures. The segment of intestine containing the fistula is resected and the ends are reapproximated. The incision is closed.

44680

The physician folds the bowel upon itself and attaches the edges with sutures for anchoring purposes. The physician makes an abdominal incision. Next, the bowel is folded upon itself and the edges are plicated with sutures without making an anastomosis to anchor the bowel in place. The incision is closed.

44700

Prior to implementing radiation therapy, the physician uses mesh, other prosthesis, ornative tissue (bladder or omentum) to lift and fix the small intestine away from the site of radiation therapy. An abdominal incision is made. If mesh or other prosthetic material is used, it is sutured into place. If native tissue is used, a sling is fashioned and sutured into place. The incision sutured closed.

44800

The physician excises a Meckel's diverticulum or an omphalomesenteric duct. The physician makes an abdominal incision. Next, the Meckel's diverticulum in the terminal ileum or the omphalomesenteric duct connecting the terminal ileum to the umbilicus is identified. The Meckel's diverticulum or omphalomesenteric duct is excised and the defect in the ileum is closed with sutures or staples or the segment of ileum may be excised and reapproximated. The incision is closed.

44820

The physician excises a lesion in the mesentery. The physician makes an abdominal incision. Next, the lesion in the mesentery is identified. The lesion is removed by shelling it out of the mesentery, resecting a portion of the mesentery with the lesion, or resecting a segment of bowel and mesentery to include the lesion with reapproximation of the bowel. The incision is closed.

44850

The physician repairs a defect in the mesentery with sutures. The physician makes an abdominal incision. Next, the mesenteric defect is identified and closed with sutures. The incision is closed.

44900

The physician drains an appendiceal abscess. The physician makes an abdominal incision. Next, the abscess near the appendix is identified and incised and drained. A drain may be left in the abscess cavity. The abdominal wall incision is closed and the skin incision may be left open to heal secondarily.

44901

The physician performs percutaneous drainage of an appendiceal abscess. The physician may create a small incision in the skin proximal to the appendiceal abscess to ease placement of drainage instruments through the skin (percutaneous). The physician uses a CAT scan or ultrasound to guide placement of a drainage needle or trocar into the appendiceal abscess. The physician advances the drainage needle or trocar through the abdominal wall into the peritoneum to gain access to the abscess cavity. The fluid is allowed to drain. Once drained, a catheter may be placed (and later removed) to maintain drainage. Sutures may be secured to hold the drainage catheter in place. The operative site is subsequently cleaned and bandaged. For radiological supervision and interpretation, see 75989.

44950

The physician removes the appendix. The physician makes an abdominal incision. Next, the appendix is identified and mobilized, its blood supply is divided and the appendix is transected and removed. The incision is closed.

44955

The physician removes the appendix at the time of another major procedure. The physician identifies and mobilizes the appendix during a major procedure for which an incision has been made. The blood supply to the appendix is divided and the appendix is transected and removed. The incision is closed.

44960

The physician removes a perforated appendix. The physician makes an abdominal incision. Next, the appendix is identified and mobilized, its blood supply is divided, and the appendix is transected and removed. The abscess cavity is debrided and the contaminated portion of the abdominal cavity is irrigated. The incision is closed.

44970

The physician performs a laparoscopic appendectomy. The physician places a trocar at the umbilicus and insufflates the abdomen. The laparoscope is placed through the umbilical port and additional trocars are placed into the abdominal cavity. The appendix is identified, dissected from surrounding structures and its blood supply divided. The appendix is transected with staples or suture and removed. The trocars are removed and the incisions are closed.

45000

The physician drains a pelvic abscess through the rectum. The physician identifies the area of abscess through the rectum by palpation or preoperative localizing studies. Next, a transanal incision is made through the rectum into the abscess cavity and the abscess is drained. The incision is left open to drain.

45005

The physician drains a submucosal rectal abscess. The physician identifies the area of abscess in the rectum. Next, a transanal incision is made through the rectal lining into the abscess cavity and the abscess is drained. The incision is left open to drain.

45020

The physician drains an abscess above the pelvic floor or behind the rectum through the rectum. The physician identifies the area of abscess by palpation or preoperative localizing studies. Next, a transanal incision is made through the rectum into the abscess cavity and the abscess is drained. The incision is left open to drain.

45100

The physician performs a biopsy of the rectal wall through the anus. The physician performs an incisional biopsy or a suction biopsy of the low rectal wall through the anus. An incisional biopsy may be closed with sutures.

45108

The physician removes a muscle tumor or a section of muscle from the anorectum. The physician identifies the anorectal muscle tumor or the area of interest. Next, a transanal incision is made through the rectal wall and the tumor or identified area of muscle is excised. The incision is closed by approximating the muscle edges and closing the incision in the rectal lining.

45110

The physician removes the entire rectum and anus and forms a colostomy. The physician makes an abdominal incision. Next, the proximal rectum is mobilized within the abdomen to the level of the sphincter muscles and the colon is divided above the pelvic brim. An incision is made around the anus from a perineal approach and the anus and distal rectum are dissected free of surrounding structures and the anus and rectum are removed. The proximal end of colon is brought out through a separate incision on the abdominal wall as a colostomy. The abdominal and perineal incisions are closed.

45111

The physician removes the proximal rectum. The physician makes an abdominal incision. Next, the distal colon and rectum are mobilized and divided proximal and distal to the segment of interest. The colon and distal rectum may be reapproximated or the proximal end of colon may be brought out through a separate incision on the abdominal wall as a colostomy and the remaining rectum closed with staples or sutures. The initial incision is closed.

45112

The physician removes the rectum and performs an anastomosis between the colon and the anus. The physician makes an abdominal incision. Next, the distal colon and rectum are mobilized within the abdomen to the level of the sphincter muscles. The colon is divided above the pelvic brim and the rectum at the level of the sphincter muscles and removed. The mucosa may be stripped from the remaining distal rectum from a perineal approach. The distal colon is pulled through the sphincter complex and approximated to the anus with sutures. The incision is closed.

45113

The physician removes the proximal rectum, strips the mucosa from the distal rectum and performs an anastomosis between an ileal pouch and the anus. The physician makes an abdominal incision. Next, the

distal colon and rectum are mobilized within the abdomen to the level of the sphincter muscles. The colon is divided above the pelvic brim and the rectum is divided above the sphincter muscles and removed. The mucosa of the distal rectum is stripped from a perineal approach. The distal ileum is folded upon itself and approximated in order to form a reservoir. The ileal pouch is pulled through the remaining muscular cuff of distal rectum and sutured to the anus. A loop ileostomy may be formed proximal to the anastomosis. The incision is closed.

45114

The physician removes a portion of the rectum through combined abdominal and transsacral approaches. The physician makes an abdominal incision. The proximal rectum and distal colon are mobilized and the colon is divided above the pelvic brim. Next, an incision is made posteriorly at the junction of the sacrum and coccyx. The coccyx is excised. Dissection is continued posteriorly to further mobilize the rectum. The rectum is divided distally and the excised segment is removed. The distal end of colon is approximated to the remaining rectal stump with sutures or staples. The incisions are closed.

45116

The physician removes a portion of the rectum through a transsacral approach. The physician makes a posterior incision at the junction of the sacrum and coccyx. The coccyx is excised. Next, dissection is continued posteriorly and the rectum and distal colon are mobilized. The rectum is transected proximally and distally and a portion of the rectum is removed. The distal end of colon is approximated to the remaining rectal stump with sutures or staples. The incision is closed.

45119

The physician performs a proctectomy. Once the physician performs an abdominal incision, the distal part of the diseased colon and rectum are mobilized down to the level of the anal sphincter muscles. The rectum is incised at the level of the sphincter muscles while the colon is incised above the pelvic brim where it is disease free. The diseased colon and rectum are removed. The free end of the distal colon is brought through the sphincter complex and approximated with the anus to form a colo-anal anastomosis. The distal colon is folded and sutured in such a way as to create a colonic reservoir pouch. The physician may elect to bring a loop or end of the colon through a separate abdominal incision to create a stoma (colostomy). The incisions are sutured closed.

45120

The physician removes or bypasses the diseased rectal segment and performs an anastomosis of the colon and anus. The physician makes an abdominal incision. Next, the rectum and distal colon are mobilized and the colon is divided just proximal to the diseased rectal segment. The rectal segment may be removed and the distal colon pulled through the sphincter complex and approximated to the anus with sutures from a perineal approach. Alternatively, the distal colon may be pulled down and approximated to the anus with sutures, bypassing the diseased rectal segment with a combined longitudinal anastomosis between the colon and the diseased rectal segment. The incision is closed.

45121

The physician removes the rectum, part or all of the colon, and performs an anastomosis of the remaining colon or ileum and anus. The physician makes an abdominal incision. Next, multiple biopsies are taken of the colon wall to determine the level of disease. The involved rectum and colon are mobilized and removed. The remaining segment of colon or ileum is pulled through the sphincter complex and approximated to the anus with sutures from a perineal approach. Alternatively, the colon or ileum may be pulled down and approximated to the anus with sutures, bypassing a small remaining rectal segment with a combined longitudinal anastomosis to the rectal segment. The incision is closed.

45123

The physician removes a portion of the rectum through a perineal approach. The physician makes an incision around the anus. Next, dissection is continued around the anus to mobilize the anus and distal rectum. The anus and distal rectum are removed. A proximal colostomy may be formed. The incision is closed.

45126

The physician removes pelvic organs, with or without a colostomy, due to cancer of the colon and rectum. The physician makes an abdominal incision. The distal colon and rectum are mobilized and divided proximal and distal to the segment of interest. The pelvic organs are dissected free of surrounding structures and removed. The colon and rectum may be reapproximated or the proximal end of the colon may be brought out through a separate incision on the abdominal wall as a colostomy and the remaining rectum closed with staples or sutures. The initial incision is closed. In males the procedure may include removal of the prostate and bladder. In a female the procedure may include removal of the bladder and also the uterus, cervix, fallopian tubes, and/or ovaries depending upon the extent of the disease.

45130

The physician removes a rectal prolapse through a perineal approach. The physician prolapses the rectum and colon through the anus. Next, a circular incision is made through the distal rectum at the anorectal junction. The mesentery and blood supply to the prolapsed rectum is divided and the segment is telescoped out through the anus. The proximal

rectum or colon is divided and the prolapsed segment is removed. The proximal end of rectum or colon is approximated to the anus with sutures or staples.

45135

The physician removes a rectal prolapse through a combined abdominal and perineal approach. The physician makes an abdominal incision. The proximal colon and rectum are mobilized. The rectum and colon are prolapsed through the anus. Next, a circular incision is made through the distal rectum at the anorectal junction from a perineal approach. The mesentery and blood supply to the prolapsed rectum is divided and the segment is telescoped out through the anus. The proximal rectum or colon is divided and the prolapsed segment is removed. The proximal end of rectum or colon is approximated the anus with sutures or staples. The incision is closed.

45136

The physician excises an ileoanal reservoir and creates an ileostomy. The physician makes an abdominal incision. Dissection is carried down to the site of the ileoanal reservoir. The reservoir is excised at the level where the ileum was previously anastomosed to the anus. The anus is closed. The loose end of the ileum may be trimmed. A disk of skin is excised from the abdominal wall and the terminal ileum is brought out through the split rectus muscle and the opening in the abdomen to form a stoma on the abdominal wall. An anastomosis is performed via the transanal approach and the full thickness of the ileum is sutured to the anal canal. Interrupted sutures complete the ileostomy construction.

45150

The physician performs division of a rectal stricture. The physician makes longitudinal incisions in the scar tissue in one or more places circumferentially around the strictured area of the rectal mucosa. A dilatation of the strictured area may be performed. In addition the internal anal sphincter may be incised as part of the procedure.

45160

The physician removes a rectal tumor through a transsacral or transcoccygeal approach. The physician makes an incision at the junction of the sacrum and coccyx. The coccyx is excised and dissection is continued posteriorly to mobilize the rectum. The tumor is identified, an incision is made in the rectum (proctotomy), and the tumor is excised. The rectum is closed with sutures or staples. The initial incision is closed.

45170

The physician removes a rectal tumor through a transanal approach. The physician explores the anal canal and exposes the tumor. The tumor is excised to include a full thickness of the rectal wall. The defect in the rectum is closed with sutures.

45190

The physician performs destruction of a rectal tumor from a transanal approach. The physician explores the anal canal and exposes the tumor. The tumor is ablated by electrosurgery, laser, or some other method.

45300

The physician performs rigid proctosigmoidoscopy and may obtain brushings or washings. The physician inserts the rigid proctosigmoidoscope through the anus and advances the scope. The sigmoid colon and rectal lumen are visualized and brushings or washings may be obtained. The proctosigmoidoscope is removed at the completion of the procedure.

45303

The physician performs rigid proctosigmoidoscopy and performs dilation of a rectal stricture. The physician inserts the rigid proctosigmoidoscope through the anus and advances the scope. The sigmoid colon and rectal lumen are visualized. The stricture is identified and dilated with a balloon or other device. The proctosigmoidoscope is removed at the completion of the procedure.

45305

The physician performs rigid proctosigmoidoscopy and obtains biopsies. The physician inserts the rigid proctosigmoidoscope through the anus and advances the scope. The sigmoid colon and rectal lumen are visualized and biopsies are obtained of suspicious areas. The proctosigmoidoscope is removed at the completion of the procedure.

45307

The physician performs rigid proctosigmoidoscopy and removes a foreign body. The physician inserts the rigid proctosigmoidoscope through the anus and advances the scope. The sigmoid colon and rectal lumen are visualized and the foreign body is identified. The foreign body is removed by a snare or forceps inserted through the scope. The proctosigmoidoscope is removed at the completion of the procedure.

45308

The physician performs rigid proctosigmoidoscopy and removes a tumor, polyp, or other lesion. The physician inserts the rigid proctosigmoidoscope through the anus and advances the scope. The sigmoid colon and rectal lumen are visualized and the tumor, polyp or other lesion is identified and removed by hot biopsy forceps or cautery. The proctosigmoidoscope is removed at the completion of the procedure.

45309

The physician performs rigid proctosigmoidoscopy and removes a tumor, polyp, or other lesion. The physician inserts the rigid proctosigmoidoscope through the anus and advances the scope. The

sigmoid colon and rectal lumen are visualized and the tumor, polyp or other lesion is identified and removed by snare technique. The proctosigmoidoscope is removed at the completion of the procedure.

45315

The physician performs rigid proctosigmoidoscopy and removes multiple tumors, polyps, or other lesions. The physician inserts the rigid proctosigmoidoscope through the anus and advances the scope. The sigmoid colon and rectal lumen are visualized and the tumors, polyps, or other lesions are identified and removed by hot biopsy forceps cautery or snare technique. The proctosigmoidoscope is removed at the completion of the procedure.

45317

The physician performs rigid proctosigmoidoscopy and controls an area of bleeding. The physician inserts the rigid proctosigmoidoscope through the anus and advances the scope. The sigmoid colon and rectal lumen are visualized and the area of bleeding is identified and controlled. The proctosigmoidoscope is removed at the completion of the procedure.

45320

The physician performs rigid proctosigmoidoscopy and ablation of a tumor polyp or other lesion. The physician inserts the proctosigmoidoscope through the anus and advances the scope. The lumen of the sigmoid colon and rectum is visualized and the tumor, polyp or other lesion is identified and ablation performed. The proctosigmoidoscope is removed at the completion of the procedure.

45321

The physician performs rigid proctosigmoidoscopy and decompresses a sigmoid volvulus. The physician inserts the proctosigmoidoscope through the anus and advances the scope. The lumen of the sigmoid colon and rectum is visualized. The proctosigmoidoscope is advanced into the volvulus, decompressing the volvulus as it passes through the bowel lumen. The proctosigmoidoscope is removed at the completion of the procedure.

45327

The physician uses a rigid proctosigmoidoscopy to examine the rectum and sigmoid colon and places a transendoscopic stent. The physician inserts the rigid proctosigmoidoscope through the anus and advances the scope. The sigmoid colon and rectal lumen are visualized. The endoscope is placed at the site of an obstruction or stricture and the necessary stent length is determined. The stent (endoprosthesis) is introduced into the site of the obstruction. Using a commercial delivery system ,a plastic covering over the stent is removed and the stent self-deploys, shoring-up the walls at a specific site in the sigmoid colon. When necessary, a balloon catheter is placed into the stent and gently inflated to more fully deploy

CPT® Lay Descriptions

the stent. The delivery system and endoscope are removed.

45330

The physician performs flexible sigmoidoscopy and may obtain brushings or washings. The physician inserts the sigmoidoscope through the anus and advances the scope into the sigmoid colon. The lumen of the sigmoid colon and rectum are visualized and brushings or washings may be obtained. The sigmoidoscope is withdrawn at the completion of the procedure.

45331

The physician performs flexible sigmoidoscopy and obtains biopsies. The physician inserts the sigmoidoscope through the anus and advances the scope into the sigmoid colon. The lumen of the sigmoid colon and rectum are visualized and biopsies are obtained with forceps placed through the scope. The sigmoidoscope is withdrawn at the completion of the procedure.

45332

The physician performs flexible sigmoidoscopy and removes a foreign body. The physician inserts the sigmoidoscope through the anus and advances the scope into the sigmoid colon. The lumen of the sigmoid colon and rectum are visualized. The foreign body is identified and removed with a snare or forceps placed through the sigmoidoscope. The sigmoidoscope is withdrawn at the completion of the procedure.

45333

The physician performs flexible sigmoidoscopy and removes a tumor, polyp, or other lesion. The physician inserts the sigmoidoscope through the anus and advances the scope into the sigmoid colon. The lumen of the sigmoid colon and rectum are visualized and the tumor, polyp, or other lesion is identified and removed with hot biopsy forceps or cautery. The sigmoidoscope is withdrawn at the completion of the procedure.

45334

The physician performs flexible sigmoidoscopy and controls an area of bleeding. The physician inserts the sigmoidoscope through the anus and advances the scope into the sigmoid colon. The lumen of the sigmoid colon and rectum are visualized and the area of bleeding is controlled. The sigmoidoscope is withdrawn at the completion of the procedure.

45337

The physician performs flexible sigmoidoscopy and decompresses a sigmoid volvulus. The physician inserts the sigmoidoscope through the anus and advances the scope into the sigmoid colon. The lumen of the sigmoid colon and rectum are visualized. The sigmoidoscope is advanced into the volvulus

decompressing the volvulus as the scope passes through the bowel lumen. The sigmoidoscope is removed at the completion of the procedure.

45338

The physician performs flexible sigmoidoscopy and removes tumors, polyps or other lesions. The physician inserts the sigmoidoscope through the anus and advances the scope into the sigmoid colon. The lumen of the sigmoid colon and rectum are visualized. The tumor, polyp, or other lesions are identified and removed by snare technique. The sigmoidoscope is withdrawn at the completion of the procedure.

45339

The physician performs flexible sigmoidoscopy and performs ablation of a tumor, polyp or other lesion. The physician inserts the sigmoidoscope through the anus and advances the scope into the sigmoid colon. The lumen of the sigmoid colon and rectum are visualized. The tumor, polyp or other lesions are identified and ablated by laser or other method. The sigmoidoscope is withdrawn at the completion of the procedure.

45341

The physician uses a flexible sigmoidoscopy to examine the rectum and sigmoid colon and performs an endoscopic ultrasound examination. The physician inserts the sigmoidoscopy through the anus and advances the scope into the sigmoid colon. The lumen of the sigmoid colon and rectum are visualized. Either the sigmoidoscope is removed and replaced with an echoendoscope, or an ultrasound probe is passed through the already placed sigmoidoscope. The echoendoscope or ultrasound probe is fitted with a water-filled balloon near the tip; the tip contains a transducer that picks-up the ultrasound frequency and relays it to a processor, outside of the body. The water-filled tip is positioned in the sigmoid colon, against the colon wall next to the area of interest. The area is scanned and an ultrasound image is projected through the processor to a monitor in real-time. When the ultrasound examination is complete the echoendoscope, or esophagoscope and ultrasound probe is removed.

45342

The physician uses a flexible sigmoidoscopy to examine the rectum and sigmoid colon and performs a transendoscopic ultrasound guided intramural or transmural fine needle aspiration/biopsy. The physician inserts the sigmoidoscopy through the anus and advances the scope into the sigmoid colon. The lumen of the sigmoid colon and rectum are visualized. The sigmoidoscope may be removed. A radial scanning echoendoscope is inserted and ultrasound scanning is performed, or an ultrasound probe is passed through the already placed endoscope. The site for a fine needle aspiration biopsy is determined. If a radial scanning echoendoscope is used it is removed and is replaced with a curvilinear array echoendoscope. The echoendoscope or ultrasound probe is fitted with a water-filled balloon near the tip; the tip contains a transducer that picks-up the ultrasound frequency and relays it to a processor, outside of the body. The water-filled tip is positioned in the sigmoid colon against the colon wall next to the predetermined fine needle aspiration (FNA) biopsy site. The area is scanned and an ultrasound image is projected through the processor to a monitor in real-time. A FNA needle is passed through the scope to the biopsy site and a biopsy is taken of the tissue or the needle is inserted through the wall of the tissue into the lesion, or other structure, such as a lymph node. The area is biopsied. When the FNA is complete the echoendoscope or sigmoidoscope and ultrasound probe is removed.

45345

The physician uses a flexible sigmoidoscope to examine the rectum and sigmoid colon and places a transendoscopic stent. The physician inserts the sigmoidoscopy through the anus and advances the scope into the sigmoid colon. The lumen of the sigmoid colon and rectum are visualized. The endoscope is placed at the site of an obstruction or stricture and the necessary stent length is determined. The stent (endoprosthesis) is introduced into the site of the obstruction. Using a commercial delivery system, a plastic covering over the stent is removed and the stent self-deploys, shoring-up the walls at a specific site in the sigmoid colon. When necessary, a balloon catheter is placed into the stent and gently inflated to more fully deploy the stent. The delivery system and endoscope are removed.

45355

The physician performs colonoscopy through an incision in the colon (colotomy). The physician makes an abdominal incision. Next, the colon may be mobilized. An incision is made in the colon in the segment of interest and the colonoscope is inserted through the colotomy and advanced to visualize the lumen of the colon. At the completion of the procedure the colonoscope is removed and the colotomy is closed with sutures or staples. The abdominal incision is closed.

45378

The physician performs colonoscopy and may obtain brushings or washings or perform colon decompression. The physician inserts the colonoscope through the anus and advances the scope through the colon past the splenic flexure. The lumen of the colon and rectum is visualized. Brushings or washings may be obtained or decompression of the colon may be performed. The colonoscope is withdrawn at the completion of the procedure.

45379

The physician performs colonoscopy and removes a foreign body. The physician inserts the colonoscope through the anus and advances the scope through the colon past the splenic flexure. The lumen of the colon and rectum is visualized. The foreign body is identified and removed by forceps or snare placed through the colonoscope. The colonoscope is withdrawn at the completion of the procedure.

45380

The physician performs colonoscopy and obtains tissue samples. The physician inserts the colonoscope through the anus and advances the scope past the splenic flexure. The lumen of the colon and rectum is visualized and biopsies are obtained. The colonoscope is withdrawn at the completion of the procedure.

45382

The physician performs colonoscopy and controls an area of bleeding. The physician inserts the colonoscope through the anus and advances the scope past the splenic flexure. The lumen of the colon and rectum is visualized and the area of bleeding is identified and controlled. The colonoscope is withdrawn at the completion of the procedure.

45383

The physician performs colonoscopy and performs ablation of a tumor, polyp, or other lesions. The physician inserts the colonoscope through the anus and advances the scope past the splenic flexure. The lumen of the colon and rectum is visualized. The tumor, polyp, or other lesions are identified and ablated by laser or other method. The colonoscope is withdrawn at the completion of the procedure.

45384

The physician performs colonscopy and removes a tumor, polyp or other lesions. The physician inserts the colonoscope through the anus and advances the scope past the splenic flexure. The lumen of the colon and rectum is visualized. The tumor, polyp or other lesions are identified and removed by hot biopsy forceps, or cautery. The colonoscope is withdrawn at the completion of the procedure.

45385

The physician performs colonoscopy and removes a tumor, polyp, or other lesions. The physician inserts the colonoscope through the anus and advances the scope past the splenic flexure. The lumen of the colon and rectum is visualized. The tumor, polyp, or other lesions are identified and removed by snare technique. The colonoscope is withdrawn at the completion of the procedure.

45387

The physician uses a colonoscope to examine the colon and places a transendoscopic stent. The physician inserts the sigmoidoscopy through the anus and advances the scope into the sigmoid colon. The lumen of the sigmoid colon and rectum are visualized. The endoscope is placed at the site of an obstruction or stricture and the necessary stent length is determined. The stent (endoprosthesis) is introduced into the site of the obstruction. Using a commercial delivery system a plastic covering over the stent is removed and the stent self-deploys, shoring-up the walls at a specific site in the colon, proximal to the splenic flexure. When necessary, a balloon catheter is placed into the stent and gently inflated to more fully deploy the stent. The delivery system and endoscope are removed.

45500

The physician performs proctoplasty for an area of stenosis. The physician makes a longitudinal incision through the scar tissue at the anorectal junction or may completely excise the scar tissue to an area of normal mucosa. The surrounding perianal skin is undermined and mobilized in one of several possible fashions as a flap. The flap is approximated to the normal mucosa at the edges of the incised or excised scar, thus closing the wound.

45505

The physician performs proctoplasty for an area of prolapse of rectal mucosa (ectropion). The physician makes a circular incision just proximal to the prolapsing mucosa and mobilizes the redundant mucosa. An incision is made out onto the perianal skin to form a flap of skin on the right and left sides of the anus adjacent to the mobilized mucosa. The mucosa is excised and the flaps of skin are advanced into the anal canal. The mucosal edges are reapproximated in their normal anatomic position with sutures. The skin incisions are closed completing the procedure.

45520

The physician performs sclerotherapy for rectal prolapse. The physician identifies the anorectal ring. Sclerosing solution is injected into the submucosa of the rectum circumferentially just above the anorectal ring.

45540

The physician approximates the rectum to the sacrum (proctopexy) for rectal prolapse. The physician makes an abdominal incision. The rectum is completely mobilized from the sacrum and placed in upward tension to remove any redundancy. The rectum is reapproximated to the sacrum with sutures or a mesh may be wrapped around the rectum and attached to the sacrum. The incision is closed.

45541

The physician approximates the rectum to the sacrum(proctopexy) for rectal prolapse through a perineal approach. The physician makes a transverse incision between the anus and coccyx. Dissection is

continued through the levator muscles to mobilize the rectum from the sacrum. The rectum is placed on upward tension to remove the redundancy and approximated to the sacrum with sutures or with a mesh wrapped around the rectum and secured to the sacrum. The incision is closed.

45550

The physician approximates the rectum to the sacrum and performs a sigmoid colon resection. The physician makes an abdominal incision. The sigmoid colon and rectum are mobilized. The redundant segment of sigmoid colon and rectum is excised and an anastomosis is created between the remaining bowel ends with sutures or staples. The rectum is approximated to the sacrum with sutures. The incision is closed.

45560

The physician repairs a rectocele. The physician makes an incision in the mucosa of the posterior vaginal wall over the rectocele. The rectocele is dissected free of surrounding structures and the levator muscles are identified. The rectum is plicated to surrounding fascia with multiple sutures and the levator muscles are reapproximated. The vaginal mucosa is excised and the incision is closed.

45562

The physician explores, repairs, and drains a rectal injury. The physician makes an abdominal incision. The rectal injury is explored and repaired with sutures if possible. An incision is made between the coccyx and anus and drains are placed in the presacral space. The abdominal incision is closed.

45563

The physician explores, repairs, and drains a rectal injury and performs a proximal colostomy. The physician makes an abdominal incision. The rectal injury is explored and repaired with sutures. A loop or end of sigmoid colon is brought through a separate incision on the abdominal wall as a colostomy. An incision is made between the sacrum and anus and drains are placed in the presacral space. The abdominal incision is closed.

45800

The physician closes a connection between the rectum and the bladder (rectovesical fistula). The physician makes an abdominal incision. The sigmoid colon and rectum are mobilized and the connection between the rectum and bladder is identified and divided. The fistulous openings in the rectum and bladder are debrided and closed with sutures.

45805

The physician closes a connection between the rectum and bladder (rectovesical fistula) and performs a proximal colostomy. The physician makes an abdominal incision. The sigmoid colon and rectum are mobilized and the connection between the rectum and bladder is identified and divided. The fistulous openings in the rectum and bladder are debrided and closed. The involved segment of colon or rectum may be excised. A loop or end of sigmoid colon proximal to the involved area is brought out through a separate incision on the abdominal wall as a colostomy. The abdominal incision is closed.

45820

The physician closes a rectourethral fistula. The physician makes an abdominal incision. The rectum is dissected from the prostate and the fistula is identified and divided. The fistulous opening in the rectum is closed with sutures and the opening in the urethra may be closed or left open. A pedicle of omentum is usually mobilized and placed between the areas of repair. The incision is closed. As an alternate method an incision may be made between the anus and urethra from a perineal approach and dissection continued between the rectum and urethra. The fistula is identified and divided and the openings in the rectum and urethra are closed. The incision is closed.

45825

The physician closes a rectourethral fistula and forms a proximal colostomy. The physician makes an abdominal incision. The rectum is dissected from the prostate and the fistula is identified and divided. The fistulous opening in the rectum is closed with sutures and the opening in the urethra may be closed or left open. A pedicle of omentum is usually mobilized and placed between the areas of repair. A loop or end of proximal colon is brought through a separate incision on the abdominal wall as a colostomy. The initial incision is closed.

45900

The physician reduces a rectal prolapse (procidentia) to a patient under general anesthesia. The physician performs a manual reduction of an incarcerated rectal prolapse by pushing the prolapsed segment back up through the anus under the relaxation of anesthesia.

45905

The physician dilates the anal sphincter under anesthesia. The physician performs dilation of the anal sphincter digitally or with a dilating instrument under the relaxation of anesthesia.

45910

The physician dilates a rectal stricture under anesthesia. The physician performs dilation of a rectal stricture digitally or with a dilating instrument under the relaxation of anesthesia.

45915

The physician removes a foreign body or fecal impaction under anesthesia. The physician performs removal of a foreign body or fecal impaction manually or with an instrument under the relaxation of anesthesia.

46020

The physician makes an incision in the anal opening. A suture is passed and the seton is securely tied using a rubber band, or similar technique. A nylon suture is threaded around the sphincter and tied loosely. An elastic band is secured to the suture and a safety pin is attached. The pin is taped to the patient's thigh and the patient is instructed to adjust the amount of pull to produce minimal discomfort until the seton cuts through.

46030

The physician removes an anal seton or other marker. The physician identifies the seton stitch or other marker at the anal verge. The seton is divided and removed. The external anal sphincter at the level of the seton may be divided.

46040

The physician drains a perirectal or ischiorectal abscess. The physician identifies the location of the abscess. The perianal skin over the abscess is incised and the abscess cavity is opened and drained. The incision is packed open for continued drainage.

46045

The physician drains a perirectal abscess in the intramural, intramuscular, or submucosal position. The physician identifies the location of the abscess in relation to the sphincter muscles. The perianal skin or rectal mucosa over the abscess is incised. Dissection is carried through muscle if necessary and the abscess cavity is opened and drained. The incision is packed open for continued drainage.

46050

The physician drains a superficial perianal abscess. The physician identifies the location of the abscess. The perianal skin over the abscess is incised and the abscess cavity is opened and drained. The incision is packed open for continued drainage.

46060

The physician drains an ischiorectal or intramural perirectal abscess with fistulectomy or fistulotomy and may place a seton. The physician identifies the location of the abscess and the internal and external openings of the anal fistula in relation to the sphincter muscles. An incision is made in the perianal skin over the abscess and the abscess cavity is opened and drained. The mucosa, skin, and internal sphincter muscle overlying the fistula is incised and the fistula is completely unroofed or may be excised. If the fistula goes beneath the external sphincter muscle a stitch (seton) may be placed through the fistula tract to allow drainage and preserve continence. The incision is left open to drain and the abscess cavity is packed open for continued drainage.

46070

The physician incises a congenital anal septum. The physician identifies the anal opening and septum in the infant. The septum is sharply incised.

46080

The physician divides the anal sphincter. The patient is placed in jackknife or lithotomy position. The physician performs digital and instrumental dilation of the anus with exposure of the patient's anal canal. A small incision is made between the muscle layers of the anus and internal muscle is divided without opening the lining of the anus.

46083

The physician performs incision of a thrombosed external hemorrhoid. The physician identifies the thrombosed external hemorrhoid. An incision is made in the skin over the hemorrhoid and the thrombus is removed. The incision is left open for continued drainage.

46200

The physician excises a fissure (fissurectomy) and may perform a sphincterotomy. The physician identifies the anal fissure and the internal sphincter muscle by palpation. An incision is made around the fissure dissecting it free of underlying sphincter muscle and the fissure is excised. The internal sphincter muscle may be incised usually in a lateral position away from the fissure. The incision is usually left open to allow drainage.

46210

The physician performs excision of an anal crypt. The physician identifies an anal crypt usually associated with the internal opening of an anal fistula. An incision is made overlying the fistula and the fistula and associated crypt are excised. The incision is usually left open to allow continued drainage.

46211

The physician performs excision of multiple anal crypts. The physician identifies the involved anal crypts usually associated with the internal openings of anal fistulas. Incisions are made overlying the fistulas. The fistulas and associated crypts are excised. The incisions are usually left open to allow continued drainage.

46220

The physician performs excision of an anal skin tag or papilloma. The physician identifies the anal skin tag or papilloma usually associated with the external edge of a fissure or fistula. An incision is made around the skin tag or papilloma and the lesion is dissected from the underlying sphincter muscle and removed. The incision is closed with sutures or may be left partially open to drain.

46221

The physician performs hemorrhoidectomy by ligation of an external hemorrhoid. The physician identifies the external hemorrhoid. The hemorrhoid is ligated at its base usually with a rubber band. The hemorrhoid tissue is allowed to slough over time.

46230

The physician performs an excision of external hemorrhoid tags or multiple papillae. Once the physician has identified the external hemorrhoid tags or papillae, incisions are made around the lesions. The lesions are dissected from the underlying sphincter muscle and removed. The incisions are closed with sutures or may be left partially open to drain.

46250

The physician performs an excision of external hemorrhoids. The physician identifies the external hemorrhoids. Incisions are made around the hemorrhoids and the lesions are dissected from the underlying sphincter muscle and removed. The incisions are closed with sutures.

46255

The physician performs excision of internal and external hemorrhoids. The physician explores the anal canal and identifies the hemorrhoid column. An incision is made in the rectal mucosa around the hemorrhoids and the lesions are dissected from the underlying sphincter muscles and removed. The incisions are closed with sutures.

46257

The physician performs excision of internal and external hemorrhoids and an associated fissure. The physician explores the anal canal and identifies the hemorrhoid columns and the fissure. An incision is made in the rectal mucosa around the hemorrhoids and the lesions are dissected from the underlying sphincter muscles and removed. An incision is made around the fissure and the fissure is dissected from the underlying sphincter muscles and excised. The incisions are closed with sutures.

46258

The physician performs excision of internal and external hemorrhoids with associated fistulectomy and possible fissurectomy. The physician explores the anal canal and identifies the hemorrhoid column and the fistula. If the fistula is in the same plane as the hemorrhoid a single incision is made in the mucosa around the lesions and the lesions are dissected from the underlying sphincter muscles and removed. If the lesions are in different planes separate incisions are used to excise the lesions. If a fissure is present it may be excised in a similar manner. The incisions are closed with sutures.

46260

The physician performs excision of complex or extensive internal and external hemorrhoids. The physician explores the anal canal and identifies the hemorrhoid columns. Incisions are made in the rectal mucosa around the hemorrhoid columns. The lesions are dissected from the underlying sphincter muscles and removed. The incisions are closed with sutures.

46261

The physician performs excision of complex or extensive internal and external hemorrhoids and an associated fissure. The physician explores the anal canal and identifies the hemorrhoid columns and the fissure. Incisions are made in the rectal mucosa around the hemorrhoid columns and around the fissure. The lesions are dissected from the underlying sphincter muscles and removed. The incisions are closed with sutures.

46262

The physician performs excision of complex or extensive internal and external hemorrhoids with an associated fistulectomy and possible fissurectomy. The physician explores the anal canal and identifies the hemorrhoid columns and the fistula. Incisions are made in the rectal mucosa around the hemorrhoid columns and around the fistula. The lesions are dissected from the underlying sphincter muscles and removed. If a fissure is present it may be excised in a similar manner. The incisions are closed with sutures.

46270

The physician excises or incises a subcutaneous anal fistula. The physician explores the anal canal and identifies the location of the fistula in relation to the sphincter muscles. The skin and subcutaneous tissue overlying the fistula is excised or incised to open the fistula tract. The incision is usually left open to allow continued drainage.

46275

The physician excises or incises a submuscular anal fistula. The physician explores the anal canal and identifies the location of the fistula in relation to the sphincter muscles. The skin, subcutaneous tissue, and internal sphincter muscle overlying the fistula is excised or incised to open the fistula tract. If the external sphincter is involved a portion of the external sphincter may also be safely incised. The incision is usually left open to allow continued drainage.

46280

The physician excises or incises a complex or multiple anal fistula. The physician explores the anal canal and identifies the location of the fistula in relation to the sphincter muscles. The tissue overlying the fistula or fistulas is excised or incised to open the fistula tract. If the external sphincter or the puborectal muscular sling is involved, only a portion of the

muscle is incised to open the fistula. A permanent suture is placed through the remainder of the fistula tract (seton) in order to allow drainage and preserve continence. The incisions are usually left open to allow continued drainage.

46285

The physician performs a second stage excision or incision or an anal fistula. The physician explores the anal canal and identifies the location of the fistula in relation to the sphincter muscles. Usually the fistula tract has been partially opened and a seton may be in place. The remainder of the fistula tract is excised or incised and a seton if present is removed. The incision is usually left open to allow continued drainage.

46288

The physician excises an anal fistula and closes the defect with a rectal advancement flap. The physician explores the anal canal and identifies the location of the fistula in relation to the sphincter muscles. The fistula tract is excised. An incision is made onto the perianal skin and a wedge of skin and subcutaneous tissue is mobilized and advanced into the defect created by the excision of the fistula. The incisions are closed with sutures.

46320

The physician performs an incision and drainage or excision of a thrombosed external hemorrhoid. The physician exposes the thrombosed external hemorrhoid. The hemorrhoid may be either incised and the thrombus removed or completely excised. The incision may be closed or left open to allow continued drainage.

46500

The physician performs sclerotherapy of internal hemorrhoids. The physician explores the anal canal and identifies the hemorrhoid columns. Sclerosing solution is injected into the submucosa of the rectal wall under the hemorrhoid columns.

46600

The physician performs anoscopy and may obtain brushings or washings. The physician inserts the anoscope through the anus and advances the scope. The anal canal and distal rectal mucosa are visualized and brushings or washings may be obtained. The anoscope is withdrawn at the completion of the procedure.

46604

The physician performs anoscopy and performs anal dilation. The physician inserts the anoscope through the anus and advances the scope. The anal canal and distal rectal mucosa are visualized. Dilation of the anal sphincter or a distal stricture is performed with the anoscope, digitally, or by some other instrument. The anoscope is withdrawn at the completion of the procedure.

CPT® Lay Descriptions

46606

The physician performs anoscopy and obtains tissue samples. The physician inserts the anoscope through the anus and advances the scope. The anal canal and distal rectal mucosa are visualized and tissue samples are obtained. The anoscope is withdrawn at the completion of the procedure.

46608

The physician performs anoscopy and removes a foreign body. The physician inserts the anoscope through the anus and advances the scope. The anal canal and distal rectal mucosa are visualized. The foreign body is identified and removed with a snare or forceps placed through the anoscope. The anoscope is withdrawn at the completion of the procedure.

46610

The physician performs anoscopy and removes a single tumor, polyp, or other lesion. The physician inserts the anoscope through the anus and advances the scope. The anal canal and distal rectal mucosa are visualized. The tumor, polyp, or other lesion is identified and removed by hot biopsy forceps or cautery. The anoscope is withdrawn at the completion of the procedure.

46611

The physician performs anoscopy and removes a single tumor, polyp, or other lesion. The physician inserts the anoscope through the anus and advances the scope. The anal canal and distal rectal mucosa are visualized. The tumor, polyp, or other lesion is identified and removed by snare technique. The anoscope is withdrawn at the completion of the procedure.

46612

The physician performs anoscopy and removes multiple tumors, polyps, or other lesions. The physician inserts the anoscope through the anus and advances the scope. The tumors, polyps or other lesions are identified and removed by hot biopsy forceps, cautery, or snare technique. The anoscope is removed at the completion of the procedure.

46614

The physician performs anoscopy and controls an area of bleeding. The physician inserts the anoscope through the anus and advances the scope. The anal canal and distal rectal mucosa are visualized. The area of bleeding is identified and controlled. The anoscope is withdrawn at the completion of the procedure.

46615

The physician performs anoscopy and performs ablation of a tumor, polyp, or other lesions. The physician inserts the anoscope through the anus and advances the scope. The anal canal and distal rectal mucosa are visualized. The tumor, polyp, or other lesions are identified and ablation of the lesions is performed. The anoscope is withdrawn at the completion of the procedure.

46700

The physician performs anoplasty for an anal stricture in an adult. The physician explores the anal canal and identifies the stricture. An incision is made in the scar of the stricture and a portion of the stricture is excised. Incisions are extended onto the perianal skin and subcutaneous tissue and skin flaps are mobilized and advanced into the defects created by the scar excision. The flaps are sutured to the surrounding skin and anoderm thus closing the defect.

46705

The physician performs anoplasty for an anal stricture in an infant. The physician explores the anal canal and identifies the stricture. An incision is made in the scar of the stricture and a portion of the stricture is excised. Incisions are extended onto the perianal skin and subcutaneous tissue and skin flaps are mobilized and advanced into the defects created by the scar excision. The flaps are sutured to the surrounding skin and anoderm thus closing the defect.

46715

The physician performs an incision to open a low imperforate anus ("cutback" procedure). The physician exposes the perineum and identifies the fistulous opening to the imperforate anus. An incision is made through the fistula into the anus onto the skin thus opening the anus. The anus is usually dilated with Hegar dilators. The incision is usually left open to heal.

46716

The physician transposes an ectopic anal orifice. The imperforate anus has usually been previously incised and opened. The physician makes an incision around the anus. Dissection is continued circumferentially up around the distal rectum. Next, a cruciate incision is made over the usual site of the anus and an opening is created through the subcutaneous tissue and what remains of the external sphincter. The rectum is tunneled down through the new orifice and sutured to the new location. The incision at the previous anal site is closed.

46730

The physician repairs a high imperforate anus through a perineal or sacroperineal approach. The physician makes an incision at the usual site of the anus. Dissection is continued through the external sphincter. The puborectalis muscle is identified and dissection is carried through the muscle to identify and mobilize the rectal stump. The rectal stump is pulled through the sphincter complex, opened, and sutured to the sphincter and skin creating an anal opening. Alternately, a posterior midline sacral incision may be made initially. Dissection is carried superiorly, the puborectalis muscle is identified and a tract is formed through the puborectalis sling to the new anal opening. A perineal incision is made and the rectal stump mobilized and pulled through the sphincter complex onto the skin as described above.

46735

The physician repairs an imperforate anus by combined transabdominal and sacroperineal approaches. The physician makes a posterior midline incision on the sacrum and removes the coccyx. The puborectalis muscle is identified and a tract is made through the puborectalis sling to the future anal site. Next, the physician makes an abdominal incision and mobilizes the distal colon and rectum. The rectum is divided and the mucosa is striped from the distal rectum. An incision is made in the bottom of the rectal muscle pouch and the proximal rectum or colon is pulled through the muscular floor and puborectalis sling to the new anal site. A skin incision is made at the new anal site and the end of the colon is sutured to the sphincter muscles and skin creating a new anus. The incisions are closed.

46740

The physician repairs a high imperforate anus with a urethral or vaginal fistula through a perineal or sacroperineal approach. The physician makes an incision at the usual site of the anus. Dissection is continued through the external sphincter. The puborectalis muscle is identified and dissection is carried through the muscle to identify and mobilize the rectal stump. The urethral or vaginal fistula is identified, divided, and closed with sutures. The rectal stump is pulled through the sphincter complex, opened and sutured to the sphincter muscles and skin creating a new anal orifice. A posterior midline sacral incision may be made initially. Dissection is carried superiorly, the puborectalis muscle is identified and a tract is formed through the puborectalis sling to the new anal opening. A perineal incision is made at the site of the new anal opening. The rectal stump is mobilized, the fistula identified and divided, and the rectum pulled through the sphincter complex onto the skin as described above.

46742

The physician repairs an imperforate anus with a urethral or vaginal fistula by combined transabdominal and sacroperineal approaches. The physician makes a posterior midline incision on the sacrum and removes the coccyx. The puborectalis muscle is identified and a tract is developed through the puborectalis sling to the future anal site. Next, the physician makes an abdominal incision and mobilizes the distal colon and rectum. The rectum is divided, the mucosa is stripped from the distal rectum and the urethral or vaginal fistula is identified and closed with sutures. An incision is made in the bottom of the rectal muscle pouch and the proximal rectum or colon is pulled through the muscular floor and puborectalis sling to the new anal site. A skin incision

is made at the new anal site end of the colon is sutured to the sphincter muscles and skin creating a new anus. The incisions are closed.

46744

The physician repairs a cloacal anomaly. The patient is placed in a lithotomy position. The physician makes a small incision in the perineum. The bladder, urethra, and vagina are dissected free of each other. A new rectum is formed by interposing muscle posterior to the rectum. The incision is closed with sutures.

46746

The physician repairs a cloacal anomaly. The physician makes a small incision, using a combined abdominal and sacroperineal approach. The bladder, urethra, and vagina are dissected free of each other. A new rectum is formed by interposing muscle posterior to the rectum. The incision is closed.

46748

The physician corrects a congenital anomaly of the cloaca. A cloacal anomaly usually involves a single opening on the anterior perineum for the urethra, vagina, and rectum. The physician enters the pelvic cavity through an incision in the lower abdomen then makes a second incision in the perineum from the clitoris to the anal area. The surgeon then creates separate openings and divides membranes for the urethra, vagina, and rectum by using intestinal grafts, pedicle flaps, and free skin grafts.

46750

The physician performs anal sphincteroplasty for prolapse or incontinence in an adult. The physician makes a transverse incision anterior to the anus. Dissection is carried through subcutaneous tissues to expose the anal canal. The external anal sphincter muscle is dissected from the internal sphincter in the anterior plane and divided in the midline. The ends of the external sphincter are wrapped around the anal canal in an overlapping fashion and approximated with sutures. The incision is closed.

46751

The physician performs anal sphincteroplasty for prolapse or incontinence in a child. The physician makes a transverse incision anterior to the anus. Dissection is carried through the subcutaneous tissues to expose the anal canal. The external anal sphincter muscle is dissected from the internal sphincter and divided in the midline. The ends of the external sphincter are wrapped around the anal canal in an overlapping fashion and approximated with sutures. The incision is closed.

46753

The physician places a wire, suture, or muscular graft around the anus for rectal prolapse or incontinence (Thiersch procedure). The physician makes incisions on opposite sides of the anus in the lateral perianal subcutaneous tissue. A wire, suture or muscular graft mobilized from the thigh is wrapped around the anus in the subcutaneous space and secured in place. The incisions are closed.

46754

The physician removes a wire or suture that has been placed around the anal canal for rectal prolapse or incontinence. The physician makes incisions in the lateral perianal subcutaneous tissue. The wire or suture that is encircling the anus is identified, divided and removed. The incisions are closed.

46760

The physician performs an anal sphincteroplasty with a muscular graft for incontinence in an adult. The physician makes a transverse incision anterior to the anus. Dissection is carried through subcutaneous tissue to expose the anal canal and the remaining external sphincter muscle is dissected from the internal sphincter. A muscle from the thigh is mobilized and tunneled to the perineum. The muscle is wrapped around the anal canal and approximated with sutures. The incisions are closed.

46761

The physician performs sphincteroplasty with levator muscle imbrication for incontinence in an adult (Park repair). The physician makes a transverse incision anterior to the anus. Dissection is carried through the subcutaneous tissue to expose the anal canal. The external sphincter muscle is dissected from the internal sphincter and dissection is continued between the sphincters to expose the puborectalis muscle (levator). The edges of the puborectalis muscle are imbricated around the anal canal with sutures. The external sphincter muscle is imbricated around the anal canal with sutures. The incision is closed.

46762

The physician makes a midline abdominal incision. The physician dissects the perineum overlying the rectal orifice. The external anal sphincter muscle is mobilized along with its fibrotic ends. Surgical repair of the defective sphincter is performed with the implantation of an artificial sphincter. The external sphincter muscle may be wrapped around the anal canal and approximated without tension. The surgeon may find it necessary to approximate the levator ani muscle to restore the anorectal angle to normal; the puborectalis and external sphincter muscles are also tightened with sutures. This procedure lengthens the anal canal. Once implantation of the artificial sphincter is complete and the sphincter is reconstructed, the perineum is closed.

46900–46916

The physician performs destruction of anal lesions with chemicals in 46900. The physician exposes the perianal skin and identifies the lesions. The lesions

are painted with destructive chemicals. In 46910, the physician performs destruction of anal lesions with electrodesiccation. The physician exposes the perianal skin and identifies the lesions. The lesions are destroyed with cautery. In 46916, the physician performs destruction of anal lesions with cryosurgery. The physician exposes the perianal skin and identifies the lesions. The lesions are frozen and destroyed, usually with liquid nitrogen.

46917–46922

The physician performs destruction of anal lesions with laser therapy in 46917. The physician exposes the perianal skin and identifies the lesions. The lesions are destroyed by laser ablation or laser excision. In 46922, the physician performs destruction of anal lesions by excision. The physician exposes the perianal skin and identifies the lesions. The lesions are surgically excised. The incisions are closed.

46924

The physician performs destruction of extensive anal lesions. The physician exposes the perianal skin and identifies the lesions. An extensive destruction of the lesions is performed by various methods, such as laser surgery, electrosurgery, cryosurgery, or chemosurgery.

46934–46936

The physician performs destruction of internal hemorrhoids in 46934. The physician explores the anal canal and identifies the hemorrhoid columns. In 46935, the physician performs destruction of external hemorrhoids. The physician exposes the perianal area and identifies the external hemorrhoids. In 46936, the physician performs destruction of internal or external hemorrhoids. The physician explores the anal canal and identifies the internal or external hemorrhoids. The hemorrhoids are destroyed by any method. The hemorrhoidal remnants may be removed.

46937–46938

The physician performs cryosurgery of a benign rectal tumor in 46937 or a malignant tumor in 46938. The physician explores the anal canal and identifies the tumor. The tumor is frozen, usually with liquid nitrogen. The tumor may be partially removed or allowed to spontaneously slough.

46940–46942

The physician performs an initial (46940) or subsequent (46942) curettage or cautery of an anal fissure with dilation of the anal sphincter. The physician exposes the perianal area and identifies the fissure. The fissure is debrided with curettage or cautery. The anal sphincter is manually dilated.

46945–46946

The physician performs ligation of internal hemorrhoids. The physician explores the anal canal and identifies the hemorrhoid columns. A single suture ligation of the hemorrhoid columns is performed in 46945. Multiple suture ligations of the hemorrhoid columns are performed in 46946.

47000–47001

The physician takes tissue from the liver for examination. In 47000, the physician uses separately reportable ultrasound guidance to place a hollow bore needle between the ribs on the patient's right side. The liver biopsy is sent for pathology for separately reportable activity. Report 47001 when the liver biopsy is performed during an open procedure.

47010

The physician incises the liver to drain an abscess or a cyst, sometimes taking one or two stages. The physician exposes the liver via an upper midline incision. The cyst is carefully incised and suctioned with care to not contaminate the abdomen with purulent matter. Cultures and pathology are sent in a separately reported activity. The incision is closed.

47011

The physician performs a hepatotomy for percutaneous drainage of abscess or cyst, one or two stages. The physician may create a small incision in the skin proximal to the liver abscess or cyst to ease placement of drainage instruments through the skin (percutaneous). The physician uses a CAT scan or ultrasound to guide placement of a drainage needle or trocar into the liver abscess or cyst. The physician advances the drainage needle or trocar through the abdominal wall into the peritoneum to gain access to the abscess or cystic cavity. The procedure sometimes requires multiple stages. The fluid is allowed to drain. Once drained, a catheter may be placed (and later removed) to maintain drainage. Sutures may be secured to hold the drainage catheter in place. The operative site is subsequently cleaned and bandaged. For radiological supervision and interpretation, see 75989.

47015

The physician performs aspiration or injection of liver parasitic cysts or abscesses. The physician makes an abdominal incision. The liver is mobilized and the parasitic cysts or abscesses are identified. The remaining abdominal contents are packed off with sponges for protection. The cysts are aspirated with a needle and syringe or unroofed and aspirated and may be injected with a hypertonic solution. The abdominal incision is closed.

47100

The physician takes a wedge-shaped section of liver tissue for biopsy. The physician exposes the abdomen via an upper abdominal incision through skin, fascia, and muscle. Interrupted mattress sutures are placed on the edge of the liver lobe. A pie-shaped wedge of the liver is resected and sent for pathology in a separately reportable activity. Electrocautery is used to

obtain hemostasis of the liver edge. The abdominal incision is closed with layered sutures.

47120–47130

The physician removes a section of liver, or lobectomy. The physician exposes the liver via an upper midline incision through skin, fascia, and muscle. The fibrous connections of the liver to the diaphragm are divided and the portal structures are controlled. The portal and hepatic vessels associated with the affected lobe are divided. The portal structures are clamped. The liver parenchyma is divided by pressure or coagulation hemostases. The portal clamp is removed and hemostasis is assured before the abdomen is closed with sutures. Report 47120 if a partial lobectomy is performed; report 47122 if a trisegmentectomy is performed; report 47125 if a total left lobectomy is performed; and report 47130 if a total right lobectomy is performed.

47133

The physician performs a liver resection with preservation in a cadaver for transplantation into a recipient. The physician makes an abdominal incision. The liver is mobilized from its attachments and the blood supply and bile ducts to the liver are dissected out and isolated. The selected segment of liver is resected with its attached blood vessels and bile ducts. The resected segment is perfused with a cold preservation solution and removed from the operative field for transplantation. Drains are placed and the abdominal incision is closed.

47134

The physician performs a partial liver resection with preservation in a living donor for transplantation into a recipient. The physician makes an abdominal incision. The liver is mobilized from its attachments and the blood supply and bile ducts to the liver are dissected out and isolated. The selected segment of liver is resected with its attached blood vessels and bile ducts. The resected segment is perfused with a cold preservation solution and removed from the operative field for transplantation. Drains are placed and the abdominal incision is closed.

47135

The physician performs partial or whole liver transplantation in a position other than normal anatomic position of the liver. The physician makes an abdominal incision. The donor liver is placed in the upper abdominal cavity. Anastomoses are created between the donor hepatic vessels and the appropriate recipient vessels. The donor bile duct is approximated to the recipient bile duct or to a limb of small bowel for drainage. Drains are placed and the abdominal incision is closed.

47136

The physician transplants a partial or whole liver to a position other than normal anatomic position of the liver. The physician makes an abdominal incision. The donor liver is placed in the upper abdominal cavity. Anastomoses are created between the donor hepatic vessels and the appropriate recipient vessels. The donor bile duct is approximated to the recipient bile duct or to a limb of small bowel for drainage. Drains are placed and the abdominal incision is closed.

47300

The physician creates a pouch with the lining of a cyst on the liver. The physician exposes the liver via an upper midline abdominal incision through skin, fascia, and muscles. The cyst is incised and suctioned with care not to contaminate the abdomen. Electrocautery is used to resect the cyst wall to allow open drainage into the abdomen. The abdominal incision is closed with sutures.

47350–47362

The physician sutures a liver wound to control the bleeding or repair damage. In 47350, the physician exposes the liver via an upper midline abdominal incision. The abdomen is packed to control bleeding. The patient is stabilized hemodynamically. The liver is systematically exposed with pressure on bleeding points. The liver tissue is divided to expose the points of bleeding and the bleeding is controlled by ligation of bleeding vessels. The abdominal incision is closed. Report 47360 if the procedure requires a complex suture of liver wound or injury, with or without hepatic artery ligation; report 47361 if procedure requires an exploration of a hepatic wound, extensive debridement, coagulation and/or suture, with or without packing of the liver; and report 47362 if the procedure is a re-exploration of hepatic wound for removal of packing.

47370–47371

The physician places a laparoscope via a small periumbilical port or through a small incision in the right upper quadrant, and an additional port is placed in the right upper quadrant under direct vision. Adhesions are lysed and ligamentous attachments divided to mobilize the liver. The physician examines all the parietal and visceral peritoneal surfaces, the lesser sac, the omentum, and the viscera. The gastrohepatic omentum is opened for inspection of the caudate lobe, followed by sequential laparoscopic ultrasonographic examination of all eight liver segments using an ultrasonic probe. Radiofrequency ablation is performed using a 15-gauge needle with a retractable curved electrode placed percutaneously into the abdomen at the place overlying the area of interest under direct vision. The needle is directed into the center of the lesion under real-time ultrasound guidance, tynes are deployed and alternating current is delivered to ablate the tumor. Upon completion of ablation, the probe tract is cauterized and the needle withdrawn. Report 47371 if

ablation is accomplished using a cool-tipped multiple probe electrode.

47380

The physician performs radiofrequency ablation of a liver tumor via an open laparotomy. Grounding pads are placed on the patient's legs. The physician performs a midline laparotomy. Dissection is carried down to the liver. Under direct visualization, a needle-electrode, with an insulated shaft and an uninsulated distal tip, is inserted into the tumor. Each treatment session has about 10 to 15 minutes of active ablation. The energy at the needle tip causes ionic agitation and frictional heat in the surrounding tissue, which, when hot enough, leads to cell death and coagulative necrosis. This results in a 3.0 to 5.5 cm sphere of dead tissue per treatment session. In large tumors, the physician may create more than one sphere next to each other to try to turn the tumor edges in three dimensions. A small margin of normal tissue next to the tumor is also burned, as a precaution to destroy all tumor cells. The tumor cells are not removed, but are gradually replaced by fibrosis and scar tissue. One method uses a needle-within-a-needle electrode system with an inner needle that expands once placed into the tumor.

47381

The physician performs cryosurgical ablation of a liver tumor. The physician performs a laparotomy. Dissection is carrier down to the liver. Special cryosurgical probes are inserted into the liver tumor. The cryosurgical probes rapidly freeze (liquid nitrogen at -196°C or nitrous oxide at -89.5°C) the area being treated, then the liver tissue is slowly thawed, and repeated cycles of freezing and thawing are immediately performed. Cryogen may also be applied directly into or on to the tumor by probe, direct application, spraying, or by pouring. The incision is closed with layered suture.

47382

Intravenous sedation is administered and grounding pads are placed on the patient's legs. A needle-electrode, with an insulated shaft and an uninsulated distal tip, is inserted through the skin and directly into the tumor. Ultrasound, CT scan, or MRI guide the needles to the correct spot and monitor treatment. Each treatment session has about 10 to 15 minutes of active ablation. The energy at the needle tip causes ionic agitation and frictional heat in the surrounding tissue, which, when hot enough, leads to cell death and coagulative necrosis. This results in a 3.0 to 5.5 cm sphere of dead tissue per treatment session. In large tumors, the physician may create more than one sphere next to each other to try to turn the tumor edges in three dimensions. A small margin of normal tissue next to the tumor is also burned, as a precaution to destroy all tumor cells. The tumor cells are not removed, but are gradually replaced by fibrosis and scar tissue. One method uses a needle-within-a-needle electrode system with an inner needle that expands once placed into the tumor.

47400

The physician makes a midline abdominal incision.The physician makes an incision into the hepatic duct and surgically creates an artificial opening. The physician performs exploration, drainage, or removal of calculus from the hepatic duct. The hepatic duct is closed either primarily or around a tube for continued drainage. If a drainage tube is placed, a separate incision is made in the abdominal wall through which the drainage tube is positioned. The abdominal incisions are closed.

47420–47425

The physician explores the common bile duct, removing calculus, draining purulent matter, and/or constructing a new duct. The physician exposes the common bile duct within the portal triad through a subcostal or upper midline incision. The common bile duct is incised, explored, and drained. The common bile duct is closed with interrupted sutures either primarily or around a drainage tube (choledochostomy). If placed, the drainage tube is brought out through the skin at a site separate from the incision. The abdominal incision is closed. Report 47425 if this procedure performed with transduodenal sphincterotomy or sphincteroplasty.

47460

The physician performs a transduodenal sphincterotomy or sphincteroplasty and may repair the duodenal sphincter or remove a stone, as needed. The physician exposes the second portion of the duodenum via a subcostal or upper midline incision through skin, fascia, and muscle. The duodenum is opened using a longitudinal incision. The ampulla of Vater is identified and an incision is made in the ampulla at the two o'clock position. The common bile duct mucosa may be reapproximated to the duodenal mucosa and the duodenum transversely closed with interrupted sutures. Stones may be removed. The abdominal incision is closed.

47480

The physician performs a cholecystotomy or cholecystostomy with exploration, drainage, or removal of calculus. The physician exposes the gallbladder through a subcostal or upper midline incision. The gallbladder is incised, explored, and may be drained. Calculi may be removed. The gallbladder is closed with interrupted sutures either primarily or around a drainage tube. If placed, the drainage tube is brought out through the skin at a site separate from the incision. The abdominal incision is closed.

47490

The physician inserts a tube into the gallbladder to allow drainage through the skin. The physician uses ultrasound guidance, separately reportable, to place a

subcostal drainage tube into the gallbladder. The physician places a needle between the ribs into the gallbladder. The needle position is checked by aspiration. A guidewire is passed through the needle. A catheter is passed over the wire into the biliary tree. The wire is removed and the tube is left in place.

47500

The physician injects a radiographic medium for diagnostic purposes. Using separately reportable computerized tomography or fluoroscopy guidance, the physician places a needle between the ribs into the lumen of the common bile duct. The needle position is checked by aspiration. Radiographic dye is injected. The needle is removed.

47505

The physician injects a radiographic medium through an existing catheter for diagnostic purposes. The physician injects a radiographic medium into the gallbladder via an existing tube while visualizing the liver under separately reportable fluoroscopy.

47510

The physician introduces a catheter into the liver to drain fluid. Using separately reportable computerized tomography or fluoroscopy guidance, the physician places a needle between the ribs into the lumen of the biliary tree. The needle position is checked by aspiration. A guidewire is passed through the needle. A catheter is passed over the wire into the biliary tree. The wire is removed and the catheter is left in place.

47511

The physician introduces a stent into a liver duct to open a stricture. Using separately reportable computerized tomography or fluoroscopy guidance, the physician places a needle between the ribs into the common bile duct across the stricture. A balloon catheter and stent is placed across the stricture. The stent is employed and the balloon and wire are removed. The stent and catheter remain in place and the catheter is sutured to the skin.

47525

The physician changes a drainage catheter in the liver. Under fluoroscopic guidance (reported separately), the physician passes a wire through the original catheter. A new catheter is passed over the guidewire. The new catheter is sutured to the skin.

47530

The physician revises or reinserts a tube to the liver. Under fluoroscopic guidance (reported separately), the physician passes a wire through the original catheter. The old catheter is removed. A new catheter is passed over the guidewire and sutured to the skin.

47550

The physician performs a biliary endoscopy during the same surgical session as other biliary procedures.

The physician advances an endoscope through the previously made abdominal incision. With the endoscope the physician is able to directly visualize portions of the biliary tract, which may be filled with contrast medium for identifying the common bile duct, biliary tree and gall bladder (including areas of abnormality, stricture, or obstruction) under separately reportable fluoroscopy.

47552

The physician makes a small incision in the abdominal wall. The physician advances an endoscope through an opening in the abdominal wall or through a T-tube inserted through the abdominal wall into the common bile duct. With the endoscope, the physician is able to directly visualize portions of the biliary tract, which may be filled with contrast medium for identifying the common bile duct, biliary tree, and gall bladder (including areas of abnormality, stricture, or obstruction) under separately reportable fluoroscopy. The physician may collect specimens by brushing and/or washing (separate procedure). The endoscope is removed. The T-tube is withdrawn and the defect in the common bile duct is sutured closed. The tract, peritoneum, and abdominal wall are closed with layered sutures.

47553

The physician makes a small incision in the abdomen. The physician advances an endoscope through an opening in the abdominal wall or through a T-tube inserted through the abdominal wall into the common bile duct. With the endoscope, the physician is able to directly visualize portions of the biliary tract, which may be filled with contrast medium for identifying the common bile duct, biliary tree, and gallbladder (including areas of abnormality, stricture, or obstruction) under separately reportable fluoroscopy. The physician advances biopsy forceps along the tract or T-tube to obtain single or multiple biopsies under direct endoscopic visualization or with the use of fluoroscopy. The endoscope is removed. The T-tube is withdrawn and the defect in the common bile duct is sutured closed. The tract, peritoneum, and abdominal wall are closed using a layered technique.

47554

The physician makes a small incision in the abdomen. The physician advances an endoscope through an opening in the abdominal wall or through a T-tube inserted through the abdominal wall into the common bile duct. With the endoscope, the physician is able to directly visualize portions of the biliary tract, which may be filled with contrast medium for identifying the common bile duct, biliary tree, and gallbladder (including areas of abnormality, stricture, or obstruction) under separately reportable fluoroscopy. Calculi are identified and removed. The endoscope is removed. The T-tube is withdrawn and the defect in the common bile duct is sutured closed. The tract,

peritoneum, and abdominal wall are closed using a layered technique.

47555

The physician makes a small incision in the abdomen. The physician advances an endoscope through an opening in the abdominal wall or through a T-tube inserted through the abdominal wall into the common bile duct. With the endoscope, the physician is able to directly visualize portions of the biliary tract, which may be filled with contrast medium for identifying the common bile duct, biliary tree, and gallbladder (including areas of abnormality, stricture, or obstruction) under fluoroscopy. The physician advances a balloon-tipped catheter through the tract or T-tube so that it is above the site of the duct stricture, inflates the balloon and draws it back through the site of stricture to achieve dilation. This procedure may be repeated until optimal dilation is obtained. The endoscope is removed and the tract, peritoneum, and abdominal wall are approximated. The endoscope is removed. The T-tube is withdrawn and the common bile duct is sutured closed. The abdomen is sutured closed.

47556

The physician makes a small incision in the abdomen. The physician advances an endoscope through an opening in the abdominal wall or through a T-tube inserted through the abdominal wall into the common bile duct. With the endoscope, the physician is able to directly visualize portions of the biliary tract, which may be filled with contrast medium for identifying the common bile duct, biliary tree, and gallbladder (including areas of abnormality, stricture, or obstruction) under separately reportable fluoroscopy. The physician advances a balloon-tipped catheter through the tract or T-tube so that it is above the site of duct stricture, inflates the balloon and draws it back through the site of stricture to achieve dilation. This procedure may be repeated until optimal dilation is obtained. The physician places a stent to prevent future stricture. The endoscope is removed. The T-tube is withdrawn and the defect in the common bile duct is sutured closed. The abdomen is sutured closed.

47560

The physician examines the peritoneal cavity and performs a contrast study of the bile ducts through the liver with the laparoscope. The physician places a trocar through a small abdominal incision and insufflates the abdominal cavity. The laparoscope is placed through the port and additional trocars are placed. The peritoneal cavity is examined. A contrast study of the bile ducts is obtained by placing a needle through the liver into an intrahepatic bile duct under fluoroscopy and injecting dye. The trocars are removed and the incisions are closed.

47561

The physician examines the peritoneal cavity, performs a contrast study of the bile ducts through the liver and obtains tissue samples with the laparoscope. The physician places a trocar through a small abdominal incision and insufflates the abdominal cavity. The laparoscope is placed through the port and additional trocars are placed. The peritoneal cavity is examined. A contrast study of the bile ducts is obtained by placing a needle through the liver into an intrahepatic bile duct under fluoroscopy and injecting dye. Tissue samples are obtained of one or more intra-abdominal structures. The trocars are removed and the incisions are closed.

47562

The physician removes the gallbladder through a laparoscope. The physician makes a 1.0-centimeter infraumbilical incision through which a trocar is inserted. Pneumoperitoneum is achieved by insufflating the abdominal cavity with carbon dioxide. A fiberoptic laparoscope fitted with a camera and light source is inserted through the trocar. Other incisions are made on right side of the abdomen and in the subxiphoid area to allow other instruments or an additional light source to be passed into the abdomen. The tip of the gallbladder is mobilized and placed in traction. The Hartmann's pouch (junction of the cystic duct and gallbladder neck) is identified. Tissue is dissected free from around the area for exposure of Calot's triangle (formed by the cystic artery, and cystic and common bile ducts). Clips are applied to the proximal area of the cystic duct and artery (close to the gallbladder) and the cystic duct and artery are cut. The gallbladder is dissected from the liver bed and removed through a trocar site. Any loose stones that have dropped into the abdominal cavity are retrieved with forceps. The intraabdominal cavity is irrigated. The trocars are removed and the incisions are closed.

47563

The physician removes the gallbladder and performs a contrast study of the bile ducts through the laparoscope. The physician places a trocar at the umbilicus and insufflates the abdominal cavity. The laparoscope is placed through the umbilical port and additional trocars are placed into the abdominal cavity. The gallbladder is mobilized and placed on traction. The neck of the gallbladder and cystic duct are dissected from surrounding structures. A contrast study of the bile ducts is obtained through the cystic duct. The cystic duct and artery are divided. The gallbladder is dissected from the liver bed and removed through a trocar site. The trocars are removed and the incisions are closed.

47564

The physician removes the gallbladder and performs a common bile duct exploration through the laparoscope. The physician places a trocar at the umbilicus and insufflates the abdominal cavity. The

laparoscope is placed through the umbilical port and additional trocars are placed into the abdominal cavity. The gallbladder is mobilized and placed on traction. The neck of the gallbladder and cystic duct are dissected from surrounding structures. A contrast study of the bile ducts is usually obtained through the cystic duct. The common bile duct may be explored with a small choledochoscope through the cystic duct or a separate incision may be made in the common bile duct. The common duct is visualized with a choledochoscope and stones may be extracted from the duct with a variety of instruments. If an incision was made in the common bile duct this is usually closed with sutures over a T-tube that is brought out through the abdominal wall. The cystic duct and artery are divided. The gallbladder is removed through a trocar site. A drain is usually placed below the liver and brought out through the abdominal wall. The trocars are removed and the incisions are closed.

47570

Through the laparoscope the physician performs an anastomosis between the gallbladder and small bowel (cholecystoenterostomy). The physician places a trocar at the umbilicus and insufflates the abdominal cavity. The laparoscope is placed through the umbilical port and additional trocars are placed into the abdominal cavity. The gallbladder and a proximal loop of small bowel are identified and mobilized. An anastomosis is created between the gallbladder and loop or limb of proximal small bowel with staples or sutures. The trocars are removed and the incisions are closed.

47600–47605

The physician removes the gallbladder. The physician exposes the liver and gallbladder via a right subcostal incision. The cystic duct and cystic artery are ligated and the gallbladder is removed using electrocautery. The incision is closed with layered sutures. Report 47605 if this is performed with a cholangiography.

47610–47620

The physician removes the gallbladder and explores the common duct. The physician exposes the liver and gallbladder via a right subcostal incision. The cystic duct and cystic artery are ligated and the gallbladder removed using electrocautery. The common bile duct is exposed in the portal triad, incised, and the stones removed. The common bile duct is closed and the abdominal incision is closed with sutures. Report 47612 if this procedure is performed with choledocheoenterostomy, establishment of communication between the intestine and the common bile duct; report 47620 if this procedure is performed with transduodenal sphincterotomy or sphincteroplasty, with or without cholangiography.

47630

The physician removes a stone from the biliary duct, percutaneous. Approximately two weeks after placement of a choledochostomy, the physician removes the choledochostomy tube (T-tube) and places a choledochoscope through the choledochostomy tract. The biliary tree, liver, and ampulla are visualized. Using a basket or snare through the choledochoscope and with fluoroscopy guidance (reported separately), the stones are removed.

47700

The physician explores a congenital atresia of the bile ducts without making a repair, with or without liver biopsy, with or without cholangiography. The physician uses an upper midline abdominal incision to expose the liver, gall bladder, and bile ducts. Inspection and evaluation of the gallbladder, common bile ducts, and duodenum is carried out to determine the status of the bile ducts. A tissue sample may be removed. Cholangiography may be performed. A biliary drainage tube may be placed.

47701

The physician performs a portoenterostomy, a procedure in which the jejunum is connected to the bile ducts and other portal structures of the liver and gallbladder. The physician exposes the liver and gallbladder via an upper midline or subcostal incision. The bile ducts are connected to the small bowel for drainage by anastomosing a Roux-en-Y hook of jejunum to the divided extravascular portal structures. The abdominal incision is closed.

47711

The physician performs excision of an extrahepatic bile duct tumor and reconstructs bile duct drainage. The physician makes an abdominal incision and explores the abdomen. The bile duct is dissected from surrounding structures and the tumor is identified and mobilized. The tumor is excised with a margin of normal bile duct tissue proximal and distal to the tumor. An anastomosis is usually created between the proximal end of the bile duct and a loop of small bowel to allow biliary drainage. The distal end of the bile duct is oversewn. The incision is closed.

47712

The physician performs excision of an intrahepatic bile duct tumor and reconstructs bile duct drainage. The physician makes an abdominal incision and explores the abdomen. The distal bile duct is isolated. The tumor is identified and dissection is continued proximally along the bile duct into the parenchyma of the liver beyond the tumor onto the left and right hepatic ducts. The tumor is excised with a normal margin of bile duct or hepatic duct proximal and distal to the tumor. An anastomosis is created between the proximal bile duct or left and right hepatic ducts and a limb of small bowel to allow biliary drainage.

The distal end of the bile duct is oversewn. The incision is closed.

47715

The physician excises a cyst in the common bile duct. The physician exposes the liver and gallbladder via an upper midline or subcostal incision made through skin, fascia, and muscle. The cyst is exposed and excised and the defect of the biliary system is repaired. The abdominal incision is closed with layered sutures.

47716

The physician connects a cyst of the common bile duct to the intestine for drainage. The physician exposes the liver and gallbladder via an upper midline or subcostal incision made through skin, fascia, and muscle. The cyst is opened and connected to the intestine for drainage. The abdominal incision is closed.

47720–47741

The physician performs a cholecystoenterostomy, in which a communication is made between the gallbladder and an artificial anus or fistula in the abdominal wall. The physician exposes the liver and gallbladder via an upper midline or subcostal incision. The cyst is opened and connected to the small intestine for drainage. The abdominal incision is closed. Report 47721 if this procedure is performed with gastroenterostomy; report 47740 if this procedure is performed with Roux-en-Y; and report 47741 if this procedure is performed with Roux-en-Y with gastroenterostomy.

47760

The physician performs an anastomosis between an extrahepatic biliary duct and the small bowel. The physician makes an abdominal incision and explores the abdomen. The extrahepatic biliary duct is divided and anastomosis is formed between an extrahepatic biliary duct and the small bowel with sutures or staples (end-to-side). The incision is closed in layers.

47765

The physician performs an anastomosis between an intrahepatic biliary duct and the small bowel. The physician makes an abdominal incision and explores the abdomen. The intrahepatic biliary duct is divided and anastomosis is formed between an intrahepatic biliary duct and the small bowel with sutures or staples (end-to-side). The incision is closed in layers.

47780

The physician performs an anastomosis between a limb of small bowel (Roux-en-Y) and the gallbladder and stomach. The physician makes an abdominal incision and explores the abdomen. The proximal small bowel is divided and anastomoses are formed between the distal limb of jejunum and the gallbladder and the stomach with sutures or staples.

The proximal end of bowel is approximated to the limb of jejunum distal to the gallbladder and stomach anastomoses. This procedure is usually performed for a mass obstructing the bile duct and stomach. The incision is closed.

47785

The physician performs an anastomosis between a limb of small bowel (Roux-en-Y) and the intrahepatic biliary ducts. The physician makes an abdominal incision. The bile duct is isolated and dissection is carried proximally along the duct into the liver parenchyma exposing the intrahepatic biliary ducts. The bile duct is divided or excised. The proximal small bowel is divided and an anastomosis is created between the distal limb of jejunum and the intrahepatic biliary ducts with sutures. The distal bile duct is oversewn. The proximal end of bowel is approximated to the limb of jejunum distal to the bile duct anastomosis. The incision is closed.

47800

The physician reconstructs the biliary ducts through anastomosis. The physician exposes the liver and gallbladder via an upper midline or subcostal incision made via skin, fascia, and muscle. The abnormal biliary tree is excised and the resected ends are reconnected. The incision is closed with layered sutures.

47801

The physician inserts a stent into the bile duct. The physician makes a small incision overlying the bile duct. Using an endoscope or percutaneous choledochostomy tube, a catheter and stent are placed to bridge a narrowing in the common bile duct. The scope or tube is removed and the incision closed.

47802

The physician establishes a communication between the hepatic ducts and the intestine. The physician exposes the liver and gallbladder via an upper midline or subcostal incision. A Silastic tube is connected between the biliary tree and the intestine for drainage of biliary obstruction. The abdominal incision is closed.

47900

The physician performs suture closure of a biliary duct injury. The physician makes an abdominal incision. The bile duct is dissected from surrounding structures and the injury of the duct is identified. The duct injury is closed with sutures. A drain is usually placed and brought out through the abdominal wall. The incision is closed.

48000

The physician places peripancreatic drains for pancreatitis and performs cholecystostomy, gastrostomy and jejunostomy. The physician makes an abdominal incision. The pancreas is exposed, necrotic

pancreatic tissue may be debrided and drains are placed around the pancreas. The gallbladder is identified and a tube is sutured into the gallbladder and brought out through the abdominal wall. An incision is made in the anterior gastric wall and a tube is sutured into the stomach and brought out through the anterior abdominal wall. An incision is made in a proximal segment of jejunum and a tube is sutured into the jejunum and brought out through the anterior abdominal wall. The abdominal incision is closed.

48001

The physician makes an upper transverse abdominal incision. The transverse colon and small intestines are retracted to reveal the underlying pancreas. Necrotic pancreatic tissue may be resected. Drains are placed circumferentially around the pancreas. The anterior gastric wall is incised and a drainage tube is inserted, sutured secure, and anchored through the abdominal wall. The jejunum is incised and a drainage tube is inserted, sutured, secured, and anchored through the abdominal wall. The gallbladder is located, incised, and a drainage tube is placed in it with the caudal end being drawn through a separate abdominal incision. The upper transverse abdominal incision is closed with sutures.

48005

The physician performs resection and debridement of the pancreas for necrotizing pancreatitis. The physician makes an abdominal incision. The pancreas is exposed and necrotic areas of the pancreas and peripancreatic tissue are debrided. Drains are usually placed around the pancreas. The incision is closed.

48020

The physician removes a stone from the pancreas. The physician exposes the pancreas via an upper midline incision through skin, fascia, and muscle. The pancreatic duct is opened and calculus removed. The pancreatic duct is connected directly to the small bowel for drainage. The abdominal incision is closed.

48100

The physician obtains a biopsy of the pancreas. The physician makes a midline epigastric incision and retracts the skin and underlying tissues laterally. The physician approaches the pancreas through the lesser sac of the omental bursa. The pancreas is palpated, the lesion is identified, and a biopsy is obtained by various methods, such as fine needle aspiration or needle core or wedge biopsy. Bleeding is controlled and the lesser sac is closed. Tissues are reapproximated to the anatomical position and the operative incision is closed in sutured layers.

48102

The physician removes tissue from the pancreas. The physician passes the biopsy needle through the skin of the upper abdomen under separately reportable

CPT® Lay Descriptions

computerized tomography guidance. The pancreatic lesion is removed and the specimen is sent for pathology for examination (reported separately).

48120

The physician excises a lesion of the pancreas. The physician makes a midline epigastric incision and retracts the skin and underlying tissues laterally. The physician approaches the pancreas through the lesser sac of the omental bursa or the through the transverse mesocolon. The pancreas is palpated, the lesion is identified and excised. Bleeding is controlled, and the lesser sac is closed. Tissues are reapproximated to anatomical position, and the operative incision is closed in sutured layers.

48140–48145

The physician removes the distal portion of the pancreas, with or without removing the spleen and jejunum. The physician makes a midline epigastric incision and retracts the skin and underlying tissues laterally. The physician approaches the pancreas through the lesser sac of the omental bursa or the through the transverse mesocolon. The pancreas is identified and freed from attachments. If the blood supply to the distal pancreas also supplies the spleen, the spleen is sacrificed in the resection. The pancreas is transected, and the distal portion is removed, with or without the spleen. In 48140, the pancreatic duct is not obstructed, permitting free drainage of pancreatic enzymes. In 48145, the duct flow is obstructed and a jejunal loop is brought up to create a fistula for enzyme flow to the digestive tract. Bleeding is controlled, and the lesser sac is closed. Tissues are reapproximated to anatomical position, and the operative incision is closed in sutured layers.

48146

The physician performs a near-total pancreatectomy. The physician makes an abdominal incision. The pancreas is exposed and the body and tail of the pancreas are mobilized. The pancreas is transected at the junction of the head and body of the pancreas over the superior mesenteric vessels. The distal pancreas is removed. Frequently the spleen is removed with the distal pancreas. The end of the proximal pancreas is closed with staples or sutures. Drains are usually placed in the pancreatic bed. The incision is closed.

48148

The physician excises the ampulla of Vater, a saccular dilation of liver and/or pancreas. The physician exposes the duodenum and pancreas via an upper midline abdominal incision. The duodenum is opened with a longitudinal incision. The ampulla of Vater is exposed and the abnormality is excised. The common bile duct and duodenal mucosa are re-approximated as needed. The duodenum is closed with transverse interrupted sutures. The abdominal incision is closed.

48150

The physician performs excision of the proximal pancreas, duodenum, distal bile duct and distal stomach with reconstruction (Whipple procedure) but with pancreaticojejunostomy. The physician makes an abdominal incision and explores the abdomen. The duodenum, proximal pancreas, and bile duct are mobilized. The distal bile duct, distal stomach, and distal duodenum are divided. The pancreas is transected at the junction of the head and body and the pancreatic head, duodenum, distal stomach, and distal bile duct are removed en bloc. The anatomy is reconstructed by performing sequential anastomoses between the proximal jejunum and the distal bile duct and distal stomach. The edge of the remaining distal pancreas is closed with sutures or staples. The incision is closed.

48152

The physician performs excision of the proximal pancreas, duodenum, distal bile duct and distal stomach with reconstruction (Whipple procedure) but without pancreaticojejunostomy. The physician makes an abdominal incision and explores the abdomen. The duodenum, proximal pancreas, and bile duct are mobilized. The distal bile duct, distal stomach, and distal duodenum are divided. The pancreas is transected at the junction of the head and body and the pancreatic head, duodenum, distal stomach, and distal bile duct are removed en bloc. The anatomy is reconstructed by performing sequential anastomoses between the proximal jejunum and the distal bile duct and distal stomach. The edge of the remaining distal pancreas is closed with sutures or staples. The incision is closed.

48153

The physician performs excision of the proximal pancreas, duodenum, and distal bile duct with reconstruction (pylorus preserving Whipple procedure). The physician makes an abdominal incision and explores the abdomen. The duodenum, proximal pancreas, and bile duct are mobilized. The distal bile duct and distal duodenum are divided. The proximal duodenum is divided just distal to the pylorus. The pancreas is transected at the junction of the head and body and the proximal pancreas, duodenum and distal bile duct are removed en bloc. The anatomy is reconstructed by performing sequential anastomoses between the proximal jejunum and the remaining pancreatic tail, distal bile duct and pylorus. The incision is closed.

48154

The physician performs excision of the proximal pancreas, duodenum and distal bile duct with reconstruction but without pancreaticojejunostomy. The physician makes an abdominal incision and explores the abdomen. The duodenum, proximal pancreas and bile duct are mobilized. The distal bile duct and distal duodenum are divided. The proximal duodenum is divided just distal to the pylorus. The pancreas is transected at the junction of the head and body and the proximal pancreas, duodenum, and distal bile duct are removed en block. The anatomy is reconstructed by performing sequential anastomoses between the proximal jejunum and the distal bile duct and the pylorus. The edge of the remaining distal pancreas is closed with sutures or staples and no anastomosis is performed to the pancreas. The incision is closed.

48155–48160

The physician removes all or part of the pancreas. The physician makes a midline epigastric incision and retracts the skin and underlying tissues laterally. The physician approaches the pancreas through the lesser sac of the omental bursa or the through the transverse mesocolon. The pancreas is identified and freed from attachments. In 48155, the entire pancreas is removed. In 48160, all or part of the pancreas is removed and pancreatic islet cells are transplanted into the abdominal tissue. Blood vessels are ligated and the affected pancreas is removed. Bleeding is controlled, and the lesser sac is closed. Tissues are reapproximated to anatomical position, and the operative incision is closed in sutured layers.

48180

The physician creates a pancreatical jejunostomy to drain pancreatic enzymes through a side-to-side anastomosis. The physician makes a midline epigastric incision and retracts the skin and underlying tissues laterally. The physician approaches the pancreas through the lesser sac of the omental bursa or the through the transverse mesocolon. A jejunal loop is brought up to create a fistula for enzyme flow to the digestive tract. Bleeding is controlled, and the lesser sac is closed. Tissues are reapproximated to anatomical position, and the operative incision is closed in sutured layers.

48400

The physician performs a contrast study of the pancreatic duct. The physician makes an abdominal incision. The pancreas is exposed and may be mobilized by dissecting it from its retroperitoneal attachments. A separately reported pancreatogram may be obtained by injecting contrast into the common bile duct thus filling the pancreatic duct in a retrograde fashion and a radiograph obtained. Alternately, the duodenum may be opened and the pancreatic duct injected directly, or the tail of the pancreas may be transected and the pancreatic duct injected directly with contrast and a radiograph obtained. The duodenum is closed or the pancreatic tail is sutured closed. The incision is closed.

48500

The physician marsupializes a pancreatic cyst. The physician approaches the pancreas through a midline abdominal incision and retracts the skin and underlying tissues laterally. The physician approaches the pancreas through the lesser sac of the omental bursa or the through the transverse mesocolon. The cyst is located, and the anterior cyst wall is incised. The cut edges of the cyst are sutured to the skin edges establishing a pouch of what was formally an enclosed cyst. The remainder of the operative site is closed in sutured layers.

48510

The physician externally drains a pancreatic cyst. The physician approaches the pancreas through a midline abdominal incision. The physician locates the cyst through an incision and approaches the pancreas through the lesser sac of the omental bursa or the through the transverse mesocolon. Once the drain is placed, the adjacent tissues are returned to anatomic position and the operative site is closed in sutured layers.

48511

The physician performs percutaneous drainage of a pseudocyst of the pancreas. The physician may create a small incision in the flank, or abdomen proximal to the pancreatic pseudocyst in order to ease placement of drainage instruments through the skin into the pseudocyst for drainage of the pseudocyst to an external fluid collection system. The physician uses a CAT scan or ultrasound to guide placement of a drainage needle or trocar into the pseudocyst. The physician advances the drainage needle or trocar through the skin into the pseudocyst. The pseudocyst is allowed to drain. Once the pseudocyst is drained a drainage catheter may be placed (and later removed) to maintain drainage. Sutures may be placed to secure the drainage catheter in place. The operative site is cleaned and bandaged. For radiological supervision and interpretation, see 75989.

48520

The physician creates an internal anastomosis of a pancreatic cyst to a portion of the gastrointestinal tract. The physician approaches the pancreas through a midline abdominal incision and retracts the skin and underlying tissues laterally. The physician approaches the pancreas through the lesser sac of the omental bursa or the through the transverse mesocolon. The cyst is located. The physician approximates the stomach wall or a loop of duodenum or jejunum and incises it. The anterior cyst wall is incised and the cyst edges are approximated with the cut edges of the gastrointestinal tract and sutured. The cyst is decompressed through the drainage tract. The surrounding tissues are returned to anatomic position and the operative site is closed in sutured layers.

48540

The physician creates a Roux-en-Y anastomosis to drain enzymes from the pancreatic duct. The physician approaches the pancreas through a midline abdominal incision and retracts the skin and underlying tissues laterally. The physician approaches the pancreas through the lesser sac of the omental bursa or the through the transverse mesocolon. The physician divides a loop of small intestine (usually the jejunum) and implants the distal end into the stomach or duodenum. The proximal end is anastomosed distal to the first anastomosis to prevent reflux. The pancreatic duct is fistulized to the proximal end to create a drain to the gastrointestinal tract for pancreatic enzymes. The surrounding tissues are returned to anatomic position and the operative site is closed in sutured layers.

48545

The physician repairs a pancreatic injury (pancreatorrhaphy). The physician makes an abdominal incision and the abdomen is explored. The pancreas is exposed and the pancreatic injury is identified and repaired with sutures. A peripancreatic drain is usually placed. The incision is closed.

48547

The physician performs duodenal exclusion and gastrojejunostomy for a pancreatic injury. The physician makes an abdominal incision and explores the abdomen. The pancreas is exposed and an injury in the duodenum or pancreas may be closed with sutures. An incision is made in the stomach (gastrotomy). The natural opening from the stomach to the duodenum is closed with sutures or staples. A limb of proximal small bowel is brought up to the stomach and an anastomosis is performed (gastrojejunostomy) at the site of the gastrotomy. The abdominal incision is closed.

48550

The physician removes the pancreas from an organ donor and prepares it for transplantation. The physician makes an abdominal incision. The pancreas and duodenum are mobilized and dissected from their retroperitoneal attachments. The segments of mesenteric and splenic arteries and portal vein supplying the pancreas and duodenum are divided. The pancreas is removed en bloc with its vascular supply. Usually a segment of duodenum is removed en block with the pancreas. The incision is closed.

48554

The physician performs pancreas transplantation. The physician makes an abdominal incision. The iliac arteries and veins in the pelvis are exposed and isolated. An anastomosis is usually performed between the artery and vein supplying the pancreas to the iliac artery and vein on one side of the pelvis. An additional anastomosis is usually performed between the attached duodenal segment and the bladder. The incision is closed.

48556

The physician removes a transplanted pancreas graft. The physician makes an abdominal incision. The pancreatic graft is mobilized. The vascular supply to the pancreatic graft is isolated, ligated and divided. The anastomosis between the duodenum and bladder is taken down and the defect in the bladder is closed with sutures. The incision is closed.

49000

To explore the intra-abdominal organs and structures, the physician makes a large incision extending from just above the pubic hairline to the rib cage. The abdominal cavity is opened for a systematic examination of all organs. The physician may take tissue samples of any or all intra-abdominal organs for diagnosis. The incision is then closed with sutures.

49002

The physician reopens the incision of a recent laparotomy before the incision has fully healed to control bleeding, remove packing, or drain a postoperative infection.

49010

The physician explores the retroperitoneum and may obtain sample tissue for separately reportable diagnostic testing. The physician may approach the retroperitoneum through a flank or an abdominal incision. The surface of the retroperitoneum is inspected and any area of interest of the retroperitoneum may be opened and the retroperitoneum explored. Tissues may be sampled. The incision is closed.

49020

The physician makes an open abdominal or flank incision (laparotomy) to gain access to the peritoneal cavity. The peritoneum is explored and the abscess or isolated area of peritoneal inflammation is identified. The abscess is incised and drained, and inflamed peritoneal tissue may be excised. Specimens are typically sent to microbiology for identification and to determine antibiotic suitability. The abscess and surrounding peritoneal cavity may be irrigated. A drain may be placed whereby a separated abdominal incision is made and the drain is drawn through it and sutured in place. The physician may completely reapproximate the abdominal incision or leave a portion of the incision open to allow further drainage. If a drain is placed it is removed at a later date. This procedure does not apply to abscess of the appendix.

49021

To avoid exposure of the abdominal cavity, the physician makes a small skin incision in the abdomen or flank. Percutaneous needle aspiration and closed catheter drainage using computer tomographic (CT) or ultrasound guidance is performed. A needle, guidewire, or pigtail catheter is placed within the abscess. Specimens are typically sent to microbiology for identification and to determine antibiotic suitability. If a drain is placed, it is removed at a later date. This procedure does not apply to abscess of the appendix.

49040

The physician drains a subdiaphragmatic or subphrenic abscess. The physician makes an abdominal incision and the abdomen is explored. The abscess beneath the diaphragm is identified and the abscess cavity is opened and drained. Irrigation of the cavity is usually performed. A drain is usually placed into the abscess cavity and brought out through the abdominal wall. The incision is closed. The superficial portion of the incision may be packed open to allow drainage.

49041

The physician performs percutaneous drainage of a subdiaphragmatic or subphrenic abscess. The physician may create a small incision in the flank, thorax or abdomen proximal to an abscess located beneath the diaphragm (subdiaphragmatic/subphrenic) in order to ease placement of drainage instruments through the skin into the subphrenic abscess for drainage of fluid. The physician uses a CAT scan or ultrasound to guide placement of a drainage needle or trocar into the subphrenic abscess. The physician advances the drainage needle or trocar through the skin into the abscess. The abscess is allowed to drain. Once emptied, a drainage catheter may be placed (and later removed) to maintain drainage. Sutures may be placed to secure the drainage catheter in place. The operative site is cleaned and bandaged. For radiological supervision and interpretation, see 75989.

49060

The physician drains a retroperitoneal abscess. The physician makes an abdominal or flank incision. The abscess is identified and the retroperitoneal space is entered. The abscess cavity is opened and drained. Irrigation of the cavity is usually performed. A drain is usually placed in the abscess cavity and brought out through the abdominal wall. The incision is closed. The superficial portion of the incision may be packed open to allow drainage.

49061

The physician performs a percutaneous drainage of a retroperitoneal abscess. The physician may create a small incision in the skin between two ribs proximal to the abscess or in the flank in order to ease placement of drainage instruments through the skin into the retroperitoneal space. The physician uses a CAT scan or ultrasound to guide placement of a drainage needle or trocar into the retroperitoneal abscess. The physician advances the drainage needle or trocar through the skin to gain access to the abscess. The fluid is allowed to drain. Once the abscess is drained, a drainage catheter may be placed

(and later removed) to maintain drainage. Sutures may be placed to secure the drainage catheter in place. The operative site is cleaned and bandaged. For radiological supervision and interpretation, see 75989.

49062

The physician drains a lymphocele to the peritoneal cavity. The physician creates an opening in a lymphatic swelling or cavity (lymphocele) located outside the abdominopelvic walls to drain the material contained within to a cavity of the peritoneum. Irrigation of the lymphocele is performed. The incision is sutured closed. For radiological supervision and interpretation, see 75989.

49080

The physician withdraws fluid from the abdominal cavity (paracentesis) or performs infusion and drainage of fluid from the abdominal cavity (peritoneal lavage). The physician inserts a needle or catheter into the abdominal cavity and withdraws and drains fluid for diagnostic or therapeutic purposes. Alternately, the physician may insert a needle or catheter into the abdominal cavity and infuse and subsequently withdraw fluid for diagnostic or therapeutic purposes. The needle or catheter is removed at the completion of the procedure.

49081

The physician withdraws fluid from the abdominal cavity (paracentesis) or performs infusion and drainage of fluid from the abdominal cavity (peritoneal lavage) subsequent to some other procedure. The physician inserts a needle or catheter into the abdominal cavity and withdraws fluid for diagnostic or therapeutic purposes. Alternately, the physician may insert a needle or catheter into the abdominal cavity and infuse and subsequently withdraw fluid for diagnostic of therapeutic purposes. This is done subsequent to some other procedure. The needle or catheter is removed at the completion of the procedure.

49085

The physician performs removal of a foreign body from the abdominal cavity. The physician makes an abdominal incision and explores the abdominal cavity. The foreign body is identified and removed. The incision is closed.

49180

Using radiological supervision, the physician locates the mass within or immediately outside the peritoneal lining of the abdominal cavity. A biopsy needle is then passed into the mass, a tissue sample is removed, and the needle is withdrawn. This may be repeated several times. No incision is necessary.

49200–49201

The physician removes or destroys tumors, cysts, or endometriomas (displaced endometrial tissue) located inside or just outside the peritoneal lining of the abdominal cavity. The physician makes a large incision extending from just above the pubic hairline to the rib cage. The growths are removed using a laser, electrical cautery, or a scalpel. The incision is then closed by suturing. 49201 is used when the procedure is extensive, involving numerous or large growths, or a significantly greater amount of time than usual.

49215

The physician performs resection of a presacral or sacrococcygeal tumor. The physician makes an abdominal incision and explores the abdomen. The tumor is identified and the rectum is mobilized from the sacrum to expose the tumor. The tumor is dissected free of surrounding structures and removed. Alternately, the tumor may be approached posteriorly through an incision between the sacrum and coccyx. The coccyx is removed, the rectum is mobilized from the sacrum and the tumor is dissected from surrounding structures and removed. A portion of the sacrum may be excised en bloc with the tumor. The incision is closed.

49220

The physician performs a staging laparotomy for Hodgkin's disease or lymphoma. The physician makes an abdominal incision and the abdomen is explored. The spleen is mobilized, divided from its vascular supply and removed. Needle or wedge tissue samples are obtained from the left and right lobes of the liver for separately reportable analyses. Abdominal and retroperitoneal lymph nodes are identified and sampled. A bone marrow biopsy may be obtained. The ovaries may be plicated out of a planned radiation field. The incision is closed.

49250

The physician performs excision of the umbilicus. The physician makes an incision around the umbilicus and dissects the umbilicus from surrounding subcutaneous tissue. The umbilical arteries and vein, the urachal remnant, and the omphalomesenteric remnant identified and divided. The umbilicus is removed. The fascial defect is closed and the umbilicus is reconstructed with small skin flaps.

49255

The physician performs resection of the omentum or epiploectomy. The physician makes an abdominal incision and the abdomen is explored. The omentum is mobilized from the stomach and colon, divided from its blood supply and removed. One or more epiploica of the colon may be removed. The incision is closed.

49320

The physician makes a 1.0-centimeter incision in the umbilicus through which the abdomen is inflated and

a fiberoptic laparoscope is inserted. Other incisions are also made through which trocars can be passed into the abdominal cavity to deliver instruments, a video camera, and when needed an additional light source. The physician manipulates the tools so that the pelvic organs, peritoneum, abdomen, and omentum can be viewed through the laparoscope and/or video monitor. Biopsy from any or all of the areas observed are obtained by brushing the surface and collecting the cells or by washing (bathing) the area with a saline solution, and then suctioning out the cell rich solution. When the procedure is complete, the laparoscope, instruments, and light source are removed and the incisions are closed with sutures. If biopsy of pelvic organs is performed, the physician may also insert an instrument through the vagina to grasp the cervix and pass another instrument through the cervix, into the uterus to manipulate the uterus.

49321

The physician makes a 1.0-centimeter incision in the umbilicus through which the abdomen is inflated and a fiberoptic laparoscope is inserted. Other incisions are also made through which trocars can be passed into the abdominal cavity to deliver instruments, a video camera, and when needed an additional light source. The physician manipulates the tools so that the pelvic organs, peritoneum, abdomen and omentum can be viewed through the laparoscope and/or video monitor. Biopsy from any or all of the areas observed are obtained by grasping a sample with a special biopsy forceps that is capable of "biting off" small pieces of tissue. When the procedure is complete, the laparoscope, instruments, and light source are removed and the incisions are closed with sutures. If biopsy of pelvic organs is performed, the physician may also insert an instrument through the vagina to grasp the cervix and pass another instrument through the cervix, into the uterus to manipulate the uterus.

49322

The physician makes a 1.0-centimeter incision in the umbilicus through which the abdomen is inflated and a fiberoptic laparoscope is inserted. A second incision is made directly below the umbilicus, just above the pubic hairline, through which a trocar can be passed into the abdominal cavity to deliver instruments. The physician manipulates the tools to view the pelvic organs through the laparoscope. An additional incision may be needed for a second light source. Once the biopsy site is viewed through the laparoscope, a 5.0-centimeter incision is made just above the site. Through this incision, the physician uses an aspirating probe to aspirate a cavity or cyst or to collect fluid for culture. The instruments are removed and the incisions are sutured.

49323

The physician drains a lymphocele to the peritoneal cavity. With the patient under anesthesia, the physician places a trocar at the umbilicus into the abdominal or retroperineal space and insufflates the abdominal cavity. The physician places a laparoscope through the umbilical incision and additional trocars are placed into the abdomen. The lymphocele is identified and instruments are passed through to open and drain the lymphocele. The trocars are removed and the incisions are closed with sutures.

49400

The physician injects air contrast into the peritoneal cavity. The physician inserts a needle or catheter into the peritoneal cavity and injects air as a diagnostic procedure. An x-ray is usually obtained to define the pattern of air in the abdomen. The needle or catheter is removed at the completion of the procedure.

49420

The physician places a temporary intraperitoneal catheter for drainage or dialysis. The physician makes a small abdominal incision, opens the peritoneum and inserts the catheter into the abdominal cavity. The proximal end of the catheter is tunneled subcutaneously away from the initial incision and brought out through the skin. The incision is closed. Alternately, the physician may percutaneously insert the catheter over a wire placed through a needle inserted into the peritoneal cavity.

49421

The physician places a permanent intraperitoneal catheter for drainage or dialysis. The physician makes a small abdominal incision, opens the peritoneum and inserts the catheter into the abdominal cavity. The proximal end of the catheter is tunneled subcutaneously away from the initial incision and brought out through the skin. The incision is closed.

49422

The physician performs removal of an intraperitoneal catheter. The physician makes an incision over the insertion site of the catheter. The catheter is dissected free of surrounding scar tissue, transected and removed from the peritoneal insertion site and skin exit site. The incision at the insertion site of the catheter is closed. The skin exit site is left open to allow drainage.

49423

The physician exchanges a previously placed drainage catheter. The physician locates the drainage catheter and removes sutures that may be holding it in place. The drainage catheter is removed. With the use of fluoroscopy the physician places a new drainage catheter, and the physician may elect to use a catheter guidewire to assist in this maneuver. Once placed and found to be patent, the new drainage catheter may be

sutured in place. For radiological supervision and interpretation, see 75984.

49424

The physician injects a radio-contrast dye through a previously placed catheter to determine the existence, nature, or size of an abscess or cyst. Once the radio-contrast dye is placed, the operative site is examined under direct fluoroscopy or with radiographic studies. The contrast dye may be aspirated and/or irrigated from the cyst or abscess. For radiological supervision and interpretation, see 76080.

49425

The physician places a peritoneal-venous shunt. The physician makes a small lateral upper abdominal incision. Dissection is carried through the abdominal wall layers, the peritoneum is entered and the peritoneal end of the catheter is inserted into the peritoneal cavity and sutured into place. A subcutaneous tunnel is created from the abdominal incision up to the neck and the catheter is pulled through the tunnel into the neck. A counter incision is made in the neck over the internal jugular vein and the venous end of the catheter is inserted into the jugular vein. The incisions are closed.

49426

The physician performs revision of a peritoneal-venous shunt. The physician may remove the shunt by incisions over the venous and peritoneal insertion sites with a subcutaneous tunnel is created from the abdominal incision up to the neck and the catheter is pulled through the tunnel into the neck. A counter incision is made in the neck over the internal jugular vein and the venous end of the catheter is inserted into the jugular vein. Alternately, the physician may make an incision over the dysfunctional end of the shunt and replace that portion of the shunt and insert it back into the peritoneal cavity or jugular vein. The incisions are closed.

49427

The physician injects contrast into a peritoneo-venous shunt. The physician injects contrast material through the skin into the reservoir of the peritoneo-venous shunt. Radiography is used to visualize the flow of contrast through the shunt into the peritoneal and venous ends for evaluation.

49428

The physician performs ligation of a previously placed peritoneo-venous shunt. The physician makes an incision over the path of the shunt. The shunt tubing under the incision is isolated and ligated with sutures. The incision is closed.

49429

The physician performs removal of a peritoneal venous shunt. An incision is made over the abdominal insertion site of the shunt. The shunt is dissected from surrounding scar tissue and removed from the abdominal cavity. The fascia and peritoneum of the abdominal insertion site is closed. Usually the venous end of the catheter can be removed by placing traction on the shunt through the abdominal incision and pulling it through the subcutaneous tunnel. If necessary a second incision is made over the venous insertion site and the catheter removed from the jugular vein. The incisions are closed.

49491–49492

The physician repairs an initial inguinal hernia in a preterm infant (less than 37 weeks gestation at birth), performed up to 50 weeks postconceptual age. The physician dissects in the preperitoneal plane to present the hernia ring. The physician applies manual pressure to the inguinal region from outside while trying to dissect the hernia sac to reduce the hernia. If that fails, which can occur when there is a discrepancy in size of the hernia compared to its contents, the physician enlarges the hernia ring by an electrocautery incision in a ventral direction. The incision is made in a ventromedial direction for medial hernias and a ventrolateral direction for lateral hernias. The hernia is reduced using pleural insufflation of carbon dioxide. If a hydrocele is present, it is incised and drained. The hernia defect is repaired by suture and reinforced either by staples or mesh. Report 49492 if, in the case of an incarcerated or strangulated hernia, the physician empties the contents of the hernia sac, places the contents in the lower abdomen, and repairs the hernia defect by suture.

49495

The physician repairs an initial inguinal hernia in a full-term infant under age six months, or a preterm infant over 50 weeks postconceptual age. The physician makes a groin incision. The hernia sac is identified and dissected free of surrounding structures. The hernia sac is ligated and resected. If a hydrocele is present it is incised and drained. The groin incision is closed.

49496

The physician repairs an incarcerated inguinal hernia in a full-term infant under age six months or a preterm infant over 50 weeks postconceptual age. The physician makes a groin incision. The hernia sac is identified and dissected free of surrounding structures. The hernia sac is opened and the contents of the sac are examined. If the hernia contents are viable, they are removed from the hernia sac into the lower abdomen and the hernia defect is repaired by suture. If a hydrocele is present it is incised and drained. The groin incision is closed.

49500

The physician repairs an inguinal hernia in a child between six months and 5 years of age. The physician makes a groin incision. The hernia sac is identified

and dissected free of surrounding structures. The hernia sac is ligated and resected. If a hydrocele is present it is incised and drained. The groin incision is closed.

49501

The physician repairs an incarcerated inguinal hernia in a child between six months and 5 years of age. The physician makes a groin incision. The hernia sac is identified and dissected free of surrounding structures. The hernia sac is opened and the contents of the sac are examined. If the hernia contents are viable the hernia is reduced and the sac ligated and resected. If a hydrocele is present it is incised and drained. The groin incision is closed.

49505

The physician repairs an inguinal hernia in a patient age 5 or over. The physician makes a groin incision. The hernia sac is identified and dissected free from surrounding structures. The hernia sac is ligated and resected. The groin incision is closed.

49507

The physician repairs an incarcerated inguinal hernia in a patient over the age of 5 years. The physician makes a groin incision. The hernia sac is identified and dissected free from surrounding structures. The hernia sac is opened and the contents of the sac are examined. If the contents of the hernia are viable the hernia is reduced and the hernia sac is ligated and resected. The groin incision is closed.

49520

The physician repairs a recurrent inguinal hernia. The physician makes a groin incision. Dissection is continued through scar tissue and the spermatic cord and the hernia sac are identified and dissected from surrounding structures. The hernia sac may be ligated and resected. The incision is closed.

49521

The physician repairs an incarcerated recurrent inguinal hernia. The physician makes a groin incision. Dissection is continued through scar tissue and the spermatic cord and hernia sac is identified and dissected from surrounding structures. The hernia sac is opened and the contents of the sac are examined. If the contents of the hernia are viable the hernia is reduced and the hernia sac may be ligated and resected. The incision is closed.

49525

The physician repairs a sliding inguinal hernia. The physician makes a groin incision. The hernia sac is identified and dissected from surrounding structures. The hernia sac is opened and the abdominal viscera attached to the sac are dissected away from the sac if possible. The hernia contents are reduced and the hernia sac is closed and a portion of the sac may be resected. The incision is closed.

49540

The physician repairs a lumbar hernia. The physician makes an incision posteriorly over the hernia. The hernia sac is identified and dissected from surrounding structures to expose the fascial defect. The hernia is reduced and the hernia sac may be resected. The fascial defect is closed with sutures. The incision is closed.

49550

The physician repairs a femoral hernia. The physician makes a femoral or groin incision. The hernia sac is identified and dissected from surrounding structures. The femoral defect is closed with a prosthetic patch or sutures by plicating the fascia and muscles to cover the defect. The incision is closed.

49553

The physician repairs an incarcerated femoral hernia. The physician makes a groin or femoral incision. The hernia sac is identified and dissected from surrounding structures. The hernia sac is opened and the contents of the sac are examined. If the contents of the hernia are viable the hernia is reduced and the hernia sac is closed and may be resected. The femoral defect is closed with sutures by plicating the fascia and muscles to cover the defect. The incision is closed.

49555

The physician repairs a recurrent femoral hernia. The physician makes a groin or femoral incision. Dissection is continued through scar tissue and the hernia sac is identified and dissected from surrounding structures. The hernia sac is reduced and may be resected. The femoral defect is closed with sutures by plicating the fascia and muscles to cover the defect. The incision is closed.

49557

The physician repairs an incarcerated recurrent femoral hernia. The physician makes a groin or femoral incision. Dissection is continued through scar tissue and the hernia sac is identified and dissected from surrounding structures. The hernia sac is opened and the contents of the sac are examined. If the hernia contents are viable the hernia is reduced and the hernia sac is closed and may be resected. The femoral defect is closed with sutures by plicating fascia and muscle to cover the defect. The incision is closed.

49560

The physician repairs an incisional or ventral hernia. The physician makes an incision over the hernia. Dissection is continued through scar tissue and the hernia sac is identified and dissected from surrounding structures. The fascial defect is identified circumferentially. The hernia is reduced and the hernia sac may be resected. The hernia defect is closed with sutures. The incision is closed.

49561

The physician repairs an incarcerated incisional hernia. The physician makes an incision over the hernia. Dissection is continued through scar tissue and the hernia sac is identified and dissected from surrounding structures. The fascial defect is identified circumferentially. The hernia sac is opened and the contents of the hernia sac are examined. If the contents of the hernia sac are viable the hernia is reduced and the hernia sac is closed and may be resected. The hernia defect is closed with sutures. The incision is closed.

49565

The physician repairs a recurrent incisional or ventral hernia. The physician makes an incision over the hernia. Dissection is continued through scar tissue and the hernia sac is identified and dissected from surrounding structures. The fascial defect is identified circumferentially. The hernia is reduced and the sac may be resected. The hernia defect is closed with sutures. The incision is closed.

49566

The physician repairs an incarcerated recurrent incisional hernia. The physician makes an incision over the hernia. Dissection is continued through scar tissue and the hernia sac is identified and dissected from surrounding structures. The fascial defect is identified circumferentially. The hernia sac is opened and the contents of the sac are examined. If the contents of the hernia sac are viable the hernia is reduced and the hernia sac is closed and may be resected. The hernia defect is closed with sutures. The incision is closed.

49568

The physician implants mesh for a separately reported incisional hernia repair. The hernia defect is closed with mesh or some other prosthetic material. The incision is closed. This code is listed "in addition to" an incisional or ventral hernia repair and is not subject to modifier -51 or reduced.

49570

The physician repairs an epigastric hernia. The physician makes an incision over the hernia. The hernia sac is identified and dissected from surrounding structures. The fascial defect is identified circumferentially. The hernia is reduced and the hernia sac may be resected. The hernia defect is closed with sutures. The incision is closed.

49572

The physician repairs an incarcerated epigastric hernia. The physician makes an incision over the hernia. The hernia sac is identified and dissected from surrounding structures. The fascial defect is identified circumferentially. The hernia sac is opened and the contents of the sac are examined. If the contents of the hernia are viable the hernia is reduced and the hernia sac may be resected. The hernia defect is closed with sutures. The incision is closed.

49580

The physician repairs an umbilical hernia in a child under 5 years of age. The physician makes an umbilical incision. The hernia sac and fascial defect are identified and dissected from surrounding structures. The hernia sac is reduced and may be resected. The hernia defect is closed with sutures. The incision is closed.

49582

The physician repairs an incarcerated umbilical hernia in a child under 5 years of age. The physician makes an umbilical incision. The hernia sac and fascial defect are identified and dissected from surrounding structures. The hernia sac is opened and the contents of the sac are examined. If the contents of the hernia sac are viable the hernia is reduced and the hernia sac may be resected. The hernia defect is closed with sutures. The incision is closed.

49585

The physician repairs an umbilical hernia in a patient over 5 years of age. The physician makes an umbilical incision. The hernia sac and fascial defect are identified and dissected from surrounding structures. The hernia is reduced and the hernia sac may be resected. The hernia defect is closed with sutures. The incision is closed.

49587

The physician repairs an incarcerated umbilical hernia in a patient over 5 years of age. The physician makes an umbilical incision. The hernia sac and fascial defect are identified and dissected from surrounding structures. The hernia sac is opened and the contents of the sac are examined. If the contents of the hernia sac are viable the hernia is reduced and the hernia sac may be resected. The hernia defect is closed with sutures. The incision is closed.

49590

The physician repairs a spigelian hernia. The physician makes an incision over the hernia. The hernia sac and fascial defect are identified and dissected from surrounding structures. The hernia is reduced and the hernia sac may be resected. The hernia defect is closed with a prosthetic patch or by plicating layers of muscle and fascia over the defect with sutures. The incision is closed.

49600

The physician repairs a small omphalocele. The physician identifies the omphalocele and dissects the peritoneal sac from the umbilicus and the abdominal wall defect. The peritoneal sac is reduced and the abdominal wall defect is closed with sutures. The umbilicus is reconstructed and the skin is loosely closed.

49605

The physician repairs a large omphalocele or gastroschisis. The peritoneal sac of the omphalocele is dissected from the umbilicus and surrounding structures and reduced or the herniated contents of the gastroschisis are reduced into the abdominal cavity if possible. The abdominal wall defect is identified. If possible the abdominal wall defect is closed with sutures and the umbilicus is reconstructed. If the defect is too large or if the herniated contents cannot be reduced a prosthetic material is used to create a patch or silo that is sutured over the defect to close the defect and accommodate the herniated contents.

49606

The physician removes a previously placed prosthesis and closes an omphalocele or gastroschisis. The physician removes the previously placed prosthetic material covering the abdominal wall defect. The herniated contents are reduced and the edges of the defect are identified. The abdominal wall defect is closed with sutures. The umbilicus is reconstructed with skin flaps if possible. The remainder of the skin incision is usually left open to allow drainage.

49610

The physician performs the first stage of an omphalocele repair (Gross type operation). The physician identifies the omphalocele. Skin flaps are widely mobilized around the omphalocele and the skin flaps are closed over the intact omphalocele with sutures. The abdominal wall defect is not addressed.

49611

The physician performs the second stage of an omphalocele repair (Gross type operation). The physician makes an incision in the previously closed skin over the omphalocele. Skin flaps are mobilized off the omphalocele and the peritoneal sac of the omphalocele is dissected from the abdominal wall defect. The abdominal wall defect is closed with sutures. The skin flaps are closed over the repair thus closing the incision.

49650

The physician performs laparoscopic repair of an inguinal hernia. The physician places a trocar at the umbilicus and insufflates the abdominal or retroperitoneal cavity. The laparoscope is placed through the umbilical port and additional trocars are placed into the peritoneal or retroperitoneal space. The hernia sac is identified and reduced into the abdominal cavity. A sheet of mesh is placed into the abdominal or retroperitoneal cavity and stapled into place on the pubis and abdominal wall covering the hernial defect. The trocars are removed and the incisions are closed.

49651

The physician performs laparoscopic repair of a recurrent inguinal hernia. The physician places a trocar at the umbilicus and insufflates the abdominal or retroperitoneal cavity. The laparoscope is placed through the umbilical port and additional trocars are placed into the peritoneal or retroperitoneal space. The hernia sac is identified and reduced into the abdominal cavity. A sheet of mesh is placed into the abdominal or retroperitoneal cavity and stapled into place on the pubis and abdominal wall covering the hernial defect. The trocars are removed and the incisions are closed.

49900

The physician performs a secondary closure of the abdominal wall for dehiscence or evisceration. The physician completely opens the former incision and removes the remaining sutures. Necrotic fascia is debrided to viable tissue. Any eviscerated abdominal contents are reduced into the abdominal cavity. The abdominal wall is closed with sutures.

49905

The physician mobilizes an omental flap for reconstruction of a defect. The physician makes an abdominal incision. The omentum is mobilized on a pedicle of its blood supply. The omental flap may be mobilized and placed in a new location to fill a defect with its blood supply intact. Alternately, the omental flap may be divided from its blood supply and placed as a free flap into a new location to fill a defect. An arterial anastomosis is performed to restore blood flow to the omental flap. The abdominal incision is closed.

49906

The physician makes an abdominal incision to gain access to the omentum. The greater omentum is dissected free of the greater curvature of the stomach and transverse colon. The blood supply is provided via the right or left gastroepiploic vessels. The freed omental flap may be transferred to satisfy a defect of the abdominal or chest wall. Using microvascular anastomosis, the physician connects arteries and veins of the omental flap with the arteries and veins surrounding the area to which the omentum is being transferred. Once this is accomplished, the omentum may be covered with a meshed split-thickness skin graft. The incisions are closed.

50010

The physician examines the kidney and renal pelvis. To access the kidney, the physician makes an incision in the skin of the flank, cuts the muscles, fat, and fibrous membranes (fascia) overlying the kidney, and sometimes removes a portion of the eleventh or twelfth rib. The physician clears away the fatty tissue surrounding the kidney, explores the area, and performs a layered closure.

50020

The physician drains an infection (abscess) on the kidney or on the surrounding renal tissue. To access the renal or perirenal abscess, the physician makes a small incision in the skin of the flank, cuts the muscles, fat, and fibrous membranes (fascia) overlying the kidney, and sometimes removes a portion of the eleventh or twelfth rib. After exploring the abscess cavity, the physician irrigates the site, inserts multiple drain tubes through separate stab wounds, and sutures the drain tube ends to the skin. The physician packs the wound with gauze and sutures the fascia and muscles. The skin and subcutaneous tissue are usually left open to prevent formation of a secondary body wall abscess.

50021

The physician performs a percutaneous drainage of a perirenal or renal abscess. The physician may create a small incision in the skin between two ribs proximal to the abscess or in the flank in order to ease placement of drainage instruments through the skin into an abscess located within the kidney or immediately adjacent to it. The physician uses a CAT scan or ultrasound to guide placement of a drainage needle or trocar into the abscess. The physician advances the drainage needle or trocar through the skin to gain access to the abscess. The fluid is allowed to drain. Once the abscess is drained a drainage catheter may be placed (and later removed) to maintain drainage. Sutures may be placed to secure the drainage catheter in place. The operative site is cleaned and bandaged. For radiological supervision and interpretation, see 75989.

50040

The physician creates an opening through the kidney to the exterior of the body by making an incision in the kidney. To access the kidney, the physician makes an incision in the skin of the flank, cuts the muscles, fat, and fibrous membranes (fascia) overlying the kidney, and sometimes removes a portion of the eleventh or twelfth rib. Using an incision to open the renal pelvis (pyelotomy), the physician passes a curved clamp into the renal pelvis, a middle or lower minor calyx, and the cortex of the kidney. The physician inserts a catheter tip through the same path as the clamp, and passes the tube through a stab incision in the skin of the flank. After suturing the incisions, the physician inserts a drain tube, bringing it out through a separate stab incision, and performs a layered closure.

50045

The physician makes a small incision in the kidney to explore the interior of the kidney. To access the kidney, the physician makes an incision in the skin of the flank, cuts the muscles, fat, and fibrous membranes (fascia) overlying the kidney, and sometimes removes a portion of the eleventh or twelfth rib. The physician makes an incision in the

CPT® Lay Descriptions

kidney (nephrotomy) and sometimes places fine traction sutures at the edges of the incision. After exploration, the physician sutures the incision, inserts a drain tube, bringing it out through a separate stab incision, and performs a layered closure.

50060–50070

The physician removes a kidney stone (calculus) by making an incision in the kidney. To access the calculus, the physician makes an incision in the skin of the flank, cuts the muscles, fat, and fibrous membranes (fascia) overlying the kidney, and sometimes removes a portion of the eleventh or twelfth rib. The physician isolates the calculus and removes it through an incision. After examining the kidney for other defects, the physician sutures the incision, inserts a drain tube, bringing it out through a separate stab incision, and performs a layered closure. Report 50065 when a previous surgery on the kidney complicates the procedure. Report 50070 if the procedure is complicated because of a congenital kidney abnormality, wherein the physician usually repairs any calyces that are obstructed or abnormally narrowed.

50075

The physician removes a stone that fills the calyces and renal pelvis (staghorn calculus) by making incisions in the kidney and renal pelvis. To access the staghorn calculus, the physician makes an incision in the skin of the flank, cuts the muscles, fat, and fibrous membranes (fascia) overlying the kidney, and sometimes removes a portion of the twelfth rib. After isolating the staghorn calculus, the physician makes an incision in the renal pelvis (pyelotomy) and may make an incision in the kidney (nephrotomy). The physician removes the staghorn calculus, irrigates the area with a sterile fluid, and examines the kidney for other defects. After closing the incisions, the physician inserts a drain tube and performs a layered closure.

50080–50081

The physician creates a percutaneous passageway to remove kidney stones (calculi). The physician makes a small incision in the skin of the back, inserts a large needle, and radiologically guides it toward the kidney or renal pelvis. After passing a guidewire through the needle, the physician dilates the passageway by inserting and removing tubes with increasingly larger diameters. The physician inserts an endoscope over the guidewire and passes an instrument through the endoscope to crush or extract calculi. The physician may pass a ureteral stent from the pelvis into the bladder. The physician removes the guidewire and allows the passageway to seal on its own, or inserts a nephrostomy or pyelostomy tube before removing the guidewire. Report 50080 for removal of calculi measuring up to 2.0 cm; use 50081 for removal of calculi measuring more than 2.0 cm.

50100

The physician corrects an obstruction by cutting across or repositioning renal vessels that deviate from proper anatomical placement. To access the kidney, the physician makes an incision in the skin of the flank, cuts the muscles, fat, and fibrous membranes (fascia) overlying the kidney, and sometimes removes a portion of the twelfth rib. After repositioning the aberrant vessels to a more functional anatomic placement, the physician performs a layered closure.

50120

The physician makes an incision in the renal pelvis to explore the calyces and renal pelvis. To access the kidney, the physician makes an incision in the skin of the flank, cuts the muscles, fat, and fibrous membranes (fascia) overlying the kidney, and sometimes removes a portion of the eleventh or twelfth rib. The physician makes an incision in the renal pelvis (pyelotomy). The physician may place fine traction sutures at the edges of the pyelotomy while exploring the calyces and renal pelvis. After closing the pyelotomy, the physician inserts a drain tube, bringing it out through a separate stab incision, and performs a layered closure.

50125

The physician makes an incision in the renal pelvis to insert a pyelostomy tube for drainage. To access the kidney, the physician makes an incision in the skin of the flank, cuts the muscles, fat, and fibrous membranes (fascia) overlying the kidney, and sometimes removes a portion of the eleventh or twelfth rib. After exposing the renal pelvis, the physician makes an incision in the renal pelvis (pyelotomy). The physician inserts the tip of a catheter into the renal pelvis and passes the tube out through a stab incision in the skin of the flank. The physician performs a layered closure.

50130

The physician removes stones (calculi) or an insoluble mass (coagulum) from the renal pelvis by making an incision into the renal pelvis. To access the kidney, the physician makes an incision in the skin of the flank, cuts the muscles, fat, and fibrous membranes (fascia) overlying the kidney, and sometimes removes a portion of the eleventh or twelfth rib. The physician makes an incision in the renal pelvis (pyelotomy) to isolate and remove the calculus. The physician irrigates the area with a sterile fluid, and examines the renal pelvis for other defects. The physician inserts a drain tube, bringing it out through a separate stab incision, and performs a layered closure.

50135

The physician makes an incision in the renal pelvis of a kidney complicated by a congenital abnormality or a previous surgery. To access the kidney, the physician makes an incision in the skin of the flank, cuts the muscles, fat, and fibrous membranes (fascia) overlying the kidney, and sometimes removes a portion of the eleventh or twelfth rib. The physician makes an incision in the renal pelvis (pyelotomy) and explores the calyces and renal pelvis. The physician may place fine traction sutures at the edges of the pyelotomy while exploring the calyces and renal pelvis or repairing defects. After closing the pyelotomy and nephrotomy, the physician inserts a drain tube, bringing it out through a separate stab incision, and performs a layered closure.

50200

The physician extracts a plug of biopsy tissue from the kidney by inserting a needle or trocar in the skin of the back. Using radiologic or ultrasonic guidance, the physician advances the instrument into the suspect tissue of the kidney. With the instrument's cutting sheath, the physician traps a specimen of renal tissue and removes the instrument. After usually repeating the process several times, the physician applies pressure to the puncture wound.

50205

The physician excises a specimen of biopsy tissue from the kidney through an incision. To access the kidney, the physician makes an incision in the skin of the flank and cuts the muscles, fat, and fibrous membranes (fascia) overlying the kidney. After excising a specimen of the diseased or damaged renal tissue, the physician sutures the incision and performs a layered closure.

50220–50225

The physician removes the kidney and upper portion of the ureter. To access the kidney and ureter, the physician usually makes an incision in the skin of the flank, cuts the muscles, fat, and fibrous membranes (fascia) overlying the kidney, and sometimes removes a portion of the eleventh or twelfth rib. After mobilizing the kidney and ureter, the physician clamps, ligates, and severs the upper ureter and major renal blood vessels (renal pedicle). The physician removes the kidney and upper ureter, but does not remove the adrenal gland, surrounding fatty tissue, or Gerota's fascia. After controlling bleeding, the physician irrigates the site with normal saline and places a drain tube, bringing it out through a separate stab incision in the skin. The physician removes the clamps and performs a layered closure. Report 50225 when a previous surgery on the kidney and/or ureter complicates the procedure.

50230

The physician removes the kidney, surrounding fat, Gerota's fascia, adrenal gland, periaortic lymph nodes, and upper ureter. To access the kidney and upper ureter, the physician usually makes an incision in the skin of the chest (transthoracic approach) or flank. After mobilizing the kidney and ureter, the physician clamps, ligates, and severs the upper ureter and major

renal blood vessels (renal pedicle). The physician removes the kidney, upper ureter, neural and vascular structures at the apex of the renal pelvis, surrounding fat, Gerota's fascia, adrenal gland, and involved renal lymph nodes. The physician irrigates the site, places a drain tube, removes the clamps, and performs a layered closure. In a transthoracic approach, the lung is re-expanded and the chest tube left in.

50234

The physician removes the kidney, ureter, and small cuff of the bladder through one excision. To access the kidney and ureter, the physician usually makes an incision in the skin of the flank, cuts the muscles, fat, and fibrous membranes (fascia) overlying the kidney, and sometimes removes a portion of the eleventh or twelfth rib. After mobilizing the kidney, ureter, and bladder, the physician clamps, ligates, and severs the ureter, major renal blood vessels (renal pedicle), and a small cuff of the bladder. The physician pulls the kidney, ureter, and bladder cuff upward through the flank incision. The physician does not remove the adrenal gland, surrounding fatty tissue, or Gerota's fascia. After controlling bleeding, the physician irrigates the site with normal saline and places a drain tube, bringing it out through a separate stab incision in the skin. The physician sutures and catheterizes the bladder, removes the clamps, and performs a layered closure.

50236

The physician removes the kidney, ureter, and small cuff of the bladder through two incisions. To access the kidney and upper ureter, the physician usually makes an incision in the skin of the flank, cuts the muscles, fat, and fibrous membranes (fascia) overlying the kidney, and sometimes removes a portion of the eleventh or twelfth rib. After mobilizing the kidney and ureter, the physician isolates, clamps, ligates, and severs the upper ureter and major renal blood vessels (renal pedicle) and removes the kidney. The physician does not remove the adrenal gland, surrounding fatty tissue, or Gerota's fascia. After controlling bleeding, the physician irrigates the site with normal saline and places a drain tube, bringing it out through a separate stab incision in the skin. To access the lower ureter and bladder, the physician makes an incision in the skin of the abdomen. After mobilizing the bladder, the physician removes the lower ureter and a small cuff of the bladder. The physician sutures and catheterizes the bladder. After placing a drain tube behind the bladder, the physician removes the clamps and performs a layered closure.

50240

The physician removes a portion of the kidney. To access the kidney and ureter, the physician usually makes an incision in the skin of the flank, cuts the muscles, fat, and fibrous membranes (fascia) overlying the kidney, and sometimes removes a portion of the eleventh or twelfth rib. After mobilizing the kidney and the major renal blood vessels (renal pedicle), the physician clamps the renal vessels, and sometimes induces hypothermia of the kidney with iced saline slush. The physician excises a wedge containing the diseased or damaged kidney tissue. After clamping and ligating the exposed arteries and veins, the physician inserts a drain tube, bringing it out through a separate stab incision in the skin, removes the clamps, and performs a layered closure.

50280–50290

The physician excises a cyst on the kidney or in the surrounding renal tissue. To access the kidney, the physician makes an incision in the skin of the flank, cuts the muscles, fat, and fibrous membranes (fascia) overlying the kidney, and sometimes removes a portion of the twelfth rib. After clearing away the fatty tissue surrounding the kidney, the physician excises the cyst from the renal surface. The physician destroys tiny vessels bordering the cyst with high-frequency electric current (fulguration) to minimize the need for sutures. If the cyst requires a deep excision, the physician usually sutures the renal tissue. The physician inserts a drain tube, bringing it out through a separate stab incision in the skin, and performs a layered closure. 50280 reports excision of a cyst (or cysts) on the kidney; 50290 reports excision of a cyst (or cysts) in the tissue surrounding the kidney.

50300

The physician removes the kidney and upper ureter from a cadaver for transplantation. To access the kidney and upper ureter, the physician usually makes a midline incision in the skin from the xiphoid process to the symphysis pubis. After cutting the muscles, fat, and fibrous membranes (fascia) overlying the kidney, the physician uses clamps, ties, suture ligatures, and electrocoagulation to control bleeding. Before clamping the major renal blood vessels (renal pedicle), the physician administers heparin sodium to prevent intravascular clotting. The physician dissects and removes the kidney, renal vessels, and ureter, usually removing sections of the inferior vena cava and aorta with both kidneys. To maintain the renal transplant (homograft), the physician places the kidney in cold saline solution and flushes it with a cold electrolyte solution to rinse any remaining donor blood from the kidney and lower its temperature.

50320

The physician removes the kidney and upper ureter from a living donor for transplantation. To access the kidney, the physician usually makes an incision in the skin of the flank, cuts the muscles, fat, and fibrous membranes (fascia) overlying the kidney, and sometimes removes a portion of the eleventh or twelfth rib. After mobilizing the kidney and ureter, the physician administers an anticlogging agent. The physician clamps, ligates, and severs the upper ureter and major renal blood vessels (renal pedicle), and removes the kidney and upper ureter. The physician

administers medication to reverse the effects of the anticlogging agent. After controlling bleeding, the physician irrigates the site, places a drain tube, and performs a layered closure. To maintain the renal transplant (homograft), the physician places the kidney in cold saline solution and flushes it with a cold electrolyte solution.

50340

The physician removes the kidney and the upper portion of the ureter in a patient who is to receive a kidney transplant. To access the kidney and ureter, the physician usually makes an incision in the skin of the flank, cuts the muscles, fat, and fibrous membranes (fascia) overlying the kidney, and sometimes removes a portion of the eleventh or twelfth rib. After mobilizing the kidney and ureter, the physician clamps, ligates, and severs the upper ureter and major renal blood vessels (renal pedicle). The physician removes the kidney and upper ureter, but does not remove the adrenal gland, surrounding fatty tissue, or Gerota's fascia. After controlling bleeding, the physician irrigates the site with normal saline and places a drain tube, bringing it out through a separate stab incision in the skin. The physician performs a layered closure.

50360

The physician surgically implants a human kidney and ureter from a living donor or cadaver into a transplant recipient. To access the transplant site, the physician usually makes a curved, right or left lower quadrant incision in the skin. After cutting the muscles, fat, and fibrous membranes (fascia), the physician controls bleeding with clamps, ties, and electrocoagulation. The physician surgically connects the renal vein and artery of the donor kidney to the recipient's clamped and dissected internal iliac vein and hypogastric artery. After removing the clamps, the physician checks for leakage, bleeding, and insufficient blood supply. To implant the donor ureter, the physician makes an incision into the bladder and passes the ureter through the bladder. The physician sutures the ureter as well as the opening in the bladder (cystotomy). The physician performs a layered closure. The drain tube may be left in.

50365

The physician implants a donor kidney and upper ureter after removing the recipient's kidney and upper ureter. To access the recipient's kidney and ureter, the physician usually makes an incision in the skin of the flank, cuts the muscles, fat, and fibrous membranes (fascia) overlying the kidney, and sometimes removes a portion of the eleventh or twelfth rib. The physician clamps, ligates, and severs the upper ureter and major renal blood vessels (renal pedicle), and removes the kidney and upper ureter. To implant the donor kidney and upper ureter, the physician usually makes a curved lower quadrant incision in the skin. The physician surgically connects the renal vein and artery of the donor kidney to the recipient's clamped and dissected internal iliac vein and hypogastric artery. After incising the bladder, the physician passes the donor ureter through the bladder and sutures the ureter and opening in the bladder (cystotomy). The physician performs a layered closure. The drain tube may be left in.

50370

The physician removes a transplanted donor kidney from the recipient. To access the rejected kidney, the physician usually reopens the original kidney transplant incision, and cuts the muscles, fat, and fibrous membranes (fascia) overlying the kidney. After mobilizing the kidney, the physician clamps, ligates, and severs the major renal blood vessels (renal pedicle). The physician removes the rejected kidney. After controlling bleeding, the physician irrigates the site with normal saline. The physician may place a drain tube, bringing it out through a separate stab incision in the skin. After removing the clamps, the physician performs a layered closure.

50380

The physician moves the kidney from its original anatomic site and revascularizes the kidney by connecting the renal and iliac vessels to a new site. To access the transplant site, the physician usually makes a midline transabdominal incision in the skin and cuts the muscles, fat, and fibrous membranes (fascia). After exposing the kidney, the physician clamps, ligates, and severs the renal vessels, keeping the ureter intact. The physician flushes the kidney with cold, anticoagulant electrolyte solution, and surgically connects the renal vessels to another appropriate arterial and venous site. The physician removes the clamps and checks for leakage, bleeding, and infarction. After placing a drain tube and bringing it out through a separate stab incision in the skin, the physician removes the clamps and performs a layered closure.

50390

The physician inserts a needle through the skin to inject or drain fluid from the renal pelvis or a renal cyst. The physician usually inserts a long, thin needle in the skin of the back. Using radiologic guidance, the physician advances the needle toward the renal pelvis or renal cyst and injects or drains fluid.

50392

The physician inserts a catheter or intracatheter into the renal pelvis for drainage of urine and/or an injection. The physician usually inserts a long, thin needle with a removable probe in the skin of the back. Using radiologic guidance, the physician advances the needle toward the renal pelvis. When urine flows back through the needle, the physician advances a catheter over the needle, and withdraws the needle.

50393

The physician inserts a catheter or stent through the renal pelvis into the ureter for drainage of urine and/or an injection. The physician usually inserts a long, thin needle with a removable probe in the skin of the back. The physician advances the needle toward the renal pelvis and into the ureter. When urine flows back through the needle, the physician advances a catheter over the needle. The physician removes the needle and leaves the catheter in place for drainage and/or injection.

50394

The physician injects a contrast agent through a tube or indwelling catheter into the renal pelvis to study the kidney and renal collecting system. The physician determines immediate allergic response to the contrast agent by injecting a small initial dose of contrast material through an existing pyelostomy or nephrostomy tube or indwelling ureteral catheter. If no allergic response occurs, a large quantity of contrast material is injected into the renal pelvis. The radiologist then produces a representation of the kidney, renal pelvis, and/or ureter with an x-ray.

50395

The physician inserts a guide into the renal pelvis and/or ureter to establish a passageway between the skin and kidney. To create the percutaneous passageway, the physician makes a small incision in the skin of the back, inserts a large needle, and ultrasonographically guides it toward the kidney. After passing a guidewire through the needle through the kidney into the renal pelvis, the physician removes the needle by passing it backward over the guidewire. The physician enlarges (dilates) the guidewire passageway by inserting and removing tubes with increasingly larger diameters. When the passageway is sufficiently dilated, the physician passes a nephrostomy tube over the guidewire, removes the guidewire, and sutures the tube to the skin.

50396

The physician connects an indwelling ureteral catheter or existing pyelostomy or nephrostomy tube to a manometer line to measure pressure and flow in the kidneys and ureters. The physician connects a ureteral catheter or pyelostomy or nephrostomy tube to a manometer line filled with sterile fluid. The physician inserts a bladder catheter that may be irrigated with sterile fluid. The physician measures intrarenal and/or extrarenal pressure. After discontinuing perfusion of fluid, the physician aspirates residual fluid from the kidney and disconnects the manometer line. The physician may remove the ureteral catheter or pyelostomy or nephrostomy tube and dress the wound.

50398

The physician changes a nephrostomy or pyelostomy tube. To remove the existing tube, the physician takes out the sutures securing the tube to the skin. The physician inserts a guidewire through the tube and passes the tube back over the guidewire. The physician passes a new tube over the guidewire, removes the guidewire, and sutures the tube to the skin.

50400–50405

The physician uses plastic surgery to correct an obstruction or defect in the renal pelvis or ureteropelvic junction. To access the renal pelvis and ureter, the physician usually makes an incision in the skin of the flank. The physician incises, trims, and shapes the renal pelvis and ureter, using absorbable sutures or soft rubber drains for traction. The physician usually inserts a slender tube into the renal pelvis to provide support during healing. In Foley Y-pyeloplasty, the physician advances a Y-shaped flap of the renal pelvis into a vertical incision in the upper ureter. The physician may surgically fixate (nephropexy) a floating or mobile kidney, and/or establish an opening between the kidney (nephrostomy) or renal pelvis (pyelostomy) and the exterior of the body. The physician places a drain tube, bringing it out through a separate stab incision in the skin, and performs a layered closure. Report 50405 if a congenital abnormality, secondary pyeloplasty, solitary kidney, or calycoplasty complicates the procedure.

50500

The physician uses sutures to surgically fixate a wound or injury of the kidney. To access the kidney, the physician makes an incision in the skin of the flank, cuts the muscles, fat, and fibrous membranes (fascia) overlying the kidney, and sometimes removes a portion of the eleventh or twelfth rib. After using sutures to close or surgically fixate a kidney wound or injury, the physician places a drain tube, bringing it out through a separate stab incision in the skin, and performs a layered closure.

50520

The physician closes a fistula that is an abnormal opening between the skin and the kidney (nephrocutaneous) or the renal pelvis (pyelocutaneous). After excising the fistula, the physician sutures the clean percutaneous tissues together to create a smooth surface.

50525–50526

The physician closes a fistula that is an abnormal opening between the kidney and an organ of the digestive, respiratory, urogenital, or endocrine system. For 50525, the physician usually makes an incision in the abdomen, cuts the muscles, fat, and fibrous membranes (fascia) overlying the kidney to access the fistula. For 50526, the physician makes an incision in the skin of the chest, opens the chest cavity, collapses the lung, and separates the leaves of the diaphragm to expose the kidney. After excising the fistula, the physician sutures the clean tissues together to create a smooth surface. The physician places a drain tube, bringing it out through a separate stab incision in the skin, and performs a layered closure. For 50526, the physician inserts a chest tube to re-expand the lung.

50540

The physician divides an abnormal union of the kidneys to correct a horseshoe kidney. To access the horseshoe kidney, the physician usually makes an incision in the skin of the lower abdomen and cuts the muscles, fat, and fibrous membranes (fascia) overlying the kidney. After incising the union and placing two rows of sutures to control bleeding, the physician usually performs pyeloplasty or another plastic procedure on one or both sides of the divided kidney. After completion of repair, the physician may rotate the kidney to effect drainage. The physician irrigates the site with normal saline, places a drain tube, bringing it out through a separate stab incision in the skin, and performs a layered closure.

50541

The physician performs a laparoscopic surgical ablation of renal cysts through the abdomen or back. With the abdominal approach, an umbilical port is created by placing a trocar at the level of the umbilicus. The abdominal wall is then insufflated. The laparoscope is placed through the umbilical port and additional trocars are placed into the abdominal cavity. In the back approach, the trocar is placed at the back proximate to the retroperitoneal space near to the kidney with additional ports placed nearby for appropriate access to the operative site. The physician uses the laparoscope fitted with a fiberoptic camera and/or an operating instrument. The renal cysts are visualized through the scope are ablated by fulguration or other method. The instruments are removed and the abdominal or back incisions are closed by staples or sutures.

50544

The physician performs a laparoscopic pyeloplasty to correct an obstruction or defect in the renal pelvis or ureteropelvic junction through the abdomen or back. With the abdominal approach, an umbilical port is created by placing a trocar at the level of the umbilicus. The abdominal wall is then insufflated. The laparoscope is placed through the umbilical port and additional trocars are placed into the abdominal cavity. In the back approach, the trocar is placed at the back proximate to the retroperitoneal space near to the kidney with additional ports placed nearby for appropriate access to the operative site. The physician uses the laparoscope fitted with a fiberoptic camera and/or an operating instrument. The physician then incises, trims, and/or shapes the renal pelvis and ureter using absorbable sutures or soft rubber drains for traction. A tube is usually inserted to promote healing. The instruments are removed and abdominal or back incisions are closed by staples or sutures.

50545

The physician performs a radical nephrectomy, including removal of Gerota's fascia and surrounding fatty tissue, regional lymph nodes, and the adrenal gland through a laparoscope. The physician makes a 1.0 centimeter periumbilical incision and inserts a trocar. The abdominal cavity is insufflated with carbon dioxide. A fiberoptic laparoscope fitted with a camera and light source is inserted through the trocar. Other incisions (ports) are made in the abdomen or flank to allow other instruments or an additional light source to be passed into the abdomen or retroperitoneum. The colon is mobilized, and the laparoscope is advanced to the operative site. The ureter is transected at the ureterovesical junction. The physician then clamps, ligates, and severs the renal vein and renal artery. The Gerota's fascia is dissected to expose the upper pole of the kidney. The adrenal gland is visualized. Clips are placed on the suprarenal vein and adrenal arteries (diaphragmatic [inferior phrenic], aortic, and renal) which are then cut. Any lymph nodes in the surrounding area are excised and removed. The kidney, adrenal gland, renal (Gerota's) fascia, and surrounding fat are dissected free; they are bagged and removed through an enlarged port site. The instruments are removed. The incisions are closed with staples or suture.

50546

The physician removes the kidney and a portion of the ureter through a laparoscope. The physician makes a 1.0-centimetersperiumbilical incision and inserts a trocar. The abdominal cavity is insufflated with carbon dioxide. A fiberoptic laparoscope fitted with a camera and light source is inserted through the trocar. Other incisions (ports) are made in the abdomen or flank to allow other instruments or an additional light source to be passed into the abdomen or retroperitoneum. The colon is mobilized and the laparoscope is advanced to the operative site. The physician mobilizes the kidney and clamps, ligates, and severs part of the ureter and major renal blood vessels (renal pedicle). The kidney and upper ureter are bagged and brought through one of the port sites (e.g., periumbilical) that has been slightly enlarged. The instruments are removed, and the small abdominal or flank incisions are closed with staples or suture.

50547

The physician performs a donor nephrectomy from a living donor by removing the kidney and upper portion of the ureter with the laparoscope through the abdomen or back. With the abdominal approach, an umbilical port is created by placing a trocar at the level of the umbilicus. The abdominal wall is then insufflated. The laparoscope is placed through the umbilical port and additional trocars are placed into the abdominal cavity. In the back approach, the trocar is placed at the back proximate to the retroperitoneal space near to the kidney with additional ports placed nearby for appropriate access to the operative site. The physician uses the laparoscope fitted with a fiberoptic camera and/or an operating instruments to explore the area. After mobilization of the kidney and ureter, an anti-clotting agent is administered. The physician then clamps, ligates, and severs the upper ureter and major renal blood vessels (renal pedicle), and removes the kidney and upper ureter. The physician administers medication to reverse the effects of the anti-clotting agent. The small abdominal or back incisions are closed by staple or suture in the usual fashion. To maintain the renal transplant (homograft), the kidney is placed in cold saline solution and flushed with a cold electrolyte solution.

50548

The physician removes the kidney and all of the ureter through a laparoscope. The physician makes a 1.0-centimeter periumbilical incision and inserts a trocar. The abdominal cavity is insufflated with carbon dioxide. A fiberoptic laparoscope fitted with a camera and light source is inserted through the trocar. Other incisions (ports) are made in the abdomen or flank to allow other instruments or an additional light source to be passed into the abdomen or retroperitoneum. The colon is mobilized and the laparoscope is advanced to the operative site. The physician then mobilizes the kidney and clamps, ligates, and severs the all of the ureter at the ureterovesical junction and major renal blood vessels (renal pedicle). The kidney and ureter are bagged and brought through one of the port sites (e.g., periumbilical) that has been slightly enlarged. The instruments are removed, and the small abdominal or flank incisions are closed with staple or suture.

50551

The physician examines the kidney and ureter with an endoscope passed through an established opening between the skin and kidney (nephrostomy) or renal pelvis (pyelostomy). After inserting a guidewire, the physician removes the nephrostomy or pyelostomy tube and passes the endoscope through the opening into the kidney or renal pelvis. To better view renal and ureteric structures, the physician may flush (irrigate) or introduce by drops (instillate) a sterile saline solution. The physician may introduce contrast medium for radiologic study of the renal pelvis and ureter (ureteropyelogram). After examination, the physician removes the endoscope and guidewire and either reinserts the nephrostomy tube or allows the surgical passageway to seal on its own.

50553

The physician examines the kidney and ureter with an endoscope passed through an established opening between the skin and kidney (nephrostomy) or renal pelvis (pyelostomy), and inserts a catheter into the ureter. After inserting a guidewire, the physician removes the nephrostomy or pyelostomy tube and passes the endoscope through the opening into the

CPT® Lay Descriptions

kidney or renal pelvis. To better view renal and ureteric structures, the physician may flush (irrigate) or introduce by drops (instillate) a sterile saline solution. The physician may introduce contrast medium for radiologic study of the renal pelvis and ureter (ureteropyelogram). After examination, the physician passes a thin tube through the endoscope into the ureter. The physician may insert a balloon catheter to dilate a ureteral constriction. The physician either reinserts the nephrostomy tube or allows the passageway to seal on its own.

50555

The physician examines the kidney and ureter with an endoscope passed through an established opening between the skin and kidney (nephrostomy) or renal pelvis (pyelostomy), and biopsies renal tissue. After inserting a guidewire, the physician removes the nephrostomy or pyelostomy tube and passes the endoscope through the opening into the kidney or renal pelvis. To better view renal and ureteric structures, the physician may flush (irrigate) or introduce by drops (instillate) a sterile saline solution. The physician may introduce contrast medium for radiologic study of the renal pelvis and ureter (ureteropyelogram). After examination, the physician passes an cutting instrument through the endoscope into the suspect renal tissue and takes a biopsy specimen. The physician removes the endoscope and either reinserts the nephrostomy or pyelostomy tube or allows the passageway to seal on its own.

50557

The physician examines the kidney and ureter with an endoscope passed through an established opening between the skin and kidney (nephrostomy) or renal pelvis (pyelostomy), and removes renal lesions by electric current (fulguration) or incision. After inserting a guidewire, the physician removes the nephrostomy or pyelostomy tube and passes the endoscope through the opening into the kidney or renal pelvis. To better view renal and ureteric structures, the physician may flush (irrigate) or introduce by drops (instillate) a sterile saline solution. The physician may introduce contrast medium for radiologic study of the renal pelvis and ureter (ureteropyelogram). After examination, the physician passes through the endoscope an instrument that destroys lesions with electric current or incises lesions. The physician may insert a cutting instrument to biopsy renal tissue. The physician removes the endoscope and either reinserts the nephrostomy/pyelostomy tube or allows the passageway to seal on its own.

50559

The physician examines the kidney and ureter with an endoscope passed through an established opening between the skin and kidney (nephrostomy) or renal pelvis (pyelostomy), and inserts radioactive substance into renal tissue. After inserting a guidewire, the

physician removes the nephrostomy or pyelostomy tube and passes the endoscope through the opening into the kidney or renal pelvis. To better view renal and ureteric structures, the physician may flush (irrigate) or introduce by drops (instillate) a sterile saline solution. The physician may introduce contrast medium for radiologic study of the renal pelvis and ureter (ureteropyelogram). After examination, the physician releases radioactive substance via an instrument passed through the endoscope. The physician may insert instruments to fulgurate renal lesions or biopsy the renal tissue. The physician removes the endoscope and either reinserts the nephrostomy or pyelostomy tube or allows the surgical passageway to seal on its own.

50561

The physician examines the kidney and ureter with an endoscope passed through an established opening between the skin and kidney (nephrostomy) or renal pelvis (pyelostomy), and removes a foreign body or calculus. After inserting a guidewire, the physician removes the nephrostomy or pyelostomy tube and passes the endoscope through the opening into the kidney or renal pelvis. To better view renal and ureteric structures, the physician may flush (irrigate) or introduce by drops (instillate) a sterile saline solution. The physician may introduce contrast medium for radiologic study of the renal pelvis and ureter (ureteropyelogram). After examination, the physician passes an instrument through the endoscope to remove a foreign body or calculus. The physician removes the endoscope and either reinserts the nephrostomy tube or allows the surgical passageway to seal on its own.

50570

The physician examines the kidney and ureter with an endoscope passed through an incision in the kidney (nephrotomy) or renal pelvis (pyelotomy). After accessing the renal and ureteric structures with an incision in the skin of the flank, the physician incises the kidney or renal pelvis and guides the endoscope through the incision. To better view renal and ureteric structures, the physician may flush (irrigate) or introduce by drops (instillate) a sterile saline solution. The physician may introduce contrast medium for radiologic study of the renal pelvis and ureter (ureteropyelogram). After examination, the physician sutures the incision, inserts a drain tube, and performs a layered closure.

50572

The physician examines the kidney and ureter with an endoscope passed through an incision in the kidney (nephrotomy) or renal pelvis (pyelotomy), and inserts a catheter into the ureter. After accessing the renal and ureteric structures with an incision in the skin of the flank, the physician incises the kidney or renal pelvis and guides the endoscope through the incision. To better view renal and ureteric structures, the physician may flush (irrigate) or introduce by drops (instillate) a sterile saline solution. The physician may introduce contrast medium for radiologic study of the renal pelvis and ureter (ureteropyelogram). After examination, the physician passes a thin tube through the endoscope into the ureter, and may insert a balloon catheter to dilate a ureteral constriction. The physician sutures the incisions, inserts a drain tube, and performs a layered closure.

50574

The physician examines the kidney and ureter with an endoscope passed through an incision in the kidney (nephrotomy) or renal pelvis (pyelotomy), and biopsies renal tissue. After accessing the renal and ureteric structures with an incision in the skin of the flank, the physician incises the kidney or renal pelvis and guides the endoscope through the incision. To better view renal and ureteric structures, the physician may flush (irrigate) or introduce by drops (instillate) a sterile saline solution. The physician may introduce contrast medium for radiologic study of the renal pelvis and ureter (ureteropyelogram). After examination, the physician passes a cutting instrument through the endoscope into the suspect renal tissue and takes a biopsy specimen. The physician removes the endoscope, sutures the incision, inserts a drain tube, and performs a layered closure.

50575

The physician examines the kidney and ureter with an endoscope passed through an incision in the kidney (nephrotomy) or renal pelvis (pyelotomy), and dilates ureter and ureteropelvic junction. After accessing the renal and ureteric structures with an incision in the skin of the flank, the physician incises the kidney or renal pelvis and guides the endoscope through the incision. To better view renal and ureteric structures, the physician may flush (irrigate) or introduce by drops (instillate) a sterile saline solution. The physician may introduce contrast medium for radiologic study of the renal pelvis and ureter (ureteropyelogram). For endopyelotomy, the physician places endoscope through the ureter and/or the pelvis, incises the pelvis, enlarges the ureteropelvic junction, and sutures the junction as in a Y-V pyeloplasty. The physician inserts the stent through the renal pelvis into the junction, sutures the incisions, inserts a drain tube, and performs a layered closure.

50576

The physician examines the kidney and ureter with an endoscope passed through an incision in the kidney (nephrotomy) or renal pelvis (pyelotomy), and removes renal lesions by electric current (fulguration) or incision. After accessing the renal and ureteric structures with an incision in the skin of the flank, the physician incises the kidney or renal pelvis and guides the endoscope through the incision. To better

view renal and ureteric structures, the physician may flush (irrigate) or introduce by drops (instillate) a sterile saline solution. The physician may introduce contrast medium for radiologic study of the renal pelvis and ureter (ureteropyelogram). After examination, the physician passes through the endoscope an instrument that destroys lesions by electric current or incision The physician may insert instrument to biopsy renal tissue. The physician removes the scope, sutures the incision, inserts a drain tube, and performs a layered closure.

50578

The physician examines the kidney and ureter with an endoscope passed through an incision in the kidney (nephrotomy) or renal pelvis (pyelotomy), and inserts a radioactive substance. After accessing the renal and ureteric structures with an incision in the skin of the flank, the physician incises the kidney or renal pelvis and guides the endoscope through the incision. To better view renal and ureteric structures, the physician may flush (irrigate) or introduce by drops (instill) a sterile saline solution. The physician may introduce contrast medium for radiologic study of the renal pelvis and ureter (ureteropyelogram). To release radioactive substance, the physician passes instruments through endoscope. The physician may insert instruments through the endoscope to fulgurate renal lesions or biopsy the renal tissue. The physician removes the endoscope, sutures the incision, inserts a drain tube, and performs a layered closure.

50580

The physician examines the kidney and ureter with an endoscope passed through an incision in the kidney (nephrotomy) or renal pelvis (pyelotomy), and removes a foreign body or calculus. After accessing the renal and ureteric structures with an incision in the skin of the flank, the physician incises the kidney or renal pelvis and guides the endoscope through the incision. To better view renal and ureteric structures, the physician may flush (irrigate) or introduce by drops (instillate) a sterile saline solution. The physician may introduce contrast medium for radiologic study of the renal pelvis and ureter (ureteropyelogram). After examination, the physician passes instruments through the endoscope to remove a foreign body or calculus, and may pass a stent through the ureter into the bladder. The physician sutures the incision, inserts a drain tube, and performs a layered closure.

50590

The physician pulverizes a kidney stone (renal calculus) by directing shock waves through a liquid medium. Two different methods are currently available to accomplish this procedure. The physician first uses radiological guidance to determine the location and size of the renal calculus. In the first method, the patient is then immersed in a liquid medium (degassed, deionized water) with shock waves directed through the liquid to the kidney stone. In the second method, the one most often used, the patient is placed on a specially designed treatment table. A series of shock waves are directed through a water-cushion, or bellow that is placed against the patient's body at the location of the kidney stone. Each shock wave is directed to the stone for only a fraction of a second, and the entire procedure generally takes from 30 to 50 minutes. The treatment table is equipped with video x-ray so the physician can view the pulverization process. Over several days or weeks, the tiny stone fragments pass harmlessly though the patient's urinary system and are discharged during urination.

50600

The physician makes an incision in the ureter (ureterotomy) for examination of the ureter or insertion of a drainage catheter (ureterostomy tube) between the ureter and skin. To access the ureter, the physician makes an incision in the skin of the flank, and cuts the muscles, fat, and fibrous membranes (fascia) overlying the ureter. The physician makes an incision in the ureter and sometimes places fine traction sutures at the edges of the incision. The physician examines the interior of the ureter or, if the incision is for drainage, the physician inserts a catheter tip into the ureter and passes the tube through a stab incision in the skin of the flank. The physician sutures the incision and performs a layered closure.

50605

The physician makes an incision in the ureter (ureterotomy) to insert a catheter (stent) in the ureter. To access the ureter, the physician makes an incision in the skin of the flank, and cuts the muscles, fat, and fibrous membranes (fascia) overlying the ureter. The physician makes an incision in the ureter and sometimes places fine traction sutures at the edges of the incision. The physician inserts a slender rod or catheter into the ureter, sutures the incision, and performs a layered closure.

50610–50630

The physician makes an incision in the ureter (ureterotomy) to remove a stone (calculus) from the ureter. To access the ureter, the physician makes an incision in the skin and cuts the muscles, fat, and fibrous membranes (fascia) overlying the ureter. For the upper or middle third of the ureter, the physician usually makes an incision in the skin of the flank; to access the lower third of the ureter, the physician usually makes a curved lower quadrant incision. The physician isolates the calculus and removes it through an incision in the ureter. After examining the ureter for other defects, the physician sutures the incision and performs a layered closure, inserting a drain tube through a stab incision in the skin. Report 50610 for calculus removal from the upper third of the ureter;

50620 for calculus removal from the middle third; and 50630 for calculus removal from the lower third.

50650

The physician removes the ureter and a small cuff of the bladder. To access the ureter, the physician usually makes a curved lower quadrant incision in the skin of the abdomen, and cuts the muscles, fat, and fibrous membranes (fascia) overlying the ureter. The physician mobilizes the bladder, dissects a small cuff of the bladder, and ligates and dissects the ureter. After removing the bladder cuff and lower ureter, the physician sutures and catheterizes the bladder. The physician places a drain tube behind the bladder and performs a layered closure.

50660

The physician removes a ureter that deviates from proper anatomical placement. To access the ureter, the physician makes an incision in the skin of the abdomen, perineum, and/or vagina. The physician cuts the muscles, fat, and fibrous membranes (fascia) overlying the ureter. After mobilizing the bladder and ureter, the physician ligates, dissects, and removes the ureter. The physician places a drain tube at the site of the incision and performs a layered closure.

50684

The physician injects a contrast agent through an opening between the skin and the ureter (ureterostomy) or via an indwelling catheter into the ureter and renal pelvis to study the renal collecting system. To determine immediate allergic response to the contrast agent, the physician injects a dose of contrast material through the ureterostomy or indwelling catheter into the ureter and renal pelvis, and takes an x-ray.

50686

The physician connects an indwelling ureteral catheter or existing ureterostomy to a manometer line to measure pressure and flow in the kidneys and ureters. The physician connects a ureteral catheter or ureterostomy to a manometer line filled with sterile fluid. The physician inserts a bladder catheter that may be irrigated with sterile fluid. The physician measures intrarenal and/or extra renal pressure. After discontinuing perfusion of fluid, the physician aspirates residual fluid from the kidney and disconnects the manometer line. The physician may remove the ureteral catheter or ureterostomy tube (if applicable) and dress the wound.

50688

The physician changes a ureterostomy tube. To remove the existing tube, the physician takes out the sutures securing the tube to the skin. The physician inserts a guidewire through the tube and passes the tube back over the guidewire. The physician passes a new tube over the guidewire, removes the guidewire, and sutures the tube to the skin.

50690

The physician injects a contrast agent into an ileal stoma by a catheter into the renal pelvis to study the ileal conduit and renal collecting system. To determine immediate allergic response to the contrast agent, the physician injects a dose of contrast material through the ureterostomy or indwelling catheter into the ureter and renal pelvis, and takes an x-ray.

50700

The physician uses plastic surgery to correct an obstruction or defect in the ureter. To access the ureter, the physician makes an incision in the skin and cuts the muscles, fat, and fibrous membranes (fascia) overlying the ureter. For the upper or middle third of the ureter, the physician usually makes an incision in the skin of the flank; to access the lower third of the ureter, the physician usually makes a curved lower quadrant incision. The physician inserts a catheter into the ureter to the point of obstruction. The balloon is inflated, sometimes using repeated inflation with increasing diameter of the catheter. The physician incises, trims, and shapes the ureter, using absorbable sutures or soft rubber drains for traction. The physician may insert a slender tube into the ureter to provide support during healing. The physician places a drain tube, bringing it out through a separate stab incision in the skin, and performs a layered closure.

50715

The physician surgically frees the ureter from localized inflammatory disease of retroperitoneal fibrous tissue. To access the ureter, the physician makes a midline incision in the skin of the abdomen and cuts the muscles, fat, and fibrous membranes (fascia) overlying the ureter. The physician incises surrounding fibrotic tissue to free the ureter, and may use sutures to reposition the ureter away from obstructive fibrous tissue. The physician places a drain tube, bringing it out through a separate stab incision in the skin, and performs a layered closure.

50722

The physician surgically frees the ureter from ureteral obstruction caused by aberrant ovarian veins (ovarian vein syndrome). To access the ureter, the physician makes an incision in the skin above the pubic hairline, and cuts the muscles, fat, and fibrous membranes (fascia) overlying the ureter. The physician incises surrounding adhesions to free the ureter from the obstructing ovarian veins. The physician places a drain tube, bringing it out through a separate stab incision in the skin, and performs a layered closure.

50725

The physician divides and reconnects a ureter aberrantly positioned behind the vena cava. To access the ureter, the physician makes a midline incision in the skin of the abdomen, and cuts the muscles, fat,

and fibrous membranes (fascia) overlying the ureter. The physician dissects the ureter on both sides of the vena cava, leaving the ureteric segment behind the vena cava in place. The physician connects (anastomosis) the distal end of the ureter to the upper ureter by fashioning a long, elliptical flap from the renal pelvis. The physician may alternatively dissect and connect the two ends of the vena cava, positioning the ureter in front. To provide support during healing, the physician may insert a slender tube into the renal pelvis. After wrapping the anastomosis with perinephric fat, the physician inserts a drain tube and performs a layered closure.

50727–50728

The physician revises any surgical opening (anastomosis) between the skin and ureter, bladder, or colon segment. The physician removes the sutures securing the anastomosis to the skin and revises the anastomosis. The physician may make a midline incision in the skin of the abdomen to access the urinary tract. For 50728, the physician repairs a defect in surrounding fibrous membranes (fascia), and/or a rupture (hernia) in ureteral tissues.

50740

The physician surgically connects the upper ureter and renal pelvis to allow for urinary drainage. To access the renal pelvis and ureter, the physician makes an incision in the skin of the flank, cuts the muscles, fat, and fibrous membranes (fascia) overlying the kidney, and sometimes removes a portion of the eleventh or twelfth rib. The physician ligates the renal pelvis and ureter at the point of blockage. After excising the obstructing part of the ureter or pelvis, the physician surgically connects (anastomosis) the two structures, bypassing the obstructing point. To provide support during healing, the physician may insert a slender tube into the renal pelvis. After wrapping the anastomosis with perinephric fat, the physician inserts a drain tube and performs a layered closure.

50750

The physician connects the upper ureter and a renal calyx to allow for urinary drainage. To access the renal calyces and ureter, the physician makes an incision in the skin of the flank, cuts the muscles, fat, and fibrous membranes (fascia) overlying the kidney, and sometimes removes a portion of the eleventh or twelfth rib. The physician ligates the appropriate renal arteries and performs a partial nephrectomy by removing a part of the kidney. The physician partially mobilizes the calyx and ureter, and places a nephrostomy tube and stent. After surgically joining (anastomosing) the calyx and ureter, the physician closes the renal pelvis and wraps the anastomosis with perinephric fat. The physician inserts a drain tube and performs a layered closure.

50760

The physician divides and reconnects the ureter to bypass a defect or obstruction. To access the ureter, the physician makes an incision in the skin of the abdomen and cuts the muscles, fat, and fibrous membranes (fascia) overlying the ureter. For the upper or middle third of the ureter, the physician usually makes an incision in the skin of the flank; to access the lower third of the ureter, the physician usually makes a curved lower quadrant incision. The physician ligates and dissects the ureter at the point of blockage, and surgically rejoins (anastomosis) the two ends, bypassing the obstructing point. To provide support during healing, the physician may insert a slender tube into the ureter. The physician inserts a drain tube and performs a layered closure.

50770

The physician divides and connects a diseased or obstructed ureter to the other ureter. To access the ureters, the physician usually makes a midline incision in the skin of the abdomen, and cuts the muscles, fat, and fibrous membranes (fascia) overlying the ureters. The physician ligates and dissects the ureter at the point of disease or blockage, and surgically attaches (anastomosis) the end of the usable ureteric portion to the other ureter. To provide support during healing, the physician may insert a slender tube into the ureter. The physician inserts a drain tube and performs a layered closure.

50780–50785

The physician connects the lower ureter and bladder to allow for urinary drainage. The physician usually makes an incision in the skin of the abdomen. After dissecting the ureter at the point of disease or obstruction, the physician brings the ureter through a stab incision in the bladder and sutures the ureter to the bladder. To provide support during healing, the physician may insert a catheter into the ureter. The physician inserts a drain tube and performs a layered duplicated ureter to the bladder. Report 50780 if this procedure is used. Report 50782 if the physician attaches a duplicated ureter to the bladder. Report 50783 if the anastomosis requires extensive urethral reconstruction. Report 50785 if the anastomosis requires suturing the bladder and psoas, or by fashioning a long, elliptical flap from the bladder.

50800

The physician connects the ureter to a segment of intestine to divert urine flow. To access the ureter and intestine, the physician makes an incision in the skin of the abdomen and cuts the corresponding muscles, fat, and fibrous membranes (fascia). The physician dissects the ureter, makes small incisions in the intestine segment, and surgically connects (anastomosis) the ureter to the intestine. To provide support during healing, the physician may insert a slender tube into the ureter. The physician inserts a drain tube and performs a layered closure.

50810

The physician connects the ureters to a segment of sigmoid colon to create a bladder with an opening to the skin. To access the ureters and sigmoid colon, the physician makes a midline incision in the skin of the abdomen and cuts the corresponding muscles, fat, and fibrous membranes (fascia). After dissecting an isolated segment of sigmoid colon, the physician reconnects (anastomosis) the divided colon to restore bowel continuity. The sigmoid section is closed by sutures on one end. The physician dissects each ureter, makes small incisions in the sigmoid segment, and surgically connects each ureter to the sigmoid segment. To provide support during healing, the physician may insert a slender tube into each ureter. The physician fashions a bladder by closing the proximal end of the sigmoid segment, and brings the distal end through an incision in the skin of the abdomen to establish an opening (colostomy) for intermittent emptying of urine. The physician inserts a drain tube and performs a layered closure.

50815–50820

The physician connects the ureters to a segment of intestine to divert urine flow through an opening in the skin. To access the ureters and intestine, the physician makes a midline incision in the skin of the abdomen and cuts the corresponding muscles, fat, and fibrous membranes (fascia). After dissecting an isolated segment of intestine, the physician reconnects (anastomosis) the divided intestine to restore bowel continuity. The colon segment is closed by sutures on one end. The physician dissects each ureter, makes small incisions in the intestine segment, and surgically connects each ureter to the colon segment. To provide support during healing, the physician may insert a slender tube into each ureter. The physician closes the proximal end of the intestine segment and brings the distal end through an incision in the skin of the abdomen to establish an opening (stoma) for direct emptying of urine. The physician inserts a drain tube and performs a layered closure. Report 50820 if the physician dissects a segment of ileal colon to divert urine flow.

50825

The physician connects the ureter(s) to loops of intestine fashioned into a reservoir with a valve opening. To access the intestine and ureters, the physician makes a midline incision in the skin of the abdomen and cuts the corresponding muscles, fat, and fibrous membranes (fascia). After dissecting an isolated segment of intestine, the physician reconnects (anastomosis) the divided intestine to restore bowel continuity. After shaping the intestine segment into a pouch, the physician dissects each ureter, makes small incisions in the intestine segment, and surgically connects each ureter to the intestine segment. To provide support during healing, the physician inserts a slender tube into each ureter, and closes the pouch. The physician brings part of the pouch out through an abdominal wall opening, or anastomosis the pouch to the male urethra. The physician inserts a drain tube and performs a layered closure.

50830

The physician restores continuity of a ureter through which urine flow was previously diverted. To access the ureter, the physician usually reopens the original ureteral diversion incision and cuts the corresponding muscles, fat, and fibrous membranes (fascia). The physician reverses the diversion by removing sutures connecting the ureter and colon, colon segment, and/or skin. The physician closes the opening in the skin used for the diversionary anastomosis. To restore ureteral continuity, the physician either reconnects the upper and lower ureter segments or connects the ureter to the other ureter (ureteroureterostomy), or reimplants the ureter into the bladder (ureteroneocystostomy). To provide support during healing, the physician inserts a slender tube into the ureter. The physician inserts a drain tube and performs a layered closure.

50840

The physician replaces part or all of the ureter with a segment of intestine. To access the ureters and intestine, the physician makes a midline incision in the skin of the abdomen and cuts the corresponding muscles, fat, and fibrous membranes (fascia). After dissecting an isolated segment of intestine, the physician reconnects (anastomosis) the divided intestine to restore bowel continuity. The physician dissects and removes the diseased or defective ureteral segment, replacing it with the intestine segment. To provide support during healing, the physician may insert a slender tube into the ureter. The physician inserts a drain tube and performs a layered closure.

50845

The physician connects a segment of cecum colon (vermiform appendix) to the bladder to directly divert urine flow through an opening in the skin (cutaneous appendico-vesicostomy). To access the bladder and cecum colon, the physician makes a midline incision in the skin of the abdomen and cuts the corresponding muscles, fat, and fibrous membranes (fascia). After dissecting vermiform appendix, the physician sutures the colon to restore bowel continuity. The physician makes an incision in the bladder and surgically connects the proximal end of the vermiform appendix to the bladder. The physician brings the distal end of vermiform appendix through an incision in the skin of the abdomen to establish an opening (stoma) for direct emptying of urine. The physician inserts a drain tube and performs a layered closure.

50860

The physician connects the ureter to the skin for urinary drainage. To access the ureter, the physician makes a midline incision in the skin of the abdomen and cuts the corresponding muscles, fat, and fibrous

membranes (fascia). The physician ligates the distal ureter and brings the proximal end to the skin. The physician splits the end of the ureter and sutures it to the skin with a double Z-plasty to prevent the ureter from narrowing. To provide support during healing, the physician may insert a slender tube into the ureter. The physician inserts a drain tube and performs a layered closure.

50900

The physician sutures a wound or defect in the ureter. To access the ureter, the physician makes an incision in the skin and cuts the muscles, fat, and fibrous membranes (fascia) overlying the ureter. For the upper or middle third of the ureter, the physician usually makes an incision in the skin of the flank; to access the lower third of the ureter, the physician usually makes a curved lower quadrant incision. The physician uses sutures to close or surgically fixate a ureteral wound or defect. To provide support during healing, the physician may insert a slender tube into the ureter. The physician inserts a drain tube and performs a layered closure.

50920

The physician closes an abnormal opening (fistula) between the skin and the ureter (ureterocutaneous). After excising the fistula, the physician sutures the clean percutaneous tissues together to create a smooth surface.

50930

The physician closes an abnormal opening (fistula) between the ureter and an organ of the digestive, respiratory, urogenital, or endocrine system. To access the ureter, the physician makes a midline incision in the skin of the abdomen and cuts the corresponding muscles, fat, and fibrous membranes (fascia). After excising the fistula, the physician sutures the clean tissues together to create a smooth surface. The physician places a drain tube, bringing it out through a separate stab incision in the skin, and performs a layered closure.

50940

The physician removes a thread, wire, or constricting band (ligature) placed on the ureter during a previous operative session. To access the ureter, the physician usually reopens the incision used for the previous operative session. After removing the ligature(s) from the ureter, the physician places a drain tube, bringing it out through a separate stab incision in the skin, and performs a layered closure.

50945

The physician performs a laparoscopic surgical removal of a stone (calculus) lodged in the ureter (ureterolithotomy). In an abdominal approach, the physician creates an umbilical port by placing a trocar at the level of the umbilicus. The abdominal wall is insufflated. The laparoscope is placed through the umbilical port and additional trocars are placed into the abdominal cavity. In the back (flank) approach, the trocar is placed at the back proximate to the retroperitoneal space near the kidney with additional ports placed nearby for appropriate access to the operative site. The physician uses the laparoscope fitted with a fiberoptic camera and/or an operating instrument to isolate the calculus and remove it through an incision in the ureter. The ureter is surgically closed. The small abdominal or back (flank) incisions are closed with staples or sutures.

50947–50948

The physician repositions the ureter on the bladder (due to an obstruction of the ureterovesical junction), using a laparoscopic approach. A stent may be placed with a cystoscope. In both procedures the physician makes a 1.0 centimeter periumbilical incision and inserts a trocar. The abdominal cavity is insufflated with carbon dioxide. A fiberoptic laparoscope fitted with a camera and light source is inserted through the trocar. Other incisions (ports) are made in the abdomen to allow other instruments or an additional light source to be passed into the abdomen. The physician manipulates the tools so the ureter and bladder can be observed through the laparoscope. The physician transects the ureter above the point of obstruction, brings the ureter through a stab incision in the bladder, and sutures the ureter to the new site on the bladder. In 50947, the physician inserts a cystoscope and places a stent in the repositioned ureter to provide support of the ureter. In 50948, the ureter is repositioned without cystoscopy or stent placement. The instruments are removed. The incisions are closed with staples or suture.

50951

The physician examines renal and ureteral structures with an endoscope passed through an established opening between the skin and ureter (ureterostomy). The physician inserts a guidewire, removes the ureterostomy tube, and passes the endoscope into the kidney or renal pelvis. The physician may flush (irrigate) or introduce by drops (instillate) a sterile saline solution to better view the renal and ureteral structures, and/or may introduce contrast medium for radiologic study of the renal pelvis and ureter (ureteropyelogram). The physician removes the endoscope and guidewire and either reinserts the ureterostomy tube or allows the passageway to seal on its own.

50953

The physician examines renal and ureteral structures with an endoscope passed through an established opening between the skin and ureter (ureterostomy), and inserts a catheter into the ureter. The physician inserts a guidewire, removes the ureterostomy tube, and passes the endoscope into the kidney or renal pelvis. The physician may flush (irrigate) or introduce by drops (instillate) a sterile saline solution to better

view the renal and ureteral structures, and/or may introduce contrast medium for radiologic study of the renal pelvis and ureter (ureteropyelogram). The physician passes a thin tube through the endoscope into the ureter, and may insert a balloon catheter to dilate a ureteral constriction. The physician removes the endoscope and guidewire and either reinserts the ureterostomy tube or allows the passageway to seal on its own.

50955

The physician examines renal and ureteral structures with an endoscope passed through an established opening between the skin and ureter (ureterostomy), and biopsies renal and/or ureteral tissue. The physician inserts a guidewire, removes the ureterostomy tube, and passes the endoscope into the kidney or renal pelvis. The physician may flush (irrigate) or introduce by drops (instillate) a sterile saline solution to better view the renal and ureteral structures, and/or may introduce contrast medium for radiologic study of the renal pelvis and ureter (ureteropyelogram). The physician passes a cutting instrument through the endoscope into the suspect tissue and takes a biopsy specimen. The physician removes the endoscope and guidewire and either reinserts the ureterostomy tube or allows the passageway to seal on its own.

50957

The physician examines renal and ureteral structures with an endoscope passed through an established opening between the skin and ureter (ureterostomy), and removes lesions by electric current (fulguration) or incision. The physician inserts a guidewire, removes the ureterostomy tube, and passes the endoscope into the kidney or renal pelvis. The physician may flush (irrigate) or introduce by drops (instillate) a sterile saline solution to better view the renal and ureteral structures, and/or may introduce contrast medium for radiologic study of the renal pelvis and ureter (ureteropyelogram). The physician passes through the endoscope an instrument that destroys lesions by electric current or incision. The physician may insert an instrument to biopsy renal tissue. The physician removes the endoscope and guidewire and either reinserts the ureterostomy tube or allows the passageway to seal on its own.

50959

The physician examines renal and ureteral structures with an endoscope passed through an established opening between the skin and ureter (ureterostomy), and inserts a radioactive substance. The physician inserts a guidewire, removes the ureterostomy tube, and passes the endoscope into the kidney or renal pelvis. The physician may flush (irrigate) or introduce by drops (instillate) a sterile saline solution to better view the renal and ureteral structures, and/or may introduce contrast medium for radiologic study of the renal pelvis and ureter (ureteropyelogram). To release radioactive substance, the physician passes an instrument through the endoscope. The physician may insert instruments through the endoscope to fulgurate renal lesions or biopsy the renal tissue. The physician removes the endoscope and guidewire and either reinserts the ureterostomy tube or allows the passageway to seal on its own.

50961

The physician examines renal and ureteral structures with an endoscope passed through an established opening between the skin and ureter (ureterostomy), and removes a foreign body or calculus. The physician inserts a guidewire, removes the ureterostomy tube, and passes the endoscope into the kidney or renal pelvis. The physician may flush (irrigate) or introduce by drops (instillate) a sterile saline solution to better view the renal and ureteral structures, and/or may introduce contrast medium for radiologic study of the renal pelvis and ureter (ureteropyelogram). The physician passes an instrument through the endoscope to remove a foreign body or calculus. The physician removes the endoscope and guidewire and either reinserts the ureterostomy tube or allows the passageway to seal on its own.

50970

The physician examines renal and ureteral structures with an endoscope passed through an incision in the ureter (ureterotomy). After accessing the ureter with an incision in the skin of the flank, the physician incises the ureter and guides the endoscope through the incision. The physician may flush (irrigate) or introduce by drops (instillate) a sterile solution to better view the renal and ureteral structures, and/or may introduce contrast medium for radiologic study of the renal pelvis and ureter (ureteropyelogram). After examination, the physician sutures the incision, inserts a drain tube, and performs a layered closure.

50972

The physician examines renal and ureteral structures with an endoscope passed through an incision in the ureter (ureterotomy), and inserts a catheter into the ureter. After accessing the ureter with an incision in the skin of the flank, the physician incises the ureter and guides the endoscope through the incision. The physician may flush (irrigate) or introduce by drops (instillate) a sterile solution to better view the renal and ureteral structures, and/or may introduce contrast medium for radiologic study of the renal pelvis and ureter (ureteropyelogram). To catheterize the ureter, the physician passes a thin tube through the endoscope into the ureter. The physician may insert a balloon catheter to dilate a ureteral constriction. The physician sutures the incision, inserts a drain tube, and performs a layered closure.

50974

The physician examines renal and ureteral structures with an endoscope passed through an incision in the

ureter (ureterotomy), and biopsies ureteral and/or renal tissue. After accessing the ureter with an incision in the skin of the flank, the physician incises the ureter and guides the endoscope through the incision. The physician may flush (irrigate) or introduce by drops (instillate) a sterile solution to better view the renal and ureteral structures, and/or may introduce contrast medium for radiologic study of the renal pelvis and ureter (ureteropyelogram). The physician passes a cutting instrument through the endoscope into the suspect tissue and take a biopsy specimen. The physician removes the endoscope, sutures the incision, inserts a drain tube, and performs a layered closure.

50976

The physician examines renal and ureteral structures with an endoscope passed through an incision in the ureter (ureterotomy), and removes renal or ureteral lesions by electric current (fulguration) or incision. After accessing the ureter with an incision in the skin of the flank, the physician incises the ureter and guides the endoscope through the incision. The physician may flush (irrigate) or introduce by drops (instillate) a sterile solution to better view the renal and ureteral structures, and/or may introduce contrast medium for radiologic study of the renal pelvis and ureter (ureteropyelogram). The physician passes through the endoscope an instrument that either destroys lesions with electric sparks, or incises lesions. The physician may insert an instrument to biopsy renal tissue. The physician removes the endoscope, sutures the incision, inserts a drain tube, and performs a layered closure.

50978

The physician examines renal and ureteral structures with an endoscope passed through an incision in the ureter (ureterotomy), and inserts a radioactive substance. After accessing the ureter with an incision in the skin of the flank, the physician incises the ureter and guides the endoscope through the incision. The physician may flush (irrigate) or introduce by drops (instillate) a sterile solution to better view the renal and ureteral structures, and/or may introduce contrast medium for radiologic study (ureteropyelogram). The physician releases radioactive substance with an instrument passed through the endoscope. The physician may insert instruments to fulgurate renal lesions or biopsy renal tissue. The physician removes the endoscope, sutures the incision, inserts a drain tube, and performs a layered closure.

50980

The physician examines renal and ureteral structures with an endoscope passed through an incision in the ureter (ureterotomy), and removes a foreign body or stone (calculus). After accessing the ureter with an incision in the skin of the flank, the physician incises the ureter and guides the endoscope through the incision. The physician may flush (irrigate) or introduce by drops (instillate) a sterile solution to better view the renal and ureteral structures, and/or may introduce contrast medium for radiologic study of the renal pelvis and ureter (ureteropyelogram). The physician passes an instrument through the endoscope to remove a foreign body or calculus, and may pass a stent through the ureter into the bladder. The physician removes the endoscope, sutures the incision, inserts a drain tube, and performs a layered closure.

51000–51010

In 51000, the physician inserts a needle through the skin into the bladder to withdraw urine. In 51005 and 51010, the physician inserts a trocar or intracatheter through the skin into the bladder. In addition, in 51010, a suprapubic catheter is placed through the incision. This procedure may also be performed after the abdomen has been surgically incised.

51020–51030

The physician makes an incision (cystotomy) or creates an opening (cystostomy) into the bladder to destroy abnormal tissue. To access the bladder, the physician makes an incision in the skin of the lower abdomen and cuts the corresponding muscles, fat, fibrous membranes (fascia), and bladder wall. Report 51020 if the physician uses electric current (fulguration) or (usually with the aid of a radiation oncologist) inserts radioactive material to destroy a lesion on the bladder. Report 51030 if the physician uses cryosurgery to destroy the lesion. The bladder wall and lower abdomen is sutured closed. If a cystostomy is made, the cystostomy tube is sutured in place and the bladder and abdominal wall is closed.

51040

The physician creates an opening into the bladder (cystostomy) through an incision in the bladder (cystotomy). To access the bladder, the physician makes an incision in the skin of the lower abdomen and cuts the corresponding muscles, fat, and fibrous membranes (fascia). The physician makes a small incision and inserts a catheter (cystostomy tube) into the bladder, passing the tube through a stab incision in the skin of the abdomen. After closing the cystotomy, the physician may insert a drain tube, bringing it out through a separate stab incision, and performs a layered closure with absorbable sutures.

51045

The physician makes an incision in the bladder to insert a catheter or slender tube (stent) into the ureter. To access the bladder and ureters, the physician makes a midline incision in the skin of the abdomen and cuts the corresponding muscles, fat, and fibrous membranes (fascia). The physician incises the bladder (cystotomy) and inserts a stent or catheter in the ureter. Insertion of a ureteral catheter requires that the physician bring the tube end out through the urethra or bladder incision. The physician inserts a drain tube and performs a layered closure.

51050

The physician makes an incision in the bladder to remove a calculus. To access the bladder, the physician makes an incision in the skin of the lower abdomen and cuts the corresponding muscles, fat, and fibrous membranes (fascia). The physician performs a cystotomy, isolates the calculus, and removes it. The bladder neck is not excised. After examining the bladder for other defects, the physician sutures the incision and performs a layered closure using absorbable sutures, inserting a drain tube through a stab incision in the skin.

51060

The physician makes an incision in the bladder to remove a calculus in the ureter. To access the bladder and ureters, the physician makes a midline incision in the skin of the abdomen and cuts the corresponding muscles, fat, and fibrous membranes (fascia). The physician isolates the calculus and removes it through incisions in the bladder (cystotomy) and ureter (ureterotomy). After examining the ureter for other defects, the physician inserts a ureteral catheter and sutures the incisions. The physician inserts a drain tube and performs a layered closure.

51065

The physician makes an incision in the bladder and inserts an instrument in the ureter to remove or destroy the calculus. To access the bladder and ureters, the physician makes a midline incision in the skin of the abdomen and cuts the corresponding muscles, fat, and fibrous membranes (fascia). After isolating the calculus, the physician makes an incision in the bladder (cystotomy). The physician inserts an instrument (e.g., a stone basket) through the bladder incision into the ureter to remove or destroy a ureteral calculus. After examining the ureter for other defects, the physician inserts a ureteral catheter and sutures the incision. The physician inserts a drain tube and performs a layered closure.

51080

The physician drains an infection (abscess) near the bladder. To access the bladder, the physician makes an incision in the skin of the lower abdomen and cuts the corresponding muscles, fat, and fibrous membranes (fascia). After exploring the abscess cavity, the physician irrigates the site, inserts multiple drain tubes through separate stab wounds, and sutures the drain tube ends to the skin. The physician inserts a urethral catheter and performs a layered closure.

51500

The physician removes a cyst or dilated urachus (the remnant of bladder development that attaches from bladder to umbilicus). To access the urachus, the physician makes an incision in the skin of the lower abdomen through the umbilicus, and cuts the corresponding muscles, fat, and fibrous membranes (fascia). After isolating the urachus with a clamp, the physician excises the urachal cyst or sinus and a small cuff of the bladder. The physician sutures the bladder and removes the urachal tissue, leaving the navel intact. The physician may also repair a rupture (hernia) of tissue in the umbilicus. After inserting a drain tube and urethral catheter, the physician performs a layered closure.

51520

The physician removes part or all of the bladder neck. The physician makes an incision in the skin of the lower abdomen and cuts the corresponding muscles, fat, and fibrous membranes (fascia). Through this incision, the physician accesses the bladder neck and removes diseased or enlarged bladder neck tissue. The bladder is sutured and the abdominal wall is closed.

51525

The physician removes a diverticulum, a herniated defect of the bladder. To access the diverticulum, the physician makes an incision in the skin of the lower abdomen and cuts the corresponding muscles, fat, and fibrous membranes (fascia). The physician makes an incision in the bladder and may insert a ureteral stent if the diverticulum is close to the ureter. After dissecting the diverticulum from surrounding tissues and arteries, the physician excises the defective tissue and closes the remaining musculature and mucosa with absorbable sutures. This process may be repeated in other diverticula. The operative incision is repaired with a layered closure.

51530

The physician makes an incision in the bladder to remove a tumor of the bladder. To access the bladder, the physician makes an incision in the skin of the lower abdomen and cuts the corresponding muscles, fat, and fibrous membranes (fascia). The bladder is incised (cystotomy). After removing the tumor and surrounding diseased vesical tissue, the physician inserts a drain tube and performs a layered closure.

51535

The physician makes an incision in the bladder to remove or repair a saccular dilation of the ureteral end (ureterocele) that protrudes into the bladder. To access the bladder and ureters, the physician makes a midline incision in the skin of the abdomen and cuts the corresponding muscles, fat, and fibrous membranes (fascia). The physician incises the bladder (cystotomy) and excises or fulgurates the ureterocele. After examining the ureter for other defects, the physician sutures the bladder incision and inserts a ureteral catheter. The physician inserts a drain tube and performs a layered closure.

51550–51555

The physician removes a portion of diseased or damaged bladder tissue. To access the bladder, the physician makes an incision in the skin above the pubic bone and cuts the corresponding muscles, fat, and fibrous membranes (fascia). The physician mobilizes the bladder and the major vesical blood vessels, and incises the bladder wall to access the diseased or damaged bladder tissue. After removing the tissue, the physician inserts catheters into the bladder and urethra and sutures the bladder tissues. The physician performs a layered closure and inserts a drain tube, bringing it out through a separate stab incision in the skin. Report 51550 if the cystectomy presents few complications; report 51555 if the procedure is complicated because of prior administration of radiation, a previous surgery, or difficult access to the diseased or damaged bladder tissue.

51565

The physician removes diseased or damaged bladder tissue close to the ureteral orifice, and reimplants ureter(s) into the bladder (ureteroneocystostomy). To access the bladder and ureters, the physician makes a midline incision in the skin of the abdomen and cuts the corresponding muscles, fat, and fibrous membranes (fascia). The physician mobilizes the bladder, ureter(s), and the major vesical blood vessels, and may incise the bladder wall to access the diseased or damaged bladder tissue. The physician removes the diseased or damaged bladder tissue, requiring removal of the ureteral orifice and/or ureteral division. The physician brings the cut end of the ureter through a stab wound in the bladder and sutures the ureter to the bladder. To provide support during healing, the physician inserts a ureteral catheter, bringing the tube end out through the urethra or bladder incision. The physician inserts a drain tube and performs a layered closure.

51570–51575

The physician removes the bladder (cystectomy). To access the bladder, the physician makes an incision in the skin of the lower abdomen and cuts the corresponding muscles, fat, and fibrous membranes (fascia). Report 51570 if the physician dissects and ties (ligates) the hypogastric and vesical vessels, and severs the bladder from the urethra, rectum, surrounding peritoneum, vas deferens, and prostate (if applicable). After removing the bladder and controlling bleeding, the physician inserts drain tubes and performs a layered closure. If the physician bilaterally removes the pelvic lymph nodes, report 51575.

51580

The physician removes the bladder (cystectomy) and connects the ureters to the skin or sigmoid colon. To access the bladder and ureters, the physician makes a midline incision in the skin of the abdomen and cuts the corresponding muscles, fat, and fibrous membranes (fascia). The physician dissects and ligates the hypogastric and vesical vessels, and severs the bladder from the ureters and urethra. Blunt dissection from adherent rectum, surrounding peritoneum, and vas deferens and prostate may be needed. After controlling bleeding, the physician diverts urine by implanting the ureters to the skin (ureterocutaneous transplant), or connecting (anastomosing) the ureters to the sigmoid colon (ureterosigmoidostomy). To provide support during healing, the physician inserts a slender tube into each ureter. After completing the urinary diversion procedure, the physician inserts drain tubes and performs a layered closure.

51585

The physician removes the bladder (cystectomy) and pelvic lymph nodes, and connects the ureters to the skin or sigmoid colon. To access the bladder and ureters, the physician makes a midline incision in the skin of the abdomen and cuts the corresponding muscles, fat, and fibrous membranes (fascia). The physician dissects and ligates the hypogastric and vesical vessels, and severs the bladder from the ureters and urethra. Blunt dissection from adherent rectum, surrounding peritoneum, and vas deferens and prostate may be needed. The physician also removes external iliac, hypogastric, and obturator lymph nodes. After controlling bleeding, the physician diverts urine by implanting the ureters to the skin (ureterocutaneous transplant), or connecting the ureters to the sigmoid colon (ureterosigmoidostomy). The physician also inserts a slender tube into each ureter for support. After completing the urinary diversion procedure, the physician inserts drain tubes and performs a layered closure.

51590

The physician removes the bladder (cystectomy) and diverts urine by connecting the ureters to a ureteroileal conduit or sigmoid bladder with an opening into the skin. To access the bladder and ureters, the physician makes a midline incision in the skin of the abdomen and cuts the corresponding muscles, fat, and fibrous membranes (fascia). The physician dissects and ligates the hypogastric and vesical vessels, and severs the bladder from the ureters and urethra. Blunt dissection from adherent rectum, surrounding peritoneum, and vas deferens and prostate may be needed. After controlling bleeding, the physician diverts urine by connecting the ureters to a segment of ileal or sigmoid colon fashioned into a conduit or bladder, respectively, with an opening into the skin. To provide support during healing, the physician inserts a slender tube into each ureter. After completing the urinary diversion procedure, the physician inserts drain tubes and performs a layered closure.

51595

The physician removes the bladder (cystectomy) and pelvic lymph nodes, and diverts urine by connecting the ureters to a ureteroileal conduit or sigmoid bladder with an opening into the skin. To access the bladder and ureters, the physician makes a midline incision in the skin of the abdomen and cuts the corresponding muscles, fat, and fibrous membranes (fascia). The physician dissects and ligates the hypogastric and vesical vessels, and severs the bladder from the ureters and urethra. Blunt dissection from adherent rectum, surrounding peritoneum, and vas deferens and prostate may be needed. The physician also removes external iliac, hypogastric, and obturator lymph nodes. After controlling bleeding, the physician diverts urine by connecting the ureters to a segment of ileal or sigmoid colon fashioned into a conduit or bladder, with an opening into the skin. The physician inserts a slender tube into each ureter. After completing the urinary diversion procedure, the physician inserts drain tubes and performs a layered closure.

51596

The physician removes the bladder (cystectomy) and diverts urine by any method, using any bowel segment to create a new bladder. To access the bladder and ureters, the physician makes a midline incision in the skin of the abdomen and cuts the corresponding muscles, fat, and fibrous membranes (fascia). The physician dissects and ligates the hypogastric and vesical vessels, and severs the bladder from the urethra. Blunt dissection from adherent rectum, surrounding peritoneum, and vas deferens and prostate may be needed. After controlling bleeding, the physician diverts urine by connecting the ureters to a segment of large or small bowel fashioned into a bladder with an opening into the skin. To provide support during healing, the physician inserts a slender tube into each ureter. After completing the urinary diversion procedure, the physician inserts drain tubes and performs a layered closure.

51597

The physician removes the bladder, lower ureters, lymph nodes, urethra, prostate (if applicable), colon, and rectum, due to a vesical, prostatic, or urethral malignancy. To access the bladder and ureters, the physician makes a midline incision in the skin of the abdomen and cuts the corresponding muscles, fat, and fibrous membranes (fascia). The physician dissects and ligates the hypogastric and vesical vessels, and severs the bladder, urethra, lower ureters, lymph nodes, and prostate (if applicable) from surrounding structures. The physician removes the bladder and diverts urine flow by transplanting the ureters to the skin or colon. The vagina and uterus (if applicable) and/or rectum and part of the colon may be removed and an artificial abdominal opening in the skin surface created for waste (colostomy). After completing the urinary diversion procedure, the physician inserts drain tubes and performs a layered closure.

51600–51610

The physician injects a radiocontrast agent through a catheter inserted in the bladder to study the lower urinary tract. Using radiologic instruments, the physician produces an image of the bladder with x-rays (cystogram). Filling, voiding, and post-voiding x-rays are obtained. The catheter is partially or completely withdrawn and the urethra is studied by x-ray. As a starred procedure, 51600 reports the radiological procedure only. Any pre- or postoperative services are reported separately. Report 51605 if the physician inserts a chain in the bladder or through the urethra as part of the injection procedure for contrast x-rays of the bladder and urethra (chain urethrocystogram). Report 51610 if contrast material is injected through a urethral catheter or catheter-tipped syringe for x-rays of the urethra and bladder (retrograde urethrocystogram).

51700

The physician irrigates the bladder with saline solution that is flushed, injected, or introduced by drops (instillation) through a catheter. The physician initially places the catheter into the bladder and irrigates by hand until the bladder is free of clots or debris. A three-way Foley catheter may be inserted for continuous bladder irrigation.

51705–51710

The physician changes a cystostomy tube. To remove the existing tube, the physician removes the sutures securing the tube to the skin. Report 51705 if the physician inserts a guidewire through the tube and passes the tube back over the guidewire. The physician passes a new tube over the guidewire, removes the guidewire, and sutures the tube to the skin. Report 51710 if complications such as infection, inflammation, hemorrhage, constriction, or dilation arise.

51715

The physician injects natural proteins or synthetic material into the urethra and bladder neck, helping to prevent urinary incontinence. Before the injection, an endoscope is placed through the urethra into the bladder. Using local anesthesia, the physician makes one to three injections into the transurethra submucous. The injections are made through the endoscope into the affected area. The procedure can also be performed through the lower abdomen.

51720

The physician introduces by drops (instillation) an anticarcinogenic agent into the bladder to treat a cancer. Prior to the instillation of the agent, a standard lavage is usually performed. The anticarcinogenic agent is then introduced through a catheter placed in the bladder. This procedure may be used in conjunction with a cystostomy (51020) or with procedures such as cystorectomy for the removal of a tumor.

51725

The physician inserts a pressure catheter into the bladder and connects it to a manometer line filed with sterile fluid to measure pressure and flow in the lower urinary tract.

51726

The physician inserts an electronic microtip pressure-transducer catheter into the bladder and connects it to electronic equipment to measure pressure and flow in the lower urinary tract.

51736

The physician assesses the rate of emptying the bladder by stopwatch, recording the volume of urine per time.

51741

The physician assesses the rate of emptying of the bladder by electronic equipment, recording the volume of urine per time.

51772

The physician measures urethral pressure by pulling a transducer through the urethra and noting the pressure change.

51784

The physician places a pad in the anal or urethral sphincter and measures the electrical activity with the bladder filled and during emptying.

51785

The physician places a pad or needle in the anal or urethral sphincter and measures the electrical activity with the bladder filled and during emptying.

51792

The physician electrically stimulates the head of the penis. The physician measures the delay time for travel of stimulation through the pelvic nerves to the pudendal nerve.

51795

The physician places a transducer in the bladder to measure urine flow rate and pressure during emptying of the bladder.

51797

The physician places a transducer in the abdomen to measure intra-abdominal pressure during emptying of the bladder.

51800

The physician uses plastic surgery to correct an obstruction or defect in the bladder or vesical neck and urethra. The bladder is distended using a Foley catheter. To access the bladder, the physician makes an incision in the skin of the lower abdomen and cuts the corresponding muscles, fat, and fibrous membranes (fascia). The physician incises, trims, and shapes the bladder or vesical neck and urethra, using absorbable sutures or soft rubber drains for traction. The physician may insert a catheter through the urethra to provide support during healing. In anterior Y-plasty, the physician makes a Y-shaped flap of the bladder extending the vertical incision into the vesical neck. The vertical part of this incision is then pulled up into the V-shaped incision, which becomes a straight line when sutured. The physician may remove a portion of the vesical neck. The physician places a drain tube, bringing it out through a separate stab incision in the skin, and performs a layered closure.

51820

The physician uses plastic surgery to correct a defect in the bladder and urethra, and reimplants one or both ureters into the bladder (ureteroneocystostomy). To access the bladder, urethra, and ureters, the physician makes a midline incision in the skin of the abdomen and cuts the corresponding muscles, fat, and fibrous membranes (fascia). The physician incises, trims, and shapes the bladder and urethra, using absorbable sutures or soft rubber drains for traction. The physician brings the cut end of one or both ureters through a stab wound in the bladder and sutures the ureter(s) to the bladder. To provide support during healing, the physician inserts a ureteral catheter, bringing the tube end out through the urethra or bladder incision. The physician inserts a drain tube and performs a layered closure.

51840–51841

The physician performs a vesicourethropexy or urethropexy in the Marshall-Marchetti-Krantz or Burch style. The physician makes a small horizontal incision in the abdomen above the symphysis pubis, which is the midline junction of the pubic bones at the front. The bladder is suspended by placing several sutures through the tissue surrounding the urethra and into the vaginal wall. The sutures are pulled tight so that the tissues are tacked up to the symphysis pubis and the urethra is moved forward. The incision is then closed by suturing. 51841 is used when the procedure is performed for the second time or if some other factor increases the time or level of complexity.

51845

The physician surgically suspends the bladder neck by suturing surrounding tissue to the fibrous membranes (fascia) of the abdomen in a female patient. After inserting a catheter through the urethra to visualize the bladder neck, the physician makes an incision in the vagina, extending it upward toward the base of the bladder. On both sides of the vesical neck, the physician passes a needle through a small incision in the skin above the pubic bone down through the

vaginal incision. The physician threads the needle in the vagina and pulls the needle back up through the suprapubic incision. Dacron tubing may be threaded onto the sutures to provide extra periurethral support. The physician repeats this process, using an endoscope to ensure proper placement of the suspending sutures. After placing sutures on both sides of the bladder neck, the physician uses moderate upward traction to tighten the bladder neck. The physician inserts a drain tube, bringing it out through a stab incision in the skin, and performs a layered closure.

51860–51865

The physician sutures a wound, injury, or rupture in the bladder. To access the bladder, urethra, and ureters, the physician makes an incision in the skin of the abdomen and cuts the corresponding muscles, fat, and fibrous membranes (fascia). To provide support during healing, the physician may insert a catheter through the urethra. The physician inserts a drain tube and performs a layered closure. Constant irrigation is provided to help prevent infection. Report 51865 if the procedure is complicated due to a previous surgery, congenital defect, or other reason.

51880

The physician closes an artificial opening into the bladder (cystostomy). To access the cystostomy, the physician uses the original incision creating the cystostomy, or makes an incision in the skin of the lower abdomen. After removing the sutures securing the cystostomy tube to the skin and bladder, the physician removes the cystostomy tube. The physician places a drain tube, bringing it out through a separate stab incision in the skin, and performs a layered closure.

51900

The physician excises a vesicovaginal fistula, which is an abnormal opening between the vagina and the bladder. The procedure is done through a vertical abdominal incision from just above the umbilicus to the pubic symphysis. The anterior bladder wall is opened and the bladder interior explored. The fistula is excised along with the surrounding tissue to assure preservation of only healthy tissue. The resulting defect is closed with layered sutures starting with the vaginal wall, then the bladder walls, and finally the abdominal incision. A catheter is left in the bladder to prevent distension of the bladder and tension to the sutured areas.

51920–51925

The physician excises the fistula, which is an abnormal opening between the uterus and the bladder, then sutures the clean tissues together closing the resulting defect and creating a smooth surface. For 51920, the procedure is done through the bladder with a small abdominal incision or during a laparotomy. For 51925, the physician completes the fistula closure and also removes the uterus through a small horizontal incision just above the pubic hairline.

51940

The physician closes a congenital defect in the front of the bladder wall, which is associated with lack of closure of the pubic bone at the symphysis pubis. The physician makes an incision around the exposed bladder and around the urethra to develop thick skin flaps. The physician brings the skin flaps together in the midline to close the roof of the urethra and allow the bladder and prostatic urethra to drop back beneath the bony pelvis (male patients), or lengthen the urethra (female patients). To invert the bladder and establish a functional vesical neck, the physician dissects the edge of the bladder from the rectus muscle, and divides the fibromuscular bar that unites the pubic bone to the bladder base. To support the urethra and bladder neck, the physician brings the muscles of the urogenital diaphragm toward the midline. The physician places drain tubes and performs a layered closure.

51960

The physician reconstructs or enlarges a bladder with a segment of intestine. To access the intestine and bladder, the physician makes a transverse or longitudinal incision on the lower abdomen and cuts the corresponding muscles, fat, and fibrous membranes (fascia). After dissecting an isolated segment of colonic intestine, the physician reconnects (anastomosis) the ileum end-to-end to the ascending colon, restoring continuity to the bowel. The colon is divided and the distal end is sutured. An incision is made at the bladder dome and the unsutured end of colonic segment is sutured to the bladder. After controlling bleeding, the physician inserts a catheter and closes the abdomen in layers over the catheter for support.

51980

The physician connects the bladder to the skin (cutaneous vesicostomy) for direct urinary drainage. The Blocksom technique is performed mostly on newborns. To access the bladder, the physician makes a suprapubic incision in the abdomen and cuts the corresponding muscles, fat, and fibrous membranes (fascia). After securing the bladder dome to the rectus fascia, the physician incises the bladder to create an opening that is sutured to a small incision in the skin. To support the opening during healing, the physician inserts a catheter or stent into the bladder. The physician inserts a drain tube and performs a layered closure. In adults, the Lapides technique differs by passing a flap of bladder beneath the skin to replace a retracted section of abdominal skin. The abdominal skin is then passed below the abdominal surface and sutured to the opening in the bladder, making a long-term tubular passage for urine. A catheter is placed through the stoma for two or three days.

51990

The physician inserts an instrument through the vagina to grasp the cervix while passing another instrument through the cervix into the uterus to manipulate the uterus. Next, the physician makes a 1.0 cm incision just below the umbilicus (belly button) through which a fiberoptic laparoscope is inserted. A second incision is made on the left or right side of the abdomen and a second instrument is passed into the abdomen. The physician then manipulates the tools so that the pelvic organs can be observed through the laparoscope. The bladder is suspended by placing several sutures through the tissue surrounding the urethra and into the vaginal wall. The sutures are pulled tight so that the tissues are tacked up to the symphysis pubis and the urethra is moved forward. The instruments are removed and incisions are closed with sutures.

51992

The physician inserts an instrument through the vagina to grasp the cervix while passing another instrument through the cervix into the uterus to manipulate the uterus. Next, the physician makes a 1.0 cm incision just below the umbilicus (belly button) through which a fiberoptic laparoscope is inserted. A second incision is made on the left or right side of the abdomen and a second instrument is passed into the abdomen. The physician then manipulates the tools so that the pelvic organs can be observed through the laparoscope. The physician places a sling under the junction of the urethra and bladder. The physician first places a catheter in the bladder, then makes an incision in the anterior wall of the vagina and folds and tacks the tissues around the urethra. A sling is formed out of synthetic material or from fascia harvested from the sheath of the rectus abdominus muscle. The loop end of the sling is sutured around the junction of the urethra. An incision is made in the lower abdomen and the ends of the sling are grasped with a clamp and pulled up into the incision and sutured to the rectus abdominus sheath. The instruments are removed and incisions are closed with sutures.

52000

The physician examines the urethra, bladder, and ureteric openings with a cystourethroscope passed through the urethra and bladder. No other procedure is performed at this time. After examination, the physician removes the cystourethroscope.

52001

The patient is placed in a dorsolithotomy position, when using a rigid scope, and the physician performs a bimanual exam of the pelvis prior to prepping and draping the perineum and external genitalia. When cystourethroscopy is performed with a flexible cystoscope, the male is examined in the supine position and the female is placed in a froglike position. The urethra is anesthetized with lidocaine jelly and the patient is sedated. The cystoscope is introduced into the meatus and the urethra is inspected before proceeding to the bladder. When the bladder is entered, the urine is evacuated using a syringe; the cystoscope is advanced further through the bladder and deflected upward. Following cystoscopic examination, and localization of the area of interest, the physician inserts a suction and irrigation probe with laser guide to evacuate any clots and to automatically remove any tissue from the operative site. The operative site is irrigated. Following completion of the procedure, the instrument is slowly removed.

52005–52007

The physician examines the urinary collecting system with a cystourethroscope passed through the urethra and bladder. The physician passes the cystourethroscope through the urethra into the bladder, moving the scope to visualize the urethra and bladder. After insertion of a catheter into the ureter, the physician may flush (irrigate) or introduce by drops (instillate) a sterile saline solution to better view structures, and/or may introduce contrast medium for radiologic study of the renal pelvis and ureter (ureteropyelogram, retrograde pyelogram). The physician removes the cystourethroscope after examination. If performing a brush biopsy of the ureter or renal pelvis, report 52007.

52010

The physician examines the urinary collecting system with a cystourethroscope passed through the urethra and bladder, and inserts a catheter into the ejaculatory duct. The physician may flush (irrigate) or introduce by drops (instillate) a sterile saline solution to better view structures, and may introduce contrast medium for radiologic study of ejaculatory duct (duct radiography). The physician removes the cystourethroscope.

52204

The physician examines the urinary collecting system with a cystourethroscope passed through the urethra and bladder, and extracts biopsy tissue from the bladder or urethra. The physician passes a cutting instrument through the endoscope to the suspect tissue and traps a specimen of tissue. The physician removes the instrument and cystourethroscope.

52214

The physician examines the urinary collecting system with a cystourethroscope passed through the urethra and bladder, and removes lesions by fulguration. The physician passes through the endoscope an instrument that uses electric current to destroy lesions on the urethra, periurethral glands, bladder neck, depression below the prostate surface (prostatic fossa), and triangular area at the base of the bladder (trigone). The physician may use liquid nitrogen or carbon dioxide (cryosurgery) or lasers to destroy

lesions. The physician removes the instruments and cystourethroscope.

52224

The physician examines the urinary collecting system with a cystourethroscope passed through the urethra and bladder, and uses electric current (fulguration) to remove small lesions on the bladder. The physician may also use liquid nitrogen or carbon dioxide (cryosurgery) or lasers to destroy lesions. The physician may insert an instrument to extract biopsy tissue from the bladder. The physician removes the instruments and cystourethroscope.

52234–52240

The physician examines the urinary collecting system with a cystourethroscope passed through the urethra and bladder, and removes tumors of the bladder by electric current (fulguration) or excision. The physician passes an instrument through the endoscope to destroy or remove tumors of the bladder by electric current (fulguration) or excision. The physician may also use liquid nitrogen or carbon dioxide (cryosurgery) or lasers to destroy lesions. The physician removes the instruments and cystourethroscope. For tumors that are 0.5–2.0 cm in size, report 52234. For tumors that are 2.0–5.0 cm in size, report 52235. For tumors that are larger than 5.0 cm, report 52240.

52250

The physician examines the urinary collecting system with a cystourethroscope passed through the urethra and bladder, and inserts a radioactive substance. To release a radioactive substance, the physician passes an instrument through the endoscope. The physician may insert instruments through the endoscope to remove lesions or extract biopsy tissue from the bladder. The physician removes the instruments and cystourethroscope.

52260–52265

The physician examines the urinary collecting system with a cystourethroscope passed through the urethra and bladder and dilates the bladder with a balloon to relieve chronic inflammation of the bladder (interstitial cystitis). The physician removes the instrument and cystourethroscope. If the physician administers general or spinal anesthesia, use 52260. If the physician administers local anesthesia, use 52265.

52270–52276

The physician examines the urinary collecting system with a cystourethroscope passed through the urethra and bladder. With a cutting instrument introduced through the cystourethroscope, the physician incises the inside of the urethral constriction. The physician removes the instrument and cystourethroscope. For incision of a male urethra, report 52275. If the physician passes a catheter through the ureters into the bladder for direct vision of the urethral lumen during the urethrotomy, report 52276.

52277

The physician examines the urinary collecting system with a cystourethroscope passed through the urethra and bladder, and makes an incision (sphincterotomy) in the musculature of the urethral closure (urethral sphincter). The physician passes a cutting instrument through the cystourethroscope for resection of the external sphincter. After the sphincterectomy, the physician removes the instrument and cystourethroscope.

52281

The physician widens the urethra. The physician examines the urinary collecting system with a cystourethroscope passed through the urethra and bladder and dilates a stricture. The physician inserts a balloon catheter to dilate a urethral stricture or stenosis. The physician may pass a cutting instrument through the cystourethroscope to make an incision (meatomy) in the opening of the urethra or inject radiocontrast for radiologic study of the bladder. After dilation, the physician removes the instrument and cystourethroscope.

52282

The physician widens the urethra. With the patient under anesthesia, the physician examines the urinary collection system with a cystourethroscope passed through the urethra and dilates a stricture. Using an instrument passed through the cystourethroscope, the physician inserts a stent to dilate the urethral stricture or stenosis. After placing the stent, the physician removes the instruments and cystourethroscope.

52283

The physician treats a stricture with steroids. The physician examines the urinary collecting system with a cystourethroscope passed through the urethra and bladder, injecting material into a stricture. The physician passes an instrument through the cystourethroscope to inject the steroid into the urethral stricture. The physician removes the instrument and cystourethroscope.

52285

The physician passes a cystourethroscope through the urethra and bladder to treat female urethral syndrome. The physician may pass special instruments through the cystourethroscope to incise the opening of the urethra (urethral meatomy), dilate the urethra, incise the inside the urethra, treat septal fibrosis of the urethra and vagina, incise the bladder neck, or destroy polyps of the urethra in the bladder neck or trigone with electric current (fulguration). The physician removes the instruments and cystourethroscope.

52290

The physician examines the urinary collecting system with a cystourethroscope passed through the urethra and bladder, and makes an incision in the opening of the ureter(s) into the bladder (ureteral meatomy). The physician passes the cystourethroscope through the urethra into the bladder, and inserts a cutting instrument through the cystourethroscope to incise the opening of one or both ureters into the bladder. The physician removes the instrument and cystourethroscope.

52300

The physician corrects an orthotopic (normally positioned) intravesical ureterocele(s). A ureterocele is a saccular dilation generally associated with single ureters. An orthotopic ureterocele is less common than an ectopic ureterocele, see 52301. The physician passes the cystourethroscope through the urethra into the bladder, and examines the urinary collecting system. An instrument is then inserted through the cystourethroscope which allows the physician the excise the ureterocele or destroy the ureterocele with electric current (fulguration). The physician removes the instrument and the cystourethroscope. The physician usually performs this procedure with local anesthesia. When an open procedure is necessary it is chosen on the basis of the anatomical location of the ureteral meatus, the position of the ureterocele, and the impairment of renal function.

52301

An ectopic (abnormally positioned) ureterocele is a saccular dilation generally located, in part, at the bladder neck or in the urethra. This type of ureterocele most often involves the upper pole of duplicated ureters. An ectopic ureterocele is four times more common than an intravesical, or orthotopic, ureterocele (52300), and in females the ectopic ureterocele may prolapse through the urethra. The physician passes the cystourethroscope through the urethra into the bladder, and examines the urinary collecting system. An instrument is then inserted through the cystourethroscope which allows the physician to excise the ureterocele with electric current (fulguration). The physician removes the instrument and the cystourethroscope.

52305

The physician corrects a diverticulum in the bladder. The physician examines the urinary collecting system with a cystourethroscope passed through the urethra and bladder, and removes a saccular opening of the bladder (diverticulum) by excision or fulguration. The physician removes the instrument and cystourethroscope.

52310–52315

The physician examines the urinary collecting system with a cystourethroscope passed through the urethra and bladder, and removes a foreign body, calculus, or ureteral stent from the urethra or bladder. The physician passes the cystourethroscope through the urethra into the bladder, and inserts a special instrument through the cystourethroscope to extract a foreign body, calculus, or ureteral stent from the urethra or bladder. The physician removes the instrument and cystourethroscope. Report 52315 if the procedure is complicated due to previous surgery or the size or condition of the foreign body, calculus, or ureteral stent.

52317–52318

The physician uses ultrasound to smash a calculus. The physician examines the urinary collecting system with a cystourethroscope passed through the urethra and bladder to remove a foreign body. The physician inserts an instrument that generates shock waves through the cystourethroscope. The physician crushes the calculus in the bladder (litholapaxy) and washes out the fragments through a catheter. Post-shockwave fragments too large to be easily suctioned may require manual crushing. For a calculus smaller than 2.5 cm, report 52317. For a calculus larger than 2.5 cm, report 52318.

52320–52330

The physician examines the urinary collecting system with a cystourethroscope passed through the urethra and bladder, and removes, fragments, or manipulates a calculus in the ureter. The physician passes the cystourethroscope through the urethra into the bladder, and inserts a special instrument through the cystourethroscope to extract, fragment, or manipulate a calculus in the ureter. The physician inserts a ureteral catheter and removes the cystourethroscope. Report 52320 if the physician uses a stone basket or other instrument to remove the calculus. Report 52325 if the physician uses ultrasound or electrohydraulics to fragment the calculus. Report 52327 if the physician uses a subureteric injection of implant material. Report 52330 if the physician uses an instrument to manipulate, not remove, the calculus.

52332

The physician examines the urinary collecting system with a cystourethroscope passed through the urethra and bladder, and inserts an indwelling catheter (stent) in the ureter. The physician passes the cystourethroscope through the urethra into the bladder, and inserts a special instrument through the cystourethroscope to insert an indwelling stent in the ureter. The stent provides support of the ureter. The physician removes the instrument and cystourethroscope.

52334

The physician examines the urinary collecting system, and creates an opening through the kidney to the exterior of the body (nephrostomy) by inserting a guidewire through a cystourethroscope. After

examining the urinary collecting system through a cystourethroscope inserted through the urethra into the bladder, the physician inserts a catheter through the cystourethroscope into the ureter. The physician passes a guidewire through the ureteral catheter into the kidney and through a small incision in the skin of the flank. The physician removes the cystourethroscope and enlarges (dilates) the percutaneous opening by passing tubes with increasingly larger diameters through the skin incision over the guidewire to the kidney. The physician passes a nephrostomy tube over the guide, removes the guide, and sutures the tube to the skin. The physician usually withdraws the ureteral catheter at the end of the procedure.

52341–52343

The physician treats a ureteral stricture by balloon dilation, laser, electrocautery, or incision through a cystourethroscope. Under direct vision, the physician passes a flexible or rigid cystourethroscope through the urethra into the bladder. A balloon catheter is placed into the ureteral stricture, and the balloon is gently inflated. After approximately five minutes, the balloon is deflated and removed. In laser treatment of a ureteral stricture, probes, in combination with laser fibers, are used to apply laser energy to the entire stricture. In electrocautery, heat is applied to eliminate the stricture. The ureteral stricture may be incised alone or in combination with balloon dilation, laser, or electrocautery to open the blocked ureter. Report 52341 when a ureteral stricture is treated, 52342 when a ureteropelvic junction stricture is treated, or 52343 when an intra-renal stricture is treated.

52344–52346

The physician treats a ureteral stricture by balloon dilation, laser, electrocautery, or incision through a cystourethroscope and ureteroscope. Under direct vision, the physician passes a flexible or rigid cystourethroscope through the urethra into the bladder and a ureteroscope into the ureter, then examines the urinary collecting system. In balloon dilation, a balloon catheter is placed into the ureteral stricture, and the balloon is gently inflated. After approximately five minutes, the balloon is deflated and removed. In laser treatment of a ureteral stricture, probes, in combination with laser fibers, are used to apply laser energy to the entire stricture. In electrocautery, heat is applied to eliminate the stricture. Alternately, the ureteral stricture may be incised alone or in combination with balloon dilation, laser, or electrocautery to open the blocked ureter. Report 52344 when a ureteral stricture is treated, 52345 when a ureteropelvic junction stricture is treated, or 52346 when an intra-renal stricture is treated.

52347

Through the urethra, the physician performs a transurethral resection or a transurethral incision of the ejaculatory ducts (TUIED). The urethra is anesthetized with lidocaine jelly and the patient is sedated. The cystourethroscope is introduced into the meatus and the urethra is inspected. Instruments are inserted through the cystourethroscope to the region of the ejaculatory ducts. The seminal vesicles are compressed and the ejaculatory ducts are incised with a hook electrode or resected in one "bite" with a loop electrode. The seminal vesicles are again compressed. The area is observed through the scope and the instruments and cystourethroscope are removed.

52351

The physician examines the urinary collecting system for diagnostic purposes with endoscopes passed through the urethra into the bladder (cystourethroscope), ureter (ureteroscope), and renal pelvis (pyeloscope). After examination, the physician removes the endoscopes.

52352–52353

The physician examines the urinary collecting system with endoscopes passed through the urethra into the bladder (cystourethroscope), ureter (ureteroscope), and renal pelvis (pyeloscope), and removes or manipulates a stone (calculus). To extract or manipulate a calculus, the physician passes a stone basket through an endoscope. The physician inserts a ureteral catheter and removes the endoscopes. Report 52352 if the physician passes a stone basket through an endoscope to extract or manipulate a calculus. Report 52353 if the physician passes an electro-hydraulic lithotriptor probe through an endoscope to pulverize a calculus.

52354

The physician examines the urinary collecting system with endoscopes passed through the urethra into the bladder (cystourethroscope), ureter (ureteroscope), and renal pelvis (pyeloscope), and takes a biopsy and/or uses electric current (fulguration) to destroy a lesion. The physician passes instruments through the endoscope to take a biopsy of suspect tissue and/or destroy a lesion with electric current. The physician removes required instruments and endoscopes.

52355

The physician examines the urinary collecting system with endoscopes passed through the urethra into the bladder (cystourethroscope), ureter (ureteroscope), and renal pelvis (pyeloscope), and excises a tumor. The physician inserts a cutting instrument through the endoscope and excises the tumor. After flushing the area with saline solution, the physician may insert a ureteral stent. The physician removes the cutting instrument and endoscopes.

52400

The physician examines the urinary collecting system with a cystourethroscope passed through the urethra and bladder, and incises, excises, or uses electric current (fulguration) to correct defects of the bladder neck or the back of the urethra.

52450

Through a cystourethroscope, the physician relieves an obstruction of the outlet of the bladder caused by the prostate gland. After the scope is passed through the urethra, instruments are inserted through the cystourethroscope to the target region and incisions are made in the capsule of the prostate gland and carried into but not through the true prostate to create a larger passage for urine. A small transurethral biopsy of the prostate is often done at the same time. The bladder is catheterized for the immediate postoperative period.

52500

Through a cystourethroscope, the physician relieves an obstruction of the outlet of the bladder. After the scope is passed up through the urethra, instruments are inserted through the cystourethroscope to the target region. The physician excises the tissue responsible for the obstruction of urine flow.

52510

The physician enlarges the diameter of the urethra that passes through the prostate by inflating a balloon catheter inside the urethra. The physician may first pass instruments through the urethra to prepare the way for the balloon catheter. The balloon portion of the catheter is positioned in the urethra surrounded by the prostate and then gently inflated to enlarge the passageway by stretching the urethra and compressing the surrounding tissues. The inflation may be repeated several times until adequate dilation of the prostatic urethra is achieved. The scope and balloon catheter are then removed.

52601

After preliminary cystourethroscopy, the physician passes the resectoscope under direct vision up the urethra to the region of the prostate. Meatotomy, cutting to enlarge the opening of the urethra, and/or dilatation of the urethra may be necessary to allow the passage of the resectoscope. The prostate gland is removed in a systematic fashion by using a series of small cuts into the glandular tissue with an electrocautery "knife." The resected tissue is removed and the area is keep clear by irrigation through the resectoscope. Bleeding is controlled by fulguration (electrocoagulation). A large catheter is passed into the bladder and left in place for the postoperative period.

52606

The physician inserts an endoscope in the urethra and uses electric current (fulguration) to control postoperative bleeding occurring after the usual follow-up time.

52612–52614

The physician uses two operative sessions to excise the prostate using an endoscope inserted in the urethra. Dilation of the urethra may be necessary to permit endoscope insertion. Work is performed on one side of the prostate at a time. Pieces of the obstruction or tumor are sliced free and suctioned from the site. All of the prostate is removed as far distant as the verumontanum.The physician may remove (resect) a hypertrophied interureteric ridge. A catheter is inserted and the incision is closed in layers. Report 52612 for the first stage of the excision. Report 52614 for the completion of the excision.

52620–52630

The physician inserts an endoscope through the urethra to postoperatively remove residual obstructive tissue resulting from a previous surgical prostate procedure. After preliminary cystourethroscopy, the physician passes the resectoscope up the urethra to the prostate. Meatotomy, cutting to enlarge the external opening of the urethra, and dilatation of the urethra may be necessary to allow the passage of the resectoscope. The physician removes residual tissue of the prostate gland through a series of small cuts. The resected tissue is removed and the area is kept clear by irrigation through the resectoscope. Bleeding is controlled by fulguration (a form of electrocoagulation). A large catheter is passed into the bladder and left in place. For removal of residual obstructive tissue after 90 days postoperative, report 52620. For removal after one year postoperative, report 52630.

52640

Contracture of the bladder neck outlet usually results from scarring after a transurethral resection of the prostate gland. After preliminary cystourethroscopy, the physician passes the resectoscope under direct vision up the urethra to the region of the bladder neck contracture. Meatotomy, cutting to enlarge the opening of the urethra, and dilation of the urethra may be necessary to allow the passage of the resectoscope. The scar tissue is either incised at one to three sites, or resected, using a cutting electrocautery "knife." The operative site is thoroughly inspected for bleeding, which is controlled by fulguration (electrocoagulation). A large catheter is passed into the bladder at the end of the procedure and let in place for the postoperative period.

52647–52648

The physician uses a laser to excise the prostate through an endoscope inserted in the urethra. Dilation of the urethra may be necessary to permit endoscope insertion. Work is performed on one side of the prostate at a time. Pieces of the prostate are treated with a non-contact laser in 52647 or a contact laser in 52648. All of the prostate is treated. To accomplish this, vasectomy, meatotomy, cycstourethroscopy, and internal urethrotomy may be

necessary. Once the laser treatment is completed, a catheter is inserted and the incision is closed in layers.

52700

The physician inserts an endoscope through the urethra to drain an abscess on or near the prostate. The physician passes a cystourethroscope through the penile urethra to the region of the prostate and identifies the area of the abscess. A needle is passed into the abscess and purulent matter is removed by aspiration. The cystourethroscope is then removed.

53000–53010

The physician makes an external incision in the urethra or creates an opening between the urethra and the skin. The physician places the patient in the lithotomy position and passes a sound into the urethra until it meets the obstructing stricture. A longitudinal incision is made down to the urethra directly over the sound. After the stricture is identified, the urethra is incised the length of the stricture so defects may be removed. The sound is removed and a catheter is passed through the urethra into the area of the incision and guided past it into the bladder. The urethra is then repaired over the catheter, using sutures. Occasionally, the urethra is not repaired by suturing but is simply allowed to grow epithelial cells (epithelize) around the catheter. In 53010, the physician meets the stricture in the perineal part of the urethra.

53020–53025

The physician makes an incision in the opening of the urethra (urethral meatus) using a small pointed knife and a meatotomy clamp. The meatus is opened on the ventral surface and the meatus may be dilated. Sutures may be required on the mucosa of the meatus. The physician often uses a hemostat to separate the tissue in the urethra prior to making his incision. Report 53020 if the patient is older than one year, or 53025 if the patient is a child under the age of one year.

53040–53060

The physician drains an abscess in the urethra resulting from a urethral infection or traumatic injury. The physician makes an incision through the skin, subcutaneous tissue, and overlying layers of muscle, fat, and tissue (fascia) over the site of the abscess. By blunt or sharp dissection, the incision is carried into the abscessed area to provide drainage. Several drains are inserted and the incision is closed in layers. Report 53040 for drainage of a deep periurethral abscess. For an abscess or cyst in Skene's or paraurethral glands in the female, report 53060.

53080–53085

The physician drains urine that has passed out of the urethra (extravasation) into the perineal tissue. The physician makes an incision through the skin over the site. The incision is carried to the extravasation for drainage. Following drainage, the incision is closed with sutures. Report 53080 for uncomplicated drainage and 53085 for a complicated drainage.

53200

The physician excises a specimen of tissue from the urethra for biopsy. At the site to be analyzed, a portion of the suspect tissue is excised by blunt or sharp dissection. The incision is closed in layers.

53210–53220

The physician removes the urethra and creates an opening between the bladder and skin for drainage of urine. The physician makes a slightly curved, suprapubic (Cherney) incision down to the ureter and bladder. The bladder is opened and the urethral orifice is circumcised and usually tied off with sutures. Tumors of the urethra are removed by partial or complete urethrectomy or by electric current (fulguration). If the bladder has been opened, it is closed in two layers or more. Report 53210 for females; use 53215 for male-specific procedure. Report 53220 for removal of malignant tumor from the urethra.

53230–53235

The physician removes a female's urethral diverticulum. A longitudinal incision is made in the anterior vaginal wall of the female and the urethral diverticulum is separated from the vaginal wall by a combination of blunt and sharp dissection. The urethra may be opened back to the orifice of the diverticulum in order to facilitate identification. A balloon catheter may be inserted and inflated. Once the diverticulum has been excised, the urethra is closed over a catheter and the vaginal wall is repaired with a layered closure. Report 53230 if performed on a female and 53235 if performed on a male. In the male, a cystourethroscope is inserted into the urethra and the diverticulum is excised through a transurethral incision. The physician may inject fluid or pass a balloon catheter into the diverticulum to allow it to be easily found and dissected. The diverticulum is isolated down to the neck, which is transected. The physician closes the urethra, leaving a catheter in place.

53240

The physician repairs a urethral diverticulum by creating a pouch (marsupialization). A longitudinal incision is made in the anterior vaginal wall of the female and the borders of the urethral diverticulum are raised and sutured to create a pouch. The interior of the sac separates and gradually closes by granulation. The urethra is closed over a catheter and the vaginal wall is repaired with a layered closure. In the male, a cystourethroscope is inserted into the urethra and the diverticulum treated in the same manner, but through the perineum.

53250

The physician excises the bulbourethral gland. The bulbourethral glands are located on each side of the prostate gland near the external sphincter and are connected to the urethra with one-inch ducts. The glands secrete what becomes part of the seminal fluid. The physician completes this procedure through transurethral or segmental resection with end-to-end sutures (anastomosis).

53260–53275

The physician removes urethral polyps. The physician separates the urethra from the vaginal wall. The urethra is incised. A circular excision is made around the lesion and the polyp resected. The urethra and vaginal mucosa are reattached in layers. The physician removes or destroys urethral polyps, urethral caruncle, or Skene's glands, respectively. Report 53265 if removing a urethral caruncle or 53270 if removing the Skene's glands. Report 53275 if treating urethral prolapse.

53400–53405

The physician reconstructs the urethra in two stages. In the first stage (53400), the area of the stricture is identified by a catheter and urethrography and its location is marked with ink or dye. All strictures distal to the perineum are handled in the same manner. The incision is made over the stricture area. When no further strictures can be identified, the area involved is removed. Otherwise, the stricture is opened widely and the normal skin of the male or female is sutured to the edge of the mucosa on each side. In those areas in which mucosa had to be removed, the skin is sutured edge-to-edge. Six to eight weeks are required for complete healing of this stage. In the second stage (53405), the physician makes parallel incisions around the defect and continues around the urethral opening both proximally and distally. The lateral skin edges are closed over an indwelling catheter to create a new urethra. The corpora and muscles are then closed, respectively, becoming the new urethra structure.

53410

The physician reconstructs the urethra. The area of the urethral stricture is identified by catheterization. The physician cuts over the stricture area through the skin, fascia, corpus, and urethra. When the stricture is so severe that the urethral lumen cannot be identified, the physician removes the entire area involved. Otherwise, the stricture is opened widely and the normal skin is sutured to the edge of the mucosa on each side. In those areas in which the mucosa had to be removed, the skin is sutured edge-to-edge.

53415

The physician repairs the urethra. The stricture of the male perineal urethra is opened through a midline perineal or transpubic incision extending from the base of the scrotum to the anal margins. The

CPT® Lay Descriptions

physician makes an incision into the normal urethra distal to the stricture and opens the entire stricture on its ventral surface. From here a wide-based skin flap is developed by a U-shaped incision in the scrotum and advanced until it can be approximated to the posterior angle of the perineal incision without tension. With fine sutures, the ends of the proximal and distal urethra are connected (anastomosis) to the extremities of the scrotal incision and anchored to the midline of the urethral bed to provide a stable urethral roof. When the urethra stricture has been opened but not excised, the edges of the longitudinal incision in the scrotal flap are sutured to the edges of the urethral wall. The outer edges of the flap are sutured to the edges of the original perineal skin incision.

53420–53425

Urethroplasties are performed to open a stricture, repair trauma, or correct a prolapse. In the first stage, the physician identifies the injured area using a catheter or a urethrograph. The incision is made over the injury and carried through the skin, fat, and other tissues (fascia). If a urethral or vaginal prolapse is involved, other incisions may be involved. The problem is repaired or excised and layered sutures are made to provide adequate support. A catheter is placed and left for at least six to 12 days. In the second stage, to close the urethra, the physician cuts around the urethral defect, using skin from the scrotal flap to make a urethra. The right size urethra must be constructed to allow a catheter and prevent obstructions. The physician pulls the loose skin around the urethra and closes the incisions. The first stage is 53420; report 53425 for the second stage.

53430

The physician uses perineal or vaginal tissue to reconstruct the female urethra. With the patient in the lithotomy position and a catheter in the urethra, the physician cuts an inverted U-shaped flap above the urethral meatus and extending on the anterior vaginal wall. This flap is undermined with sharp dissection and spreading of the scissors around the upper portion of the urethral meatus, leaving a strip attached. The flap is sutured into a tube shape, reconstructing the distal urethra. The vaginal wall on each side is brought together in several layers to cover the new urethra. Small submucosal vessels are sealed using a cautery and a small drain may be placed under the vaginal closure and removed in one to two days.

53431

In the Tenago, Leadbetter procedure, the physician elongates the urethra by using bladder musculature. Continence is achieved due to contraction of the bladder musculature. The physician exposes the bladder through a suprapubic incision. The bladder is opened and the bladder neck incision is made 2.0 cm lateral to the urethra on each side. The musculature is

drawn together in a tube and attached to the urethra. The urethral canal is closed in a two-layer technique. For the Tenago procedure, they are moved laterally.

53440

The physician produces a mechanical obstruction in the male urethra that prevents leakage but past which the patient can still force urine. Under endoscopic control, the physician may inject a solution of polytetrafluoroethylene (PTFE) into the region of the distal sphincter. A silicone gel prosthesis can be inserted into the area of the urethra via a perineal incision.

53442

The physician removes a prosthetic device introduced to induce continence in a male. A Foley catheter is placed in the urethra. The physician enters through a midline scrotal or a penile incision. An incision is made into the urethra and corporal cavernosa are exposed. The cylinders are removed and the corpal incisions closed. The endopelvic fascia is carefully examined to make sure that the external inguinal prosthetic ring did not do any damage. Incisions are closed over a drain or catheter in layers.

53444

A urethral retention catheter is placed in the bladder and a midline lower abdominal incision is made to gain access to the space of Retzius. The bladder neck and urethra are exposed and the plane between the bladder neck and urethra is dissected and the urethrovaginal septum is dissected at the midline attachment at the distance required for accommodating the tandem cuff. Having freed the bladder neck, the physician measures its circumference and the tandem cuff is placed in position around the bladder neck and the tubing brought up to the suprapubic area.

53445

The physician implants an artificial sphincter to stem urinary incontinence. In male patients where the incontinence is caused by anything other than prostatic surgery, the entire prosthesis is inserted through a subpubic incision. In female patients, the sphincter is inserted through a suprapubic incision. The space of Retzius (between the bladder and the pubis) is opened and the bladder neck is cut free, making space for the device. The bladder neck circumference is measured and a cuff of slightly larger size is chosen and sutured around the bladder neck. A space is created below the skin low in the scrotum, and the control pump passed into this position from the subpubic incision. The pressure balloon is placed in a pocket behind the rectus muscle on the same side as the control pump. The physician injects fluid into the pressure balloon. In females, the plane between the bladder neck and vagina is dissected to serve the same purpose as the scrotum.

53446

In females, the vagina is prepared preoperatively and a urethral retention catheter is placed in the bladder. The patient is administered general anesthesia and placed supine. The physician makes a midline lower abdominal incision to gain access to the space of Retzius. The artificial urinary sphincter is exposed and the plane between the bladder neck and vagina is dissected. The device is removed and the opening is closed using suture for the rectus fascia. The subcutaneous tissues are closed and staples are used for skin closure. In males, the patient is placed under general anesthesia in the lithotomy position. The urethral bulb is exposed and the bulbospongiosus muscles are left intact over the urethra. The strap of the prosthesis is grasped under the crus and the muscle and the procedure is repeated distally to grasp the second lateral strap. The same maneuvers are repeated on the opposite site. The proximal straps are untied, as are the lateral straps. The incision is closed and a Foley catheter is left indwelling for several days.

53447

The physician removes and replaces an artifical sphincter (including pump, reservoir, and cuff) used to Stem urinary incontinence. In male patients where the incontinence is caused by anything other than prostatic surgery, the entire prothesis is accessed through a subpubic incision. In female patients, the sphincter is accessed through a suprapubic incision. The sphincter and pump are examined, removed, and replaced. The bladder neck circumference is measured and a cuff of slightly larger size is chosen and positioned around the bladder neck. A space is created below the skin low in the scrotum and the control pump passed into this position from the subpubic incision. The pressure balloon is placed in a pocket behind the rectus muscle on the same side as the control pump. The physician injects fluid into the pressure balloon and the connections are then permanently established. In females, the plane between the bladder neck and vagina is dissected.

53449

The physician repairs an inability of an inflatable sphincter device to stem incontinence. The rectus muscles are separated bluntly and a space created behind the muscle of one side large enough to gain access to the reservoir of the prosthesis. The physician checks the reservoir for any malfunctions or abnormalities. The physician then follows the tubing (this may require a second incision in the rectus sheath). A space is dilated within the spongy corpal tissue where the cylinder tubing is checked. After both cylinders are examined, they are test-inflated to ensure that they reach into the glans portion of the corpora and that there is no buckling when they are inflated. The physician closes the incisions. The reservoir is filled and all connections are made. Several test inflations and deflations are performed

during closure. The physician places a catheter in the bladder for about one day.

53450

The physician performs this surgery to open or reconstruct the urethra, improving voiding or allowing insertion of an instrument. The meatus, which may be congenitally small or narrowed as the result of infection, is opened and a mucosal flap is advanced and sutured to the glans.

53460

The physician widens the meatus to enhance voiding. The physician makes an incision on the ventral surface of the penis and skin is freed from the shaft. Fibrous tissue is removed. An erection is artificially induced to confirm all fibrous tissue has been removed.

53502–53515

The physician repairs a urethral wound or injury, including the skin and even more traumatic wounds requiring more than a layered closure. Examples include debridement of cuts (lacerations) or tears (avulsion). Suturing of the urethra is done in layers to prevent later complications and fistula formations. The tissue can be constructed around a catheter. Report 53502 if the patient is female, report 53505 if the patient is male, report 53510 if the wound is perineal, and report 53515 if repair is prostatomembranous.

53520

The physician closes a urethrostomy or urethrocutaneous fistula. An elliptical incision is made around the opening of the urocutaneous fistula and carried deeper into the supporting tissue towards the urethra. The entire tract is freed up and excised unless it involves other important structures, such as the external sphincters. When the tract cannot be completely removed, the remaining part is cut. The defect of the urethra is closed in layers over a catheter.

53600–53605

When the physician examines the patient, a soft rubbery urethral catheter is passed and the stricture is noted. If a stricture is found, a dilator is used. Report 53600 for the first visit and 53601 for subsequent visits. Report 53605 if spinal anesthesia is administered.

53620–53621

The physician uses fine tools to dilate the urethra. A filiform (a small silk-like instrument with woven spiral tips, to which followers made of a similar material can be attached by a screw-like mechanism) is used when a stricture cannot be passed. With a filiform as a guide, the follower is passed through the urethra. Increasing sizes of followers are introduced, dilating the stricture. The filiform is manipulated up a lubricated urethra to the stricture. The physician attaches a follower to the filiform and the stricture is widened. Report 53621 if it is a subsequent procedure.

53660–53665

The physician uses dilators of increasing size to widen the urethra. A suppository or instillation of a saline solution may be used. Report 53660 for initial dilation, and 53661 for subsequent dilation. Use 53665 if general or spinal anesthesia is administered for dilation of female urethral stricture.

53670–53675

The physician places a catheter (catheterizes) in the urethra or bladder to treat chronic or interstitial inflammation. A soft rubbery urethral catheter is passed with an inflatable balloon secured to the top. The balloon is inflated. Report 53675 if catheter removal is difficult.

53850

The physician performs transurethral destruction of prostate tissue by microwave thermotherapy. The physician inserts an endoscope in the penile urethra, prior to endoscope placement the urethra may need to be dilated to allow instrument passage. After the endoscope is passed, a microwave thermotherapy stylet is inserted in the urethra and the diseased prostate is treated with electromagnetic radiation. The treated prostate is examined for evidence of bleeding which may be controlled with electrocoagulation. The endoscope and instruments are removed. A urinary catheter is inserted into the bladder and left in place postoperatively.

53852

The physician performs transurethral destruction of prostate tissue by radiofrequency thermotherapy. The physician inserts an endoscope in the penile urethra, prior to endoscope placement. The urethra may be dilated to allow instrument passage. After the endoscope is placed a radio frequency thermotherapy stylet is inserted in the urethra and the diseased prostate is treated with radiant energy. The treated prostate is examined for evidence of bleeding, which may be controlled with electrocoagulation. The endoscope and instruments are removed. A urinary catheter is inserted into the bladder and left in place postoperatively.

53853

The physician performs transurethral destruction of prostate tissue by water-induced thermotherapy (WIT) using a topical urethral anesthetic. A specialized catheter with a balloon tip is inserted through the penis to the prostatic urethra. The catheter shaft is insulated to protect the urethra. The other end of the catheter is connected to a console that heats water. Hot water (40 degrees centigrade) is then circulated through the balloon for 45 minutes.

The conductive heat transmitted by the balloon (generated by the hot water) to a specific area destroys (necrotizes) some of the prostatic tissue, effectively reducing the size of the prostate and relieving symptoms of urinary obstruction. At the end of the procedure the special catheter is removed and a urinary catheter is left in place.

54000–54001

The prepuce is the fold of penile skin commonly called the foreskin. The physician makes a cut or slit in the prepuce to relieve a constriction that prevents the retraction of the foreskin back over the head of the penis. A segment of foreskin on either the dorsal or the side of the penis is crushed with forceps. Using scissors, the physician makes a cut through the crushed tissue and sutures the divided skin to control bleeding. The prepuce of a newborn is slit in 54000, while 54001 reports the slitting of the prepuce of any male other than a newborn.

54015

The physician drains a deep abscess or hematoma (pocket of blood) by incising penile tissue. After instilling a local anesthesia, the physician makes an incision through the skin and deeper tissues into the abscessed cavity. The urethra and the main arteries and nerves are avoided. Often a drain is left in place to assure adequate drainage.

54050–54055

The physician treats skin lesions of the penis by local application of a chemical (54050) or local electrodesiccation (54055) to kill the diseased tissue or organism. Using a cotton-tipped applicator soaked in the chemical or an electrodesiccator, the physician applies the treatment to the specific lesions only, taking care to avoid touching normal skin with the chemical or the electrodesiccator. Using either method, no tissue is removed and no closure is required.

54056–54057

The physician treats skin lesions of the penis by local application of liquid nitrogen or the use of a cryothermal instrument (54056) or by laser beam (54057) to kill the diseased tissue or the organism. Using a cotton-tipped applicator dipped in liquid nitrogen (-78 degrees Celsius), the physician carefully freezes or burns with the laser only the specific lesions, taking care to avoid normal skin. No tissue is removed and no closure is required.

54060

The physician excises selected large lesions of the penis not removable by other methods. After adequate local anesthesia has been administered, the physician cuts out an elliptical piece of skin that includes the lesion and a rim of normal tissue. With a forceps or hemostat clamp, the physician grasps and elongates the involved skin containing the lesion, causing the tissue to tent. Using either a scalpel or scissors, an ellipse of tissue containing the lesion is excised. The resulting defect is closed with sutures.

54065

The physician destroys extensive lesions of the penis using one or more of several methods. Extensive destruction generally means the procedure took more time or was more difficult than usual due to such factors as the size and number of lesions involved. The methods used by the physician include local application of a chemical, freezing, electrodesiccation, laser vaporization to kill the diseased tissue, or excision. Local anesthesia may be used for these procedures. The physician carefully applies the method only to the specific lesions, taking care to avoid normal skin.

54100

The physician removes a portion of a skin lesion on the penis by punch biopsy or by excising a small portion of the lesion with scalpel or scissors. The resulting defect may require simple repair with sutures.

54105

The physician removes a portion of a penile mass by deep punch biopsy or by making an incision in the penis and dissecting tissues to the deep mass and excising a portion of the lesion. The incision may be repaired with layered sutures.

54110–54112

Peyronie's disease is a toughening of the spongy body of the penis. The physician corrects Peyronie's disease by excising abnormal fibrous tissue on the dorsal aspect of the penis. After an incision is made around the penis, the physician retracts the skin to expose the abnormal tissue on the underlying normal spongy tissue. Avoiding critical nerves and blood vessels, with the penis erect the defective tissue is excised. The skin is closed by suturing. Report 54111 if a graft measuring 5.0 cm or less in length is required; report 54112 if a graft greater than 5.0 cm is required.

54115

The physician removes a foreign body from deep within the shaft of the penis by making an incision and carefully dissecting the tissues to avoid damaging important nerves and blood vessels. The foreign body, usually a penile implant, is localized and then removed. The resulting defect is closed with layered sutures.

54120

The physician removes a portion of the penis due to disease or mutilating injury. The distal penis is enclosed in a rubber glove and a tourniquet is applied at the base of the penis. An incision is made completely around the penile shaft. The various structures of the penis are isolated and then divided

with care to leave enough of the urethra to form an opening for the passage of urine. The remaining tissues and skin are closed with layered sutures.

54125

The physician removes the penis due to disease or mutilating injury. The distal penis is enclosed in a rubber glove. An incision is made from above the penis and carried around the base of the penile shaft and down through the midline of the scrotum. The various structures of the penis are isolated and then divided with care to leave enough of the urethra for drainage. The urethra is brought through the perineum below the scrotum and an opening is created for the passage of urine. The remaining tissue and skin are closed in layered sutures with drains placed in the scrotum and a catheter in the bladder.

54130

The physician removes the entire penis and surrounding lymph nodes to treat invasive cancer. The distal penis is enclosed in a rubber glove. An incision is made from above the base of the penis and carried around the base of the penile shaft and down through the midline of the scrotum. The various structures of the penis are isolated and then divided with care to leave enough of the urethra for drainage. The urethra is brought through the perineum below the scrotum and an opening is created for the passage of urine. The remaining tissues and skin are closed in layered sutures with drains placed in the scrotum and a catheter in the bladder. The physician also removes the lymph nodes in the groin areas. An incision is made from the pubic bone to the lateral pelvic bone exposing the area for dissection. The fatty tissues bearing the lymph nodes are removed. The defect is covered by rotating one of the thigh muscles over the area and suturing it in place. The subcutaneous tissues and the skin are closed in layered sutures over drains placed in the region.

54135

The physician removes the entire penis and surrounding lymph nodes to treat invasive cancer. The distal penis is enclosed in a rubber glove. An incision is made from above the base of the penis and carried around the base of the penile shaft and down through the midline of the scrotum. The various structures of the penis are isolated and then divided leaving enough of the urethra for drainage. The urethra is brought through the perineum below the scrotum and an opening is created for the passage of urine. The remaining tissues and skin are closed in layered sutures with drains placed in the scrotum and a catheter in the bladder. The physician also removes the lymph nodes in the groin areas. An incision is made from the pubic bone to the lateral pelvic bone exposing the area for dissection. The fatty tissues bearing the lymph nodes are removed. The defect is covered by rotating one of the thigh muscles over the area and suturing it in place. The subcutaneous tissues and the skin are closed in layered sutures over drains placed in the region. A lower midline abdominal incision is made and the pelvic cavity is entered and the lymph nodes deep in the pelvis are removed. The abdominal incision is also closed in multiple layers of sutures.

54150–54152

The physician removes the foreskin of the penis in the newborn (54150) or older male (54152) by clamping the foreskin in a plastic device and trimming the excess protruding skin. A segment of foreskin on either the dorsal or the side of the penis is crushed with a forceps. A cut is made through the crushed tissue with scissors and the divided foreskin is fitted in a plastic bell-shaped clamp. The clamp crushes a ring of the foreskin and holds the skin edges together while the excess skin is trimmed from the top of the device. The clamp is left in place and simply falls off when healing has finished days later.

54160–54161

The physician removes the foreskin of the penis in the newborn (54160) or older male (54161) by excision of the skin. A segment of foreskin on either the dorsal or the side of the penis is crushed with a forceps. A cut is made through the crushed tissue with scissors and the divided foreskin is pulled down over the head of the penis while the excess skin is trimmed from around the head of the penis. Bleeding is controlled by chemical cautery or suture ligatures. The skin edges created are sutured together with absorbable suture material.

54162

Under general anesthesia, the physician retracts the foreskin, releases the preputial post-circumcision adhesions, and cleanses the glans. If retraction of the foreskin reveals a fibrous ring, the physician places two vertical incisions directly over the fibrous ring and the transversely running fibrous bands are divided to expose the underlying Bucks' fascia. With the foreskin retracted, the defect is closed horizontally with interrupted sutures.

54163

A repeat circumcision may be performed if there is circumferential scarring of excessive residual skin or incomplete removal of the preputial skin during the initial circumcision. First, the skin at the base of the penis is cleansed with alcohol and allowed to dry. The physician uses an index finger to palpate the lateral side of the penis to determine the position of the root of the penis. With a tuberculin syringe and needle, the anesthetic is injected parallel to the root of the penis. While the penis is stabilized by gentle downward or ventral traction, the needle is inserted at the base of the penis and inserted beneath the skin surface. The anesthetic is injected and the needle withdrawn. An incision is made around the base of the foreskin, the foreskin is pulled back, and it is cut away from the

penis. Stitches are usually used to close the skin edges.

54164

The physician performs an incision of the membrane that attaches the foreskin to the glans and shaft of the penis (frenulum). A dorsal penile nerve block is administered with a needle directed through the fascia of the symphysis pubis and into the frenum space where the anesthetic is deposited to block the dorsal nerves of the penis. A longitudinal incision is made ventrally though the outer layer of the prepuce. After retracting the prepuce, the physician extends the incision along the inner layer. Bleeding is controlled with an electrocoagulator. The resultant wound is closed.

54200–54205

Peyronie's disease is a toughening of the spongy body of the penis. The physician injects medication into the abnormal fibrous tissue of the penis to correct painful curvature of the penis caused by Peyronie's disease. In 54200, no incision is made. The medication is injected into the dorsal area of the penis through the skin. In 54205, the physician makes an incision in the dorsum of the penis and identifies the abnormal fibrous tissue. An injection is then made directly into the abnormal fibrous tissue under direct visualization through the incision.

54220

Corpora cavernosa is the spongy tissue of the penis. In priapism, this spongy tissue is in a state of persistent erection. The physician treats priapism by irrigating the corpora cavernosa. After adequate local anesthesia, the physician passes a large bore needle into the body of the penis and aspirates a quantity of blood and then irrigates the space with 20.0 ml to 30.0 ml of saline solution. This may be accompanied by injecting medication into the same region, repeating it several times to get the abnormal erection to resolve.

54230

Corpora cavernosa is the spongy tissue of the penis. The physician injects medication into the penis for x-ray studies to evaluate erectile dysfunction. After placing a constricting rubber band around the penis, the physician passes a needle into the body of the penis and aspirates a small quantity of blood. X-ray contrast medication is then injected directly into the body of the penis. The constricting band is removed and x-rays are taken to demonstrate the function and integrity of the corpora cavernosa and the blood flow of the penis.

54231

Corpora cavernosa is the spongy tissue of the penis. The physician injects vasoactive drugs into the corpora cavernosa for studies to evaluate erectile dysfunction. A rubber band is placed around the base of the penis and the intracavernous pressure is measured using instrumentation. The physician evaluates the penis for leakage between the diastolic and the systolic pressures. A swift rate of decay between the two indicates arterial and/or venous insufficiency of the penis. After the test, the band is removed and the instrumentation removed.

54235

Corpora cavernosa is the spongy tissue of the penis. The physician injects medication into the penis to treat erectile dysfunction. After placing a constricting rubber band around the penis, the physician passes a needle into the body of the penis and aspirates a small quantity of blood. The selected medication is then injected directly into the body of the penis. This produces an erection in most patients that may last from minutes to hours.

54240

A plethysmograph is an instrument that measures variations in the volume of an organ and in the amount of blood in it or passing through it. The physician measures the physiological potential of the penis to attain and maintain an erection using plethysmography. The volume change of the penis is measured in response to external stimuli.

54250

The physician monitors nighttime erections in impotent patients during rapid eye movement sleep. Testing can be performed in a sleep center or in the patient's home. During the test, the patient's penis is wired to a strain gauge monitor and recordings are made of the strength and duration of any erections occurring while the patient sleeps.

54300

The physician corrects and repairs chordee, which is the abnormal curvature of the penis. To assist in planning the surgery, an artificial erection may be produced by placing a band around the base of the penis and injecting saline into the body of the penis. The area of deformity is determined and by using a combination of incisions and excisions of abnormal fibrous tissue and sometimes normal tissue, the defect is corrected. Care is taken to dissect around nerves and blood vessels. Sometimes the urethra is dissected free of its position and retracted temporarily away from the operative site. The separate tissues of the penis are closed in layers with absorbable suture material. An artificial erection may again be produced to test and demonstrate the adequacy of the repair.

54304

The physician corrects and repairs chordee, which is the abnormal curvature of the penis. The physician also prepares the penis for correction of hypospadias, an abnormal opening of the urethra on the underside of the penis or on the perineum. To assist in planning the surgery, an artificial erection may be produced by

placing a band around the base of the penis and injecting saline into the body of the penis. The area of deformity is determined and the defect is corrected using a combination of incisions and excisions of the prepuce (foreskin). Care is taken to dissect around the nerves and blood vessels. Often the foreskin is used in either a free graft or a flap graft to cover the ventral skin defects created to correct the chordee. The separate tissues of the penis are closed in layers with absorbable suture material. An artificial erection may again be produced to test and demonstrate the adequacy of the repair. The urethral opening is left on the ventral shaft of the penis for repair during a later stage.

54308–54312

The physician completes the repair of chordee (abnormal curvature of the penis) and hypospadias (an abnormal opening of the urethra on the underside of the penis or on the perineum) by creating a urethral opening in the end of the penis. The urethra is dissected free of the surrounding tissues to mobilize it. A distal urethra, less than 3.0 cm in 54308 or greater than 3.0 cm in 54312, is formed from the prepuce (foreskin) and an opening is created at or near the tip of the head of the penis. Urine may be diverted by the use of a catheter in the bladder. The skin is closed with sutures.

54316

The physician completes the repair of chordee (abnormal curvature of the penis) and hypospadias (abnormal opening of the urethra on the underside of the penis or on the perineum) by creating a urethral opening in the end of the penis. The urethra is mobilized by dissecting it free from the surrounding tissues. A distal urethra is formed from skin obtained from a site other than the genitalia and sutured to the existing urethra and to an opening created at or near the tip of the head of the penis. Urine may be diverted using a catheter in the bladder. The skin and tissues are closed with fine absorbable sutures.

54318

The physician completes the repair of chordee (abnormal curvature of the penis) and hypospadias (an abnormal opening of the urethra on the underside of the penis or on the perineum) by separating the temporary attachments sutured between the penis and scrotum during a previous stage of the repair. Urine may be diverted using a catheter in the bladder. The skin is closed with fine sutures.

54322

The physician corrects and repairs a chordee, which is an abnormal curvature of the penis. The physician also prepares the penis for correction of hypospadias, an abnormal opening of the urethra on the underside of the penis or on the perineum. The physician corrects hypospadias in the distal penis at the base of the head of the penis in a one-stage procedure. An incision is made around the shaft of the penis next to the glans (head) and the skin is dissected from the penile shaft taking care to avoid injury to the urethra. An erection is artificially produced to evaluate any chordee before and after the correction. Any chordee present is corrected by excising the responsible fibrous band. A second incision is made in the groove on the under side of the glans. Skin in the area is pulled up to the glans and fashioned into an opening by suturing in the head of the penis. A circumcision, or excision of some foreskin, may be performed. The original incision around the penis is closed by suturing.

54324

In a one-stage procedure, the physician corrects hypospadias, which is an abnormal opening of the urethra on the underside of the penis, in the distal or end portion of the penile shaft. An incision is made from the head of the penis around the urethral opening. An erection is artificially produced to evaluate the chordee before and after the correction. Any chordee present is corrected by excising the responsible fibrous band. A flap is created from the skin below the urethral opening and flipped up and over the opening of the urethra and sutured together forming a tube extension of the urethra. The foreskin is divided and sutured over the defect left by the flap on the ventral surface of the penis. A circumcision is usually the result of the procedure.

54326

In a one-stage procedure, the physician corrects hypospadias, which is an abnormal opening of the urethra on the underside of the penis, in the distal or end portion of the penile shaft. An incision is made on the ventral surface of the penis and around the urethral opening. An erection is artificially produced to evaluate any chordee before and after the correction. Any chordee present is corrected by excising the responsible fibrous band. The urethra is dissected free of the shaft to mobilize it. A flap of skin is created from the foreskin and sutured together to form a tube to be used as a segment of urethra. The foreskin is further divided and sutured over the defect left by the flap on the ventral surface of the penis. Foreskin excision (circumcision) may be part of this procedure.

54328

Hypospadias is an abnormal opening of the urethra on the underside of the penis or on the perineum. The physician corrects hypospadias in the distal or end portion of the penile shaft in a one-stage procedure. An incision is made on the ventral surface of the penis and around the urethral opening. An erection is artificially produced to evaluate the chordee before and after the correction. Any chordee present is corrected by excising the responsible fibrous band. The urethra is dissected free of the shaft to mobilize it. An island flap of skin is created from the foreskin

and sutured together to form a tube to be used as a segment of urethra. This formed urethral tube flap is sutured in place between the urethral opening in the shaft of the penis and an opening created in the head of the penis. The foreskin is further divided and sutured over the defect left by the flap on the ventral surface of the penis. Foreskin removal (circumcision) may be part of this procedure.

54332

Hypospadias is an abnormal opening of the urethra on the underside of the penis or on the perineum. The physician corrects hypospadias in the base portion of the penis in a one-stage procedure. An incision is made on the ventral surface of the penis and around the urethral opening. An erection is artificially produced to evaluate the chordee before and after the correction. Chordee is corrected by excising the responsible fibrous band. Considerable dissection is required to mobilize the urethra. An island flap of skin is created from the foreskin and sutured together to form a tube to be used as a segment of urethra. This formed urethral tube flap is sutured in place between the urethral opening at the base of the shaft of the penis and an opening created in the head of the penis. The foreskin and skin overlying the shaft are further divided and dissected free and sutured over the defect left by the flap on the ventral surface of the penis. A circumcision is usually the result of the procedure.

54336

Hypospadias is an abnormal opening of the urethra on the underside of the penis or on the perineum. The physician corrects hypospadias in the perineal portion of the penis in a one-stage procedure. An incision is made on the ventral surface of the penis and around the urethral opening. An erection is artificially produced to evaluate the chordee before and after the correction. Any chordee present is corrected by excising the responsible fibrous band. Considerable dissection is required to mobilize the urethra in preparation for repair of the hypospadias. An island flap of skin is created from the foreskin and sutured together to form a tube to be used as a segment of urethra. This formed urethral tube flap is sutured in place between the urethral opening at the base of the scrotum in the perineum and an opening created in the head of the penis. The foreskin and skin overlying the shaft are further divided and dissected free and sutured over the defect left by the flap and dissections on the ventral surface of the penis. Circumcision is usually the result of the procedure.

54340

Hypospadias is an abnormal opening of the urethra on the underside of the penis or on the perineum. The physician repairs a fistula, stricture, and/or diverticula resulting from a former hypospadias repair. The fistula (abnormal passage) or diverticula (pouch or sac) is identified and excised, often using microsurgical techniques. The defect in the urethra is repaired by suturing and the skin is also closed with sutures. A stricture (narrowing) is corrected by dilating the area with dilating catheters or by incision and suture closure.

54344

Hypospadias is an abnormal opening of the urethra on the underside of the penis or on the perineum. The physician repairs a fistula, diverticula, and/or stricture resulting from a former hypospadias repair. The fistula (abnormal passage) or diverticula (pouch or sac) is identified and excised, often using microsurgical techniques. The defect in the urethra is repaired by closure with a free patch graft or flap graft. The skin defect is closed by simple suturing or by the use of a flap skin graft. A stricture (narrowing) is corrected by dilating the area with dilating catheters or by incision and suture repair.

54348

Hypospadias is an abnormal opening of the urethra on the underside of the penis or on the perineum. The physician repairs a fistula, diverticula, and/or stricture resulting from a former hypospadias repair. The fistula (abnormal passage) or diverticula (pouch or sac) is identified and excised, often using microsurgical techniques. The defect in the urethra is repaired by closure with a free patch graft or a flap graft that both require extensive dissection, mobilization of tissues, and the creation of complicated grafts such as a tube graft. The skin defect is closed by simple suturing or by use of a flap skin graft. A stricture (narrowing) is corrected by dilating the area with dilating catheters or by incision and suture repair. The urine may be diverted through a catheter left in the bladder. The catheter can be passed through the urethra or placed directly in the bladder through the lower abdominal wall just above the pubic bone.

54352

Hypospadias is an abnormal opening of the urethra on the underside of the penis or on the perineum. The physician repairs severe, disabling complications from former hypospadias repairs. Often using microsurgical techniques and considerable excision of scarred and damaged tissues, the deformities and malfunctions of the urethra and penis are corrected. Two or three stages may be necessary to complete this complicated task. A new urethral segment is created with a free patch graft, a flap graft, or by the use of a tube graft. Extensive dissection and mobilization of tissues are generally required to complete the process. Skin defects are closed using flap or free skin grafts. Any strictures (narrowing of hollow structures) are corrected by dilating the area with dilating catheters or by incision and suture repair. Urine may be diverted through a catheter left in the bladder. The catheter can be passed through the urethra or placed in the bladder through an incision in the lower abdominal wall just above the pubic bone.

54360

The physician corrects an abnormal curvature of the penis using a series of excisions of tissue on the side of the penis. To assist in planning the surgery, an erection may be artificially produced by placing a band around the base of the penis and injecting saline into the body of the penis. The area of deformity is determined and using a combination of incisions and excisions of tissue, the defect is corrected. An incision is made in the skin of the penis just proximal to the glans (head of the penis) and the skin is pulled to the base of the penis, exposing the underlying tissues. Further dissection is done to expose the thick connective tissue on one side of the shaft. A series of parallel excisions are made and the resulting defects are closed by suturing. The separate tissues and the skin of the penis are closed in a layered fashion with absorbable suture material. An erection may again be induced to test the adequacy of the repair.

54380

The physician corrects epispadias, which is the congenital absence of the upper wall of the urethra. The urethra has its opening anywhere on the top surface of the penis. A closed urethra is created by reapproximating the tissues, and by using skin grafts, tube grafts, free tissue grafts, or a combination of techniques depending on the extent of the defect.

54385

The physician corrects epispadias and associated urinary incontinence in one or more stages. Epispadias with incontinence is the congenital absence of the upper wall of the urethra and the lack of function of the muscles that control the bladder neck. Through an incision in the lower abdomen, the surgeon reconstructs the bladder neck and reimplants the ureters from the kidneys away from the bladder neck outlet. A closed urethra is created by reapproximating the tissues and by using skin grafts, tube grafts, free tissue grafts, or a combination of techniques depending on the extent of the defect.

54390

The physician corrects epispadias and exstrophy of the bladder in stages. Epispadias is the congenital absence of the upper wall of the urethra. Bladder exstrophy is the turning inside out of the bladder so that the bladder is open directly to the outside and as such, urine does not collect in the bladder but simply drains without any control to the outside onto the lower abdomen. The first stage is to close the bladder through incisions in the lower abdomen. The surgeon frees the bladder from the abdominal wall and proceeds to close the bladder and reimplant the ureters from the kidneys away from the bladder neck outlet. In the second stage, a closed urethra is created by reapproximating the tissues and by using skin grafts, tube grafts, free tissue grafts, or a combination of techniques depending on the extent of the defect. In the following stages, the physician reconstructs the bladder neck to provide urinary control and, if necessary, does additional surgery on the penis and urethra.

54400–54401

The physician inserts a semi-rigid penile prosthesis in 54400, which is either a hinged or malleable device, or a self-contained inflatable penile prosthesis in 54401, which is a one piece, paired hydraulic device that allows fluid to be pumped from one portion of the device to another. A transverse incision is made just above the penis over the pubic bone. With care to avoid important nerves and blood vessels, dissection is carried down to the erectile tissues at the base of the penis. Incisions are made in the thick fibrous membranes surrounding the two main erectile tissues to allow the insertion of dilators to create space for the prostheses. The paired prosthetic devices are inserted one at a time into the two erectile tissue compartments down the length of the penis. The incisions and tissues are closed by suturing. The operation can also be done in similar fashion using an incision just below the scrotum in the perineum to enter the erectile tissue or in the upper scrotum at the base of the penis.

54405

The physician inserts an inflatable penile prosthesis made up of three components-the reservoir, the pump, and two inflatable cylinders. A transverse incision is made at the base of the penis in the upper scrotum. With care to avoid the urethra and important nerves and blood vessels, dissection is carried down to the erectile tissues at the base of the penis. The thick fibrous membranes surrounding the two main erectile tissues are incised and dilators are inserted to create space for the prostheses. Two prosthetic devices are inserted into the two erectile tissue compartments down the length of the penis. A pouch is made in one side of the scrotum, and the pump mechanism and tubing are inserted into the space created. Using an index finger, the surgeon creates a tunnel from the pump to the space behind the pubic bone. The reservoir is placed behind the pubic bone with tubing running from it through the tunnel to the pump in the scrotum. The incisions and tissues are closed by suturing. The operation can also be done in similar fashion using an incision just below the scrotum in the perineum to enter the erectile tissue and in the area above the pubic bone to gain access to place the reservoir

54406

The patient is taken to the operating room, placed in a supine or lithotomy position, and the physician makes an incision using the same penoscrotal or infrapubic approach as the original procedure to remove the multi-component, inflatable penile prosthesis. The physician makes an incision into the corpus cavernosum and the prosthesis is withdrawn. The corporotomy is closed by suture. The

subcutaneous tissue is closed by suture and a dressing is applied to the incision. The bladder is emptied with a catheter. An indwelling urethral catheter, if used, is removed on the first postoperative day.

54408

Under general anesthesia, the patient is taken to the operating room, placed in a supine or lithotomy position, and the physician makes an incision using the same penoscrotal or infrapubic approach as the original procedure to repair the previously placed multi-component, inflatable penile prosthesis. The physician makes an incision into the corpus cavernosum to inspect the previously placed prosthesis. Repairs are made. The corporotomy is closed by suture. The subcutaneous tissue is closed by suture and a dressing is applied to the incision. The bladder is emptied with a catheter. An indwelling urethral catheter, if used, is removed on the first postoperative day.

54410

Under general anesthesia, the patient is taken to the operating room, placed in a supine or lithotomy position, and the physician makes an incision using the same penoscrotal or infrapubic approach as the original procedure to remove the previously placed multi-component, inflatable penile prosthesis and to insert a replacement during the same operative session. The physician makes an incision into the corpus cavernosum and the prosthesis is withdrawn. The replacement prosthesis is brought through the glans and the deflated cylinder is drawn into the distal corporal body for insertion into the curs of the penis. The corpotomy is closed and the cylinders are inflated and deflated several times to check the flow of the fluid to and from the cylinders. The reservoir is brought through the external inguinal ring and the bladder is emptied by catheter. The existing subfascial pocket in used to place the reservoir, as well as the pump/activator mechanism, which is placed in the existing scrotal pocket. Sutures are placed to prevent upward migration, the tubing is filled with fluid, and the physician makes the connections between the tubing of the pump and reservoir and the tubing of the pump and cylinders. Before the wound is closed, the prosthesis is cycled to check proper functioning. The corporotomy is closed by suture. The subcutaneous tissue is closed by suture and a dressing is applied to the incision. The bladder is emptied with a catheter. An indwelling urethral catheter, if used, is removed on the first postoperative day.

54411

The physician removes and replaces a multi-component inflatable penile prosthesis and irrigates and debrides infected tissue. The patient is taken to the operating room and placed under general anesthesia. The physician makes an incision using the same penoscrotal or infrapubic approach as the original procedure. The physician makes an incision into the corpus cavernosum and the prosthesis is withdrawn. Any infected tissue is debrided and irrigated with an antibiotic solution. The replacement prosthesis is brought through the glans and the deflated cylinder is drawn into the distal corporal body for insertion into the curs of the penis. The corpotomy is closed and the cylinders are inflated and deflated several times to check the flow of the fluid to and from the cylinders. The reservoir is brought through the external inguinal ring and the bladder is emptied by catheter. The existing subfascial pocket is used to place the reservoir, as well as the pump/activator mechanism, which is placed in the existing scrotal pocket. Any infected tissue is debrided and irrigated with an antibiotic solution. Sutures are placed to prevent upward migration, the tubing is filled with fluid, and the physician makes the connections between the tubing of the pump and reservoir and the tubing of the pump and cylinders. Before the wound is closed, the prosthesis is cycled to check proper functioning. The corporotomy is closed by suture. The subcutaneous tissue is closed by suture and a dressing is applied to the incision. The bladder is emptied with a catheter. An indwelling urethral catheter, if used, is removed on the first postoperative day.

54415

Under general anesthesia, the patient is taken to the operating room and the physician makes an incision using the same approach (i.e., penoscrotal or distal penile) as the original procedure to remove the non-inflatable or self-contained inflatable penile prosthesis. An incision is made into the corpus cavernosum, the corporal tissue is dissected, and the prosthesis is removed from the corporal body. The wound is irrigated with antibiotics, and the corporotomy is closed by suture. The subcutaneous tissue is closed by suture and a dressing is applied to the incision. The bladder is emptied with a catheter.

54416

Under general anesthesia, the patient is taken to the operating room, placed in a supine or lithotomy position, and the physician makes an incision using the same approach (i.e., penoscrotal or distal penile) as the original procedure to remove the non-inflatable or self-contained inflatable penile prosthesis and to insert a replacement prosthesis. An incision is made into the corpus cavernosum, the corporal tissue is dissected, and the prosthesis is removed from the corporal body. The wound is irrigated with antibiotics and the replacement prosthesis is advanced to the mid-glans and introduced into the corporal space. Once implanted, the wound is again irrigated with antibiotics, and the corporotomy is closed by suture. The subcutaneous tissue is closed by suture and a dressing is applied to the incision. The bladder is emptied with a catheter. An indwelling urethral catheter, if used, is removed on the first postoperative day.

54417

The physician removes and replaces a non-inflatable (semi-rigid) or inflatable (self-contained) penile prosthesis, and irrigates and debrides infected tissue. The physician makes an incision using the same intrapubic, penoscrotal, or distal penile approach as the original procedure to remove the prosthesis and to insert a replacement non-inflatable or inflatable penile prosthesis at the same operative session. Using corporal incisions, the physician is able to remove the prosthesis. A corposcopy may be performed to ensure all fibrous elements are excised, and a replacement prosthesis is implanted. Any infected tissue is debrided and irrigated with an antibiotic solution. The corporotomy is closed by suture. The subcutaneous tissue is closed by suture and a dressing is applied to the incision. The bladder is emptied with a catheter. An indwelling urethral catheter, if used, is removed on the first postoperative day.

54420

The physician treats priapism, an abnormally sustained erection, by creating a shunt for the diversion of blood from the penis to the femoral vein. An incision is made in the groin area of the thigh and the saphenous vein is cut and dissected free of its attachments creating a mobile segment about 10.0 cm long. A second incision is made at the base of the penis and the saphenous vein is tunneled through the subcutaneous tissues to the base of the penis. A 1.0 cm in diameter piece of the thick fibrous tissue of the corpus cavernosum (erectile tissue) is excised and the free end of the saphenous vein is sutured to the defect. The erection resolves as blood flows from the penis to the femoral vein through this saphenous vein segment. The incisions are closed by suturing. The procedure is sometimes repeated on the opposite side.

54430

The physician treats priapism, an abnormally sustained erection, by creating a shunt for the diversion of blood from one region of the penis to an adjacent region. With a catheter in the urethra into the bladder, an incision is made in the side of the penis. Dissection is carried to the thick fibrous tissues surrounding one of the corpus cavernosum (erectile tissue) and to the corpus spongiosum, which is the erectile tissue around the urethra. Oval discs of the fibrous tissue are excised from the adjacent surfaces of these two structures. The excisional defects are sutured together creating a shunt (passageway) for the flow of blood from the engorged corpus cavernosum to the corpus spongiosum thus relieving the erection. The tissues and the skin are sutured closed. The procedure is sometimes repeated on the opposite side.

54435

The physician treats priapism, an abnormally sustained erection, by creating a shunt for the diversion of blood from the one region of the penis to an adjacent region. With adequate local anesthesia,

CPT ® Lay Descriptions

the head of the penis is punctured with a biopsy needle and advanced into the tip of the corpus cavernosum (erectile tissue). A portion of tissue from the head of the penis to the corpus cavernosum is removed as if taking a biopsy. This creates a passageway for blood trapped in the cavernosum to escape through the circulation to the head of the penis. The procedure is repeated to the opposite corpus cavernosum. The two puncture sites in the head of the penis are closed by suturing.

54440

The physician repairs an injury of the penis using one or more of plastic surgery techniques. The repair may require skin grafts, tissue grafts, urethral repair, extensive debridement, microsurgical repairs, or any combination.

54450

The physician treats adhesions between the uncircumcised foreskin and the head of the penis that prevent the retraction of the foreskin. Adhesions are broken either by stretching the foreskin back over the head of the penis onto the shaft, or by inserting a clamp between the foreskin and the head of the penis and spreading the jaws of the clamp.

54500

The physician obtains a sample of testicular tissue by needle biopsy. While the testis is held firmly with the scrotal skin stretched tightly over the testis and the epididymis positioned away from the biopsy site, a biopsy needle is inserted into the testis at the area of concern. The needle biopsy sheath is advanced over the needle and twisted to shear off the enclosed sample and then withdrawn with the sample enclosed. The scrotal wound may be closed by suturing.

54505

The physician obtains a sample of testicular tissue by direct incisional biopsy. The procedure is done under either local or regional anesthesia. While the testis is held firmly with the scrotal skin stretched tightly over the testis and the epididymis positioned away from the biopsy site, a small incision is made through the skin of the scrotum. The underlying tissues are incised and dissected to expose the testis. The testis is stabilized by two sutures and an ellipse of tissue is removed between the two sutures. The incisions are closed by suturing.

54512

The physician excises an extraparenchymal lesion of the testis. The physician makes an inguinal incision, incising the skin and subcutaneous fat. The testicle is delivered through the incision, the tunica vaginalis is opened, and the lesion is excised. The incision is closed with suture.

54520

An incision is made in one side of the scrotum and the tissues are separated to expose the spermatic cord. The spermatic cord is opened and the individual bundles making up the cord are cross-clamped, cut, and secured with nonabsorbable suture material. The testis is removed through the scrotal incision. If the patient so chooses, and if no contraindications are present, a prosthetic testis is inserted into the scrotum before the wound is closed in layers by suturing. An alternative method uses an incision in the groin. The testis is pulled up through the incision after cutting and tying the cord in a fashion similar to the scrotal approach.

54522

The physician performs a partial excision of one testis or both testes. The surgeon makes a longitudinal incision midline in the scrotum to expose the testis. The tunica vaginalis is incised, and the testicular vessels and vas deferens are identified, clamped separately, and divided. The cords are ligated at a level slightly above the area of infection, abscess, neoplasm, or trauma and the spermatic cord is isolated for manipulation of the testicle. The testis is delivered to the wound and dissected below the ligated cords. The wound is closed by suture and a pressure dressing and scrotal supporter are applied.

54530

The physician performs a radial orchiectomy by removing en bloc the contents of half of the scrotum. An incision is made in the inguinal area from the pubic bone up towards the lateral pelvic bone. The incision made deep into the tissues and the spermatic cord is dissected free and cross-clamped. The testis and all its associated structures are pushed up from the scrotum into the incision and removed. Packing is then placed in the empty scrotum. When the spermatic cord is opened and the individual bundles making up the cord are cross-clamped, cut, and secured with nonabsorbable suture material, care is taken to avoid important nerves and vessels in the area. The packing is removed and bleeding controlled. A prosthetic testis may be placed in the scrotum before the incision is closed in layers by suturing. This procedure results in complete removal of the testis.

54535

The physician performs a radical orchiectomy by removing en bloc the entire contents of half of the scrotum and also explores the inside of the abdomen for evidence of tumor spread. An incision is made in the inguinal area from the pubic bone up towards the lateral pelvic bone. The incision made deep into the tissues and the spermatic cord is dissected free and cross-clamped. The testis and all its associated structures are pushed up from the scrotum and delivered into the incision and then removed. Packing is placed in the empty scrotum. Care is taken to avoid important nerves and vessels in the area, when the spermatic cord is opened and the individual bundles making up the cord are cross-clamped, cut and secured with nonabsorbable suture material. This results in complete removal of the testis. The packing is removed and bleeding controlled. A prosthetic testis may be placed in the scrotum before the incision is closed in layers by suturing. A midline incision is made from the upper to the lower abdomen and the abdominal cavity is entered. The back wall of the abdomen is exposed and the lymph nodes are checked for spread of tumor. Some may be removed and/or biopsied and the abdominal wound is closed in multiple layers by suturing.

54550

The physician searches for a testis that failed to descend into the scrotum during development. An incision is made either in the scrotum or the inguinal area from the pubic bone to the upper lateral pelvic area in the skin fold made by the thigh and the lower abdomen. The tissues are separated by dissection to find the testis in the area. No other procedure is performed. The incision is closed in layers by suturing.

54560

The physician searches the abdominal cavity for a testis that failed to descend in to the scrotum during development. An incision is made either in the inguinal area from the pubic bone to the upper lateral pelvic area or in the skin fold made by the thigh and the lower abdomen. The tissues are separated by dissection and the incision is extended into the abdominal cavity. No other procedure is performed at this time. The incision is closed in layers by suturing.

54600

The physician treats a torsion of the testis, which is a twisting of the testis upon itself so that its blood supply is compromised. The physician makes an incision in the scrotum and exposes the twisted testis. The testis and spermatic cord is untwisted to restore blood flow to the organ. If the testis is viable, the surgeon anchors the testis to the inside wall of the scrotum with three or more sutures. The incision is closed in layers by suturing. Because the problem that allowed the testis to twist may affect the other testis (contralateral testis), a second procedure is commonly performed to anchor it in similar fashion.

54620

The physician makes an incision in the scrotum and exposes the testis on side opposite to the one that had previously been twisted. The surgeon anchors the testis to the inside wall of the scrotum with three or more sutures to prevent the twisting of the cord and the testis. The incision is closed in layers by suturing.

54640

Orchiopexy is the surgical fixation of an undescended testicle into the scrotum. An incision is made either in the scrotum or the inguinal area from the pubic bone to the upper lateral pelvic area in the skin crease made by the thigh and the lower abdomen. The physician searches for a testis that failed to descend in to the scrotum during development. The tissues are separated by dissection to find the testis in the inguinal canal area. The spermatic cord is mobilized to allow positioning of the testis in the scrotum. In the scrotum, a small pouch is created for the testis where the testis is sutured in place to prevent retraction back in to the inguinal canal. If there is a concomitant hernia it is often repaired at the same time through the same incision. The hernia present in the inguinal canal is repaired by folding and suturing of tissues to strengthen the abdominal wall and correct the weakness responsible for the hernia. The incision is closed in layers by suturing.

54650

Orchiopexy is the surgical fixation of an undescended testicle into the scrotum. An incision is made either in the inguinal area from the pubic bone to the upper lateral pelvic area in the skin fold made by the thigh and the lower abdomen. The physician searches the abdominal cavity for a testis that failed to descend in to the scrotum during development. The tissues are separated by dissection and the incision is extended into the abdominal cavity to find the testis in the abdominal area. The tissues are separated by dissection to find the testis in the area. At this point several surgical options are available. The one chosen will depend on the mobility of the testis and how far it can be brought down through the inguinal canal and into the scrotum. The procedure may take two stages approximately six to 12 months apart. Eventually, the spermatic cord is mobilized sufficiently to allow positioning of the testis in the scrotum. In the scrotum a small pouch is created for the testis where the testis is sutured in place to prevent retraction back in to the inguinal canal or into the abdominal cavity. The incision is closed in layers by suturing.

54660

For cosmetic reasons, the physician places an artificial testis in the scrotum of a patient. After adequate local anesthesia, an incision is made in the inguinal area and the empty scrotal sac is carefully dilated by passing a dissecting finger or a moist gauze sponge through the inguinal canal into the scrotum. A prosthetic testis is inserted into the scrotal sac and the neck of the scrotum is closed by suturing. The inguinal incision is closed in layers by suturing.

54670

The physician repairs injury (laceration or traumatic rupture) to the testis that occurs as a result of either a blunt or penetrating injury. Often a laceration is present in the scrotum and the testis is explored and repaired through the open wound. Otherwise, an incision is made in the scrotum to expose the testis. Any devitalized testicular tissue is removed by sharp dissection and the thick tough fibrous tissue encasing the testis is closed by suturing. The scrotum is closed in layers by suturing. Often a rubber drain is placed to prevent the accumulation of fluid and blood in the scrotum.

54680

The physician transplants the testis(es) under the skin of the thigh to preserve function and viability following massive injury or surgical loss of the scrotal skin. The thigh is chosen because the temperature just under the skin is approximately the same as in the scrotum, a condition to normal testicular function. Incisions are made in the skin of the thigh adjacent to the scrotum and the testis is carefully sutured in place with attention to preserving blood flow to the organ. The thigh incisions are closed in layers over a rubber drain brought out through the skin. In four to six weeks scrotal reconstruction is begun.

54690

The physician removes one or both testicles, which may be undescended, injured or diseased using a laparoscope. The physician places a trocar at the umbilicus into the abdominal or retroperitoneal space and insufflates the abdominal cavity. The physician places a laparoscope through the umbilical incision and additional trocars are placed into the abdomen. The testis and all its associated structures are pushed up from the scrotum or freed from their undescended intra-abdominal location and removed through the abdominal or retroperitoneal space via the trocar port. Packing may be placed in the empty scrotum. Care is taken to avoid important nerves and vessels in the area. A prosthetic testis may be placed in the scrotum before the incision is closed in layers by suturing. The trocars are removed and the incisions are closed with sutures.

54692

The physician performs a orchiopexy (the surgical fixation of an undescended testicle into the scrotum) with the assistance of a fiber optic laparoscope. A para-umbilical port is created by placing a trocar at the level of the umbilicus. The abdominal wall is then insufflated. The laparoscope is placed through the umbilical port and additional trocars are placed into the abdominal cavity. The physician uses the laparoscope fitted with a fiberoptic camera and/or an operating instruments to search the abdominal cavity for the undescended testes. The physician may have several surgical options depending on the mobility of the testis and how far it can be brought down through the inguinal canal and into the scrotum. The procedure may take two stages approximately three to 12 months apart. Once, the spermatic cord is mobilized sufficiently to allow positioning of the testis

in the scrotum (which often occurs during the first and perhaps only operative session). A small pouch is created for the testis where the testis is sutured in place to prevent retraction back in to the inguinal canal or into the abdominal cavity. The small abdominal incisions are closed by staple or suture in the usual fashion.

54700

The physician drains a collection of blood or an abscess within the scrotum. If the testis is the target of the drainage, it is held firmly with the scrotal skin stretched tightly over the testis and the epididymis positioned away from the site. A small incision is made through the skin of the scrotum. The underlying tissues are incised and dissected to expose the testis and the site to be drained. The testis may be stabilized by two sutures as an incision is made into the abscess or hematoma and fluid is expressed. Packing or a rubber drain may be placed to promote drainage. The incisions are usually not closed by suturing. Similar procedures are followed if the target is the epididymis or the scrotal space.

54800

The physician obtains a sample of epididymal tissues by needle biopsy. While the testis is held firmly with the scrotal skin stretched tightly over the testis and the epididymis positioned just under the taut skin, a biopsy needle is inserted into the area of concern in the epididymis. The needle biopsy sheath is advanced over the needle and twisted to shear off the enclosed sample and then withdrawn containing the sample. The scrotal wound may be closed by suturing.

54820

The physician explores the epididymis by making an incision in scrotum. The procedure is done under either local or regional anesthesia. While the testis is held firmly with the scrotal skin stretched tightly over the testis and the epididymis positioned just under the taught skin, a small incision is made through the skin of the scrotum. The underlying tissues are incised and dissected to expose the epididymis. The epididymis may be biopsied by placing two sutures on each side of the area of concern and an ellipse of tissue is removed from the epididymis containing the lesion between the two sutures. The stabilizing sutures are tied across the excision site to close it. The scrotal incision is closed by suturing. Alternatively, if a biopsy is done, it may be done by needle puncture under direct vision.

54830

The physician removes a local lesion of the epididymis by direct incision. The procedure is done under either local or regional anesthesia. While the testis is held firmly with the scrotal skin stretched tightly over the testis and the epididymis positioned just under the taut skin, a small incision is made through the skin of the scrotum. The underlying tissues are incised and dissected to expose the epididymis and the area of concern. The epididymis may be stabilized by two sutures placed on each side of the lesion and an ellipse of tissue is removed from the epididymis containing the lesion between the two sutures. The stabilizing sutures are tied across the excision site to close it. The scrotal incision is closed by suturing.

54840

The physician removes a spermatocele, which is a small cyst, filled with fluid and spermatozoa, between the body of the testis and the epididymis. After adequate local anesthesia, an incision is made in the scrotum and the testis with its attached epididymis is brought out of the wound. The cyst is dissected free of the testis and excised. The involved area of the epididymis is sutured to the underlying testis and the scrotal wound is closed by suturing. Alternately the epididymis may be dissected free of all of its attachments to the testis. The blood vessels involved are tied and cut and/or cauterized to control bleeding. The freed epididymis is thus removed, a rubber drain is placed in the scrotum and the incision is closed by suturing.

54860–54861

The physician removes the epididymis. After adequate local anesthesia, an incision is made in the scrotum and the testis with its attached epididymis is brought out of the wound. The epididymis is dissected free of all of its attachments to the testis. The blood vessels involved are tied and cut and/or cauterized to control bleeding. The freed epididymis is thus removed, a rubber drain is left in the scrotum and the incision is closed by suturing. The epididymectomy is performed on one side in 54860, or both sides in 54861.

54900–54901

The physician treats obstruction of the flow of spermatozoa from the epididymis to vas deferens, the tube that carries the semen. After adequate anesthesia, an incision is made in the scrotum and the testis with its attached epididymis and the vas deferens is brought out of the wound. The vas deferens is transected and the selected area of the epididymis is opened and the appropriate tubule in the area is brought out of the surrounding tissues and then transected. The cut ends of these two tubes are sutured together and the vas deferens is sutured to the epididymis. A rubber drain is often placed in the scrotum and the incision is closed by suturing. In 54900, the procedure is performed on one side; in 54901, the procedure is bilateral.

55000

A hydrocele is a sac of fluid in the tunica vaginalis or along the spermatic cord. The physician treats a hydrocele by aspirating the fluid. After injecting a small area with local anesthetic, the physician inserts a needle on an aspirating syringe into the fluid filled

hydrocele sac and withdraws the fluid into the syringe. After the aspiration and with the needle still in place, the sac may be injected with sclerosing medication to prevent accumulation of new fluid by stimulating scarring and hardening of the empty sac.

55040–55041

A hydrocele is a sac of fluid in the tunica vaginalis or along the spermatic cord. The physician treats a hydrocele by removing it. After injecting an area with local anesthetic and using aseptic techniques, the physician makes an incision in the scrotum or in the inguinal area. Care is taken to keep the hydrocele intact while it is dissected free of its attachments to the testis and other structures. The sac is opened, drained and partially excised leaving a remnant of tissue. The remaining tissue is swung back behind the epididymis and the spermatic cord and closed by suturing the edges together. The testis is anchored to the inside of the scrotum with three sutures to prevent later torsion or twisting of the testis. A rubber drain may be left in the scrotum and the incision closed in layers by suturing. The hydrocele is on one side in 55040. In 55041, each side side is treated for hydrocele.

55060

The physician treats a hydrocele by removing the abnormal fluid filled sac in the scrotum or in the inguinal canal. After injecting an area with local anesthetic and using aseptic techniques, the physician makes an incision in the scrotum or in the inguinal area. Care is taken to keep the hydrocele intact while it is dissected free of its attachments to the testis and other structures. The sac is opened high along its front surface and the testis is pushed up through the sac and out through the incision. This inverts the hydrocele sac which is tacked by suturing to the spermatic cord structures behind the testis. The testis is returned to the scrotum and is anchored to the inside of the scrotum with three sutures to prevent later torsion or twisting of the testis. A rubber drain may be left in the scrotum and the incision closed in layers by suturing.

55100

After adequate local anesthesia, the physician makes an incision directly into the abscess of the scrotal wall. Pus is expressed and a drain or medicated gauze packing placed in the abscess cavity.

55110

The physician makes an incision in the scrotum for the purpose of direct visual inspection of the contents of the scrotum. This may involve one or both sides of the scrotum and may be done through one or two incisions and require incisions through the various layers of tissues to expose the testis and other structures. A drain may be left in the scrotum and the incisions closed in successive layers of sutures.

CPT® Lay Descriptions

55120

The physician makes an incision in the scrotum for the purpose of foreign body removal. This may involve one or both sides of the scrotum and may be done through one or two incisions and may require incisions through the various layers of tissues to expose and locate the object. The foreign body is identified and isolated and removed with care to avoid damaging tissues in the scrotum. A drain may be placed in the scrotum and the incisions closed in successive layers of sutures.

55150

The physician removes excessive or diseased scrotal skin by excision. The extent of the procedure is dependent upon the disease process and the degree of involvement. The physician makes incisions in the scrotal skin, taking care to avoid injury to the underlying scrotal contents. In the simple case, the excess skin is removed and the defects closed in layers by suturing. In the more involved cases the testes and spermatic cords must be mobilized and removed from the scrotum and swung out of the way by making incisions in the inguinal areas. The affected scrotal skin is excised and the testes and cord structures returned to their anatomic positions. If not enough scrotal skin remains, flaps of skin are raised from the adjacent thighs and rotated to cover the testes. These grafts or flaps are separately reported. Rubber drains may be left in the scrotum and the operative site closed in layers by suturing.

55175–55180

The physician repairs defects and developmental abnormalities of the scrotum by wound revisions or the creation and suturing of simple scrotal skin flaps in 55175. In 55180, the reconstruction is more complex and the physician uses either free skin grafts, mesh grafts and/or the extensive use of rotational pedicle grafts from adjacent skin. These flaps or grafts are separately reported.

55200

The physician enters the vas deferens (the tube that carries spermatozoa from the testis) for purpose of obtaining a sample of semen or testing the patency of the tubes. Under local anesthesia, an incision is made in the upper outer scrotum overlying the spermatic cord. The tissues are dissected to expose the vas deferens. The tube is entered by puncturing with a small needle and fluid samples removed or solution injected to check for blockages. An alternate method involves the tube being cut open with a scalpel. A blunt needle is placed in the tube under direct vision and fluid samples removed or the tube checked for patency. If an incision is made in the tube, the tube must be repaired using microsurgical techniques before the scrotal incisions are closed in layers by suturing.

55250

The physician grasps the upper scrotum near the inguinal area and holds the spermatic cord between the thumb and the index finger. The skin overlying the immobilized cord is injected with local anesthetic and an incision is made through the scrotal wall to expose the tubular structures. Another incision is made to expose the vas deferens (spermatic tube) and the tissues dissected to free it from the adjacent vessels and supporting tissues. The isolated vas deferens is cut in two places and the intervening section of tube is removed. The cut ends of the vas deferens are cauterized and tied with suture material. The incisions are closed in layers by suturing. The procedure is usually repeated on the opposite side.

55300

The physician enters the vas deferens (the tube that carries spermatozoa from the testis) for purpose of testing the patency of the spermatozoa collecting system. An incision is made in the upper outer scrotum overlying the spermatic cord and the tissues dissected to expose the vas deferens.

55400

The physician treats a blockage in the vas deferens, the tube that carries semen. After anesthesia, an incision is made in the scrotum. The testis with its attached epididymis and the vas deferens are brought out of the wound. Dye injection studies and semen sampling is often done during the operation to determine the site of the blockage and to accurately choose the segment of tube for excision. The vas deferens is transected in two places, one on each side of the blocked area and the abnormal segment removed. The created cut ends are sutured together in either one or two layers with care to align accurately the lumens of the tubes. The testis and associated structures are returned to the scrotum. A rubber drain is often placed in the scrotum and the incisions closed by suturing.

55450

The physician performs a ligation of the vas deferens (vasectomy) without cutting an incision in the skin. The procedure is done under local anesthesia. With thumb and index finger the surgeon grasps the spermatic cord beneath the skin, high in the scrotum near the inguinal area. The skin is pulled taught with the spermatic cord just underneath the skin. An instrument is pressed against the structures and activated sequentially. The instrument punctures the skin and cuts the spermatic cord, then clips the cord on each side of the cut area. The procedure may be repeated on the opposite side. The resulting puncture wounds are bandaged.

55500

A hydrocele is an abnormal fluid-filled sac. The physician treats a hydrocele of the spermatic cord by removing from the spermatic cord above the testis in the scrotum or in the inguinal canal. After injecting the area with local anesthetic, the physician makes an incision in the scrotum or in the inguinal area. The hydrocele is kept intact while it is freed of its attachments to the spermatic cord. The sac is opened, drained,and excised all the way to the internal inguinal ring in the upper groin area. The remaining tissues are repaired and closed by suturing. The testis is anchored to the inside of the scrotum with three sutures to prevent later torsion or twisting of the testis. A rubber drain may be placed in the scrotum and the incision closed in layers by suturing.

55520

The physician removes a lesion of the spermatic cord by dissection and excision. After injecting the area with local anesthetic, the physician makes an incision in the scrotum or in the inguinal area and dissects the tissues to expose the lesion. Care is taken to keep the lesion intact while it is dissected free of its attachments to the spermatic cord. This may involve mobilization of the testis. The lesion is removed by cutting all of its attachments. The tissues damaged during the dissection are repaired and closed by suturing. If the testis has been mobilized, it is anchored to the inside of the scrotum with three sutures to prevent later torsion or twisting. A drain may be placed in the scrotum and the incision is closed in layers by suturing.

55530

A varicocele is an abnormal dilation of the veins of the spermatic cord in the scrotum. The physician ligates the spermatic veins and/or excises a varicocele. An incision is made in the pubic area on the affected side and carried down to the spermatic cord as passes through the inguinal canal. The cord is brought up into the incision and the structures of the cord are dissected, the veins identified, and ligated with suture material. Alternately, an incision is made in the scrotum and the dilated veins ligated separately may be removed. The operative incision is closed in layers by suturing.

55535

The physician ligates the spermatic veins and/or excises a varicocele which is an abnormal dilation of the veins of the spermatic cord in the scrotum. An incision is made in lateral lower abdomen just medial to the bony prominence of the pelvic bone on the affected side and carried down through the abdominal musculature to the spermatic vein and artery. The vein is identified and ligated (tied off) with suture material. The abdominal incision is closed in multiple layers by suturing.

55540

The physician repairs an inguinal hernia and ligates the spermatic veins or excises a varicocele (an abnormal dilation of the veins of the spermatic cord in the scrotum). An incision is made in the pubic area

on the affected side to expose the spermatic cord as it passes through the inguinal canal. The cord is brought up into the incision and the structures of the cord are carefully dissected, the veins identified and ligated (tied off) with suture material. The hernia is repaired through the same incision by folding and suturing of tissues to strengthen the abdominal wall and correct the weakness responsible for the hernia. Alternately, an incision is made in the scrotum and the dilated veins ligated separately and may be removed (excision) and a second incision made for hernia repair. All incisions are closed in layers by suturing.

55550

The physician ligates (ties or binds with suture) the spermatic veins and/or excises a varicocele which is an abnormal dilation of the veins of the spermatic cord in the scrotum. An umbilical port is created by placing a trocar at the level of the umbilicus. The abdominal wall is then insufflated. The laparoscope is placed through the umbilical port and additional trocars are placed into the abdominal or pelvic cavity. The physician uses the laparoscope fitted with a fiberoptic camera and/or an operating instrument to explore and surgically ligate the spermatic veins to repair or remove the varicocele. The structures of the cord are dissected, the veins identified, and ligated with suture. The abdomen is then deflated, the trocars removed and the incisions are closed with sutures.

55600–55605

The physician incises or punctures one of the seminal vesicles, paired glands that lie behind the urinary bladder and produce fluid that is mixed with the semen produced in the testis. The seminal vesicle is approached through an incision in the lower abdomen or an incision in the perineum (area between the base of the scrotum and the anus). In the abdominal method, the physician either retracts the bladder forward toward the pubic bone to expose the back of the bladder where the seminal vesicles are positioned, or the surgeon cuts through the front and back walls to gain access to the gland. The operative wounds are closed in layers by suturing. If the procedure does not require extensive dissection, report 55600; if extensive, report 55605.

55650

The physician removes one of the seminal vesicles, paired glands that lie behind the urinary bladder and produce a fluid that is mixed with semen from the testis. Through an incision in the lower abdomen or an incision in the perineum (area between the base of the scrotum and the anus) the seminal vesicle is approached. If the abdominal method is used the surgeon either retracts the bladder forward toward the pubic bone to expose the back of the bladder where the seminal vesicles are positioned or the surgeon cuts through the front and back walls to gain access to the glands. The surgeon dissects the gland free of its attachments and clips it at its joint with the ejaculatory duct and removes it. The operative wounds are closed in layers by suturing.

55680

The physician excises a Mullerian duct cyst, a remnant of the prenatal development of the seminal vesicle. The seminal vesicles are paired glands that lie behind the urinary bladder and produce a fluid that is mixed with the semen from the testis. Through an incision in the lower abdomen or an incision in the perineum (area between the base of the scrotum and the anus) the seminal vesicle is approached. If the abdominal method is used, the surgeon either retracts the bladder forward toward the pubic bone to expose the back of the bladder where the seminal vesicles are positioned or the surgeon cuts through the front and back walls to gain access to the glands. The surgeon dissects the cyst free of its attachments and clips it at the attachment to the seminal vesicle and removes it. The operative wounds are closed in layers by suturing.

55700

The physician obtains tissue from the prostate for analysis by needle or punch biopsy through one or more of three approaches. The biopsy needle is passed into the suspect area of the prostate either by puncturing through skin of the perineum (the area between the base of the scrotum and the anus), by advancing the needle into the rectum by guidance with the index finger and then puncturing through the rectal mucosa, or by advancing a biopsy instrument up the urethra. The biopsy needle is inserted into the prostate guided by an index finger or by ultrasound and the needle biopsy sheath is advanced over the needle and twisted to shear off the enclosed sample. The needle is withdrawn, containing the sample. This may be repeated two or more times to assure adequate sampling and then the puncture site is bandaged.

55705

The physician obtains tissue from the prostate for analysis by direct incisional sampling. The prostate is usually approached in one of three ways: through skin of the perineum (the area between the base of the scrotum and the anus), through the rectal mucosa, or by advancing a biopsy instrument up the urethra. In any case, an incision is made and the tissues dissected to expose the prostate. The area of concern is identified and an excision is performed to remove tissue for analysis. Bleeding is controlled and the dissected tissues and skin incision are closed in layers by suturing.

55720–55725

The physician performs a simple prostatotomy (cutting or puncturing the prostate) through one of two usual approaches. An aspirating needle is passed into the abscessed area of the prostate either by puncturing through skin of the perineum (the area

between the base of the scrotum and the anus), or by advancing the needle up into the rectum by guidance with the index finger and then puncturing through the rectal mucosa. The needle is inserted into the abscess in the prostate guided by an index finger or by ultrasound and the contents of the abscess removed by aspiration. The needle is withdrawn and the puncture site bandaged. Report 55720 for simple drainage, or 55725 if the procedure is complicated by excessive bleeding, infection, or other problem.

55801

The physician performs a prostatectomy (removal of the prostate gland) through an incision made in the perineum. The caliber (internal diameter) of the urethra is measured and if it is not adequate, the opening of the urethra is enlarged (meatotomy) and the diameter of the penile urethra is enlarged with an instrument (internal urethrotomy). A curved instrument (Lowery Tractor) is advanced up the urethra to the prostate to help to identify the structures and aid in the dissection. Through the perineal incision and with manipulation of the tractor, the tissues are dissected to expose the prostate. The curved tractor instrument in the urethra is replaced with a straight tractor. A portion of the prostate or the entire gland is removed with care to preserve the seminal vesicles. The operation is "subtotal" because the seminal vesicles remain intact. The bladder outlet is revised and the vas deferens is ligated and may be partially removed (vasectomy). Bleeding is controlled by ligation or cautery. A Foley catheter is placed in the bladder. A rubber drain may be placed in the site of the operative wound and brought out through a separate stab wound. The dissected tissues and the skin incision are closed in layers by suturing.

55810–55812

The physician performs a radical prostatectomy through an incision made in the the skin between the base of the scrotum and the anus. If the internal diameter of the urethra is not adequate, the opening of the urethra is enlarged (meatotomy) and the diameter of the penile urethra is enlarged with an instrument (internal urethrotomy). A curved instrument (Lowery Tractor) is advanced up the urethra to the prostate to aid in the dissection. Through the perineal incision and with manipulation of the tractor, the tissues are dissected to expose the prostate. The curved tractor instrument in the urethra is replaced with a straight tractor. The entire gland is removed along with the seminal vesicles and the vas deferens. The bladder outlet is revised and bleeding controlled by ligation or cautery. For 55812, local lymph nodes are also removed for analysis. A Foley catheter is placed and left in the bladder. A rubber drain may be placed in the site of the operative wound and brought out through a separate stab wound. The dissected tissues and the skin incision are closed in layers by suturing.

55815

The physician removes the prostate gland through an incision made in the perineum and also a pelvic lymphadenectomy through a separate lower abdominal incision. A midline abdominal incision is made from the upper to the lower abdomen and the back wall of the abdomen is exposed. All lymph nodes along back wall of the pelvic and abdominal cavities are removed. The abdominal wound is closed in multiple layers by suturing. In preparation for removal of the prostate, the caliber (internal diameter) of the urethra is measured and if it is not adequate the opening of the urethra is enlarged (meatotomy) and the diameter of the penile urethra is enlarged with an instrument (internal urethrotomy). A curved instrument (Lowery Tractor) is advanced up the urethra to aid in the dissection. Through the perineal incision and with manipulation of the tractor, the tissues are dissected to expose the prostate. The curved tractor instrument in the urethra is replaced with a straight tractor. The entire gland is removed along with the seminal vesicles and the vas deferens. The bladder outlet is revised and bleeding controlled by ligation or cautery. A Foley catheter is placed and left in the bladder. A rubber drain may be placed in the site of the operative wound and brought out through a separate stab wound. The dissected tissues and the skin incision are closed in layers by suturing.

55821

The physician removes the prostate gland through an incision made in the lower abdomen just above the pubic area. In preparation for removal of the prostate, the caliber (internal diameter) of the urethra is measured and if it is not adequate the opening of the urethra is enlarged (meatotomy) and the diameter of the penile urethra is enlarged with an instrument (internal urethrotomy) and a catheter is passed up the urethra into the bladder. Through the lower abdominal incision the urinary bladder is exposed and opened by an incision in the region just above the bladder neck. During the dissection to expose the bladder a vasectomy may be performed. The bladder mucosa over the prostate is removed by excision to expose the prostate. The entire gland is removed by "shelling it out" by blunt dissection with the surgeon's index finger. The bladder outlet and the bladder wall are revised and bleeding controlled by packing with rolls of gauze, by ligation or cautery of bleeding vessels. A second catheter is placed and left in the bladder through the incision in the lower abdomen. A rubber drain is placed in the space between the pubic bone and the bladder and brought out through a separate stab wound. The dissected tissues and the skin incision are closed in layers by suturing.

55831

The physician removes the prostate gland through an incision made in the lower abdomen just above the pubic area. In preparation for removal of the prostate, the caliber (internal diameter) of the urethra is

measured and if it is not adequate the opening of the urethra is enlarged (meatotomy) and the diameter of the penile urethra is enlarged with an instrument (internal urethrotomy) and a catheter is passed up the urethra into the bladder. Through the lower abdominal incision the urinary bladder is exposed and opened by an incision in the region just above the bladder neck. During the dissection to expose the bladder a vasectomy may be performed. The bladder mucosa over the prostate is removed by excision to expose the prostate. The entire gland is removed by "shelling it out" by blunt dissection with the surgeon's index finger. The bladder outlet and the bladder wall are revised and bleeding controlled by packing with rolls of gauze, by ligation or cautery of bleeding vessels. A second catheter is placed and left in the bladder through the incision in the lower abdomen. A rubber drain is placed between the pubic bone and the bladder and brought out through a separate stab wound. The dissected tissues and the skin incision are closed in layers by suturing.

55840

The physician performs a radical prostatectomy (removal of the prostate gland) through an incision made in the lower abdomen just above the pubic area. In preparation for removal of the prostate, a catheter is passed up the urethra into the bladder. Through a lower abdominal incision, with or without care to spare the nerves in the area, the urinary bladder is exposed and displaced backwards to enter the space behind the pubic bone and expose the area of the prostate. The entire gland with the capsule intact and the seminal vesicles and the portions of the vas deferens in the area are removed by freeing the the prostate by blunt dissection and by transecting the urethra and by cutting through the bladder outlet. The urinary catheter is brought up into the operative site and used to create traction for the dissection. A second catheter is place in the bladder after the first one is removed along with the prostate. The transected urethra is repaired by suturing to the newly created bladder outlet. A rubber drain is placed in the space between the pubic bone and the bladder and brought out through a separate stab wound. The dissected tissues and the skin incision are closed in layers by suturing.

55842

The physician performs a radical prostatectomy and a pelvic lymph node biopsy(ies) through a midline abdominal incision (this may be done in two stages within 7 to 10 days). A midline incision is made from the upper to the lower abdomen and the abdominal cavity is entered. The back wall of the abdomen is exposed and the lymph nodes are checked for spread of tumor. Some may be removed and/or biopsied. Through the abdominal incision, with or with out sparing the nerves in the area, the urinary bladder is exposed and displaced backwards to enter the space behind the pubic bone and expose the area of the prostate. The entire gland with the capsule intact and the seminal vesicles and the portions of the vas deferens in the area are removed by freeing the the prostate by blunt dissection and by transecting the urethra and by cutting through the bladder outlet. The urinary catheter is brought up into the operative site and used to create traction for the dissection. A second catheter is place in the bladder after the first one is removed along with the prostate. The transected urethra is repaired by sutured to the newly created bladder outlet. A rubber drain is placed between the pubic bone and the bladder and brought out through a separate stab wound.

55845

The physician performs a radical prostatectomy and a pelvic lymph node biopsy(ies) through a midline abdominal incision (this may be done in two stages within 7 to 10 days). A midline incision is made from the upper to the lower abdomen and the abdominal cavity is entered. The back wall of the abdomen is exposed and all the lymph nodes along back wall of the pelvic and abdominal cavities are removed. In preparation for removal of the prostate, a catheter is passed up the urethra into the bladder. Through the abdominal incision, with or without care to spare the nerves in the area, the urinary bladder is exposed and displaced backwards to enter the space behind the pubic bone and expose the area of the prostate. The entire gland with the capsule intact and the seminal vesicles and the portions of the vas deferens in the area are removed by freeing the the prostate by blunt dissection and by transecting the urethra and by cutting through the bladder outlet. The urinary catheter is brought up into the operative site and used to create traction for the dissection. A second catheter is place in the bladder after the first one is removed along with the prostate. The dissected tissues and the skin incision are closed in layers by suturing.

55860

Through an incision made in the lower abdomen just above the pubic area, the physician inserts radioactive materials in the prostate. In preparation for the radiation treatment, a catheter is passed up the urethra into the bladder and a sterile sheath is inserted into the rectum. Through the lower abdominal incision the urinary bladder is exposed and displaced backwards to enter the space behind the pubic bone and expose the prostate gland. With a finger in the rectum to guide the placement, the physician passes a hollow needle into the prostate through the abdominal incision. The needle is positioned in the prostate tumor and radioactive seeds are introduced into the needle and implanted in the prostate using an applicator. The needle is withdrawn a few millimeters and another seed is placed. This is repeated several times through multiple needle insertions. A rubber drain(s) is placed in the space between the pubic bone and the bladder and brought out through the operative incision wound. The dissected tissues and the skin incision are closed in

layers by suturing. Alternatively, other approaches may be used in a similar fashion.

55862

Through an incision made in the abdomen, the physician inserts radioactive materials in the prostate and examines the pelvic and abdominal lymph nodes. A midline incision is made from the upper to the lower abdomen and the abdominal cavity is entered. The back wall of the abdomen is exposed and the lymph nodes are checked for spread of tumor. Some may be removed and/or biopsied. In preparation for the radiation treatment, a catheter is passed up the urethra into the bladder and a sterile sheath is inserted into the rectum. Through the lower abdominal incision the urinary bladder is exposed and displaced backwards to enter the space behind the pubic bone and expose the prostate gland. With a finger in the rectum to guide the placement, the physician passes a hollow needle into the prostate through the abdominal incision. The needle is positioned in the prostate tumor and radioactive seeds are introduced into the needle and implanted in the prostate using an applicator. The needle is withdrawn a few millimeters and another seed is placed. This is repeated several times through multiple needle insertions. A rubber drain(s) is placed between the pubic bone and the bladder and brought out through the operative incision wound. The dissected tissues and the skin incision are closed in layers by suturing. Alternatively, other approaches may be used in a similar fashion.

55865

Through an incision made in the abdomen, the physician inserts radioactive materials in the prostate and examines the pelvic and abdominal lymph nodes. A midline incision is made from the upper to the lower abdomen and the abdominal cavity is entered. The back wall of the abdomen is exposed and all the lymph nodes along back wall of the pelvic and abdominal cavities are removed. In preparation for the radiation treatment, a catheter is passed up the urethra into the bladder and a sterile sheath is inserted into the rectum. Through the lower abdominal incision the urinary bladder is exposed and displaced backwards to enter the space behind the pubic bone and expose the prostate gland. With a finger in the rectum to guide the placement, the physician passes a hollow needle into the prostate through the abdominal incision. The needle is positioned in the prostate tumor and radioactive seeds are introduced into the needle and implanted in the prostate using an applicator. The needle is withdrawn a few millimeters and another seed is placed. This is repeated several times through multiple needle insertions. A rubber drain(s) is placed between the pubic bone and the bladder and brought out through the operative incision wound. The dissected tissues and the skin incision are closed in layers by suturing. Alternatively, other approaches may be used in a similar fashion.

55870

The physician uses an electrovibratory device that stimulates ejaculation. The electrostimulator probe is placed in the rectum and positioned adjacent to the prostate gland and a current of electricity is passed into the region of the prostate, seminal vesicles and the vas deferens. The stimulation excites the nerves of the area, causing ejaculation. The semen is collected and used for artificial insemination.

55873

The physician performs cryosurgical ablation of the prostate with ultrasonic guidance for interstitial cryosurgical probe placement. The physician places a suprapubic catheter into the bladder through a stab incision just above the pubic hairline. Next, the physician inserts a warming catheter through the urethra and into the bladder. The scrotum is elevated out of the operative field using a gauze sling. An ultrasound probe is inserted into the rectum to monitor the freezing process, and to view in real-time the probe placement during the procedure. Under ultrasonic guidance, the surgeon inserts from three to eight needles into the perineum and advances the needles into the prostate. Into each needle the surgeon advances a guidewire used to facilitate instrumentation. The skin is incised and a dilator is inserted over each guidewire to dilate the channels. Saline is injected to aid visibility of the ultrasound, the guidewire is removed, and a cryoprobe (three-millimeter diameter) is inserted through each dilator for direct contact with the prostate tissue. The cryoprobe's, which delivers super-cooled liquid nitrogen or argon gas (both inert materials) to the prostate, are turned on at -70°C. Up to five cryoprobes can be running simultaneously at any one time. The five cryoprobes are turned on, taking the temperature down to -190°C, while the warming catheter guards against freezing the ureter. If the prostate thaws, the probes may be re-positioned, and a second freeze may be performed. Once the prostate gland is completely frozen (resembling an ice ball) and all of the visible prostate tissue is destroyed, the surgeon removes the probes and applies pressure to the perineum to prevent hematoma formation. The punctures are sutured shut and the urethral warming catheter is removed.

55970

In a series of staged procedures, the physician removes portions of the male genitalia and forms female external genitals. The penis is dissected and portions are removed with care to preserve vital nerves and vessels in order to fashion a clitoris-like structure. The urethral opening is moved to a position similar to that of a normal female. A vagina is made by dissecting and opening the perineum. This opening is then lined using either pedicle or split thickness grafts. Labia are created out of skin from the scrotum and adjacent tissue. A stent or obturator is usually left in place in the newly created vagina for three weeks or longer.

55980

In a series of staged procedures, the physician forms a penis and scrotum using pedicle flap grafts and free skin grafts. Portions of the clitoris are used as well as the adjacent skin. Prostheses are often placed in the penis in order to have a sexually functional organ. Prosthetic testicles are fixed in the scrotum. The vagina is either closed or removed.

56405

The vulva includes the labia majora, labia minora, mons pubis, bulb of the vestibule, vestibule of the vagina, greater and lesser vestibular glands, and vaginal orifice. The perineum is the area between the vulva and the anus. The physician makes an incision into the abscess at its softest point and drains the purulent contents. The cavity of the abscess is flushed and often packed with medicated gauze to facilitate drainage.

56420

The physician incises and drains a Bartholin's gland abscess. Bartholin's gland is at the end of the bulb of the vestibule of the vagina and is connected by a duct to the mucosa at the opening of the vagina. The physician makes an incision just inside the opening of the vagina through the mucosal surface into the cavity of the abscess to flush and drain it. A small wick or catheter may be left in the cavity to facilitate drainage.

56440

The physician treats a Bartholin's gland cyst with marsupialization. Bartholin's gland is at the end of the bulb of the vestibule of the vagina and is connected by a duct to the mucosa at the opening of the vagina. The physician makes an elliptical excision over the center of the Bartholin's gland cyst and then drains it. The lining of the cyst is everted and approximated to the vaginal mucosa with sutures creating a pouch. Marsupialization prevents recurrent cysts and infections.

56441

The labia majora and minora are the greater and lesser folds of skin on the pudendum on either side of the vagina. The physician separates the labia majora from the labia minora, which are fused by fibrous bands of scar tissue. Using a blunt instrument and/or scissors, the labia are separated by breaking or cutting the fibrous tissue. The procedure is accomplished using general or local anesthesia.

56501–56515

The vulva includes the labia majora, labia minora, mons pubis, bulb of the vestibule, vestibule of the vagina, greater and lesser vestibular glands, and vaginal orifice. The physician destroys one or more lesions of the vulva. After examining the lower genital tract and perianal are with a colposcope, the physician destroys any lesions of the vulva by laser surgery, electrosurgery, chemosurgery, cryosurgery, or excision. Use 56501 to report single, simple lesion destruction, or 56515 to report multiple or complicated destruction of extensive vulvar lesions.

56605–56606

The vulva includes the labia majora, labia minora, mons pubis, bulb of the vestibule, vestibule of the vagina, greater and lesser vestibular glands, and vaginal orifice. The perineum is the area between the vulva and the anus. The physician removes a sample of tissue from the vulva or perineum. After injecting a local anesthetic around the suspect tissue, the physician obtains a sample using a skin punch or sharp scalpel. A clip or suture can be used to control bleeding if pressure is not successful. Use 56605 for the biopsy of one lesion and 56606 for each additional lesion.

56620

The physician removes part of the vulva to treat premalignant or malignant lesions. A simple, partial vulvectomy may include removal of part or all of the labia majora and the labia minora on one side and the clitoris. After examining the lower genital tract and the perianal skin with a colposcope, the physician makes a wide semi-elliptical incision which contains the diseased area. The underlying subcutaneous fatty tissue is removed along with the large portion of excised skin. Vessels are clamped and tied off with sutures or are electrocoagulated to control bleeding. The resulting defect is usually closed in layers using separately reportable plastic techniques. Vaginal gauze packing may be placed in the vagina.

56625

The physician removes all of the vulva to treat premalignant or malignant lesions. A simple vulvectomy includes removal of all of the labia majora, labia minora, and clitoris. After examining the lower genital tract and the perianal skin with a colposcope, the physician makes two wide elliptical incisions encompassing the entire vulvar area. One elliptical incision extends from well above the clitoris around both labia majora to a point just in front of the anus. The second elliptical incision starts at a point between the clitoris and the opening of the urethra and is carried around both sides of the opening of the vagina. The underlying subcutaneous fatty tissue is removed along with the large portion of excised skin. Vessels are clamped and tied off with sutures or are electrocoagulated to control bleeding. The resulting sizable defect is usually closed in layers using separately reportable plastic techniques. Vaginal gauze packing may be placed in the vagina.

56630

The physician removes part of the vulva to treat malignancy. A partial radical vulvectomy includes partial or complete removal of a large, deep segment of skin from the following structures: abdomen and groin, labia majora, labia minora, clitoris, mons veneris, and terminal portions of the urethra, vagina, and other vulvar organs. Through incisions in the lower abdomen, thighs, and vulvar area, the physician removes skin, subcutaneous fatty tissue, and deeper tissue. Also included in the en bloc removal of tissue are portions of the saphenous veins and ligaments and the target lesion. The resulting large and disfiguring defect is usually closed using separately reported plastic surgical techniques, which may include pedicle flaps or free skin grafts. Subcutaneous rubber drains may be left in the surgical site, and vaginal gauze packing may be placed in the vagina.

56631

The physician removes part of the vulva to treat malignancy. A partial radical vulvectomy includes the partial or complete removal of a large, deep segment of skin and tissue from the following structures: abdomen and groin, labia majora, labia minora, clitoris, mons veneris, and terminal portions of the urethra, vagina, and other vulvar organs. Through incisions in the lower abdomen, thighs, and vulvar area, the physician removes skin, subcutaneous fatty tissue, and deeper tissue. The physician also removes superficial and deep inguinal lymph nodes and adjacent femoral lymph nodes on one side. Also included in the en bloc removal of tissue are portions of the saphenous veins and ligaments and the target lesion. The resulting large and disfiguring defect is usually closed in multiple layers using separately reported plastic surgical techniques, which may include pedicle flaps or free skin grafts. Subcutaneous rubber drains may be left in the surgical site, and vaginal gauze packing may be placed in the vagina.

56632

The physician removes part of the vulva to treat malignancy. A radical vulvectomy includes the partial or complete removal of a large, deep segment of skin and tissue from the following structures: abdomen and groin, labia majora, labia minora, clitoris, mons veneris, and terminal portions of the urethra, vagina, and other vulvar organs. Deep tissue from less than 80 percent of the vulva is removed. Through the lower abdomen, thighs, and the vulva, the physician removes skin, subcutaneous fatty tissue, and deeper tissue. The physician also removes superficial and deep inguinal lymph nodes and adjacent femoral lymph nodes on both sides. Also included in the en bloc removal of tissue are portions of the saphenous veins and ligaments and the target lesion. The resulting large and disfiguring defect is usually closed in multiple layers using separately reported plastic surgical techniques, which may include pedicle flaps or free skin grafts. Subcutaneous rubber drains may be left in the surgical site, and vaginal gauze packing may be placed in the vagina.

56633

The physician removes the vulva to treat malignancy. A complete radical vulvectomy includes the removal of a large, deep segment of skin and tissue from the following structures: abdomen and groin, labia majora, labia minora, clitoris, mons veneris, and terminal portions of the urethra, vagina, and other vulvar organs. Deep tissue from more than 80 percent of the vulva is excised. Through incisions in the lower abdomen, thighs, and vulvar area, the physician removes skin, subcutaneous fatty tissue, and deeper tissues. Also included in the en bloc removal of tissue are portions of the saphenous veins and ligaments and the target lesion. The resulting large and disfiguring defect is usually closed in multiple layers using separately reported plastic surgical techniques, which may include pedicle flaps or free skin grafts. Subcutaneous rubber drains may be used, and vaginal gauze packing may be placed in the vagina.

56634

The physician removes the vulva to treat malignancy. A complete radical vulvectomy includes the removal of a large, deep segment of skin and tissue from the following structures: lower abdomen and groin, labia majora, labia minora, clitoris, mons veneris, and terminal portions of the urethra, vagina, and other vulvar organs. Deep tissue from more than 80 percent of the vulva is removed. Through in the lower abdomen, thighs, and vulvar area, the physician removes skin, subcutaneous fatty tissue, and deeper tissues. The physician also removes the inguinal and femoral lymph nodes on one side. Also included in the en bloc removal of tissue are portions of the saphenous veins and ligaments and the target lesion. The resulting large and disfiguring defect is usually closed in multiple layers using separately reported plastic surgical techniques, which may include pedicle flaps or free skin grafts. Subcutaneous rubber drains may be used, and vaginal gauze packing may be placed in the vagina.

56637

The physician removes the vulva to treat malignancy. A complete radical vulvectomy includes the removal of a large, deep segment of skin and tissues from the following structures: lower abdomen and groin, labia majora, labia minora, clitoris, mons veneris, and terminal portions of the urethra, vagina, and other vulvar organs. Deep tissue from more than 80 percent of the vulva is removed. Through in the lower abdomen, thighs, and vulvar area, the physician removes skin, subcutaneous fatty tissue, and deeper tissues. The physician also removes the inguinal and femoral lymph nodes on both sides. Also included in the en bloc removal of tissue are portions of the saphenous veins and ligaments and the target lesion. The resulting large and disfiguring defect is usually closed in multiple layers using separately reported plastic surgical techniques, which may include pedicle flaps or free skin grafts. Subcutaneous rubber drains

may be used, and vaginal gauze packing may be placed in the vagina.

56640

The physician removes the vulva to treat malignancy. A complete radical vulvectomy includes the removal of a large, deep segment of skin and tissue from the following structures: lower abdomen and groin, labia majora, labia minora, clitoris, mons veneris, and terminal portions of the urethra, vagina, and other vulvar organs. Deep tissue from more than 80 percent of the vulva is removed. Through in the lower abdomen, thighs, and vulvar area, the physician removes skin, subcutaneous fatty tissue, and deeper tissue. The physician also removes the inguinal and femoral lymph nodes on both sides as well as the iliac and pelvic lymph nodes in the pelvic cavity, which is entered through an abdominal incision. Also included in the en bloc removal of tissue are portions of the saphenous veins and ligaments and the target lesion. The resulting large and disfiguring defect is usually closed in multiple layers using separately reported plastic surgical techniques, which may include pedicle flaps or free skin grafts. Subcutaneous rubber drains may be used, and vaginal gauze packing may be placed in the vagina.

56700

A hymen is a membrane that partially or wholly occludes the vaginal opening. Following local injection of an anesthetic, the physician excises a portion of the hymenal membrane. Using either a scalpel or scissors, the membrane is removed at its junction with the opening of the vagina. The cut margins of the vaginal mucosa are sutured with fine, absorbable material.

56720

A hymen is a membrane that partially or wholly occludes the vaginal opening. Following local injection of an anesthetic, the physician incises the hymenal membrane with a stellate (star-shaped) incision. This procedure is sometimes preceded by aspiration of the intact membrane with a needle and syringe.

56740

The physician removes a cystic Bartholin's gland, which lies at the tail end of the bulb of the vestibular opening just inside of the vagina. The physician makes an incision through the vaginal mucosa. The cyst is isolated through the vaginal incision by dissecting the deeper fatty tissues and excised. The remaining cavity and skin are closed in layers using absorbable material.

56800

The physician repairs and restores the anatomy of the opening of the vagina by excising scar tissue and strengthening the supporting tissues using tissue flaps and suturing techniques. This procedure varies greatly from patient to patient, depending on the defect to be corrected.

56805

The physician reduces the size of an enlarged clitoris, which has been masculinized by the production of male hormones from an abnormal adrenal gland. A portion of the body of the clitoris is resected with care to ensure preservation of vital nerves and blood vessels to the glans of the clitoris. The incisions are closed using plastic surgical techniques.

56810

With upward traction on the vagina, the physician makes an incision from the lower vaginal opening to a point just in front of the anus. The underlying weakened tissues are dissected and then repaired and tightened by suturing. This restores strength to the pelvic floor, closes tissue defects, and improves function of the perineal muscles.

57000

Colpotomy is an incision in the wall of the vagina, usually to access a recess between the rectum and uterus formed by a fold in the peritoneum (cul de sac). Through a speculum inserted in the vagina, the physician grasps the posterior lip of the cervix with a toothed instrument called a tenaculum. The cervix is lifted up exposing the posterior vaginal pouch. An incision is made through the back wall of the vagina into the posterior pelvic cavity. Through this opening, the pelvic cavity can be explored using instruments. After exploration, the physician closes the incision with absorbable sutures.

57010

Colpotomy is an incision in the wall of the vagina, usually to access a recess between the rectum and uterus formed by a fold in the peritoneum (cul de sac). Through a speculum inserted in the vagina, the physician grasps the posterior lip of the cervix with a toothed instrument called a tenaculum. The cervix is lifted up exposing the posterior vaginal pouch. An incision is made through the back wall of the vagina into the posterior pelvic cavity. Through this opening, the pelvic cavity can be explored. The abscess in the cavity is located, entered, and drained through the vaginal incision. Rubber drains are often inserted and left in place for several days. The physician closes the incision with absorbable sutures.

57020

Colpocentesis is the aspiration of fluid in the peritoneum through the wall of the vagina. Through a speculum inserted in the vagina, the physician grasps the posterior lip of the cervix with a toothed instrument called a tenaculum. The cervix is lifted up exposing the posterior vaginal pouch and deep back wall of the vagina. A long needle attached to a syringe is inserted through the exposed vaginal wall and the posterior pelvic cavity is entered. Fluid is then aspirated through the needle into the syringe.

57022–57023

The physician incises and drains a vaginal hematoma in an obstetrical or postpartum patient. The patient is placed in a dorso-lithotomy position. The physician inserts a sterile speculum into the vagina. The hematoma is visualized, and incised. Blood and clot are drained from the hematoma. Electrocautery or suture is used to control bleeding. When needed, a Hemovac drain is placed. The vagina is irrigated, and the area of hematoma is sponged with dressings. When hemostatis is achieved, the speculum is removed. Report 57022 when the procedure is performed on an obstetrical patient and 57023 when the procedure is performed on a non-obstetrical patient. Hemovac drains may be placed if the hematoma bed is still oozing.

57061–57065

Using a colposcope, which is a binocular microscope used for direct visualization of the vagina and cervix, the physician identifies lesion(s) in and/or around the vagina. The physician destroys the abnormal tissue by chemosurgery, electrosurgery, laser surgery, or cryotherapy. Use 57061 if the lesions are few in number, small, or simple. Use 57065 if the lesions are numerous, large, or difficult.

57100

The physician takes a sample of vaginal mucosa for examination. After injecting a local anesthetic into the area, the physician obtains a sample with a skin punch or sharp scalpel.

57105

The physician takes a sample of vaginal tissue for examination. After injecting a local anesthetic around a small suspicious area, the physician obtains a sample with a skin punch or sharp scalpel. This code should be used if the procedure is extensive and bleeding must be controlled with a clip or suture.

57106–57109

The physician excises part of the vagina. This is sometimes proceeded by injection of medication to constrict blood vessels to control bleeding. The vagina is everted and sizeable sections are removed by sharp and blunt dissection. In 57107, the physician removes surrounding diseased and/or damaged tissue. In 57109, the physician removes surrounding diseased and/or damaged tissue, in addition to removing the pelvic lymph nodes, and performing biopsy of the lymph nodes of the aorta to check for the extent of disease. Remaining vaginal and/or support tissue is inverted and sutured in place to obliterate some or all of the space formerly occupied by the vagina. The perineum is closed over the former vaginal opening.

57110–57112

The physician performs a complete removal of the vaginal wall. This is sometimes proceeded by injection of medication to constrict blood vessels to control bleeding. The vagina is everted. An incision circumscribes the hymen, and the vagina is marked into four quadrants. Each quadrant of vaginal wall is removed by sharp and blunt dissection. In 57111, the physician removes surrounding diseased and/or damaged tissue. In 57112, the physician removes surrounding diseased and/or damaged tissue, in addition to removing the pelvic lymph nodes, and performs biopsy of the lymph nodes the aorta to check for the extent of disease. The remaining support tissues are inverted and sutured in place obliterating the space formerly occupied by the vagina. The perineum is closed over the former vaginal opening.

57120

Under a local or general anesthesia, the physician grasps the deepest portion of the vaginal vault and everts the vagina. Two large flaps of vaginal wall are removed from opposite sides of the prolapsed vagina. The vaginal walls are sutured to one another and this structure is inverted back inside the body. The former vaginal opening is closed with sutures obliterating the vagina and preventing uterine prolapse.

57130

The physician excises a vaginal septum, an anomaly that separates the vagina into two portions. The septum can be longitudinal, creating two vaginal canals; or transverse, blocking the vagina and preventing menstrual flow. For a small, thin septum, the procedure is often done by injecting a local anesthetic in the tissues around the septum and then making an incision through the narrowest portion of the septum. The divided tissue is then tied off with suture material and the tissue is excised. For a thicker and more extensive septum, the procedure may be done under general anesthesia. The tissue is excised, and the resulting vaginal lining defects are closed. The vagina is packed with medicated gauze or a support device.

57135

Through a speculum inserted in the vagina, the physician uses a forceps or hemostat clamp to grasp and elongate the vaginal tissue containing the cyst or tumor, causing the mucosa to tent. With either a scalpel or scissors, the physician excises an ellipse of tissue containing the lesion. The defect is closed with absorbable sutures.

57150

The physician passes a catheter or similar tube high into the vaginal canal and flushes the canal with medicated solution from a large syringe. The physician also paints infected areas with medication using a cotton-tipped applicator or similar device.

57155

Preoperative radiation may be prescribed for patients who have endometrial cancer with major cervical involvement that precludes initial hysterectomy. Vaginal brachytherapy is administered using low-dose rate (LDR) or high-dose rate (HDR) radiotherapy. The upper half to two-thirds of the vagina is treated. HDR vaginal brachytherapy is delivered using intracavitary vaginal insertion with a Fletcher applicator, consisting of a uterine tandem and vaginal cylinders. HDR treatments require multiple insertions, generally with one insertion done every week for three to six weeks; hospitalization is not required, and each insertion takes only a brief amount of time. LDR treatments are delivered once but do require hospitalization for two to three days. Hysterectomy follows in four to six weeks.

57160

The physician inserts a pessary into the vagina. A pessary is a prosthesis that comes in different shapes and styles and is used to support the uterus, cervical stump, or hernias of the pelvic floor.

57170

The physician fits a diaphragm or cervical cap and provides instructions for use. A diaphragm is a device that acts as a mechanical barrier between the vagina and the cervical canal. Cervical caps are larger cup-like diaphragms placed over the cervix and held in place by suction. Either device is used to prevent pregnancy.

57180

The physician pushes gauze packing into the vagina to put pressure on bleeding. The packing may be coated with a chemical to make the blood clot stop hemorrhaging.

57200

The physician inserts a speculum into the vagina and identifies the extent of the vaginal laceration or wound. Usually a local anesthetic is used; however, some instances may require general anesthesia. The wound is closed with absorbable sutures.

57210

The physician inserts a speculum into the vagina and identifies the extent of the vaginal laceration or wound. Usually a local anesthetic is used; however, some instances may require general anesthesia. The vaginal wound is closed with sutures made of absorbable material. The speculum is removed and perineal laceration is closed in layers with sutures.

57220

The physician accesses the urethral sphincter from the vagina. With a catheter in the urethra, the physician dissects the midline vaginal wall separating it from the bladder and the proximal urethra. Sutures are placed at the junction of the bladder and urethra on each

CPT® Lay Descriptions

side of the urethra. This pushes up the urethrovesical junctions and supports the area. Excess vaginal tissue is excised and the vaginal wall is closed.

57230

The physician repairs a urethrocele, which is a sagging or prolapse of the urethra through its opening or a bulging of the posterior wall of the urethra into the vaginal canal. The prolapsed urethral tissue is excised from the meatus in a circular manner. The cut edges of urethral mucosa and vaginal mucosa are then sutured.

57240

The physician repairs a cystocele, which is a herniation of the bladder through its support tissues into the anterior vaginal wall causing it to bulge downward. The physician may also repair a urethrocele, which is a prolapse of the urethra. An incision is made from the apex of the vagina to within 1.0 cm of the urethral meatus. Plication sutures are placed along the urethral course from the meatus to the bladder neck. A suture is placed through the pubourethral ligament to the posterior symphysis pubis on each side of the urethra. The sutures are tied (ligated) and the posterior urethra is pulled upward to a retropubic position. If a cystococele is repaired, mattress sutures are placed in the mobilized paravesical tissue. The vaginal mucosa is closed.

57250

The physician repairs a rectocele by colporrhaphy. A rectocele is a protrusion of part of the rectum through its supporting tissues into the vagina causing a bulging in the vagina. Colporrhaphy involves a plastic repair of the vagina and the fibrous tissue separating the vagina and rectum. The physician makes a posterior midline incision that includes the perineum and posterior vaginal wall. In order to strengthen the area, the rectovaginal fascia are plicated by folding and tacking them, then they are closed with layered sutures. The physician may also perform a perineorrhapy, which is a plastic repair of the perineum, including midline approximation of the levator and perineal muscles. Excess fascia in the posterior vaginal wall is excised. The incisions are closed with sutures.

57260

The physician repairs both a cystocele and rectocele by colporrhaphy. Colporrhaphy involves a plastic repair of the vagina and the fibrous tissue separating the bladder, vagina, and rectum. A cystocele is a herniation of the bladder through its support tissues causing the anterior vaginal wall to bulge downward. A rectocele is a protrusion of part of the rectum through its support tissues causing the posterior vaginal wall to bulge. Using a combined vaginal approach and a posterior midline incision that includes the perineum and posterior vaginal wall, the physician dissects the tissues between the bladder,

urethra, vagina, and rectum. The specific tissue weaknesses are repaired and strengthened using tissue transfer techniques and layered and plication suturing. The physician may also repair a urethrocele, which is a prolapse of the urethra, and perform a perineorrhaphy, which is a plastic repair of the perineum, including midline approximation of the levator and perineal muscles. The incisions are closed with sutures.

57265

The physician repairs both a cystocele and rectocele by colporrhaphy. Colporrhaphy involves a plastic repair of the vagina and the fibrous tissue separating the bladder, vagina, and rectum. A cystocele is a herniation of the bladder through its support tissues causing the anterior vaginal wall to bulge downward. A rectocele is a protrusion of part of the rectum through its support tissues causing the posterior vaginal wall to bulge. Using a combined vaginal approach and a posterior midline incision that includes the perineum and posterior vaginal wall, the physician dissects the tissue between the bladder, urethra, vagina, and rectum. The specific tissue weaknesses are repaired and strengthened using tissue transfer techniques and layered and plication suturing. The physician also repairs an enterocele, which is a herniation of the bowel contents of the rectouterine pouch that protrudes into the septum of tissue either between the bladder and vagina or between the vagina and rectum. Through the vagina, the enterocele sac is incised and ligated and the uterosacral ligaments and endopelvic fascia anterior to the rectum are approximated. The physician may also repair a urethrocele, which is a prolapse of the urethra, and perform a perineorrhaphy, which is a plastic repair of the perineum, including midline approximation of the levator and perineal muscles. The incisions are closed with sutures.

57268

The physician repairs an enterocele, which is a herniation of the bowel contents of the rectouterine pouch that protrudes into the septum of tissue either between the bladder and vagina or between the vagina and rectum. Through the vagina, the physician incises and ligates the enterocele sac and approximates the uterosacral ligaments and endopelvic fascia anterior to the rectum. A vaginal hysterectomy, anterior (cystocele) and posterior (rectocele) colporrhaphy, and perineorrhaphy may also be performed to augment the support.

57270

The physician repairs an enterocele, which is a herniation of the bowel contents of the rectouterine pouch that protrudes into the septum of tissue either between the bladder and vagina or between the vagina and rectum. Through a lower abdominal wall incision, the physician incises and ligates the enterocele sac and approximates the uterosacral ligaments and endopelvic fascia anterior to the rectum. The abdominal incision is closed with sutures. A vaginal hysterectomy, anterior (cystocele) and posterior (rectocele) colporrhapy, and perineorrhaphy may also be performed to augment the support.

57280

Through a lower abdominal incision, the physician attaches the vault of the vagina to the prominent point of the sacrum. This is accomplished by suturing surgical fabric or a strip of abdominal wall fascia to the tissue in front of the internal sacral wall inside the pelvic cavity forming a bridge. The apex of the vagina is then firmly sutured to this bridge. This stabilizes the vaginal vault and prevents prolapse of the vagina. The abdominal incision is closed with sutures.

57282

Using a transvaginal approach, the physician makes an incision in the apex of the posterior vaginal wall and enters the space between the rectum and vagina. The prolapsed vaginal vault is sewn to the internal ligament between the sacrum and the right pelvic bone. The vaginal incision is closed with sutures.

57284

Using a vaginal approach, the physician dissects the tissues between the vagina and the bladder and urethra. The specific tissue weaknesses are found and then repaired and strengthened using tissue transfer techniques and plication suturing. The physician repairs a cystocele, (a herniation of the bladder through its support tissues into the anterior vaginal wall causing it to bulge downward). The physician then treats stress urinary incontinence and may also correct sagging and bulging (incomplete vaginal prolapse) of the area. These procedures help restore the normal anatomic relationships of the urethra, bladder, and vagina.

57287

The physician removes or revises a fascial or synthetic sling previously placed to correct urinary stress incontinence. To remove a sling, the physician makes a small abdominal skin incision to the level of the rectus fascia and releases the arm of the sling from the rectus abdominus. The physician releases the sling's attachment to the junction of the urethra via canals or tunnels formed by an instrument or a finger placed through a vertical or flap incision in the vaginal wall. In revision of a sling the physician may remove and partially or completely replace the sling using fascia or a synthetic graft through an abdominal and vaginal approach. The sling may be revised by increasing the tension on the sling using suture at one or both of the attachment sites at the junction of the urethra and/or to the rectus abdominus muscle. At the end of the procedure the area is irrigated, and hemostasis is achieved. The abdominal and/or vaginal incisions are closed with layered suture.

57288

Through vaginal and abdominal incisions, the physician places a sling under the junction of the urethra and bladder. The physician first places a catheter in the bladder, then makes an incision in the anterior wall of the vagina and folds and tacks the tissues around the urethra. A sling is formed out of synthetic material or from fascia harvested from the sheath of the rectus abdominus muscle. The loop end of the sling is sutured around the junction of the urethra. An incision is made in the lower abdomen and the ends of the sling are grasped with a clamp and pulled up into the incision and sutured to the rectus abdominus sheath. The abdominal and vaginal incisions are closed in layers by suturing.

57289

The physician makes an inverted U-shaped incision in the area between the vagina and the urethra. By blunt and sharp dissection, the physician creates an opening in the space on each side of the urethra as it passes into the bladder. Using a continuous suture for each side, the physician stitches the fascial tissues along the urethra to the urethrovesical junction. The physician then makes an incision in the abdomen above the pubis and, doing each side in turn, drives a special Pereyra ligature carrier through the tissues just lateral to the midline and takes it down to the sutured tissue. The sutures are threaded into the instrument and brought back through the abdominal incision. The urethrovesical junction is elevated by pulling up on the sutures and fixing them around the rectus abdominus muscle. In addition, the physician performs an anterior colporrhaphy using a vaginal approach, which corrects a cystocele and repairs the tissues between the vagina, bladder, and urethra.

57291

The physician develops a vagina by a program of perineal pressure using progressively longer and wider firm obturators. Pressure is applied to the soft area between the urethra and rectum with an obturator. Over several months of consistent, daily use by the patient, a sexually functional vagina can be created.

57292

The physician creates or enlarges the vagina using one or more skin grafts. Through a midline episiotomy incision, the physician creates a space between the urethra and rectum. Using either split thickness or full thickness skin grafts, the space is lined and the vagina created. An obturator or mold is inserted into the vagina and a catheter is passed into the bladder and left for several days. The full thickness skin donor sites are closed using plastic surgical techniques. The split thickness sites are dressed with medicated gauze.

57300

The physician closes a rectovaginal fistula, which is an abnormal passage between the rectum and the vagina. The physician also repairs the perineum, fascia, and muscle-supporting structures between the rectum and vagina. The scar tissue and tract between the rectum and vagina are excised and the clean edges sutured together. Often a flap of tissue is transplanted in between the vagina and the rectum and the area is closed in multiple layers. The rectal wall opening is closed by inverting the mucosa into the rectal canal. The vaginal wall opening is closed by inverting the mucosal layer into the vaginal wall. Sometimes the vaginal side is left open for drainage.

57305

Through a lower abdominal incision, the physician closes a rectovaginal fistula, which is an abnormal passage between the rectum and the vagina. The physician also repairs the perineum, fascia, and muscle-supporting structures between the rectum and vagina. The scar tissue and tract between the rectum and vagina are excised and the clean edges sutured together. Often a flap of tissue is transplanted in between the vagina and the rectum and the area is closed in multiple layers. The rectal wall opening is closed by inverting the mucosa into the rectal canal. The vaginal wall opening is closed by inverting the mucosal layer into the vaginal wall. Sometimes the vaginal side is left open for drainage. The abdominal incision is closed with sutures.

57307–57308

Through a lower abdominal incision, the physician closes a rectovaginal fistula, which is an abnormal passage between the rectum and vagina. The physician also repairs the perineum, fascia, and muscle-supporting structures between the rectum and vagina. The scar tissue and tract between the rectum and vagina are excised and the clean edges sutured together. Often a flap of tissue is transplanted in between the vagina and rectum and the area is closed in multiple layers. The rectal wall opening created during the excision is closed by inverting the mucosa into the rectal canal. The vaginal wall opening is closed by inverting the mucosal layer into the vaginal canal. Sometimes the vaginal side is left open for drainage. A transverse colostomy is also done to divert the flow of feces and to allow healing of the rectal colon repair. The abdominal incision is closed with sutures. Report 57308 if the physician takes a transperineal approach, reconstructing the perineal body, with or without a levator plication.

57310–57311

Through a vaginal speculum, the physician closes a urethrovaginal fistula, which is an abnormal passage between the urethra and vagina. With a catheter in the urethra, the fistula tract is excised and the defect in the urethra is sutured closed. A pad of fatty tissue is sutured between the repaired urethral defect and the vaginal defect in 57310. In 57311, a pad of fatty tissue and a strip of the bulbocavernosus muscle are brought through a tunnel created between the vagina and one labium. The fat and muscle flap are sutured

between the repaired urethral defect and the vaginal defect. In either case, the involved area in the vagina is excised and the defect is sutured closed using the healthy tissues. The catheter is left in place for several days to allow healing of the urethra.

57320

The physician closes a vesicovaginal fistula, which is an abnormal passage between the bladder and the vagina. This procedure is done through the vagina with catheters via the urethra into both ureters. The fistula and surrounding scar tissue of the vaginal wall are usually excised. The bladder wall is opened and the bladder interior is explored. The fistula is excised along with the surrounding tissue to assure preservation of only healthy tissue. The resulting defect is closed with sutures in multiple layers, starting with the bladder wall and ending with the vaginal mucosa. In some cases, a pedicle graft of tissue may be sutured in between the bladder and the vagina. A urethral or suprapubic catheter is left in the bladder to prevent distension of the bladder and tension to the sutured areas.

57330

The physician closes a vesicovaginal fistula, which is an abnormal passage between the bladder and the vagina. The procedure is done through the vagina and through the lower abdomen, with catheters through the urethra into both ureters. The physician opens the bladder wall through the lower abdominal incision and excises the fistula. The resulting defect is closed with sutures in multiple layers, starting with the bladder wall and ending with the abdominal wall. Through the vagina, the physician excises the fistula and surrounding scar tissue of the vaginal wall. In some cases, a pedicle graft of tissue may be sutured in between the bladder and the vagina. A urethral or suprapubic catheter is left in the bladder to prevent distension of the bladder and tension to the sutured areas.

57335

The physician uses various plastic surgical techniques to correct a small, underdeveloped vagina due to the overproduction of male hormones from the adrenal glands. The physician constructs a larger and more functional vagina using carefully placed incisions and skin grafts.

57400

Under general anesthesia, the physician enlarges the vagina by using a set of progressively longer and wider vaginal obturator dilators. The physician inserts the vaginal dilators sequentially from smaller to larger with firm and gentle pressure.

57410

The physician performs a manual examination of the vagina including the cervix, uterus, tubes, and ovaries. During the examination, the patient is under a general anesthesia because of the patient's inability to tolerate the procedure while awake.

57415

Using a vaginal speculum, the physician removes a foreign body that is lodged in the vagina. During the procedure, the patient is under general anesthesia because of the patient's inability to tolerate the procedure while awake as in the case of a young child or due to the type or size of the object being removed.

57452

The physician views the vagina through a colposcope, which is a binocular microscope used for direct visualization of the vagina and cervix.

57454

The physician views the vagina and cervix through a colposcope, which is a binocular microscope used for direct visualization of the vagina and cervix or performs endocervical curettage. The physician inserts a biopsy instrument through the vagina and takes one or more small biopsies of the cervix. In endocervical curettage the physician passes a curet or a suction tube through the cervix and endocervical canal, and into the uterus. The physician either suctions or gently scrapes the endometrial lining of the uterus. The instruments are removed.

57460

The physician views the vagina and cervix through a colposcope, which is a binocular microscope used for direct visualization of the vagina and cervix. A section of the cervix is removed with the loop electrosurgical excision procedure (LEEP), which uses a hot cautery wire to cut off a cone or section of cervical tissue and cauterize the area at the same time.

57500

The physician inserts a speculum into the vagina to view the cervix. A small cut is made in the cervix and biopsy forceps are used to remove a piece or multiple pieces of tissue, or to completely remove a lesion. Bleeding, usually minimal, may be stopped by electric current (fulguration).

57505

The physician inserts a speculum into the vagina to view the cervix. A small curet is used to scrape tissue from the endocervix, which is the region of the opening of the cervix into the uterine cavity.

57510–57513

The physician inserts a speculum into the vagina to view the cervix. For 57510, electric current or heat is used to destroy the outer layers of the cervix causing them to slough off. For 57511, the outer layers of the cervix are destroyed by freezing using a liquid such as carbon dioxide, freon, nitrous oxide, or nitrogen, or a low temperature instrument. The outer layers of the cervix slough off. This code can be used for either a

first-time or repeat procedure. For 57513, a laser is directed at the cervix to vaporize the outer cells.

57520–57522

The physician inserts a speculum into the vagina to view the cervix. A cone or slice of tissue including both endocervical and exocervical cells is then cut from the end of the cervix. Bleeding may be stopped by electric current. The cervix may need to be dilated if tissue is to be taken from farther up inside the uterus. The physician also may need to repair the incision by suturing, or by using any method of cautery (electro, thermal, cryocautery, laser). Report 57520 if a cold knife or laser is used. Report 57522 if a loop electrode is used to make the excision.

57530–57531

The physician inserts a speculum into the vagina to view the cervix. A tool is used to pull sown the cervix. A scalpel is then used to divide the cervix from the uterus just after it enters the vagina. The physician removes the cervix through the vagina and sops the bleeding with cautery. In 57531, the physician also removes the pelvic lymph nodes bilaterally, performs a para-aortic lymph node biopsy, and may remove a tube and/or ovary.

57540–57545

The physician makes an incision horizontally just within the pubic hairline. For 57540, the physician removes the cervical stump, which is the part of the cervix left after the supracervical uterus has been removed. The incision is closed by suturing. For 57545, the physician removes the cervical stump and repairs the muscular floor of the pelvis where the cervix rests using suture plication. This involves folding the tissues on top of each other and suturing. The incision is sutured.

57550

Through an incision at the apex of the vagina, the physician removes the cervical stump, which is the part of the cervix left after the supracervical uterus has been removed. The vaginal incision is closed with sutures.

57555–57556

Through an incision in the apex of the vagina, the physician removes the cervical stump. For code 57555, the physician also repairs the relaxed or herniated tissues in the front or back wall of the vagina. Through the vaginal incision, the physician dissects the tissues between the bladder, urethra, vagina, and rectum. The specific tissue weaknesses are repaired and strengthened using tissue transfer techniques and layered and plication suturing. The incisions are closed with sutures. For code 57556, the physician also repairs an enterocele, which is a herniation of the bowel contents of the rectouterine pouch. Through the vaginal incision, the physician incises and ligates the enterocele sac and approximates the uterosacral ligaments and endopelvic fascia anterior to the rectum. The incisions are closed with sutures.

57700

The physician inserts a speculum into the vagina to view the cervix. Heavy suture material or wire is threaded around the cervix and pulled tight to make the opening smaller.

57720

The physician inserts a speculum into the vagina to view the cervix. The physician performs a plastic suture repair of a laceration or wound on the cervix. A plastic repair also can encompass excising scar tissue or tightening an incompetent cervix.

57800

The physician inserts a speculum into the vagina to view the cervix. A tool is used to grasp the cervix and pull it down. A dilator or series of dilators is then inserted into the endocervix and passed up through the cervical canal.

57820

The physician inserts a speculum into the vagina to view the cervix. The physician enlarges the cervix using a dilator and scrapes tissue from the lining of the cervical stump, which is the part of the cervix left after removal of the uterus.

58100

The physician passes a small curet through the vagina into the endocervical canal. The physician may firmly stroke each of the four walls of the endocervical canal with the curet and/or may pass the curet into the uterus and scrape tissue from each of the four endometrial walls.

58120

The physician inserts a speculum into the vagina to view the cervix. A tool is used to grasp the cervix and pull it down. A dilator is then inserted into the endocervix and up through the cervical canal to enlarge the opening. The physician places a curet in the endocervical canal and passes it into the uterus. The entire endometrial lining of the uterus is thoroughly scraped on all sides to obtain tissue for diagnosis or to remove unhealthy tissue.

58140

Through a horizontal incision just below the top of the pubic hairline, the physician removes a leiomyomata or multiple leiomyomata from the wall of the uterus. The leiomyomata may be on the outside of the wall, within the wall, or on the inner surface of the uterine wall. The rectus muscles and the uterus are incised and the leiomyomata removed. The uterus is closed and the abdominal incision is sutured.

58145

The physician removes a leiomyomata or multiple leiomyomata from the uterus. The procedure is performed vaginally by dilating the cervix and passing a snare-like device into the uterus. The physician uses this device as a lasso to encircle the leiomyomata, cut it from its stalk, and remove it vaginally.

58150

Through a horizontal incision just within the pubic hairline, the physician removes the uterus including the cervix and may elect to remove one or both of the ovaries and one or both of the fallopian tubes (salpingo-oophorectomy). The supporting pedicles containing the tubes, ligaments, and arteries are clamped and cut free. The uterus and cervix are removed along with a narrow rim or cuff of vaginal lining. The vaginal defect is often left open for drainage. The abdominal incision is closed by suturing.

58152

Through a horizontal incision just within the pubic hairline, the physician removes the uterus including the cervix and may elect to remove one or both of the ovaries and one or both of the fallopian tubes (salpingo-oophorectomy). The supporting pedicles containing the tubes, ligaments, and arteries are clamped and cut free. The uterus and cervix are removed. The bladder neck is suspended by placing sutures through the tissue surrounding the urethra and into the back of the symphysis pubis, which is the midline junction of the pubic bones in the front (Marshall-Marchetti-Krantz). The sutures are pulled tight so that the tissues are tacked up to the symphysis pubis and the urethra is moved forward. The abdominal incision is then closed by suturing.

58180

Through a horizontal incision just within the pubic hairline, the physician removes the uterus above the cervix and may elect to remove one or both of the ovaries and one or both of the fallopian tubes (salpingo-oophorectomy). The supporting pedicles containing the tubes, ligaments, and arteries are clamped and cut free. The uterus is cut free from the cervix leaving the cervix still attached to the vagina. The abdominal incision is then closed by suturing.

58200

Through a horizontal incision just within the pubic hairline, the physician removes the entire uterus, including the cervix and part of the vagina. The supporting pedicles containing the tubes, ligaments and arteries are clamped and cut free and the uterus, cervix, and part of the vagina are removed. A sample or biopsy is taken of the para-aortic and pelvic lymph nodes. The physician may elect to remove one or both of the ovaries and one or both of the fallopian tubes (salpingo-oophorectomy). The abdominal incision is then closed by suturing.

58210

Through a horizontal incision just within the pubic hairline, the physician removes the uterus, including the cervix and the pelvic lymph nodes on both sides and takes a sample or biopsy of the para-aortic lymph nodes. The supporting pedicles containing the tubes, ligaments, and arteries are clamped and cut free and the uterus, cervix, all or part of the vagina, and the pelvic lymph nodes are removed. The physician may elect to remove one or both of the ovaries and one or both of the fallopian tubes (salpingo-oophorectomy). The abdominal incision is then closed by suturing.

58240

Through a horizontal incision just within the pubic hairline, the physician removes all of the organs and adjacent structures of the pelvis including the cervix, uterus, and all or part of the vagina. The supporting pedicles containing the tubes, ligaments, and arteries are clamped and cut free and the uterus, cervix, and all or part of the vagina are removed. The physician may remove one or both of the ovaries and one or both of the fallopian tubes (salpingo-oophorectomy). The physician removes the bladder and diverts urine flow by transplanting the ureters to the skin or colon. The rectum and part of the colon may be removed and an artificial abdominal opening in the skin surface created for waste (colostomy). The abdominal incision is closed by suturing.

58260

The physician removes the uterus and cervix through an incision in the vagina around the cervix. The uterus is pulled outward and downward exposing the supporting pedicles containing the tubes, ligaments, and arteries. The pedicles are clamped and cut free, and the uterus and cervix are removed through the vagina. The vaginal cuff is closed with sutures.

58262

Through an incision in the vagina around the cervix, the physician removes the uterus including the cervix and may elect to remove one or both of the ovaries and the fallopian tubes (salpingo-oophorectomy). The uterus is pulled outward and downward exposing the supporting pedicles containing the tubes, ligaments, and arteries. The pedicles are clamped and cut free, and the uterus, cervix, tube(s) and/or ovary(ies) are removed through the vagina. The vaginal cuff is closed with sutures.

58263

Through an incision in the vagina around the cervix, the physician removes the uterus including the cervix and may elect to remove one or both of the ovaries and the fallopian tubes (salpingo-oophorectomy). The uterus is pulled outward and downward exposing the supporting pedicles containing the tubes, ligaments, and arteries. The pedicles are clamped and cut free, and the uterus, cervix, and the tube(s) and/or ovary(ies) are removed through the vagina. The

enterocele, which is a hernia of the intestine that is protruding through the posterior vaginal wall, is also repaired. The hernia sac is excised and ligated, and the surrounding tissues are strengthened and sutured. The vaginal incision is closed with sutures.

58267

Through an incision in the vagina around the cervix, the physician removes the uterus including the cervix. The uterus is pulled outward and downward exposing the supporting pedicles containing the tubes, ligaments, and arteries. The pedicles are clamped and cut free, and the uterus and cervix are removed through the vagina. The bladder is suspended by threading several sutures through the tissue surrounding the urethra and into the vaginal wall. An endoscope may be placed in the bladder to ensure no sutures pass through the lining of the bladder. The sutures are then pulled tight so that the tissues are tacked up to the symphysis pubis, which is the midline junction of the pubic bones at the front, and the urethra is moved forward. The vaginal incision is closed with sutures.

58270

Through an incision in the vagina around the cervix, the physician removes the uterus, including the cervix. The uterus is pulled outward and downward exposing the supporting pedicles containing the tubes, ligaments, and arteries. The pedicles are clamped and cut free leaving the fallopian tubes and ovaries in the pelvic cavity. The uterus and cervix are removed. The physician also repairs the enterocele, which is a herniation of the bowel contents of the rectouterine pouch that protrudes into the septum of tissue either between the bladder and vagina or between the vagina and rectum. Through the vaginal incision, the physician incises and ligates the enterocele sac and approximates the uterosacral ligaments and endopelvic fascia anterior to the rectum. The incisions are closed with sutures.

58275

Through an incision in the vagina at some distance from the cervix, the physician removes the uterus including the cervix. The uterus is pulled outward and downward exposing the supporting pedicles containing the tubes, ligaments, and arteries. The pedicles are clamped and cut free leaving the fallopian tubes and ovaries in the pelvic cavity. The uterus, cervix, and a portion or all of the vagina are removed. This is sometimes preceded by injection of a medication to constrict blood vessels to control bleeding. After removing the uterus and cervix, the vagina is everted out through its opening and totally or partially removed by blunt and sharp dissection. The remaining vaginal tissue and support tissues are inverted into the resulting defect and are sutured in place, obliterating the space formerly occupied by the vagina. The perineum is closed over the vaginal opening.

58280

Through an incision in the vagina at some distance from the cervix, the physician removes the uterus, including the cervix and a portion of the vagina. The uterus is pulled outward and downward exposing the supporting pedicles containing the tubes, ligaments, and arteries. The pedicles are clamped and cut free leaving the fallopian tubes and ovaries in the pelvic cavity. The uterus, cervix, and a portion or all of the vagina are removed. This is sometimes preceded by injection of a medication to constrict blood vessels to control bleeding. After removing the uterus and cervix, the vagina is everted out through its opening and sizable sections are removed by blunt and sharp dissection. Any remaining vaginal tissue and support tissues are inverted into the resulting defect and are sutured in place. Through the vaginal incision, the physician incises and ligates the enterocele sac and approximates the uterosacral ligaments and endopelvic fascia anterior to the rectum. The incisions are closed with sutures.

58285

This is an extensive procedure where the physician removes the uterus, all immediately adjacent tissue, and the pelvic lymph nodes through an incision in the vagina around the cervix. The uterus is pulled outward and downward exposing the supporting pedicles containing the tubes, ligaments, and arteries. The pedicles are clamped and cut free, and the uterus and cervix are removed. The physician also removes the surrounding tissues, the pelvic lymph nodes, and part or all of the vagina. Any incisions are closed by suturing.

58300

The physician inserts a speculum into the vagina to visualize the cervix. A tool is used to gently pull down the cervix; then it is dilated. An intrauterine device (IUD), any of a variety of shapes (coil, loop, T, 7), is guided into the uterus through an insertion tube.

58301

The physician removes an intrauterine device (IUD), any of a variety of shapes (coil, loop, T, 7), from the uterus. A speculum is inserted into the vagina to visualize the cervix. The cervix is then dilated and a device is used to grasp and remove the IUD.

58321

The physician injects semen into the endocervical canal by applying the blunt tip of a plastic syringe to the external os (opening) of the cervix. Sometimes a cervical cap is used to keep the semen in and around the cervix for eight to 16 hours.

58322

The physician dilates the cervix and inserts a long plastic tube into the cavity of the uterus. Semen is then injected into the uterus by a syringe connected to the plastic tubing.

58323

Sperm are spun in a centrifuge that removes the superficial antibodies on the sperm in order to facilitate fertilization. The sperm are first washed in a medium three times the volume of the collected semen. This mixture is then spun in a centrifuge and the layer of liquid is discarded. The sperm are resuspended in a fresh medium. This method removes debris, bacteria, antibodies, and abnormal spermatazoa.

58340

A small catheter is introduced into the cervical opening and a saline or liquid radiographic contrast material is injected into the endometrial cavity with mild pressure to force the material into the fallopian tubes. The shadow of this contrast material on x-ray film permits examination of the uterus and tubes for any abnormalities or blockages. The physician may, instead, use an ultrasound unit to perform the same examination. Report radiology services separately, using 76831 for the hysterosonography and 74740 for hysterosalpingography.

58345

The physician introduces a catheter into the cervix, then takes it up into the uterus and through the fallopian tube. The catheter must be made of a material that will show up on x-ray film so that any blockages or abnormalities in the tube can be seen. The physician may elect to inject liquid radiographic contrast material into the endometrial cavity with mild pressure to force the material into the tubes. The shadow of this material on x-ray film permits examination of the uterus and tubes for any abnormalities or blockages. Report radiology services separately.

58346

Radiotherapy is often the prescribed treatment for patients who are medically inoperable for endometrial carcinoma. Brachytherapy is administered via low dose radiation (LDR) or high dose radiation (HDR) technique, with the goal of achieving coverage of the fundal region of the intact uterus. For low-dose treatment, Heyman capsules are used for patients with a large uterus to help expand the uterine cavity and cover the entire uterus. Heyman capsules also may be prescribed for patients with early-stage disease and low-grade histology, when radiation alone is the preferred therapy. Both an intrauterine intracavity insertion and external pelvic irradiation may be performed for patients with more advanced disease, a large uterus, or aggressive histology.

58350

The physician injects a liquid medication or saline solution into the uterine cavity and fallopian tubes.

This procedure is frequently performed during surgery open or laparoscopically verify patency of tubes.

58353

The physician performs an endometrial ablation, using heat without hysteroscopic guidance. The physician inserts a soft, flexible balloon attached to a thin catheter into the vagina through the cervix and into the uterus. The balloon is inflated with a sterile fluid, which expands to fit the size and shape of the patient's uterus. The fluid in the balloon is heated to 87°C or 188°F and maintained for eight to nine minutes while the uterine lining is treated. When the treatment cycle is complete, all the fluid is withdrawn from the balloon and the catheter is removed.

58400

The physician plicates the stretched broad ligaments that suspend the uterus, bringing it back into place. Plication shortens the ligament by folding and tacking it. The physician may elect to plicate the round and sacrouterine ligaments as well. This procedure may be done through a small abdominal incision or through the vagina.

58410

The physician plicates the stretched broad ligaments that suspend the uterus, bringing it back into place. Plication shortens the ligament by folding and tacking it. The physician may elect to plicate the round and sacrouterine ligaments as well. A portion of the presacral sympathetic nerve is removed or destroyed to alleviate pelvic pain. The procedure may be done through a small abdominal incision or through the vagina.

58520

The physician repairs a lacerated or ruptured uterus by suturing. A large incision is made in the abdomen and the uterus is sutured in multiple layers. The abdominal incision is then closed.

58540

Through a small incision in the lower abdomen, the physician performs a plastic repair of a malformed uterus. This often is an extensive procedure that involves removing abnormal tissues, rearranging the uterine walls, and suturing.

58550

The physician performs a surgical removal of the uterus through the vagina with the assistance of a laparoscope and possible removal of the ovary(s) and tube(s). The physician first inserts an instrument through the vagina to grasp the cervix and manipulate the uterus during surgery. Next, the physician makes a small incision just below the umbilicus through which a fiberoptic laparoscope is inserted. A second incision is made on the left or right side of the abdomen with additional instruments placed through these incisions into the abdomen or pelvis. The physician then manipulates the tools so the pelvic organs can be observed, manipulated and surgically excised through the laparoscope. The uterus, tubes, and ovaries are identified and freed through the laparoscope. The physician then makes an incision in the vaginal lining around the cervix. The uterus and cervix are freed and removed through the vagina. Additionally, the physician may remove one or both ovaries and tubes along with the uterus. The vaginal incision is sutured closed. The abdomen is then deflated, the trocars removed and the incisions are closed with sutures.

58551

The physician performs a laparoscopic surgical removal of a leiomyomata (uterine fibroid tumor) with the assistance of a laparoscope. The physician makes a small incision just below the umbilicus through which a fiberoptic laparoscope is inserted. A second incision is made on the left or right side of the abdomen with additional instruments being placed through these incisions into the abdomen or pelvis. The physician then manipulates the tools so that the pelvic organs can be observed. The uterus with its leiomyomata is identified. The uterus is incised and the fibroids mobilized. Through this incision, the physician removes the leiomyomata, single or multiple. The abdomen is deflated, the trocars removed and the abdominal incisions are closed with sutures.

58555

The physician performs a diagnostic inspection of the uerus using a hysteroscope. The physician advances the hysteroscope through the vagina and into the cervical os to gain entry into the uterine cavity. The physician inspects the uterine cavity with the fiberoptic scope for diagnostic purposes.

58558

The physician performs a diagnostic inspection of the uterus using a hysteroscope and may remove a uterine polyp take a uterine biopsy and perform cervical dilation and uterine curettage (D&C). The physician advances the hysteroscope through the vagina and into the cervical os to gain entry into the uterine cavity. The physician inspects the uterine cavity with the fiberoptic scope and removes a sample of the uterine lining and/or removes a growth (polypectomy) within the uterus and may perform a cervical dilation and uterine curettage, scraping (D&C) to take a complete sampling of the uterine lining.

58559

The physician removes scar tissue (adhesions) from within the uterus using a fiber optic hysteroscope. The physician advances the hysteroscope through the vagina and into the cervical os to gain entry into the uterine cavity. The physician inspects the uterine cavity with the fiberoptic scope and removes or divides adhesions (fibrous scar tissue) that are artificially connecting the walls of the uterus.

58560

The physician removes tissue abnormally dividing the intrauterine cavity using a fiber optic hysteroscope. The physician advances the hysteroscope through the vagina and into the cervical os to gain entry into the uterine cavity. The physician inspects the uterine cavity with the fiberoptic scope and resects an intrauterine septum (tissue creating an abnormal partition in the uterus).

58561

The physician surgically removes a leiomyomata (uterine fibroid tumor) with the assistance of a fiber optic hysteroscope. The physician advances the hysteroscope through the vagina and into the cervical os to gain entry into the uterine cavity. The physician inspects the uterine cavity with the fiberoptic scope and removes uterine leiomyomata with the assistance of the fiber optic scope.

58562

The physician surgically removes an impacted foreign body with the assistance of a fiber optic hysteroscope. The physician advances the hysteroscope through the vagina and into the cervical os to gain entry into the uterine cavity. The physician inspects the uterine cavity with the fiberoptic scope and removes an impacted foreign body from the uterine wall with the assistance of the hysteroscope.

58563

The physician surgically removes (ablates) the inner lining of the uterus with the assistance of a fiberoptic hysteroscope. The physician advances the hysteroscope through the vagina and into the cervical os to gain entry into the uterine cavity. The physician inspects the uterine cavity with the fiberoptic scope and ablates the endometrium by various methods, such as resection, electrosurgical ablation, or thermoablation.

58600

The physician ties off the fallopian tube or removes a portion of it on one side or both. The procedure may be done through the vagina or through a small incision just above the pubic hairline.

58605

The physician ties off the fallopian tube or removes a portion of it on one side or both. This procedure is done through a small incision just above the pubic hairline or vaginally during the same hospital stay as the delivery of a baby.

58611

The physician ties off the fallopian tube or removes a portion of it on one side or both. This procedure is done at the time of a cesarean section or during intra-abdominal surgery.

58615

The physician blocks one or both of the fallopian tubes with a band, clip, or Falope ring. The physician may elect to do the procedure through the vagina or through a small incision just above the pubic hairline.

58660

The physician performs a laparoscopic surgical cutting/releasing (lysis) of scar tissue (adhesions) surrounding the ovaries and/or fallopian tubes with the assistance of a fiber optic laparoscope. The physician may first insert an instrument through the vagina to grasp the cervix and manipulate the uterus during surgery. Next, the physician makes a small incision just below the umbilicus through which a fiberoptic laparoscope is inserted. A second incision is made on the left or right side of the abdomen with additional instruments being placed through these incisions into the abdomen or pelvis. The physician then manipulates the tools so that the pelvic organs can be observed, manipulated and lysis of adhesions can be performed. The abdomen is then deflated, the trocars removed and the incisions are closed with sutures.

58661

The physician performs a laparoscopic surgical removal of one or both ovaries and their accompanying fallopian tubes with the assistance of a fiber optic laparoscope. The physician may first insert an instrument through the vagina to grasp the cervix and manipulate the uterus during surgery. Next, the physician makes a small incision just below the umbilicus through which a fiberoptic laparoscope is inserted. A second incision is made on the left or right side of the abdomen with additional instruments being placed through these incisions into the abdomen or pelvis. The physician then manipulates the tools so that the pelvic organs can be observed, manipulated and removal of one or both ovaries and fallopian tubes can be performed with the laparoscope. The abdomen is then deflated, the trocars removed and the incisions are closed with sutures.

58662

The physician performs a laparoscopic electrical cautery destruction of an ovarian, pelvic or peritoneal lesion with the assistance of a fiber optic laparoscope. The physician may first inserts an instrument through the vagina to grasp the cervix and manipulate the uterus during surgery. Next, the physician makes a small incision just below the umbilicus through which a fiberoptic laparoscope is inserted. A second incision is made on the left or right side of the abdomen with additional instruments being placed through these incisions into the abdomen or pelvis. The physician then manipulates the tools so that the pelvic organs can be observed, manipulated and operated upon with the laparoscope. Once lesions are identified with the laparoscope third incision is typically made adjacent to the lesion through which an electric cautery tool, knife or laser is inserted for lesion fulguration. The abdomen is then deflated, the trocars removed and the incisions are closed with sutures.

58670

The physician performs a laparoscopic electrical cautery destruction of an oviduct (the uterine tube) with or without complete cutting through the fallopian tubes (transection) with the assistance of a fiber optic laparoscope. The physician may first inserts an instrument through the vagina to grasp the cervix and manipulate the uterus during surgery. Next, the physician makes a small incision just below the umbilicus through which a fiberoptic laparoscope is inserted. A second incision is made on the left or right side of the abdomen with additional instruments being placed through these incisions into the abdomen or pelvis. The physician then manipulates the tools so that the pelvic organs can be observed, manipulated and operated upon with the laparoscope. A third incision is typically made adjacent to the fallopian tubes. To fulgurate the fallopian tube the physician inserts either an electric cautery tool or a laser. The physician may cut the tubes and fulgurate or burn the ends. Additionally, the physician may transect (cut through) the fallopian tubes. The abdomen is then deflated, the trocars removed and the incisions are closed with sutures.

58671

The physician performs a laparoscopic occlusion of the oviduct (the uterine tube) with the assistance of a fiber optic laparoscope. The physician may first insert an instrument through the vagina to grasp the cervix and manipulate the uterus during surgery. Next, the physician makes a small incision just below the umbilicus through which a fiberoptic laparoscope is inserted. A second incision is made on the left or right side of the abdomen with additional instruments being placed through these incisions into the abdomen or pelvis. The physician then manipulates the tools so that the pelvic organs can be observed, manipulated and operated upon with the laparoscope. A third incision is typically made adjacent to the fallopian tubes. To occlude the fallopian tubes, the physician places silicone rings or clips around the tubes through this incision. The abdomen is then deflated, the trocars removed and the incisions are closed with sutures.

58672

The physician performs a laparoscopic surgical repair of the ovarian fimbria (fingerlike processes on the distal part of the infundibulum of the uterine tube) with the assistance of a fiber optic laparoscope. The physician may first insert an instrument through the

vagina to grasp the cervix and manipulate the uterus during surgery. Next, the physician makes a small incision just below the umbilicus through which a fiberoptic laparoscope is inserted. A second incision is made on the left or right side of the abdomen with additional instruments being placed through these incisions into the abdomen or pelvis. The physician then manipulates the tools so that the pelvic organs can be observed, manipulated and operated upon with the laparoscope. A third incision is typically made adjacent to the fallopian tubes. The physician performs surgical repair of the ovarian fimbria using instruments placed through the abdomen and pelvic trocars. The abdomen is then deflated, the trocars removed and the incisions are closed with sutures.

58673

The physician performs a laparoscopic surgical restoration of the patency of the uterine tube damaged typically by infection, tumor or endometriosis. The physician may first insert an instrument through the vagina to grasp the cervix and manipulate the uterus during surgery. Next, the physician makes a small incision just below the umbilicus through which a fiberoptic laparoscope is inserted. A second incision is made on the left or right side of the abdomen with additional instruments being placed through these incisions into the abdomen or pelvis. The physician then manipulates the tools so that the pelvic organs can be observed, manipulated and operated upon with the laparoscope. A third incision is typically made adjacent to the fallopian tubes. The physician performs surgical restoration of the fallopian tube (salpingostomy) using instruments placed through the abdomen and pelvic trocars. The abdomen is then deflated, the trocars removed and the incisions are closed with sutures.

58700

Through a small incision in the lower abdomen just above the pubic hairline, the physician removes part or all of the fallopian tube on one or both sides. The incision is closed by suturing.

58720

Through a small incision in the abdomen just above the pubic hairline, the physician removes part or all of the ovary and part or all of its fallopian tube on one or both sides. The incision is closed by suturing.

58740

The physician cuts free any fibrous tissue adhering to the ovaries or tubes through a small incision just above the pubic hairline.

58750

Through a small incision just above the pubic hairline, the physician excises the closed or blocked portion of the tube and sutures the clean edges together. The procedure is generally performed microsurgically in order to do an accurate repair.

58752

Through a small incision just above the pubic hairline, the physician removes a blocked portion of the tube near its junction with the uterus and reimplants the tube into the uterus in the same place.

58760

Through a small incision just above the pubic hairline, the physician reconstructs the existing fimbriae in a partially or totally obstructed (occluded) or closed off oviduct. Fimbriae are the hairlike fringes at the end of the fallopian tubes. Depending on the nature of the blockage, the physician may separate the fimbriae by gentle dilation or by electrosurgical dissection. The procedure is generally performed microsurgically in order to do an accurate repair.

58770

Through a small incision just above the pubic hairline, the physician creates a new opening in the fallopian tube where the fimbrial end has been closed by inflammation, infection, or injury. The procedure is generally performed microsurgically in order to do an accurate repair.

58800

The physician drains a cyst or cysts on one or both ovaries through an incision in the vagina. A cyst is a sac containing fluid or semisolid material. The cyst is ruptured with a surgical instrument, electrocautery, or a laser, and the fluid is removed.

58805

Through a small incision just above the pubic hairline, the physician drains a cyst or cysts on one or both ovaries. A cyst is a sac containing fluid or semisolid material. The cyst is ruptured with a surgical instrument, electrocautery, or a laser, and the fluid is removed.

58820

The physician drains an abscess (infection) on the ovary through an incision in the vagina. The abscess is drained, cleaned out, and irrigated with antibiotics. Temporary catheters and tubes are often left in place to help drainage.

58822

Through a small abdominal incision just above the pubic hairline, the physician drains an abscess (infection) on the ovary. The abscess is drained, cleaned out, and irrigated with antibiotics. Temporary catheters and tubes are often left in place to help drainage.

58823

The physician drains an abscess (infection) in the pelvis percutaneously. The abscess is drained, cleaned out, and irrigated with antibiotics. Temporary catheters and tubes are often left in place to help

drainage. For radiological supervision and interpretation, see 75989.

58825

The ovaries are placed behind the uterus and sutured in place prior to radiation therapy of the pelvis. The uterus acts as a shield protecting the ovaries from the radiation. The procedure is done through a small abdominal incision just above the pubic hairline.

58900

The physician takes a tissue sample from one or both ovaries for diagnosis. This procedure may be done through the vagina or abdominally through a small incision just above the pubic hairline.

58920

Through a small abdominal incision just above the pubic hairline, the physician takes a pie-shaped section or half of one or both of the ovaries to reduce the size and then sutures the edges together.

58925

Through a small abdominal incision just above the pubic hairline, the physician removes a cyst or cysts on one or both of the ovaries.

58940

Through a small abdominal incision just above the top of the pubic hairline, the physician removes part or all of one or both of the ovaries.

58943

Through a full abdominal incision extending from the top of the pubic hairline to the rib cage, the physician removes part or all of one or both ovaries depending on the extent of the malignancy. The physician takes a sampling of the lymph nodes surrounding the lower aorta within the pelvis and flushes the peritoneum, which is the lining of the abdominal cavity. The liquid is removed from the peritoneum to check for cancerous cells and multiple tissue samples are taken. The physician also examines and takes tissue samples of the diaphragm. The physician may elect to remove one or both fallopian tubes and the omentum. The abdominal incision is closed with layered suture.

58950

The physician resects an ovarian, tubal or primary peritoneal malignancy. Through a full abdominal, the physician removes both tubes, both ovaries and the omentum, which is an apron of peritoneum and fat that extends from the stomach to the transverse colon. The abdominal incision is closed with layered suture.

58951

Through a full abdominal incision extending from just above the pubic hairline to the rib cage. The physician treats an ovarian, tubal, or peritoneal malignancy by taking out both tubes, both ovaries, and the omentum, which is an apron of peritoneum and fat extending from the stomach to the transverse colon. The physician also removes the uterus, the pelvic lymph nodes, and a portion of the lymph nodes surrounding the lower aorta. The abdominal incision is closed with layered suture.

58952

Through a full abdominal incision extending from just above the pubic hairline to the rib cage, the physician treats an ovarian, tubal, or peritoneal malignancy by excising both tubes, both ovaries, the uterus, and the omentum, which is an apron of peritoneum and fat extending from the stomach to the transverse colon. The physician also reduces the size of a tumor that has grown large enough to cause discomfort or problems. Due to the size and location, it may not be possible to remove the entire tumor. The abdominal incision is closed with layered sutures.

58953–58954

Through a full abdominal incision extending from just above the pubic hairline to the rib cage, the physician treats an ovarian malignancy. Additionally, the physician may excise pelvic lymph nodes and partially remove par-aortic lymph nodes. In either procedure, the physician makes a full abdominal incision and carries dissection down to the abdominal cavity. The physician excises the fallopian tubes, both ovaries, the uterus and the omentum, an apron of peritoneum, and fat that extends from the stomach to the transverse colon. The physician removes (debulks) metastatic ovarian cancer implants from the abdominal cavity. In 58954, the physician additionally removes pelvic lymph nodes and a portion of the lymph nodes that surrounds the lower aorta within the pelvis. The abdominal incision is closed with layered suture.

58960

This procedure is the second operation to check for a recurrence of the ovarian malignancy. Through a full abdominal incision extending from just above the pubic hairline to the rib cage, the physician may elect to remove the omentum, which is an apron of peritoneum and fat that extends from the stomach to the transverse colon. The physician may flush the lining of the abdominal cavity (peritoneum) and remove the liquid to check for cancerous cells. A tissue sample of the abdominal and pelvic peritoneum may be taken. The physician also may examine and take tissue samples of the diaphragm. The pelvic lymph nodes are removed and a portion of the lymph nodes that surrounds the lower aorta within the pelvis is removed. The abdominal incision is closed with layered suture.

58970

The physician aspirates a mature or nearly mature egg from its follicle for in vitro fertilization. Visualization of the aspiration may be done laparoscopically or by ultrasound. The laparoscopic method uses three puncture sites in the lower abdomen — one for the laparoscope, one for the holding forceps, and one for the aspirating needle. The ultrasound guided technique involves using a transabdominal ultrasound transducer for guidance. The aspirating needle is either passed through the bladder wall to the ovary or through the urethra and then into the pelvic cavity. Another ultrasound method uses transvaginal ultrasound and transvaginal needle aspiration of the ovary. In all methods, the ovary and preovulatory follicle are visualized and then punctured with a needle to withdraw the follicular fluid containing the egg.

58974

After approximately 48 hours to 72 hours of laboratory culture, the physician places the fertilized eggs in the uterus. The embryos are aspirated into a small catheter. The catheter is passed through the cervix and into the uterus. The eggs are then injected into the uterus.

58976

In a gamete intrafallopian transfer (GIFT), the physician mixes previously captured eggs with sperm and draws the mixture into a catheter. The catheter is then either passed through the cervix and uterus and into the tubes or through an abdominal incision and directly into the fimbrial end of the fallopian tube. The physician deposits the eggs and sperm in the tubes, permitting fertilization. In a zygote intrafallopian transfer (ZIFT), a physician draws an already fertilized egg up into a catheter. The catheter is then passed through the cervix and uterus and into the tube where the egg is deposited. GIFT is a one-step procedure while ZIFT is a two-step process. In ZIFT, the egg is collected and fertilized then transferred to the fallopian tube at a later time. GIFT and ZIFT can be done laparoscopically or hysteroscopically.

59000

Using ultrasonic guidance, the physician inserts an amniocentesis needle through the abdominal wall into the interior of the pregnant uterus and directly into the amniotic sac to collect amniotic fluid for diagnostic analysis. Amniocentesis is usually done between 16 weeks and 18 weeks of gestation, but it can be performed as early as 12 weeks and up to term.

59001

The physician performs a therapeutic amniotic fluid reduction. Using ultrasonic guidance, the physician inserts an 18- or 20-guage amniocentesis needle through the abdominal wall into the interior of the pregnant uterus and directly into the amniotic sac to remove excess levels of amniotic fluid (amnioreduction). Serial amniotic fluid volume reduction may be accomplished on an ongoing basis by repeating the procedure. The amount of fluid drained at a single procedure can range from one liter to seven liters.

59012

Using ultrasonic guidance, the physician inserts an amniocentesis needle through the abdominal wall into the cavity of the pregnant uterus and into the umbilical vessels to obtain fetal blood. It may be accomplished with a transplacental or transamniotic approach. This procedure is done in the second or third trimester.

59015

This procedure uses ultrasonic guidance and can be done by any one of three methods. In the transcervical method, the physician inserts a sterile catheter through the cervix and into the uterine cavity toward the placental site. A sample of the placenta (chorionic villus) is aspirated to obtain placental cells for analysis for chromosomal abnormalities. The procedure may also be performed transvaginally or transabdominally. The transabdominal approach can be performed throughout pregnancy. The other approaches are usually done between nine and 12 weeks of gestation.

59020

The physician applies external fetal monitors to the maternal abdominal wall. Pitocin is given intravenously to the mother to cause uterine contractions. The fetal heart rate and uterine contractions are monitored and recorded for 20 minutes to determine the effects on the fetus. This procedure is usually performed during the third trimester.

59025

The patient reports fetal movements as an external monitor records fetal heart rate changes. The procedure is noninvasive and takes 20 to 40 minutes to perform.

59030

This test, which assesses fetal distress during labor, must be done when the cervix is dilated more than 2.0 cm and the fetal vertex is low in the pelvis. The physician breaks the amniotic sac in patients whose water has not broken spontaneously and inserts an amnioscope through the vagina. The fetal scalp is wiped clean. An incision is made in the scalp with a special narrow blade that penetrates no more than 2.0 mm. Blood is aspirated into a heparinized capillary tube. The incision must be closely watched to ensure bleeding stops.

59050–59051

In 59050, a consultant other than the attending physician attaches an electrode directly to the presenting fetus' scalp via the cervix. The electrocardiographic impulses are then transmitted to a cardiotachometer which converts the fetal electrocardiographic pattern into recorded electronic impulses. A catheter is inserted through the dilated cervix into the amniotic sac to measure and record the intervals between contractions. The procedure is supervised during labor until delivery. The recordings are analyzed and accompanied by an interpretive written report. In 59051, the consultant initiates the monitoring, provides the analysis and interpretive report, but does not supervise the patient during labor.

59100

The physician removes an embryo or hydatidiform mole through an incision in the abdominal wall and uterus. The surgery is similar to a cesarean section but the abdominal and uterine incisions are smaller. First, the lower abdominal wall is opened with either a vertical or horizontal incision, and then the uterus is entered through the lower uterine segment. The physician removes the embryo or hydatidiform mole and may also remove any remaining membranes and placenta from the uterine cavity. Curettage of the uterine cavity may also be performed. The abdominal and uterine incisions are closed by suturing.

59120

The physician treats a tubal or ovarian ectopic pregnancy by removing the fallopian tube and/or ovary. Through the vagina or through an incision in the lower abdomen, the physician explores the pelvic cavity, inspects the gestation site for bleeding, and removes all products of conception, clots, and free blood. If the tube is affected, it may be excised by cutting a small wedge of the uterine wall at the junction of the fallopian tube and body of the uterus. If the ovary is affected, it may be removed. Lysis of adhesions may be indicated and the pelvis lavaged with saline solution. If an abdominal approach is used, the incision is closed with sutures.

59121

The physician treats a tubal or ovarian ectopic pregnancy by removing the embryo from the tube or ovary. Through an incision in the lower abdomen, the physician explores the pelvic cavity, inspects the gestation site for bleeding, and removes all products of conception, clots, and free blood. If the embryo is implanted in the fallopian tube, the physician may do one of the following: manually remove the embryo from the tube, make an incision to remove the embryo, or excise the section of the tube containing the embryo. If the embryo is implanted in the ovary, the physician resects the ovary to remove the embryo. Lysis of adhesions may be indicated and the pelvis lavaged with saline solution. The incision is closed with sutures.

59130

The physician removes an embryo or fetus implanted in the abdomen. The fertilized ovum may have implanted directly in the abdomen (primary) or it may have implanted after escaping from the tube through a rupture or through the fimbriated end (secondary). After making an abdominal incision, the physician surgically removes the fetus from the abdomen. The membranes are also removed and the cord is ligated near the placenta. The placenta is usually not removed unless attached to the fallopian tube, ovary, or uterine broad ligament. Abdominal lavage may also be indicated. The abdominal incision is then closed with sutures. Although this procedure is rare, it can be done any time during gestation, even at or near term.

59135

The physician treats an interstitial pregnancy where the fertilized ovum has implanted in the portion of the tube that transverses the uterine wall by removing the uterus and cervix. Through an incision extending from just above the pubic hairline to the rib cage, the physician clamps and cuts free the supporting pedicles containing the tubes, ligaments, and arteries. The physician then removes the uterus and cervix and may elect to remove the tubes and/or ovaries. Abdominal or pelvic lavage may also be indicated. The abdominal incision is closed with sutures.

59136

The physician treats an interstitial ectopic pregnancy where the fertilized ovum has implanted in the portion of the tube that transverses the uterine wall by partially resecting the uterus. Through an incision extending from just above the pubic hairline to the rib cage, the physician resects then reconstructs the uterine wall. The physician may also remove a portion or all of the fallopian tube. Abdominal or pelvic lavage may be indicated. The abdominal incision is closed with sutures.

59140

The physician treats an ectopic pregnancy where the embryo has implanted in the cervix. If the pregnancy is less than 12 weeks gestation, the physician usually removes the embryo through the vagina. The physician ligates the hypogastric arteries or the cervical branches of the uterus to control bleeding. Curettage of the endocervix and endometrium may stop heavy bleeding. Sutures and gauze packing may also be necessary. If later than 12 weeks gestation, the physician may treat the cervical pregnancy by performing an abdominal hysterectomy. Through a horizontal incision just within the pubic hairline, the physician clamps and cuts free the supporting pedicles containing the tubes, ligaments, and arteries. The uterus is removed above the cervix, and the incision is closed by suturing.

59150

The physician treats an ectopic pregnancy by laparoscopy without salpingectomy and/or oophorectomy. The physician inserts an instrument through the vagina to grasp the cervix while passing another instrument through the cervix and into the uterus to manipulate the uterus. Next, the physician makes a 1.0 cm incision in the umbilicus through which the abdomen is inflated and a fiberoptic laparoscope is inserted. A second incision is made on the left or right side of the abdomen. After locating the site of the gestation, another small incision is made above the site. Instruments are then passed into the abdomen through the incisions. The physician removes the ectopic pregnancy by making an incision in the tube or ovary or by segmental excision. The abdominal incisions are then closed with sutures.

59151

The physician treats an ectopic pregnancy by laparoscopy with salpingectomy and/or oophorectomy. The physician inserts an instrument through the vagina to grasp the cervix while passing another instrument through the cervix and into the uterus to manipulate the uterus. Next, the physician makes a 1.0 cm incision in the umbilicus through which the abdomen is inflated and a fiberoptic laparoscope is inserted. A second incision is made on the left or right side of the abdomen. After locating the site of the gestation, another small incision is made above the site. Instruments are then passed into the abdomen through the incisions. The physician removes the tube and/or ovary containing the embryo and closes the abdominal incisions with sutures.

59160

The physician scrapes the endometrial lining of the uterus following childbirth. The physician passes a curet through the cervix and endocervical canal, and into the uterus. Due to the large, soft postpartum uterus that is especially susceptible to perforation, a large blunt curet, also known as a "banjo" curet, is preferable to the suction curet. The physician gently scrapes the endometrial lining of the uterus to control bleeding, treat obstetric lacerations, or remove any remaining placental tissue.

59200

The physician inserts a cervical dilator, such as a laminaria or prostaglandin, into the endocervix to chemically stimulate and dilate the cervical canal. Using a speculum, the physician views the cervix then uses a tool to grasp it and pull it down. A laminaria, which is a sterile applicator made of kelp or synthetic material, may be placed in the cervical canal where it absorbs moisture, swells, and gradually dilates the cervix prior to inducing labor. Or the physician may insert prostaglandin in the form of gel or suppositories into the cervix in order to prime it six to 12 hours before induction.

59300

A physician other than the physician who performed the delivery repairs an episiotomy or a vaginal tear or laceration. To repair an episiotomy, the physician sutures an incision made in the external genital area to widen the vulvar opening, avoid tearing, and permit easier passage of the fetus. To repair a vaginal tear, the physician approximates and sutures any vaginal tears or lacerations resulting from delivery.

59320

The physician threads suture material or wraps banding around the cervix to close an incompetent cervix. An incompetent cervix is one that dilates during the second trimester and will eventually allow the pregnancy to fall out. After inserting a speculum into the vagina to view the cervix, heavy suture material or wire is threaded around the cervix using purse-string sutures. The sutures are pulled tight to make the opening smaller and prevent spontaneous abortion.

59325

Through a small abdominal incision just above the pubic hairline, the physician places a band around the cervix at the level of the internal os (opening) to make the cervical opening smaller and prevent spontaneous abortion from an incompetent cervix. An incompetent cervix is one that dilates during the second trimester and will eventually allow the pregnancy to fall out. The abdominal incision is then closed with sutures.

59350

The physician repairs a uterus that is lacerated or ruptured during pregnancy. A large incision is made in the abdomen and the uterus is sutured in multiple layers. The abdominal incision is then closed with sutures.

59400

The physician delivers an infant and placenta through the uterus and vagina. The physician may elect to assist the delivery with the use of forceps, vacuum extraction, or rupture of membranes. The physician may also elect to do an episiotomy, which is an incision in the perineum to widen the external opening. Episiotomy and laceration repair are included as well. This procedure covers both antepartum and postpartum care. Antepartum or prenatal care includes the initial and subsequent histories, physical examinations, recording of weight, blood pressures, fetal heart tones, and routine chemical urinalysis. It includes monthly visits up to 28 weeks gestation, biweekly visits to 36 weeks gestation, and weekly visits until delivery. Postpartum care includes hospital and office visits following delivery.

59409

The physician delivers an infant and placenta through the uterus and vagina. The physician may elect to assist the delivery with the use of forceps, vacuum extraction, or rupture of membranes. The physician may also elect to do an episiotomy, which is an incision in the perineum to widen the external opening. Episiotomy and laceration repair are included as well.

59410

The physician delivers an infant and placenta through the uterus and vagina. The physician may elect to assist the delivery with the use of forceps, vacuum extraction, or rupture of membranes. The physician may also elect to do an episiotomy, which is an incision in the perineum to widen the external opening. Episiotomy and laceration repair are included as well. This procedure also covers postpartum care, which includes hospital and office visits following delivery.

59412

The physician turns the fetus from a breech presenting position to a cephalic presenting position. External cephalic version is performed by manipulating the fetus from the outside of the abdominal wall. The physician places both hands on the patient's abdomen and locates each pole of the fetus by palpation. The fetus is then shifted so that the breech or rear end of the fetus is moved upward and the head downward. The physician may elect to use tocolytic drug therapy to suppress uterine contractions during the manipulation.

59414

The physician removes a retained placenta following delivery of the fetus, usually unattended, and after separation of the placenta from its intrauterine attachment. The physician places abdominal pressure just above the symphysis to elevate the uterus into the abdomen and prevent inversion of the uterus. This also helps move the placenta downward into the vagina. The umbilical cord is then very gently pulled to help guide the placenta out of the birth canal. If the placenta cannot be removed by this technique or there is brisk bleeding, manual removal of the placenta may be indicated. Manual removal requires adequate analgesia or anesthesia. It is accomplished by grasping the fundus of the uterus with a hand on the abdomen. The other hand, wearing an elbow-length glove, is passed up through the vagina into the uterus to separate the placenta and then remove it.

59425–59426

Antepartum or prenatal care includes the initial and subsequent histories, physical examinations, recording of weight, blood pressures, fetal heart tones, and routine chemical urinalysis. It includes monthly visits up to 28 weeks gestation, biweekly visits to 36 weeks gestation, and weekly visits until delivery. 59425 includes four to six visits. 59426 covers seven or more visits.

59430

Postpartum care includes hospital and office visits following vaginal or cesarean section delivery.

59510

The physician delivers an infant through a horizontal or vertical incision in the abdomen and uterus. Once the incisions are made, the infant is delivered and the placenta separated and removed. The uterine and abdominal incisions are then closed with sutures. This procedure includes both antepartum and postpartum care. Antepartum or prenatal care includes the initial and subsequent histories, physical examinations, recording of weight, blood pressures, fetal heart tones, and routine chemical urinalysis. It includes monthly visits up to 28 weeks gestation, biweekly visits to 36 weeks gestation, and weekly visits until delivery. Postpartum care includes hospital and office visits following delivery.

59514

The physician delivers an infant through a horizontal or vertical incision in the abdomen and uterus. Once the incisions are made, the infant is delivered and the placenta separated and removed. The uterine and abdominal incisions are then closed with sutures.

59515

The physician delivers an infant through a horizontal or vertical incision in the abdomen and uterus. Once the incisions are made, the infant is delivered and the placenta separated and removed. The uterine and abdominal incisions are then closed with sutures. This procedure includes postpartum care, which consists of hospital and office visits following delivery.

59525

The physician performs a hysterectomy immediately following cesarean delivery. Through the abdominal incision, the physician clamps and cuts free the supporting pedicles containing the tubes, ligaments, and arteries. The uterus is removed and the physician may elect to remove the cervix as well. In a subtotal hysterectomy, just the uterus is removed. In a total hysterectomy, both the uterus and cervix are removed. The abdominal incision is closed with sutures.

59610

The physician delivers an infant and placenta through the vagina. The patient has previously delivered by cesarean section. The physician may elect to assist the delivery with the use of forceps, vacuum extraction, or rupture of membranes. The physician may also elect to do an episiotomy, which is an incision in the perineum to widen the external opening. Episiotomy and laceration repair are included as well. This procedure covers both antepartum and postpartum care. Antepartum or prenatal care includes the initial and subsequent histories, physical examinations, recording of weight, blood pressures, fetal heart tones, and routine chemical urinalysis. It includes monthly visits up to 28 weeks gestation, biweekly visits to 36 weeks gestation, and weekly visits until delivery (approximately 12-15 visits). Because of the previous cesarean delivery, the physician monitors the patient

carefully during labor and delivery. Postpartum care includes hospital and office visits following delivery.

59612–59614

The physician delivers an infant and placenta through the vagina. The patient has previously delivered by cesarean section. The physician may elect to assist the delivery with the use of forceps. The physician may also elect to do an episiotomy, which is an incision in the perineum to widen the external opening. Episiotomy and laceration repair are included. Because of the previous cesaren delivery, the physician monitors the patient carefully during labor and delivery. Code 59614 includes postpartum care, hospital office visits following delivery.

59618

After first attempting a vaginal delivery, the physician delivers an infant through a horizontal or vertical incision in the abdomen and uterus. The patient has previously delivered by cesarean section. Once the incisions are made, the infant is delivered and the placenta separated and removed. The uterine and abdominal incisions are then closed with layered sutures. This procedure includes both antepartum and postpartum care. Antepartum or prenatal care includes the initial and subsequent histories, physical examinations, recording of weight, blood pressures, fetal heart tones, and routine chemical urinalysis. It includes monthly visits up to 28 weeks gestation, biweekly visits to 36 weeks gestation, and weekly visits until delivery (approximately 13-15 visits). Because of the previous cesarean delivery and the attempted vaginal delivery, the physician monitors the patient carefully during labor and delivery. Postpartum care includes hospital and office visits following delivery.

59620–59622

After first attempting a vaginal delivery, the physician delivers an infant through a horizontal or vertical incision in the abdomen and uterus. The patient has previously delivered by cesarean section. Once the incisions are made, the infant is delivered and the placenta separated and removed. The uterine and abdominal incisions are then closed with layered sutures because of the previous cesarean delivery and the attempted vaginal delivery, the physician monitors the patient carefully during labor and delivery. Only delivery is included in 59620. Postpartum care is included in 59622. Postpartum care includes hospital and office visits following delivery.

59812

The physician removes the products of conception remaining after an incomplete spontaneous abortion in any trimester. To evacuate the uterus, the physician performs a dilation and suction curettage. The physician inserts a speculum into the vagina to view the cervix. A tenaculum is used to grasp the cervix, pull it down, and exert traction. If the cervix is not sufficiently dilated, a dilator is then inserted into the endocervix and up through the cervical canal to enlarge the opening. The physician places a cannula in the endocervical canal and passes it into the uterus. The suction machine is then activated and the uterine contents are evacuated by rotation of the cannula. After suction curettage, a sharp curet may be used to gently scrape the uterus to ensure that it is empty.

59820

The physician treats a missed abortion in the first trimester by suction curettage. In missed abortion, the fetus remains in the uterus four to eight weeks following its death. Ultrasonography may be needed to determine the size of the fetus prior to the procedure. The physician inserts a speculum into the vagina to view the cervix. A tenaculum is used to grasp the cervix, pull it down, and exert traction. A dilator is then inserted into the endocervix and up through the cervical canal to enlarge the opening. The physician places a cannula in the endocervical canal and passes it into the uterus. The suction machine is then activated and the uterine contents are evacuated by rotation of the cannula. After suction curettage, a sharp curet may be used to gently scrape the uterus to ensure that it is empty.

59821

The physician treats a missed abortion in the second trimester by suction curettage. Ultrasonography may be needed to determine the size of the fetus prior to the procedure. The physician inserts a speculum into the vagina to view the cervix. A tenaculum is used to grasp the cervix, pull it down, and exert traction. A dilator is then inserted into the endocervix and up through the cervical canal to enlarge the opening. The physician places a cannula in the endocervical canal and passes it into the uterus. The suction machine is then activated and the uterine contents are evacuated by rotation of the cannula. After suction curettage, a sharp curet may be used to gently scrape the uterus to ensure that it is empty.

59830

The physician treats a septic abortion with prompt evacuation of the uterus and vigorous medical treatment of the patient. A septic abortion is one complicated by generalized fever and infection. There is also inflammation and infection of the endometrium and in the cellular tissue around the uterus. The physician treats the infection with intravenous antibiotics and blood transfusions as necessary. To evacuate the uterus, the physician inserts a speculum into the vagina to view the cervix. A tenaculum is used to grasp the cervix, pull it down, and exert traction. A dilator is then inserted into the endocervix and up through the cervical canal to enlarge the opening. The physician places a cannula in the endocervical canal and passes it into the uterus. The suction machine is then activated and the uterine contents are evacuated by rotation of the cannula.

After suction curettage, a sharp curet may be used to gently scrape the uterus to ensure that it is empty.

59840

The physician terminates a pregnancy by dilation and curettage. The physician inserts a speculum into the vagina to view the cervix. A tenaculum is used to grasp the cervix, pull it down, and exert traction. A dilator is then inserted into the endocervix and up through the cervical canal to enlarge the opening. The physician places a curet in the endocervical canal and passes it into the uterus. The uterine contents are removed by rotating the curet and gently scraping the uterus until all the products of conception are removed.

59841

The physician terminates a pregnancy by dilation and evacuation (D&E). Because D&E requires wider cervical dilation than curettage, the physician may dilate the cervix with a laminaria several hours to several days before the procedure. At the time of the procedure, the physician inserts a speculum into the vagina to view the cervix. A tenaculum is used to grasp the cervix, pull it down, and exert traction. The physician places a cannula in the dilated endocervical canal and passes it into the uterus. The suction machine is then activated and the uterine contents are evacuated by rotation of the cannula. For pregnancies through 16 weeks, the cannula will usually evacuate the pregnancy. For later pregnancies, the cannula is used to drain amniotic fluid and to draw tissue into the lower uterus for extraction by forceps. In either case, a sharp curet may be used to gently scrape the uterus to ensure that it is empty.

59850

The physician terminates a pregnancy by inducing labor with amniocentesis and intra-amniotic injections. This method is usually used after the first trimester (13 weeks or more). The physician inserts an amniocentesis needle into the abdomen to obtain a free flow of clear amniotic fluid. A hypertonic solution is then administered by gravity drip. The hypertonic solution results in fetal death and labor usually results. The fetus and placenta are then delivered through the vagina.

59851

The physician begins the termination of a pregnancy by inducing labor with amniocentesis and intra-amniotic injections. This method is usually used after the first trimester (13 weeks or more). The physician inserts an amniocentesis needle into the abdomen to obtain a free flow of clear amniotic fluid. A hypertonic solution is then administered by gravity drip. The hypertonic solution results in fetal death and labor usually results. 59851 is used when this method fails to expel all products of conception, and a dilation and curettage and/or evacuation is used to remove the remaining tissue.

59852

The physician begins the termination of a pregnancy by inducing labor with amniocentesis and intra-amniotic injections. This method is usually used after the first trimester (13 weeks or more). The physician inserts an amniocentesis needle into the abdomen to obtain a free flow of clear amniotic fluid. A hypertonic solution is then administered by gravity drip. The hypertonic solution results in fetal death and labor usually results. 59852 is used when this method fails to expel all products of conception, and a hysterotomy, through an incision in the abdominal wall and uterus, is used to remove the remaining tissue. Following removal, the incision is closed with sutures.

59855

The physician terminates a pregnancy by inducing labor with vaginal suppositories. Before using the suppositories, a laminaria, which is an applicator made of kelp or synthetic material, may be inserted in the cervix to soften and expand the cervical canal. Once the cervix is ready, the physician inserts the vaginal suppositories and labor usually results. The fetus and placenta are then delivered through the vagina.

59856

The physician begins the termination of a pregnancy by inducing labor with vaginal suppositories. Before using the suppositories, a laminaria, which is an applicator made of kelp or synthetic material, may be inserted in the cervix to soften and expand the cervical canal. Once the cervix is ready, the physician inserts the vaginal suppositories and labor usually results. 59856 is used when this method fails to expel all products of conception, and a dilation and curettage and/or evacuation is used to remove the remaining tissue.

59857

The physician begins the termination of a pregnancy by inducing labor with vaginal suppositories. Before using the suppositories, a laminaria, which is an applicator made of kelp or synthetic material, may be inserted in the cervix to soften and expand the cervical canal. Once the cervix is ready, the physician inserts the vaginal suppositories and labor usually results. 59857 is used when this method fails to expel all products of conception, and a hysterotomy, through an incision in the abdominal wall and uterus, is used to remove the remaining tissue. Following removal, the incision is closed with sutures.

59866

Selective reduction is performed to eliminate one or more fetuses of a multiple pregnancy in an attempt to increase the viability of the remaining fetuses. Fetuses are usually eliminated in this procedure until only a twin or triplet pregnancy remains. Physicians most often use ultrasound guided intracardiac injection of potassium chloride to reduce the number of fetuses, although injection of potassium chloride in any part of the fetal body accomplishes the same result. When an intracardiac injection is performed, a 22 gauge spinal needle is advanced through the abdominal and uterine walls towards a cardiac echo using high-resolution ultrasound as a guide. With the needle position in the heart, a solution of potassium chloride is injected at intervals until prolonged cardiac standstill is observed. The physician then withdraws the needle and redirects it into another gestational sac, as needed. The embryo(s) or fetus(es) that have been injected shrivel and decompose, leaving the remaining fetuses in utero an increased chance of surviving to term. Any sacs that remain intact are removed during delivery of the surviving fetus(es).

59870

The physician treats a hydatidiform mole (molar pregnancy) by evacuation and curettage of the uterus. The physician inserts a speculum into the vagina to view the cervix. A tenaculum is used to grasp the cervix, pull it down, and exert traction. A dilator is then inserted into the endocervix and up through the cervical canal to enlarge the opening. The physician places a cannula in the endocervical canal and passes it into the uterus. The suction machine is then activated and the hydatidiform mole is evacuated by rotation of the cannula. After suction curettage, a sharp curet may be used to thoroughly scrape the uterus and confirm that it is empty.

59871

The physician removes a cervical cerclage, a suture that had been placed to hold the cervix closed. A cerclage is most often placed when a cervix dilates too early during pregnancy and risks a miscarriage. The physician severs the sutures and removes them. This code includes anesthesia other than local.

60000

The physician incises and drains an infected thyroglossal duct cyst. The physician localizes the cyst either by palpation or separately reportable ultrasound. An incision is made through the skin overlying the cyst. The cyst is incised and drained. A temporary drain may be placed in the wound and the incision may be closed in layers.

60001

The physician aspirates or injects a thyroid cyst. The physician localizes the thyroid cyst either by palpation or separately reportable ultrasound. A needle is passed through the skin into the cyst. The cyst is aspirated and tissue captured is sent for separately reportable analysis, or the cyst is injected with therapeutic or diagnostic matter.

60100

The physician removes tissue from the thyroid for examination. The physician localizes the area to be biopsied either by palpation or separately reportable ultrasound. A large, hollow bore needle is passed through the skin into the thyroid. The tissue is removed and sent for separately reportable analysis.

60200

The physician removes a cyst or adenoma from a thyroid, or transects the isthmus. The physician exposes the thyroid via a transverse cervical incision in the skin line. The platysmas is divided and the strap muscles separated in the midline. The thyroid mass is identified. Blood supply to and from the lesion is controlled and the mass is locally excised. The skin and platysmas are closed.

60210

The physician removes part of the lobe of a thyroid, with or without an isthmusectomy. The physician exposes the thyroid via a transverse cervical incision in the skin line. The platysmas is divided and the strap muscles separated in the midline. The superior and inferior thyroid vessels are divided in the area for resection. The thyroid parenchyma is divided and dissected with cautery dissection. The skin and platysmas are closed.

60212

The physician removes part of the lobe of a thyroid, with contralateral subtotal lobectomy, including isthmusectomy. The physician exposes the thyroid via a transverse cervical incision in the skin line. The platysmas is divided and the strap muscles separated in the midline. The superior and inferior thyroid vessels are divided in the area for resection. The thyroid is divided and dissected with cautery dissection. The isthmus is dissected. The lobe is removed The skin and platysmas are closed. Report 60212 if with contralateral subtotal lobectomy, including isthmusectomy.

60220

The physician removes all of a lobe of a thyroid with or without isthmusectomy. The physician exposes the thyroid via a transverse cervical incision in the skin line. The platysmas is divided and the strap muscles separated in the midline. The thyroid lobe to be excised is isolated and superior and inferior thyroid vessels serving that lobe are ligated. Parathyroid glands are preserved. The thyroid gland is divided in the midline of the isthmus over the anterior trachea. The entire thyroid lobe is resected. The platysmas and skin are closed.

60225

The physician removes all of a lobe of a thyroid with contralateral subtotal lobectomy, including isthmusectomy. The physician exposes the thyroid via a transverse cervical incision in the skin line. The platysmas is divided and the strap muscles separated in the midline. The thyroid lobe to be excised is isolated and superior and inferior thyroid vessels

serving that lobe are ligated. The isthmus is severed. Parathyroid glands are preserved. The thyroid gland is divided in the midline of the isthmus over the anterior trachea. The entire thyroid lobe is resected. The platysmas and skin are closed. Report 60225 if performed with contralateral subtotal lobectomy, including isthmusectomy.

60240

The physician removes all of the thyroid. The physician exposes the thyroid via a transverse cervical incision in the skin line. The platysmas is divided and the strap muscles separated in the midline. The thyroid gland is mobilized and the superior and inferior thyroid vessels are ligated. The parathyroid glands are preserved and the thyroid is resected free of the trachea and removed. The platysmas and skin are closed.

60252–60254

The physician removes a malignant thyroid and some lymph nodes. The physician exposes the thyroid via a transverse cervical incision in the skin line. The platysmas is divided and the strap muscles separated in the midline. The thyroid gland is mobilized and the superior and inferior thyroid vessels are ligated. The parathyroid glands are preserved and the thyroid is resected free of the trachea and removed. All enlarged lymph nodes are identified and excised. The platysmas and skin are closed. Report 60254 if a radical neck dissection is included in the procedure.

60260

The physician removes thyroid tissue remaining following a partial thyroidectomy. The physician enters through the previous incision scar. The platysmas and scar tissue are divided and the strap muscles are divided in the midline. While preserving the parathyroid glands, all the remaining scar tissue is resected. The platysmas and skin are closed.

60270–60271

The physician removes the thyroid, including the substernal thyroid gland. The physician exposes the thyroid via sternal split/transthoracic approach in 60270 or via a transverse cervical incision in the skin line in 60271. The platysmas is divided and the strap muscles separated in the midline. The thyroid gland is mobilized and the superior and inferior thyroid vessels are ligated. The parathyroid glands are preserved and the thyroid is resected free of the trachea and removed. Any substernal thyroid is bluntly dissected. Upper sternal incision may be necessary for complete excision of substernal thyroid. The platysmas and skin are closed. Report 60271 if with cervical approach.

60280–60281

The physician excises a thyroglossal duct cyst or sinus. The physician circumferentially incises the skin around the cyst or sinus and extends the incision along the tract to its origin. The midpart of the hyoid bone is excised. The wound is packed and allowed to heal by secondary intention. Report 60281 if thyroglossal duct cyst or sinus is recurrent.

60500

The physician removes or explores the parathyroids, glands adjacent to the thyroids. The physician exposes the thyroid via a transverse cervical incision in the skin line. The platysmas is divided and the strap muscles separated in the midline. The parathyroid glands are identified and tissue is excised for separately reportable pathological examination. The parathyroid may be removed; usually a port remains following excision. The platysmas and skin are closed.

60502

The physician re-explores the parathyroids, glands adjacent to the thyroids. The physician exposes the thyroid via the previous incision. The parathyroid glands are identified and tissue is excised for separately reportable pathological examination. The parathyroid may be removed; usually a port remains following excision. The platysmas and skin are closed.

60505

The physician removes or explores the parathyroids, glands adjacent to the thyroids with mediastinal exploration, sternal split or transthoracic approach. The physician exposes the thyroid via a sternal split or transthoracic approach. The parathyroid glands are identified and tissue is excised for separately reportable pathological examination. The mediastinum is explored. The parathyroid may be removed; usually a port remains following excision. The platysmas and skin are closed.

60512

The physician excises and reimplants a portion of the parathyroid. The physician exposes the thyroid via a transverse cervical incision in the skin line. The platysmas is divided and the strap muscles separated in the midline. Tissue is excised for separately reportable pathological examination. All four parathyroid glands are completely removed. One half of one gland is secured to either the muscle of the sternocleidomastoid or upper arm. The platysmas and skin of the neck and transplant site are closed.

60520–60522

The physician removes part or all of the thymus gland. The physician exposes the thymus via a cervical incision in the skin line in 60520. The sternum is retracted and strap muscles separated. The superior lobe of the thymus is separated from the inferior aspect of the thyroid. The blood supply to the thymus is divided and the thymus is dissected free from the pericardium and removed. The incision is closed. Report 60521 if performed with a sternal split or transthoracic approach without radical mediastinal dissection; report 60522 if performed with a sternal

split or transthoracic approach, with radical mediastinal dissection.

60540–60545

The physician removes part or all of the adrenal gland with or without biopsy. The physician exposes the adrenal gland via an upper anterior midline abdominal or posterior incision. The retroperitoneal space is explored. The capsule of the kidney is incised and the adrenal capsule is opened. Blood supply to the adrenal gland is ligated and the gland is removed. The physician may remove tissue from the site for separately reportable pathological study. The physician closes the incision with sutures. Report 60545 if this procedure is performed with excision of an adjacent retroperitoneal tumor.

60600–60605

This physician removes a tumor from a small epithelioid structure just above the bifurcation of the carotid. The physician exposes the carotid body via an incision anterior to the sternocleidomastoid. After dissection down to the carotid sheath, the vein is retracted and the carotid bifurcation exposed. The blood supply to the tumor is ligated and the tumor resected. The incision is closed. Report 60605 if the carotid body tumor excision is performed with excision of the carotid artery.

60650

The physician performs a laparoscopic excision (removal) of the adrenal gland, or performs and laparoscopic exploration of the adrenal gland through the abdomen or back. In the abdominal approach, a trocar is placed at the level of the umbilicus and the abdomen is insufflated. The laparoscope is placed through the umbilical port and additional trocars are placed into the abdominal cavity as needed. In the back approach, the trocar is placed at the back proximal to the retroperitoneal space superior to the kidney, adjacent to the adrenal gland. The physician uses the laparoscope fitted with a fiberoptic camera and/or an operating tool to explore, biopsy, or removal of all or part of the adrenal gland. The abdomen is the deflated, the trocars are removed and the incisions are closed with sutures.

61000–61001

The physician draws off cerebral spinal fluid through a cranial or fontanel suture in an infant in response to hydrocephalus or diagnosed meningitis. The physician places a needle through the fontanel at the suture line until cerebral spinal fluid is obtained. The needle is withdrawn and the area is bandaged. Report 61001 for subsequent taps for cerebral spinal fluid.

61020–61026

The physician drains cerebral spinal fluid for study. In 61020, The physician places a ventricular catheter through a previously formed bur hole or fontanel suture and withdraws fluid for study. In 61026, the catheter is used to inject a medication or other substance for diagnosis or treatment.

61050–61055

The physician performs a spinal puncture in the high cervical region (C1-2) or at the base of the skull in the cisterna magna (cerebellomedullary cistern) for diagnostic or therapeutic procedures. For lateral cervical puncture, the physician uses a paramedian approach. For cisternal punctures, the needle is placed at the base of the skull. In 61050, the physician inserts a needle through the tissues to obtain fluid from the spine or cisterna magna. In 61055, a diagnostic or therapeutic injection of a medication or other substance is performed.

61070

The physician injects or aspirates the shunt tubing or reservoir with a needle to determine function. Shunt tubing is a drain to eliminate excess cerebral spinal fluid in cases of hydrocephalus. The tubing runs behind the ear through the neck area and into the gut. The physician places a needle into the tube or reservoir and injects radiologic dye or aspirates to check for effective drainage.

61105–61108

The physician uses a twist drill to create an opening in the skull for subdural or ventricle puncture, implanting of a device, or evacuation of subdural hematoma. A twist drill is manually operated. The physician places the drill over the affected area of the skull and twists until the drill pierces the periosteum and the dura is exposed. Fluid may be drawn off from the subdural space or from the ventricles. In 61105, the hole is made to alleviate pressure, and is used for subsequent surgery. In 61107, the hole is used to implant a ventricular catheter to facilitate drainage or a pressure recording device to determine the amount of excess fluid. In 61108, the hole is used to access and evacuate or drain a subdural hematoma.

61120

The physician uses a bur drill to create a ventricular puncture to inject diagnostic fluid. A bur drill is electrically operated. The physician places the drill over the area to be injected, and drills until the periosteum is reached. Then a ventricular puncture is made. The ventricles may be injected with gas, contrast media, dye, or radioactive material for diagnostic purposes.

61140–61151

The physician uses a bur drill or trephine to create a hole in the cranium through which a brain or intracranial lesion or abscess is located. An abscess or cyst may be drained. In 61140, a lesion biopsy is obtained using a forceps or curet. In 61150, a catheter is placed through the hole and into a brain abscess or cyst for drainage. Report 61151 for subsequent

drainage of the abscess or cyst through the original bur hole.

61154

The physician drills a bur hole in the cranium to drain a hematoma. The hematoma is identified using separately reportable computerized axial tomography (CT) scan. The physician incises the scalp and peels it away from the area to be drilled. The physician uses a bur drill to access the hematoma. An extradural (epidural) hematoma is located outside the dura, just under the periosteum. A subdural hematoma is located under the dura mater, which must be incised to reach the hematoma. The hematoma is decompressed and bleeding is controlled. For subdural hematomas, the dura is sutured closed. The scalp is repositioned and sutured into place.

61156–61210

The physician drills a bur hole in the cranium to aspirate a hematoma or cyst located in the brain. The hematoma or cyst is identified using a CT scan. The physician incises the scalp and peels the it away from the area to be drilled. The physician drills through the cranium to the dura mater, which is incised. The brain is dissected and gently retracted until the hematoma or cyst is located. The hematoma or cyst is then aspirated using a syringe if the fluid is to be sent to pathology. Otherwise, the fluid is irrigated and suctioned. The dura mater is sutured closed and the scalp is repositioned and sutured into place. In 61210, a ventricular catheter, reservoir, EEG electrodes or a pressure recording device is placed through the bur hole following aspiration of the hematoma. These devices or monitors are used to follow intracranial pressure and cerebral function following surgery.

61215

The physician places a device for administering chemotherapy or other medication into the cerebral spinal fluid. The physician makes a skin incision at the level where the catheter will be inserted into the reservoir. A dermal or subdermal pocket is created with blunt dissection. The reservoir is connected to the catheter and tested to ensure function. The pocket is closed in sutured layers.

61250–61253

The physician drills a bur hole or trephine. In 61250 the hole is made to access the supratentorial area of the brain. In 61253, the infratentorial, unilateral, or bilateral area of the brain is accessed. The physician makes an incision in the scalp over the area to be drilled, and uses a bur hole drill or a trephine to create an opening to the brain. The physician explores the area then closes the wound. No other procedures are reported at this time.

61304–61305

The physician performs an exploratory craniectomy or craniotomy. In 61304, the supratentorial area of the brain (above the tentorium of the cerebellum) is accessed. In 61305, the infratentorial (below the tentorium of the cerebellum) area of the brain is accessed. A craniectomy involves removal of skull bone. A craniotomy involves incision without bone removal. The physician incises the scalp and retracts it. The physician drills or cuts the cranium to access the area to be explored. Bone is removed and the area of the brain is explored. If performing a craniotomy, the bone is replaced. The skull pieces are screwed together and the scalp is closed in sutured layers.

61312–61315

The physician performs craniectomy or craniotomy to drain a hematoma. In 61312, the supratentorial hematoma is located in the epidural or subdural space. In 61313, the supratentorial hematoma is located within the brain. In 61314, the infratentorial hematoma is located in the epidural or subdural space. In 61315, the infratentorial hematoma is located in the cerebellum. The hematoma is identified using a CT scan. The physician incises the scalp and retracts it. The physician drills or cuts the cranium to access the hematoma. Bone is removed. Epidural and subdural hematomas are identified and evacuated under direct visualization. Hematomas within the brain are located using CT verified coordinates and directed dissection. After locating the hematoma, the physician evacuates it with suction and irrigates the area while monitoring for hemorrhage. The dura is sutured closed. The skull pieces are screwed together and the scalp is closed in sutured layers.

61320–61321

The physician performs craniectomy or craniotomy to drain an abscess. In 61320, the abscess is located in the supratentorial region. In 61321, the abscess is located infratentorial region. The abscess is identified using separately reportable CT scan. The physician incises the scalp and retracts it. The physician drills or cuts the cranium to access the abscess. Bone is removed. Epidural and subdural abscesses are identified and evacuated under direct visualization. Abscesses within the brain are located using CT verified coordinates and directed dissection. After locating the abscess, the physician evacuates it with suction and irrigates the area while monitoring for hemorrhage. The dura is sutured closed. The skull pieces are screwed together and the scalp is closed in sutured layers.

61330

The physician decompresses an orbital roof fracture. The physician incises the frontal scalp area and retracts the scalp posteriorly and the forehead anteriorly. The frontal bone is cut and removed. The forebrain is retracted until the superior margins of the orbit are visualized. The roof of the orbit is decompressed after ensuring freedom of movement of extraocular eye muscles. The dura is closed, and the

bone is replaced. The forehead and scalp are reanastomosed and closed in sutured layers.

61332–61334

The physician explores the orbit, and removes lesions or foreign bodies. The physician incises the frontal scalp area and retracts the scalp posteriorly and the forehead anteriorly. The frontal bone is cut and removed. The forebrain is retracted until the superior margins of the orbit are visualized. In 61332, suspect tissue is biopsied. In 61333, a lesion is excised. In 61334, a foreign body is removed. The roof of the orbit is reconstructed and freedom of movement of extraocular eye muscles is ensured. The dura is closed, and the skull is replaced. The forehead and scalp are reanastomosed and closed in sutured layers.

61340

The physician decompresses a skull fracture or defect located in the supratentorial region. The physician incises and retracts the scalp over the area to be decompressed. The bone is cut and reshaped for appearance if necessary. The bone is replaced and secured to neighboring bone. The scalp is reanastomosed and closed in sutured layers.

61343

The physician removes the posterior inferior occipital scalp and the posterior aspects of the cervical vertebrae to decompress the brain stem. A dural graft may be necessary. The physician makes a longitudinal incision from the occipital through the cervical spine and retracts laterally. Decompression is achieved when the inferior occiput is cut and removed and the posterior elements of the upper cervical vertebrae are removed. If a dural graft is needed to cover the resulting defect, fascia is harvested from the thigh or a cadaveric dural graft is used. The graft is positioned over the defect and sutured to the surrounding dura. The operative incision is closed in sutured layers.

61345

The physician lowers pressure in the brain caused by excess fluid. The patient is placed in a seated position or prone. The physician makes an incision in the midline extending from the posterior mid-scalp to the midcervical region. Dissection is continued to the skull. Drills and saws are used to open the occipital bone to enter the posterior fossa of the skull. The brain is decompressed by removal of blood and pathological tissue. The occipital bone is secured with sutures, wires, or plates and screws. The scalp and neck are sutured closed in layers.

61440

The physician cuts the tentorium. The tentorium supports the occipital lobes and covers the cerebellum. The physician incises and retracts the scalp then removes bone from the occiput. The tentorium is identified. The tissue that supports the

CPT® Lay Descriptions

occipital lobes is incised to loosen the tissue, releasing tension in the posterior brain.

61450

The physician applies or releases pressure on the sensory root of the gasserian ganglion. The gasserian ganglion supplies sensory innervation to the face via the trigeminal nerve. The physician makes a periauricular incision and retracts the scalp and raises a bone flap. The gasserian ganglion is located and decompressed or stimulated. If indicated, the nerve or a nerve branch is sectioned. The bone flap is replaced and fastened. The scalp is reanastomosed and closed in sutured layers.

61458–61480

The physician preforms a suboccipital craniectomy to explore or release pressure from the cranial nerves or tracts in the brain stem. In 61458, the physician explores and frees affected cranial nerves from the surrounding tissue. In 61460, the physician, resects one or more cranial nerves. The nerves are freed before resection. In 61470, the physician resects a nerve tract as it passes through the medulla. In 61480, the physician resects a nerve tract as it passes through the mesencephalon or the cerebellar or cerebral peduncle. The physician incises and retracts the scalp then removes bone from the occiput. The brain is retracted to reveal the brain stem. The affected nerve tract is explored, decompressed, or resected. The bone is replaced and stabilized. The scalp is anastomosed and closed in sutured layers.

61490

The physician performs a lobotomy and a cingulotomy. The physician incises and retracts the scalp then removes bone in the frontal or parietal region. For a midline lobotomy, the physician dissects between the two cerebral hemispheres and creates a lesion through the gyrus cinguli. The bone is replaced and stabilized. The scalp is anastomosed and closed in sutured layers.

61500–61501

The physician removes a portion of the skull invaded by tumor or infection. In 61500, the physician removes a tumor or bony lesion. In 61501, the physician removes infected bone. The physician incises and retracts the scalp then removes bone from the affected area. A bone graft or plastic replacement may be used to reconstruct the skull. The scalp is anastomosed and closed in sutured layers.

61510–61516

The physician removes a supratentorial abscess or cyst. Supratentorial structures are those located above the tentorium cerebelli, the membrane that separates the cerebellum from the basal surface of the occipital and temporal lobes of the cerebrum. The physician incises and retracts the scalp then removes bone over the area of the tumor, meningioma, abscess, or cyst.

The tumor, meningioma, abscess or cyst is identified and excised. The bone is replaced and stabilized. The scalp is anastomosed and closed in sutured layers. In 61510, the physician removes a brain tumor. In 61512, a meningioma is removed. A meningioma is a tumor of the lining of the brain. In 61514, an abscess is excised. In 61516, a cyst is excised or fenestrated. Fenestration is the surgical creation of an opening or window in the cyst to allow it to drain.

61518–61519

The physician removes an infratentorial or posterior fossa brain tumor or meningioma. Infratentorial structures are those located below the tentorium cerebelli, the membrane that separates the cerebellum from the basal surface of the occipital and temporal lobes of the cerebrum. The physician incises and retracts the scalp then removes bone from the affected area. The tumor is identified and excised. The bone is replaced and stabilized. The scalp is anastomosed and closed in sutured layers.In 61518, the physician removes a brain tumor other than a meningioma, cerebellopontine angle tumor, or midline tumor of skull base. In 61519, a meningioma is removed.

61520

The physician removes a brain tumor at the cerebellopontine angle. The physician makes a lateral posterior incision and removes an occipital bone flap. The cerebellum is retracted and brain stem is examined. The tumor at the cerebellopontine angle is resected. The bone is replaced and stabilized. The scalp is anastomosed and closed in sutured layers.

61521

The physician removes a midline brain tumor at the base of the skull. The physician uses a posterior auricular or transmastoid approach. The physician incises and retracts the scalp then removes a bone flap. The lateral cerebellum is retracted and the tumor, located near the brain stem, is identified and resected. The bone is replaced and stabilized. The scalp is anastomosed and closed in sutured layers.

61522–61524

The physician removes an abscess or cyst located in the infratentorium or posterior fossa. Infratentorial structures are those located below the tentorium cerebelli, the membrane that separates the cerebellum from basal surface of the occipital and temporal lobes of the cerebrum. The physician incises and retracts the scalp then removes bone over the area of the abscess or cyst. The abscess or cyst is identified and excised the bone is replaced and stabilized. The scalp is anastomosed and closed in sutured layers. In 61522, an abscess is excised. In 61524 the cyst is excised or fenestrated. Fenestration is the surgical creation of an opening or window in the cyst to allow it to drain.

61526–61530

The physician excises a tumor at the cerebellopontine angle. Cerebellopontine angle tumors are benign neoplasms of the 8th cranial nerve and are more often referred to as acoustic neuromas. Other terms include: acoustic tumor, vestibular schwannoma, or angle tumor. Using a transmastoid approach, the physician incises the scalp, then removes a bone flap. The tumor is identified and excised. The bone is replaced and stabilized. The scalp is anastomosed and closed in sutured layers. In 61530, a multiple approach technique is used with the tumor being accessed from both a transtemporal and a middle or posterior fossa approach.

61531

The physician implants electrodes in the subdural layer for long term seizure monitoring. The physician uses a bur drill or trephine to reach the subdural layer and implants linear strip electrodes in each hole. Subdural electrodes are placed just below the dura and do not penetrate the cerebral tissue. The scalp is sutured to close the incisions.

61533–61534

The physician implants electrodes in the subdural layer for long term seizure monitoring. A bone flap is elevated to implant a subdural electrode array along the cerebral hemispheres. The bone is replaced and stabilized. The scalp is anastomosed and closed in sutured layers. Report 61534 if the eliptogenic focus (the seizure center) is excised.

61535–61536

The physician removes an electrode array located in the subdural layer. The bone flap covering the electrode array is elevated and the array is removed. The bone is replaced and stabilized. The scalp is anastomosed and closed in sutured layers. Report 61536 if the array is removed in addition to excision of the eliptogenic focus (the seizure center).

61538–61539

The physician performs a craniotomy to resect a lobe of the brain, primarily to control seizure activity. The bone flap covering the lobe is removed. An electrode array is placed to monitor brain activity and/or provide intraoperative cortical stimulation for mapping of cortical function. The lobe responsible for seizure activity is either partially or completely removed. The electrode array may be removed or left in place for postoperative monitoring. The bone is replaced and stabilized. The scalp is anastomosed and closed in sutured layers. In 61538, either the right or left temporal lobe is resected. In the dominant hemisphere, removal extends back at least 4.5-5 cm behind the temporal tip or to the level of the central sulcus. In the non-dominant hemisphere, the lobectomy will extend at least 7-8 cm. Mesial temporal structures including the hippocampus are also removed. In 61539, a resection is performed on

either the frontal, parietal or occipital lobe(s), the most common site being the in the frontal lobe.

61541–61543

The physician cuts the fibers within the corpus callosum or removes all or part of a brain hemisphere. An electrode array is used to monitor brain function during surgery. In 61541, the physician transects the corpus callosum. In 61542, an entire hemisphere is removed. Report 61543 if a partial or subtotal hemispherectomy is performed. The dura is sutured around the remaining brain tissue. The bone flap is replaced and stabilized. The scalp is anastomosed and closed in sutured layers.

61544

The physician excises or destroys the choroid plexus. The choroid plexus produces spinal fluid. The physician cuts and retracts the scalp in the affected region. A bone flap is raised and tissues are dissected to the ventricle where the affected choroid plexus is located. The choroid plexus is resected, or destroyed using electrocautery. The bone is replaced and stabilized. The scalp is anastomosed and closed in sutured layers.

61545

The physician excises a craniopharyngioma through a craniotomy. The physician cuts and retracts the frontal scalp and raises a bone flap. The tissues are dissected to the sella turcica, and the craniopharyngioma is resected. The bone is replaced and fastened. The scalp is anastomosed and closed in sutured layers.

61546

The physician uses a craniotomy to remove a pituitary tumor or resect a portion of the gland. The physician cuts and retracts the frontal scalp and raises a bone flap. The tissues are dissected to the sella turcica, and the pituitary is identified. The tumor or hypertrophic gland is resected. The bone is replaced and fastened. The scalp is anastomosed and closed in sutured layers.

61548

The physician uses a transnasal or transseptal approach to remove a pituitary tumor or resect a portion of the gland. The physician accesses the base of the sella turcica through the nose. The incision may be made in the mouth underneath the upper lip to avoid facial scarring (transeptal approach). A small hole is drilled in the skull base through the inferior aspect of the sella turcica. The pituitary is identified and the tumor or hypertrophic gland is resected. The hole is packed with Gelfoam, with or without bone chips. The nasal and oral mucosa are sutured closed.

61550–61552

The physician performs a craniectomy for craniosynostosis. Craniosynostosis is a premature closure of the sutures of the skull. The physician incises and retracts the scalp over the fused suture line. The bones are cut to reshape the skull into an anatomically correct position. The recreated suture line is left open and the scalp is reanastomosed and closed in sutured layers. Report 61550 if a single suture is reformed. Report 61552 for multiple suture lines.

61556–61557

The physician performs a craniotomy for craniosynostosis. Craniosynostosis is a premature closure of the sutures of the skull. The physician incises and retracts the scalp over the fused suture lines. In 61556, the frontal or parietal bones are removed. In 61557, bifrontal bone flaps are raised. The bones are reshaped and a bone flap is created from the harvested bones to enlarge and reshape the skull. If the dura mater was damaged during bone harvest, it is sutured closed. The reshaped bone flap is positioned and secured to neighboring bone. The scalp is reanastomosed and closed in sutured layers.

61558–61559

The physician performs an extensive craniectomy for craniosynostosis affecting many suture lines. Craniosynostosis is a premature closure of the sutures of the skull. In 61558, no bone grafts are used to reshape the skull. In 61559, the physician harvests bone grafts to aid in reshaping. The physician retracts most or all of the scalp to expose the entire skull. The cranium is removed as a single unit. The physician breaks the skull and restores correct anatomical shape. If the cranium will not supply bone necessary to provide adequate room for brain growth, bone grafts are obtained and used for skull reshaping. If the dura mater was damaged during cranium harvest, it is primarily closed, or closed with a dural graft. The reshaped cranium pieces are replaced and secured to neighboring bone. The scalp is reapproximated and closed in sutured layers.

61563–61564

The physician removes an intra and extracranial bone tumor. In 61563, the optic nerve is not decompressed. In 61564, the optic nerve is decompressed. The physician cuts and retracts the scalp overlying the affected bone. The affected bone is resected and removed. Grafts may be necessary for reconstruction. The bone is fastened into place and the scalp is reanastomosed and closed in sutured layers.

61570–61571

The physician removes a foreign body from the brain. The physician incises the scalp and cuts the bone or creates a bone flap as necessary to reach the foreign body. The object is identified and removed. In 61571, the brain tissue damaged by the foreign object is debrided and irrigated. The dura is sutured closed and the bone is fastened into place.

61575–61576

The physician approaches the skull base, brain stem, or upper spinal cord and obtains a biopsy, decompresses the brain stem or spinal cord, or excises a lesion. In 61575, the physician access the affected area through the patient's mouth. In 61576, the physician performs a tracheostomy and then cuts through the mandible and tongue to reach an extensive defect. The physician places a gag retractor in the patient's mouth and makes a posterior pharyngeal wall incision. The mucosa is retracted to the deep muscle layers which are dissected to reach the skull base or superior spinal cord. The bone is removed to expose the area of interest. A lesion may be biopsied or excised. Decompression is accomplished by removing bone from around the structure. If incised, the dura is closed, then the posterior pharyngeal wall is reapproximated and closed in sutured layers.

61580

In this approach procedure, the physician exposes the anterior cranial fossa using a craniofacial approach to an extradural (outside the dura) lesion or defect at the skull base. To adequately expose the lesion or defect, the physician performs a lateral rhinotomy, ethmoidectomy, and sphenoidectomy all of which are included in the approach procedure. For full exposure of the lesion, the brain may need to be retracted from the skull base.

61581

In this approach procedure, the physician exposes the anterior cranial fossa using a craniofacial approach to an extradural (outside the dura) lesion or defect at the skull base. To adequately expose the lesion or defect, the physician performs an orbital exenteration, a lateral rhinotomy, ethmoidectomy, sphenoidectomy and/or maxillectomy all of which are included in the approach procedure. For full exposure of the lesion, the brain may need to be retracted from the skull base.

61582

In this approach procedure, the physician exposes the anterior cranial fossa using a craniofacial approach to an extradural (outside the dura) lesion or defect at the skull base. To adequately expose the lesion or defect, the physician performs a unilateral or bilateral craniotomy which is included in the approach procedure. For full exposure of the lesion, the frontal lobe is elevated and retracted from the skull base. If skull base lesions extend into the bones of the face, an osteotomy of the anterior cranial fossa may be required.

61583

In this approach procedure, the physician exposes the anterior cranial fossa using a craniofacial approach to an intradural (inside the dura) lesion or defect at the skull base. To adequately expose the lesion or defect, the physician performs a unilateral or bilateral craniotomy which is included in the approach procedure. For full exposure of the lesion, the frontal lobe is elevated and retracted from the skull base. If skull base lesions extend into the bones of the face, an osteotomy of the anterior cranial fossa may be required.

61584

In this approach procedure, the physician exposes the anterior cranial fossa using a orbitocranial (transorbital) approach to an extradural (outside the dura) lesion or defect at the skull base. To adequately expose the lesion or defect, the physician performs a supraorbital ridge osteotomy which is included in the approach procedure. For full exposure of the lesion, the frontal and/or temporal lobes are elevated and retracted from the skull base.

61585

In this approach procedure, the physician exposes the anterior cranial fossa using a orbitocranial (transorbital) approach to an extradural (outside the dura) lesion or defect at the skull base. To adequately expose the lesion or defect, the physician performs a supraorbital ridge osteotomy which is included in the approach procedure. The orbital contents are completely removed. For full exposure of the lesion, the frontal and/or temporal lobes are elevated and retracted from the skull base.

61586

In this approach procedure, the physician exposes the anterior cranial fossa using a bicoronal, transzygomatic and/or LeFort I osteotomy approach to a lesion or defect at the skull base. To enter the anterior cranial fossa, the surgeon may use a bicoronal scalp incision to expose the zygoma bone. The zygoma is removed with burs and saws to enter the anterior skull. If visualization is inadequate, the surgeon may use an intraoral approach to fracture the maxilla and enter the skull. Once the lesion is adequately exposed, a separately reportable surgical procedure is performed which may include biopsy, excision, or other treatment of the lesion. At the conclusion, of this separately reportable procedure, the surgeon responsible for the approach will replace and secure the bony structures using wires, plates or screws as needed.

61590

In this approach procedure, the physician exposes the middle cranial fossa using an infratemporal (below the temporal fossa) pre-auricular (in front of the external ear) approach to a lesion at the skull base. This is also sometimes referred to as a transparotid approach. The transparotid approach allows access to the parapharyngeal space. First, the parotid gland is mobilized. This is followed by identification and dissection of the facial nerve. Parotidectomy with facial nerve preservation is then performed. If

adequate exposure has not been accomplished, the muscle overlying the mandible is divided and the mandible is displaced anteriorly. This approach may be combined with a transtemporal approach to improve exposure to lesions which extend posteriorly to involve the temporal bone.

61591

In this approach, the physician exposes the middle cranial fossa using a infratemporal (below temporal fossa), post-auricular (behind the external ear) approach. To adequately expose the lesion or defect, it may be necessary to perform a mastoidectomy, resect the sigmoid sinus and/or decompress/mobilize the contents of the auditory canal or petrous carotid artery.

61592

In this approach procedure, an orbitocranial approach to the middle cranial fossa is performed. Skin incisions are made over the zygoma, and the frontal branches of the facial nerve and infraorbital nerve are identified, tagged, and divided. Soft tissue flaps are raised from the maxilla and zygoma, and osteotomies are performed with removal of the orbitozygomaticomaxillary complex. The temporalis muscle is then displaced inferiorly exposing the skull base. If intracranial access is required a subtemporal craniectomy, or frontal or temporal craniotomy is performed. Following separately reportable lesion removal, bone segments are replaced and neurorrhaphy is performed along with meticulous reconstruction and closure.

61595

In this approach code, a transtemporal approach to the posterior cranial fossa, jugular foramen, or midline skull base is used. To obtain adequate exposure of the lesion or defect, the physician performs a mastoidectomy, decompression of sigmoid sinus and/or facial nerve, with or without mobilization. The temple, anterior and posterior ear, orbits, mandible, and mastoid may be resected to reach the affected area of the posterior cranial fossa.

61596

In this approach code, a transcochlear approach is used to expose the posterior cranial fossa, jugular foramen, or midline skull base. A postauricular incision is made and the ear is reflected anteriorly. A labyrinthectomy is performed and the internal auditory canal is skeletonized. The incus is removed, the facial nerve is completely decompressed, and opened widely into the hypotympanum. The greater superficial petrosal nerve is transected and the facial nerve is completely removed from the stylomastoid foramen to the internal auditory canal and rerouted posteriorly. The fallopian canal, stapedius muscle, and the turns of the cochlea are completely exenterated, carrying the dissection forward until the internal carotid artery wall is identified.

61597

In this approach, a transcondylar approach is used to expose the posterior cranial fossa, jugular foramen, or midline skull base. This far lateral suboccipital approach is used to expose the vertebral artery and lower cranial nerve complex in the posterior fossa. A post-auricular incision is made approximately 3 cm lateral to the midline, curving back toward the mastoid eminance. The skin flap created by the incision is retracted laterally exposing the greater occipital nerve and the greater occipital artery and vein. The sternocleidomastoid is incised parallel to its attatchment. The suboccipital musculature is also incised and retracted. A suboccipital craniectomy is performed. The C1-C3 vertebral bodies are resected to further expose the cerebellum and a portion of the occipital condyle is removed. The vertebral artery is identified, decompressed and mobilized

61598

In this approach code, a transpetrosal approach is used to expose the posterior cranial fossa, jugular foramen, or midline skull base. A craniotomy is performed posterior to the sigmoid sinus. The cerebellum is retracted posteriorly, allowing access to the petrosal and sigmoid sinuses which are ligated.

61600–61601

The physician uses a separately reportable anterior cranial fossa approach to resect a neoplastic, vascular, or infectious lesion at the base of the anterior cranial fossa. The physician incises and retracts the scalp or nasal mucosa and removes a bone flap to access the anterior cranial fossa. In 61600, the extradural lesion is identified and resected. Unaffected bone is replaced and fastened to neighboring bone. Bone defects are replaced with bone grafts. In 61601, the intradural lesion is identified and resected. The dura is primarily closed, with or without a dural graft. The bone flap is replaced and fastened to neighboring bone. The scalp is reapproximated and closed in sutured layers.

61605–61606

The physician uses a middle cranial fossa approach to resect a neoplastic, vascular, or infectious lesion located at the base of the middle cranial fossa (infratemporal fossa, peripharyngeal space, petrous apex). The approach is reported separately. The physician makes a pre- or post-auricular incision or an orbital zygomatic incision to access the middle cranial fossa. The physician retracts the tissues and performs an osteotomy to access the lesion. In 61605, the extradural lesion is identified and resected. Unaffected bone is replaced and fastened to neighboring bone. Bone defects are replaced with bone grafts. In 61606, the intradural lesion is identified and resected. The dura is primarily closed, with or without a dural graft. The bone flap is replaced and fastened to neighboring bone. The scalp is reapproximated and closed in sutured layers.

61607–61608

The physician uses a middle cranial fossa approach to resect a neoplastic, vascular, or infectious lesion located at the base of the middle cranial fossa (parasellar area, cavernous sinus, clivus, or midline skull base). The approach is reported separately. The physician makes a pre- or post auricular incision or an orbital zygomatic incision to access the middle cranial fossa. The physician retracts the tissues and performs an osteotomy to access the lesion. In 61607, the extradural lesion is identified and resected. Unaffected bone is replaced and fastened to neighboring bone. Bone defects are replaced with bone grafts. In 61608, the intradural lesion is identified and resected. The dura is primarily closed, with or without a dural graft. The bone flap is replaced and fastened to neighboring bone. The scalp is reapproximated and closed in sutured layers.

61609–61612

The physician transects or ligates a carotid artery in the cavernous sinus or petrous canal. Report 61609 for transection or ligation without repair in the cavernous sinus. Report 61610 if the carotid artery in the cavernous sinus is repaired by reanastomosis or graft placement. Report 61611 for transection or ligation without repair in the petrous canal. Report 61612 if the carotid artery in the petrous canal is repaired by reanastomosis or graft placement. These procedures are reported in addition to 61605 through 61608 (the primary definitive procedure).

61613

The physician uses a middle cranial fossa approach to access and obliterate a carotid aneurysm, arteriovenous malformation, or carotid-cavernous fistula. The approach is reported separately. Using a orbitocranial zygomatic approach, the physician incises and retracts the skin over the zygoma. The zygoma and the base of the skull are osteotomized to reach the cavernous sinus. The aneurysm, defect, or fistula is dissected and ligated. The skull and zygoma are packed with Gelfoam or bone pieces. The skin is reanastomosed and closed in sutured layers.

61615–61616

The physician uses a separately reportable skull base approach to resect or excise a neoplastic, vascular, or infectious lesion in the posterior cranial fossa, jugular foramen, foramen magnum, or C1-C3 vertebral bodies. The physician incises and retracts the scalp overlying the posterior cranial fossa and uses a transtemporal, transcochlear, transcondylar, or transpetrosal approach to reach the lesion. In 61615, the extradural lesion is identified and resected. Unaffected bone is replaced and fastened to neighboring bone. Bone defects are replaced with bone grafts. In 61616, the intradural lesion is identified and resected. The dura is primarily closed, with or without a dural graft. The bone flap is replaced and fastened to neighboring bone. The scalp is reapproximated and closed in sutured layers.

61618–61619

The physician repairs a cerebrospinal fluid leak in the dura following a craniotomy of the skull base. The approach is dependent on the location of the dural leak. In 61618, the physician uses a dural graft obtained from fascia, tensor fascia lata, or pericranium. In 61619, a vascularized pedicle flap is rotated over the dural defect. The temporalis, frontalis, or occipitalis muscle is used. The dural leak is closed by suturing the flap to the dura. Following anastomosis, intracranial pressure may be increased to test repair success under direct visualization. The bone flap is replaced and the scalp incision is closed in sutured layers.

61624

The physician uses a percutaneous catheter to access an arterial venous malformation, tumor, or bleeding aneurysm. The physician places a catheter in a peripheral artery (e.g., femoral artery). Using fluoroscopic guidance, the physician locates the lesion with the catheter. The defect is occluded or embolized with materials placed through the catheter to aid clotting.

61626

The physician uses a percutaneous catheter to access an arterial venous malformation, tumor, or bleeding aneurysm. The defect lies outside the central nervous system, in the head or neck regions (common carotid, external carotid, vertebral and their branches). The physician places a catheter in a peripheral artery (e.g., femoral artery). Using fluoroscopic guidance, the physician locates the lesion with the catheter. The defect is occluded or embolized with materials placed through the catheter to aid clotting.

61680–61692

The physician resects an arteriovenous malformation in the brain. This malformation is a tumor-like growth of blood vessels. After using angiography to locate the malformation, the physician performs a craniotomy in the affected area. The arteriovenous malformation is located and the blood vessels feeding the tumor are ligated. The tumor is resected and bleeding is controlled. The bone flap is repositioned and secured; the scalp is reanastomosed and closed in sutured layers. Report according to tumor location and ease of access: Report 61680 if the tumor is located in the supratentorial region and is easily accessible; in 61682 the supratentorial tumor is more difficult to access and remove. Report 61684 if the tumor is located in the infratentorial region and is easily accessible; in 61686 the infratentorial region and is more difficult to access and remove. Report 61690 if the tumor is located in the dural layer; in 61692 the dural tumor is more difficult to access and remove.

61697

An open middle cranial fossa approach is used to locate a complex aneurysm of the internal carotid circulation. Complex aneurysms include those that are larger than 15 millimeters as well as those that contain calcifications or incorporate normal vessels at the aneurysm neck. The surgical technique used is dependent on the specific anatomic characteristics of the aneurysm. One technique involves direct treatment of the aneurysm with clipping and resection of the mass lesion. However, clipping of the aneurysm neck may not be possible if a thick, calcified wall is present. In this instance, aneurysmorrhaphy (opening of the aneurysm) and resection may be necessary. When critical perforating vessels arise from the aneurysm, the patient may not be able to tolerate occlusion of the parent vessel. If this is the case, an extracranial or intracranial bypass procedure must first be performed with subsequent trapping or proximal occlusion of the vessel. In some instances, adjunctive techniques are utilized to aid in direct surgery. Techniques include cardiopulmonary bypass with cardiac arrest to allow for a slack aneurysm, which can be dissected from surrounding cerebral tissue. Another adjunctive technique is temporary occlusion of the parent vessel to allow decompression of the aneurysm. Once the aneurysm has been occluded, resected, and/or bypassed, the physician checks to make sure that the repairs are secure and that there is no bleeding. The dura is closed and the bone flap repositioned and secured. The scalp is closed in sutured layers.

61698

An open posterior cranial fossa approach is used to locate a complex aneurysm of the vertebrobasilar circulation. Complex aneurysms include those that are larger than 15 millimeters as well as those that contain calcifications or incorporate normal vessels at the aneurysm neck. The surgical technique used is dependent on the specific anatomic characteristics of the aneurysm. One technique involves direct treatment of the aneurysm with clipping and resection of the mass lesion. However, clipping of the aneurysm neck may not be possible if a thick, calcified wall is present. In this instance, aneurysmorrhaphy (opening of the aneurysm) and resection may be necessary. When critical perforating vessels arise from the aneurysm, the patient may not be able to tolerate occlusion of the parent vessel. If this is the case, an extracranial or intracranial bypass procedure must first be performed with subsequent trapping or proximal occlusion of the vessel. In some instances, adjunctive techniques are utilized to aid in direct surgery. Techniques include cardiopulmonary bypass with cardiac arrest to allow for a slack aneurysm, which can be dissected from surrounding cerebral tissue. Another adjunctive technique is temporary occlusion of the parent vessel to allow decompression of the aneurysm. Once the aneurysm has been occluded, resected, and/or bypassed, the physician checks to make sure that the repairs are secure and

CPT® Lay Descriptions

that there is no bleeding. The dura is closed and the bone flap repositioned and secured. The scalp is closed in sutured layers.

61700

The physician resects a simple carotid aneurysm. Simple aneurysms include those that are 15 millimeters or less in size and contain no anatomical features that will complicate the surgery such as calcifications or critical perforating vessels at the aneurysm neck. After using angiography to locate the aneurysm, the physician uses a middle cranial fossa approach for access. The aneurysm is located and clipped under direct visualization. After making sure the clip is secure and there is no bleeding, the physician closes the dura. The bone flap is repositioned and secured and the scalp is closed in sutured layers.

61702

The physician resects a simple vertebrobasilar aneurysm. Simple aneurysms include those that are 15 millimeters or less in size and contain no anatomical features that will complicate the surgery such as calcifications or critical perforating vessels at the aneurysm neck. After using angiography to locate the aneurysm, the physician uses a posterior cranial fossa approach for access. The aneurysm is located and clipped under direct visualization. After making sure the clip is secure and there is no bleeding, the physician closes the dura. The bone flap is repositioned and secured and the scalp is closed in sutured layers.

61703

The physician resects an aneurysm after clamping the carotid artery to control bleeding. The physician makes a high neck incision and locates the ipsilateral carotid artery. Next, the physician performs a craniotomy to access the intracranial aneurysm. When the aneurysm is located, the carotid artery is occluded with a clamp. The physician then places a clip on the aneurysm under direct visualization. Once the aneurysm has been clipped and bleeding is controlled, the carotid clamp is released. The aneurysm site is reexamined for bleeding. The physician closes the dura. The bone flap is repositioned and secured; the scalp is reanastomosed and closed in sutured layers. The neck incision is closed in sutured layers.

61705–61710

The physician clips an aneurysm, vascular malformation, or carotid-cavernous fistula. The physician makes a high neck incision and locates the ipsilateral carotid artery. Next, the physician performs a craniotomy to access the defect. In 61705, the physician performs a craniotomy to access the intracranial aneurysm, vascular malformation or carotid -cavernous fistula. Once the lesion is located, the cervical carotid is clamped and the carotid artery proximal and distal to the lesion is ligated to prevent

blood flow to the lesion. The cervical carotid is unclamped while monitoring for bleeding in the craniotomy site. In 61708, the lesion is obliterated using electrothrombosis. In 61710, the physician embolizes the lesion with an intraarterial balloon catheter or injects material to form a regional clot to obliterate the blood supply to the lesion. After the lesion has been obliterated, the dura is closed. The bone flap is repositioned and secured; the scalp is reanastomosed and closed in sutured layers.

61711

The physician anastomoses the arterial and extracranial-intracranial arteries. The physician performs a craniotomy in the affected area and locates the arteries to be anastomosed and dissects them from the surrounding tissue. The feeding artery is clamped and ligated and the proximal limb is sutured to the receiving artery. After verifying successful anastomosis and adequate blood flow, the dura is closed. The bone flap is repositioned and secured; the scalp is reanastomosed and closed in sutured layers.

61720–61735

The physician creates a lesion of the brain through stereotactic methods. The tissue to be lesioned is mapped by using a CT or MRI scanning technique. The physician uses the coordinates obtained from the scans to locate the area of interest. The physician incises and retracts the scalp. A bur hole is drilled. Then an electrocautery unit or surgical knife is directed to the area of interest. When the precise location is reached and confirmed by the coordinates, the lesion is made. In 61720, a lesion is made in the globus pallidus or in the thalamus. In 61735, a lesion is made in subcortical structures other than the globus pallidus or the thalamus. After the lesion is made, the dura is sutured and the scalp is reapproximated and closed in sutured layers.

61750–61751

The physician biopsies, aspirates, or excises an intracranial lesion stereotactically. The lesion is mapped using a CT or MRI scanning technique. The physician uses the coordinates obtained from the scans to locate the area of interest. The physician incises and retracts the scalp. A burr hole is drilled. The physician inserts a biopsy needle into the area of interest to aspirate or biopsy the tissue. If the lesion is to be destroyed the physician inserts an electrocautery unit, knife or curet into the lesion. In 61751, the physician utilizes CT or MRI scanning intraoperatively to confirm lesion location and accurate placement of surgical instruments. The physician closes the dura and reapproximates the scalp and closes it in sutured layers.

61760

The physician implants depth electrodes into the cerebrum for long-term monitoring of seizures. After the desired locations of the electrodes have been mapped by CT or MRI scanning techniques, the physician incises and retracts the scalp. The physician drills a bur hole(s) and the electrodes are placed into the desired area of the brain by following the coordinates established by the scans. The dura is sutured closed and the scalp is reapproximated and closed in sutured layers.

61770

The physician implants catheters or probes into a lesion of the brain for radiation therapy. After using CT or MRI scanning techniques to map the desired locations of the catheters or probes, the physician incises and retracts the scalp. The physician drills a bur hole and the catheters or probes are placed into the desired area of the brain by following the coordinates established by the scans. The dura is sutured closed and the scalp is reapproximated and closed in sutured layers.

61790–61791

The physician under stereotactic guidance percutaneously creates a neurolytic lesion in the gasserian ganglion or the medullary trigeminal tract. The area of interest is located and mapped by CT or MRI scanning techniques. The physician guides a needle into the region to be destroyed. After reaffirming position by checking the coordinates of the needle, the physician injects, or electrically destroys the tissue. In 61790, the physician destroys the gasserian ganglion. In 61791, the physician destroys the medullary trigeminal tracts.

61793

Prior to imaging, patients undergo application of a stereotactic head frame (20660). Using stereotactic techniques, a precise 3-dimensional location of the brain lesion is identified using CT, MRI, or angiogram. The physician uses the coordinates obtained from the images to focus gamma ray or proton beam energy onto the lesion, thereby destroying it. This is a non-invasive procedure that does not require incision of the scalp or drilling into the skull. Use this code for one or more sessions.

61795

Use this code in addition to the procedure code when the physician uses a computer to assist with coordinate determination established with a CT or MRI scan.

61850

The physician uses a twist or burr drill to reach the cortex or subcortex and implant neurostimulator electrodes. The physician incises the scalp and uses a twist or bur drill to expose the cortex for neurostimulator electrode placement. The physician places an electrode through an introducer needle into the tissue to be stimulated. The electrodes are tested to verify placement, then the incision is closed in sutured layers.

61860

The physician performs a craniectomy or craniotomy to reach the cortex and implant neurostimulator electrodes to affect the cerebrum. The cerebrum occupies the frontal portion of the cranial cavity. Its two hemispheres joined by the corpus callosum supply the majority of brain function. The physician incises the scalp and retracts it. The physician drills or cuts the cranium to expose the cortex for neurostimulator electrode placement. Bone is removed. The physician places an electrode through an introducer needle into the tissue to be stimulated, and the electrodes are tested to verify placement.

61862

The physician drills a hole in the cranium to implant a neurostimulator in a subcortical site. The site to be implanted is mapped by using CT or MRI scanning. Coordinates obtained from the brain imaging studies are used to locate the subcortical site. The physician incises the scalp and retracts it away from the site to be drilled. The physician cuts into the cranium (craniotomy) or removes a portion of the cranium (craniotomy) or drills through the cranium to reach the dura mater (burr hole) which is incised and retracted. When the exact region within the subcortical space is reached and identified by stereotactic coordinates the physician places an inducer needle into the tissue to be stimulated. The electrodes are tested to verify proper placement. The dura is sutured closed. If performing a craniotomy, the bone is replaced. The skull pieces are screwed together and the scalp is closed with sutures or staples.

61870–61875

The physician performs a craniectomy to reach the cortex or subcortex and implant neurostimulator electrodes to affect the cerebellum. The cerebellum is located behind the brain stem and supplies coordination of movements. The physician incises the scalp and retracts it. The physician drills or cuts the cranium to expose the area for neurostimulator electrode placement. Bone is removed. The physician places an electrode through an introducer needle into the tissue to be stimulated, and the electrodes are tested to verify placement. In 61870, the electrodes are placed in the cortex. In 61875, the electrodes are placed in the subcortex (the area near the cortex). The dura is sutured closed. The skull stabilized and the scalp is closed in sutured layers.

61880

The physician removes or revises neurostimulator electrodes. The physician incises and retracts the scalp and drills a bur hole in the cranium to locate the electrode. The electrode is removed or revised. If necessary, the electrode is replaced. The dura is closed and the scalp is reapproximated and closed in sutured layers.

CPT® Lay Descriptions

61885–61886

The physician places a cranial neurostimulator pulse generator or receiver in the subcutaneous tissue. The physician selects a location site, usually the infraclavicular area, and incises the skin. Using blunt dissection, the physician creates a pocket for the generator or receiver. The unit is connected with the previously placed and separately reportable single electrode array and placed in the pocket. The operative incision is closed in layered sutures. In 61886, the pulse generator or receiver is implanted and connected to two or more electrode arrays.

61888

The physician removes or revises a pulse generator or receiver in the subcutaneous tissue. The physician incises the skin above the unit. After locating the generator or receiver, the physician removes or revises it. The operative incision is closed in sutured layers.

62000–62010

The physician elevates a depressed skull fracture to restore anatomical position. The physician incises and retracts the scalp to expose the skull depression. In 62000, the physician drills a bur hole and pulls up on the skull to elevate the bone. In 62005, there are multiple fracture lines. The bony pieces are stabilized in anatomic position. In 62010, the fracture has damaged the dura and brain. The physician removes the bony fragments and debrides the brain and dura. The dura is sutured closed and the bony fragments are approximated and stabilized in anatomic position. The scalp is reapproximated and closed in sutured layers.

62100

The physician repairs a dural/cerebrospinal fluid leak. The physician determines the location of the skull fracture using an MRI scan. The skin over the damaged area is incised. A bone flap is removed to access the dura which is sutured closed. The bone flap is replaced and stabilized. The scalp is reapproximated and closed in sutured layers.

62115–62117

The physician reduces an enlarged skull (e.g., secondary to hydrocephalus). The physician incises and retracts the scalp to expose the cranium. In 62115, the skull is cut and the bone is reshaped. In 62116, bone flaps are raised. After reshaping, the bony fragments are replaced and stabilized. In 62117, bone flaps are cut and raised. The bones are removed and reshaped; bone grafts may be used to shape the cranium. This code includes bone harvest.

62120–62121

The physician corrects an encephalocele. An encephalocele is a herniation in the brain into or through a defect in the cranium. In 62120, the defect is located in the skull vault. In 62121, the defect is in the skull base. The physician incises and retracts the

scalp and raises a bone flap. The bone is reshaped to increase skull size. The skull is stabilized and the scalp is reapproximated and closed in sutured layers.

62140–62141

The physician corrects a defect in the cranium. In 62140, the defect is less than 5.0 cm. In 62141, the defect is greater than 5.0 cm. The physician incises and retracts the scalp. The bone flaps are lifted and remodeled. A prosthesis may be used to reapproximate the bony edges. The skull is stabilized and the scalp is reapproximated and closed in sutured layers.

62142

The physician removes a bone flap or prosthetic plate of the skull. The physician incises the scalp above the area to be resected and retracts it. The stabilizers are removed and the bone flap lifted. The scalp is reapproximated over the dura and closed in sutured layers.

62143

The physician replaces a bone flap or prosthetic plate of the skull. The physician incises the scalp and retracts it to expose the dura. The bone graft or prosthetic plate is placed over dura to correct the defect. The bone or prosthetic plate is stabilized and the scalp is reapproximated and closed in sutured layers.

62145

The physician reshapes or reconstructs the cranium in addition to reparative brain surgery. The physician incises the scalp above the defect area. A bone flap is raised and the physician inspects the dura and the underlying brain. Any dural defects are corrected. The bone flaps are reshaped, reapproximated and stabilized. The scalp is closed in sutured layers.

62146–62147

The physician reshapes or reconstructs the cranium using bone grafts obtained from the patient. The physician incises the scalp above the defect area. The scalp is retracted and the defect is located. The physician incises the cranium and reshapes available skull bone. The physician then obtains bone grafts from the patient. The harvested bone is reshaped to supplement the cranium. The bones are approximated and stabilized. The scalp is reanastomosed and closed in sutured layers. In 62146 the defect is less than 5.0 cm in size. In 62147, the defect is greater than 5.0 cm.

62180

The physician performs a ventriculocisternostomy to form a communicating duct from the lateral ventricles to the cisterna magna to drain excess CSF into the spinal cord where it can be absorbed. The scalp is incised and retracted posterior to the ear. The physician drills a bur hole and inserts the proximal portion of the shunt toward the lateral ventricles, with or without the aid of an endoscope until CSF flows through the shunt. The distal end of the shunt is directed toward the cisterna magna until CSF flows through the shunt. The two ends are connected and tested. The dura is sutured closed and the scalp is reapproximated and closed in sutured layers.

62190–62192

The physician creates a shunt to form a communicating duct from the subdural or subarachnoid to the atria, jugular veins, auricular processes, pleural space, peritoneal space, or another area to drain excess CSF. The scalp is incised over the affected area. The physician drills a bur hole and inserts the proximal portion of the shunt into the subdural or subarachnoid space. The distal end of the shunt is directed and tunneled subcutaneously toward the selected drain site. The two ends are connected and tested. The dura is sutured closed and the scalp is reapproximated and closed in sutured layers. In an incision is required at the distal end, the operative incision is closed in sutured layers. Report 62190 if the distal end is located at the atria, jugular veins, or auricular processes. Report 62192 if it is located at the pleural space, peritoneal space, or another area.

62194

The physician irrigates or replaces a subarachnoid or subdural shunt system catheter. The physician incises and retracts the scalp over the placement origin. The dura is incised, and the catheter is irrigated to verify function. If the catheter is inoperative, it is replaced. The dura is sutured closed and the scalp is reapproximated and closed in sutured layers.

62200–62201

The physician performs a ventriculocisternostomy to form a communicating duct from the third ventricle to the cisterna magna to drain excess CSF into the spinal cord where it can be absorbed. The scalp is incised and retracted posterior to the ear. The physician drills a bur hole and inserts the proximal portion of the shunt toward the third ventricle, with or without the aid of an endoscope until CSF flows through the shunt. The distal end of the shunt is directed toward the cisterna magna until CSF flows through the shunt. The two ends are connected and tested. The dura is sutured closed and the scalp is reapproximated and closed in sutured layers. In 62201, the physician additionally uses MRI or CT guided stereotechniques.

62220–62223

The physician creates a shunt to form a communicating duct from the lateral ventricles to the atria, jugular veins, auricular processes, pleural space, peritoneal space, or another area, to drain excess CSF. The scalp is incised and retracted posterior to the ear. The physician drills a bur hole and inserts the proximal portion of the shunt toward the lateral ventricles, with or without the aid of an endoscope until CSF flows through the shunt. The distal end of the shunt is directed and tunneled subcutaneously toward the selected drain site. The two ends are connected and tested. The dura is sutured closed and the scalp is reapproximated and closed in sutured layers. If an incision is required at the distal end, the operative incision is closed in sutured layers. Report 62220 if the distal end is located at the atria, jugular veins, or auricular processes. Report 62223 if it is located at the pleural space, peritoneal space, or another area.

62225–62230

The physician replaces or revises an inoperative cerebrospinal fluid shunt system or component. The physician incises and retracts the scalp over the placement origin. The dura is incised, and the inoperative portion of the shunt system is located and replaced or revised. In 62225, the ventricular catheter is irrigated or replaced. In 62230, a cerebrospinal fluid shunt, valve, or distal catheter is revised or replaced. The shunt system is reconnected and tested. The dura is sutured closed; the scalp is reapproximated and sutured in layers.

62252

An adjustable cerebrospinal fluid (CSF) shunt is reprogrammed. Adjustable shunts have a pressure differential valve that alters resistance using a magnetic field transmitted through the skin. During a routine office visit, the valve setting is changed using an antenna whose emitted magnetic field rotates the stepper valve to the desired position. The stepper adjusts the tension of the spring, which in turn imposes resistance on the ball valve altering the flow of CSF fluid from the ventricles.

62256–62258

The physician removes a complete cerebrospinal fluid shunt system without replacement in 62256, and with replacement by a similar or other shunt in 62258. The physician incises and retracts the scalp over the placement origin. The dura is incised, and the shunt is located and removed. The dura is sutured closed; the scalp is reapproximated and sutured in layers. Report 62256 if the shunt system is only removed. Report 62258 if the shunt system is replaced during the same operation.

62263

The patient is placed in the sitting or lateral decubitus position for insertion of a needle into a vertebral interspace. The site to be entered is sterilized, local anesthesia is administered and the needle is inserted. Contrast media with fluoroscopy may be injected to confirm proper needle placement and to identify epidural adhesions. The physician injects solution or performs mechanical adhesion destruction to relieve epidural adhesions. With the procedure completed the needle is removed and the wound is dressed.

CPT® Lay Descriptions

62268

The physician removes the contents of a cyst or syrinx with a needle. A C-arm x-ray machine verifies placement of the needle (separately reportable). A spinal needle is inserted once the cyst or syrinx is located. The contents of the cyst are aspirated and the needle is removed. The wound is dressed.

62269

This procedure is performed to determine the nature and extent of a suspected lesion. The patient is placed in a spinal tap position. The affected vertebrae are located and local anesthesia is administered. The biopsy needle is inserted. In some cases, blood is drawn through the needle for testing. Imaging equipment is used to confirm placement, and samples are drawn from the lesion for inspection. When the procedure is completed, the needle is removed and the wound is dressed.

62270

The patient is placed in a spinal tap position. The biopsy needle is inserted. Fluid is drawn through the needle for separately reportable testing. When the procedure is completed, the needle is removed and the wound is dressed.

62272

This procedure is performed to lessen cerebrospinal fluid pressure. The patient is placed in a spinal tap position. The L3 and L4 vertebrae are located and local anesthesia is administered. The lumbar puncture needle is inserted. In some cases, spinal fluid is drawn through the needle as in a lumbar puncture test. In other cases, a catheter is inserted and the fluid empties into a reservoir. Pressure reading is performed with a manometer. When the procedure is completed, the needle is removed and the wound is dressed. In many cases, the patient lies prone to prevent fluid leakage.

62273

This procedure is performed following a spinal puncture to prevent spinal fluid leakage. The patient remains in a spinal tap position. The patient's blood is injected outside the dura to clot and plug the wound, preventing spinal fluid leakage. The wound is dressed and monitored.

62280–62282

This procedure is performed to destroy nerve tissue or adhesions. The patient is placed in a spinal tap position. The site is sterilized, and the needle is inserted under separately reportable fluoroscopic guidance. The needle is placed at the proper level and the neurolytic substance is administered. Once the injection/infusion is completed, the needle is removed and the wound dressed. Report 62280 if the substance is administered to the subarachnoid level. Report 62281 if the needle is inserted in the epidural region of a cervical or thoracic level. Report 62882 if the

needle is inserted in the epidural region of a lumbar or sacral (caudal) level.

62284

The physician injects dye into the epidural or intrathecal space for myelography and or computerized axial tomography (CT scan), reported separately. The patient is placed in a spinal tap position. The site is sterilized, and the needle is inserted. The needle is placed to the proper level and the dye is administered. The needle is removed and the wound dressed.

62287

This procedure corrects a bulge in an intervertebral disk. It is commonly referred to as percutaneous diskectomy and may be accomplished by several techniques including non-automated (manual), automated, or laser. For all techniques, the patient is placed in a spinal tap position on the left side. In a separately reportable procedure, a C-arm x-ray verifies placement of the needle in the disk. Once the disk is located, local anesthesia is injected and a small stab wound is made. A spinal needle is inserted with additional monitoring of placement and injection of anesthesia. Using a manual technique, the physician inserts one or two needles into the disk without puncturing the dura. The patient is placed on pure oxygen and the nucleus pulposus is suctioned out until the desired decompression is accomplished. The needle(s) are removed and the wound is dressed. The automated technique makes use of a probe that can simultaneously dissect the disc and suck it into the probe. Laser diskectomy accomplishes the decompression by vaporizing the protruding disc.

62290

This procedure is performed to gauge the amount of damage suffered by an intervertebral disk. The patient is placed on an image intensification table in a left lateral decubitus position with hips and knees are flexed. The injection site is determined and marked on the sterilized surface, and local anesthesia is injected. A small stab wound is made in the tissue overlying the vertebrae. The physician directs a needle at a 45 degree angle to the center line toward the spine. In a separately reported procedure, the needle is monitored radiographically. A small needle is inserted through original needle once the needle reaches the lamina. The physician pushes this needle to the disk and injects 1.0 ml to 2.0 ml of contrast medium. In separately reported procedures, radiographs are made and the procedure may be performed again on another level. The wound is dressed.

62291

This procedure is performed to gauge the amount of damage suffered by an intervertebral disk. The patient is placed on an image intensification table in a supine position with the head extended. The proper injection site is determined and marked on the sterilized surface, and local anesthesia is injected. A small stab wound is made in the tissue overlying the vertebrae. The physician directs a needle at a 35 degree angle to the sagittal plane toward the spine. In a separately reported procedure, the needle is monitored radiographically. A small needle is inserted through original needle once the needle reaches the lamina. The physician pushes this needle to the disk and injects 1.0 ml to 2.0 ml of contrast medium. In separately reported procedures, radiographs are made and the procedure may be performed again on another level. The wound is dressed.

62292

This procedure introduces a corrective chemical enzyme into a herniated disk. The patient is placed in a spinal tap position on the left side. In a separately reported procedure, a C-arm x-ray machine is used to verify location of the disk. Once the disk is located, local anesthesia is injected and a small stab wound is made. A spinal needle is inserted with additional monitoring of placement and injection of anesthesia. Without puncturing the dura, the physician inserts the needle into the disk. This procedure can be performed with one or two needles. A separately reportable saline acceptance test is performed to verify correct placement. Diskography is then performed with an opaque substance to verify location of the herniated disk.. A reparative enzyme is injected. The needles are removed and the wound is dressed.

62294

This procedure is performed to locate and occlude an arteriovenous malformation in the spinal cord. A separately reportable image intensifying x-ray is used to position the patient and identify the artery to be injected. The physician directs a needle at the feeder arteries of the arteriovenous malformation and causes an occlusion by embolization. The needle is monitored radiographically. Once the occlusion of the malformation is completed and needle is removed, the wound is dressed.

62310

The patient is placed in a sitting or lateral decubitus position for the physician to insert a needle into the vertebral interspace of the thoracic or cervical region. The site to be entered is sterilized, local anesthesia is administered and the needle is inserted. Contrast media with fluoroscopy may be injected to confirm proper needle placement. The physician injects a solution to provide either a therapeutic or diagnostic outcome. The solution is injected into the epidural or subarachnoid space. With the procedure complete the needle is removed and the wound is dressed.

62311

The patient is placed in a sitting or lateral decubitus position for the physician to insert a needle into the vertebral interspace of the lumbar or sacral region.

The site to be entered is sterilized, local anesthesia is administered and the needle is inserted. Contrast media may be injected to confirm proper needle placement under fluoroscopy. The physician injects a solution to provide either a therapeutic or diagnostic outcome. The solution is injected into the epidural or subarachnoid space. With the procedure complete the needle is removed and the wound is dressed.

62318

The patient is placed in the sitting or lateral decubitus position for the physician to insert a catheter into the vertebral interspace of the cervical or thoracic region for continuous or intermittent infusion of material. The site to be entered is sterilized, local anesthesia is administered and the infusion catheter is inserted. Contrast media with fluoroscopy may be injected to confirm proper catheter placement. The physician provides continuous infusion or intermittent bolus injection of solution to provide either a therapeutic or diagnostic outcome. The solution is injected into the epidural or subarachnoid space. With the procedure complete the needle is removed and the wound is dressed.

62319

The patient is placed in the sitting or lateral decubitus position for the physician to insert a catheter into the vertebral interspace of the lumbar or sacral region for continuous or intermittent infusion of material. The site to be entered is sterilized, local anesthesia is administered and the infusion catheter is inserted. Contrast media may be injected to confirm proper catheter placement. The physician provides continuous infusion or intermittent bolus injection of solution to provide either a therapeutic or diagnostic outcome. The solution is injected into the epidural or subarachnoid space. With the procedure complete the needle is removed and the wound is dressed.

62350–62355

This procedure is performed to allow direct instillation of medication via the cerebrospinal fluid. If the catheter is to be implanted the patient is placed in a spinal tap position and and the fascia, paravertebral muscles, and ligaments are incised and separated. The physician inserts the catheter tip into the epidural space (the space outside the dura) or through the dura placing the catheter tip into the subarachnoid space. Tissue around the catheter may be sutured to hold the catheter in place. The catheter end is tunneled to the site where an implantable reservoir or implantable infusion pump has been previously placed or where a pump or reservoir is to be placed (subcutaneously) in a separately reportable procedure. This procedure also includes the revision of a intrathecal or epidural catheter, which may include replacing or repositioning a catheter. In 62351, the physician performs a laminectomy, making an incision and removing the lamina of the vertebra to access the dura through which the catheter is inserted. In 62355, the catheter is removed.

62360–62365

This procedure is performed to allow medication (e.g., cancer chemotherapy, pain management drugs) to be placed into a subcutaneous reservoir for intrathecal or epidural drug infusion. The patient is placed prone. The physician makes a midline incision overlying the placement site. The reservoir is placed in the subcutaneous tissues and attached to a previously placed catheter. Layered sutures are used to close the incision. Report 62360 for subcutaneous reservoir implantation or replacement, 62361 for non-progmammable pump implantation or replacement, 62362 for a programmable pump implantation or replacement, and 62365 for removal of the reservoir or pump.

62367–62368

The physician, physician's assistant, nurse, or physical therapist places electrodes over the site of the programmable pump and reviews performance of the generator on a computer. Report 62637 if the pump is not reprogrammed; report 62368 if it is reprogrammed.

63001–63011

The patient is placed prone and the physician makes a posterior midline incision overlying the vertebrae. The paravertebral muscles are retracted. The physician removes the appropriate spinous process and interspinous ligament with a rongeur. The physician excises the lamina and the attached ligamentum flavum may be removed. Decompression is continued by removal of bony overgrowths or tissue until the dural sac and nerve roots are free from any compression. Free-fat grafts or Gelfoam may be placed over the exposed nerve roots. If the ligamentum flavum has not been removed or if only portions of it were removed, it may be closed over the fat graft. A drain is placed superficial to the fat graft; the fascia, subcutaneous tissue, and skin are closed in layers. Report 63003 if vertebrae are thoracic; report 63005 if vertebrae are lumbar, except in the case of spondylolisthesis; and report 63011 if vertebrae are sacral.

63012

The physician performs the laminectomy to correct spondylolisthesis, the slipping of the lumbar vertebrae forward where they join the sacral vertebrae. The patient is placed prone. The physician makes a midline incision overlying the lumbar vertebrae to facilitate repair of the spondylolisthesis. The fascia are incised and the paravertebral muscles are retracted. The physician resects the spinous processes of all three vertebrae and the middle part of the loose fifth lumbar neural arch. The ligamentum flavum is freed or excised at various levels of vertebrae. The fifth lumbar nerve root is carefully retracted.

Decompression is carried out to include the facets as well as other bony or soft tissue structures that may be applying pressure to the spinal cord, nerve roots, or cauda equina. The procedure is then repeated on the opposite side. The incision is closed with layered sutures.

63015–63017

The patient is placed prone and the physician makes a posterior midline incision overlying the vertebrae. The paravertebral muscles are retracted. A rongeur is used to remove the appropriate spinous processes and interspinous ligaments. The physician excises the affected laminae and the attached ligamentum flavum may be removed. Decompression is continued by removal of bony overgrowths or tissue until the dural sac and nerve roots are free from any compression. Free-fat grafts or Gelfoam may be placed over the exposed nerve roots. If the ligamentum flavum has not been removed or if only portions of it were removed it may be closed over the fat graft. A drain is placed superficial to the fat graft; the fascia, subcutaneous tissue, and skin are closed in layers. Report 63015 if vertebrae are cervical; report 63016 if the laminae are thoracic; report 63017 if lumbar.

63020–63035

Through a posterior (back) approach a midline incision is made overlying the vertebrae. The incision is carried down through the tissue to the paravertebral muscles, which are retracted. The ligamentum flavum, which attaches the lamina from one vertebra to the lamina of another may be partially or completely removed. Part of the lamina is removed on one side to allow access to the spinal cord. If a disk has ruptured, fragments or the part of the disk compressing the nerves are removed. A partial removal of a facet (facetectomy) or removal of bone around the foramen (foraminotomy) may also be performed to relieve pressure on the nerve. When decompression is complete, a free-fat graft may be placed to protect the nerve root. If the ligamentum flavum was not entirely removed, it is placed over the fat graft. Paravertebral muscles are repositioned and the tissue is closed in layers. Report 63020 if the disks are cervical. Report 63030 if lumbar. Note that lumbar approaches may be performed using either an open approach as described above or an endoscopically assisted approach. In an endoscopically assisted approach, a small guide probe is inserted under fluoroscopic guidance. Using magnified video as well as fluoroscopic guidance, the endoscope is manipulated through the foramen and into the spinal canal. Once the guide probe has been advanced to the surgical site, a slightly larger tube is manipulated over the guide probe. Surgical instruments are advanced through the hollow center of the tube. Herniated disk fragments are removed and the disk is reconfigured to eliminate pressure on the nerve root(s). The endoscope is withdrawn. The incision is sutured or simply dressed with an adhesive bandage. Report 63035 for additional interspaces, cervical or lumbar.

63040–63044

Through a posterior approach, a midline incision is made overlying the vertebrae. The incision is carried through the tissue to the paravertebral muscles, which are retracted. If the ligamentum flavum (which attaches lamina from one vertebrae to the lamina of another) is still present, it may be partially or completely removed. The lamina may be removed on the opposite side or more of the lamina may be removed from the previous site to allow access to the spinal cord. If ruptured intervertebral disk fragments or part of the disk continues to compress the nerve, they are removed. A partial removal of a facet or removal of bone around the foramen may also be performed if they are causing pressure on the nerve. When decompression is complete, a previously placed free-fat graft may be replaced over the nerve root. If the ligamentum flavum was not entirely removed in the first surgery or in the exploration it is placed over the fat graft. Paravertebral muscles are repositioned and the tissue is closed in layers. Report 63040 if performed on a single cervical interspace; report 63042 if performed on a single lumbar interspace; report 63043 for each additional cervical interspace; report 63044 for each additional lumbar interspace.

63045–63048

The patient is placed prone. Magnification may be used during the procedure. The physician makes a midline incision overlying the affected vertebrae. Fascia is incised. Paravertebral muscles are retracted. The physician removes the spinous processes with ronguers. If the stenosis is central, the physician removes the lamina out to the articular facets using a burr. If the compression is in the lateral recess, only half of the lamina is removed. A Penfield elevator is used to peel the ligamentum flavum away from the dura. Nerve root canals are freed by additional resection of the facet, and compression is relieved by removal of any bony or tissue overgrowth around the foramen. Removal of the lamina, facets, and bony tissue or overgrowths may be performed bilaterally when indicated. The ronguer, retractor, and microscope are removed. A free-fat graft may be placed over the nerve root(s) for protection. If the ligamentum flavum was spared, it is placed over the free-fat graft. Paravertebral muscles are repositioned and the deeper tissues and skin are closed with layered sutures. Report 63046 if the procedure affects a thoracic vertebra; report 63047 if the procedure affects a lumbar vertebra; and 63048 for procedures affecting each additional vertebra.

63055–63057

This procedure is performed to relieve pressure on the spinal cord, equina, and nerve roots caused by a herniated disk. The physician approaches the herniated disk through the pedicle on the side of the disk's bulge. Additional exposure is made by removing the lamina and facet joint. The physician removes the disk fragments and closes the wound in layers. Report

63055 if the segment is thoracic. Report 63056 if the segment is lumbar. A far lateral herniated lumbar intervertebral disc may require an alternative approach either through the facet joint (transfacet) or foramina (transforaminal). Report 63057 for each additional segment, thoracic or lumbar.

63064–63066

The physician makes an incision two inches to three inches lateral to the spine through fascia, muscles, and a section of a rib. The physician enters anterior to the transverse process and the pedicle using a Kerrington rongeur or burr. Exposure may be increased by removal of the transverse process. The spinal cord or nerve root is decompressed by removing the herniated disk. The wound is filled with saline and radiographs (separately reported) are made to assure no air is leading into the lungs. The muscles are allowed to fall over a drain and the tissue is closed with layered sutures. Report 63064 if a single segment is repaired. Report 63066 for additional segments.

63075–63076

The physician performs a cervical diskectomy to remove all or part of a herniated intervertebral disk. The patient is placed supine with a head halter on the jawbone (mandible). The physician makes a transverse incision overlying the intervertebral disk. The sternocleidomastoid muscle and the carotid artery are retracted. The physician excises the anterior anulus of the disk and uses pituitary forceps to remove as much disk material as possible. A spreader and microscope are used to enhance the evacuation. A drill is used to remove the transverse bar above and below. Graft material is obtained from the ilium and fashioned into a T-shape. The graft is placed into the disk space and traction is released. The muscles are allowed to fall back into place and the incision is closed with layered sutures. Report 63075 if the diskectomy is in a single interspace. Report 63076 for each additional cervical interspace.

63077–63078

The physician makes an incision along the rib corresponding to the second thoracic vertebra above the involved intervertebral disk, except in cases involving the top five disks. The rib is removed for access and eventually used in the graft, which is obtained through an extrapleural or transpleural approach. Vessels are tied away from the spine. The disk is removed to the posterior ligament using a microscope and nibbling instruments. The end plates are stripped of their cartilage. The physician makes a slot in one vertebral body and a hole in the other to accept the graft, which is made of several sections of rib. The physician ties the grafts together with heavy suture material and closes the tissue with layered sutures. A chest drain may be inserted. Report 63077 for a single thoracic interspace. Report 63078 for each additional thoracic interspace.

63081–63082

The patient is placed supine with traction-producing tongs. The physician makes a right transverse incision at mid position of the planned surgical procedure, and longitudinally between the thyroid gland and the carotid sheath. The disks above and below the vertebrae are excised using a curet. Cartilaginous endplates are removed using a high-speed burr. The crushed part of the vertebral body is partially or completely removed, and the section is prepared for the graft. The anterior surfaces of the vertebrae above and below the fusion are debrided. The physician prepares a separately reportable, tricortical iliac graft and inserts it into the site, tapping it into place with a Moe impacter. Traction is released. Bone chips are packed in and, if needed, a metal plate is screwed to the spine over the graft. The muscles are allowed to fall back into place and the wound is closed with layered sutures. Report 63081 if one segment is involved; report 63082 for each additional cervical segment.

63085–63088

This procedure corrects compression on the spinal cord resulting from an anterior fracture of the vertebra. The patient is placed in a swimmer's position. The physician makes an incision through the fascia, muscles, and organs. The disks above and below the vertebrae are excised using a curet. Cartilaginous endplates are removed using a high-speed burr. The crushed part of the vertebral body is partially or completely removed, and the section is prepared for the graft. The anterior surfaces of the vertebrae above and below the fusion are debrided. The physician prepares a tricortical iliac graft and inserts it into the site, tapping it into place with a Moe impacter. Traction is released. Bone chips are packed in and, if needed, a metal plate is screwed to the spine over the graft. The muscles are allowed to fall back into place and the wound is closed with layered sutures. Report 63085 if one thoracic segment is involved; report 63086 if more than one is involved; report 63087 if caudal equina, lower thoracic, or lumbar, single segment is involved; report 65088 for each additional segment.

63090–63091

The physician makes a transperitoneal or retroperitoneal approach through skin, fascia, muscles, and ligaments. The physician incises the anterior longitudinal ligament above and below the vertebral body. Using magnification, the physician removes the disk to the posterior longitudinal ligament using nipper instruments. The physician may choose to use dowel or tricortical iliac grafts and prepares the site as appropriate using an osteotome. Usually three grafts can be inserted. They are tapped into place and surrounded with bone chips. The physician sutures the anterior longitudinal ligament. The peritoneum and abdomen are closed in the usual manner. Report 63090 for a single segment. Report 63091 for each additional segment.

63170

This procedure is performed to alleviate peripheral pain caused by avulsion of parts of the spinal cord's white matter. The patient is placed prone. The physician makes a midline incision. The fascia are incised. The paravertebral muscles and ligaments are retracted. Following a laminectomy, the physician incises the dura to gain access to the spinal cord. Without disturbing the central grey matter, the physician incises the outer white matter of the spinal cord, using a laser or a a radio frequency electrode to thermally coagulate the white matter. Fascia, muscles, and ligaments are allowed to fall back into place. The physician closes the incision with layered sutures.

63172–63173

This procedure is performed to alleviate the effects of a spinal cyst or syrinx. The patient is placed prone. The physician makes a midline incision overlying the affected vertebrae. The fascia are incised. The paravertebral muscles are retracted. Laminectomy is performed. The spinal needle is placed in the intramedullary cyst or syrinx, and the cyst or syrinx is drained to the subarachnoid space. Fascia, muscles, and ligaments are allowed to fall back into place. The incision is closed with layered sutures. Report 63172 if the drainage is to the subarachnoid space. Report 63173 if the drainage is to the peritoneal space.

63180–63182

The patient is placed prone. The physician makes a midline incision overlying the affected vertebrae. The fascia are incised. The paravertebral muscles are retracted. The physician incises the dura and locates the dentate ligaments. With the aid of magnification, the physician sections the affected ligaments. The dura is closed with sutures or a graft to assure competency. The incision is closed with layered sutures. Report 63180 if the one or two vertebra is affected; report 63182 if more than two vertebrae are affected.

63185–63190

A rhizotomy is performed on the anterior nerve roots to stop involuntary spasmodic movements associated with paraplegia or torticollis. It is also performed on the posterior nerve roots to eliminate pain in a restricted area. The patient is placed prone. The physician makes a midline incision overlying the affected vertebrae. The fascia are incised. The paravertebral muscles are retracted. Laminectomy is performed. The physician identifies the anterior or posterior nerve roots to be divided. Each is lifted with a nerve hook and severed. Fascia, muscles, and ligaments are allowed to fall back into place. The incision is closed with layered sutures. Report 63185 if the procedure includes one or two segments; report 63190 if the procedure includes two or more segments.

63191

This procedure is performed to alleviate chronic pain. The patient is placed prone. The physician makes a midline incision overlying the affected vertebrae. The fascia are incised. The paravertebral muscles are retracted. The physician removes the lamina. The physician identifies and incises the spinal accessory nerve. The lesion is removed and sutures are placed in the perineurium of the nerves. The sutures are approximated and tied. Fascia, muscles, and ligaments are allowed to fall back into place. The incision is closed with layered sutures.

63194–63195

This procedure is performed to alleviate pain. The patient is placed prone. The physician makes a midline incision overlying the affected vertebrae. The fascia are incised. The paravertebral muscles are retracted. A laminectomy is performed. The physician identifies the anterolateral tracts in the appropriate level on the side opposite the pain. The dentate ligament is divided at the level of the cordotomy. The ligament is drawn posteriorly toward the midline to expose the anterolateral part of the cord. A cordotomy knife is introduced into the spinal cord anterior to the dentate ligament and directed toward the anterior spinal artery. The tissue in front of this artery is divided with the knife. The incision is closed with layered sutures. Report 63194 if the affected vertebrae are cervical; report 63195 if the affected vertebrae are thoracic.

63196–63197

This procedure is performed to alleviate pain. The patient is placed prone. The physician makes a midline incision overlying the site of the cordotomy. The fascia are incised. The paravertebral muscles are retracted. A laminectomy is performed. The physician identifies the spinothalamic tracts in the appropriate levels. The dentate ligament is divided at the level of the cordotomy. The ligament is drawn posteriorly toward the midline to expose the anterolateral part of the cord. A cordotomy knife is introduced into the spinal cord anterior to the dentate ligament and directed toward the anterior spinal artery. The tissue in front of this artery is divided with the knife. The incision is closed with layered sutures. Report 63196 if the affected vertebrae are cervical; report 63197 if the affected vertebrae are thoracic.

63198–63199

This procedure is performed to stop chronic pain or spasms. The patient is placed prone. The physician makes a midline incision overlying the affected vertebrae. The fascia are incised. The paravertebral muscles are retracted. The physician identifies the spinothalamic tracts in the appropriate level. The dentate ligament is divided at the level of the cordotomy. The ligament is drawn posteriorly toward the midline to expose the anterolateral part of the cord. A cordotomy knife is introduced into the spinal

cord anterior to the dentate ligament and directed toward the anterior spinal artery. The tissue in front of this artery is divided with the knife. Muscles, fascia, and ligaments are allowed to fall back into place. The incision is closed with layered sutures. The procedure is performed on the opposite side of the spinal cord within 14 days. Report 63198 if the cervical vertebrae are affected; report 63199 if the thoracic vertebrae are affected.

63200

This procedure is performed to correct neurological deficits in the lower extremities and sphincter dysfunctions caused by a spinal cord shortened by adhesions to the dura. The patient is placed prone. The physician makes a midline incision over the lumbar vertebrae. The fascia are incised. The paravertebral muscles are retracted. A laminectomy is performed. The physician may choose from a number of techniques, but generally requires a dural opening. A surgical microscope is used to dissect the adhesions and fibrous bands. The filum is identified and transected. Care is taken to avoid severing the nerves tangled with the adhesions. If no spina bifida or myelomeningocele is present, the dura is closed to make a "sac." Muscles, fascia, and ligaments are closed. The incision is closed with a layered sutures.

63250–63252

This procedure is performed for excision or purposeful occlusion of an arteriovenous malformation of the spinal cord. The patient is placed prone. The physician makes an incision overlying the cervical vertebra in the area of the arteriovenous malformation. The fascia and paraspinal muscles are retracted and a laminectomy is performed to to access the spinal cord. Microsurgical techniques are used to excise or occlude the arteriovenous malformation. After muscles, fascia, and ligaments are repaired, the incision is closed with layered sutures. Report 63251 if thoracic; report 63252 if thoracolumbar.

63265–63268

This procedure removes a growth in the spine. The patient is placed prone. The physician makes a midline incision. Fascia are incised. Paravertebral muscles are retracted. The physician removes the laminae and the spinous processes of the vertebrae to expose the outside of the dura. The extradural intraspinal lesion is excised or evacuated. The incision is closed with layered sutures. Report 63265 if the lesion is in the cervical region; report 63266 if the lesion is in the thoracic region; report 63267 if the lesion is in the lumbar region. Report 63268 if the lesion is in the sacral region.

63270–63273

This procedure removes a growth in the spine. The patient is placed prone. The physician makes a midline incision. The fascia are incised. The paravertebral muscles are retracted. The physician removes the laminae and the spinous processes of the vertebrae to be exposed. The dura is exposed and incised. The pia-arachnoid is incised as necessary. The lesion is removed. The incision is closed with layered sutures. Report 63270 if the lesion is located in the cervical region; report 63271 if the lesion is in the thoracic region; report 63272 if the lesion is in the lumbar region; report 63273 if the lesion is in the sacral region.

63275–63278

The patient is placed prone. The physician makes a midline incision. Fascia are incised. Paravertebral muscles are retracted. The physician removes the laminae and the spinous processes of the vertebrae to the dura. A biopsy is taken of the neoplasm and the neoplasm is removed. Muscles, fascia, and ligaments are repaired. The incision is closed with layered sutures. Report 63275 if the neoplasm is in the cervical area; report 63276 if it is in the thoracic area; report 63277 if it is in the lumbar area; and report 63278 if it is in the sacral area.

63280

This procedure is performed to remove a growth in the spine. The patient is placed in a prone position. The physician makes a midline incision. Fascia are incised. Paravertebral muscles are retracted. The physician removes the laminae and the spinous processes of the vertebrae to be exposed. The dura is exposed and incised. The neoplasm is identified and a biopsy is taken. The neoplasm is removed. The dura is sutured with silk sutures, and the incision is closed with layered sutures.

63281

The patient is placed in a prone position. The physician makes a midline incision. Fascia are incised. Paravertebral muscles are retracted. The physician removes the laminae and the spinous processes of the vertebrae to be exposed. The dura is exposed and incised. The neoplasm is identified and a biopsy is taken. The neoplasm is removed. The dura is sutured with silk sutures, and the incision is closed with layered sutures.

63282

This procedure is performed to remove a growth in the spine. The patient is placed in a prone position. The physician makes a midline incision. Fascia are incised. Paravertebral muscles are retracted. The physician removes the laminae and the spinous processes of the vertebrae to be exposed. The dura is exposed and incised. The neoplasm is identified and a biopsy is taken. The neoplasm is removed. The dura is sutured with silk sutures, and the incision is closed with layered sutures.

63283

This procedure is performed to remove a growth in the spine. The patient is placed in a prone position.

The physician makes a midline incision. Fascia are incised. Paravertebral muscles are retracted. The physician removes the laminae and the spinous processes of the vertebrae to be exposed. The dura is exposed and incised. The neoplasm is identified and a biopsy is taken. The neoplasm is removed. The dura is sutured with silk sutures, and the incision is closed with layered sutures.

63285

This procedure is performed to remove a growth in the spine. The patient is placed in a prone position. The physician makes a midline incision. Fascia are incised. Paravertebral muscles are retracted. The physician removes the laminae and the spinous processes of the vertebrae to be exposed. The dura is exposed and incised. The neoplasm is identified and a biopsy is taken. The neoplasm is removed. The dura is sutured with silk sutures, and the incision is closed with layered sutures.

63286

This procedure is performed to remove a growth in the spine. The patient is placed in a prone position. The physician makes a midline incision. Fascia are incised. Paravertebral muscles are retracted. The physician removes the laminae and the spinous processes of the vertebrae to be exposed. The dura is exposed and incised. The neoplasm is identified and a biopsy is taken. The neoplasm is removed. The dura is sutured with silk sutures, and the incision is closed with layered sutures.

63287

This procedure is performed to remove a growth in the spine. The patient is placed in a prone position. The physician makes a midline incision. Fascia are incised. Paravertebral muscles are retracted. The physician removes the laminae and the spinous processes of the vertebrae to be exposed. The dura is exposed and incised. The neoplasm is identified and a biopsy is taken. The neoplasm is removed. The dura is sutured with silk sutures, and the incision is closed with layered sutures.

63290

This procedure is performed to remove a growth in the spine. The patient is placed in a prone position. The physician makes a midline incision. Fascia are incised. Paravertebral muscles are retracted. The physician removes the laminae and the spinous processes of the vertebrae to be exposed. The dura is exposed and incised. The neoplasm is identified and a biopsy is taken. The neoplasm is removed. The dura is sutured with silk sutures, and the incision is closed with layered sutures.

63300

This procedure is performed to remove an intraspinal lesion in the extradural space of the spinal canal. The patient is placed supine with the head extended by tongs and traction. Either a right transverse incision or right vertical incision is made in the lateral neck. The muscles and fascia are incised and retracted. Entering between the trachea and the carotid sheath, the physician resects the vertebral body and the intraspinal lesion is excised by the physician. After repair of the muscles, fascia, and ligaments, the wound closed with layered sutures.

63301

This procedure is performed to remove a lesion from a vertebra. The patient is placed in a lateral decubitus position and the physician makes a transthoracic approach overlying the rib corresponding to the affected vertebrae. The physician removes the rib and retracts muscles, fascia, and organs to expose the spine. The tumor mass is completely excised. Following repair of the muscles, fascia, and ligaments, the wound is closed in a routine fashion over suction drains.

63302

This procedure is performed to remove a lesion of the vertebral body, which compresses the spinal cord. The patient is placed in a lateral decubitus position with supports under the buttocks and shoulder, and the muscle, fascia, ribs, and organs are incised or retracted. An incision is made in the diaphragm to purchase access to the spine. The tumor mass is completely excised. After muscles, fascia, and ligaments are repaired, the wound is closed in a routine fashion over suction drains.

63303

This procedure is performed to remove a lesion of the vertebral body, which compresses the spinal cord. The patient is placed in a lateral decubitus position with approach from the left side, and the muscle, fascia, ribs, and organs are incised or retracted. The physician makes a groove in the vertebral bodies above and below the crushed vertebra and removes the disks above and below. Tricortical iliac crest grafts are obtained, prepared, and tapped into the grooves with a Moe impactor. An AO plate is screwed to the vertebra above and below the injured level to maintain fusion. A separately reported radiograph is obtained to assure proper placement, and the wound closed with layered sutures.

63304

This procedure is performed to correct a fracture or growth of the vertebral body, which compresses the spinal cord. The patient is placed supine with the head extended by tongs and traction. Either a right transverse incision or right vertical incision is made in the lateral neck. The muscles and fascia are incised and retracted. The dura may be incised. Entering between the trachea and the carotid sheath, the physician makes a groove in the vertebral bodies above and below the crushed vertebra and removes the disks above and below. Tricortical iliac crest grafts

are obtained, prepared, and tapped into the grooves with a Moe impactor. Traction is removed. An AO plate is screwed to the vertebra above and below the injured level to maintain fusion. A separately reported radiograph is obtained to assure proper placement, and the wound closed with layered sutures.

63305

This procedure is performed to correct a fracture or growth of the vertebral body, which compresses the spinal cord. The patient is placed in a lateral decubitus position and the muscle, fascia, ribs, and organs are incised or retracted. The dura may be incised.The physician makes a groove in the vertebral bodies above and below the crushed vertebra and removes the disks above and below. Tricortical iliac crest grafts are obtained, prepared, and tapped into the grooves with a Moe impactor. An AO plate is screwed to the vertebra above and below the injured level to maintain fusion. A separately reported radiograph is obtained to assure proper placement, and the wound closed with layered sutures.

63306

This procedure is performed to remove a lesion of the vertebral body, which compresses the spinal cord. The patient is placed in a lateral decubitus position with supports under the buttocks and shoulder, and the muscle, fascia, ribs, and organs are incised or retracted. The dura may be incised. An incision is made in the diaphragm to purchase access to the spine. The physician makes a groove in the vertebral bodies above and below the crushed vertebra and removes the disks above and below. Tricortical iliac crest grafts are obtained, prepared, and tapped into the grooves with a Moe impactor. An AO plate is screwed to the vertebra above and below the injured level to maintain fusion. A separately reported radiograph is obtained to assure proper placement, and the wound closed with layered sutures.

63307

This procedure is performed to remove a lesion of the vertebral body, which compresses the spinal cord. The patient is placed in a lateral decubitus position with approach from the left side, and the muscle, fascia, ribs, and organs are incised or retracted. The dura may be incised. The physician makes a groove in the vertebral bodies above and below the crushed vertebra and removes the disks above and below. Tricortical iliac crest grafts are obtained, prepared, and tapped into the grooves with a Moe impactor. An AO plate is screwed to the vertebra above and below the injured level to maintain fusion. A separately reported radiograph is obtained to assure proper placement, and the wound closed with layered sutures.

63308

This procedure is performed to remove a lesion of the vertebral body, which compresses the spinal cord. The patient is placed in a lateral decubitus position with approach from the left side, and the muscle, fascia, ribs, and organs are incised or retracted. The physician makes a groove in the vertebral bodies above and below the crushed vertebra and removes the disks above and below. Tricortical iliac crest grafts are obtained, prepared, and tapped into the grooves with a Moe impactor. An AO plate is screwed to the vertebra above and below the injured level to maintain fusion. A separately reported radiograph is obtained to assure proper placement, and the wound closed with layered sutures.

63600–63615

Lesions in the spinal cord are produced to alleviate chronic pain in a particular area of the body. A common surgery involves creating a lesion in the spinothalamic tracts for pain relief. In this procedure, a stereotactic guidance system is used to enable a physician to conceptualize a position in three-dimensional space. The stereotactic frame is applied to the head with full neck flexion and fixed to the operating table with the patient in the sitting position. Following previously determined coordinates, needles are placed through the C1–C2 interspace. Electrical stimulation and other methods are applied to create a lesion that will block the pain. The needles and the frame are removed. Wounds are dressed. Report 63610 if the stereotactic method is used for a procedure not followed by another; report 63615 if the stereotactic method is used to biopsy, aspirate, or excise a lesion from the spinal cord.

63650

This procedure is performed to alleviate pain or control spasms. The patient is placed prone. A standard epidural puncture is made. A thin-walled needle is placed at the appropriate segment. A flexible wire electrode is threaded through the needle under fluoroscopic control. Intraoperative testing is carried out to assure correct electrode positioning creating maximum parasthesia in the pain region. The needle is removed and a dressing applied. A transmitter (pulse generator or receiver) is inserted in a separately reportable procedure. Stimulation may be applied as soon as four days following the procedure.

63655

This procedure is performed to alleviate pain or control spasms. The patient is placed prone. The physician makes a midline incision overlying the affected vertebra. The fascia are incised. The paravertebral muscles are retracted. The lamina is removed to expose the epidural space. The physician places passive electrodes or plates or paddles in the epidural space proximate to the desired spine segment. Paravertebral muscles are reapproximated and the incision is closed with layered sutures. A transmitter (pulse generator or receiver) is inserted in a separately reportable procedure. Stimulation may be applied as soon as four days following the procedures.

63660

This procedure is performed to remove or revise neurostimulator electrodesor plates or paddles. The patient is placed prone. The physician makes a midline incision overlying the affected vertebrae. The fascia are incised. The paravertebral muscles are retracted. If the original electrodes were placed percutaneously, a laminectomy of the vertebra would not be performed. If moved to a new segment, a laminectomy may be performed to gain access to the epidural space. The physician removes the electrodes or plates or paddles in the epidural space proximate to the spine segment or moves them to a new vertebral segment. Stimulation is applied.

63685

This procedure is performed to promote nerve regeneration. The patient is placed in a prone position. The physician makes a midline incision overlying the affected vertebrae. The fascia is incised. The paravertebral muscles are retracted. The physician places the direct electrode needles or inductive electrode pads in or on the epidural space proximate to the damaged spine segment, placing them in the right plane. The generator or receiver is placed over sutured muscles but below the skin. Layered sutures are used to close the incision.

63688

This procedure is performed to promote nerve regeneration. The patient is placed in a prone. The physician makes a midline incision overlying the affected vertebrae. The fascia is incised. The paravertebral muscles are retracted. The physician moves or removes the direct electrode needles or inductive electrode pads in or on the epidural space proximate to the damaged spine segment, placing them in the right plane. The generator or receiver is moved or removed over sutured muscles but below the skin. Layered sutures are used to close the incision.

63700–63702

The physician corrects a defect in which the outer coverings of the spinal cord, meninges, and (sometimes) nervous tissue bulge through a bony defect. The patient is placed prone, and the physician makes a midline incision and retraction through the skin, muscles, and paravertebral ligaments. The dura is incised to avoid herniated neural tissue. The physician places the neural tissue in the spinal canal. In the lumbar region, filum terminale are often identified tethering the cord and divided. The dural defect, subcutaneous tissues, and skin are closed with layered sutures. Report 63700 for meningoceles less than 5.0 cm diameter; report 63702 for meningoceles greater than 5.0 cm.

63704–63706

The physician corrects a defect in which the spinal cord, malformed nerve roots, and meninges all protrude through the defect, often directly exposed to the outside of the body. Surgery can be performed in one of many ways, though most require fusion from the thoracic region to the sacrum. The physician places the patient prone and incises the defect to the subarachnoid space. Using a microscope, the edges of the neural placode are trimmed of skin, dural remnants, and fat. The lateral edges of the placode are sutured together to form a tube. The dura is then incised and closed. Skin is closed with sutures. Report 63704 if the myelomeningocele is less than 5.0 cm in diameter; report 63706 if the defect is more than 5.0 cm in diameter.

63707–63709

This procedure is performed to mend an opening in the dura, preventing a dangerous infection. The patient is placed prone, and the physician makes a midline incision, retracting the skin, muscles, and paravertebral ligaments. The physician removes and prepares a graft of subcutaneous fat, freeze-dried dura, fascia, or muscle. Suction is used to keep the incision free of cerebrospinal fluid. Single dural stitches are used to achieve closure. A second needle is attached to the free suture ends and the needles are passed through the graft, which is tied down over the outside of the repaired tear to achieve watertight closure. If the dural defect is small and difficult to access, the graft can be placed inside the dura. After verifying that the repair is watertight, the physician proceeds with closure. Report 63709 if a laminectomy is required to correct a dural/cerebrospinal fluid leak or pseudomeningocele.

63710

At the end of a procedure where the dura has been incised, the physician sometimes prepares a graft of subcutaneous fat, freeze-dried dura, fascia, or muscle. Suction is used to keep the incision free of cerebral spinal fluid. Single dural stitches are used to achieve closure. A second needle is attached to the free suture ends and the needles are passed through the graft, which is tied down outside of the repaired tear to achieve watertight closure. If the dural defect is small and difficult to access, the graft can be placed inside the dura. After verifying that the repair is watertight, the physician proceeds with closure.

63740–63741

This procedure drains excess cerebral spinal fluid that may cause hydrocephalus. The patient is placed in a spinal tap position and the fascia, paravertebral muscles, and ligaments are incised and separated. The physician removes the lamina, inserting the shunt through the dura into the subarachnoid space. The shunt is passed around the flank to the peritoneal, pleural, or other space for drainage. The incisions are closed with layered sutures. Report 63740 if a laminectomy is needed to place the shunt. Report 63741 if the shunt is placed without excising the lamina.

63744

The physician makes an incision at the site of the original incision. Scar tissue, colloidal tissues, and adhesions are removed. The physician may irrigate the shunt with saline or other substances. If it is malfunctioning, the shunt is freed and replaced. A new shunt is placed in the site. Incisions are closed using layered sutures.

63746

The physician makes an incision at the site of the original incision. Scar tissue, colloidal tissues, and adhesions are removed. The shunt is freed and removed. Incisions are closed using layered sutures.

64400–64405

The physician anesthetizes a branch of the trigeminal nerve in 64400, the facial nerve in 64402, or the greater occipital nerve in 64405. The trigeminal nerve supplies sensory and motor fibers to the face, and is usually blocked superficially. The facial nerve supplies motor fibers to the muscles of facial expression. The greater occipital nerve supplies sensory fibers to the scalp. The physician draws a local anesthetic into a syringe and injects it into the branch of the nerve to be anesthetized.

64408

The physician anesthetizes the vagus nerve. The vagus nerve supplies sensory fibers to the pharynx and glottis, and carries parasympathetic fibers to the digestive system and heart. The physician draws a local anesthetic into a syringe and injects it in the branch of the nerve proximal to the area to be anesthetized.

64410

The physician anesthetizes the phrenic nerve to limit motor control of the diaphragm. The physician draws a local anesthetic into a syringe and injects it in the nerve. This anesthesia would be supplied in cases of unending hiccups, or diagnostically to predict the effect of nerve loss.

64412

The physician anesthetizes the spinal accessory nerve to limit sensation in the trapezius and lower neck. The physician draws a local anesthetic into the syringe and injects it into the branch of the nerve proximal to the area to be anesthetized.

64413

The physician anesthetizes the cervical plexus for sympathetically mediated pain and anesthesia to the back of the neck and head. The physician draws a local anesthetic into three syringes and injects near the transverse processes of C2 to C4, avoiding vascular injection.

64415–64417

The physician anesthetizes the brachial plexus to provide anesthesia to the arm. In 64415, the entire brachial plexus is blocked. In 64417, the block is limited to the axillary nerve, which supplies sensory innervation to the shoulder. The physician draws a local anesthetic into a syringe and approaches the brachial plexus in one of three locations: intrascalene, supraclavicular, or axillary.

64418

The physician anesthetizes the suprascapular nerve to relax the supraspinatus and infraspinatus muscles and differentiate between brachial plexus mediated or C5 or C6 mediated pain. The physician draws a local anesthetic into the syringe and injects it into the suprascapular nerve.

64420–64421

The physician anesthetizes the intercostal nerve to block chest wall pain. In 64420, a single injection is performed. In 64421, multiple nerves are injected to provide pain relief to a larger area (regional block).

64425

The physician anesthetizes the ilioinguinal and iliohypogastric nerves to block the inguinal and lower abdomen for pain control. The physician draws a local anesthetic into the syringe and injects it in a fan-like manner medial to the hip bone toward the umbilicus.

64430–64435

The physician anesthetizes the pudendal nerve for anesthesia of the vaginal vault, perineum, rectum, and parts of the bladder. In 64430, the pudendal nerve is blocked typically for perineal pain control during vaginal delivery. In 64435, the area around the cervix is injected with a local anesthetic to supply pain control for the first stage of labor.

64445

The physician anesthetizes the sciatic nerve to provide anesthesia to the distal lower extremity. The physician draws a local anesthetic into the syringe and injects it into the sciatic nerve.

64450

The physician anesthetizes a nerve to provide pain control or blockage. The physician draws a local anesthetic into the syringe and injects it into the branch of the nerve to be anesthetized. This code is used to report nerve blocks of other nerves not specifically listed in this section.

64470–64472

The paravertebral facet joint consists of the bony surfaces between the vertebrae that articulate with each other. The physician injects anesthetic and/or steroid into this joint or the facet joint nerve using separately reportable fluoroscopic direction. The injection may be performed on a single or multiple cervical or thoracic level. Report 64470 for a single level; report 64472 for each additional level.

64475–64476

The paravertebral facet joint consists of the bony surfaces between the vertebrae that articulate with each other. The physician injects anesthetic and/or steroid into this joint or the facet joint nerve using separately reportable fluoroscopic direction. The injection may be performed on a single or multiple lumbar or sacral level. Report 64475 for a single level, report 64476 for each additional level.

64479–64480

The physician injects anesthetic and/or steroid into the epidural space using a transforaminal approach. This approach is used primarily in the treatment of herniated discs and requires the use of separately reportable fluoroscopic direction. The injection may be performed on a single or multiple cervical or thoracic level. Report 64479 for a single level; report 64480 for each additional level.

64483–64484

The physician injects anesthetic and/or steroid into the epidural space using a transforaminal approach. This approach is used primarily in the treatment of herniated discs and requires the use of separately reportable fluoroscopic direction. The injection may be performed on a single or multiple lumbar or sacral level. Report 64483 for a single level, report 64484 for each additional level.

64505

The physician injects the sphenopalatine ganglion nerve with an anesthetic agent to provide anesthesia to the nasal mucosa. The anesthesia is applied by entering through the nares and injecting cocaine posterior to the middle turbinate.

64508

The physician injects the carotid sinus nerve with an anesthetic agent to block sympathetically mediated pain or cardiovascular responses. Injection location is chosen carefully to avoid the carotid artery.

64510–64520

The physician injects the stellate ganglion, lumbar, or thoracic sympathetic chains with an anesthetic agent to block sympathetically mediated pain. In 64510, the stellate ganglion block is used to provide anesthesia to the face, neck, and upper extremity. In 64520, the lumbar or thoracic block provides anesthesia to the torso, pelvis, and lower extremities. In a separately reportable procedure, the physician uses fluoroscopy to guide needle placement.

64530

The physician injects the celiac plexus with an anesthetic to block sympathetically mediated or visceral pain. Anesthesia is provided with or without radiologic monitoring.

64550

The physician places electrode pads over the area to be stimulated and connects a transmitter box to the electrodes (e.g., TENS unit). Current is transmitted through the skin to sensory fibers which helps decrease the pain sensation at the brain level.

64553–64565

The physician places an electrode percutaneously (through the skin) through an introducer needle into the tissue to be stimulated. Electrodes placed over sensory nerves decrease pain sensation in the distribution of the nerve. Electrodes placed over motor nerves stimulate paralyzed muscles to prevent atrophy. In 64553, the electrodes are placed over the motor or sensory points of cranial nerves. In 64555, the electrodes are placed over peripheral motor or sensory nerves, excluding sacral nerves. In 64560, the electrodes are placed over the autonomic nerves contributing to sympathetically mediated pain. Report 64561 when stimulators are placed near sacral nerves, which control the behavior of the bladder, sphincter, and pelvic floor muscles. In 64565, the electrodes are placed at the neuromuscular junction to stimulate a specific area of muscle tissue.

64573–64581

The physician makes an incision to place the electrode. The physician uses a scalpel to incise the skin and dissects the to the anatomical location. The incision aides the physician in accurately placing and testing the electrode while visualizing results. After stimulating the area, the incision is closed with layered sutures. Electrodes placed over sensory nerves decrease pain sensation in the distribution of the nerve. Electrodes placed over motor nerves stimulate paralyzed muscles to prevent atrophy. In 64573, the incision is placed in the region of a specific sensory or motor cranial nerve. In 64575, the electrodes are placed over peripheral motor or sensory nerves. In 64577, the electrodes are placed over autonomic nerves contributing to sympathetically mediated pain. In 64580, the electrodes are placed at the neuromuscular junction to stimulate a specific area of muscle tissue. In 64581, the electrodes are placed at the sacral nerve for urinary control.

64585

The physician revises or removes previously placed neurostimulator electrodes. The physician makes an incision overlying the electrodes. If the initial placement has not resulted in optimal pain control or motor stimulation, the electrodes are moved to optimize results. If the neurostimulator device is no longer required, the electrodes are removed. The incision is closed with layered sutures.

64590

The physician places a peripheral neurostimulator pulse generator or receiver to be connected to neurostimulator electrodes. The generator or receiver can be placed anywhere in the patient's subcutaneous tissue; however, size usually dictates placement. The physician makes an incision overlying the placement area and dissects the subcutaneous tissues to form a pocket. The unit is placed in the pocket and the electrodes are connected. After verification of nerve stimulation, the incision is closed in sutured layers.

64595

The physician revises or removes a peripheral neurostimulator pulse generator or receiver with or without replacement. The placement incision is reopened and tissues are dissected to the transmitter pocket. If the procedure is performed because the device is malfunctioning, the unit is checked and repairs made or a new unit is inserted. If the device is no longer required, it is removed. The incision is closed in layered sutures.

64600–64610

The physician destroys a portion of the trigeminal nerve to block pain or motor control to the face or scalp. Destruction is accomplished by injecting the nerve with alcohol or phenol. In 64600, a supraorbital, infraorbital, mental, or inferior alveolar branch of the trigeminal nerve is destroyed. In 64605, the second and third division branches at the foramen ovale are destroyed. Report 64610 if the second and third division branches at the foramen ovale are destroyed under radiologic monitoring.

64612

Chemodenervation paralyzes dysfunctional muscle tissue innervated by the facial nerve. The physician destroys the ends of the nerve closest to the muscle by injecting the endplate of the muscle with botulinum toxin type A (BTX-A). The physician identifies the muscle either by direct surgical exposure or through the insertion of an electromyographic needle into the muscle. A small amount BTX-A is injected into the muscle belly, which causes muscle paralysis within 24 hours to 48 hours. Gradually, blocked nerves form new neuromuscular junctions resulting in the return of muscle function, usually within six weeks to eight weeks. BTX-A injections are an effective treatment for a variety of disorders of abnormal muscle tone, including muscle overactivity or spasticity.

64613

Chemodenervation paralyzes dysfunctional muscle tissue innervated by cervical spinal nerves. The physician destroys the ends of the nerve closest to the muscle by injecting the nerve or muscle endplate with alcohol, phenol, and/or botulinum toxin type A (BTX-A). The physician identifies the nerve or muscle endplate either by direct surgical exposure or through the insertion of an electromyographic needle into the muscle. A small amount of the selected agent is injected into nerve or muscle endplate, which causes muscle paralysis. Gradually, blocked nerves form new neuromuscular junctions resulting in the return of muscle function. The duration of the effect is variable, usually one month to 12 months when phenol or alcohol is used and six weeks to eight weeks when BTX-A is used.

64614

Chemodenervation paralyzes dysfunctional muscle tissue in the extremities or trunk. The physician destroys the ends of the nerve closest to the muscle by injecting the nerve or muscle endplate with alcohol, phenol, and/or botulinum toxin type A (BTX-A). The physician identifies the nerve or muscle endplate either by direct surgical exposure or through the insertion of an electromyographic needle into the muscle. A small amount of the selected agent is injected into nerve or muscle endplate, which causes muscle paralysis. Gradually, blocked nerves form new neuromuscular junctions resulting in the return of muscle function. The duration of the effect is variable, usually one to 12 months when phenol or alcohol is used and six weeks to eight weeks when BTX-A is used.

64620–64640

These procedures are performed to treat chronic pain. The affected nerve is destroyed using chemical, thermal, electrical, or radiofrequency techniques. These techniques may be used singley or in combination. These procedures are designed to destroy the specific site(s) in the nerve root that produce(s) the pain while leaving sensation intact. Generally intravenous conscious sedation is utilized during the initial phase of the procedure so that the patient can assist the physician in identifying the site of pain and the correct placement of the neurolytic agent and local anesthesia is administered during the destruction phase of the procedure. Using separately reportable fluoroscopic guidance, a needle is inserted into the affected nerve root. An electrode is then inserted through the needle and a mild electrical current is passed through the electrode. The current produces a tingling sensation at a site on the nerve. The electrode is manipulated until the tingling sensation is felt at the same site as the pain. Once the physician has determined that the electrode is positioned at the site responsible for the pain, a local anesthetic is administered and a neurolytic agent applied. Chemical destruction involves injection of a neurolytic substance (eg, alcohol, phenol, glycerol) into the affected nerve root. Thermal techniques utilize heat. Electrical techniques utilize an electrical current. Radiofrequency, also referred to as radiofrequency rhizotomy, utilizes a solar or microwave current. Report 64620 when the site is the intercostal nerve. Report 64622–64623 when one or more lumbar/sacral paravertebral facet joint nerve are treated and 64626–64627 when the treatment is at the

cervical/thoracic facet joint level. Report 64630 for the pudendal nerve and 64640 for other peripheral nerves or branches.

64680

The physician destroys the celiac plexus by applying a neurolytic agent to the celiac plexus. The celiac plexus is a network of nervous tissue that mediates sympathetic pain from the abdomen. This block is often performed for pain relief of unresectable cancer in the upper abdomen. The celiac plexus is destroyed usually by chemodenervation, injecting either phenol or alcohol to paralyze the network of nervous tissue. This procedure is normally performed under CT guidance.

64702–64704

The physician releases a compressed nerve in a finger, hand, or foot. The physician makes an incision overlying the nerve. Surrounding tissues are dissected from the nerve freeing it from scar tissue or adhesions. The incision is repaired in multiple layers. In 64702, one or both of the digital nerves in a single finger are decompressed. In 64704, a nerve in the hand or foot is decompressed.

64708–64714

The physician repairs a compressed major peripheral nerve in the arm or leg. Repair is accomplished by decompressing the nerve from the surrounding tissue. Report 64708 if repair was done on a nerve other than the following: if sciatic nerve, report 64712; if brachial plexus, report 64713; and lumbar plexus, report 64714.

64716

The physician frees an intact cranial nerve from scar tissue (neuroplasty) or moves an intact nerve to a new position (transposition). The physician makes an incision overlying the nerve, dissects it free of the surrounding tissue and, if necessary, moves the nerve to a new position. If the nerve is in bone and must be decompressed, freed, or moved, the overlying bone is first removed using drills and/or osteotomes.

64718

The physician decompresses a stressed ulnar nerve by freeing the nerve and the tissue surrounding the nerve. The physician makes an incision at the lateral epicondyle and locates the nerve. Surrounding tissues are dissected from the nerve and the nerve is freed from the underlying bed. The nerve is moved over the epicondyle and stabilized with sutures in the surrounding tissue. The incision is closed in sutured layers.

64719–64721

The physician decompresses or transposes a portion of the ulnar or median nerve to restore feeling to the hand. The physician makes a horizontal incision in the wrist at the metacarpal joints and locates the nerve. In 64719, the ulnar nerve is located and freed. In 64721, the median nerve is decompressed by freeing the nerve inside the carpal tunnel. Soft tissues are resected and the nerve is freed from the underlying bed. Care is taken to ensure tension is released and the incision is closed in sutured layers.

64722–64726

The physician decompresses a nerve. In 64722, the nerve is unspecified. In 64726 the nerve is located at the base of the foot and supplies sensory fibers to one of the toes. The physician makes an incision in the area of nerve tension and locates the nerve. Surrounding soft tissues are dissected from the nerve to release pressure on the nerve.

64727

The physician makes an incision over the affected nerve and locates the nerve. The physician then resects the nerve sheath parallel to the fibers and releases scar tissue within the nerve.

64732–64736

The physician transects or removes a nerve that supplies motor or sensory innervation to the affected head and neck area to eliminate pain. For supraorbital nerve, report 64732, for infraorbital nerve report 64734, for the mental nerve report 64736.

64738

The physician transects or removes a nerve that supplies sensory innervation to the lower jaw and teeth. The physician makes a small osteotomy into the bone and locates the nerve. The nerve is transected to eliminate pain.

64740–64744

The physician transects or removes a nerve that supplies motor or sensory innervation to the affected head and neck area to eliminate pain. For lingual nerve, report 64740. For facial nerve (complete or any branches) report 64742. For the greater occipital nerve, report 64744. The physician incises the area at the most proximal portion of the nerve innervating the problem area. The nerve is located, and transected and the proximal portion of the nerve is buried in the surrounding tissue or bone to prevent neuroma formation.

64746

The physician transects or removes a portion of the phrenic nerve. The phrenic nerve supplies innervation to the diaphragm. The physician makes a horizontal neck incision and dissects the surrounding tissue and locates the nerve. The nerve is transected and the proximal portion of the nerve is buried in the surrounding tissue to prevent neuroma formation.

64752–64760

The physician transects or removes a portion of the vagus nerve. The vagus nerves supplies

parasympathetic fibers to the heart and gastrointestinal tract. In 64752, the physician performs a left thoracotomy and locates the vagus nerve inferior to the cardiac branches. The nerve is transected to decrease gut motility and acid production in the stomach. In 64755, the physician makes a vertical midline epigastric incision and locates specific branches of the vagus nerve responsible for acid production in the stomach. In 64760, the physician makes a vertical midline epigastric incision and locates the vagus nerve. After locating the nerve or nerve branches, the physician transects them. The incision is closed in sutured layers.

64761

The physician transects or removes a portion of the pudendal nerve. The pudendal nerve supplies sensory innervation to the groin. The physician makes a incision over the ischial spine and dissects the tissues to locate the nerve. The nerve is transected and the proximal portion of the nerve is buried in the surrounding tissue to prevent neuroma formation. This block may be performed for chronic pelvic pain or cancer pain. The incision is closed in sutured layers.

64763–64766

The physician transects (cuts) or avulses (pulls out) the obturator nerve. The physician makes an incision overlying the adductor muscles. The adductor muscles are separated from each other and the obturator nerve is located. The physician accesses the nerve by an extrapelvic approach in 64763 or by an intrapelvic approach in 64766. The nerve is then transected or avulsed and the incision repaired in multiple layers.

64771

The physician cuts or avulses another cranial nerve, such as branch nerves of major nerves not listed in previous codes. The physician makes an incision on the face or neck overlying the extradural portion of the other cranial nerve. The tissues are dissected and the nerve is exposed. The nerve is destroyed. The incision is closed in sutured layers.

64772

The physician cuts or avulses another spinal nerve, such as branch nerves of major nerves not listed in other codes. The physician incises the skin overlying the nerve from C1 to S4. The tissues are dissected and the nerve is exposed. The nerve is destroyed. The incision is closed in sutured layers.

64774–64778

The physician excises a neuroma of a peripheral nerve. A neuroma is a tumor formed secondarily by trauma to the nerve. In 64744, the physician incises the skin and locates and excises the neuroma in the subcutaneous tissue. In 64776, the physician incises the skin over the digital nerve and excises the neuroma. Report 64778 for each additional neuroma of a separate digit.

64782–64783

The physician excises a neuroma of a peripheral nerve (except digital nerve) of the hand or foot. A neuroma is a benign tumor formed secondarily by trauma to the nerve. The physician incises the affected area in a hand or foot. After locating the nerve with the symptomatic neuroma, the physician excises the tumor. The incision is closed in sutured layers. Report 64783 for additional neuromas of the hand or foot.

64784–64786

The physician excises a neuroma of a major peripheral nerve. A neuroma is a benign tumor formed secondarily by trauma to the nerve. In 64784, the physician incises the area over the affected major peripheral nerve except sciatic. After locating the nerve with the symptomatic neuroma, the physician excises the tumor. The incision is closed in sutured layers. In 64786, the physician incises the skin at the back of the upper leg or buttocks near the symptomatic neuroma and locates the tumor on the sciatic nerve. After locating the nerve with the symptomatic neuroma, the physician excises the tumor. The incision is closed in sutured layers.

64787

The physician implants a nerve into a bone or muscle to prevent neuroma formation after excision of a neuroma. In bony implantation, the physician drills a small hole in the bone to implant the nerve. The surrounding tissue is brought together around the nerve to secure the nerve to the bone. In muscle implantation the nerve is sutured into muscle bed. The surrounding tissue is brought together and sutured to secure the nerve in the muscle.

64788–64792

The physician excises a neurofibroma or a neurolemmoma. A neurofibroma is a tumor of peripheral nerves caused by abnormal proliferation of Schwann cells. A neurolemmoma is a tumor of a peripheral nerve sheath. To remove the tumor, the physician incises the skin over the tumor and dissects the surrounding tissue. The tumor is freed and excised from the nerve, without damaging the nerve when possible. The incision is closed in sutured layers. In 64788, the tumor is located on a cutaneous nerve. In 64790, the tumor lies on a major peripheral nerve. In 64792, an extensive excision is required due to size or malignancy.

64795

The physician biopsies a nerve. The physician makes an incision overlying the suspect nerve. The tissues are dissected to locate the nerve, and a biopsy specimen is obtained. The incision is closed in sutured layers.

64802–64804

The physician performs a cervical sympathectomy or cervical thoracic sympathectomy. The cervical sympathetic chain supplies sympathetic innervation to the head, neck, and upper extremities. The thoracic chain supplies sympathetic innervation to the chest and its contents. In 64802, the physician makes a midlateral incision of the neck and dissects the tissues to locate the sympathetic chain. In 64804, the physician makes a thoracotomy and dissects the tissues to locate the sympathetic chain along the vertebral bodies. The ganglia (nerve cell bodies which lay outside the spinal cord) are identified and resected. The incision is closed in sutured layers.

64809

The physician performs a sympathectomy on the thoracolumbar sympathetic nerves. The physician makes a lateral incision through the thoracic area to reach the sympathetic ganglia, which lie on the lateral border of the vertebral column. The physician determines at which level to remove the ganglia, and dissects to the vertebral bodies. The sympathetic plexus is located and resected. The wound is closed in sutured layers.

64818

The physician performs a sympathectomy on the lumbar sympathetic nerves. The physician makes a lateral incision through the lumbar area to reach the sympathetic ganglia, which lie on the lateral border of the vertebral column. The physician determines at which level to remove the ganglia, and dissects to the vertebral bodies. The sympathetic plexus is located and resected. The wound is closed in sutured layers.

64820

The physician performs a digital sympathectomy. The physician makes an incision along the digital artery in the medial and lateral aspects of the digit. The artery is identified and the adventitia is stripped from the blood vessel. Peripherally, the sympathetic nerves follow the arteries and lie in the adventitia layer. The incision is closed in sutured layers.

64820–64823

In 64820, the physician performs a digital sympathectomy using a microscope for visualization. The physician makes an incision along the digital artery in the medial and lateral aspects of the digit. The artery is identified and the adventitia is stripped from the blood vessel. Peripherally, the sympathetic nerves follow the arteries and lie in the adventitia layer. The incision is closed in layers. Report 64821 when the procedure is performed on the radial artery. Report 64822 when the procedure is performed on the ulnar artery. Report 64823 when the procedure is performed on the superficial palmar arch.

64831–64832

The physician repairs a digital (finger or toe) nerve. The physician locates the damaged nerve in a previously opened incision or wound of a finger or toe. The nerve is sutured to restore sensory or motor function. Report 64831 for a single nerve, report 64832 for each additional nerve repaired.

64834–64840

The physician repairs a sensory or motor nerve in the hand or foot. The physician locates the damaged nerve in a previously opened incision or wound of the hand or foot. The nerve is sutured to restore sensory function. In 64834, a common sensory nerve is repaired. In 64835, the median motor thenar nerve is repaired. This nerve supplies motor innervation to the thenar eminence (proximal thumb). In 64836, the ulnar motor nerve is repaired. This nerve supplies motor innervation to the extensor muscles of the forearm and hand. Report 64837 for repair of additional nerves in the hand or foot. In 64840, the tibial nerve is repaired. The tibial nerve supplies sensory innervation to the sole of the foot. Closure or reconstruction is separately reported.

64856–64859

The physician repairs a major peripheral nerve in the arm or leg, except for the sciatic nerve. The physician locates the damaged nerve in a previously opened incision or wound of the arm or leg. The nerve is sutured to restore sensory and/or motor innervation. The nerve may be moved (transposed) to decrease tension on the nerve. 64856 covers all peripheral nerves of the arm or leg except the sciatic nerve. Report 64857 if no transposition is necessary for repair. Report 64858 for repair of the sciatic nerve. When repairing more than one nerve, report 64859 for each addition nerve. Closure or reconstruction is separately reported.

64861–64862

The physician repairs the brachial plexus nerve or the lumbar plexus nerve. The brachial plexus supplies sensory and motor innervation to the arm. The lumbar plexus supplies sensory and motor innervation to the lower back, buttocks, and legs. The physician locates the damaged nerve in a previously opened incision or wound. In 64861, the nerve damage is in the neck or axilla. In 64862, the nerve damage is in the pelvis. The nerve is sutured to restore sensory and/or motor innervation. Closure or reconstruction is separately reported.

64864–64865

The physician repairs a nerve of the face or exterior head. The physician locates the damaged nerve in a previously opened incision or wound. In 64864, the damaged nerve is located on the face or the external cranium. In 64865, the damaged nerve is located in the temple area and grafting may be required. If a nerve is grafted, the sural nerve is often the donor nerve. Graft harvest is separately reported. The nerve is sutured to restore sensory and/or motor innervation. Closure or reconstruction is separately reported.

64866–64870

The physician creates an anastomosis (connection of two nerves that are not normally connected) to restore motor innervation to the face. In 64866, the facial nerve is anastomosed with the spinal accessory nerve. The physician makes a horizontal incision in the posterior lateral neck and isolates the spinal accessory nerve. The nerve is isolated and brought forward and sutured to the facial nerve. In 64868, the physician makes a horizontal lateral neck incision and isolates the hypoglossal nerve. The nerve is brought forward and sutured to the facial nerve. In 64870, the physician makes a horizontal anterior neck incision and isolates the phrenic nerve. The nerve is rotated toward the facial nerve and sutured into place.

64872–64876

The physician repairs a nerve where repair was delayed because the initial wound was contaminated. The wound is explored to locate the distal portion of the nerve. In 64872, the proximal and distal nerves are sutured together to restore innervation. In 64874, the nerve was shortened during damage. To reanastomose the nerve, the distal and proximal portions of the nerve are freed from surrounding tissues, approximated, and sutured to restore innervation. Report 64876 if excessive trauma caused loss of a significant section of a major nerve. For this procedure, a portion of the parallel bone is resected in order to approximate the distal and proximal ends of the nerve.

64885–64886

The physician obtains and places a nerve graft to restore innervation to the head or neck. In 64885, the graft is less than 4.0 cm long, in 64886, the graft is greater than 4.0 cm. A typical graft harvest is obtained from the sural nerve. To harvest the graft, the physician makes a lateral incision of the lateral mallelous of the ankle. The nerve is identified and freed. The physician cuts the nerve to obtain the length needed for the graft, elongating the incision as necessary. The proximal and distal sural nerve endings are anastomosed. The physician makes an incision over the damaged nerve and dissects the tissues to locate the nerve. The damaged area of the nerve is resected and removed. Then, innervation is restored by suturing the graft is sutured to the proximal and distal ends of the damaged nerve.

64890–64891

The physician obtains and places a nerve graft to restore innervation to the hand or foot. In 64890, the graft is up to 4.0 cm long; in 64891, the graft is greater than 4.0 cm. A typical graft harvest is obtained from the sural nerve. To harvest the graft, the physician makes a lateral incision of the lateral mallelous of the ankle. The nerve is identified and freed. The physician cuts the nerve to obtain the length needed for the graft, elongating the incision as necessary. The proximal and distal sural nerve endings are anastomosed. The physician makes an incision over the damaged nerve and dissects the tissues to locate the nerve. The damaged area of the nerve is resected and removed. Then, innervation is restored by suturing the graft to the proximal and distal ends of the damaged nerve.

64892–64893

The physician obtains and places a nerve graft to restore innervation to the arm or leg. In 64892, the graft is up to 4.0 cm long; in 64893, the graft is greater than 4.0 cm. A typical graft harvest is obtained from the sural nerve. To harvest the graft, the physician makes a lateral incision of the lateral mallelous of the ankle. The nerve is identified and freed. The physician cuts the nerve to obtain the length needed for the graft, elongating the incision as necessary. The proximal and distal sural nerve endings are anastomosed. The physician makes an incision over the damaged nerve and dissects the tissues to locate the nerve. The damaged area of the nerve is resected and removed. Then, innervation is restored by suturing the graft to the proximal and distal ends of the damaged nerve.

64895–64896

The physician obtains and places a nerve graft to restore innervation where a cable nerve of the hand or foot is damaged. In 64895, the graft is up to 4.0 cm long, and in 64896, the graft is greater than 4.0 cm. A typical graft harvest is obtained by taking multiple sections of the sural nerve. To harvest the graft, the physician makes an incision near the lateral malleolus of the ankle. The nerve is identified and freed. The physician cuts the nerve to obtain the length needed for the graft, elongating the incision as necessary. The proximal and distal sural nerve endings are anastomosed. The physician makes an incision over the damaged nerve and dissects the tissues to locate the nerve. The damaged area of the nerve is resected and removed. Then, innervation is restored by suturing graft strands to multiple proximal and distal ends of the damaged nerve cable.

64897–64898

The physician obtains and places a nerve graft to restore innervation where a cable nerve of the arm or leg is damaged (e.g., sciatic nerve or lumbar plexus nerve). In 64897, the graft is less than 4.0 cm long, and in 64898, the graft is greater than 4.0 cm. A typical graft harvest is obtained by taking multiple sections of the sural nerve. To harvest the graft, the physician makes an incision near the lateral malleolus of the ankle. The nerve is identified and freed. The physician cuts the nerve to obtain the length needed for the graft, elongating the incision as necessary. The

proximal and distal sural nerve endings are anastomosed. The physician makes an incision over the damaged nerve and dissects the tissues to locate the nerve. The damaged area of the nerve is resected and removed. Then, innervation is restored by suturing graft strands to multiple proximal and distal ends of the damaged nerve cable.

64901–64902

The physician grafts additional nerves. This code is used in addition to initial nerve graft codes, and includes graft harvest. Report 64901 for each additional single strand graft, report 64902 for each additional multiple strand graft.

64905–64907

The physician transfers a nerve pedicle from an intact nerve to a damaged nerve. A pedicle is an intact nerve used as a donor for regeneration of axons in the damaged nerve. In 64905 the first stage is completed. The physician makes an incision over the donor nerve site and locates the nerve. The nerve is freed from surrounding tissues and cut. The proximal portion of the donor nerve is transferred to the distal portion of the recipient nerve. The incision is closed in sutured layers. In 64907, the second stage is completed. The physician reopens the surgical incision and locates the donor and recipient nerves. The donor nerve is resected from the recipient nerve and primarily reanastomosed to its distal end. The distal end of the recipient nerve is reanastomosed to its proximal end. The nerves may be freed from surrounding tissues if necessary to complete anastomosis. The incision is closed in sutured layers.

65091–65093

The physician removes the contents of the eyeball: the vitreous, retina, choroid, lens, iris, and ciliary muscles. Retained is the tough, white outer shell (the sclera). After an ocular speculum has been inserted, the physician dissects the conjunctiva free from the sclera. An elliptical incision is made in the sclera surrounding the cornea, and the contents of the anterior chamber are removed. The physician uses a spoon to remove the contents of the posterior chamber, and then scrapes the inside of the sclera with gauze on a curet. Only the scleral shell remains. The conjunctiva may be removed. A temporary (e.g., for 65091) or permanent (e.g., for 65093) implant is inserted into the scleral shell at this time. The sclera is attached to the implant, usually with sutures.

65101–65105

The physician severs the eyeball from the extraorbital muscles and optic nerve and removes it. After an ocular speculum has been inserted, the physician dissects the conjunctiva free at the corneal-scleral juncture (the limbus). The physician cuts each extraocular muscle at its juncture to the eyeball and severs the optic nerve. The eyeball, and sometimes the conjunctiva, is removed but the extraocular muscles remain attached at the back of the eye socket. A spherical implant is placed in the eye socket. This implant, if unattached to the extraocular muscles, may be temporary (e.g., 65101) or permanent (e.g., 65103). The extraocular muscles may be attached to the permanent implant to allow normal movement of the prosthesis (e.g., 65105).

65110–65112

The physician sutures the eyelids closed. An elliptical incision is cut through the skin, subcutaneous tissue, muscle and periosteum to the bone beginning at the upper nasal orbital rim and is carried below the brow to the lateral canthus. The incision is extended from the upper nasal quadrant along the nasal and inferior orbit rim to the lateral canthus, terminating in a wide canthotomy. The periosteum is freed around the orbital rim with a periosteum elevator, beginning in the upper temporal quadrant. The trochlea is detached with a sharp dissection. In the upper temporal quadrant, the lacrimal gland is removed. The lacrimal sac is separated from its attachments and removed. The medial and lateral canthal ligaments are cut with a blunt dissection. A blunt dissection is also used to separate the periorbital to the apex, and the firm attachment of the periosteum is cut from the bone with scissors. The orbital contents are removed. Pieces of orbital bone may be excised (e.g., for 65112). The orbit is packed with dry gauze and pressure is applied to control bleeding.

65114

The physician splits the upper and lower eyelids at the gray line throughout their length, leaving the cilia and the skin anteriorly, and the tarsus, the orbicularis muscle, the conjunctiva, the palpebral muscle and the fascial planes posteriorly. The margins of the posterior halves of the lids are sutured together. The lateral bony wall and the temporal fossa are exposed by lateral canthotomy and dissection of the skin, continuous with both lids. The orbital septum is incised. The trochlea is detached with a sharp dissection. The lacrimal gland and lacrimal sac are removed. The medial and lateral canthal ligaments are cut with a blunt dissection. A blunt dissection is also used to separate the periorbital to the apex. The firm attachment of the periosteum is cut from the bone with scissors. The orbital contents are removed. An incision is made in the fascia at the origin of the temporalis muscle. Fascia and muscle are reflected from the temporal fossa. Adherent fascia is excised from the upper margin of the zygomatic process. The muscle is dissected beneath the process. The temporalis muscle and its fascia are taken through the opening into the orbit. After the muscle and the fascia are spread to fill the orbit, they are sutured to the periosteum.

65125

The physician modifies an ocular implant that has been created elsewhere. The modifications may

include the addition of screws or other prosthetic appendages to alter the shape of the prosthesis so that it better fits the patient's eye. The physician may drill holes to accommodate the screws.

65130–65140

The physician inserts a permanent ocular prosthesis into a patient's orbit. In each case, an ocular speculum is placed in the eye, any conjunctiva is retracted, and any temporary prosthesis is removed. In a patient whose eye has been eviscerated, the implant is attached to the remaining sclera (e.g., 65130). In a patient following enucleation, the implant is otherwise secured (e.g., 65135). In some cases, eye muscles are attached to corresponding niches in the prosthesis to provide for more natural movement of the artificial eye following enucleation (e.g., 65140).

65150–65155

The physician returns an ocular prosthesis to the patient's eye socket. After an ocular speculum is inserted, the physician places the ocular prosthesis back into an eye from which it had been previously removed. The prosthesis is attached to the sclera in an eviscerated eye, or otherwise secured in an enucleated eye (e.g., 65150). In 65155, foreign material may be required to better secure the prosthesis and/or the prosthesis may be reattached to extraocular muscles. In either procedure, conjunctival tissue may be grafted over the prosthesis once it is secured.

65175

The physician removes the ocular implant from the eye socket. After placing an ocular speculum, the physician cuts and retracts any conjunctival tissue or Tenon's capsule overlying the prosthesis. Any connection between the implant and extraocular muscle or sclera is severed and the ocular implant is removed.

65205–65210

The physician picks the foreign body or mineral deposit from the conjunctiva with the side of the beveled edge of a needle (e.g., 65205). A small incision may be required to remove an embedded foreign body (e.g., 65210). In this case, the physician may cut a V-shaped incision to access the defect through a flap, or a straight incision may be made. The incision may penetrate the conjunctiva, but it does not penetrate the sclera. Generally, a slit lamp is used when removing any embedded foreign body. After the removal, the physician may apply a broad spectrum antibiotic and a moderate pressure patch over the closed lid for 24–48 hours.

65220–65222

The physician may remove a superficial foreign body or mineral deposit from the cornea with the side of the beveled edge of a needle (e.g., 65220). An incision may be required to remove an embedded foreign body (e.g., 65222). If so, the physician may cut a V-shaped incision to access the defect through a flap, or a straight incision may be made. The incision does not penetrate the cornea. Generally, a slit lamp is used with any embedded foreign body. After the removal, the physician may apply a broad spectrum antibiotic and a moderate pressure patch over the closed lid for 24–48 hours.

65235

The physician removes a foreign body, intraocular, from the anterior chamber of the eye or lens. The physician makes a small incision in the connective tissue between the cornea and the sclera (the limbus) and retrieves the foreign body through the opening with intraocular forceps or another small instrument. Generally, foreign bodies that pierce the lens are self-sealing and removal is not attempted. The incision is sutured. The physician applies an antibiotic ointment. Sometimes a pressure patch is placed on the eye for 24-48 hours.

65260

Diagnostic tests locate the foreign body before surgery is attempted. The physician will use an electromagnetic or magnetic probe to retrieve a metallic foreign body from the area behind the lens (the posterior segment). In the anterior route, the physician first dilates the patient's pupil. In a series of moves aligning the magnet to the metallic foreign body, the physician draws the foreign body to the front of the eye and around the lens into the anterior chamber. The physician then makes an incision in the connective tissue between the cornea and the sclera (the limbus) and retrieves the foreign body. In the posterior route, the physician makes a small incision in the conjunctiva over the site of the foreign body. A magnet is applied and the foreign body removed. The incision from either is repaired, and an injection may be required to reestablish proper fluid levels in the anterior and/or posterior chamber of the eye. A broad spectrum antibiotic or a pressure patch may be applied. Among the tools common to this procedure are Gruning's, Haab's, or Hirschberg's magnets.

65265

Diagnostic tests locate the foreign body before surgery is attempted. The physician will use intraocular forceps to retrieve the nonmetallic foreign body from the area behind the lens (the posterior segment). The physician makes an incision through the conjunctiva overlying the site of the foreign body. The foreign body is retrieved with intraocular forceps. Nonmetallic foreign bodies in the vitreous or retina may be removed through a pars plana approach. Either incision is repaired with a layered closure, and an injection may be required to reestablish proper fluid levels in the anterior or posterior chambers of eye. A broad spectrum antibiotic or a pressure patch may be applied.

65270–65273

An ocular speculum may be placed in the patient's eye. The physician irrigates the laceration and sutures the conjunctival wound (e.g., 65270). In mobilization and rearrangement (e.g., 65272), an extensive conjunctival laceration requires the creation of a flap or graft sutured over the wound, and the eyes are patched to limit their movement while the injury heals. A graft may be obtained from conjunctival tissue of the upper eyelid or from a sliding flap formed following a circumcorneal incision. Extensive repair or repair of the eye of a child may require hospitalization to further limit eye movement (e.g., 65273).

65275–65285

The physician removes any foreign body from the cornea with a hollow needle or forceps and the wound is irrigated. The nonperforating tear in the cornea (e.g., 65275) is repaired with sutures. In 65280 and 65285, the perforating tear in the cornea and any tear in the sclera may be sutured. The cornea may be splinted using a soft contact lens bandage. An air or saline injection may be required to reestablish proper ocular pressure in the anterior chamber. If the laceration involves the uveal tissue (the vascular layer beneath the sclera), injured tissue may be cut out or repositioned before the uvea is sutured (e.g., 65285), and the sclera and conjunctiva may each require separate closure. In any of the three procedures, topical antibiotic or a pressure patch may be applied.

65286

Tissue glue, also called medical adhesive or Cyanoacrylate tissue adhesive, acts as a suture in laceration repairs of the cornea and/or sclera. If the cornea is perforated, the physician may seal the perforation with tissue adhesive after debriding the outermost layer of cornea (the epithelium) to enhance adhesion. The patient may be fitted with a soft contact lens to be worn during the healing process. Antibiotic ointment is applied. A pressure patch may be used.

65290

The physician repairs a deep laceration to the orbital complex. This laceration extends through the extraocular muscles that aid the eye in directional movement. The laceration extends through tendinous attachment of the muscles to the bony orbit and may include the deep connective tissue envelope encasing the eyeball. Each anatomic structure is identified and reapproximated with sutures. The wound is closed in multiple layers.

65400–65410

The physician removes the entire corneal lesion (e.g., 65400) using a blade and forceps or scleral scissors. The edges of the lesion are undermined following a superficial incision in the cornea. Sutures are not required. Antibiotic ointment and possibly a 24-hour pressure patch is applied. The lesion is superficial; the cornea is not perforated by the excision. Sometimes, only a portion of the lesion is removed for diagnostic purposes (e.g., 65410).

65420–65426

A pterygium is a fleshy, wedge of the bulbar conjunctiva covering a portion of the medial cornea. The physician excises the pterygium with a blade and forceps or scleral scissors. The edges of the pterygium are undermined following a superficial incision in the clear cornea. Forceps retract the freed pterygium and it is excised as gentle pressure pulls it away from the corneal tissue and across the limbus and sclera. The physician applies sutures to the sclera and conjunctiva as needed. Often, no graft or tissue rearrangement is needed (e.g., 65420). However, the physician may transpose the pterygium with normal conjunctival tissue to move it out of the field of vision in what is sometimes called McReynold's operation, or may make a circumcorneal incision and use a conjunctival flap to repair the pterygium site (e.g., 65426). A topical antibiotic and a pressure patch may be applied in either procedure.

65430

In the office, the physician scrapes the surface of the corneal defect with a spatula. The scrapings will be cultured to determine a diagnosis.

65435–65436

In cases of corneal erosion or degeneration, the physician may attempt to stimulate new growth of the cornea's outermost layer by essentially "wounding" it. The physician removes the outermost layer of the cornea (epithelium) by scraping or cutting it with a spatula or curet (e.g., 65435). Chemical cauterization may then be applied. An alternative to cutting or scraping is the application by swab of EDTA (ethylenediaminetetraacetic acid), an acid that destroys the corneal epithelium. (e.g., 65436). In either case, an antibiotic ointment or pressure patch may be applied once the procedure is complete.

65450

The physician applies a freezing probe, a laser beam, or a heat probe directly to a corneal defect to destroy it. Freezing is the most common method used for this procedure. The physician then applies antibiotic ointment and sometimes, a pressure patch.

65600

In cases of corneal erosion or degeneration, the physician may attempt to stimulate new growth of the cornea's outermost layer by essentially "wounding" it. The physician places a speculum in the eye and uses a fine needle to create hundreds of tiny pricks in the surface of the outermost layer of the cornea (the epithelium). A topical antibiotic and patch may be applied. This procedure is sometimes called a corneal "tattoo."

65710

"Lamellar" means thin layer, and refers to the outermost layers of the cornea. The physician measures the patient's cornea to select the size of trephine that will be used to excise corneal tissue. The physician punches a circular hole in the outermost layers of the cornea of a donor eye, using the trephine. The physician removes the round layer of corneal tissue, threads it with sutures, and sets it aside. The trephine is used to repeat this process in the cornea of the patient, removing the defective corneal tissue. The donor cornea is of similar diameter and thickness as the removed tissue. The donor cornea is positioned with the preplaced sutures, and then additional sutures secure it to the cornea. The physician may use a saline or air injection into the anterior chamber during the procedure. When the procedure is completed, the speculum is removed. Antibiotic ointment and a pressure patch may be applied.

65730–65755

Penetrating refers to the thickness of the donor cornea, indicating its full thickness. The physician measures the patient's cornea to select the size of trephine that will be used to excise corneal tissue. The physician punches a circular hole in the cornea of the donor eye using the trephine. The physician removes the disk of corneal tissue, threads it with preplaced sutures, and sets it aside. In aphakic patients, vitreous and/or aqueous may be withdrawn from the eye before the cornea is removed. A metal ring may be sutured to the sclera of an aphakic patient to stabilize the operative field. The defective cornea of the patient is removed with the trephine. The donor cornea is positioned with sutures, and then additional sutures secure it to the cornea. The physician may use a saline or air injection to restore proper intraocular pressure. The difference in these three codes is the lens status of the patient. 65730 is for those patients who still have a natural lens: these patients are phakic — with lens. 65750 is for those patients who have had cataract surgery: these patients are aphakic — without lens. 65755 is for patients who have an artificial lens: these patients are pseudoaphakic — without natural lens.

65760

The cornea is one of several structures in the eye that contributes to refraction. Altering the shape of the cornea therefore alters visual acuity. The physician retracts the patient's eyelids with an ocular speculum. Using a planing device, the physician removes a partial-thickness central portion of the patient's cornea, freezes it and then reshapes it on an electronic lathe. The revised cornea is positioned and secured with sutures. This is done to correct optical error. The physician may use a saline or air injection into the anterior chamber during the procedure. The speculum is removed. Antibiotic ointment and a pressure patch may be applied.

CPT® Lay Descriptions

65765

The cornea is one of several structures in the eye that contributes to refraction. Altering the shape of the cornea therefore alters visual acuity. The physician retracts the patient's eyelids with an ocular speculum, then measures the patient's cornea to select the size of trephine that will be used to excise corneal tissue. The physician punches a circular hole in the cornea of the donor eye using the trephine. The physician removes the disk of corneal tissue and sets it aside. An incision is made at the juncture of the cornea and the sclera (the limbus) and the patient's cornea is separated into two layers. The physician inserts the donor cornea between layers of the recipient's cornea. The resulting change in the corneal curvature alters the refractive properties of the cornea to correct the preexisting refractive error. The speculum is removed. Antibiotic ointment and a pressure patch may be applied.

65767

The cornea is one of several structures in the eye that contributes to refraction. Altering the shape of the cornea therefore alters visual acuity. The physician retracts the patient's eyelids with an ocular speculum, then measures the patient's cornea to select the size of trephine that will be used to excise corneal tissue. The physician punches a circular hole in the cornea of the donor eye using the trephine. The physician removes the disk of corneal tissue and sets it aside. On a lathe, the physician shapes a lens made of two layers from a donor cornea, the stroma and Bowman's membrane. The physician sutures this donor cornea to the surface of the patient's cornea. The resulting change in corneal curvature alters the refractive properties of the cornea to correct the preexisting refractive error. The speculum is removed. Antibiotic ointment and a pressure patch may be applied.

65770

The physician creates a new anterior chamber with a plastic optical implant that replaces a severely damaged cornea that cannot be repaired. Sometimes the corneal prosthesis is sutured to the sclera; other times, extensive damage to the eye requires the implant be sutured to the closed and incised eyelid.

65771

The cornea is one of several structures in the eye that contributes to refraction. Altering the shape of the cornea therefore alters visual acuity. The physician retracts the patient's eyelids with an ocular speculum, then measures the patient's cornea. The physician places multiple nonpenetrating cuts in the cornea in a bicycle spoke on the patient's corneal to reduce myopia, or a variety of peripheral cornea tangential cuts for astigmatic correction. There are two basic surgical approaches: Russian, in which the incisions are made from the edges to the center of the cornea; and American, in which the incisions are made from the center to the periphery. The number and length of the incisions depend upon the patient's age and degree

of myopia. The resulting change in the corneal curvature alters the refractive properties of the cornea to correct the preexisting refractive error. The speculum is removed. Antibiotic ointment and a pressure patch may be applied.

65772–65775

The cornea is one of several structures in the eye that contributes to refraction. Altering the shape of the cornea therefore alters visual acuity. When a previous surgery (e.g., for insertion of an intraocular lens or a corneal procedure) results in astigmatism, the physician at a later date returns the patient to the operating room to correct the problem. The physician retracts the patient's eyelids with an ocular speculum. In corneal relaxing (65772), an "X" cut is made on the cornea to repair the error. Slices along the "X" are removed and its edges are sutured. In the corneal wedge resection (65775), a wedge is cut from the cornea and the edges sutured. The resulting change in the corneal curvature alters the refractive properties of the cornea to correct the preexisting refractive error. The speculum is removed. Antibiotic ointment and a pressure patch may be applied.

65800–65805

Though constantly flushed and renewed, the overall pressure of aqueous is constant in a healthy eye's anterior chamber. Too little or too much fluid can cause permanent damage. The physician aspirates aqueous from between the iris and the cornea (the anterior chamber) with a needle in what is typically called an "anterior chamber tap." The needle usually enters the anterior chamber through the corneal-scleral juncture (the limbus). In some cases, the removal of the fluid is diagnostic (e.g., 65800). The physician may inject air to normalize eye pressure after fluid has been removed. If ocular pressure is high, a therapeutic removal of aqueous may be performed (e.g., 65805).

65810

The physician aspirates the gel-like vitreous that has pushed forward into the space between the iris and the cornea (the anterior chamber). Using a needle that enters the eye through the corneal-scleral juncture (the limbus), the prolapsed vitreous is removed. A laser might be used to destroy part of the membrane between the lens and the vitreous (the anterior hyaloid membrane). The physician may inject air to normalize eye pressure after fluid has been removed.

65815

Blood in the anterior chamber can coagulate and block the flow of aqueous. It can also cause cornea staining. The physician aspirates blood from between the iris and the cornea (the anterior chamber) with a needle that enters the eye through the corneal-scleral juncture (the limbus). In some cases, the physician may inject saline to flush the blood and make its removal easier. The physician may inject air to normalize eye pressure after fluid has been removed.

65820

To improve drainage of fluids in the eye, the physician enters the anterior chamber through an incision in the scleral-corneal juncture (the limbus) and cuts with a gonioknife. The blade passes across the anterior to the opposite limbus and a sweep is made to open the angle of the ring of meshlike tissue at the iris-scleral junction (the trabecular meshwork) of the opposite portion of the eye. De Vincentiis operation and Barkan's operation are both goniotomy procedures.

65850

To improve drainage of fluids in the eye, the physician inserts a special tool called a trabeculotome into Schlemm's canal and rotates it into the anterior chamber to open the ring of meshlike tissue (the trabecular meshwork). The name (ab) externo, meaning outside the eye, refers to the surgical approach from outside the eye cutting toward the anterior chamber.

65855

The physician uses an argon laser to selectively burn the ring of meshlike tissue at the iris-scleral junction (the trabecular meshwork) to improve the drainage of fluids in the anterior segment. The physician begins by placing a special contact on the eye to be treated. This lens allows the physician to view the angle structures of the eye and the trabecular network while using the laser. Though the trabecular network runs along the entire circumference of the iris, the physician burns holes in only a portion of that circumference during a single treatment session. In this way, the physician can measure the effects of each treatment upon the eye's fluid, and suspend treatment once the proper intraocular fluid pressure is reached. No incision is made during this procedure.

65860

Sometimes scar tissue or adhesions bind structures within the eye, interfering with vision or with intraocular pressure. The physician uses a YAG laser to selectively sever vitreal, corneal, or ciliary strands or adhesions binding the iris to adjunct structures and interfering with vision. The physician begins by placing a special contact on the eye to be treated. This lens allows the physician to view the angle structures of the eye and the trabecular network while using the laser. The strands or adhesions are not removed; they simply fall out of the visual field.

65865

Sometimes scar tissue or adhesions bind structures within the eye, interfering with vision or with intraocular pressure. Through an incision in the corneal-scleral juncture (the limbus) the physician enters the anterior segment to sever vitreal, corneal, or ciliary strands or adhesions binding the iris to

adjunct structures interfering with vision. The strands or adhesions are not removed; they simply fall out of the visual field.

65870–65875

The physician enters the anterior segment through the limbus to sever strands or adhesions binding the iris to adjunct structures interfering with vision. In the anterior synechiae (e.g., for 65870) the physician severs adhesions of the base of the iris to the cornea. For posterior synechiae (e.g., for 65875), the adhesions between the iris to the capsule of the lens or to the surface of the vitreous body are severed. Once the adhesions have been severed, the intraocular pressure may be restored with an injection of fluid or air. The incision is closed and an antibiotic and pressure patch may be applied.

65880

The physician enters the anterior segment through the limbus to sever strands or adhesions binding the cornea to the gel-like vitreous that has prolapsed into the anterior chamber. Once the adhesions have been severed, the intraocular pressure may be restored with an injection of fluid or air. The incision is closed and an antibiotic and pressure patch may be applied.

65900

Epithelial downgrowth describes the improper healing of surgical or traumatic wound to the cornea. The outer lining of the cornea (the epithelium) fails to close properly over the wound, instead growing around to the inner side of the cornea, sometimes continuing its growth to other structures of the eye. Disturbances in intraocular pressure and vision can result. The physician retracts the patient's eyelids with an ocular speculum. The physician locates and excises the extraneous epithelial tissue from where it has spread into the anterior chamber. The original wound may be trimmed and revised. Injections may be required to restore pressure in the anterior or posterior chambers. The procedure may require sutures or tissue glue, antibiotic ointment or a pressure patch.

65920

The clouding of the lens capsule (cataract) causes visual loss. To correct this problem, a bad lens is replaced with an artificial one. Sometimes complications require the removal of the artificial lens. The physician retracts the patient's eyelids with an ocular speculum. The physician cuts and retracts the conjunctiva and makes an incision at the juncture of the cornea and sclera (the limbus). The physician removes from the anterior segment the previously placed artificial lens (called an intraocular lens or IOL). It is not replaced. The limbus and the conjunctiva are closed with sutures. Antibiotic or a pressure patch may be applied.

65930

A blood clot in the anterior segment can block the flow of aqueous, thereby elevating intraocular pressure. It can also stain the cornea. Either condition can lead to permanent visual loss. The physician retracts the patient's eyelids with an ocular speculum. The physician uses a needle to aspirate a blood clot which has pooled in the anterior section between the iris and the cornea. The needle may enter the anterior segment through the cornea or through the limbus (the juncture of the cornea and sclera). Topical antibiotic or a patch may be applied when the procedure is complete.

66020–66030

Too little or too much fluid can cause permanent damage. The physician administers a needle injection of air or liquid (e.g., 66020) or medication (e.g., 66030) to the anterior of the eye. The needle may enter the anterior segment through the cornea or through the limbus (the juncture of the cornea and sclera).

66130

The sclera, coming from the Greek word for "hard," is the tough, white, outer coat of the eye. To remove a scleral lesion, the physician cuts through the thin, transparent conjunctiva and then snips the lesion with scleral scissors. The scleral and conjunctival wounds may not require sutures. The physician then applies antibiotic ointment and possibly a 24-hour pressure patch.

66150–66155

To create a new pathway for fluids in the eye, the physician makes an incision in the conjunctiva near the limbus (the corneal-scleral juncture). Either by using a trephine to remove a circular portion of sclera and iris (e.g., 66150), or by destroying a portion of the sclera and iris by burning it with a hot probe (e.g., 66155), the physician creates a collection area to improve the flow of aqueous. One method of this procedure is called Elliot's operation. The physician closes the incision with sutures and may restore the intraocular pressure with an injection of water or saline. A topical antibiotic or pressure patch may be applied.

66160

To improve the flow of aqueous, the physician makes an incision in the conjunctiva near the limbus (the corneal-scleral juncture). By using a punch or scleral scissors, the physician removes a portion of sclera and iris, creating a collection area for fluids in the anterior chamber. Various methods of sclerectomy include Lindner's, LaGrange, Knapp's, Holth's and Herbert's operations. The physician closes the incision with sutures and may restore the intraocular pressure with an injection of water or saline. A topical antibiotic or pressure patch may be applied.

66165

To improve the flow of fluids in the eye, the physician places an ocular speculum in the patient's eye, and accesses the anterior chamber through an incision through the limbus (the corneal-scleral juncture). The physician creates a permanent drainage route through the anterior chamber by taking a piece of iris tissue clipped with scleral scissors from the edge of the iris and wedging it into an incision in the iris so that it will act as a wick to draw aqueous from one side of the iris to the other. The physician closes the incision with sutures and may restore the intraocular pressure with an injection of water or saline. A topical antibiotic or pressure patch may be applied.

66170–66172

Though constantly flushed and renewed, the overall pressure of aqueous is constant in a healthy eye's anterior chamber. Too little or too much fluid can cause permanent damage. The physician places an ocular speculum in the patient's eye, and accesses the anterior chamber through an incision through the limbus (the corneal-scleral juncture).To promote better drainage of fluid, the physician removes a partial thickness portion of the ring of meshlike tissue at the iris-scleral junction (the trabecular meshwork), and a scleral trap door is left open so that aqueous may flow through the new channel into the space between the conjunctival and the sclera or cornea (bleb). The physician closes the incision with sutures and may restore the intraocular pressure with an injection of water or saline. A topical antibiotic or pressure patch may be applied. This procedure is performed in absence of previous surgery (e.g., for 66170) or as a repeated surgery where adhesions are reduced (e.g., for 66172). The adhesions may also have been caused by trauma.

66180–66185

Though constantly flushed and renewed, the overall pressure of aqueous is constant in a healthy eye's anterior chamber. Too little or too much fluid can cause permanent damage. To enhance drainage, the physician places an ocular speculum in the patient's eye and makes an incision in the conjunctiva and sutures tubing to the sclera. The tubing enters the anterior portion of the eye at the juncture of the sclera and cornea (the limbus). This improves the aqueous flow in the anterior chamber. The tube implant connects to a reservoir plate (a bleb) sutured into place behind the pars plana between the extraocular muscles. The physician stretches conjunctival tissue over the shunt and reservoir and sutures it into place. The physician closes the incision with sutures and may restore the intraocular pressure with an injection of water or saline. A topical antibiotic or pressure patch may be applied. A revision is done and 66185 reported if the first procedure is unsuccessful and must be altered.

66220–66225

A staphyloma is a bulging protrusion of the vascular coating of the eyeball (uvea) into a thin, stretched portion of the sclera. To repair the staphyloma, the physician places an ocular speculum in the patient's eye, and makes an incision in the conjunctiva and sclera over the site of a staphyloma. The physician excises the full-thickness staphyloma. A piece of stretched sclera may also be removed. The physician uses sutures or tissue glue in the layered repair. Antibiotic ointment and a patch may be applied. A graft (e.g., 66225) usually indicates that size of the staphyloma required that donor sclera tissue be grafted across the wound.

66250

The physician reexplores an eye wound that is the site of previous surgery to revise post-operative defects. The physician uses a number of techniques, based on the wound and previous surgery. Surgery may be major or minor.

66500–66505

Though constantly flushed and renewed, the overall pressure of aqueous is constant in a healthy eye's anterior chamber. Too little or too much fluid can cause permanent damage. To enhance the flow of fluids in the anterior chamber, the physician makes an incision in the corneal-scleral juncture (the limbus). The physician slices through the iris in a side-to-side motion in an effort to increase the flow of aqueous hampered by a pupilary block (e.g., 66500). No tissue is removed. In the iris bombe, where the iris balloons forward blocking aqueous outflow channels, the surgeon pierces the iris in two places (e.g., 66505). The physician closes the incision with sutures and may restore intraocular pressure with an injection of water or saline. A topical antibiotic or pressure patch may be applied.

66600–66605

The physician places a contact lens on the patient's eye to help direct the laser's beam. The excision of a full-thickness piece of the iris is usually accomplished with an argon laser. The physician uses the "chipping away technique" until the iris is penetrated for the excision. With cyclectomy (e.g., 66605), the burn is deeper, going through the iris into the ciliary body.

66625

After placing an ocular speculum in the patient's eye, the physician makes an incision at the juncture of the cornea and sclera (the limbus). The physician then removes a piece of iris, providing a direct passageway for aqueous. This causes the intraocular pressure to fall as aqueous from behind the iris can then flow forward and drain from the eye. This procedure is also called basal, buttonhole, or stenopeic iridectomy. The physician may close the incision with sutures and may restore the intraocular pressure with an injection

of water or saline. A topical antibiotic or pressure patch may be applied.

66630

Though constantly flushed and renewed, the overall pressure of aqueous is constant in a healthy eye's anterior chamber. Too little or too much fluid can cause permanent damage. To enhance the flow of fluids in the eye, the physician makes an incision at the juncture of the cornea and sclera (the limbus). The physician then removes a wedge piece from the iris leaving what is often referred to as a keyhole pupil. This causes the intraocular pressure to fall as aqueous from behind the iris can then flow forward and drain from the eye. The physician may close the incision with sutures and may restore the intraocular pressure with an injection of water or saline. A topical antibiotic or pressure patch may be applied.

66635

After placing an ocular speculum in the patient's eye, the physician makes an incision at the juncture of the cornea and sclera (the limbus). The physician then trims an inner ring of iris as a means of widening an abnormally small pupil and improving vision. The physician may close the incision with sutures and may restore the intraocular pressure with an injection of water or saline. A topical antibiotic or pressure patch may be applied.

66680–66682

After placing an ocular speculum in the patient's eye, the physician makes an incision at the juncture of the cornea and sclera (the limbus) to approach and repair a trauma-caused tear of the iris from from the ciliary body. The wedge shaped tear is affixed to the ciliary body with dissolving sutures, or with stitches that can be removed through an incision prepared for that retrieval. This procedure includes the later removal of the McCannel suture. The physician may close the incision with sutures and may restore the intraocular pressure with an injection of water or saline. A topical antibiotic or pressure patch may be applied. Report 66682 for a suture of the iris or ciliary body.

66700–66710

The ciliary body supplies the anterior chamber with aqueous. In cases where high intraocular pressure cannot otherwise be controlled, portions of the ciliary body are destroyed to reduce the production of aqueous. The physician makes an incision in the conjunctiva and sclera in the pars plana opposite from the site to be treated. The physician uses a heat probe (diathermy) or laser (cyclophotocoagulation) to burn holes in the ciliary body. The physician closes the incision with layered sutures and may restore the intraocular pressure with an anterior and/or posterior injection. A topical antibiotic or pressure patch may be applied. Report 66710 if cyclophotocoagulation be used.

CPT® Lay Descriptions

66720

The ciliary body supplies the anterior chamber with aqueous. In cases where high intraocular pressure cannot otherwise be controlled, portions of the ciliary body are destroyed to reduce the production of aqueous. The physician applies a freezing probe to the sclera over the ciliary body with the purpose of destroying the ciliary process. This is especially useful in aphakic patients.

66740

The ciliary body supplies the anterior chamber with aqueous. In cases where high intraocular pressure cannot otherwise be controlled, portions of the ciliary body are destroyed to reduce the production of aqueous. The physician makes an incision in the conjunctiva and sclera in the pars plana adjacent to the portion of ciliary body to be treated. The physician passes a spatula through the incision and into the suprachoroidal space of the anterior chamber. The spatula separates the ciliary body from the scleral spur. This may result in a lowering of intraocular pressure either by a decrease in aqueous humor formation from the now detached ciliary body or or by increasing uveovascular scleral outflow of aqueous. The physician closes the incision with layered sutures and may restore the intraocular pressure with an anterior and/or posterior injection. A topical antibiotic or pressure patch may be applied.

66761

After applying a topical anesthetic, the physician places a special contact lens on the eye of the patient. The argon or YAG laser is focused on the iris and multiple short bursts of laser light create holes in the iris. This procedure allows fluids in the eye to pass from behind the iris through the openings into the space between the iris and the cornea (the anterior chamber). This lowers intraocular pressure.

66762

The physician places a special contact lens on the eye of the patient and uses multiple bursts of light from an argon laser to create an additional hole in the iris.

66770

The physician places a special contact lens on the eye of the patient. The YAG or Argon laser is focused on the cyst or lesion and multiple short bursts of light destroy the abnormal tissue.

66820

The patient initially had extracapsular cataract surgery in which the posterior shell of the lens was not removed from the eye. But the capsule and/or the membrane adjacent to it (the anterior hyaloid) has since become opaque and must be opened in this new surgery. After placing an ocular speculum in the patient's eye, the pupil is dilated. The physician inserts a small needle, a Ziegler or Wheeler knife or special scissors into the corneal-scleral juncture (the limbus) and advances it to the edge of the capsule and through to the membrane, cutting a flap in the opaque membrane in the field of vision. The physician maneuvers the instrument around any artificial lens. No tissue is removed from the eye; the flap simply opens a window of vision. The physician may close the incision with sutures and may restore the intraocular pressure with an injection of water or saline. A topical antibiotic or pressure patch may be applied.

66821

The patient initially had extracapsular cataract surgery in which the posterior shell of the lens was not removed from the eye. But the capsule and/or the membrane adjacent to it (the anterior hyaloid) has since become opaque and must be destroyed in this new surgery. After a topical anesthetic is applied to the eye, the pupil is dilated. A number of YAG laser shots are focused to a point on the capsule, cutting it. Bursts from the YAG open a flap in the capsule, resulting in immediate improvement in vision. Multiple sessions may be needed to create an adequate opening in the lens capsule.

66825

The physician inserts a lid speculum between the patient's eyelids and the eye is secured by a suture. The physician cuts an opening at the juncture of the cornea and sclera (limbus) to access the artificial lens. The physician adjusts the artificial lens so that the attachments (haptics) of the implant are secured. The physician may close the incision with sutures and may restore the intraocular pressure with an injection of water or saline. A topical antibiotic or pressure patch may be applied.

66830

The patient initially had extracapsular cataract surgery, in which the posterior shell of the lens was not removed from the eye. But the capsule and/or the membrane adjacent to it (the anterior hyaloid) has since become opaque and must be removed in this new surgery. The physician inserts an ocular speculum into the patient's orbit, and makes an incision at the juncture of the cornea and sclera (the limbus). A small cutting needle and suction device (an irrigating cystotome) is inserted to chip away the posterior lens capsule. In some cases, the iris must be cut or a piece of iris removed to access the lens capsule. The adjacent membrane (the anterior hyaloid) may also removed. The physician irrigates the area during aspiration. The physician may close the incision with sutures and may restore the intraocular pressure with an injection of water or saline. A topical antibiotic or pressure patch may be applied.

66840

The physician makes an incision at the juncture of the cornea and sclera (the limbus). The anterior wall of the lens is incised. A probe attached to an irrigating/aspirating machine is inserted into the lens and the lens is destroyed and sucked away. The physician may close the incision with sutures and may restore the intraocular pressure with an injection of water or saline. A topical antibiotic or pressure patch may be applied.

66850

The physician makes an incision in the cornea or the pars plana. The anterior wall of the lens is cut out. The same type of irrigating/aspirating machine used for extracapsular surgery is used for phacofragmentation, but this time the probe is a needle that vibrates 40,000 times per second (phacofragmentation), or sound waves (phacoemulsification, ultrasound) that break up the lens. The physician uses irrigation and suction to remove the once hard nucleus, now liquefied by mechanical or sound vibrations. The physician may close the incision with sutures or may design a sutureless "self-sealing" incision. The physician may restore the intraocular pressure with an injection of water or saline. A topical antibiotic or pressure patch may be applied.

66852

To remove a cataract obstructing the view of the retina during retinal surgery, or to remove a piece of natural lens retained following cataract surgery, the physician makes an incision in the conjunctiva, sclera, and choroid of the pars plana. The physician approaches the lens capsule from behind. If the entire lens is being removed, the wall of the posterior lens capsule is removed and a small suction device is inserted into the lens. The lens material is sucked out. The physician irrigates the area during aspiration. If a retained portion of the lens is removed, a portion of the clear gel in the back of the eye may be removed as well (vitrectomy). The incision is closed with layered sutures. The physician may restore anterior or posterior intraocular pressure with an injection of water or saline. A topical antibiotic or pressure patch may be applied.

66920–66930

Intracapsular cataract extraction (ICCE) is when the lens and capsule are removed intact. The physician inserts an ocular speculum. An incision is made in the corneal-scleral juncture (the limbus). To enhance the flow of fluids in the eye, the physician may punch a hole in the iris before inserting a surgical instrument filled with coolant (cryoprobe) into the anterior chamber. The lens adheres to the cryoprobe as it freezes, and when the cryoprobe is removed, the lens comes with it (e.g., for 66920). The same technique is used to removed a dislocated lens (e.g., for 66930). The physician may close the incision with sutures and may restore intraocular pressure with an injection of water or saline. A topical antibiotic or pressure patch may be applied.

66940

Extracapsular cataract extraction (ECCE) is when the anterior shell and the nucleus of the lens capsule are both removed, leaving the posterior shell of the lens capsule in place. The physician inserts a lid speculum between the patient's eyelids and makes an incision in the corneal-scleral juncture (the limbus). To enhance the flow of fluids in the eye, the physician may punch a hole in the iris. Using a method other than aspiration or phacofragmentation, the physician removes the lens in parts: first the anterior lens, then the inner, hard nucleus. The clear, posterior capsule remains. The physician may close the incision with sutures and may restore the intraocular pressure with an injection of water or saline. A topical antibiotic or pressure patch may be applied.

66982

The physician performs a complex extracapsular cataract removal with insertion of an intraocular lens prothesis in a one-stage procedure. A local anesthetic is injected into the periorbital area. The physician makes a small horizontal incision where the cornea and sclera meet and, upon entering the eye through the incision, gently opens the front of the capsule and removes the hard center, or nucleus, of the lens. Using a microscope, the ophthalmologist suctions out the soft lens cortex, leaving the capsule in place. The area is irrigated and aspirated and an intraocular lens (IOL) (plastic disc that replaces the natural lens) is inserted. The ophthalmologist sutures the incision and instills antibiotic ointment and applies an eye patch. A metal shield is secured over the eye with tape. Standard phacoemulsification may be performed if the lens capsule is intact and sufficient zonular support remains. In capsulorrhexis, the ophthalmologist shatters the cataract nucleus with an ultrasonic oscillating probe. After fragmentation, the phaco probe is inserted into the eye and the cataract suctioned out through an irrigation-aspiration probe. An IOL is inserted once all of the material is removed. Suture fixation is chosen if both capsular and zonular supports are insufficient and the angle is minimally damaged.

66983

Intracapsular cataract extraction (ICCE) is when the lens and capsule are removed intact. The physician inserts an ocular speculum. An incision is made in the corneal-scleral juncture (the limbus). To enhance the flow of fluids in the eye, the physician may punch a hole in the iris before inserting a surgical instrument filled with coolant (cryoprobe) into the anterior chamber. The lens adheres to the cryoprobe as it freezes, and when the cryoprobe is removed, the lens comes with it. The physician injects a bubble of air into the anterior chamber to protect the cornea. The physician places an intraocular lens in the anterior chamber. The optic, or center, of the implant lies centered at the pupil and the haptics (securing attachments) of the implant are wedged in the anterior chamber, fixating the implant so it cannot move. The physician may close the incision with sutures and may restore the intraocular pressure with an injection of water or saline. A topical antibiotic or pressure patch may be applied.

66984

Extracapsular cataract extraction (ECCE) is when the anterior shell and the nucleus of the lens capsule are both removed, leaving the posterior shell of the lens capsule in place. The physician inserts a lid speculum between the patient's eyelids and makes an incision in the corneal-scleral juncture (the limbus). To enhance the flow of fluids in the eye, the physician may punch a hole in the iris. Using a cutting and suction or ultrasonic device, the physician removes the lens in parts: first the anterior lens, then the inner, hard nucleus. The clear, posterior capsule remains. The physician injects a bubble of air into the anterior chamber to protect the cornea. The physician then guides the intraocular implant into the eye. The haptics (securing attachments) lodge into the ciliary sulcus or the lens capsule, occupying the exact position of the original cataract. The physician may close the incision with sutures and may restore the intraocular pressure with an injection of water or saline. A topical antibiotic or pressure patch may be applied.

66985

The physician inserts an ocular speculum. An incision is made in the corneal-scleral juncture (the limbus). For an anterior lens, the physician places an intraocular lens in the fluid-filled space between the iris and cornea (the anterior chamber). The optic, or center, of the implant lies just in front of the pupil and the haptics (securing attachments) of the implant are wedged between the iris and cornea, fixating the implant so it cannot move. For a posterior lens, the physician injects a bubble of air into the anterior chamber to protect the cornea. The physician then guides the intraocular implant into the eye. The haptics lodge into the ciliary sulcus or the lens capsule. The physician may close the incision with sutures and may restore the intraocular pressure with an injection of water or saline. A topical antibiotic or pressure patch may be applied.

66986

Early models of intraocular lens (IOL) implants sometimes cause irritation in the patient's eye. They can also become dislocated. Here, the physician exchanges the problematic lens for a newer one. For anterior IOL, the physician replaces an intraocular lens in the fluid-filled space between the iris and cornea (the anterior chamber). The optic, or center, of the implant lies just in front of the pupil and the haptics (securing attachments) of the implant are lodged between the iris and cornea, fixating the implant so it cannot move. For posterior IOL, the physician injects a bubble of air into the anterior

chamber through a syringe to protect the cornea. The physician then replaces the intraocular implant in the eye. The haptics lodge into the ciliary sulcus or the lens capsule. The physician may close the incision with sutures and may restore the intraocular pressure with an injection of water or saline. A topical antibiotic or pressure patch may be applied.

67005–67010

The physician inserts a needle at the limbus or through the cornea (open sky technique) and passes the needle to the back of the anterior segment where a portion of displaced vitreous humor is aspirated (e.g., 67005). If most or all of the vitreous is extracted, mechanical tools are used (e.g., 67010). When this is done, the physician extracts the vitreous, using a mechanical cutting and suctioning process that may involve a special instrument like a rotoextractor or vitreous infusion suction cutter (VICS). In either case the aspirated vitreous is usually replaced by an injection of a vitreous substitute or aqueous. Any incision is closed with sutures.

67015

The physician inserts a needle into the posterior chamber through the pars plana to aspirate vitreous. Sometimes a posterior sclerotomy is made to release the fluid. When this is done, the physician extracts the vitreous, using a mechanical cutting and suctioning process that may involve a special instrument like a rotoextractor or vitreous infusion suction cutter (VICS). This is often called a vitreous chamber tap in operative reports. Once completed, the incision is repaired with sutures. Intraocular pressure may be adjusted with an injection. A pressure patch may be applied.

67025

The physician inserts a syringe in the pars plana to inject a material like healon or silicone. The injection may be required to replace vitreous that has been aspirated as part of this procedure, to restore intraocular pressure lost in another manner.

67027–67028

The physician implants an intravitreal drug delivery system to provide consistent delivery of a drug to an area of the eye affect by disease. Implants are capable of releasing a controlled amount of a specific drug for months; avoiding drug toxicity and other problems associated with prolonged intravenous therapies. Using a scalpel the physician makes an inferotemporal pars plana incision. Approximately one-half a milliliter of vitreous is removed. The implant (e. g., ganciclovir) in the form of a small pellet is placed through the wound, implanted into the vitreous, and sutured to the sclera. In 67028, the physician introduces medication into the posterior segment. The wound is closed and intraocular pressure is restored.

67030

The physician makes a small incision in the conjunctiva, sclera, and choroid in the pars plana. A narrow knife is inserted to cut vitreous strands that obstruct the patient's vision (e.g., 67030). The strands generally fall away from the visual field and are not retrieved. The physician repairs the pars plana incision with a layered closure and may restore the intraocular pressure with an injection of aqueous or vitreal substitute. A cataract specialist might approach the discussion through a limbal incision (at the corneal-scleral juncture), instead of through the pars plana. A topical antibiotic or pressure patch may be applied after either approach.

67031

The vitreous is the clear gel filling the posterior cavity of the eyeball. After applying a topical anesthetic and dilating the patient's pupil, the physician applies a special contact lens to the cornea of the patient. The physician uses a YAG laser to cut vitreous strands, adhesions or opacities that obstruct the patient's vision. No tissue is removed and no incision is made. More than one treatment may be required.

67036–67038

The vitreous is the clear gel filling the posterior cavity of the eyeball. The physician applies a special contact lens to the cornea to better visualize the back of the eye. Three small incisions are made in the eyeball, each about 4.0 mm from the juncture of the cornea and sclera. (This is the pars plana approach.) One incision is for a light cannula, one for an infusion cannula, and one for the cutting or suction instruments. The physician extracts the vitreous, using a mechanical cutting and suctioning process that may involve a special instrument like a rotoextractor or vitreous infusion suction cutter (VICS). This is often called a posterior sclerotomy in operative reports. To strip the epiretinal membrane (e.g., 67038), the physician uses a retinal cutting instrument to peel membrane or scar tissue creating tension on the retinal surface. The cannulas are extracted and the incisions repaired with layered closures. Injections may be required to reestablish intraocular pressure. A topical antibiotic or pressure patch may be applied.

67039–67040

The vitreous is the clear gel filling the posterior cavity of the eyeball. The physician applies a special contact lens to the cornea to better visualize the back of the eye. Three small incisions are made in the eyeball, each about 4.0 mm from the juncture of the cornea and sclera. (This is the pars plana approach.) One incision is for a light cannula, one for an infusion cannula and one for the laser. The physician extracts the vitreous, using a mechanical cutting and suctioning process that may involve a special instrument like a rotoextractor or vitreous infusion suction cutter (VICS). Then, with focal endolaser

photocoagulation (e.g., 67039), the physician uses a laser to treat minor retinal disorders. If the physician performs endolaser panretinal photocoagulation (e.g., 67040), a stronger laser treats larger retinal problems, like retinal detachments, diabetic retinopathy, or retinal holes. The cannulas are extracted and the incisions repaired with layered closures. Injections may be required to reestablish the intraocular pressure. A topical antibiotic or pressure patch may be applied.

67101

When the retina detaches, it separates from its nourishing blood supply and falls into the posterior cavity of the eye. Loss of vision results. The physician reattaches the retina by freezing (cryotherapy) and thus sealing the retinal tissue to the back of the eye, or by diathermy, where heat is used for the same purpose. The physician explores the sclera and stay sutures are placed under the involved rectus muscles so the eye can be rotated to expose the area to be treated. Sometimes, a rectus muscle is temporarily detached to permit adequate exposure. Cryotherapy and diathermy are performed without entering the posterior chamber; either probe is pressed against the sclera overlying the site of the retinal defect, sealing it against the choroid. If subretinal fluid must be drained, the physician makes an incision in the sclera (sclerotomy) to permit access to the middle layer of the eye's shell (the choroid), which is perforated so that fluid drains out. Any incisions are repaired with layered closures. Injections may be required to reestablish proper intraocular pressure. A topical antibiotic or pressure patch may be applied.

67105

When the retina detaches, it separates from its nourishing blood supply and falls into the posterior cavity of the eye. Loss of vision results. Using a laser light or xenon arc that goes through a dilated pupil without an incision, the physician burns spots at the site of the retinal detachment or retinal tear to seal the retina back into place against the choroid (vascular, middle layer of the eye's shell). If subretinal fluid must be drained, the physician cuts through the conjunctiva and into the sclera (sclerotomy) to access to the choroid, which is perforated so that fluid drains out. Any incisions are repaired with layered closures. Injections may be required to reestablish the intraocular pressure. A topical antibiotic or pressure patch may be applied.

67107

The physician explores the sclera to locate the site overlying a retinal detachment. Stay sutures are placed under involves rectus muscles so the eye may be exposed to area that will be treated. The physician treats the retinal tear externally, by placing a cold or hot probe over the scleral and depressing it. The burn seals the choroid to the retina at the site of the tear. The physician cuts a groove in the sclera and mattress

CPT® Lay Descriptions

sutures are places across this incision. Any subretinal fluid is drained. A Silastic band is laid in the scleral bed and sutured in place. Sometimes, a silicone patch is placed under the band. Additional cryotherapy or diathermy may be accomplished at this time. When the tear has been adequately repaired and supported, the rectus muscle sutures are removed.

67108

When the retina detaches, it separates from its nourishing blood supply and falls into the posterior cavity of the eye. Loss of vision results. The physician reattaches the retina by freezing (cryotherapy) and thus sealing the retinal tissue to the back of the eye, by diathermy, where heat is used for the same purpose, or by laser. Cryotherapy and diathermy are performed without entering the posterior chamber; either probe is pressed against the sclera overlying the site of the retinal defect, sealing it against the choroid. If a laser is used, the light goes through a dilated pupil without an incision to burn spots at the site of the retinal detachment or retinal tear to seal the retina back into place against the choroid (vascular, middle layer of the eye's shell). A scleral buckle may be placed. The physician removes any vitreous opacity or vitreous traction. The lens may also be removed if it interferes with the physician's view of the retina or if the lens is in the way of the removal of scar tissue. Any incisions may be repaired with sutures. Antibiotic ointment and a pressure patch may be applied.

67110

When the retina detaches, it separates from its nourishing blood supply and falls into the posterior cavity of the eye. Loss of vision results. The physician uses a needle to inject expandable gas into the eye to flatten the retinal tear, then applies laser or cryotherapy to seal the retinal tear. The physician explores the sclera to locate the site overlying a retinal detachment. Stay sutures are placed under involved rectus muscles so the eye may be exposed to area that will be treated. Air or other gas is injected through the sclera into the posterior segment of the eye to flatten the retinal detachment against the choroid (The patient is instructed to maintain a posture that will position the bubble against the detachment.). The physician treats the retinal tear externally, by placing a cold (cryotherapy) or hot (diathermy) probe over the sclera and depressing it. The burn seals the choroid to the retina at the site of the tear. This procedure is often called pneumatic retinopexy.

67112

The physician performs a reoperative procedure to correct retinal detachment following failed surgery. Making an incision, the physician isolates the site of retinal detachment. The physician reseals the retinal tissues to the back of the eye with diathermy or cryotherapy, and uses alloplastic materials to reinforce the sclera. Any vitreous opacities and retractions are removed. Incisions are closed with sutures.

67115

The physician inserts an ocular speculum. To release tension of a previously placed scleral buckle, the physician makes an incision in the conjunctiva and sclera, adjusts the buckle and repairs the surgical wound with sutures.

67120

The physician inserts an ocular speculum. The physician removes a previously implanted extraocular tube, reservoir, buckle, or other prosthetic device from the eye. The physician may close the incision with sutures and may restore the intraocular pressure with an injection of water or saline. A topical antibiotic or pressure patch may be applied.

67121

An incision is made in the pars plana near the site of an intraocular lens that has fallen into the posterior segment of the eye. The physician then removes the extracapsular IOL from the eye. The physician closes the incision with sutures and may restore the intraocular pressure with an injection of vitreous substitute. A topical antibiotic or pressure patch may be applied.

67141

When the retina detaches, it separates from its nourishing blood supply and falls into the posterior cavity of the eye. Loss of vision results. The physician secures a degenerating retina by freezing (cryotherapy) and thus sealing the retinal tissue to the back of the eye, or by diathermy, where heat is used for the same purpose. The physician explores the sclera and stay sutures are placed under the involved rectus muscles so the eye can be rotated to expose the area to be treated. Sometimes, a rectus muscle is temporarily detached to permit adequate exposure. Cryotherapy and diathermy are performed without entering the posterior chamber; either probe is pressed against the sclera overlying the site of the retinal defect, sealing it against the choroid.

67145

Using a laser light or xenon arc that goes through a dilated pupil without an incision, the physician burns spots at the site of the retinal weakness to seal the retina into place against the choroid (vascular, middle layer of the eye's shell). No incision is made. Multiple sessions may be required.

67208

The physician destroys a lesion of the retina by freezing (cryotherapy), or by heat (diathermy). The physician explores the sclera and stay sutures are placed under the involves rectus muscles so the eye can be rotated to expose the area to be treated. Sometimes, a rectus muscle is temporarily detached to permit adequate exposure. Cryotherapy and diathermy are performed without entering the posterior chamber; either probe is pressed against the sclera overlying the site of the retinal lesion until it is destroyed or until the session is completed. Any muscle incision is repaired and any stay sutures removed. A topical antibiotic or pressure patch may be applied.

67210

The physician destroys a lesion of the retina using a laser or xenon arc. After the patient's eye has been dilated, the physician places a special contact on the eye of the patient. Photocoagulation by laser or xenon arc is performed without entering the posterior chamber; the destructive light beam is guided through the contact and to the retinal lesion, which is destroyed in one session or in a series of sessions. A topical antibiotic or pressure patch may be applied.

67218

The physician treats a malignancy by exposing it to a radioactive implant. The plaque-like implant is secured with sutures to the sclera overlying the site of a malignancy. At a future time, the physician recovers the implant. The incision is repaired. An antibiotic ointment and pressure patch may be applied.

67220

The physician destroys a lesion of the choroid using photocoagulation. In one or more sessions the physician directs short spots of a laser's beam at new blood vessels that have grown beneath the macula to seal leaking blood or fluid that can damage vision. Or, the physician may scatter the laser spots through the sides of the retina to reduce abnormal blood vessel growth (choroidal neovascularization) and help seal the retina to the back of the eye.

67220–67225

In a two-step procedure, the physician performs photodynamic therapy. First, the physician injects the drug Visudyne(r) (Verteporfin) intravenously into the patient's arm. Then using a standard ophthalmic slit lamp, the physician identifies the treatment site. Following a specific time frame, the ophthalmologist shines a non-thermal 689-nanometer laser light into the patient's eye to activate the drug. The photosensitive chemical accumulates in the tissues of diseased and damaged areas and, upon light activation, destroys the target cells, while sparing the surrounding healthy tissue. Report 67225 when photodynamic therapy is performed on the second eye during a single session.

67221

In a two step procedure the physician performs photodynamic therapy. First, the physician injects the drug Visudyne(r) (Verteporfin) intravenously into the patient's arm. Then using a standard ophthalmic slit lamp, the physician identifies the treatment site. Following a specific time frame, the ophthalmologist shines a non-thermal 689-nanometer laser light into the patient's eye to activate the drug. The

photosensitive chemical accumulates in the tissues of diseased and damaged areas and, upon light activation, destroys the target cells, while sparing the surrounding healthy tissue.

67221–67225

In a two-step procedure, the physician performs photodynamic therapy. First, the physician injects the drug Visudyne(r) (Verteporfin) intravenously into the patient's arm. Using a standard ophthalmic slit lamp, the physician identifies the treatment site. Following a specific time frame, the ophthalmologist shines a non-thermal 689-nanometer laser light into the patient's eye to activate the drug. The photosensitive chemical accumulates in the tissues of diseased and damaged areas and, upon light activation, destroys the target cells, while sparing the surrounding healthy tissue. Report 67221 when photodynamic therapy is performed on one eye and 67225 when photodynamic therapy is performed on the second eye during the same session.

67227–67228

The physician destroys small vessels that are leaking blood on the retina by freezing (cryotherapy), or by heat (diathermy) (e.g., 67227), or by laser (e.g., 67228). Cryotherapy and diathermy may be performed without entering the posterior chamber; either probe is pressed against the sclera overlying the site of the retinopathy until it is destroyed. With a laser light or xenon arc aimed through a dilated pupil without an incision, the physician may burn spots at the site of diabetic retinopathy to seal vessels that have been leaking into the retina. At least 500 Xenon arc burns or 2000 burns from an argon laser are applied. This procedure is often referred to as "scattered destruction." Multiple sessions may be required.

67250–67255

To repair a thin, weakened sclera, the physician places an ocular speculum in the patient's eye, and makes an incision in the conjunctiva and sclera over the site of the defect. The sclera may be cinched and overlapped for reinforcement (e.g., for 67250) or a patch of donor sclera may be sutured over the weakened area (e.g., 67255). A piece of stretched sclera may also be removed. The physician uses sutures or tissue glue in the layered repair. Antibiotic ointment and a patch may be applied.

67311–67312

Strabismus is an imbalance in the muscles of the eyeball that control eyeball movement. Surgery can sometimes correct this imbalance. A speculum is placed in the patient's eye (no previous surgery). The physician makes incisions in the conjunctiva at the juncture of the sclera and cornea (the limbus) or in the cul-de-sac (Parks incision). Radial relaxing incisions in the conjunctiva are made and the muscle (either medial or lateral rectus) is isolated with a

CPT® Lay Descriptions

muscle hook. The muscle is then either strengthened by resection (removal of a measured segment) or weakened by recession (retroplacement of the muscle attachment). The muscles are secured with sutures. The operative wound is closed with sutures. In 67311, one horizontal muscle is treated; in 67312 two horizontal muscles in the same eye are treated.

67314–67316

Strabismus is an imbalance in the muscles of the eyeball that control eyeball movement. Surgery can sometimes correct this imbalance. A speculum is placed in the patient's eye, the physician makes incisions in the conjunctiva at the juncture of the sclera and cornea (the limbus) or in the cul-de-sac (Parks incision). Radial relaxing incisions in the conjunctiva are made and the muscle (either superior or inferior rectus) is isolated with a muscle hook. The muscle is then either strengthened by resection (removal of a measured segment) or weakened by recession (retroplacement of the muscle attachment). The muscles are secured with sutures. The operative wound is closed with sutures. In 67314, one vertical muscle is treated; in 67316 two vertical muscles in the same eye or in different eyes are treated.

67318

Strabismus is an imbalance in the muscles of the eyeball that control eyeball movement. Surgery can sometimes correct this imbalance. A speculum is placed in the patient's eye (no previous surgery). The physician makes incisions in the conjunctiva about 7.0 mm posterior to the juncture of the sclera and cornea (the limbus) in the superior nasal quadrant of the globe. An incision is made to expose the sclera and a muscle hook is used to engage the superior rectus muscle initially. The tendon of the superior oblique may be located about 12.0 mm behind the medial or nasal edge of the insertion of the superior rectus. The physician repairs, recesses, or resects the superior oblique muscle. The operative would is closed with layered sutures.

67320

A speculum is placed in the patient's eye, the physician makes incisions in the conjunctiva at the juncture of the sclera and cornea (the limbus) to expose the muscle. The extraocular muscle or muscles to be transposed are isolated, and the physician exposes the area of sclera to which the transposed muscles are to be attached. The insertions of the transposed muscles are then relocated generally adjacent to the paretic or weak muscle. They are attached to the sclera with sutures, and the surgical wound is closed with sutures. Occasionally, the transposed muscle may be split and one-half of the muscle relocated.

67331

Strabismus is an imbalance in the muscles of the eyeball that control eyeball movement. Surgery can sometimes correct this imbalance. A speculum is placed in the patient's eye, the physician makes incisions in the conjunctiva at the juncture of the sclera and cornea (the limbus) to expose the muscle. The extraocular muscle is isolated, and the physician uses a scalpel to free the muscle from surrounding fibrotic or scarred tissues. The muscle or muscles are then dissected posteriorly to ensure lack of incarceration and then repositioned if necessary. The surgical wound is closed with sutures.

67332

Strabismus is an imbalance in the muscles of the eyeball that control eyeball movement. Surgery can sometimes correct this imbalance. A speculum is placed in the eye of a patient and the physician makes incisions in the conjunctiva at the juncture of the sclera and cornea (the limbus) to expose the muscle. The extraocular muscle is isolated, and the physician uses a scalpel to free the muscle from surrounding fibrotic or scarred tissues. The muscle or muscles are then dissected posteriorly to ensure lack of incarceration and then repositioned if necessary. The surgical wound is closed with sutures.

67334

Strabismus is an imbalance in the muscles of the eyeball that control eyeball movement. Surgery can sometimes correct this imbalance. A speculum is placed in the patient's eye, the physician makes incisions in the conjunctiva and sclera to expose the muscle. The extraocular muscle is isolated far posterior to its insertion. The borders or edges of the muscle are sutured to the eye far back of the insertion in what is commonly called the Faden procedure. The surgical wound is closed with sutures.

67335

Strabismus is an imbalance in the muscles of the eyeball that control eyeball movement. Surgery can sometimes correct this imbalance. The muscle or muscles to be placed on an adjustable suture are isolated in the usual fashion during separately reportable strabismus surgery. Instead of permanently suturing the muscle to the eyeball by tying and cutting the suture distal to the knot, the sutures are tied and brought out through the overlying conjunctiva. Tension on the muscle is adjusted later when the anesthetic is no longer affecting the position of the globe.

67340

Strabismus is an imbalance in the muscles of the eyeball that control eyeball movement. Surgery can sometimes correct this imbalance. The physician makes an extensive incision of the conjunctiva at the juncture of the cornea and the sclera (the limbus). This is called a peritomy. In the plane of the detached muscle, retractors afford increased visibility and extensive posterior dissection may be necessary in an effort to locate the severed, lost, or detached muscle and reapproximate it to the eyeball with sutures. Once the repair is completed, the incision is repaired.

67343

During the performance of separately reported horizontal muscle surgery, scar tissue from a vertical muscle is excised. Or, during the performance of separately reported vertical muscle surgery, horizontal muscle scar tissue is excised. The scar tissue of the extraocular muscle is isolated, and the physician uses a scalpel to dissect the scars and fibrotic tissue from the muscle affecting the muscle itself. The surgical wound is closed with sutures.

67345

The extraocular muscle is identified through this direct surgical exposure or through the insertion of an electromyographic needle into the muscle. A small quantity of botulin toxin is then injected into the belly of the muscle. Onset of paralysis takes 24 to 48 hours and lasts from four to eight weeks.

67350

A speculum is placed in the patient's eye, the physician makes incisions in the conjunctiva and sclera to expose the muscle. The extraocular muscle to be tested is isolated, and the physician uses a scalpel to remove a small portion of the muscle. The excision will not affect overall action of the eye muscle. The surgical wound is closed with sutures.

67400–67405

The physician accesses the orbit through a subciliary, extraperiosteal, or transconjunctival incision. In the subciliary incision, an incision is made in the upper eyelid. In the extraperiosteal incision, the approach is through an incision anterior, superior, interior, or medial to the eye allowing access to the bone beneath the periosteum. In the transconjunctival approach, the lower lid is everted and an incision is made over the infraorbital rim through the inferior cul-de-sac. In 67400, soft tissue or bone may be excised for examination, but no other tissue is removed or repaired. In 67405, fluid is drained from the orbit. In either case, the operative incision is closed with layered sutures.

67412–67413

The physician removes a lesion or a foreign body from the orbit through a subciliary, frontal, or transconjunctival incision. In the subciliary incision, an incision is made in the lower eyelid. In the frontal approach, an incision is made in the lid crease with a further postseptal dissection for removal of a lesion or foreign body in this portion of the orbit. In the transconjunctival approach, the lower lid is everted and an incision is made over the infraorbital rim through the inferior cul-de-sac. In 67412, the lesion is excised. In 67413, the foreign body is removed. In either case, the operative incision is closed with layered sutures.

67414

The physician removes bone from the orbit through a subciliary or transconjunctival incision. In the subciliary incision, an incision is made in the lower eyelid. In the transconjunctival approach, the lower lid is everted and an incision is made over the infraorbital rim through the inferior cul-de-sac. Bone is excised for decompression. The operative incision is closed with layered sutures.

67415

With the aid of a separately reported fluoroscope or x-ray visualization, the physician directs the needle toward the targeted area and aspirates a small amount. No incision is made and no repair is required.

67420–67430

The physician makes an incision in the lateral aspect of the orbit. A C-shaped incision is made down to the periosteum overlying the lateral orbital rim. The periosteum is incised posterior to the rim itself. The temporalis muscle is moved aside and the globe is protected with pliable retractors. A vibrating saw removes the bone of the lateral orbital rim. In 67420 the lesion is excised from the orbit. In 67430, a foreign body is removed. In either case, the bone is replaced and wired into position and the operative wound is closed in layers.

67440

The physician makes an incision in the lateral aspect of the orbit. A C-shaped incision is made down to the periosteum overlying the lateral orbital rim. The periosteum is incised posterior to the rim itself. The temporalis muscle is moved aside and the globe is protected with pliable retractors. A vibrating saw is used to remove the bone from the lateral orbital rim. Fluid is then excised from the orbit and the bone is replaced and wired into position. The operative wound is closed in layers.

67445

The physician makes an incision in the lateral aspect of the orbit. A C-shaped incision is made down to the periosteum overlying the lateral orbital rim. The periosteum is incised posterior to the rim itself. The temporalis muscle is moved aside and the globe is protected with pliable retractors. A vibrating saw removes the bone of the lateral orbital rim. A piece of orbital bone is removed for decompression. The bone flap is then replaced and wired into position. The operative wound is closed in layers.

67450

The physician makes an incision in the lateral aspect of the orbit. A C-shaped incision is made down to the periosteum overlying the lateral orbital rim. The periosteum is incised posterior to the rim itself. The temporalis muscle is moved aside and the globe is protected with pliable retractors. A vibrating saw removes the bone of the lateral orbital rim. The physician explores the orbit and may remove tissue for examination. No other procedure is performed. The bone is replaced and wired into position. The operative wound is closed in layers.

67500–67505

The physician injects a therapeutic or anesthetic medication (e.g., for 67500) or alcohol (e.g., for 67505) into the orbit through the lower eyelid or in a transconjunctival method.

67515

A blunt or sharp-tipped needle is guided along the surface of the globe beneath the conjunctiva and between the sclera and Tenon's capsule. When the tip of the needle is in the appropriate location, medication or other substance is injected into the Tenon's capsule.

67550–67560

The physician inserts a prosthesis in the eye in 67550 or revises or removes an orbital implant in 67560. An orbital implant lies outside the boundaries of the orbit; it is usually secured with sutures.

67570

The physician makes an incision in the lateral or medial aspect of the fornix. In a lateral approach, a C-shaped incision is made down to the periosteum overlying the lateral orbital rim. The periosteum is incised posterior to the rim itself. The temporalis muscle is moved aside and the globe is protected with pliable retractors. The bone is removed to access the optic nerve. In a medial approach, the conjunctiva is incised and the medial rectus muscle is temporarily disinserted. Sutures are passed through the terminal portion of the medial rectus muscle and its insertion into the globe is noted. The eye is rotated laterally to gain access to the optic nerve medially. In either case, once the nerve has been identified, several small fenestrations are made. A dissection is carried down through the outer meningeal layer covering the optic nerve until the subarachnoid space is reached. An egress of cerebral spinal fluid indicates decompression of the nerve sheath. The operative wound is closed in layers.

67700

The eyelid is prepped and draped and local anesthetic is applied. A transverse incision is made to drain the abscess in the lid. The wound is irrigated and may be closed with sutures.

67710

This procedure generally follows a previously performed tarsorrhaphy (closure of the eyelid), usually attempted to protect the cornea. The eyelid is prepped and draped, and local anesthetic is applied. The previously formed seam or union between the upper and lower lid is then carefully delineated and divided using sharp scissors.

67715

Under local anesthesia, the face and eyelids are draped and prepped. Scissors cut the lateral canthus to further divide the upper and lower lid to extend the division.

67800–67808

A chalazion is a small mass in the eyelid that results in chronic inflammation. The face and eye are prepped and draped and local anesthesia (e.g., for 67800, 67801 and 67805) or general anesthesia (e.g., for 67808) is administered. Usually, general anesthesia is reserved for very young or otherwise uncooperative patients. The physician applies a chalazion clamp to expose the posterior surface of the eyelid. The chalazion is incised with a blade and a curet is used to explore the lid after the incision has been drained. Any pockets of infection are drained. The lips of the wound are generally cauterized to prevent excessive bleeding. The clamp is released.

67810

A local anesthetic is applied and the face and eyelid are prepped and draped. A small amount of tissue is excised from the suspect portion of the eyelid. Sutures may be required to repair the incision.

67820

Trichiasis is a condition wherein eyelashes are ingrown or misdirected in their growth so that they irritate the tissues of the eye. Using a biomicroscope, the physician plucks the offending eyelashes with forceps. The lash follicles are not treated.

67825

Trichiasis is a condition wherein eyelashes are ingrown or misdirected in their growth so that they irritate the tissues of the eye. The physician treats the area of trichiasis with local anesthetic. In cryotherapy, the freezing probe is applied to the area of trichiasis. After a period of repeated freezing and thawing, the lash follicles are usually destroyed. In electrosurgery, electrolysis directed at the follicles destroys them.

67830–67835

Trichiasis is a condition wherein eyelashes are ingrown or misdirected in their growth so that they irritate the tissues of the eye. The physician treats the area of trichiasis with a local anesthetic and preps and drapes the face and eye. The physician uses a scalpel to split the eyelid margin at the gray line (the junction of the palpebral mucosa and skin). The area of abnormal eyelash growth is excised in both 67830 and 67835. Additionally in 67835, tissue for a split-thickness graft is harvested from the buccal mucosa inside the patient's mouth. No repair is required at the graft harvest site. The graft is inlaid between the palpebral conjunctiva and the skin. In either case, sutures may be required.

67840

The physician administers a local anesthetic and the face and eyelid are draped and prepped for surgery. The eyelid lesion is outlined in a marking pen. The lesion is incised and the surgical wound is repaired with sutures if necessary.

67850

The physician administers a local anesthetic and the face and eyelid are draped and prepped for surgery. An electrocautery tool or photocoagulation is used to destroy the small eyelid lesion.

67875

The constant action of the eyelid opening and closing against the cornea can cause problems in patients with chronic corneal conditions. Temporary closure of the eyelid may provide relief for an eroded or painful cornea. The physician administers local anesthetic to the eyelids. A permanent suture is passed through the skin and eyelid margin at the gray line of the upper lid and corresponding portion of the lower lid. This process is repeated several times in each eye, creating a permanent marginal adhesion. The sutures are usually tied over a bolster to prevent erosion of the suture through the lid.

67880

The constant action of the eyelid opening and closing against the cornea can cause problems in patients with chronic corneal conditions. Temporary closure of the eyelid may provide relief for an eroded or painful cornea. The physician administers a local anesthetic and preps and drapes the face and eyelids for surgery. Tissue along the mucocutaneous junction at the margins of the eyelids is excised. A suture is passed through the skin and eyelid margin at the gray line of the upper lid and corresponding portion of the lower lid. This process is repeated several times in each eye, creating a permanent marginal adhesion. The sutures are usually tied over a bolster to prevent erosion of the suture through the lid. The sutures are removed a week to 10 days later, after the lid margins have adhered.

67882

The constant action of the eyelid opening and closing against the cornea can cause problems in patients with chronic corneal conditions. Temporary closure of the eyelid may provide relief for an eroded or painful cornea. The physician administers a local anesthetic and preps and drapes the face and eyelids for surgery. Tissue along the mucocutaneous junction at the margins of the eyelids is excised. A tongue of tarsal plate is isolated from above the upper or lower lid. The tarsal plate is sutured into a corresponding area of the opposite lid. The physician then passes a suture through the skin and eyelid margin at the gray line of the upper lid and corresponding portion of the lower lid. This process is repeated several times in each eye, creating a permanent marginal adhesion. The sutures

are usually tied over a bolster to prevent erosion of the suture through the lid. The sutures are removed a week to 10 days later, after the lid margins have adhered.

67900

Ptosis refers to a droop or displacement resulting from paralysis. The physician makes an incision directly above the brow (supraciliary), through the mid-forehead or near the hairline (coronal). A dissection is carried down to the area of the brow. The skin is pulled superiorly and the brow approximated to its proper position above the supraorbital rim. The operative incision is repaired with sutures.

67901

Blepharoptosis refers to a droop or displacement of the upper eyelid resulting from paralysis. The physician makes an incision directly above the brow (supraciliary). The frontalis fixation technique is a mechanical suspension that transfers the movement of the upper lid to the frontalis muscle above the eyelid. It is sutured in place. The operative incision is repaired with sutures.

67902

Blepharoptosis refers to a droop or displacement of the upper eyelid resulting from paralysis. The physician makes an incision directly above the brow (supraciliary). The frontalis fixation technique is a mechanical suspension that transfers the movement of the upper lid to the frontalis muscle above the eyelid. It is sutured in place. The physician obtains fascia from the patient's thigh and uses this fascia to create a sling to the frontalis muscle. This sling helps suspend the lid. The operative incisions are repaired with sutures.

67903

Blepharoptosis refers to a droop or displacement of the upper eyelid resulting from paralysis. The physician administers local anesthetic and the patient's face and eyelid are draped and prepped for surgery. The eyelid is everted and the physician makes an incision along the upper posterior edge of the tarsus. The levator complex, including Mueller's muscle, is then isolated for a distance superiorly to correspond with the amount of ptosis to be corrected. The levator aponeurosis is then advanced onto the tarsal plate internally until the eyelid margin falls at the appropriate location below the limbus. The incision is repaired.

67904

Blepharoptosis refers to a droop or displacement of the upper eyelid resulting from paralysis. The physician administers local anesthetic and the patient's face and eyelid are draped and prepped for surgery. An incision line is outlined along the crease of the upper eyelid. A dissection is carried down the normal insertion point of the distal point of the levator tendon. The levator tendon is then isolated. The physician uses sutures to advance the levator tendon onto the tarsal plate in an adjustable fashion. If the patient is old enough to undergo the procedure under local anesthetic, the patient is placed in a sitting position and eyelid height and contour are evaluated under the effect of gravity. The amount that the levator tendon is advanced corresponds to the degree of preoperative ptosis. If the patient is not able to undergo the procedure under local anesthetic, general anesthesia is used and a predetermined amount of advancement is performed. In either case, the incision is repaired with sutures once the tendon has been secured in its new location.

67906

Blepharoptosis refers to a droop or displacement of the upper eyelid resulting from paralysis. The physician administers local anesthetic and the patient's face and eyelid are draped and prepped for surgery. The physician performs a repair that provides a mechanical suspension of the upper lid, transferring the movement of the upper lid to the frontalis muscle action of the eyebrow. The most common technique involves the creation of three horizontal incisions extending to the level of the tarsal plate approximately 3.0 mm above the upper eyelid margin in the midline, nasal, and lateral quarters. Three corresponding incisions are made just above the brow down to the periosteum of the bone. The lid is suspended in a double rhomboid configuration as the physician passes the suspending material deep in the lid tissue at the depth of the anterior surface of the levator aponeurosis through the orbital septum in front of the bone and out through the medial and lateral brow incisions. The knots are pulled up and tied to elevate the eyelid margin to the level of the superior limbus. The ends of the sutures are burned in the wound. The incisions are repaired with sutures.

67908

The physician administers local anesthetic and the patient's face and eyelid are draped and prepped for surgery. The physician everts the upper eyelid and a series of curved clamps are placed across the everted undersurface of the upper lid. All of the tissue distal to the clamps is removed or resected. This includes conjunctiva, tarsus, Muller's muscle, and the distal insertion of the levator aponeurosis. A running suture or purse string suture is used to consolidate the remaining tissues.

67909

The physician administers local anesthetic and the patient's face and eyelid are draped and prepped for surgery. With an incision usually at the previous incision line, the physician attempts to reduce a previous overcorrection of ptosis. The levator aponeurosis is either cut free of disinserted from its attachment to the levator aponeurosis, and the operative incision is repaired with sutures.

67911

The physician administers local anesthetic and the patient's face and eyelid are draped and prepped for surgery. The physician outlines the incision line, usually in the crease of the upper lid. The distal portion of the tendon responsible for elevating the lid (levator aponeurosis) is isolated from its attachment to the tarsal plate. The levator aponeurosis is then allowed to retract itself posteriorly or autogenous graft materials are inserted between the levator aponeurosis and the tarsal plate. The patient is generally placed in a sitting position and the amount of the retraction of the levator aponeurosis is judged by the position of the eyelid while the patient is sitting on the table. Alternatively, the eyelid margin may be placed approximately 2.0 mm below the limbus. When the lid is positioned satisfactorily, it is affixed. The operative incision is closed with sutures.

67914

An ectropion is a turning outward of the margin of the lower eyelid. The physician administers local anesthetic and the patient's face and eyelid are draped and prepped for surgery. The physician uses absorbable sutures to foreshorten the posterior tissues of the eyelid in an effort to redirect the rotation of the eyelid posteriorly. No incisions are required for this treatment of ectropion.

67915

An ectropion is a turning outward of the margin of the lower eyelid. The physician administers local anesthetic and the patient's face and eyelid are draped and prepped for surgery. Either bipolar or unipolar cautery is employed to shrink the posterior tissues of the eyelid margin in an effort to rotate the lid margin posteriorly toward the globe. No incision is made.

67916

An ectropion is a turning outward of the margin of the lower eyelid. The physician administers local anesthetic and the patient's face and eyelid are draped and prepped for surgery. A section of tarsus and conjunctiva in the configuration of a diamond or rhomboid is taken from the posterior or back surface of the lower lid. Incisions are then closed with interrupted absorbable sutures to rotate the eyelid margin posteriorly toward the globe.

67917

An ectropion is a turning outward of the margin of the lower eyelid. The physician administers local anesthetic and the patient's face and eyelid are draped and prepped for surgery. The physician makes an incision in the lower lid and isolates a tongue or strip of tarsus in the lateral one third of the lower lid. Nonabsorbable sutures are passed through the tarsal strip. The periosteum of tough fibrous tissue which lines the bone of the lateral orbital rim is then isolated. The sutures from the tarsal strip are passed through the periosteum overlying the bone of the lateral orbital rim. The physician tightens the sutures. Eyelid margin tension and contour are evaluated and adjusted. The incision or incisions are repaired with sutures.

67921

An entropion is an inversion of the margin of the eyelid. The physician administers local anesthetic and the patient's face and eyelid are draped and prepped for surgery. The physician threads sutures through the inferior fornix or inferior cul-de-sac externally to the lash line. The sutures are placed in the medial, middle, and lateral third of the eyelid in a mattress fashion. These absorbable sutures are tied on the skin side. The sutures act to evert the eyelid margin anteriorly, correcting the malposition of the eyelid. No incision is made in this procedure.

67922

An entropion is an inversion of the margin of the eyelid. The physician administers local anesthetic and the patient's face and eyelid are draped and prepped for surgery. The physician uses bipolar or monopolar cautery to create a central tissue shrinkage to rotate the eyelid margin anteriorly. This corrects the malposition of the eyelid. No incisions are made in this procedure.

67923

An entropion is an inversion of the margin of the eyelid. The physician administers local anesthetic and the patient's face and eyelid are draped and prepped for surgery. A triangular section of tarsus is excised from the lower eyelid. A large chalazion clamp may be used to evert the lid and excise the triangle of tarsus, which usually measures 8.0 mm to 10.0 mm at the base. A piece of exposed orbicularis muscle is removed with the wedge. The edges of the excision site are approximated and repaired with sutures.

67924

An entropion is an inversion of the margin of the eyelid. The physician administers local anesthetic and the patient's face and eyelid are draped and prepped for surgery. The physician makes the incision along approximately 80 percent of the width of the eyelid. The physician uses deep sutures to sever the eyelid margin outwardly. A triangular section of tarsus may also be excised from the lower eyelid. All incisions are repaired with sutures. This procedure is sometimes performed under general anesthesia.

67930–67935

The physician administers local anesthetic and the patient's face and eyelid is draped and prepped for surgery. The physician irrigates the wound and approximates its edges. The wound is repaired in layered sutures. In 67930, the wound is through a partial thickness of eyelid; in 67935, the wound is through the full thickness of the eyelid.

67938

The physician administers local anesthetic and the patient's face and eyelid are draped and prepped for surgery. The physician locates the foreign body through palpation. An incision is made through the anterior surface if the foreign body is principally on the anterior of the lid; the lid is everted if the foreign body is near the posterior surface. An attempt is made to conceal the incision line in the crease of the upper lid, or through a subciliary incision, when possible. The foreign body is removed and the wound is irrigated. The wound is repaired with layered sutures.

67950

The physician administers local anesthetic and the patient's face and eyelid are draped and prepped for surgery. The physician increases the lid margin by cutting the medial or lateral canthus (juncture of upper and lower eyelid). The physician rearranges the anterior tissues of the lids to prevent adherence.

67961–67966

The physician administers local anesthetic and the patient's face and eyelid are draped and prepped for surgery. A section of full-thickness eyelid is excised from the upper or lower eyelid. The section includes the defect and a margin of normal tissue. The edges of the excision site are approximated to reconstitute the eyelid contour and the wound is closed with layered sutures. Sometimes, a separately reported skin graft or pedicle flap is required to achieve proper cosmetic results. In 67961, up to one-fourth of the lid margin is removed; in 67966, more than one-fourth is removed.

67971

The patient's face and eyelid are draped and prepped for surgery. Local or general anesthesia may be administered. The patient has already undergone a separately reported excision that has created a significant eyelid defect requiring reconstruction of up to two-thirds of the eyelid. Because the defect is too large for direct closure, portions of the opposing eyelid are excised and grafted to reconstruct the eyelid. The opposite lid is everted and a horizontal incision through the tarsus and conjunctival approximately 4.0 mm from the eyelid margin is performed. Vertical incisions are then made through the conjunctiva to match the width of the flap. The dissection is carried down through Muller's muscle toward the fornix or cul-de-sac. The advancing tarsal conjunctival flap is then grafted to the opposing lid and secured with sutures. A separately reportable free, full-thickness skin graft may be applied to complete the reconstruction.

67973–67974

The patient's face and eyelid are draped and prepped for surgery. Local or general anesthesia may be administered. The patient has already undergone a separately reported excision that has created a significant eyelid defect requiring reconstruction.

Because the defect is too large (e.g., total lower lid for 67973 and total upper lid for 67974), portions of the opposing eyelid are excised and grafted to reconstruct the eyelid. The opposite lid is everted and a horizontal incision through the tarsus and conjunctival approximately 4.0 mm from the eyelid margin is performed. Vertical incisions are then made through the conjunctiva to match the width of the flap. The dissection is carried down through Muller's muscle toward the fornix or cul-de-sac. The advancing tarsal conjunctival flap is then grafted to the opposing lid and secured with sutures. A separately reported free, full-thickness skin graft may be applied to complete the reconstruction.

67975

The patient's face and eyelid are draped and prepped for surgery. Local or general anesthesia may be administered. Approximately six weeks after a separately reported reconstruction of the eyelid, the tissue is divided to create an upper and lower lid. Any redundant tissue is trimmed.

68020

The patient's face and eyelid are draped and prepped for surgery. Local anesthesia is administered. A vertical or horizontal incision is made in the posterior surface of the eyelid margin. The incision does not extend to the eyelid margin itself. The contents of the cyst are drained either with a cotton-tipped probe or a curet.

68040

Trachoma is a chronic inflammation of the eye causing granulations to form on conjunctival tissue. The patient's face and eyelid are draped and prepped for surgery. Local anesthesia may be administered. Under biomicroscopic guidance, the physician everts the eyelid margin and removes the conjunctival follicles with a cotton-tipped swab or a curet. No incision is required.

68100

The patient's face and eyelid are draped and prepped for surgery. Local anesthesia may be administered. A portion of the bulbar or palpebral conjunctival is excised with a curet. Sutures may be required to repair the wound.

68110–68115

The patient's face and eyelid are draped and prepped for surgery. Local anesthesia is administered. A lesion on the bulbar or palpebral conjunctival is excised with a curet. Sutures may be required to repair the wound. The lesion is up to 1.0 cm in size in 68110 and larger than 1.0 cm in 68115.

68130

The patient's face and eyelid are draped and prepped for surgery. Local anesthesia is administered and a lid speculum is inserted. A lesion on the conjunctiva and adjacent superficial sclera is excised with a curet. No sutures usually are required.

68135

The patient's face and eyelid are draped and prepped for surgery. Local anesthesia is administered and a lid speculum is inserted. A freezing probe (cryotherapy) is applied to a lesion on the conjunctiva. No repair is required.

68200

The physician applies a drop of topical anesthetic to the eye. A small gauge needle is inserted to deliver a medication such as a cortical steroid or antibiotic into the subconjunctival space.

68320

The patient's face and eyelid are draped and prepped for surgery. Local anesthesia is administered. With the aid of an operating microscope, the physician separates the conjunctival epithelial tissue from the underlying Tenon's capsule. The site to which the harvested tissue is to be grafted is then prepared to accept the tissue. Its margins are freshened and the conjunctival graft is arranged and sutured into place. The tissue for graft can be a free graft or extensive rearrangement of existing tissue.

68325

The patient's face and eyelid are draped and prepped for surgery. Local anesthesia is administered. The physician separates the buccal mucous membrane that will be used for the graft from its location within the patient's mouth. The site to which the donor tissue is to be grafted is then prepared to accept the tissue. Its margins are freshened and the conjunctival graft is arranged and sutured into place. The donor graft site does not usually require a repair.

68326

The patient's face and eyelid are draped and prepped for surgery. Local anesthesia is administered. With the aid of an operating microscope, the physician separates the conjunctival epithelial tissue from the underlying Tenon's capsule. The tissue for graft can be a free graft or extensive rearrangement of existing tissue. The site to which the donor tissue is to be grafted is then prepared to accept the tissue. Its margins are freshened and the conjunctival graft is sutured into a foreshortened, or scarred inferior cul-de-sac or fornix. The fornix can be reformed with the use of a cul-de-sac suture fixation or with the use of a silicon stent attached to the orbital rim. The stent is used to mold the fornix and is sutured into place securely and left for up to two weeks.

68328

The patient's face and eyelid are draped and prepped for surgery. Local anesthesia is administered. The physician separates the buccal mucous membrane that will be used for the graft from its location within the patient's mouth. The donor graft site does not usually require a repair. The site to which the donor tissue is to be grafted is then prepared to accept the tissue. Its margins are freshened and the conjunctival graft is sutured into a foreshortened, or scarred inferior cul-de-sac or fornix. The fornix can be reformed with the use of a cul-de-sac suture fixation or with the use of a silicon stent attached to the orbital rim. The stent is used to mold the fornix and is sutured into place securely and left for up to two weeks.

68330

A symblepharon is an adhesion between the conjunctiva on the eyeball (bulbar conjunctiva) and the conjunctiva on the inner eyelid (tarsal conjunctiva). The patient's face and eyelid are draped and prepped for surgery. Local anesthesia is administered. The physician divides the adhesions between the globe and palpebral conjunctiva and repairs the conjunctival wound with adjacent tissue transfer. Sutures are required, and a silicon stent may be placed in the eye to prevent the development of further adhesions during the healing process.

68335

A symblepharon is an adhesion between the conjunctiva on the eyeball (bulbar conjunctiva) and the conjunctiva on the inner eyelid (tarsal conjunctiva). The patient's face and eyelid are draped and prepped for surgery. Local anesthesia is administered. The physician separates the conjunctival adhesions and grafts replacement tissue over the site of the symblepharon. The tissue for graft can be a free graft of conjunctival tissue from the same or other eye, or buccal mucosa obtained from inside the patient's mouth. The site to which the donor tissue is to be grafted is then prepared to accept the tissue. Its margins are freshened and the conjunctival graft is sutured in place. A silicon stent or contact lens may be placed in the eye to prevent the development of further adhesions during the healing process.

68340

A symblepharon is an adhesion between the conjunctiva on the eyeball (bulbar conjunctiva) and the conjunctiva on the inner eyelid (tarsal conjunctiva). The patient's face and eyelid are draped and prepped for surgery. Local anesthesia is administered. The physician divides the adhesions between the globe and palpebral conjunctiva. No other repair is usually needed, although a conformer or contact lens may be placed in the eye to prevent the development of further adhesions during the healing process.

68360

The patient's face and eyelid are draped and prepped for surgery. Local anesthesia is administered. The physician elevates the conjunctiva from the Tenon's capsule and a small tongue of free conjunctiva is advanced via a flap to another site where it is secured with sutures.

68362

The patient's face and eyelid are draped and prepped for surgery. Local anesthesia is administered. The physician elevates the conjunctiva from the Tenon's capsule and the conjunctiva is advanced cover the de-epithelialized cornea. The leading edge of the conjunctival flap is sutured along the medial extent of the corneal defect.

68400

The lacrimal system serves to keep the conjunctiva and cornea moist through the production, distribution, and elimination of tears. The physician administers a local anesthetic along the edge of the supratemporal portion of the orbital rim over the lacrimal gland. An incision is made either beneath the superior orbital rim or in the lid crease of the upper lid. The incision is extended to the lacrimal fossa where the abscess is drained. The wound is irrigated and then repaired with layered sutures.

68420

The lacrimal system serves to keep the conjunctiva and cornea moist through the production, distribution, and elimination of tears. The lacrimal sac is an enlarged portion of the lacrimal duct that drains these tears. The physician administers a local anesthetic along the medical canthal tendon. A stab incision is made directly into the lacrimal sac and pressure created by the sequestered abscess is relieved. The wound may be irrigated and then repaired with layered sutures.

68440

The lacrimal system serves to keep the conjunctiva and cornea moist through the production, distribution, and elimination of tears. Tears produced by the lacrimal gland are eliminated through the lacrimal punctum, a small openings in the inner canthus. The physician administers a local anesthetic at the lacrimal punctum then uses sharp scissors to snip the lacrimal punctum, usually posteriorly. A dilating probe is introduced to ensure that enlargement of the punctum has been achieved.

68500–68505

The lacrimal system serves to keep the conjunctiva and cornea moist through the production, distribution, and elimination of tears. The tears are produced in the lacrimal gland. The physician makes an incision either beneath the superior orbital rim or in the lid crease of the upper lid. The incision is extended to the periosteum overlying the bone of the superorbital rim. A periosteal elevator is used to isolate and dissect the lacrimal gland from its position in the lacrimal fossa. The gland is removed in total in 68500 and a part of the gland is removed in 68505. In

Lay descriptions ©2001 Ingenix, Inc.
CPT® only ©2001 American Medical Association. All Rights Reserved.

CPT® Lay Descriptions

either case, the wound is repaired with layered sutures.

68510

The lacrimal system serves to keep the conjunctiva and cornea moist through the production, distribution, and elimination of tears. The tears are produced in the lacrimal gland. The physician makes an incision either beneath the superior orbital rim or in the lid crease of the upper lid. The incision is extended to lacrimal fossa. A previously determined portion of the lacrimal gland is excised for analysis. The wound is repaired with layered sutures.

68520

The lacrimal system serves to keep the conjunctiva and cornea moist through the production, distribution, and elimination of tears. The lacrimal sac is an enlarged portion of the lacrimal duct that eliminates these tears. The physician administers a local anesthetic along the medial canthal tendon. An incision is made midway between the bridge of the nose and the medial canthal tendon. The dissection is carried down to the periosteum overlying the bone of the superior lacrimal crest. A periosteal elevator is used to separate the lacrimal sac from its normal location. The sac is removed. The wound is repaired with layered sutures.

68525

The lacrimal system serves to keep the conjunctiva and cornea moist through the production, distribution, and elimination of tears. The lacrimal sac is an enlarged portion of the lacrimal duct that eliminates these tears. The physician administers a local anesthetic along the medial canthal tendon. An incision is made midway between the bridge of the nose and the medial canthal tendon. The dissection is carried down to the periosteum overlying the bone of the superior lacrimal crest. A portion of the lacrimal sac is removed. The wound is repaired with layered sutures.

68530

The lacrimal system serves to keep the conjunctiva and cornea moist through the production, distribution, and elimination of tears. Ducts distribute the tears to the eye and nose. The physician administers a local anesthetic along the medial canthal tendon. An incision is made midway between the bride of the nose and the medial canthal tendon. The dissection is carried down to the foreign body or lacrimal stone. It is removed, and the wound is repaired with layered sutures.

68540

The lacrimal system serves to keep the conjunctiva and cornea moist through the production, distribution, and elimination of tears. The tears are produced in the lacrimal gland. The physician makes an incision either beneath the superior orbital rim or in the lid crease of the upper lid. The incision is extended to the periosteum overlying the bone of the superorbital rim or to the lacrimal fossa. The tumor is isolated and removed with a rim of normal lacrimal gland tissue. The wound is repaired with layered sutures.

68550

The lacrimal system serves to keep the conjunctiva and cornea moist through the production, distribution, and elimination of tears. The tears are produced in the lacrimal gland. The physician makes an incision either beneath the superior orbital rim or in the lid crease of the upper lid. The incision is extended to the periosteum overlying the bone of the superorbital rim or to the lacrimal fossa. The tumor has invaded the lacrimal fossa, so an osteotome is used to remove the portion of affected bone. The wound is repaired with layered sutures.

68700

The lacrimal system serves to keep the conjunctiva and cornea moist through the production, distribution, and elimination of tears. Lacrimal canaliculi are the ducts that carry the tears from the lacrimal gland where they are produced to the nose. The physician uses a probe to locate the distal and proximal ends of the canaliculi in the injured eye of patient. The ends are freshened and reattached with sutures. The wound is closed with layered sutures.

68705

The lacrimal system serves to keep the conjunctiva and cornea moist through the production, distribution, and elimination of tears. Tears produced by the lacrimal gland are released into the eye through the lacrimal punctum, a small opening in the inner canthus. The physician administers a local anesthetic at the lacrimal punctum then applies bipolar or monopolar cautery to the palpebral conjunctiva just below the level of the inferior punctum. The result is a repositioning of the punctum itself. No incisions are made and no repairs required in this procedure.

68720

The lacrimal system serves to keep the conjunctiva and cornea moist through the production and distribution of tears. The lacrimal sac is an enlarged portion of the lacrimal duct that distributes these tears. The physician administers a local anesthetic along the medial canthal tendon. A 1.0 cm incision is made in the skin midway between the bridge of the nose and the medial canthal tendon. The dissection is carried down to the periosteum overlying the bone of the superior lacrimal crest. The lacrimal sac is opened and a communication is established been the lacrimal sac and underlying bone and nasal mucosa. The lacrimal mucosa is exposed and a connection between the medial portion of the lacrimal sac and the nasal mucosa is created and secured with sutures. The incision is repaired with layered sutures.

68745–68750

The lacrimal system serves to keep the conjunctiva and cornea moist through the production and distribution of tears. The lacrimal sac is an enlarged portion of the lacrimal duct that distributes these tears. The physician administers a local anesthetic along the medial canthal tendon. A 1.0 cm incision is made in the skin midway between the bridge of the nose and the medial canthal tendon. The dissection is carried down to the periosteum overlying the bone of the superior lacrimal crest. The lateral portion of lacrimal sac is connected by a series of interrupted sutures to the nasal mucosa. A glass tube is inserted to create a connection from the lacrimal system to the nasal mucosa in 68750. The incision is repaired with layered sutures.

68760

The lacrimal system serves to keep the conjunctiva and cornea moist through the production, distribution, and elimination of tears. Tears produced by the lacrimal gland are drained from the eye through the lacrimal punctum, a small opening in the inner canthus. The physician administers a local anesthetic at the lacrimal punctum and then uses a heat source such as cautery or argon laser to close the proximal portion of the canalicular and lacrimal system including the lacrimal punctum.

68761

The lacrimal system serves to keep the conjunctiva and cornea moist through the production, distribution, and elimination of tears. Tears produced by the lacrimal gland are drained from the eye through the lacrimal punctum, a small opening in the inner canthus. The physician administers a local anesthetic at the lacrimal punctum and then closes the punctum by inserting a plug. The plug may be a permanent silicone plug or a temporary collagen plug.

68770

The lacrimal system serves to keep the conjunctiva and cornea moist through the production, distribution, and elimination of tears. Tears produced by the lacrimal gland are drained from the eye through the lacrimal punctum, a small opening in the inner canthus. The physician administers a local anesthetic at the lacrimal punctum and then uses a probe to locate the lacrimal fistula. The fistula is dissected and its core is removed. The incision is repaired with layered sutures.

68801

The physician treats a suspected injury or blockage of the lacrimal punctum, the opening on the medial eyelids, to assist in drainage of secretions. The physician inserts a plastic probe, catheter, or large suture. The physician may irrigate the punctum to evaluate the patency of lacrimal drainage system.

68810–68811

The lacrimal system keeps the conjunctiva and cornea moist through the production, distribution, and elimination of the watery lacrimal secretion, called tears. Tears produced by the lacrimal gland are drained from the eye through the lacrimal punctum, a small opening near the margin of each eyelid. The physician dilates the proximal portion of the lacrimal system and threads a probe along the canaliculus to the lacrimal sac. No incisions are made and no repairs are necessary. This is performed with the patient under local anesthetic in 68810. In 68825, less patent ducts or a less cooperative patient requires the use of general anesthesia.

68815

The lacrimal system keeps the conjunctiva and cornea moist through the production, distribution, and elimination of the watery lacrimal secretion, called tears. Ducts distribute the tears to the eye and nose. The physician dilates the proximal portion of the lacrimal system and threads a probe along the canaliculus to the lacrimal sac. Canalicular stents are passed through the duct and placed in the distal portion of the lacrimal system. The tubes remain in place for three to six months before they are removed. No incisions are made and no repairs are necessary.

68840

The lacrimal system serves to keep the conjunctiva and cornea moist through the production, distribution, and elimination of tears. Ducts distribute the tears to the eye and nose. The physician threads a probe along the canaliculi. No incisions are made and no repairs are necessary. The canaliculi may be irrigated during the procedure.

68850

The lacrimal system serves to keep the conjunctiva and cornea moist through the production, distribution, and elimination of tears. A cannula is inserted into the lacrimal duct. Under radiographic guidance, radiopaque dye is introduced into the lacrimal system the the cannula. The supervision and interpretation of the radiographic results of the injection are reported separately; this code reports only the injection of the contrast medium.

69000–69005

Through a small incision in the skin or at times into the perichondrium external ear at the site of the abscess or hematoma (collection of blood), the physician drains the contents of the abscess in a simple procedure (e.g., 69000). Occasionally, a small drain tube is inserted and packing is placed to facilitate healing. A bolster with through-and-through sutures is placed to help prevent accumulation of fluid. In a complicated procedure (e.g., 69005), the physician also devotes more time to cleaning the abscess cavity, and a soft sponge is placed in the canal after antibiotic ear drops have been applied.

CPT® Lay Descriptions

69020

The physician makes an incision in the skin and drains an abscess in the external auditory canal. Occasionally, packing is inserted to absorb the drainage and facilitate healing. Usually no further treatment is needed and no closure is required.

69090

The physician or technician uses a sharp instrument such as a sterile needle or a piercing gun to form an opening in the ear lobe. After the puncture is complete, the area is cleaned with a disinfectant and an earring is inserted to keep the opening patent. No further treatment is usually necessary.

69100

The physician uses a scalpel or punch forceps to excise a portion of a lesion on the external ear for diagnostic purposes. Unless the incision is large, a sutured closure is usually unnecessary.

69105

The physician uses a scalpel, curet, or small biopsy forceps to excise a portion of a lesion on the external ear for diagnostic purposes. Ear canal packing may be required.

69110

The physician removes a full-thickness section of the external ear, often as a triangular wedge. The portion of the ear removed will vary from case to case, but most frequently it is in the curved upper portion of the ear. A small portion of normal tissue surrounding the defect is also removed. The wound is closed with layered sutures.

69120

Using a scalpel or electric knife, the physician amputates the external ear. The wound is closed during a second procedure involving a skin graft or flap.

69140

Entering through the external opening of the ear, the physician makes an incision in the skin covering the exostosis to expose the bone beneath it. The bony growth is removed with a curet or drill. The skin is replaced over the site and the canal is packed with hemostasis to hold the skin in position.

69145

Through the external opening of the ear, the physician uses a knife to excise an entire soft tissue lesion with surrounding margin or normal tissue. Some limited drilling of the ear canal may be done. The external ear canal may be packed. If extensive skin is removed, a separate grafting procedure may be required at this time.

69150

Through a postauricular incision, the physician uses a scalpel to remove an extensive lesion in the ear canal. Depending upon whether the lesion involves bone, a section of supporting hard tissue may be excised. The tympanic membrane, parotid gland, facial nerve, and portions of the mandible and mastoid may also be removed. A separately reported graft or flap may be performed at this time, or the surgical wound may be repaired with a layered closure.

69155

Through a postauricular incision, the physician uses a scalpel to remove an extensive lesion of the ear canal. A section of supporting hard tissue may be excised as well as the tympanic membrane, parotid gland, facial nerve, and portions of the mandible and mastoid. The physician performs a neck dissection, removing the lymph nodes from that side of the neck. The jugular vein, spinal accessory nerve, or sternocleidomastoid muscle may be removed as well. The carotid artery, vagus, sympathetic, phrenic, brachial plexus, hypoglossal and lingual nerves are spared. A separately reported graft or flap may be performed at this time, or the surgical wound may be repaired with a layered closure.

69200–69205

Under direct visualization, the physician or technician removes a foreign body from the external auditory canal using delicate forceps, a cerumen spoon, or suction. In the case of a live insect, oil is dropped into the ear to immobilize it before it is removed. No anesthetic or local anesthetic is used in 69200. If a child or an adult cannot tolerate the procedure while awake, it is performed under general anesthesia in 69205. Code 69205 is also reported in cases where the foreign body is so large, an incision is made in the external meatus to enlarge the opening before the the foreign body can be extracted.

69210

Under direct visualization, the physician removes impacted cerumen (ear wax) using suction, a cerumen spoon or delicate forceps. If no infection is present, the ear canal may then be irrigated.

69220–69222

Routine mastoid cavity debridement is required every three to six months in patients who have undergone a radical or modified radical mastoidectomy. Under direct visualization, the physician uses suction, a cerumen spoon, and delicate forceps to remove skin debris and drainage from the mastoid cavity, a bony extension of the ear canal. The cavity is cleaned simply in 69220. The cavity may require more extensive cleaning, as in the case of infection or extensive debris, in 69222. Sometimes this extensive cleaning requires general anesthesia or the use of a laser to remove granulation tissue.

69300

The physician corrects a protruding ear. The physician makes an incision on the posterior auricle and raises the posterior skin off the cartilage. A new antihelical fold is created with multiple sutures through the cartilage. Some techniques employ limited cartilage cutting. A small ellipse of posterior skin is removed and the skin is closed with sutures. Packing corresponding to the anterior ear contours is placed. The size of the auricle may be reduced.

69310

The physician makes a postauricular incision and removes the thick, stenotic plug of soft tissue from the external auditory canal. Some drilling of the bony canal may be needed to enlarge the bony canal. Thin skin grafts are used to reline the canal and are held in place by packing. The posterior incision is repaired with sutures.

69320

The physician makes a postauricular incision and drills just behind and above the temporomandibular joint region. Drilling is continued until the ossicles are identified. The new bony canal is carefully enlarged. The eardrum is reconstructed and split thickness skin grafts are used to line the new canal. A large canal opening is made by removing skin and soft tissue. The canal is packed and the incision is repaired with sutures.

69400

The physician topically decongests and anesthetizes the nose and nasopharynx. The eustachian tube is cannulated with a small catheter through the nose, often with the aid of a nasopharyngoscope. Air is forced into the catheter to inflate the eustachian tube. The catheter is then removed.

69401

The physician inflates a blocked or collapsed eustachian tube by increasing the air pressure in the nasopharynx. One method is to blow air against the resistance of the closed mouth and nose. Another method is to close one side of the nose and force air into the other nostril with a Politzer bag as the patient swallows.

69405

The physician makes an incision in the posterior ear canal skin and raises the eardrum. The eustachian tube opening in the middle ear is visualized and a small catheter is inserted into the eustachian tube to stent it open. This can be left in place indefinitely. No repair is made.

69410

Focal application of phase control substance, middle ear (baffle technique). The middle ear is the portion of the ear from the connection of the eardrum to the inner ear (cochlea) that contains the ossicles (three bones; malleus, incus and stapes). The three bones oscillate back and forth in the patterns of the sound just heard. The focal application of phase control substances focus on a measurement technique that circumvents the problem of standing waves in the ear canal using a wideband (125-10,700 Hz) analysis of middle ear function. The technique improves diagnostic methods, provides more specific assessment of middle ear disease, and more effective intervention.

69420–69421

After the application of a local anesthetic (e.g., for 69420) or a general anesthetic (e.g., for 69421) and using a microscope for guidance, the physician makes an incision in the patient's tympanic membrane. Fluid is suctioned from the middle ear space and may be reserved for analysis. The eustachian tube may be inflated. No closure is required.

69424

Assisted by microscopic visualization and using delicate forceps or hook, the physician removes from the tympanic membrane a previously placed ventilating tube. No other treatment is required.

69433–69436

In a patient who has received a local or topical anesthetic (e.g., for 69433) or a general anesthetic (e.g., for 69436), the physician inserts a ventilating tube. Under direct visualization with a microscope, the physician makes a small incision in the tympanum (eardrum). Any middle ear fluid is suctioned and may be reserved for analysis. The physician inserts a ventilating tube into the opening in the tympanum. No other treatment is required.

69440

Entering either through the external ear canal opening or through a postauricular incision (behind the ear) and into the ear canal, the physician performs exploratory surgery of the middle ear. The eardrum is lifted posteriorly and the middle ear is explored including testing the mobility of the ossicular chain. No major treatment is rendered at this time. The eardrum and canal skin are repositioned and the canal is packed. Any postauricular incision is sutured.

69450

Through the external ear canal opening, the physician treats a lesion or other irritation to the tympanic membrane. The physician makes an incision in the posterior canal skin and reflects the eardrum forward. Under microscopic guidance, the physician removes adhesions from the tympanic membrane (tympanolysis). When tympanolysis is complete, the eardrum and canal skin are repositioned and packing is placed in the ear canal.

69501

Through a postaural or endaural incision, the physician removes the mastoid cortex (outer bone) and drills out some of the mastoid air cells to enter the mastoid antrum. This is usually done as a drainage procedure for mastoid disease limited to the antrum region. A myringotomy with or without tube placement may be performed. A temporary drain may be placed and the incision is sutured.

69502

Through a postaural or endaural incision, the physician drills out the mastoid cavity. The mastoid sinus is exposed posteriorly. The tegmen (bony plate separating the mastoid and middle cranial fossa) is exposed superiorly. The posterior ear canal wall remains intact. The horizontal semicircular canal and part of the incus are visualized. Cholesteatoma or diseased mastoid mucosa is removed. The incision is sutured. A temporary drain may be placed a dressing is applied.

69505

The physician makes incisions in the ear canal to develop a posterior tympanomeatal flap that is reflected forward. Through a postaural or endaural incision, the physician drills out the mastoid cortex. The mastoid antrum is identified. Granulations and any cholesteatoma are removed. The posterior bony canal wall is taken down to the level of the facial nerve. If cholesteatoma involves the ossicles, they are removed. The posterior skin flap and eardrum are repositioned to cover the facial ridge and part of the mastoid cavity. A meatoplasty is performed. The mastoid cavity and ear canal are packed, the incision sutured, and a dressing placed.

69511

The physician makes incisions in the ear canal to develop a posterior tympanomeatal flap that is reflected forward. Through a postaural or endaural incision, the physician drills out the mastoid cells. The posterior and superior bony canal walls are taken down to the level of the facial nerve. The ossicles, except for the stapes if possible, are removed as well as the eustachian tube orifice muscosa, middle ear mucosa, granulations, and cholesteatoma. The middle ear and mastoid are exposed to the exterior through the ear canal. A large meatoplasty is performed. Packing is placed, the incision is sutured, and a dressing is applied.

69530

Through a postaural or endaural incision, the physician drills out the mastoid cavity. The mastoid sinus is exposed posteriorly. The tegmen (bony plate separating the mastoid and middle cranial fossa) is exposed superiorly. The posterior ear canal wall remains intact. The horizontal semicircular canal and part of the incus are visualized. Various cell tracts around the semicircular canals are carefully explored

in an attempt to drain the petrous apex. If this is unsuccessful, the posterior and superior bony canal walls are taken down to the level of the facial nerve. The ossicles, except for the stapes if possible, are removed as well as the eustachian tube orifice mucosa, middle ear mucosa, granulations, and cholesteatoma. Cell tracts between the carotid artery and cochlea or the jugular bulb and cochlea are followed to open the petrous apex and drain any infection. A meatoplasty is performed. A temporary drain may be placed. The incision is sutured and a dressing is applied.

69535

The physician elevates the auricle with a superior flap. If the auricle and surrounding skin is involved, a wide excision of the skin and subcutaneous tissues is performed. The sternocleidomastoid muscle is separated from the mastoid tip, exposing the internal jugular vein. The seventh nerve is sacrificed. The zygomatic arch is divided. The middle fossa dura is exposed and elevated from the temporal bone. The head of the mandible is removed to expose the internal carotid artery. With a drill and chisel, the carotid canal is opened. The sigmoid sinus is skeletonized and a chisel is used to make the final bony cuts through the medial temporal bone. Hemostasis is obtained with cautery and packing. A parotidectomy and/or neck dissection may also be required. A separately reportable reconstructive procedure may be performed at this time. Otherwise, the incisions are repaired with a layered closure.

69540

Through the external ear canal opening, the physician removes the aural polyp with a cup forceps or an ear snare. Bleeding is controlled with packing or epinephrine on a cotton ball. Antibiotic drops may be instilled.

69550

Through the external auditory canal, the physician makes an incision in the posterior canal skin and reflects the skin flap and eardrum forward. Under microscopic visualization, the small vascular tumor is grasped with a cup forceps and gently removed. Hemostasis is obtained with packing soaked in epinephrine. Once bleeding is controlled, the middle ear is packed with absorbable material. The eardrum and skin flap are repositioned and the ear canal is packed.

69552

Through a postaural incision, the physician drills out the mastoid cavity. The mastoid sinus is exposed posteriorly. The tegmen (bony plate separating the mastoid and middle cranial fossa) is exposed superiorly. The posterior ear canal wall remains intact. An extended facial recess is sometimes needed to completely visualize the tumor. The vascular tumor is grasped and removed with cup forceps. Hemostasis is obtained using absorbable packing. Usually, the ossicles can be left undisturbed. For larger tumors, the posterior canal wall and ossicles may be removed. The incision is repaired with sutures and a dressing is applied.

69554

The surgeon makes an incision in front of the ear. The facial nerve, hypoglossal nerve, spinal accessory nerve, internal jugular vein, and carotid artery are identified in the neck. A complete mastoidectomy with extended facial recess is performed. The tip of the mastoid is removed and the jugular bulb is exposed and ligated inferiorly. The mastoid sinus is skeletonized, opened, and packed. Hemostasis is obtained with packing. If the tumor extends intracranially, a craniotomy may be necessary. A parotidectomy may also be needed if further mobilization of the facial nerve is required. The ear canal and ossicles may be removed. The incision is repair with a layered closure. Dressings are applied.

69601

Using a postaural incision, the physician revises a perviously performed simple mastoidectomy with a complete mastoidectomy. The physician drills out the mastoid cavity. The mastoid sinus is exposed posteriorly. The tegmen (bony plate separating the mastoid and middle cranial fossa) is exposed superiorly. The posterior ear canal wall remains intact. The horizontal semicircular canal and part of the incus are visualized. Cholesteatoma or diseased mastoid mucosa are removed. The incision is sutured. A temporary drain may be placed and a dressing is applied.

69602

Using a postaural incision, the physician revises a previously performed simple or complete mastoidectomy with a modified radical mastoidectomy by removing all the mastoid cells, granulations, pus, and the bony partitions of the mastoid cavity. A tympanomeatal flap is developed and reflected anteriorly. The posterior and superior bony canal walls are taken down to the level of the facial nerve. If cholesteatoma is present around the ossicles, the ossicles are removed. The tympanomeatal flap is repositioned over the facial ridge and into the mastoid cavity. Some middle ear space is thus maintained. A large mataoplasty is made. The ear canal and mastoid cavity are packed and the incision is closed with sutures.

69603

Using an endaural or postauricular incision, the physician revises a previously performed complete or modified radical mastoidectomy with a radical mastoidectomy. The posterior and superior bony canal walls are taken down to the level of the facial nerve. The ossicles, except for the stapes if possible, are removed as well as the eustachian tube orifice

muscosa, middle ear mucosa, granulations, and cholesteatoma. The middle ear and mastoid are exposed to the exterior through the ear canal. A large meatoplasty is performed. Packing is placed, the incision is sutured, and a dressing is applied.

69604

Through a postauricular or endaural incision, the physician revises the site of a previous mastoidectomy. The posterior canal may be taken down. Ossicles may be removed. The physician performs a tympanoplasty in conjunction with the revision mastoidectomy. The edges of the tympanic membrane perforation are roughened ("rimming the perforation") and a fascia graft is placed under or over the tympanic membrane remnant. No ossicular reconstruction is done. Absorbable packing may be placed in the middle ear. The canal and mastoid cavity are packed, and the incision is sutured. A dressing is applied.

69605

The physician revises a previously performed mastoidectomy with an apicectomy. Through a postural or endaural incision, the physician drills out the remaining mastoid cavity. The mastoid sinus is exposed posteriorly. The tegmen (bony plate separating the mastoid and middle cranial fossa) is exposed superiorly. The posterior ear canal wall remains intact. The horizontal semicircular canal and part of the incus are visualized. Various cell tracts around the semicircular canals are carefully explored in an attempt to drain the petrous apex. If this is unsuccessful, the posterior and superior bony canal walls are taken down to the level of the facial nerve. The ossicles, except for the stapes if possible, are removed as well as the eustachian tube orifice muscosa, middle ear mucosa, granulations, and cholesteatoma. Cell tracts between the carotid artery and cochlea or the jugular bulb and cochlea are followed to open the petrous apex and drain any infection. A meatoplasty is performed. A temporary drain may be placed. The incision is sutured and a dressing is applied.

69610

Under microscopic visualization, the physician roughens the tympanic membrane perforation ("rimming the perforation") and applies a paper patch. In some cases, the edges of a traumatic perforation of the eardrum may need to be elevated from the middle ear with a delicate hook.

69620

Through the external ear canal, the physician visualizes the tympanic membrane and the eardrum defect. The edges of the eardrum perforation are roughened ("rimming the perforation"). Some dissolvable packing may be placed through the perforation into the middle ear space. A fat graft plug may be placed in the perforation or a piece of fascia may be placed medial to the eardrum over the dissolvable packing. A tympanomeatal flap may be raised. Any incisions are sutured and a dressing is applied.

69631

The physician makes an incision in the ear canal skin through a postauricular or transcanal approach. The edges of the tympanic membrane are roughened ("rimming the perforation"). The physician reflects the eardrum forward. The middle ear is explored, and lysis of any adhesions is performed. Any squamous debris or middle ear cholesteatoma is removed and the physician inspects and palpates the ossicles. No ossicular reconstruction is done at this time. Some drilling or curetting of the canal wall may be necessary. Some fascia from the temporalis muscle or other tissues is harvested as a graft to repair the tympanic membrane perforation. Some packing may be placed in the middle ear to support the graft. The graft may be placed under (underlay or medial graft technique) or on top of the remaining eardrum (overlay or lateral graft technique). The canal skin is repositioned and the canal is packed. Any external incisions are sutured, and a dressing is applied.

69632

The physician makes an incision in the ear canal skin through a postauricular or transcanal approach. The edges of the tympanic membrane are roughened ("rimming the perforation"). The physician reflects the eardrum forward. The middle ear is explored, and lysis of any adhesions is performed. Any squamous debris or middle ear cholesteatoma is removed and the physician inspects and palpates the ossicles. The ossicular chain can also be reconstructed by sculpting and repositioning the patient's own ossicles. The natural ossicle may be replaced with a donor cadaver ossicle, or a sculpted bone strut or piece of cartilage. Some packing may be placed in the middle ear to support the reconstructed ossicle prior to final positioning of the eardrum graft. Some drilling or curetting of the canal wall may be necessary. Some fascia from the temporalis muscle or other tissues is harvested as a graft to repair the tympanic membrane perforation. The graft may be placed under (underlay or medial graft technique) or on top of the remaining eardrum (overlay or lateral graft technique). The canal skin is repositioned and the canal is packed. Any external incisions are sutured, and a dressing is applied.

69633

The physician makes an incision in the ear canal skin through a postauricular or transcanal approach. The edges of the tympanic membrane are roughened ("rimming the perforation"). The physician reflects the eardrum forward. The middle ear is explored, and lysis of any adhesions is performed. Any squamous debris or middle ear cholesteatoma is removed and the physician inspects and palpates the ossicles. The ossicular chain is reconstructed using a synthetic

reconstructive prosthesis. A partial ossicular prosthesis (PORP) is used when the stapes suprastructure is present. If the stapes suprastructure is absent, a total ossicular replacement prosthesis (TORP) is used. A piece of cartilage may be placed between the eardrum and prosthesis. Some packing may be placed in the middle ear to support the reconstructed ossicle prior to final positioning of the eardrum graft. Some drilling or curetting of the canal wall may be necessary. Some fascia from the temporalis muscle or other tissues is harvested as a graft to repair the tympanic membrane perforation. The graft may be placed under (underlay or medial graft technique) or on top of the remaining eardrum (overlay or lateral graft technique). The canal skin is repositioned and the canal is packed.

69635

Through a postauricular incision, the physician removes the mastoid cortex (outer bone) and drills out some of the mastoid air cells to enter the mastoid antrum. The edges of the tympanic membrane are then roughened ("rimming the perforation"). The physician reflects the eardrum forward. The middle ear is explored, and lysis of any adhesions is performed. Any squamous debris or middle ear cholesteatoma is removed and the physician inspects and palpates the ossicles. No ossicular reconstruction is done at this time. Some drilling or curetting of the canal wall may be necessary. Some fascia from the temporalis muscle or other tissues is harvested as a graft to repair the tympanic membrane perforation. Some packing may be placed in the middle ear to support the graft. The graft may be placed under (underlay or medial graft technique) or on top of the remaining eardrum (overlay or lateral graft technique). The canal skin is repositioned and the canal is packed. Any external incisions are sutured, and a dressing is applied.

69636

Through a postauricular incision, the physician removes the mastoid cortex (outer bone) and drills out some of the mastoid air cells to enter the mastoid antrum. The edges of the tympanic membrane are then roughened ("rimming the perforation"). The physician reflects the eardrum forward. The middle ear is explored, and lysis of any adhesions is performed. Any squamous debris or middle ear cholesteatoma is removed and the physician inspects and palpates the ossicles. The ossicular chain can be reconstructed by sculpting and repositioning the patient's own ossicles. The natural ossicle may also be replaced with a donor cadaver ossicle, or a sculpted bone strut or piece of cartilage. Some packing may be placed in the middle ear to support the reconstructed ossicle prior to final positioning of the eardrum graft. Some drilling or curetting of the canal wall may be necessary. Some fascia from the temporalis muscle or other tissues is harvested as a graft to repair the tympanic membrane perforation. The graft may be placed under (underlay or medial graft technique) or on top of the remaining eardrum (overlay or lateral graft technique). The canal skin is repositioned and the canal is packed. Any external incisions are sutured, and a dressing is applied.

69637

Through a postauricular incision, the physician removes the mastoid cortex (outer bone) and drills out some of the mastoid air cells to enter the mastoid antrum. The edges of the tympanic membrane are then roughened ("rimming the perforation"). The physician reflects the eardrum forward. The middle ear is explored, and lysis of any adhesions is performed. Any squamous debris or middle ear cholesteatoma is removed and the physician inspects and palpates the ossicles. The ossicular chain is reconstructed using a synthetic reconstructive prosthesis. A partial ossicular prosthesis (PORP) is used when the stapes suprastructure is present. If the stapes suprastructure is absent, a total ossicular replacement prosthesis (TORP) is used. A piece of cartilage may be placed between the eardrum and prosthesis. Some packing may be placed to support the reconstructed ossicle prior to positioning of the eardrum graft. Some drilling or cureting of the canal wall may be necessary. Some fascia from the temporalis muscle or other tissues is harvested as a graft to repair the perforation. The graft may be placed under (underlay or medial graft technique) or on top of the remaining eardrum (overlay or lateral graft technique). The canal skin is repositioned and the canal is packed.

69641

The physician makes incisions in the ear canal to develop a posterior tympanomeatal flap that is reflected forward. Through a postaural or endaural incision, the physician drills out the mastoid cortex. The mastoid antrum is identified. Granulations and any cholesteatoma are removed. The posterior bony canal wall is taken down to the level of the facial nerve. The middle ear is explored, and lysis of any adhesions is performed. Any squamous debris or middle ear cholesteatoma is removed and the physician inspects and palpates the ossicles. No ossicular reconstruction is done at this time. Some fascia from the temporalis muscle or other tissues is harvested as a graft to repair the tympanic membrane perforation. Some packing may be placed in the middle ear to support the graft. The graft may be placed under (underlay or medial graft technique) or on top of the remaining eardrum (overlay or lateral graft technique). The posterior skin flap and reconstructed eardrum are repositioned to cover the facial ridge and part of the mastoid cavity. A meatoplasty is performed. The mastoid cavity and ear canal are packed, the incision sutured, and a dressing placed.

69642

The physician makes incisions in the ear canal to develop a posterior tympanomeatal flap that is reflected forward. Through a postaural or endaural incision, the physician drills out the mastoid cortex. The mastoid antrum is identified. Granulations and any cholesteatoma are removed. The posterior bony canal wall is taken down to the level of the facial nerve. The middle ear is explored, and lysis of any adhesions is performed. Any squamous debris or middle ear cholesteatoma is removed and the physician inspects and palpates the ossicles. The ossicular chain can be reconstructed by sculpting and repositioning the patient's own ossicles. The natural ossicle also may be replaced with a donor cadaver ossicle, or a sculpted bone strut or piece of cartilage. Some packing may be placed in the middle ear to support the reconstructed ossicle prior to final positioning of the eardrum graft. Some fascia from the temporalis muscle or other tissues is harvested as a graft to repair the tympanic membrane perforation. Some packing may be placed in the middle ear to support the graft. The graft may be placed under (underlay or medial graft technique) or on top of the remaining eardrum (overlay or lateral graft technique). The posterior skin flap and reconstructed eardrum are repositioned to cover the facial ridge and part of the mastoid cavity. A meatoplasty is performed. The mastoid cavity and ear canal are packed, the incision sutured, and a dressing placed.

69643

Through a postauricular incision, the physician removes the mastoid cortex (outer bone) and drills out the mastoid air cells. The edges of the tympanic membrane are then roughened ("rimming the perforation"). The physician reflects the eardrum forward. The middle ear is explored, and lysis of any adhesions is performed. Any squamous debris or middle ear cholesteatoma is removed and the physician inspects and palpates the ossicles. No ossicular reconstruction is done at this time. If the posterior canal wall is taken down, it is reconstructed with cartilage, bone, or hydroxyapatite (i.e., Wehr's canal wall reconstruction). Some fascia from the temporalis muscle or other tissues is harvested as a graft to repair the tympanic membrane perforation. Some packing may be placed in the middle ear to support the graft. The graft may be placed under (underlay or medial graft technique) or on top of the remaining eardrum (overlay or lateral graft technique). The canal skin is repositioned and the canal and mastoid cavity are packed. Any external incisions are sutured, and a dressing is applied.

69644

Through a postauricular incision, the physician removes the mastoid cortex (outer bone) and drills out the mastoid air cells. The edges of the tympanic membrane are then roughened ("rimming the perforation"). The physician reflects the eardrum forward. The middle ear is explored, and lysis of any adhesions is performed. Any squamous debris or middle ear cholesteatoma is removed and the physician inspects and palpates the ossicles. The ossicular chain may be reconstructed by sculpting and repositioning the patient's own ossicles. The natural ossicle also may be replaced with a donor cadaver ossicle, or a sculpted bone strut or piece of cartilage. Some packing may be placed in the middle ear to support the reconstructed ossicle prior to final positioning of the eardrum graft. If the posterior canal wall is taken down, it is reconstructed with cartilage, bone, or hydroxyapatite (i.e., Wehr's canal wall reconstruction). Some fascia from the temporalis muscle or other tissues is harvested as a graft to repair the tympanic membrane perforation. Some packing may be placed in the middle ear to support the graft. The graft may be placed under (underlay or medial graft technique) or on top of the remaining eardrum (overlay or lateral graft technique). The canal skin is repositioned and the canal and mastoid cavity are packed. Any external incisions are sutured, and a dressing is applied.

69645

Through a postauricular incision, the physician removes the mastoid cortex (outer bone) and drills out the mastoid air cells. A posterior canal skin flap and remaining eardrum are preserved and reflected forward. The middle ear is explored, and lysis of any adhesions is performed. Any squamous debris or middle ear cholesteatoma is removed and the physician inspects and palpates the ossicles. The posterior canal wall is taken down to the level of the facial nerve. All or part of the ossicles are removed in addition to the middle ear mucosa. No ossicular reconstruction is attempted. Some fascia from the temporalis muscle or other tissues is harvested as a graft to repair the tympanic membrane perforation. Some packing may be placed in the middle ear to support the graft. The graft may be placed under (underlay or medial graft technique) or on top of the remaining eardrum (overlay or lateral graft technique). A piece of silastic may be placed in the middle ear to help develop an air-containing space. The canal skin is repositioned and the canal and mastoid cavity are packed. Any external incisions are sutured, and a dressing is applied.

69646

Through a postauricular incision, the physician removes the mastoid cortex (outer bone) and drills out the mastoid air cells. A posterior canal skin flap and remaining eardrum are preserved and reflected forward. The middle ear is explored, and lysis of any adhesions is performed. Any squamous debris or middle ear cholesteatoma is removed and the physician inspects and palpates the ossicles. The posterior canal wall is taken down to the level of the facial nerve. All or part of the ossicles are removed in addition to the middle ear mucosa. Reconstruction is accomplished with the sculpting of the patient's own

ossicle, or through the placement of a donor cadaver ossicle, cartilage, or bone graft, or prosthetic device. A reconstructed eardrum is positioned over the reconstructed ossicular chain. Some packing may be placed in the middle ear to support the graft. The graft may be placed under (underlay or medial graft technique) or on top of the remaining eardrum (overlay or lateral graft technique). Some fascia from the temporalis muscle or other tissues is harvested as a graft to repair the tympanic membrane perforation. Some packing may be placed in the middle ear to support the graft. The graft may be placed under (underlay or medial graft technique) or on top of the remaining eardrum (overlay or lateral graft technique). The canal skin is repositioned and the canal and mastoid cavity are packed. Any external incisions are sutured, and a dressing is applied. The canal skin is repositioned and the canal and mastoid cavity are packed. Any external incisions are sutured, and a dressing is applied.

69650

The physician makes an incision in the posterior canal skin through the external ear canal opening. Under microscopic visualization, the physician reflects the skin flap and posterior eardrum forward. A small amount of the posterior bony canal may need to be removed with a curet or drill. The incus and stapes are visualized and palpated. If the stapes is fixated it can be mobilized by applying pressure to it with delicate instruments. The canal skin and eardrum are repositioned and the ear canal is packed.

69660

The surgeon makes an incision in the posterior canal skin through the external canal opening. Occasionally, a postauricular incision may be substituted. Under microscopic guidance, the physician reflects the canal skin flap and posterior eardrum forward. Some posterior canal bone may be removed with a curet or drill. The ossicular chain is palpated. If the stapes is fixed, it is separated from the incus. The stapes can be removed (stapedectomy) or an opening can be made in the stapes footplate with a laser or drill (stapedotomy). A prosthesis is placed on the incus to replace the stapes. A piece of fascia, vein, perichondrium, or fat might be applied around or under the prosthesis. The skin and eardrum are repositioned, and the ear canal is packed.

69661

The surgeon makes an incision in the posterior canal skin through the external canal opening. Occasionally, a postauricular incision may be substituted. Under microscopic guidance, the physician reflects the canal skin flap and posterior eardrum forward. Some posterior canal bone may be removed with a curet or drill. The ossicular chain is palpated. If the stapes is fixed, it is separated from the incus. The stapes is removed (stapedectomy). The physician drills an opening in the markedly thickened footplate through which the prosthesis is inserted and attached to the incus. A piece of fascia, vein, perichondrium, or fat might be applied around or under the prosthesis. The skin and eardrum are repositioned, and the ear canal is packed.

69662

The physician revises a stapedectomy or stapedotomy. The physician makes an incision over the previous incision site in the posterior canal or through the external canal opening. Alternately a previous postauricular incision may be reincised. Under microscopic guidance, the physician reflects the canal skin flap and posterior eardrum forward. Some posterior canal bone may be removed with a curet or drill. The ossicular chain is palpated. If the stapes has become fixed since the previous surgery it is separated from the incus. The footplate may be opened with a laser or drilled out. The prosthesis may be repositioned, revised, or removed and replaced. A piece of fascia, vein, perichondrium, or fat previously placed may be removed and replaced around or under the prosthesis. The skin and eardrum are repositioned, and the ear canal is packed.

69666

The physician makes a posterior canal incision through the external ear canal opening. Sometimes, a postauricular incision is performed instead. Under microscopic guidance, the physician reflects the skin flap and posterior eardrum forward. The oval window area is inspected for fluid leak from the inner ear. The lining around the oval window is gently roughened. The area is packed with fat, fascia or muscle tissue. The eardrum and skin flap are replaced and the canal is packed. If a postauricular incision is made, it is sutured.

69667

The physician makes a posterior canal incision through the external ear canal opening. Sometimes, a postauricular incision is performed instead. Under microscopic guidance, the physician reflects the skin flap and posterior eardrum forward. The round window area is inspected for fluid leak from the inner ear. The lining around the round window is gently roughened. The area is packed with fat, fascia or muscle tissue. The eardrum and skin flap are replaced and the canal is packed. If a postauricular incision is made, it is sutured.

69670

Through a postauricular incision, the physician accesses the mastoid cavity of a previous mastoidectomy. Any remaining mastoid disease is removed. To lessen the size of a large mastoid cavity or to stop a cerebrospinal leak, the cavity is obliterated with a rotation flap of fascia or muscle and/or free fat graft and skin. The flap is sutured into place, and the incision is sutured.

69676

The physician makes an incision in the posterior canal wall skin and raises a skin flap and the eardrum forward. Jacobson's nerve is identified in the middle ear and is divided. The eardrum and canal skin are repositioned and packing is placed in the ear canal.

69700

The physician makes an incision around the postauricular fistula, a skin-lined tunnel. The fistula tract is excised, and the incision site is repaired with sutures.

69710

Through a postauricular incision, the physician drills a circular depression in the outer skull cortex behind the mastoid cavity. The internal coil is seated in the circular depression and secured to the skull with titanium screws. The subcutaneous tissue over the internal coil may be thinned. The wound is irrigated and repaired with sutures. A dressing is applied.

69711

Through a postauricular incision, the physician accesses a previously implanted electromagnetic bone conduction hearing device. The device is repaired or removed. The wound is irrigated and repaired with sutures. A dressing is applied.

69714–69715

The physician uses a percutaneous connector system based on a skin penetrating bone anchored titanium pedestal, housing a multichannel electrode array to implant a cochlear implant system. The physician makes a small break in the skin at the temporal bone and angles and places the stem of a titanium pedestal towards the cochlea, leaving a bridge of bone between it and the cortical mastoid. A tunnel is drilled to create a passage for the electrode array and the stem of the titanium pedestal is tapped into a tapered hole in the mastoid. The soft tissue surrounding the pedestal is thinned to prevent local movement and minimize the incidence of infection at the site. The internal collector plate of the pedestal holds platinum-iridium pins for the electrode array. The external collector plate, attached by a spring latching mechanism to the internal plate, contains a multielectrode array that provides a number of independent channels of stimulation. Report 69714 when the procedure is performed without mastoidectomy. Report 69715 when the physician drills out the mastoid cavity to remove diseased tissue.

69717–69718

Generally, titanium fixation plates are not removed after osteosynthesis because they have high biocompatibility and high corrosion resistance characteristics. However, various problems (i.e., improper electrode insertion or migration, device failure, serious flap complication) may require removal and replacement surgery of the osseointegrated implant. To remove the implant, the physician opens the skin at the temporal bone at the site of the original implant and removes any fibrous tissue sheathing the implant. The existing pedestal and electrode array are removed and replaced. Report 69717 when the procedure is performed without mastoidectomy. Report 69718 when the physician drills out the mastoid cavity to remove diseased tissue.

69720

Through a postauricular incision, the physician drills out the mastoid cavity. The sigmoid sinus is exposed posteriorly. The posterior ear canal wall remains intact. The horizontal semicircular canal and part of the incus are visualized. The vertical portion of the facial nerve is exposed. The facial recess is opened and the bone over the horizontal portion (middle ear) of the facial nerve is removed. The incus may be separated from the stapes. The incus and part of the malleus may be removed. The facial nerve sheath is incised from the stylomastoid foramen to the geniculate ganglion. The postauricular wound is sutured and a dressing is applied.

69725

Through a postauricular incision, the physician drills out the mastoid cavity. The sigmoid sinus is exposed posteriorly. The posterior ear canal wall remains intact. The horizontal semicircular canal and part of the incus are visualized. The vertical portion of the facial nerve is exposed. The facial recess is opened and the bone over the horizontal portion (middle ear) of the facial nerve is removed. Decompression continues medial to the geniculate ganglion. The incus and part of the malleus are usually removed. Sometimes, a combined transmastoid and middle fossa approach is required to access the nerve adequately, in which case, a piece of temporal bone is excised to access the middle cranial fossa.

69740

Through a postauricular incision, the physician drills out the mastoid cavity. The posterior ear canal wall remains intact. The horizontal semicircular canal and part of the incus are visualized. The vertical portion of the facial nerve is exposed. The facial recess is opened and the bone over the horizontal portion (middle ear) of the facial nerve is removed. The incus may be separated from the stapes. The incus and part of the malleus may be removed. The nerve defect is identified, and the nerve is decompressed. Cut ends of the facial nerve are sutured to each other, or grafted to a harvested nerve in an end-to-end fashion. The postauricular wound is sutured and a dressing is applied.

69745

Through a postauricular incision, the physician drills out the mastoid cavity. The posterior ear canal wall

remains intact. The horizontal semicircular canal and part of the incus are visualized. The vertical portion of the facial nerve is exposed. The facial recess is opened and the bone over the horizontal portion (middle ear) of the facial nerve is removed. The incus and part of the malleus are usually removed. The nerve defect is identified, and the nerve is decompressed. Cut ends of the facial nerve are sutured to each other, or grafted to a harvested nerve in an end-to-end fashion. Sometimes, a combined transmastoid and middle fossa approach is required to access the nerve adequately, in which case, a piece of temporal bone is excised to access the middle cranial fossa.

69801–69802

In a transcanal approach (69801), the physician makes an incision in the posterior ear canal skin through the external ear opening and reflects the skin flap and posterior tympanic membrane forward. For a mastoid approach (69802), the physician drills out the mastoid cavity. In either case, the posterior ear canal wall remains intact. The horizontal semicircular canal is visualized. Under microscopic guidance, a variety of procedures may be performed, including placement of a small, temporary or permanent tack through the stapes footplate; placement of a hook through the round window or ultrasonography or cryotherapy of the round window. In 69801, the canal is packed. In 69802, the mastoid cavity is packed and the incision is closed with sutures.

69805–69806

Through a postauricular incision, the physician drills out the mastoid cavity. The posterior ear canal wall remains intact. The horizontal and posterior semicircular canals are visualized. Drilling is continued until the endolymphatic sac is identified. The physician uses a diamond bur and fine picks to remove the bone around the sack (decompression) in 69805. A shunt is inserted into the sac in 69806. In either case, the mastoid cavity is packed with absorbable packing and the outer incision is sutured and a pressure dressing is applied.

69820

Through an endaural incision, the physical performs a partial mastoidectomy. The mastoid antrum and horizontal semicircular canal are identified. The posterior ear canal wall is removed down to the level of the facial nerve after elevating and protecting the posterior canal wall and eardrum. The incus and head of the malleus are removed. A small opening is created in the horizontal canal. The eardrum and canal skin are repositioned to cover the opening (fenestration). The mastoid is packed, the incision is repaired, and a dressing is placed.

69840

Through an endaural incision, the physician revises a previous fenestration of the lateral semicircular canal. The physician drills through the mastoid bone to reach the lateral semicircular canal. Additional canal bone is removed, leaving the inner membrane intact. The eardrum and canal skin are repositioned to cover the opening (fenestration). The mastoid is packed, the incision is repaired, and a dressing is placed.

69905

The physician makes an incision in the posterior canal skin and reflects the skin flap and posterior eardrum forward. Under microscopic visualization through the external ear opening, the incus and stapes are removed. A right angle hook is fed through the oval window to remove the contents of the vestibule. The physician may drill a connection between the oval and round windows. The middle ear is packed with gelatin foam. The eardrum and canal skin are repositioned, and the ear canal is packed.

69910

Through a postauricular incision, the physician drills out the mastoid cavity. The posterior ear canal wall remains intact. The horizontal, posterior, and superior semicircular canals are removed along with the lining of the labyrinth. The incision is repaired with sutures and a dressing is applied.

69915

Through a postauricular incision, the physician drills out the mastoid cavity. The posterior ear canal wall remains intact. The horizontal, posterior, and superior semicircular canals are removed along with the lining of the labyrinth. The internal auditory canal is identified. The bone over the internal auditory canal is removed, exposing the dura. The dura is opened and the vestibular nerve is identified and cut. The facial nerve is preserved. The dura is closed and the mastoid cavity is packed. The incision is repaired with sutures and a dressing is applied.

69930

The physician makes a U-shaped incision, creating a skin flap well behind the mastoid, and drills a circular depression in the squamous portion of the temporal bone in which the internal coil will be housed. The mastoid air cells are removed with a drill, and a facial recess approach is used. The bony ear canal is preserved. The internal coil is secured in the depressed area of the temporal bone, and the electrode is introduced through the facial recess and the round window into the cochlea. The ground wire attached to the internal coil is introduced into the temporalis muscle. The incision is sutured.

69950

A vertical incision is made just anterior to the auricle and is extended superiorly to expose the temporalis muscle. The muscle is divided. A section of the skull (craniotomy) is removed to expose the dura over the temporal lobe of the brain. The dura is elevated off the floor of the middle fossa. The physician drills to thin the bone over the floor of the middle fossa to

identify the facial nerve. The facial nerve is followed to the internal auditory canal. The canal is decompressed with the drill and the dura covering the vestibular nerves is opened. The vestibular nerves are cut while preserving the facial and cochlear nerves. A muscle graft is placed over the internal auditory canal, and the bone is replaced in the skull defect. The incision is sutured and a dressing is applied.

69955

A vertical incision is made just anterior to the auricle and is extended superiorly to expose the temporalis muscle. The muscle is divided. A section of the skull (craniotomy) is removed to expose the dura over the temporal lobe of the brain. The dura is elevated off the floor of the middle fossa. The bone over the facial nerve is carefully removed with the drill (decompression). If there is a tumor of the facial nerve, it is resected. If the nerve has been transected because of trauma, it can be repaired with sutures. A nerve graft may be needed when the ends of the nerve cannot be approximated without tension. A transmastoid approach may also be needed if extensive decompression is required. A muscle graft is placed over the floor of the middle cranial fossa. The bone plug is replaced in the skull defect. The incision is sutured and a dressing is applied.

69960

A vertical incision is made just anterior to the auricle and is extended superiorly to expose the temporalis muscle. The muscle is divided. A section of the skull (craniotomy) is removed to expose the dura over the temporal lobe of the brain. The dura is elevated off the floor of the middle fossa. The physician identifies the internal auditory canal. A drill is used to remove bone to open the canal (decompression). A muscle graft is placed over the internal auditory canal and the bone is replaced in the skull defect. The incision is sutured and a dressing is applied.

69970

A vertical incision is made just anterior to the auricle and is extended superiorly to expose the temporalis muscle. The muscle is divided. A section of the skull (craniotomy) is removed to expose the dura over the temporal lobe of the brain. The dura is elevated off the floor of the middle fossa. The physician isolates and dissects a tumor of the temporal bone. The internal auditory canal may be decompressed. A muscle graft is placed over the internal auditory canal. The bone plug is returned to the skull, the incision is sutured, and a dressing is applied.

69990

The physician uses a surgical microscope when the services are performed using the techniques of microsurgery, except when the microscopy is part of the procedure (such as in 15756). This code is reported in addition to the primary procedure.

70010

A radiographic study using fluoroscopy is performed on the posterior fossa when a lesion is suspected. Contrast medium, usually barium sulfate, may be used to enhance visibility and is instilled in the patient through a lumbar area puncture into the subarachnoid space. The radiologist takes a series of pictures by sending an x-ray beam through the body, using fluoroscopy to view the enhanced structure on a television camera. The patient is angled from an erect position through a recumbent position with the body tilted so as to maintain feet higher than the head to help the flow of contrast into the study area.

70010–70110

The lower jaw bone is x-rayed. In 70100, three or less projections are taken for a partial view of the bone structure and in 70110, four or more projections are taken for a complete view of the bone structure.

70015

A radiographic study that helps map the tumor pathology of a mass within the posterior fossa. The brainstem and cerebellum are contained within the posterior fossa and the cerebellopontine angle cistern is often the location of a mass such as a schwannoma or meningioma. Images are taken sequentially over a period of hours and days after introducing a radiotracer intrathecally by lumbar puncture.

70030

X-rays of the eyes are obtained to determine the location of a foreign body in the eye. After positioning the patient, either a one or two view x-ray is obtained. Transparent objects such as glass may not be good candidates for x-ray visualization. The physician supervises the procedure and interprets and reports the findings.

70120

Films are taken of the mastoid processes, or lower portion of the temporal bone of the skull, which protrudes just behind the ear. Both mastoid processes are always examined for comparison purposes, and it is essential that the radiographs be exact duplicates in both positioning of the site and technical quality. Several varying views may be taken, but the key element of this procedure is that it reports less than three views per side.

70130

Films are taken of the mastoid processes, or lower portion of the temporal bone of the skull, which protrudes just behind the ear. Both mastoid processes are always examined for comparison purposes, and it is essential that the radiographs be exact duplicates in both positioning of the site and technical quality. Several varying views may be taken, but the key element of this procedure is that it reports a complete exam, or minimum of three views per side.

70134

Films are taken of the petrous portions of the skull to demonstrate internal auditory meati, or organs of hearing. Several different views may be taken, both with varying angulation of the x-ray beam, as well as varying the position of the patient's skull.

70140

X-rays of the facial bones are obtained to determine an injury, fracture, or neoplasm. After positioning the patient, less than three views of the facial bones are obtained. The physician supervises the procedure and interprets and reports the findings.

70150

X-rays of the facial bones are obtained to determine an injury, fracture, or neoplasm. After positioning the patient, a complete series of x-rays of the facial bones, with a minimum of three views, is obtained. The physician supervises the procedure and interprets and reports the findings.

70160

Films are taken of the nasal bones to include a complete exam, or minimum of three views. Typically, this exam would consist of both right and left lateral (side to side) for comparison, as well as a tangential projection in which the x-ray beam is directed from a position above the patient's head down through the nose. This view is primarily used to demonstrate the medial or lateral (side to side) displacement of nasal fractures.

70170

Dacryocystography is the radiographic evaluation of the lacrimal system to localize the site of an obstruction. One cc of a water-soluble contrast medium is injected through the lower canaliculus and x-rays of the excretory system are obtained. The physician supervises the procedure and interprets and reports the findings.

70190

Radiological examination of the optic foramina is useful in the evaluation of trauma, tumors, or foreign bodies. After positioning the patient, the radiologist obtains x-rays of the optic foramina. The physician supervises the procedure and interprets and reports the findings.

70200

Radiological examination of the orbits is useful in the evaluation of trauma, tumors, or foreign bodies. After positioning the patient, the radiologist obtains a minimum of four x-ray views of the orbits. Standard methods include posteroanterior (PA) exposures from two different positions, lateral views, optic canal projections, and oblique views of each side for comparison. The physician supervises the procedure and interprets and reports the findings.

70210

Films are taken of the paranasal sinuses in one or two views. Although there are several sinus projections, each serving a specific purpose, many of them are used only when required to visualize a specific lesion. Typically, but not necessarily, this code would call for a side to side (lateral) view and a back to front (PA) view, depending on the specific sinus in question. The projections are routinely taken with the patient in an erect position to demonstrate presence or absence of fluid.

70220

Films are taken of the paranasal sinuses for a complete study, with a minimum of three views. There are several sinus projections used when required to visualize a specific lesion. Projections routinely taken consist of four to five standard views of the skull, which adequately demonstrate all of the paranasal sinuses on a majority of patients. Specific exams may be included to test a particular sinus, e.g., frontal sinus, maxillary sinus, and sphenoid or ethmoid sinuses. These projections are routinely taken with the patient in an erect position to demonstrate presence or absence of fluid.

70240

Films are taken of the sella turcica, the depression within the sphenoid bone that houses the pituitary gland. The patient is placed in the prone semioblique position and the x-ray beam is directed to a spot slightly anterior and superior to the external auditory meatus while the patient's head is maintained in a lateral position.

70250–70260

Films are taken of the skull bones. In 70250, three or less views are taken, and in 70260, a complete exam with a four view minimum is performed. The most common projections for routine skull series are AP axial (front to back), lateral, and PA axial (back to front). X-rays may be taken with the patient placed erect, prone, or supine and either code may include stereoradiography, which is a technique that produces three-dimensional images.

70300–70320

Films are taken of the mouth to show teeth and/or surrounding bone. In dental radiography, the film may be placed either inside or outside the mouth. Code 70300 reports a single view only, 73010 reports a partial examination, and 70320 reports a complete full mouth exam.

70328–70330

The temporomandibular joint is x-rayed in two projections on one side only in 70328 and in two projections on both sides in 70330. One film is taken with the mouth open and one with the mouth closed.

70332

A radiographic contrast study is performed on the temporomandibular joint. A contrast material is injected into the joint spaces, followed by x-ray examination of the joint. This allows the physician to see the position of the structures not normally seen on conventional x-rays.

70336

Magnetic resonance imaging (MRI) is a radiation-free, noninvasive, technique to produce high quality sectional images of the inside of the body in multiple planes. MRI uses the natural magnetic properties of the hydrogen atoms in our bodies that emit radiofrequency signals when exposed to radio waves within a strong electro-magnetic field. These signals are then processed and converted by the computer into high-resolution, three-dimensional, tomographic images. Patients with metallic or electronic implants or foreign bodies cannot be exposed to MRI. The patient must remain still while lying on a motorized table within the large, circular MRI tunnel. A sedative may be administered as well as contrast material for image enhancement. This code reports an exam of the temporomandibular joint(s).

70350

A lateral or frontal x-ray projection is taken to examine the entire skull, jaw, and related tooth positions. The machine holds the patient's head in the same position each time so that a series of cephalograms can be directly compared for growth and development over time.

70355

A panoramic radiographic study is performed on the mandibular arch and its supporting structures. A single image is produced of the entire mandible for diagnostic purposes. The physician evaluates trauma, third molar, and other unique disease conditions. Tooth development and anomalies may also be studied.

70360

The technologist uses x-rays to obtain soft tissue images of the patient's neck rather than bone. The radiologist obtains two views, typically front to back (AP), and side to side (lateral). This procedure is performed to visualize abnormal air patterns or suspected foreign bodies or obstructions within the throat or neck.

70370

A radiologic examination is performed to visualize the pharynx, which serves as passage for both food and air, and larynx, or the organ of voice. Films are typically taken to show soft tissues of the neck. The films are often taken while the patient inhales or makes phonetic sounds. The key element of this code is that it includes x-ray fluoroscopy and/or

CPT® Lay Descriptions

magnification technique in addition to the radiologic exam.

70371

A radiologic study is performed for pharyngeal and speech evaluation. Cineradiography, or video recording, is employed, as the physiologic event of speech and swallowing occur too rapidly for normal fluoroscopic viewing. High-speed frame rates are used to evaluate speech and swallowing, and later reviewed and interpreted by the radiologist.

70373

A radiographic contrast study is performed of the larynx, or organ of voice. Iodized oil is given in conjunction with the examination via tubing, which allows oil to drip down the patient's throat at the radiologists discretion. The radiologist, via x-ray fluoroscopy, simultaneously watches the image amplified and displayed on a TV monitor. Rapid film sequencing must be used to record the image, which may then be studied and interpreted by the radiologist.

70380

Films are taken to visualize a salivary gland for possible calculus (calcium deposit). Typically, a front to back (AP) or back to front (PA) view is taken of the side in question. The patient is asked to fill his cheek with air, if possible, to enhance detail of the x-ray, particularly for demonstration of calcific deposits. A lateral, or side to side view, as well as an intra-oral projection, may also be taken.

70390

A radiographic contrast study is performed to visualize the salivary glands and ducts, typically to demonstrate possible lesions or tumors, salivary fistulae, or to localize calcium deposits within the gland. The radiologist injects the main salivary duct with radiopaque dye (contrast), after which it flows into the duct system and is examined with x-ray fluoroscopy. The projected image is amplified and displayed on a TV monitor for the radiologist to review and interpret.

70450–70470

Computerized axial tomography directs multiple narrow beams of x-rays around the body structure being studied and uses computer imaging to produce thin cross-sectional views of various layers (or slices) of the body. It is useful for the evaluation of trauma, tumor, and foreign bodies as CT is able to visualize soft tissue as well as bones. Patients are required to remain motionless during the study and sedation may need to be administered as well as a contrast medium for image enhancement. These codes report an exam of the head or brain. Report 70450 if no contrast is used. Report 70460 if performed with contrast and 70470 if performed first without contrast and then again following the injection of contrast.

70480–70482

Computerized axial tomography directs multiple narrow beams of x-rays around the body structure being studied and uses computer imaging to produce thin cross-sectional views of various layers (or slices) of the body. It is useful for the evaluation of trauma, tumor, and foreign bodies as CT is able to visualize soft tissue as well as bones. Patients are required to remain motionless during the study and sedation may need to be administered as well as a contrast medium for image enhancement. These codes report an exam of the orbit, sella, posterior fossa, or outer, middle, or inner ear. Report 70480 if no contrast is used. Report 70481 if performed with contrast and 70482 if performed first without contrast and then again following the injection of contrast.

70486–70488

Computerized axial tomography directs multiple narrow beams of x-rays around the body structure being studied and uses computer imaging to produce thin cross-sectional views of various layers (or slices) of the body. It is useful for the evaluation of trauma, tumor, and foreign bodies as CT is able to visualize soft tissue as well as bones. Patients are required to remain motionless during the study and sedation may need to be administered as well as a contrast medium for image enhancement. These codes report an exam of the maxillofacial area. Report 70486 if no contrast is used. Report 70487 if performed with contrast and 70488 if performed first without contrast and then again following the injection of contrast.

70490–70492

Computerized axial tomography directs multiple narrow beams of x-rays around the body structure being studied and uses computer imaging to produce thin cross-sectional views of various layers (or slices) of the body. It is useful for the evaluation of trauma, tumor, and foreign bodies as CT is able to visualize soft tissue as well as bones. Patients are required to remain motionless during the study and sedation may need to be administered as well as a contrast medium for image enhancement. These codes report an exam of the soft tissue of the neck. Report 70490 if no contrast is used. Report 70491 if performed with contrast and 70492 if performed first without contrast and then again following the injection of contrast.

70496–70498

Computed tomographic angiography (CTA) is a procedure used for the imaging of vessels to detect aneurysms, blood clots, and other vascular irregularities. The physician inserts a needle and then a guidewire into the artery through the skin. The physician feeds the guidewire to the area requiring study with the use of fluoroscopic guidance. The needle is removed and a catheter is threaded over the guidewire until it too reaches the study area. The guidewire is removed. Contrast medium is then rapidly infused at intervals, usually with an automatic injector, and the patient is scanned with thin section axial or spiral mode x-ray beams. Three-dimensional images are generated and postprocessing reconstruction is done at a workstation on the scanner. CTA also provides information unavailable with conventional angiography such as vessel wall thickness (mural thrombus) and the venous anatomy of a target organ and/or associated organs within the scan range. Report 70496 for an exam of the head without contrast, followed by contrast and further sections. Report 70498 for an exam of the neck without contrast, followed by contrast and further sections.

70540–70543

Magnetic resonance imaging (MRI) is a radiation-free, noninvasive, technique to produce high quality sectional images of the inside of the body in multiple planes. MRI uses the natural magnetic properties of the hydrogen atoms in our bodies that emit radiofrequency signals when exposed to radio waves within a strong electro-magnetic field. These signals are then processed and converted by the computer into high-resolution, three-dimensional, tomographic images. Patients with metallic or electronic implants or foreign bodies cannot be exposed to MRI. The patient must remain still while lying on a motorized table within the large, circular MRI tunnel. A sedative may be administered as well as contrast material for image enhancement. These codes report an exam of the orbit, face, and neck. Report 70540 if no contrast is used. Report 70542 if performed with contrast and 70543 if performed first without contrast and then again following the injection of contrast.

70544–70546

Magnetic Resonance Angiography (MRA) is a special type of magnetic resonance imaging (MRI) that specifically visualizes blood vessels and blood flow to evaluate vascular disorders within the structure being studied. Unlike CT, it does not rely on the absorption of x-ray energy. Magnetic resonance imaging uses the natural magnetic properties of the hydrogen atoms in our bodies that emit radiofrequency signals when exposed to radio waves within a strong electro-magnetic field. These signals are then processed and converted by the computer into high-resolution, three-dimensional tomographic images. Patients with metallic or electronic implants or foreign bodies cannot be exposed to MRI. The patient must remain still while lying on a motorized table within the large, circular MRI tunnel. A sedative may be administered as well as contrast material for image enhancement. These codes report an exam of the head. Report 70544 if no contrast is used. Report 70545 if performed with contrast and 70546 if performed first without contrast and then again following the injection of contrast.

70547–70549

Magnetic Resonance Angiography (MRA) is a special type of magnetic resonance imaging (MRI) that specifically visualizes blood vessels and blood flow to evaluate vascular disorders within the structure being studied. Unlike CT, it does not rely on the absorption of x-ray energy. Magnetic resonance imaging uses the natural magnetic properties of the hydrogen atoms in our bodies that emit radiofrequency signals when exposed to radio waves within a strong electro-magnetic field. These signals are then processed and converted by the computer into high-resolution, three-dimensional tomographic images. Patients with metallic or electronic implants or foreign bodies cannot be exposed to MRI. The patient must remain still while lying on a motorized table within the large, circular MRI tunnel. A sedative may be administered as well as contrast material for image enhancement. These codes report and exam of the neck. Report 70547 if no contrast is used. Report 70548 if performed with contrast and 70549 if performed first without contrast and then again following the injection of contrast.

70551–70553

Magnetic resonance imaging (MRI) is a radiation-free, noninvasive, technique to produce high quality sectional images of the inside of the body in multiple planes. MRI uses the natural magnetic properties of the hydrogen atoms in our bodies that emit radiofrequency signals when exposed to radio waves within a strong electro-magnetic field. These signals are then processed and converted by the computer into high-resolution, three-dimensional, tomographic images. Patients with metallic or electronic implants or foreign bodies cannot be exposed to MRI. The patient must remain still while lying on a motorized table within the large, circular MRI tunnel. A sedative may be administered as well as contrast material for image enhancement. These codes report an exam of the brain, including the brain stem. Report 70551 if no contrast is used. Report 70552 if performed with contrast and 70553 if performed first without contrast and then again following the injection of contrast.

71010

A radiograph is taken of the patient's chest from front to back (AP). Typically, this is done when the patient is too ill to stand or be turned to the prone position. The key element of this code is that it reports a single, frontal view.

71015

A stereoradiograph is taken of the patient's chest from the frontal view. Stereoradiography is a technique that produces the image in three dimensions for viewing.

71020

Films are taken of the patient's chest to include a frontal and side to side (lateral) view. This code specifically reports these two views.

71021

Films are taken of the patient's chest with the patient placed in a side to side (lateral) position, as well as a standard front to back position (AP). Another front to back (AP) film is also taken with the patient leaning back resting shoulders against the wall/film tray in a lordotic (arched back) position. This projection produces x-rays that demonstrate the top, or apices, of the lungs.

71022

Radiographs are taken of the patient's chest with the patient in a standard front to back (AP) position, as well as side to side (laterally). In addition, right and left obliques, or angled views, are taken. The key element of this code is that it reports specifically frontal, lateral, and oblique views.

71023

Films are taken of the patient's chest, which include a frontal and side to side (lateral) view, using fluoroscopy to follow an opaque medium as it is swallowed. The patient holds the cup of contrast medium and swallows as directed, during or immediately before exposure. Frontal and lateral views are taken, both of which require the patient to be either erect or recumbent. For the lateral view, the arms must be placed over the head.

71030

Films are taken of the patient's chest, specifically a complete exam, with a minimum of four views. Typically, this would include a back to front (PA), side to side (lateral), and right and left obliques, but may include any number of specialized projections, e.g., axial (angulated) views or lateral decubitus views for fluid levels.

71034

Films are taken of the patient's chest to make a complete exam with four or more views, using fluoroscopy to follow an opaque medium as it is swallowed. The patient holds the cup of contrast medium and swallows as directed, during or immediately before exposure. Contrast medium, usually barium sulfate, enhances visibility of internal organs, such as the esophagus and stomach. The radiologist takes a series of pictures by sending an x-ray beam through the body, using fluoroscopy to view the enhanced structures on a television camera.

71035

Radiographs are taken of the patient's chest. This code reports special views, but does not specify number of films allowed. Specific examples may include Bucky studies and/or lateral decubitus studies, wherein the patient is prone or supine and the x-ray beam is directed through the side of the chest. This lateral projection shows change in position of fluid and reveals areas that are obscured by the fluid in standard, upright projections.

71040–71060

In bronchography, x-rays are taken of the bronchial tree and the trachea to help locate obstructions. The patient is place supine and administered a local anesthetic. A catheter is threaded down the windpipe after being introduced through the nose or mouth. More anesthesia and the contrast medium are administered through the catheter and the x-rays are then taken. In 71040, unilateral pictures are taken and in 71060, both right and left sides are viewed.

71090

A pacemaker is inserted in the chest under fluoroscopy and radiography. An incision is made in the chest below the collarbone to create a pocket under the skin. The wire(s), called lead(s), of the pacemaker are threaded through a vein and placed in either the right atrium or right ventricle, using fluoroscopy to visually guide the wires for correct placement. The lead(s) is attached to the heart chamber on the inside surface (endocardial) and the generator is inserted into the pocket created under the collarbone. Leads may also be implanted on the outer heart surface (epicardial) and the generator inserted in a pocket created in the upper abdomen in cases of congenital heart disease. This code reports the fluoroscopy, radiography, radiological supervision and interpretation for a pacemaker insertion.

71100

Films are taken unilaterally of the affected side of the ribs with two views in either AP (front to back) or PA (back to front) views.

71101

Films are taken unilaterally of the affected side of the ribs for a minimum of three views, including the posterior ribs.

71110

Films are taken bilaterally of the ribs for three views of the ribcage, with the patient placed supine and the x-ray directed at the thorax midpoint, above or below the xiphoid process for a bilateral view.

71111

A minimum of four films are taken bilaterally of the ribcage, including the posterior ribs, with the patient placed supine for AP and PA views and the x-ray directed at the thorax midpoint, above or below the xiphoid process for a bilateral view.

71120

Films are taken of the sternum with a minimum of two views from an anterior oblique and lateral position.

71130

Films are taken of the sternoclavicular joint or joints with a minimum of three views from posteroanterior and oblique projections.

71250–71270

Computerized axial tomography directs multiple narrow beams of x-rays around the body structure being studied and uses computer imaging to produce thin cross-sectional views of various layers (or slices) of the body. It is useful for the evaluation of trauma, tumor, and foreign bodies as CT is able to visualize soft tissue as well as bones. Patients are required to remain motionless during the study and sedation may need to be administered as well as a contrast medium for image enhancement. These codes report an exam of the thorax. Report 71250 if no contrast is used. Report 71260 if performed with contrast and 71270 if performed first without contrast and then again following the injection of contrast.

71275

Computed tomographic angiography (CTA) is a procedure used for the imaging of vessels to detect aneurysms, blood clots, and other vascular irregularities. The physician inserts a needle and then a guidewire into the artery through the skin. The physician feeds the guidewire to the area requiring study with the use of fluoroscopic guidance. The needle is removed and a catheter is threaded over the guidewire until it too reaches the study area. The guidewire is removed. Contrast medium is then rapidly infused at intervals, usually with an automatic injector, and the patient is scanned with thin section axial or spiral mode x-ray beams. Three-dimensional images are generated and postprocessing reconstruction is done at a workstation on the scanner. CTA provides information unavailable with conventional angiography such as vessel wall thickness and the venous anatomy of the target organ. This code reports an exam of the chest first with contrast and then again following the injection of contrast.

71550–71552

Magnetic resonance imaging (MRI) is a radiation-free, noninvasive, technique to produce high quality sectional images of the inside of the body in multiple planes. MRI uses the natural magnetic properties of the hydrogen atoms in our bodies that emit radiofrequency signals when exposed to radio waves within a strong electro-magnetic field. These signals are then processed and converted by the computer into high-resolution, three-dimensional, tomographic images. Patients with metallic or electronic implants or foreign bodies cannot be exposed to MRI. The patient must remain still while lying on a motorized table within the large, circular MRI tunnel. A sedative may be administered as well as contrast material for image enhancement. These codes report an exam of the chest. Report 71550 if no contrast is used. Report 71551 if performed with contrast and 71552 if performed first without contrast and then again following the injection of contrast.

71555

Magnetic Resonance Angiography (MRA) is a special type of magnetic resonance imaging (MRI) that specifically visualizes blood vessels and blood flow to evaluate vascular disorders within the structure being studied. Unlike CT, it does not rely on the absorption of x-ray energy. Magnetic resonance imaging uses the natural magnetic properties of the hydrogen atoms in our bodies that emit radiofrequency signals when exposed to radio waves within a strong electro-magnetic field. These signals are then processed and converted by the computer into high-resolution, three-dimensional tomographic images. Patients with metallic or electronic implants or foreign bodies cannot be exposed to MRI. The patient must remain still while lying on a motorized table within the large, circular MRI tunnel. A sedative may be administered as well as contrast material for image enhancement. This code reports an exam of the chest.

72010

The entire spine is surveyed in a radiologic exam that includes anteroposterior views, with the patient supine, knees flexed, and feet flat on the table; and lateral views, either recumbent or erect. Right and left posterior obliques may be performed with the patient in the semi-supine position with the spine at a 45 degree angle to the table.

72020

One film is taken of the spine that requires specification of the level examined.

72040–72052

A radiologic examination of the cervical spine is performed that includes a minimum of two views in 72040, a minimum of four views in 72050, and a complete study in 72052. The complete study includes films taken in oblique (angled) positions and in flexion and/or extension positioning.

72069

Typically a film is taken of the thoracolumbar spine from front to back (AP) while the patient is standing erect. This film is used to detect any curvature of the spine when scoliosis or other pathology may be present.

72070–72074

A radiologic examination of the thoracic spine is performed that includes two views in 72070, three views in 72072, and a minimum of four views in 72074. These procedures do not specify that a certain view must be performed.

72080

Films are taken of the thoracolumbar area of the spine in two views not specifically stated.

CPT® Lay Descriptions

72090

A typical scoliosis series consists of four views of the thoracic and lumbar spine: one from front to back (AP) with the patient standing; one from front to back (AP) with the patient supine, or lying down; and finally, two views with alternate right and left flexion in the supine position. In addition, a lateral, or side to side projection made with the patient standing to show spondylolisthesis or to demonstrate exaggerated degrees of kyphosis or lordosis is often recommended. The key element to this code is that it includes supine and erect studies. The number of films allowed is not specified.

72100–72110

A radiologic examination of the lumbosacral spine is performed that includes two or three views in 72100, and a minimum of four views in 72110. These procedures do not specify that a certain view must be performed.

72114

Films are taken of the lumbosacral spine, or lower back, for a complete radiologic study. A complete lumbar spine series typically includes x-rays taken from front to back (AP), side to side (lateral), and oblique, or angled right and left views. In addition, this code includes bending views, films taken with the patient bending to the left and right to demonstrate mobility of the intervertebral joints, and/or films taken with the patient in both flexion and extension, typically in cases of disc protrusion to localize the involved joint.

72120

Films are taken of the lumbar spine, or lower back, with the patient bending to the left and right to demonstrate the mobility of the intervertebral joints and/or films with the patient in both flexion and extension, typically in cases of disc protrusion to localize the involved joint. The key element to this code is that a minimum of four films in bending views only are taken.

72125–72127

Computerized axial tomography directs multiple narrow beams of x-rays around the body structure being studied and uses computer imaging to produce thin cross-sectional views of various layers (or slices) of the body. It is useful for the evaluation of trauma, tumor, and foreign bodies as CT is able to visualize soft tissue as well as bones. Patients are required to remain motionless during the study and sedation may need to be administered. These codes report an exam of the cervical spine. For CT of the spine, contrast material may be administered either intravenously (part of the procedure)or intrathecally (reported separately). These codes report and exam of the cervical spine. Report 72125 if no contrast is used. Report 72126 if performed with contrast and 72127 if

performed first without contrast and then again following the injection of contrast.

72128–72130

Computerized axial tomography directs multiple narrow beams of x-rays around the body structure being studied and uses computer imaging to produce thin cross-sectional views of various layers (or slices) of the body. It is useful for the evaluation of trauma, tumor, and foreign bodies as CT is able to visualize soft tissue as well as bones. Patients are required to remain motionless during the study and sedation may need to be administered. These codes report an exam of the thoracic spine. For CT of the spine, contrast material may be administered either intravenously (part of the procedure)or intrathecally (reported separately). These codes report an exam of the thoracic spine. Report 72128 if no contrast is used. Report 72129 if performed with contrast and 72130 if performed first without contrast and then again following the injection of contrast.

72131–72133

Computerized axial tomography directs multiple thin beams of x-rays at the body structure being studied and uses computer imaging to produce thin cross-sectional views of various layers (or slices) of the body. It is useful for the evaluation of trauma, tumor, and foreign bodies as CT is able to visualize soft tissue as well as bones. Patients are required to remain motionless during the study and sedation may need to be administered. These codes report an exam of the lumbar spine. For CT of the spine, contrast material may be administered either intravenously (part of the procedure)or intrathecally (reported separately). These codes report an exam of the lumbar spine. Report 72131 if no contrast is used. Report 72132 if performed with contrast and 72133 if performed first without contrast and then again following the injection of contrast.

72141, 72142, 72156

Magnetic resonance imaging (MRI) is a radiation-free, noninvasive, technique to produce high quality sectional images of the inside of the body in multiple planes. MRI uses the natural magnetic properties of the hydrogen atoms in our bodies that emit radiofrequency signals when exposed to radio waves within a strong electro-magnetic field. These signals are then processed and converted by the computer into high-resolution, three-dimensional, tomographic images. Patients with metallic or electronic implants or foreign bodies cannot be exposed to MRI. The patient must remain still while lying on a motorized table within the large, circular MRI tunnel. A sedative may be administered as well as contrast material for image enhancement. For cervical spinal canal and contents, report 72141 if no contrast is used; report 72142 if performed with contrast and 72156 if performed first without contrast and then again following the injection of contrast.

72146, 72147, 72157

Magnetic resonance imaging (MRI) is a radiation-free, noninvasive, technique to produce high quality sectional images of the inside of the body in multiple planes. MRI uses the natural magnetic properties of the hydrogen atoms in our bodies that emit radiofrequency signals when exposed to radio waves within a strong electro-magnetic field. These signals are then processed and converted by the computer into high-resolution, three-dimensional, tomographic images. Patients with metallic or electronic implants or foreign bodies cannot be exposed to MRI. The patient must remain still while lying on a motorized table within the large, circular MRI tunnel. A sedative may be administered as well as contrast material for image enhancement. For thoracic spinal canal and contents, report 72146 if no contrast is used; report 72147 if performed with contrast and 72157 if performed first without contrast and then again following the injection of contrast.

72148, 72149, 72158

Magnetic resonance imaging (MRI) is a radiation-free, noninvasive, technique to produce high quality sectional images of the inside of the body in multiple planes. MRI uses the natural magnetic properties of the hydrogen atoms in our bodies that emit radiofrequency signals when exposed to radio waves within a strong electro-magnetic field. These signals are then processed and converted by the computer into high-resolution, three-dimensional, tomographic images. Patients with metallic or electronic implants or foreign bodies cannot be exposed to MRI. The patient must remain still while lying on a motorized table within the large, circular MRI tunnel. A sedative may be administered as well as contrast material for image enhancement. For lumbar spinal canal and contents, report 72148 if no contrast is used; report 72149 if performed with contrast and 72158 if performed first without contrast and then again following the injection of contrast.

72159

Magnetic Resonance Angiography (MRA) is a special type of magnetic resonance imaging (MRI) that specifically visualizes blood vessels and blood flow to evaluate vascular disorders within the structure being studied. Unlike CT, it does not rely on the absorption of x-ray energy. Magnetic resonance imaging uses the natural magnetic properties of the hydrogen atoms in our bodies that emit radiofrequency signals when exposed to radio waves within a strong electro-magnetic field. These signals are then processed and converted by the computer into high-resolution, three-dimensional tomographic images. Patients with metallic or electronic implants or foreign bodies cannot be exposed to MRI. The patient must remain still while lying on a motorized table within the large, circular MRI tunnel. A sedative may be administered as well as contrast material for image enhancement.

This code reports an exam of the spinal canal and contents.

72170

One or two views are taken of the pelvis. The most common view is from front to back (AP) with the patient lying supine with feet inverted 15 degrees to overcome the anteversion (or rotation) of the femoral necks. The pelvic girdle, femoral head, neck, trochanters, and upper femurs are also shown.

72190

A minimum of three films are taken of the pelvis, typically front to back (AP) with the patient lying supine. The patient's legs are in what is termed a "frogleg" lateral position, wherein the patient's feet are drawn up toward the buttocks, at which point the knees are allowed to drop down to the table with feet together. A third film may be taken with the patient lying on his or her side for a lateral view of the pelvis, as well as unilateral views of the hips, if necessary.

72191

Computed tomographic angiography (CTA) is a procedure used for the imaging of vessels to detect aneurysms, blood clots, and other vascular irregularities. The physician inserts a needle and then a guidewire into the artery through the skin. The physician feeds the guidewire to the area requiring study with the use of fluoroscopic guidance. The needle is removed and a catheter is threaded over the guidewire until it too reaches the study area. The guidewire is removed. Contrast medium is then rapidly infused at intervals, usually with an automatic injector, and the patient is scanned with thin section axial or spiral mode x-ray beams. Three-dimensional images are generated and postprocessing reconstruction is done at a workstation on the scanner. CTA also provides information unavailable with conventional angiography such as vessel wall thickness (mural thrombus) and the venous anatomy of a target organ and/or associated organs within the scan range. This code reports an exam of the pelvis first without contrast material and then again following contrast injection, including image post-processing.

72192–72194

Computerized axial tomography directs multiple narrow beams of x-rays around the body structure being studied and uses computer imaging to produce thin cross-sectional views of various layers (or slices) of the body. It is useful for the evaluation of trauma, tumor, and foreign bodies as CT is able to visualize soft tissue as well as bones. Patients are required to remain motionless during the study and sedation may need to be administered as well as a contrast medium for image enhancement. These codes report an exam of the pelvis. Report 72192 if no contrast is used. Report 72193 if performed with contrast and 72194 if performed first without contrast and then again following the injection of contrast.

72195–72197

Magnetic resonance imaging (MRI) is a radiation-free, noninvasive, technique to produce high quality sectional images of the inside of the body in multiple planes. MRI uses the natural magnetic properties of the hydrogen atoms in our bodies that emit radiofrequency signals when exposed to radio waves within a strong electro-magnetic field. These signals are then processed and converted by the computer into high-resolution, three-dimensional, tomographic images. Patients with metallic or electronic implants or foreign bodies cannot be exposed to MRI. The patient must remain still while lying on a motorized table within the large, circular MRI tunnel. A sedative may be administered as well as contrast material for image enhancement. These codes report an exam of the pelvis. Report 72195 if no contrast is used. Report 72196 if performed with contrast and 72197 if performed first without contrast and then again following the injection of contrast.

72198

Magnetic Resonance Angiography (MRA) is a special type of magnetic resonance imaging (MRI) that specifically visualizes blood vessels and blood flow to evaluate vascular disorders within the structure being studied. Unlike CT, it does not rely on the absorption of x-ray energy. Magnetic resonance imaging uses the natural magnetic properties of the hydrogen atoms in our bodies that emit radiofrequency signals when exposed to radio waves within a strong electro-magnetic field. These signals are then processed and converted by the computer into high-resolution, three-dimensional tomographic images. Patients with metallic or electronic implants or foreign bodies cannot be exposed to MRI. The patient must remain still while lying on a motorized table within the large, circular MRI tunnel. A sedative may be administered as well as contrast material for image enhancement. This code reports an exam of the pelvis.

72200–72202

Films are taken of the articulation between the sacrum, the triangular bone beneath the lumbar vertebrae, and the ilium, or upper portion of the hip bone. The exam may be performed in both anteroposterior and right and left posterior oblique views. Code 72200 reports one or two views and 72202 reports three or more views.

72220

Films are taken (minimum of two views) of the sacrum and the coccyx. The sacrum is a triangular bone located between the fifth lumbar vertebra and the coccyx. It is formed by five connected vertebrae and is wedged between the two innominate bones. The coccyx is the small bone at the very base of the spinal column, and is formed by the fusion of four

vertebrae. The sacrum and the coccyx form the posterior (back) boundary of the pelvis. While anteroposterior (AP; front to back) and lateral (side) views are the most common views taken, this procedure is used for any two or more views reported.

72240–72270

In myelography, a radiographic study using fluoroscopy is performed on the spinal cord and nerve root branches when a lesion is suspected. Contrast medium, usually barium sulfate, is used to enhance visibility and is instilled in the patient through a lumbar or cervical area puncture into the subarachnoid space. The radiologist takes a series of pictures by sending an x-ray beam through the body, using fluoroscopy to view the enhanced structure on a television camera. The patient is angled from an erect position through a recumbent position with the body tilted so as to maintain feet higher than the head to help the flow of contrast into the study area. Code 72240 reports a cervical myelogram; 72255 reports a thoracic myelogram; 72265 reports lumbosacral myelogram; and 72270 reports a myelogram of the entire spinal canal.

72275

A radiologic imaging examination is performed on the veins lining the spinal canal. Contrast is injected into the epidural space under direct fluoroscopy. Examining the flow of contrast in the epidural space around the nerves to be studied aids in the diagnosis of intervertebral disc herniations, narrowing and swelling around the nerve and/or nerve roots, and compressive lesions.

72285–72295

Individual intervertebral discs are imaged and examined in diskography, also known as nucleography. Iodinated contrast medium is injected into the center of the disc. A series of images is taken by the radiologist and then interpreted and reported. This technique is used to determine the extent of the target disc(s) disease. Code 72285 refers to the cervical or thoracic discs and 72295 refers to the lumbar discs.

73000

Films are taken of the clavicle for a complete radiologic examination. The number of films is not specified. The patient is placed supine for a front to back (AP) view and the x-ray is directed to the midpoint and perpendicular to the clavicle.

73010

Films are taken of the scapula for a complete examination. The number of films is not specified. Anteroposterior (AP) and lateral views may be taken. The patient is placed supine for a front to back (AP) view and may be erect or recumbent for a lateral view. The arm is abducted to make a 90 degree angle to the body with the elbow flexed.

73020–73030

Films are taken of the shoulder. The patient is supine with the arm extended to a 90 degree angle from the body and externally rotated while the head is turned to face opposite the affected side. Code 73020 is for reporting one view only and 73030 specifies a minimum of two views.

73040

The synovial joint of the shoulder is visualized internally through arthrography, the direct injection of air and/or contrast material into the joint for radiological examination. Local anesthesia in injected into the joint followed by the contrast material and/or air. A series of images are taken and interpreted. Fluoroscopic films and guidance for needle localization is included. Arthrography helps diagnose conditions of cartilage abnormalities, arthritis and bursitis, rotator cuff tear, and frozen joint. AP (front to back) views are taken with the affected arm rotated externally and internally and with the arm in a neutral, flexed position lying over the abdomen.

73050

A radiologic examination is made of the acromioclavicular joints bilaterally, with no specified amount of views. The patient is placed in a sitting or standing upright position with arms at the side for an anteroposterior view. The patient may also be given weights to hold in each hand for weighted distraction radiographs of each joint.

73060

Two or more films are taken of the humerus with the x-ray beam aimed midshaft. The patient is supine with the hand also supinated for an AP view and with the hand rotated internally for an oblique view.

73070–73080

A radiologic examination of the elbow joint is made. Films of the elbow may be taken in the AP position with the hand supinated, oblique positioning with the hand pronated and/or externally rotated, and in the lateral position with the wrist lateral and the elbow flexed at 90 degrees. Code 73070 reports two views and 73080 reports a complete exam with a minimum of three views.

73085

The synovial joint of the elbow is visualized internally through arthrography, the direct injection of air and/or contrast material into the joint for radiological examination. Local anesthesia in injected into the joint followed by the contrast material and/or air. A series of images are taken by the radiologist and interpreted. Fluoroscopic films and guidance for needle localization is included. Arthrography helps diagnose conditions of cartilage abnormalities, arthritis and bursitis, and frozen joint.

73090

Two films of the forearm are taken with the x-ray beam aimed at the midforearm. Films may be taken in the AP position with the hand supinated, in the true lateral position and in oblique positioning.

73092

A minimum of two films of an infant's forearm are taken with the x-ray beam aimed at the midforearm. The infant or child must first be immobilized to prevent movement during the film taking. Films may be taken in the AP position with the hand supinated, in the true lateral position and in oblique positioning.

73100–73110

A radiologic examination of the wrist is made in either posteroanterior, oblique, or lateral views. Code 73100 reports two views only and code 73110 reports three or more views.

73115

The wrist is visualized internally through arthrography, the direct injection of air and/or contrast material into the joint for radiological examination. Local anesthesia in injected into the joint followed by the contrast material and/or air. A series of images are taken and interpreted. Fluoroscopic films and guidance for needle localization is included. Arthrography helps diagnose conditions of cartilage abnormalities, arthritis and bursitis, and frozen joint. The hand and wrist is placed in the posteroanterior (PA) position with the hand rotated outward and the x-ray beam aimed vertically at the wrist or with the hand and wrist in PA position with the beam aimed at the wrist from a few degrees below the elbow.

73120–73130

A radiologic exam of the hand is made with films being taken in either the PA (posteroanterior), internal or external oblique, or lateral positions. Code 73120 reports two views only. Code 73130 reports three or more views.

73140

Two or more views of the fingers (second through fifth digits, not thumb) are taken. The x-ray beam is aimed at the proximal interphalangeal joint for all positions, either back to front, external or internal oblique, or lateral views.

73200–73202

Computerized axial tomography directs multiple narrow beams of x-rays around the body structure being studied and uses computer imaging to produce thin cross-sectional views of various layers (or slices) of the body. It is useful for the evaluation of trauma, tumor, and foreign bodies as CT is able to visualize soft tissue as well as bones. Patients are required to remain motionless during the study and sedation may need to be administered as well as a contrast medium for image enhancement. These codes report an exam of the upper extremity. Report 73200 if no contrast is used. Report 73201 if performed with contrast and 73202 if performed first without contrast and then again following the injection of contrast.

73206

Computed tomographic angiography (CTA) is a procedure used for the imaging of vessels to detect aneurysms, blood clots, and other vascular irregularities. The physician inserts a needle and then a guidewire into the artery through the skin. The physician feeds the guidewire to the area requiring study with the use of fluoroscopic guidance. The needle is removed and a catheter is threaded over the guidewire until it too reaches the study area. The guidewire is removed. Contrast medium is then rapidly infused at intervals, usually with an automatic injector, and the patient is scanned with thin section axial or spiral mode x-ray beams. Three-dimensional images are generated and postprocessing reconstruction is done at a workstation on the scanner. CTA also provides information unavailable with conventional angiography such as vessel wall thickness (mural thrombus) and the venous anatomy of a target organ and/or associated organs within the scan range. This code reports an exam of the upper extremity first without contrast material and then again following contrast injection, including image post-processing.

73218–73220

Magnetic resonance imaging (MRI) is a radiation-free, noninvasive, technique to produce high quality sectional images of the inside of the body in multiple planes. MRI uses the natural magnetic properties of the hydrogen atoms in our bodies that emit radiofrequency signals when exposed to radio waves within a strong electro-magnetic field. These signals are then processed and converted by the computer into high-resolution, three-dimensional, tomographic images. Patients with metallic or electronic implants or foreign bodies cannot be exposed to MRI. The patient must remain still while lying on a motorized table within the large, circular MRI tunnel. A sedative may be administered as well as contrast material for image enhancement. For upper extremity other than joint, report 73218 if no contrast is used; 73219 if performed with contrast; and 73220 if performed first without contrast and then again following the injection of contrast.

73221–73223

Magnetic resonance imaging (MRI) is a radiation-free, noninvasive, technique to produce high quality sectional images of the inside of the body in multiple planes. MRI uses the natural magnetic properties of the hydrogen atoms in our bodies that emit radiofrequency signals when exposed to radio waves within a strong electro-magnetic field. These signals are then processed and converted by the computer

into high-resolution, three-dimensional, tomographic images. Patients with metallic or electronic implants or foreign bodies cannot be exposed to MRI. The patient must remain still while lying on a motorized table within the large, circular MRI tunnel. A sedative may be administered as well as contrast material for image enhancement. For any joint of the upper extremity. Report 73221 if no contrast is used; 73222 if performed with contrast; and 73223 if performed first without contrast and then again following the injection of contrast.

73225

Magnetic Resonance Angiography (MRA) is a special type of magnetic resonance imaging (MRI) that specifically visualizes blood vessels and blood flow to evaluate vascular disorders within the structure being studied. Unlike CT, it does not rely on the absorption of x-ray energy. Magnetic resonance imaging uses the natural magnetic properties of the hydrogen atoms in our bodies that emit radiofrequency signals when exposed to radio waves within a strong electro-magnetic field. These signals are then processed and converted by the computer into high-resolution, three-dimensional tomographic images. Patients with metallic or electronic implants or foreign bodies cannot be exposed to MRI. The patient must remain still while lying on a motorized table within the large, circular MRI tunnel. A sedative may be administered as well as contrast material for image enhancement. This code reports an exam of the upper extremity.

73500–73510

One film only is taken of either the right or the left hip in 73500. Two or more films are taken for a complete study of either the right or the left hip in 73510. For a front to back (AP) view, the patient is placed supine with the toes on the affected side inverted. For a frogleg view, the affected hip is flexed with the knee bent.

73520

A minimum of two views are taken of each hip that includes a front to back view of the pelvic area. For a front to back (AP) view, the patient is placed supine with toes inverted. For a frogleg view, the knees are bent as much as possible with the soles of the feet touching each other.

73525

This code reports the radiological supervision and interpretation for hip arthrography. Using a fluoroscope, the physician marks the point of the femoral neck on the skin with ink. The femoral artery is palpated and marked as well to avoid inadvertent puncture. Skin traction may be applied to increase the space between the femoral head and acetabulum. The physician inserts a needle into the capsule (located by fluoroscope) and aspirates the synovial fluid for a culture check. After aspiration, a contrast agent is injected into the hip joint and the needle is removed.

X-rays are then taken with the hip in neutral, external, and internal rotation. A second set of x-rays may be taken following the hip movements.

73530

An x-ray is taken of the hip while on the operating table. The patient is supine with the knee on the unaffected side flexed and abducted away from the side to be studied.

73540

Two or more films are taken of an infant or child's pelvis and hips. The infant or child must first be immobilized to prevent movement during the film taking.

73542

Films are taken of the sacroiliac joint following arthrography, which involves injecting gas into the joint to visualize the cartilage and ligaments. This code reports only the radiological supervision and interpretation. If formal arthrography is not performed, recorded, and a formal radiologic report is not issued, use 76005 for fluoroscopic guidance for sacroiliac joint injections.

73550

Two films only are taken of the femur, or thigh bone, the longest and largest in the body. In either the front to back or lateral views, the x-ray beam is aimed at the midshaft. For the AP (front to back) view, the patient is supine with the foot turned inward a few degrees. For a lateral view, the patient is placed laterally with the knee flexed and the affected side down.

73560–73564

A radiologic examination of the knee is made in an AP (front to back) or lateral view. For an AP view, the patient is placed supine (lying on the back) and for a lateral view, the patient is placed in the lateral, lying position with the affected side down and the knee flexed. Code 73560 reports one or two views only. Use code 73562 to report three views and 73564 for a complete exam of the knee with a minimum of four views.

73565

An x-ray is taken of the knees bilaterally in a front to back (anteroposterior) projection while the patient is standing.

73580

The patient is placed supine (lying on the back) on an x-ray table with the knee flexed over a small pillow. The knee is cleansed with Betadine and covered with a sterile drape. A skin anesthetic may be applied. The physician then passes a 20-gauge needle into the femoropatellar space. Air and a contrast agent is then injected. After the injection, the patient is asked to move the knee to produce an even coating of the joint

structures. Multiple x-rays are then taken of the knee. This code reports the radiological supervision and interpretation only. Use a separately reportable code for the arthrography.

73590

Two films of the lower leg bones are taken. The physician interprets and reports the findings.

73592

Two or more films are taken of an infant's right or left lower extremity. The infant or child must first be immobilized to prevent movement during the film taking. The physician interprets and reports the findings.

73600–73610

Two films are taken of the ankle in 73600 and a complete radiologic exam of the ankle is performed in 73610 with three or more films taken. The codes do not specify that a specific view must be performed. The physician interprets and reports the findings.

73615

The physician injects radiopaque fluid into the ankle for arthrography. The physician inserts a needle into the joint and aspirates if necessary. Opaque contrast solution is injected into the ankle and the needle is removed. Films are then taken of the ankle. This code reports the radiological supervision and interpretation only. Use a separately reportable code for the injection.

73620–73630

Two films are taken of the foot in 73620 and a complete radiologic exam of the foot is performed in 73630 with three or more films taken. The codes do not specify that a specific view must be performed. The physician interprets and reports the findings.

73650

Two or more films are taken of the calcaneous or heel bone. The physician interprets and reports the findings.

73660

Two or more films are taken of the toes. The physician interprets and reports the findings.

73700–73702

Computerized axial tomography directs multiple narrow beams of x-rays around the body structure being studied and uses computer imaging to produce thin cross-sectional views of various layers (or slices) of the body. It is useful for the evaluation of trauma, tumor, and foreign bodies as CT is able to visualize soft tissue as well as bones. Patients are required to remain motionless during the study and sedation may need to be administered as well as a contrast medium for image enhancement. These codes report an exam of the lower extremity. Report 73700 if no contrast is used. Report 73701 if performed with contrast and 73702 if performed first without contrast and then again following the injection of contrast.

73706
Computed tomographic angiography (CTA) is a procedure used for the imaging of vessels to detect aneurysms, blood clots, and other vascular irregularities. The physician inserts a needle and then a guidewire into the artery through the skin. The physician feeds the guidewire to the area requiring study with the use of fluoroscopic guidance. The needle is removed and a catheter is threaded over the guidewire until it too reaches the study area. The guidewire is removed. Contrast medium is then rapidly infused at intervals, usually with an automatic injector, and the patient is scanned with thin section axial or spiral mode x-ray beams. Three-dimensional images are generated and postprocessing reconstruction is done at a workstation on the scanner. CTA also provides information unavailable with conventional angiography such as vessel wall thickness (mural thrombus) and the venous anatomy of a target organ and/or associated organs within the scan range. This code reports an exam of the lower extremity first without contrast material and then again following contrast injection, including image post-processing.

73718–73720
Magnetic resonance imaging (MRI) is a radiation-free, noninvasive, technique to produce high quality sectional images of the inside of the body in multiple planes. MRI uses the natural magnetic properties of the hydrogen atoms in our bodies that emit radiofrequency signals when exposed to radio waves within a strong electro-magnetic field. These signals are then processed and converted by the computer into high-resolution, three-dimensional, tomographic images. Patients with metallic or electronic implants or foreign bodies cannot be exposed to MRI. The patient must remain still while lying on a motorized table within the large, circular MRI tunnel. A sedative may be administered as well as contrast material for image enhancement. For lower extremity other than joint, report 73718 if no contrast is used; 73719 if performed with contrast; and 73720 if performed first without contrast and then again following the injection of contrast.

73721–73723
Magnetic resonance imaging (MRI) is a radiation-free, noninvasive, technique to produce high quality sectional images of the inside of the body in multiple planes. MRI uses the natural magnetic properties of the hydrogen atoms in our bodies that emit radiofrequency signals when exposed to radio waves within a strong electro-magnetic field. These signals are then processed and converted by the computer into high-resolution, three-dimensional, tomographic images. Patients with metallic or electronic implants

or foreign bodies cannot be exposed to MRI. The patient must remain still while lying on a motorized table within the large, circular MRI tunnel. A sedative may be administered as well as contrast material for image enhancement. For any joint of the lower extremity, report 73721 if no contrast is used; 73722 if performed with contrast; and 73723 if performed first without contrast and then again following the injection of contrast.

73725
Magnetic Resonance Angiography (MRA) is a special type of magnetic resonance imaging (MRI) that specifically visualizes blood vessels and blood flow to evaluate vascular disorders within the structure being studied. Unlike CT, it does not rely on the absorption of x-ray energy. Magnetic resonance imaging uses the natural magnetic properties of the hydrogen atoms in our bodies that emit radiofrequency signals when exposed to radio waves within a strong electro-magnetic field. These signals are then processed and converted by the computer into high-resolution, three-dimensional tomographic images. Patients with metallic or electronic implants or foreign bodies cannot be exposed to MRI. The patient must remain still while lying on a motorized table within the large, circular MRI tunnel. A sedative may be administered as well as contrast material for image enhancement. This code reports an exam of the lower extremity.

74000
Films are taken of the abdominal cavity in one view from front to back. Because an abdominal x-ray usually precedes another diagnostic imaging procedure, it is not coded separately unless performed as a separately identifiable examination.

74010
Films are taken of the abdominal cavity from front to back, with an oblique view and a focused (coned down or spot) view. Because an abdominal x-ray usually precedes another diagnostic imaging procedure, it is not coded separately unless performed as a separately identifiable examination.

74020
Films are taken of the abdominal cavity from front to back, back to front, or front to back with the patient lying on the side and/or standing. Because an abdominal x-ray usually precedes another diagnostic imaging procedure, it is not coded separately unless performed as a separately identifiable examination.

74022
Films are taken of the abdominal cavity with the patient lying flat, standing, and/or lying on the side. This procedure includes an upright chest x-ray. Because an abdominal x-ray usually precedes another diagnostic imaging procedure, it is not coded separately unless performed as a separately identifiable examination.

74150–74170

Computerized axial tomography directs multiple thin beams of x-rays at the body structure being studied and uses computer imaging to produce thin cross-sectional views of various layers (or slices) of the body. It is useful for the evaluation of trauma, tumor, and foreign bodies as CT is able to visualize soft tissue as well as bones. Patients are required to remain motionless during the study and sedation may need to be administered as well as a contrast medium for image enhancement. These codes report an exam of the abdomen. Report 74150 if no contrast is used. Report 74160 if performed with contrast and 74170 if performed first without contrast and then again following the injection of contrast.

74175

Computed tomographic angiography (CTA) is a procedure used for the imaging of vessels. CTA of the abdomen may detect aneurysms, thrombosis, and ischemia in the arteries supplying blood to the digestive system as well as locate gastrointestinal bleeding. The physician inserts a needle and then a guidewire into the artery through the skin. The physician feeds the guidewire to the area requiring study with the use of fluoroscopic guidance. The needle is removed and a catheter is threaded over the guidewire until it too reaches the study area. The guidewire is removed. Contrast medium is then rapidly and regularly infused, usually with an automatic injector, and the patient is scanned with thin section axial or spiral mode x-ray beams. Three-dimensional images are generated and postprocessing reconstruction is done at a workstation on the scanner. This code reports an exam of the abdomen first without contrast material and then again following contrast injection, including image post-processing.

74181–74183

Magnetic resonance imaging (MRI) is a radiation-free, noninvasive, technique to produce high quality sectional images of the inside of the body in multiple planes. MRI uses the natural magnetic properties of the hydrogen atoms in our bodies that emit radiofrequency signals when exposed to radio waves within a strong electro-magnetic field. These signals are then processed and converted by the computer into high-resolution, three-dimensional, tomographic images. Patients with metallic or electronic implants or foreign bodies cannot be exposed to MRI. The patient must remain still while lying on a motorized table within the large, circular MRI tunnel. A sedative may be administered as well as contrast material for image enhancement. These codes report an exam of the abdomen. Report 74181 if no contrast is used; 74182 if performed with contrast; and 74183 if performed first without contrast and then again following the injection of contrast.

74185

Magnetic Resonance Angiography (MRA) is a special type of magnetic resonance imaging (MRI) that specifically visualizes blood vessels and blood flow to evaluate vascular disorders within the structure being studied. Unlike CT, it does not rely on the absorption of x-ray energy. Magnetic resonance imaging uses the natural magnetic properties of the hydrogen atoms in our bodies that emit radiofrequency signals when exposed to radio waves within a strong electro-magnetic field. These signals are then processed and converted by the computer into high-resolution, three-dimensional tomographic images. Patients with metallic or electronic implants or foreign bodies cannot be exposed to MRI. The patient must remain still while lying on a motorized table within the large, circular MRI tunnel. A sedative may be administered as well as contrast material for image enhancement. This code reports an exam of the abdomen.

74190

A radiographic exam is done on the peritoneal cavity to define the pattern of air in the cavity after injection of air or contrast. The physician inserts a needle or catheter in to the peritoneal cavity and injects air or contrast as a diagnostic procedure. X-rays are then taken. The needle or catheter is removed. This code reports the radiological supervision and interpretation for a peritoneogram. Use a separately reportable code for the procedure.

74210

Films are taken of the pharynx, which is a muscular, membrane-type tube that extends from the base of the skull to the level of the sixth cervical vertebra, where it becomes one with the esophagus. It is the passageway for air from the nasal cavity to the larynx or voice box, and for food from the mouth to the esophagus. The pharynx is also referred to as the cervical esophagus. There are no number or type of views associated with this procedure.

74220

Films are taken of the esophagus, which is the muscular tube, about nine inches long, that carries swallowed foods and liquids from the pharynx to the stomach. Films are taken both before and after introduction of a contrast material consisting of barium sulfate. Hence, this study is also commonly referred to as a "barium swallow." Structural abnormalities of the esophagus and vessels, such as esophageal varices, may be diagnosed by use of this study. There are no number or type of views associated with this procedure.

74230

The pressure and duration of esophageal action, including that of the esophageal sphincter, is measured. The esophagus is the muscular tube, about nine inches long, that carries swallowed foods and liquids from the pharynx to the stomach and the sphincter prevents reflux of gastric acid into the esophagus. A topical anesthetic is applied to the patient's nose and a catheter is threaded into the nose and down through the esophagus. Pressure measurements are taken along the tube and recorded. The tube is then pulled slowly back into the esophagus and the lower esophageal sphincter pressure zone is measured. The patient swallows when the tube is in the esophagus and the contraction waves of the swallowing action are recorded.

74235

The physician uses an esophagoscope to locate and remove a foreign body from the esophagus. The physician passes either a rigid or flexible esophagoscope through the patient's mouth and into the esophagus. The foreign body is located. It may be suctioned, or grasped with forceps ad retracted through the scope. An alternative technique that may be used for objects too large to grasp is to pass a deflated balloon beyond the foreign body. The balloon is then inflated and withdrawn simultaneously with the scope and the foreign body. This code reports the radiological supervision and interpretation. Use a separately reportable code for the procedure.

74240–74245

Films are taken of the upper gastrointestinal tract in either an anterior oblique or lateral view. Breath is held during the film taking for either view positioning. This radiological exam helps diagnose neoplasms, ulcers, obstructions, and other diseases. 72420 is performed with or without delayed films and with or without KUB. 74241 is performed with KUB, which is a general x-ray of the midabdominal section. 74245 includes a radiologic exam of the small intestine in addition to the upper GI tract and multiple films taken in a series. The patient is placed prone (face down) for the small intestine films.

74246–74249

A radiologic exam is made of the upper gastrointestinal tract using fluoroscopy with a contrast material, known as barium swallow or barium "milkshake." This exam aids in diagnosing neoplasms, ulcers, obstructions, hiatal hernias and enteritis. The patient is strapped to the table and swallows the barium while standing upright in the vertical position. Throughout the exam, the table is then tilted at various angles for differing views from the fluoroscope. 74246 is done without KUB and 74247 is done with KUB, which is a general x-ray of the midabdominal section. For the small intestine follow-through reported in 74249, several hours must go by before the contrast medium reaches the point of study in the intestine. All codes may be performed with or without glucagon, which relaxes smooth muscle found in the GI tract and inhibits the muscle motility, thereby making better quality of images.

74250

A radiologic exam of the small intestine is done for which the patient is placed prone (face down) and x-rays are taken in a series of multiple films. The patient holds his or her breath during film taking.

74251

A radiologic exam of the small bowel is done by enteroclysis and taken in a series of multiple films. For enteroclysis, the physician inserts a tube through the patient's mouth and passes it down into the stomach and the small intestine. The tube is connected to a pump that sends barium through the tube for visualizing the GI tract and small bowel.

74260

X-ray films are taken of the duodenum and the pancreas to help diagnose tumors or lesions. A tube is passed through the nose, into the stomach, and on into the duodenum with guidance help from fluoroscopy. A drug for relaxing the duodenum is given and a contrast medium is pumped through the tube. Air may also be injected. X-rays are taken and the tube removed.

74270

A radiological exam of the large intestine is carried out after the administration of a barium enema to instill contrast into the colon. Fluoroscopy and x-rays are used to observe the image as the contrast fills the colon. This test helps to diagnose cancer, colitis, and other diseases. After the patient has emptied the colon, more films are taken. A general x-ray of the abdomen, known as KUB, may or may not be done.

74280

A radiological exam of the large intestine is carried out after giving the patient carbon dioxide producing granules and then barium to swallow. Fluoroscopy is used to observe the flow of the contrast medium and glucagon may or may not be administered. Glucagon relaxes smooth muscle found in the GI tract and inhibits the muscle motility, thereby making better quality of images.

74283

An enema of air or barium contrast is administered to reduce an intussusception or obstruction. An intussusception is a section of bowel that has slipped into another loop of bowel and can cause necrosis of the tissue, perforation and infection, even death. With the patient in position, the air or contrast is instilled into the colon through the anus to reduce the intussusception or clear the intraluminal obstruction.

74290

Oral cholecystography provides radiographic visualization of the gallbladder after the oral ingestion of a radiopaque, iodinated dye that comes in the form of pills. Adequate visualization of the gallbladder requires concentration of this dye within the

CPT® Lay Descriptions

gallbladder. On x-ray film, the biliary calculi (gallstones) are visualized as radiolucent shadows within a dye-filled gallbladder. Gallbladder polyps and tumors occasionally also can be seen as filling defects.

74291

Oral cholecystography provides radiographic visualization of the gallbladder after the oral ingestion of a radiopaque, iodinated dye that comes in the form of pills. Adequate visualization of the gallbladder requires concentration of this dye within the gallbladder. Occasionally, the gallbladder will not visualize after a single dose of dye tablets is ingested. In this case, the test should be repeated using a double dose, either on the same day or on another day. Should this situation occur, report this procedure for the additional or repeat study.

74300–74301

In intraoperative cholangiography, the common bile duct is directly injected with radiopaque material. The surgeon performs a cholecystectomy (removal of the gallbladder). Stones appear as radiolucent shadows. Gallstones, tumors, or strictures cause partial or total obstruction of the flow of dye into the duodenum. This code reports only the radiological supervision and interpretation. Since the surgeon performs the dye injection in an intraoperative cholangiogram, this is the only code that the radiologist can report for this procedure. 74301 is an add-on code and can not stand-alone. This code is used in conjunction with 74300, in the event that the surgeon would request another set of plain x-ray films to be taken during the operative session.

74305

Postoperative cholangiography is done through an existing catheter and is used to detect retained common bile duct stones after the gallbladder has been removed, and to demonstrate good flow of bile contrast into the duodenum. Radiopaque dye is injected through a T-tube, which is a device inserted into the biliary duct and brought out through the abdominal wall after bile duct exploration and removal of the gallbladder. It allows for drainage of the bile duct and for introduction of contrast medium for postoperative radiological study of the bile duct. This code reports only the radiological supervision and interpretation. The injection of the dye through the T-tube is reported separately.

74320

In percutaneous cholangiography, a radiographic medium is injected into the common bile duct for diagnostic purposes. The physician inserts a needle between the ribs into the lumen of the common bile duct and checks positioning by aspiration. This code reports only the radiological supervision and interpretation required in performing this procedure.

74327

The physician removes a stone from the biliary duct after previous surgery. The common bile duct is approached by placing a scope into the tract through a previously placed drainage tube (T-tube). Manipulating basket or snare tools through the scope, the physician removes the stone(s). This code reports only the radiological supervision and interpretation required in performing this procedure.

74328–74330

The physician performs an endoscopic retrograde cholangiopancreatography (ERCP) for diagnostic or therapeutic reasons. The physician passes the endoscope through the patient's oropharynx, esophagus, stomach, and into the small intestine. A smaller subscope may be fed up the sphincter of Oddi into the system of ducts that drain the pancreas (74329) or into the biliary ductal system that drains the gallbladder (74328), or both (74330). These codes report only the radiological supervision and interpretation required in performing this procedure to the respective extent of catheterization.

74340

A long, Miller-Abbott style gastrointestinal tube with a mercury-filled balloon at the bottom is introduced, usually nasally, and used to clear gastrointestinal strictures. The patient is seated lower than the person performing the procedure and the dilator is placed in the posterior pharynx. The patient swallows and the tube and balloon are carried into the small intestine. The balloon is then inflated and withdrawn until resistance is encountered. The balloon is then partially deflated, withdrawn a little more and re-inflated. This process is repeated several times to achieve dilation of the stricture. This procedure may be done without fluoroscopy or with fluoroscopy by instilling a diluted contrast into the balloon. This code includes the fluoroscopies, films, and radiological supervision and interpretation. Use a separately reportable code for the tube placement.

74350

A large needle with a suture is delivered percutaneously into the stomach through a small incision. The needle and suture material are snared endoscopically and withdrawn through the mouth. A gastrostomy tube is attached to the suture, drawn down to the stomach, and out the original incision. This code reports only the radiological supervision and interpretation required in performing this procedure.

74355

The physician places a tube in the jejunum for feeding through an abdominal incision. A section of proximal jejunum is selected and a tube is placed in the jejunum and brought out through the abdominal wall. This segment of jejunum is securely tacked to the inside of the abdominal wall. This code reports only the radiological supervision and interpretation required in performing this procedure.

74360

The physician passes a balloon dilator into the patient's mouth and uses a fluoroscope to place the dilator at the point of constriction. The balloon is briefly inflated several times until the area of narrowing is sufficiently enlarged. It is possible to use a guide wire to place the balloon. This code reports only the radiological supervision and interpretation required in performing this procedure.

74363

The physician advances an endoscope through an incision in the abdominal wall or an existing T-tube into the common bile duct. The biliary tract may be filled with contrast medium for identifying areas of abnormality, stricture, or obstruction in the common bile duct, biliary tree, and gallbladder. The physician advances a balloon-tipped catheter through the tract or T-tube so that it is above the site of the duct stricture, inflates the balloon, and draws it back through the stricture to achieve dilation. This may be repeated until optimum dilation is achieved. The physician may place a stent to prevent future stricture. This code reports only the radiological supervision and interpretation required in performing this procedure.

74400

Radiographic imaging of the kidneys and ureters is done before and after the administration of an intravenous contrast material to identify abnormalities of the kidneys and urinary tract. Abdominal films are first obtained and then the contrast medium is injected into a vein. Radiographs are again obtained while the contrast material is being excreted. This is also known as intravenous pyelography or IVP. This procedure may be done with or without KUB, a general abdominal x-ray, or with or without tomography, x-rays taken onto film moving opposite the beams to yield a single plane shadowless image.

74410–74415

Radiographic imaging of the kidneys and ureters is done immediately following either an infused intravenous drip or a rapid bolus injection of contrast agent. A front to back film of the abdomen is taken after contrast administration. Report code 74415 if done with nephrotomography, x-rays taken onto film moving opposite the beams to yield a single plane shadowless image. This can be used to check the patency of a nephrostomy tube.

74420

Radiographic imaging of the kidneys and ureters is done following retrograde (against the normal flow) administration of a radiopaque contrast material, usually barium sulfate. A catheter is passed up into the bladder and on through a ureter into the kidney.

The contrast material in injected through the catheter or tube. Films are taken to show the flow of contrast as it moves through the urethra and into the upper urinary tract. This may be performed with KUB, a general x-ray of the abdomen.

74425

A radiographic exam of the urinary tract is performed with injection or instillation of a contrast medium. This test is done to follow the normal flow of urine through the tract (antegrade) and may identify obstructions, abnormalities in the urinary tract, or asses function following surgery. Contrast medium is introduced percutaneously with a needle or though an existing tube, catheter, or stoma. For percutaneous needle injection, the skin is anesthetized and the needle inserted under fluoroscopic guidance into a calyx of the kidney. Contrast medium is injected and radiographs are taken. This code reports the radiological supervision and interpretation. Use a separately reportable code for the surgical procedure.

74430

A radiographic exam of the bladder with a minimum of three views is performed using contrast material to diagnose rupture, injury, or stress incontinence. A catheter is inserted into the bladder and contrast medium is then instilled using mild pressure injection. The catheter is clamped after the contrast medium has filled the bladder and the bladder is fully expanded. Films are then taken to observe any medium that is outside the bladder. The bladder is next drained and more films may be taken to look for other evidence of rupture following the flow of contrast outside the bladder. This code reports the radiological supervision and interpretation. Use a separately reportable code for the surgical procedure.

74440

A radiographic exam is done to determine obstruction in the epididymis, seminal vesicle duct, or vas deferens. Methylene blue is injected into the vas to test for obstruction of the ejaculatory duct. If during cystoscopy, dye is seen, the ducts are patent and vesiculography may be obtained to further determine obstruction. The vas is approached through an incision in the scrotum. The testis is freed and the vas separated. After a catheter is threaded into the vas, saline or lactated Ringers are instilled to determine patency or blockage. Flow resistance may require more formal vasography, with water-soluble contrast media instilled through a ureteral catheter fed to the seminal vesicles through a dilated vas.
Epididymography requires taking images of the coiled tube connecting the testis to the vas deferens. This code reports the radiological supervision and interpretation for epididymography, vesiculography, or vasography.

74445

Corpora cavernosography is performed to determine the area and degree of a venous leakage. The penis is anesthetized and prepped with sterile tubing attached to a pressure transducer that is connected to an infusion pump. Needles are inserted into the cavernosa and contrast material injected at a rate that will maintain a certain pressure so the penis can remain erect while the x-rays are taken. Fluoroscopy help to locate the leakage which is determined to be minimal, moderate, or diffuse. This code reports the radiological supervision and interpretation for the procedure.

74450

A radiographic exam of the urethra and bladder is performed using contrast material to diagnose strictures, obstructions and abnormalities, or as postoperative function assessments. It is most often performed on males. A balloon catheter is threaded into the urethra and the balloon is inflated. Fluoroscopy is used to aid in injecting the contrast medium through the catheter. Films are taken to show the flow of contrast as it moves retrograde (against the normal flow) through the urethra and into certain parts of the bladder. The bladder is next drained and more images may be taken of the urethra. This code reports the radiological supervision and interpretation. Use a separately reportable code for the surgical procedure.

74455

A radiographic exam of the urethra and bladder is performed using contrast material to evaluate voiding function. The patient first empties the bladder. A catheter is inserted through the urethra up into the bladder and any excess fluid is drained. Contrast medium is slowly instilled until it fills the bladder while the flow is observed via fluoroscopy. Films may be taken if reflux of medium is seen backing up into the ureters. Once voiding commences, the catheter is removed and the voiding function is imaged on films or video. This code reports the radiological supervision and interpretation. Use a separately reportable code for the surgical procedure.

74470

A renal cyst is studied using contrast medium by inserting a spinal needle into the affected kidney. With the patient placed prone (face down), the site for the puncture is identified with separate radiographic localization of the cyst and kidney. The skin of the puncture site is anesthetized and the needle is inserted and advanced to the kidney, while being observed on a fluoroscopic video monitor. Some of the cyst's contents are removed and a small amount of contrast is injected. This is repeated with films being taken intermittently throughout the process. When the entire cyst is filled with the contrast medium, more images are taken with the patient in various positions. This code reports the radiological

supervision and interpretation. Use a separately reportable code for the surgical procedure.

74475

The physician inserts a catheter or intracatheter percutaneously into the renal pelvis for drainage and/or contrast injection for radiographic studies. With the patient placed prone (face down)and the puncture site having been identified by separately reportable means, a local anesthetic is injected. A needle with a guidewire is slowly advanced into the kidney under fluoroscopic guidance. The needle is removed and the tract may be dilated to accommodate the catheter or nephrostomy tube which is fixed in place and secured also under fluoroscopic control. This code reports the radiological supervision and interpretation. Use a separately reportable code for the surgical procedure.

74480

The physician inserts a ureteral catheter or stent percutaneously into the ureter through the renal pelvis for drainage and/or contrast injection for radiographic studies. With the patient placed prone (face down)and the puncture site having been identified by separately reportable means, a local anesthetic is injected. A needle with a guidewire is slowly advanced into the kidney under fluoroscopic guidance. The needle is removed and the tract may be dilated to accommodate the ureteral catheter which is then inserted into the kidney pelvis and manipulated into and down the ureter until it reaches the bladder also under fluoroscopic monitoring. An internal stent will reside in the ureter and an external stent will have one end that remains outside the body. This code reports the radiological supervision and interpretation. Use a separately reportable code for the surgical procedure.

74485

A previously existing nephrostomy tract to the kidney and/or ureters, or urethra is dilated under fluoroscopic control. A series of dilators in increasing size are inserted into the nephrostomy opening, usually over a guidewire. A balloon may also be used. The ureters may be dilated by advancing the dilators through the nephrostomy tract or inserting them into the ureters from the bladder. For urethral dilation, a guidewire may be advanced through the urethral stricture and one or more catheters of increasing size placed over the guidewire. A balloon is then inserted and inflated until the stricture is dilated. This code reports the radiological supervision and interpretation. Use a separately reportable code for the surgical procedure.

74710

Although most abnormalities of the pelvis can be suspected by using clinical measurements, x-ray pelvimetry is the most accurate means of determining adequacy of the pelvic bony structures for a normal

CPT® Lay Descriptions

vaginal delivery. With pelvimetry, comparison is made with the capacity of the pelvis to the size of the infant's head, in order to discover any disproportion. However, radiographic pelvimetry is not used often in modern obstetrics because of the risks associated with radiation. This code is reported with or without locating the placenta.

74740

In hysterosalpingography, the uterine cavity and fallopian tubes are visualized radiographically after the injection of contrast material through the cervix. Uterine tumors, intrauterine adhesions, and developmental anomalies can be seen. Tubal obstruction caused by internal scarring, tumor, or kinking also can be detected. This code reports only the radiological supervision and interpretation. The injection portion of this study is reported separately.

74742

The physician introduces a catheter into the cervix, then takes it up into the uterus and through the fallopian tube to diagnose any blockages or to re-establish patency. The physician may elect to inject liquid radiographic contrast material into the endometrial cavity with mild pressure to force the material into the tubes (hysterosalpingogram). The shadow of this material on x-ray film permits examination of the uterus and tubes for any abnormalities or blockages. This code reports only the radiological supervision and interpretation. The introduction of the catheter into the fallopian tube is reported separately.

74775

The perineum, which is the area between the vulva and the anus in the female, is viewed to determine the sex of the patient. It is used mainly in cases where an infant is born with ambiguous genitalia. The procedure also may be used to check for an abnormal opening (fistula) between the vagina and bladder or the vagina and rectum. When locating a fistula, the use of contrast material is included.

75552–75553

Cardiac magnetic resonance imaging (MRI) is a radiation-free, noninvasive technique that produces high quality, detailed, three-dimensional imaging of complex congenital heart defects as well as functional cardiac analysis. MRI uses the natural magnetic properties of the hydrogen atoms in our bodies that emit radiofrequency signals when exposed to radio waves within a strong electro-magnetic field. These signals are then processed and converted by the computer into high-resolution images. Patients with metallic or electronic implants or foreign bodies cannot be exposed to MRI. The patient must remain still while lying on a motorized table within the large, circular MRI tunnel. A sedative may be administered as well as contrast material for image enhancement. Report 75552 for morphology imaging without

contrast and 75553 for morphology imaging with contrast.

75554–75555

Cardiac magnetic resonance imaging (MRI) is a radiation-free, noninvasive technique that produces high quality, detailed, three-dimensional imaging of complex congenital heart defects as well as functional cardiac analysis. MRI uses the natural magnetic properties of the hydrogen atoms in our bodies that emit radiofrequency signals when exposed to radio waves within a strong electro-magnetic field. These signals are then processed and converted by the computer into high-resolution images. Patients with metallic or electronic implants or foreign bodies cannot be exposed to MRI. The patient must remain still while lying on a motorized table within the large, circular MRI tunnel. A sedative may be administered as well as contrast material for image enhancement. Use 75554 to report a complete study for cardiac function, with or without morphology and 75555 for a limited study.

75556

Cardiac magnetic resonance imaging (MRI) is a radiation-free, noninvasive technique that produces high quality, detailed, three-dimensional imaging of complex congenital heart defects as well as functional cardiac analysis and blood flow. MRI uses the natural magnetic properties of the hydrogen atoms in our bodies that emit radiofrequency signals when exposed to radio waves within a strong electro-magnetic field. These signals are then processed and converted by the computer into high-resolution images. Patients with metallic or electronic implants or foreign bodies cannot be exposed to MRI. The patient must remain still while lying on a motorized table within the large, circular MRI tunnel. A sedative may be administered as well as contrast material for image enhancement. Use 75556 for reporting cardiac imaging to map the velocity of blood flow.

75600

A local anesthetic is applied over the common femoral artery. The artery is percutaneously punctured with a needle and a guidewire inserted and fed through the artery into the thoracic aorta. A catheter is threaded over the guidewire to the point of study and the guidewire removed. Contrast medium is injected and films are taken. This code reports the radiological supervision and interpretation. Use separately reportable code for the catheterization.

75605

A local anesthetic is applied over the common femoral artery. The artery is percutaneously punctured with a needle and a guidewire is inserted and fed through the artery into the thoracic aorta. A catheter is threaded over the guidewire to the point of study and the guidewire is removed. Contrast medium is injected and films are taken by serialography, producing a series of individual x-ray films. This code reports the radiological supervision and interpretation. Use a separately reportable code for the catheterization.

75625

A local anesthetic is applied over the common femoral artery. The artery is percutaneously punctured with a needle and a guidewire is inserted and fed through the artery into the abdominal aorta. A catheter is threaded over the guidewire to the point of study and the guidewire is removed. Contrast medium is injected and films are taken by serialography, producing a series of individual x-ray films. This code reports the radiological supervision and interpretation. Use a separately reportable code for the catheterization.

75630

A local anesthetic is applied over the common femoral artery. The artery is percutaneously punctured with a needle and a guidewire is inserted and fed through the artery into the abdominal aorta. A catheter is threaded over the guidewire to the point of study and the guidewire is removed. Contrast medium is injected into the abdominal aorta and a series of continuous films are taken of the contrast flow through the aorta and its runoff into the arteries of both legs. This code reports the radiological supervision and interpretation. Use a separately reportable code for the catheterization.

75635

Computed tomographic angiography (CTA) is a procedure used for the imaging of vessels to detect aneurysms, blood clots, and other vascular irregularities. The physician inserts a needle and then a guidewire into the artery through the skin. The physician feeds the guidewire into the abdominal aorta with the use of fluoroscopic guidance. The needle is removed and a catheter is threaded over the guidewire until it too reaches the aorta. The guidewire is removed. Contrast medium is then rapidly and regularly infused, usually with an automatic injector, and the patient is scanned by CT for images of the aorta and both lower extremities as the contrast runs down through the iliofemoral pathway. Three-dimensional images are generated and postprocessing reconstruction is done at a workstation on the scanner. This code is used to report the radiological supervision and interpretation for this procedure.

75650

A local anesthetic is applied over the common femoral artery, although other approaches may be used. The artery is percutaneously punctured with a needle and a guidewire inserted and fed through the artery into the aortic arch near the great vessels branching from it. A catheter is threaded over the guidewire to the point of study and the guidewire removed. Contrast medium is injected using a power injector into the aortic arch and a very rapid sequence of films are taken during the injection of the contrast flow

through the arch and the origin of the cervicocerebral arteries (left common carotid and common carotid and brachiocephalic on the right). This code reports the radiological supervision and interpretation. Use separately reportable code for the catheterization.

75658

A local anesthetic is applied over the puncture site. The artery is percutaneously punctured with a needle and a guidewire inserted and fed into the brachial artery. A catheter is threaded over the guidewire to the point of study and the guidewire removed. A retrograde (against normal flow) injection of contrast medium is done into the brachial artery and films are obtained. This code reports the radiological supervision and interpretation. Use separately reportable code for the catheterization.

75660

A local anesthetic is applied over the femoral, brachial, subclavian, or axillary artery. The artery is percutaneously punctured with a needle and a guidewire is inserted and selectively fed through the artery into the right or left external carotid. A catheter is threaded over the guidewire to the point of study and the guidewire removed. Contrast medium is injected and a series of x-rays is performed to visualize the vessels and evaluate any abnormalities, such as blockages, narrowing, or aneurysms. This code reports the radiological supervision and interpretation only. Use a separately reportable code for the catheterization.

75662

A local anesthetic is applied over the femoral, brachial, subclavian, or axillary artery. The artery is percutaneously punctured with a needle and a guidewire is inserted and selectively fed through the artery into the external carotid. A catheter is threaded over the guidewire to the point of study and the guidewire removed. Contrast medium is injected and a series of x-rays performed bilaterally to visualize the vessels and evaluate any abnormalities, such as blockages, narrowing, or aneurysms. This code reports the radiological supervision and interpretation only. Use a separately reportable code for the catheterization.

75665

A local anesthetic is applied over the femoral, brachial, subclavian, or axillary artery. The artery is percutaneously punctured with a needle and a guidewire is inserted and fed through the artery into the right or left (cerebral) carotid. A catheter is threaded over the guidewire to the point of study and the guidewire removed. Contrast medium is injected into the cerebral arterial system and a series of x-rays is performed to visualize the vessels and evaluate any abnormalities, such as blockages, narrowing, or aneurysms. This code reports the radiological

CPT® Lay Descriptions

supervision and interpretation only. Use a separately reportable code for the catheterization.

75671
A local anesthetic is applied over the femoral, brachial, subclavian, or axillary artery. The artery is percutaneously punctured with a needle and a guidewire is inserted and fed through the artery into the (cerebral) carotid. A catheter is threaded over the guidewire to the point of study and the guidewire removed. Contrast medium is injected into the cerebral arterial system and a series of x-rays performed bilaterally to visualize the vessels and evaluate any abnormalities, such as blockages, narrowing, or aneurysms. This code reports the radiological supervision and interpretation only. Use a separately reportable code for the catheterization.

75676
A local anesthetic is applied over the femoral, brachial, subclavian, or axillary artery. The artery is percutaneously punctured with a needle and a guidewire is inserted and fed through the artery into the right or left (cervical) carotid. A catheter is threaded over the guidewire to the point of study and the guidewire removed. Contrast medium is injected and a series of x-rays is performed to visualize the vessels and evaluate any abnormalities, such as blockages, narrowing, or aneurysms. This code reports the radiological supervision and interpretation only. Use a separately reportable code for the catheterization.

75680
A local anesthetic is applied over the femoral, brachial, subclavian, or axillary artery. The artery is percutaneously punctured with a needle and a guidewire is inserted and fed through the artery into the (cervical) carotid. A catheter is threaded over the guidewire to the point of study and the guidewire removed. Contrast medium is injected and a series of x-rays performed bilaterally to visualize the vessels and evaluate any abnormalities, such as blockages, narrowing, or aneurysms. This code reports the radiological supervision and interpretation only. Use a separately reportable code for the catheterization.

75685
A local anesthetic is applied over the femoral, brachial, subclavian, or axillary artery. The artery is percutaneously punctured with a needle and a guidewire is inserted and fed through the artery to the point of study suitable for imaging vertebral, cervical, and/or intracranial arteries. A catheter is threaded over the guidewire until it, too, reaches the point of study and the guidewire is removed. Contrast medium is injected and a series of x-rays performed to visualize the vessels and evaluate any abnormalities, such as blockages, narrowing, or aneurysms. This code reports the radiological supervision and

interpretation only. Use a separately reportable code for the catheterization.

75705
A local anesthetic is applied over the artery of access, usually the common femoral artery. The artery is percutaneously punctured with a needle and a guidewire is inserted and fed through the artery into the aorta. Under fluoroscopic guidance, a catheter is threaded over the guidewire to the aorta and advanced directly into a spinal artery suitable for viewing the study area. The guidewire is removed. Contrast medium is then injected in the lowest level first and then just above that in sequence and films are taken until the study has covered the entire area of interest. This code reports the radiological supervision and interpretation only. Use a separately reportable code for the catheterization.

75710
The arteries of one arm, leg, hand, or foot that are not normally seen in an x-ray are examined radiologically by injecting contrast material. A local anesthetic is applied over the area of access which could be femoral, brachial, subclavian, or axillary artery. The artery is percutaneously punctured with a needle and a guidewire inserted and fed through the artery to the point of study. A catheter is threaded over the guidewire until it, too, reaches the point of study and the guidewire is removed. Contrast medium is injected through the catheter and a series of x-rays or fluoroscopic images taken to visualize the vessels and evaluate any abnormalities such as blockages, narrowing, or aneurysms. The catheter is removed and pressure applied to the site. This code reports the radiological supervision and interpretation. Use a separately reportable code for the catheterization.

75716
The arteries of bilateral extremities such as both arms or legs, that are not normally seen in an x-ray are examined radiologically by injecting contrast material. A local anesthetic is applied over the area of access which could be femoral, brachial, subclavian, or axillary artery. The artery is percutaneously punctured with a needle and a guidewire inserted and fed through the artery to the point of study. A catheter is threaded over the guidewire until it, too, reaches the point of study and the guidewire is removed. Contrast medium is injected through the catheter and a series of x-rays or fluoroscopic images taken to visualize the vessels and evaluate any abnormalities such as blockages, narrowing, or aneurysms. The catheter is removed and pressure applied to the site. This code reports the radiological supervision and interpretation. Use a separately reportable code for the catheterization.

75722–75724
The renal artery on either the right or left side is radiologically examined using contrast material in

75722 and both renal arteries are examined in 75724. Patients with a renal complication are first well hydrated with a drip and given medications to protect the kidney from further damage by the contrast agent. A local anesthetic is applied over the access artery, usually the common femoral artery, which is percutaneously punctured with a needle. A guidewire is inserted and fed through until it reaches the renal artery. A catheter is threaded over the guidewire and the guidewire is removed. Contrast medium is injected and a series of x-rays or fluoroscopic images are taken to visualize the vessels and evaluate any abnormalities. If a flush aortogram is performed, the catheter is directed to the aorta and dye is injected as x-rays are taken to look for plaque build-up. The catheter is removed and pressure applied to the site. These codes report only the radiological supervision and interpretation for the procedure.

75726

An artery supplying the abdominal organ of concern is examined radiologically by injecting contrast material. A local anesthetic is applied over the area of access, usually the common femoral artery. The artery is percutaneously punctured with a needle and a guidewire inserted and fed through the artery to the point of study. A catheter is threaded over the guidewire until it, too, reaches the point of study and the guidewire is removed. Contrast medium is injected through the catheter and a series of x-rays or fluoroscopic images taken to visualize the vessels and evaluate any abnormalities such as blockages, narrowing, or aneurysms. If an aortogram is performed, the catheter is directed to the origin of the coronary arteries and dye is injected into them as x-rays are taken to look for plaque build-up. The catheter is removed and pressure applied to the site. This code reports the radiological supervision and interpretation. Use separately reportable code for the catheterization.

75731

The left or right adrenal gland, located on top of the upper end of each kidney is examined radiologically by injecting contrast material. A local anesthetic is applied over the common femoral artery. The artery is percutaneously punctured with a needle and a guidewire inserted and fed through the artery, the aorta, and then further into the renal artery. A catheter is threaded over the guidewire until it, too, reaches the point of study and the guidewire is removed. Contrast medium is injected through the catheter and a series of x-rays or fluoroscopic images taken to visualize the vessels and evaluate any abnormalities such as blockages, narrowing, or aneurysms. The catheter is removed and pressure applied to the site. This code reports the radiological supervision and interpretation. Use separately reportable code for the catheterization.

75733

The adrenal glands located on top of the upper end of each kidney are examined radiologically by injecting contrast material. A local anesthetic is applied over the common femoral artery. The artery is percutaneously punctured with a needle and a guidewire inserted and fed through the artery, the aorta, and then further into the renal arteries. A catheter is threaded over the guidewire until it, too, reaches the point of study and the guidewire is removed. Contrast medium is injected through the catheter and a series of x-rays or fluoroscopic images taken to visualize the vessels and evaluate any abnormalities such as blockages, narrowing, or aneurysms. The catheter is removed and pressure applied to the site. This code reports the radiological supervision and interpretation. Use separately reportable code for the catheterization.

75736

An angiogram is done on operative candidates for pelvic fixation to rule out retroperitoneal arterial bleeding. A local anesthetic is applied over the common femoral artery. The artery is percutaneously punctured with a needle and a guidewire inserted and fed through the artery into the study area in the pelvic region. A catheter is threaded over the guidewire until it, too, reaches the point of study and the guidewire is removed. Contrast medium is injected through the catheter and a series of x-rays or fluoroscopic images taken to visualize the vessels and evaluate for any transected or bleeding arteries. Embolization may be dictated by angiography results to hemorrhaging for definitive stabilization treatment. The catheter is removed and pressure applied to the site. This code reports the radiological supervision and interpretation. Use separately reportable code for the catheterization.

75741

A local anesthetic is applied over the site where the catheter is to be introduced; this is most often either the common femoral or internal jugular vein. The vein is percutaneously punctured and the catheter selectively manipulated through the vena cava, right atrium, and right ventricle into the left or right pulmonary artery. Contrast medium is injected and films are taken to visualize the vessels and evaluate any abnormalities, such as blockages, narrowing, or aneurysms. This code reports the radiological supervision and interpretation only. Use a separately reportable code for the catheterization.

75743

A local anesthetic is applied over the site where the catheter is to be introduced; this is most often either the common femoral or internal jugular vein. The vein is percutaneously punctured and the catheter selectively manipulated through the vena cava, right atrium, and right ventricle into the pulmonary arteries. Contrast medium is injected and films taken bilaterally to visualize the vessels and evaluate any abnormalities, such as blockages, narrowing, or aneurysms. This code reports the radiological supervision and interpretation only. Use a separately reportable code for the catheterization.

75746

A local anesthetic is applied over the site where the catheter is to be introduced; this is most often either the common femoral or internal jugular vein. The vein is percutaneously punctured and the catheter manipulated through to a point where the pulmonary arteries may be studied. Contrast medium is injected and films are taken to visualize the vessels and evaluate any abnormalities such as blockages, narrowing, or aneurysms. This code reports the radiological supervision and interpretation only. Use a separately reportable code for the catheterization.

75756

A local anesthetic is applied over the site where the catheter is to be introduced; this is most often either the common femoral or brachial artery. The artery is percutaneously punctured with a needle and a guidewire is inserted and fed through the artery to the internal mammary. A catheter is threaded over the guidewire to the point of study and the guidewire is removed. Contrast medium is injected and a series of x-rays performed to visualize the vessels and evaluate any abnormalities, such as blockages, narrowing, or aneurysms. This code reports the radiological supervision and interpretation only. Use a separately reportable code for the catheterization.

75774

This procedure reports each additional vessel studied after the basic, initial study. It involves manipulating the catheter into additional second, third, or higher order vessels within a vascular family and performing injection of contrast and taking additional films. This code is an add-on code and can not stand alone.

75790

A local anesthetic is applied over the site where the catheter is to be introduced; this is most often either the common femoral or brachial artery. The artery is percutaneously punctured with a needle and a guidewire is inserted and fed through the artery until it reaches the arteriovenous shunt created in the patient, usually in the upper extremity. A catheter is threaded over the guidewire to the point of study and the guidewire is removed. Contrast medium is injected and a series of x-rays taken to visualize the shunt and evaluate its function. This code reports the radiological supervision and interpretation only. Use a separately reportable code for the catheterization.

75801–75803

Vital blue dye is injected into the subcutaneous tissues for outlining of skin lymphatics. As soon as the lymphatic vessels are visualized by their blue color, the physician makes a small incision to gain access. The lymph vessel is cannulated with a needle and a fine catheter is attached. A small amount of dye is injected to ensure correct placement and the needle is advanced a few millimeters into the vessel. The needle and catheter are secured and dye is injected with a syringe. X-rays are made. 75801 reports the radiological supervision and interpretation for lymphangiography of an extremity on one side only; 75803 reports the radiological supervision and interpretation for lymphangiography of extremities on both sides. Use a separately reportable code for the injection procedure.

75805–75807

Vital blue dye is injected into the subcutaneous tissues for outlining of skin lymphatics. As soon as the lymphatic vessels are visualized by their blue color, the physician makes a small incision to gain access. The lymph vessel is cannulated with a needle and a fine catheter is attached. A small amount of dye is injected to ensure correct placement and the needle is advanced a few millimeters into the vessel. The needle and catheter are secured and dye is injected with a syringe. X-rays are made. 75805 reports the radiological supervision and interpretation for lymphangiography on one side only of the pelvic/abdominal region. 75807 reports the radiological supervision and interpretation for lymphangiography on both sides of the pelvic/abdominal region. Use a separately reportable code for the injection procedure.

75809

The physician injects contrast material through the skin into the reservoir of a peritoneal-venous shunt or directly into shunt tubing or reservoir with a needle. Shunt tubing is a drain to eliminate excess cerebral spinal fluid in cases of hydrocephalus. The tubing of a peritoneal-venous shunt drains the accumulation of fluids in cases of ascites into a major vein. The physician places the needle and injects radiologic dye. Pictures are taken to visualize the flow of contrast and check for effective drainage. This code reports the radiological supervision and interpretation only. Use a separately reportable code for the shuntogram injection procedure.

75810

The physician makes an incision in the lower left axilla. An 18 or 20-gauge sheath catheter is inserted into the middle of the soft, sponge-like tissue of the spleen. The splenic vein is visualized and the catheter is placed. 2.0-3.0 cc of radiopaque dye is injected per second, totaling about 15.0-20.0 cc of dye. X-rays are taken every second for about 12 seconds. The catheter is removed and the incision covered with a dressing. This code reports the radiological supervision and interpretation only. Use a separately reportable code for the splenoportography injection procedure.

75820–75822

The physician performs a radiographic study on the veins of either the left or right lower extremity in 75820 and of both lower extremities in 75822. A local anesthetic is applied over the site where the catheter is to be introduced; this is most often the common femoral vein. The vein is percutaneously punctured with a needle and a guidewire is inserted and fed through the vein to the point where dye will be injected. A catheter is threaded over the guidewire and the guidewire is removed. Contrast medium is injected and a series of x-rays performed to visualize the vessels and evaluate any abnormalities, such as blockages, narrowing, or aneurysms. In venography, contrast medium is injected into the catheter that has traveled to an area upstream of the site under investigation. These codes report the radiological supervision and interpretation only. Use a separately reportable code for the catheterization.

75825–75827

A local anesthetic is applied over a distal vein (typically antecubital, internal jugular, subclavian, or femoral) and the vein is percutaneously punctured with a needle. A guidewire is inserted and fed through the vein to the inferior vena cava in 75825 and the superior vena cava in 75827. The physician may slide an introducer sheath over the guidewire into the venous lumen before inserting a catheter. The catheter is inserted into the vein and threaded over the guidewire to the inferior (75825) or superior (75827) vena cava. The guidewire is removed. Contrast medium is injected and a series of x-rays performed to visualize and evaluate any abnormalities, such as blockages, narrowing, or aneurysms. In venography, contrast medium is injected into the catheter that has traveled to an area upstream of the site under investigation. These codes report the radiological supervision and interpretation only. Use a separately reportable code for the catheterization.

75831–75833

A local anesthetic is applied over the site where the catheter is to be introduced; this is most often the common femoral vein. The vein is percutaneously punctured with a needle and a guidewire is inserted and selectively fed through the vein until it reaches the desired location in the venous system. A catheter is threaded over the guidewire into the selected point in the vein and the wire is removed. Contrast medium for venography is injected through the catheter that has traveled to an area upstream of the site under investigation. X-rays are taken. Code 75831 reports the radiological supervision and interpretation only for venography of either the left or right renal vein and 75833 is used for both renal veins. Use a separately reportable code for the catheterization.

75840–75842

A local anesthetic is applied over the site where the catheter is to be introduced; this is most often the

common femoral vein. The vein is percutaneously punctured with a needle and a guidewire is inserted and selectively fed through the vein until it reaches the desired location in the venous system. A catheter is threaded over the guidewire into the selected point in the vein and the wire is removed. Contrast medium for venography is injected through the catheter that has traveled to an area upstream of the site under investigation. X-rays are taken. Code 75840 reports the radiological supervision and interpretation only for venography of either the left or right adrenal vein and 75842 is used for both adrenal veins. Use a separately reportable code for the catheterization.

75860

A local anesthetic is applied over the site where the catheter is to be introduced and the access vein is percutaneously punctured with a needle. A guidewire is inserted and advanced through the vein until it reaches the desired location in the venous system for imaging the sinus or jugular vein. A catheter is threaded over the guidewire into the selected point in the vein and the wire is removed. Non-ionic diluted contrast medium injected over approximately 30 seconds through the catheter that has traveled to an area upstream of the site under investigation. Images are acquired. This code reports the radiological supervision and interpretation only. Use a separately reportable code for the catheterization.

75870

A local anesthetic is applied over the site where the catheter is to be introduced and the access vein is percutaneously punctured with a needle. A guidewire is inserted and advanced through the dominant jugular vein until it reaches the desired location for studying the superior sagittal sinus, which is the primary venous drainage for the cranial vasculature. A catheter is threaded over the guidewire into the selected point in the vein and the wire is removed. Non-ionic diluted contrast medium is injected through the catheter that has traveled to an area upstream of the site under investigation. Images are acquired. This code reports the radiological supervision and interpretation only. Use a separately reportable code for the catheterization.

75872

In epidural venography, a needle is inserted into the epidural space of the spine while the patient is sitting in a position with the chin on the chest and the knees pulled up or positioned on the left side. A catheter is threaded over the needle until it reaches the epidural space around the spinal cord and the needle is removed. Contrast is injected into the catheter and radiographic pictures are taken. This is done on patients with a penetrating trauma to the area, or subarachnoid or parenchymal hemorrhage. This code reports the radiological supervision and interpretation only. Use a separately reportable code for the catheterization.

CPT® Lay Descriptions

75880

The physician introduces a needle or catheter through a puncture site in the skin into a peripheral vein. A guidewire is inserted and selectively fed through the vein until it reaches the desired location in the venous system for imaging the orbital veins. A catheter is threaded over the guidewire into the selected point in the vein and the wire is removed. Radiopaque dye is administered into the facial or frontal veins, and x-rays are taken to visualize the orbital veins and cavernous sinuses. This code reports the radiological supervision and interpretation only. Use a separately reportable code for the catheterization.

75885

A radiographic exam of the portal vein of the liver is done by inserting a needle through the abdomen. The patient's right side is cleansed and a local anesthetic given at the puncture site. A needle is inserted into the skin just under the ribs and diaphragm and advanced to the liver under fluoroscopic guidance. The needle is aimed at the portal vein and when blood returns from the needle, a small amount of contrast is injected to help confirm placement into the portal vein. When in place, a guidewire is inserted and a catheter follows. More contrast is injected, radiographs taken and intravenous, hemodynamic pressures in the portal vein are recorded. This code reports the radiological supervision and interpretation only. Use a separately reportable code for the catheterization.

75887

A radiographic exam of the portal vein of the liver is done by inserting a needle through the abdomen. The patient's right side is cleansed and a local anesthetic given at the puncture site. A needle is inserted into the skin just under the ribs and diaphragm and advanced to the liver under fluoroscopic guidance. The needle is aimed at the portal vein and when blood returns from the needle, a small amount of contrast is injected to help confirm placement into the portal vein. When in place, a guidewire is inserted and a catheter follows. More contrast is injected and radiographs are taken. This code reports the radiological supervision and interpretation only. Use a separately reportable code for the catheterization.

75889–75891

A local anesthetic is applied over the common femoral vein and a guidewire is then inserted and fed through until it reaches the hepatic vein. A catheter is threaded over the guidewire and the guidewire is removed. For wedged hepatic venography, the catheter is wedged into a small hepatic vein branch to approximate the portal pressure occurring in liver disease. For free hepatic venography, the catheter tip lies free in the hepatic vein. Correct positioning of the catheter is monitored by fluoroscopy. Contrast medium is injected into the vein and x-rays are taken. Report 75889 if this is done together with

hemodynamic evaluation in which blood movement through the liver is monitored by indwelling catheters connected to transducers. The pressure forces within the arteries and veins are then converted to electrical signals and displayed on screen. Report 75891 if hepatic venography is performed without the hemodynamic evaluation. These codes report the radiological supervision and interpretation only.

75893

Venous sampling involves withdrawing blood from a patient's vein into a vacuum tube. For parathyroid hormone or renin testing, a catheter is used for sampling. The catheter must be advanced through the abdominal aorta and into the renal arteries from an outside access point, usually the common femoral vein. When the catheter is correctly placed, several samples are withdrawn. This code reports the radiological supervision and interpretation only.

75894

A blood vessel is blocked by inserting an occlusive agent under fluoroscopic monitoring to stop or restrict the blood flow. This is done to restrict blood supply to a tumor, treat vascular malformations, or control hemorrhaging. A local anesthetic is given at the puncture site and a needle is inserted into the selected vessel followed by a guidewire. The needle is removed. A catheter is then inserted over the guidewire and advanced to the vessel requiring treatment. A blocking agent is carefully injected or inserted and monitored for the occlusion or restriction desired. The effect may remain permanent or require another transcatheter embolization with time. This code reports the radiological supervision and interpretation only. Use a separately reportable code for the catheterization.

75896

Blood flow in a vessel clogged by an obstruction such as a blood clot is re-established by transcatheter infusion. A local anesthetic is given at the puncture site and a needle is inserted into the selected vessel followed by a special catheter advanced within the blocked artery until its tip lies within the clot. A thrombolytic substance is infused continuously over intervals and the progress monitored using fluoroscopic images. Additional separate angiography may be done to assess vessel patency. This code reports the radiological supervision and interpretation only. Use a separately reportable code for the catheterization.

75898

Angiography is performed during or following transcatheter infusion or embolization through the existing catheter to reassess the therapy's effectiveness. A radiopaque contrast medium is injected through the catheter and by fluoroscopic images recorded of the vessel, the radiologist interprets the status of the blood vessel and the effectiveness of treatment rendered.

75900

During thrombolytic infusion therapy, the existing catheter is removed and replaced under fluoroscopic control. Contrast medium is injected for guidance. A guidewire is inserted over which the existing catheter is removed and the replacement catheter is threaded. The guidewire may then be removed or left in place. This code reports the radiological supervision and interpretation only.

75940

A filter is placed into the inferior vena cava percutaneously, usually through the right internal jugular vein. Fluoroscopy is used to monitor and guide the process. An incision is made just above the clavicle and then another small incision is made into the vein once it is identified. A catheter loaded with the filter is inserted into the vein and threaded through until it reaches the inferior vena cava. The filter is released from the catheter and opens to fill the diameter and grip the walls of the vena cava. The filter-loaded catheter may also be advanced over a guidewire to the vena cava after needle puncture of the internal jugular vein. This code reports the radiological supervision and interpretation only for this procedure.

75945–75946

An ultrasound is performed on the inside of a blood vessel previously treated for an obstruction or stricture. The ultrasound may be done during or after a therapeutic procedure such as dilation, stent deployment, or atherectomy. A special intravascular ultrasound catheter is threaded over an already placed guidewire to the study area and its external end is connected to the display monitor. Ultrasonic images of the vessel are displayed on the monitor and if satisfactory, the catheter is removed and the therapeutic procedure completed. Report 75945 for ultrasound on the initial, non-coronary vessel and 75946 for each additional (non-coronary) vessel studied beyond the initial. These codes report the radiological supervision and interpretation only.

75952

An infrarenal abdominal aortic aneurysm is repaired endovascularly using the skills of both a vascular surgeon and a radiologist. A small incision is made in the groin over one or both femoral arteries. Under separately reportable fluoroscopy, a synthetic stent graft contained inside a long plastic holding capsule is then threaded over a guidewire to the infrarenal aneurysm. Once the stent is in place, the holding capsule is released and the stent graft expands like a spring and anchors itself to the artery wall. A balloon catheter may be threaded to the graft site and inflated to help fully expand the prosthesis. The catheter is removed and the site closed. The aneurysm, excluded

from the blood flow, typically shrinks over time. This code reports the radiological supervision and interpretation only for this procedure.

75953

A leak, called an endoleak, may occur at fixation sites of a grafted aneurysm through the body of the graft or from patent arteries within the aneurysm sac and may require addition endovascular reparation. A proper extension prosthesis, contained within a long plastic holding capsule is threaded through the arteries over a guidewire to the site of the leak. Once the extension prosthesis is in place, the holding capsule is released and the extension prosthesis expands like a spring and anchors itself to the artery wall. A balloon catheter may be threaded to the graft site and inflated to help fully expand the prosthesis. The catheter is removed and the site closed. This code reports the radiological supervision and interpretation only for this procedure.

75960

A stent is introduced into a vessel requiring endovascular support either percutaneously or openly. For a percutaneous approach, a local anesthetic is applied over the puncture site and the skin is percutaneously punctured with a needle. A guidewire is inserted and fed through the blood vessel and the needle removed. A catheter with a stent-supporting tip is then advanced over the guidewire to the point where the vessel needs additional support. The compressed stent is passed off the catheter into the vessel where it deploys to support the walls. The catheter is removed and pressure applied. In an open approach, the skin overlying the vessel is incised and the stent-transporting catheter is inserted into the vessel after it is dissected and opened with a knife. After the stent is deployed and the catheter removed, the skin is closed in layers. This code reports the radiological supervision and interpretation only for this procedure.

75961

A foreign body such as the broken tip of a catheter within a blood vessel is retrieved. A local anesthetic is applied over the puncture site and the skin is percutaneously punctured with a needle. A guidewire is inserted and fed through the blood vessel and the needle is removed. A catheter with a grasping instrument (e.g., hook, loop, basket) is then advanced over the guidewire to the site of the foreign body. The instrument grasps the foreign body and it is withdrawn with the catheter. Pressure is applied over the puncture site. This code reports the radiological supervision and interpretation only for this procedure.

75962–75964

A narrowing or stricture of a peripheral artery is stretched to allow a normal flow of blood. A local anesthetic is applied over the access site, usually the femoral artery, and the skin is percutaneously punctured with a needle. A guidewire is inserted and fed through the blood vessel and the needle is removed. A catheter with a deflated balloon is then advanced over the guidewire to the narrowed portion of the vessel. The balloon is inflated to stretch the vessel to a larger diameter allowing a more normal flow of blood. Several inflations may be performed along the narrowed area. Transluminal angioplasty may be done through an incision in the skin overlying the artery of access. Vessel clamps are applied and then the artery is nicked to create an opening for the balloon catheter. Report 75962 for transluminal balloon angioplasty on one peripheral artery and 75964 for each additional peripheral artery treated after the first artery. These codes report the radiological supervision and interpretation only.

75966–75968

A narrowing or stricture of a renal or visceral artery (supplying organs in the abdominal/pelvic area) is stretched to allow a normal flow of blood. A local anesthetic is applied over the access site, usually the femoral artery, and the skin is percutaneously punctured with a needle. A guidewire is inserted and fed through the blood vessel and the needle removed. A catheter with a deflated balloon is then advanced over the guidewire to the narrowed portion of the vessel. The balloon is inflated to stretch the vessel to a larger diameter allowing a more normal flow of blood. Several inflations may be performed along the narrowed area. Transluminal angioplasty may be done through an incision in the skin overlying the artery of access. Vessel clamps are applied and then the artery is nicked to create an opening for the balloon catheter. Report 75966 for transluminal balloon angioplasty on a renal or other visceral artery and 75968 for each additional renal or visceral artery treated after the first artery. These codes report the radiological supervision and interpretation only.

75970

A biopsy specimen is obtained through a catheter. The biopsy catheter may be inserted through an already existing drainage tube or catheter, through a tract or pathway, such as the urethra during cystourethroscopy, or through the skin and into the access artery. Fluoroscopy is used to help guide the catheter through its course from whatever entry to the point of study to be biopsied. A biopsy brush, a fine biopsy needle, or biting forceps may be used through the catheter to obtain the cells or tissue for examination. This code reports the radiological supervision and interpretation only.

75978

A narrowing or stricture of a vein is stretched to allow a normal flow of blood. A local anesthetic is applied over the access site and the skin is percutaneously punctured with a needle. A guidewire is inserted and fed through the blood vessel and the needle is removed. A catheter with a deflated balloon is then

advanced over the guidewire to the narrowed portion of the vessel. The balloon is inflated to stretch the vessel to a larger diameter allowing a more normal flow of blood. Several inflations may be performed along the narrowed area. Transluminal angioplasty may be done through an incision in the skin overlying the access vein. Vessel clamps are applied and then the vein is nicked to create an opening for the balloon catheter. This code reports the radiological supervision and interpretation only for venous transluminal balloon angioplasty.

75980

The physician introduces a catheter into the liver to drain fluid using fluoroscopy and contrast to guide the process. The puncture site on the right side of the body is incised, the needle inserted between the ribs, advanced into the liver, and into the bile duct. Contrast medium is injected to visualize the intrahepatic bile ducts. A guidewire is inserted and advanced to the point of obstruction through an optimal duct permitting access and drainage. A catheter is threaded over the guidewire and dilators may be used to enlarge both the opening and the tract from the skin to the bile duct. The drainage catheter is then inserted and positioned at the obstruction and secured to the skin. This code reports the radiological supervision and interpretation only for this procedure.

75982

The physician introduces a catheter into the liver to drain fluid both internally and externally, usually on patients with inoperable bile duct obstruction. The puncture site on the right side of the body is incised. A needle is inserted between the ribs, advanced into the liver, and into the bile duct. Contrast medium is injected to visualize the intrahepatic bile ducts by fluoroscopy. A guidewire is inserted and advanced into the duodenum to bypass the inoperable obstruction. A catheter is threaded over the guidewire and dilators may be used to enlarge both the opening and the tract from the skin to the bile duct. The drainage catheter is then inserted and positioned so that openings for drainage are both above and below the obstruction and then secured in place. This allows bile to flow to an external drainage system as well as into the duodenum. This code reports the radiological supervision and interpretation only for this procedure.

75984

An existing percutaneous drainage tube or catheter is replaced with contrast monitoring. A guidewire is usually inserted into the existing catheter to guide the new one. The old catheter is removed and the replacement catheter is threaded back over the guidewire. Contrast injection allows for correct positioning to be visualized with fluoroscopic images displayed on screen. This code reports the radiological supervision and interpretation only for this procedure.

75989

Fluoroscopic, ultrasonic, or CT guidance may be used to locate and drain an abscess or obtain a specimen percutaneously and place an indwelling tube or catheter. Once the abscess is located, the skin is punctured with a needle to begin draining. A catheter may be advanced over a guidewire inserted through the needle and into the abscess cavity. The tract to the outside is dilated to facilitate placing a percutaneous drainage tube. The cavity is aspirated and the drainage tube placed at the lowest point to ensure complete drainage. The drainage tube is then secured to suction drainage. This code reports the radiological supervision and interpretation only for this procedure.

75992–75993

A stenosed peripheral artery is treated intraluminally to relieve blockage. A needle punctures the skin at the access site and is followed by a guidewire and an introducer sheath to protect and enclose the opening. A series of special catheters and guidewires are inserted until the narrowed, stenosed area has been transversed. Finally a special atherectomy catheter is manipulated to the study area and activated to cut or drill a channel through the plaque lesion and reopen the artery. Contrast medium is injected to fluoroscopically visualize the degree of luminal opening. The process may be repeated with a larger diameter catheter. Use code 75992 to report transluminal atherectomy on one peripheral artery and 75993 for each additional peripheral artery treated. These codes report the radiological supervision and interpretation only.

75994

A stenosed renal artery is treated intraluminally to relieve blockage. A needle punctures the skin at the access site and is followed by a guidewire and an introducer sheath to protect and enclose the opening. A series of special catheters and guidewires are inserted until the narrowed, stenosed area has been transversed. Finally a special atherectomy catheter is manipulated to the renal artery and activated to cut or drill a channel through the plaque lesion and reopen the artery. Contrast medium is injected to fluoroscopically visualize the degree of luminal opening. The process may be repeated with a larger diameter catheter. This code reports the radiological supervision and interpretation only for this procedure.

75995–75996

A stenosed visceral artery (supplying abdominal organs) is treated intraluminally to relieve blockage. A needle punctures the skin at the access site and is followed by a guidewire and an introducer sheath to protect and enclose the opening. A series of special catheters and guidewires are inserted until the narrowed, stenosed area has been transversed. Finally a special atherectomy catheter is manipulated to the study area and activated to cut or drill a channel through the plaque lesion and reopen the artery.

Contrast medium is injected to fluoroscopically visualize the degree of luminal opening. The process may be repeated with a larger diameter catheter. Use code 75995 to report transluminal atherectomy of one visceral artery and 75996 for each additional visceral artery treated. These codes report the radiological supervision and interpretation only.

76000

A radiologist provides separate fluoroscopic monitoring of the body for up to one hour for procedures that do not always include fluoroscopy as an integral component of the procedure. This is reported separately to describe the physician work entailed in providing fluoroscopic monitoring. If formal contrast x-ray studies are done and included as a part of the procedure to produce films with written interpretation and report, then fluoroscopy is already included and can not be separately reported.

76001

A radiologist provides fluoroscopic monitoring of the body for more than one hour while assisting a non-radiologic physician (e.g., nephrologist, pulmonologist). This is reported to describe the physician work entailed in providing fluoroscopic during procedures such as nephrostolithotomy and bronchoscopy. If formal contrast x-ray studies are done and included as a part of the procedure to produce films with written interpretation and report, then fluoroscopy is already included and can not be separately reported.

76003

Needle biopsy or fine needle aspiration is guided by fluoroscopic visualization. The entry point is anesthetized and punctured. A small incision may need to be made. A cutting biopsy or fine needle is inserted into the target area and the position reaffirmed by fluoroscopy. This is done for an internal mass or lesion that has been positively identified by other diagnostic imaging performed earlier.

76005

Spinal and certain paraspinal diagnostic or therapeutic nerve injection procedures (e.g., paravertebral facet joint nerve destruction, epidural or subarachnoid injections) are guided by fluoroscopy before and during catheter or needle insertion. The target structure is localized, the needle is placed and advanced, and the contrast injection is visualized under fluoroscopic monitoring.

76006

Films are taken of any joint under stress conditions applied by the physician to visualize characteristics of the joint that would not normally be seen on films taken in routine positioning. The physician puts on lead-lined gloves and forcibly holds the body part in the desired position to maintain stress on the joint while x-rays are taken.

76010

Children frequently ingest foreign objects that can be diagnosed by plain film radiography. A single view is taken of the gastrointestinal pathway from nose to rectum to locate a foreign body.

76012–76013

Percutaneous vertebroplasty is the procedure of injecting a substance, methyl methacrylate, into collapsed or diseased vertebra. This acts as a kind of bone cement to relieve debilitating pain resulting from osteoporosis, bone metastases, and hemangiomas. These codes report the radiological supervision and interpretation only for this procedure per vertebral body. Report 76012 if performed under fluoroscopic guidance and 76013 if done under CT guidance.

76020

Bone age studies are a way of estimating the stage of development or skeletal decline of a child based on an x-ray, usually of the nondominant hand and wrist. The x-ray is then compared to the bone structure standards equal to the child's chronological age. This allows for identifying growth failure and the need for treatment before the child's bones fuse, after which additional growth is not possible. For children under 3, films of multiple areas (e.g., wrist, knee, and foot) lead to greater accuracy.

76040

Bone length studies accurately measure the length of the long bones in the skeleton. Typically, four film exposures are performed during a scanogram, as it is usually called. Views of the hip, leg, knee, and ankle are usually taken. However, there are no number or type of views specified for this code.

76061

Various bones in the body are x-rayed. A limited study is reported when specific symptomatic sites are examined. This procedure is rarely performed to determine any spread of cancer, having been replaced by nuclear bone scanning, a more precise study for diagnosing metastases.

76062

A radiologic exam is performed in which the entire axial (head and trunk) and appendicular (extremities) skeleton is surveyed for evidence of metastatic disease. It may also be performed on children to identify current and/or old healed fractures in the case of suspected child abuse. This procedure is rarely performed for metastatic disease, having been replaced by nuclear bone scanning, a more precise study for diagnosing metastases.

76065

A radiologic exam is performed in which an infant's entire axial (head and trunk) and appendicular (extremities) skeleton is surveyed for evidence of current and/or old healed fractures in the case of

suspected child abuse or to identify signs of lesions due to leukemic infiltrates.

76066

A radiologic exam is done in which two or more joints are surveyed. A single view only is taken of the joints being examined. The joints surveyed require specification and are not delineated in the code.

76070

Bone mineral density studies are used to evaluate diseases of bone and/or the responses of bone disease to treatment. Densities are measured at the wrist, hip, spine, or calcaneous. The studies assess bone mass or density associated with such diseases as osteoporosis, osteomalacia, and renal osteodystrophy. This particular bone density study uses computerized axial tomography (CT) for the imaging modality.

76075–76076

Bone mineral density studies are used to evaluate diseases of bone and/or the responses of bone disease to treatment. Densities are measured at the wrist, hip, spine, or calcaneous. The studies assess bone mass or density associated with such diseases as osteoporosis, osteomalacia, and renal osteodystrophy. Dual energy x-ray absorptiometry (DEXA) is a two-dimensional projection system that involves two x-ray beams with different levels of energy. The results are given in two scores, which are reported as standard deviations from bone density of a person 30 years old, which is the age of peak bone mass. Use code 76075 to report DEXA of the hips, pelvis, or spine (axial skeleton) and code 76076 to report DEXA of peripheral bones such as the wrist or heel bone (appendicular skeleton).

76078

Bone mineral density studies are used to evaluate diseases of bone and/or the responses of bone disease to treatment. Densities are measured at the wrist, hip, spine, or calcaneous. The studies assess bone mass or density associated with such diseases as osteoporosis, osteomalacia, and renal osteodystrophy. Photodensitometry, or radiographic absorptiometry, provides a quantitative measurement of the bone mineral density of the cortical bone (outer layer) by taking two radiographs with direct exposure film at different settings. This procedure is done to monitor for gross bone changes as occurs with osteoporosis.

76080

An injection of radiopaque material is made directly into a sinus tract (a canal or passage leading to an abscess) or through a previously placed catheter, to determine the existence, nature, or size of an abscess or fistula (an abnormal tube-like passage from a normal body cavity to a free surface or to another body cavity). This code reports the radiological supervision and interpretation only.

76085

Digital mammography stores the electronic image on a computer. Images are recorded digitally, without film, and can be magnified and enhanced, providing better images of the breast tissues. For example, a radiologist can enhance a computerized image for a better view of a suspicious spot on a standard mammogram x-ray film. The result is that small tumors and other early signs of cancer can be detected when treatment may be more effective.

76086–76088

The physician performs an injection procedure for mammary ductogram or galactogram. A needle and cannula are inserted into the duct of the breast. Contrast medium is introduced into the breast duct for the radiographic visualization. A dissecting microscope may be used to aid in placing the cannula. The needle and cannula are removed when the study is completed. Report code 76086 for a single duct studied and code 76088 for multiple ducts. These codes report the radiological supervision and interpretation only for this procedure.

76090–76092

Mammography is a radiographic technique used to diagnose breast cysts or tumors in women with symptoms of breast disease or detect them before they are palpable in women who are asymptomatic. Mammography is done using a different type of x-ray than is used for routine exams that does not penetrate tissue as easily. The breast is compressed firmly between two planes and pictures are taken. This spreads the tissue and allows for a lower x-ray dose. Use code 76090 for a single breast and code 76091 for both breasts. Report code 76092 for both breasts done in an asymptomatic screening with two views taken of each breast.

76093–76094

Magnetic resonance imaging (MRI) is a radiation-free, noninvasive, technique to produce high quality sectional images of the inside of the body in multiple planes. MRI uses the natural magnetic properties of the hydrogen atoms in our bodies that emit radiofrequency signals when exposed to radio waves within a strong electro-magnetic field. These signals are then processed and converted by the computer into high-resolution, three-dimensional, tomographic images. Patients with metallic or electronic implants or foreign bodies cannot be exposed to MRI. The patient must remain still while lying on a motorized table within the large, circular MRI tunnel. A sedative may be administered as well as an IV injected contrast material for image enhancement. Report code 76093 for magnetic resonance imaging of either the left or right breast and 76094 for both breasts.

76095

A lesion in the breast is localized for biopsy. For the localization process, a movable arm holding the needle works together with the mammography unit that images the lesion from different angles at different fixed points. The mammogram information tells a computer where the coordinates are to correctly align the biopsy needle. Needle position is confirmed with more views taken and a stab incision made in the skin. The needle is then advanced to the lesion and additional stereotactic views confirm needle placement. This code reports the radiological supervision and interpretation only for this procedure.

76096

A needle localization wire is inserted into a breast lesion preoperatively under radiologic visualization in preparation for biopsy or removal. The skin is marked over the area of the lesion and mammograms performed. A needle with a hooked wire is inserted into the lesion from a perpendicular angle and advanced deep enough to remain within the lesion when the patient moves. X-rays are again taken to confirm needle placement within the lesion. Adjustments may need to be made. The needle is withdrawn while the hooked wire remains anchored. A short length of wire extends beyond the skin surface of the breast which is taped and covered. This code reports the radiological supervision and interpretation only for this procedure.

76098

Immediately after removal of the suspected breast lesion and the localization wire, the specimen is sent to be examined so the surgeon may complete the operative procedure. The sample is compressed and an x-ray taken to identify that it is the suspected lesion and the information is immediately returned to the surgeon.

76100

A radiological exam is done on a body section in a single plane by scanning an x-ray beam across the body in one direction to take pictures of the structures under study in the selected plane. The films show detailed images of the structures within the single selected plane by blurring out the images above and below. Use this code for a single plane radiological exam of a single body section other than urography.

76120–76125

Cineradiography uses high speed x-ray films to take a series of images of an organ or system in motion such as the vocal cords or heart. These images taken in exposure ranges of nanoseconds to milliseconds are like the individual frames of a motion picture. This allows the movement to be frozen and tracked very minutely to gather information about time-varying characteristics. Use code 76120 when performed alone and not specifically included as part of the procedure. Use code 76125 when cineradiography is performed in conjunction with a routine exam.

76140

A radiologist provides a consultation on an x-ray exam that was taken elsewhere and provides a written report.

76150

Xeroradiography produces an image on paper instead of on film. An electrically charged photosensitive plate is placed on one side of the patient and the x-ray beam is directed from the other. After exposure, charge patterns of tissue density and absorption are left on the plate which is then dusted with a colored, negatively-charged powdered toner. A blue-on-white picture is then able to be transferred to a sheet of paper covered with plastic. This test aids in detecting foreign bodies within soft tissue.

76350

Subtraction in conjunction with contrast studies is a technique whereby any subsequent images visualized after introduction of a contrast material are taken out or subtracted from the main picture or data to be studied, such as subtracting out bone in order to enhance the vasculature in angiogram studies.

76355

For stereotactic localization, a movable arm holding a needle is guided by computerized tomography (CT) to locate the lesion from different angles at different fixed points. The CT images tell the computer where the coordinates are to correctly align the needle.

76360

Computerized axial tomography (CT) is used for guiding needle biopsies. CT scanning directs multiple narrow beams of x-rays around the body structure(s) being studied and uses computer imaging to produce thin cross-sectional views of various layers (or slices) of the body. It is able to visualize soft tissue as well as bones. Patients are required to remain motionless during the study. Once the exact needle entry site is determined along with the depth of the lesion, the optimal route from the skin to the lesion is decided. The needle is inserted and advanced to the lesion and another CT scan image is done to confirm placement for the biopsy. This code reports the radiological supervision and interpretation only for this procedure.

76362

The patient receives intravenous pain medication and sedation. Grounding pads are placed on the patient's thigh. A needle-electrode with an insulated shaft and a noninsulated distal tip is inserted through the skin and directly into the tissue to be ablated. Computerized axial tomography (CT) is used to guide the needle to the correct spot and to monitor treatment. Each treatment session has about 10 to 15 minutes of active ablation. The energy at the needle tip causes ionic agitation and frictional heat in the surrounding tissue which leads to cell death and coagulative necrosis. This results in a 3 to 5

centimeter sphere of dead tissue per treatment session. In large tumors, the physician may create more than one sphere next to each other to try to turn the tumor edges in three dimensions. A small margin of normal tissue next to tumors is also burned. The dead tumor cells are not removed, but are gradually replaced by fibrosis and scar tissue. This code reports the CT guidance and monitoring of the ablation procedure.

76370

Computerized axial tomography (CT) is used in guiding the placement of radiation therapy fields. CT scanning directs multiple narrow beams of x-rays around the body structure(s) being studied and uses computer imaging to produce thin cross-sectional views of various layers (or slices) of the body. It is able to visualize soft tissue as well as bones. Patients are required to remain motionless during the study. Cross-sectional images of both normal and abnormal tissue structures are obtained and the treatment field area volume is determined. The normal tissues surrounding the treatment area are also defined. Acquiring this data is an important step in planning the patient's radiation treatment.

76375

In CT scanning, when multiple thin beams of x-rays are directed around the body structure(s) being studied, thin cross-sectional views of various layers (or slices) of the body are produced. These different slices through the study area must be combined using a computerized algorithm to reconstruct them into a three-dimensional image. In MRI, cross-sectional planes of data through the study area are acquired by signals that different tissues send back when exposed to a strong electro-magnetic field. All of these planes must be stacked back together to produce the complete picture of the tissue being studied. This code reports the reconstruction of CT, MRI, or tomographic imaging modalities.

76380

Computerized axial tomography (CT) scanning directs multiple narrow beams of x-rays around the body structure(s) being studied and uses computer imaging to produce thin cross-sectional views of various layers (or slices) of the body. It is able to visualize soft tissue as well as bones. This code reports a limited or a localized follow-up study.

76390

Magnetic resonance spectroscopy (MRS) is used for diagnosing several types of brain disorders including epilepsy, age degeneration, neoplasms, and stroke. MRS differs from MRI in that spectroscopy provides information about metabolic and biochemical processes occurring in the tissue as opposed to the anatomical or physiological conditions. A sample of tissue is placed in a spectrometer, a container filled with liquid nitrogen and liquid helium, and is spun while a generator sends bursts of short radio waves into the sample. The waves are absorbed, sent through the sample, and transmitted to a receiver into a computer which then translates and analyzes the signal.

76393

Magnetic resonance is used for guiding needle placement required for procedures such as breast biopsies, needle aspirations, injections, or placing localizing devices. Magnetic resonance imaging (MRI) is a radiation-free, noninvasive, technique that produces high quality images. MRI uses the natural magnetic properties of the hydrogen atoms in our bodies that emit radiofrequency signals when exposed to radio waves within a strong electro-magnetic field. These signals are then processed and converted by the computer into high-resolution, three-dimensional, tomographic images. Some methods for magnetic resonance needle placement include coating the needle with contrast material, placing metallic ringlets along the needle, or using a receiving coil in the tip of the needle. This code reports the radiological supervision and interpretation only for this procedure.

76394

The patient receives intravenous pain medication and sedation. Grounding pads are placed on the patient's thigh. A needle-electrode with an insulated shaft and a noninsulated distal tip is inserted through the skin and directly into the tissue to be ablated. Magnetic resonance imaging (MRI) is used to guide the needle to the correct spot and to monitor treatment. Each treatment session has about 10 to 15 minutes of active ablation. The energy at the needle tip causes ionic agitation and frictional heat in the surrounding tissue which leads to cell death and coagulative necrosis. This results in a 3 to 5 centimeter sphere of dead tissue per treatment session. In large tumors, the physician may create more than one sphere next to each other to try to turn the tumor edges in three dimensions. A small margin of normal tissue next to tumors is also burned. The dead tumor cells are not removed, but are gradually replaced by fibrosis and scar tissue. This code reports the magnetic resonance guidance and monitoring of the ablation procedure.

76400

Magnetic resonance imaging (MRI) is a radiation-free, noninvasive, technique to produce high quality sectional images of the inside of the body in multiple planes. MRI uses the natural magnetic properties of the hydrogen atoms in our bodies that emit radiofrequency signals when exposed to radio waves within a strong electro-magnetic field. The signals are transformed into images based on the differing densities of tissues. Bone marrow contains fat cells, with a high water content, and nonfat cells. MRI can give information about early changes in the marrow of the bone and the medullary cavity's composition and distribution of red and yellow marrow cells to

evaluate for avascular necrosis of bone. Metastatic tumors are visualized directly because of the differences in signal intensity between normal bone marrow and tumor tissue.

76490

The patient receives intravenous pain medication and sedation. Grounding pads are placed on the patient's thigh. A needle-electrode with an insulated shaft and a noninsulated distal tip is inserted through the skin and directly into the tissue to be ablated. Ultrasound is used to guide the needle to the correct spot and to monitor treatment. Each treatment session has about 10 to 15 minutes of active ablation. The energy at the needle tip causes ionic agitation and frictional heat in the surrounding tissue which leads to cell death and coagulative necrosis. This results in a 3 to 5 centimeter sphere of dead tissue per treatment session. In large tumors, the physician may create more than one sphere next to each other to try to turn the tumor edges in three dimensions. A small margin of normal tissue next to tumors is also burned. The dead tumor cells are not removed, but are gradually replaced by fibrosis and scar tissue. This code reports the ultrasound guidance and monitoring of the ablation procedure.

76506

Echoencephalography is done to determine ventricular size, investigate suspected fluid masses or other intracranial abnormalities, and define cerebral contents. During the test, the radiation technician guides the transducer over the area of the brain to be examined. The transducer sends an ultrasound beam through the tissue. The reflected sound waves are converted into electrical impulses and displayed on a video screen for interpretation or photographing for later interpretation. Abnormal results may indicate cerebral edema, lesions, or subdural and extradural hemorrhage. The gray (Gy) scale refers to the amount of energy absorbed by the tissue. The terms real-time, A-mode, B-scan, and M-mode describe the imaging methods used in performing the procedures. B-scan is a two-dimensional scanning procedure with two-dimensional display. Real-time scan is a two-dimensional scanning procedure with display of both two-dimensional structure and motion with time. A-mode is a one-dimensional measurement procedure.

76511

A-scan uses ultrasonography, or echography, to image intraocular anatomy or to differentiate orbital disease. High-frequency sound waves are introduced into the eye in a straight line by a transducer placed on the eye. As the waves reflect off the eye tissue, they are also picked up by the same transducer, converted to electrical pulses and displayed on screen. The resulting single-dimensional image is composed of vertical spikes that vary according to the tissue density. This code reports diagnostic ophthalmic ultrasound with amplitude quantification.

76512

B-scan utilizes sound waves in a two-dimensional scanning procedure to display a two-dimensional image of the internal ocular structures. A transducer placed on the eye sends high-frequency sound waves into the eye which reflect back to a receiver, are converted into electrical pulses, and displayed on screen. B-scan can locate structures in the eye that may be obscured by cataract, hemorrhages, or opacities.

76513

B-scan utilizes sound waves in a two-dimensional scanning procedure to display a two-dimensional image of the internal ocular structures. A transducer sends high-frequency sound waves into the eye which reflect back to a receiver, are converted into electrical pulses, and displayed on screen. In the immersion method, the eye is maintained in direct contact with a water bath and the tip of the transducer is held just beneath the surface of the water, but not in contact with the eye.

76516–76519

A-scan uses ultrasonography, or echography, to image intraocular anatomy to determine the axial length of the eye (from the cornea to the retina) for calculating the power required for an intraocular lens implant. High-frequency sound waves are introduced into the eye in a straight line by a transducer placed on the eye. As the waves reflect off the eye tissue, they are also picked up by the same transducer, converted to electrical pulses and displayed on screen. The resulting single-dimensional image is composed of vertical spikes that vary according to the tissue density. Report 76516 for ophthalmic measurements by ultrasound echography and 76519 if intraocular power lens calculation is done.

76529

B-scan utilizes sound waves in a two-dimensional scanning procedure to display a two-dimensional image of the internal ocular structures and ultrasonically locate a foreign body in the eye. A transducer placed on the eye sends high-frequency sound waves into the eye which reflect back to a receiver, are converted into electrical pulses, and displayed on screen. B-scan can also locate structures or objects in the eye that may be obscured by cataract, hemorrhages, or opacities.

76536

Diagnostic ultrasound is an imaging technique bouncing sound waves far above the level of human perception through interior body structures. The sound waves pass through different densities of tissue and reflect back to a receiving unit at varying speeds. The unit then converts the waves to electrical pulses that are immediately displayed in picture form on screen. B-scan utilizes sound waves in a two-dimensional scanning procedure to display a two-dimensional image and real time scanning displays both two-dimensional structure images and movement with time. This code reports ultrasound, B scan and/or real time with image documentation, for the soft tissues of the head and neck (e.g., thyroid, parathyroid).

76604

Diagnostic ultrasound is an imaging technique bouncing sound waves far above the level of human perception through interior body structures. The sound waves pass through different densities of tissue and reflect back to a receiving unit at varying speeds. The unit then converts the waves to electrical pulses that are immediately displayed in picture form on screen. B-scan utilizes sound waves in a two-dimensional scanning procedure to display a two-dimensional image and real time scanning displays both two-dimensional structure images and movement with time. This code reports ultrasound, B scan and/or real time, for the chest, including the mediastinum.

76645

Diagnostic ultrasound is an imaging technique bouncing sound waves far above the level of human perception through interior body structures. The sound waves pass through different densities of tissue and reflect back to a receiving unit at varying speeds. The unit then converts the waves to electrical pulses that are immediately displayed in picture form on screen. B-scan utilizes sound waves in a two-dimensional scanning procedure to display a two-dimensional image and real time scanning displays both two-dimensional structure images and movement with time. This code reports ultrasound, B scan and/or real time, for the breast(s), unilateral or bilateral.

76700–76705

Diagnostic ultrasound is an imaging technique bouncing sound waves far above the level of human perception through interior body structures. The sound waves pass through different densities of tissue and reflect back to a receiving unit at varying speeds. The unit then converts the waves to electrical pulses that are immediately displayed in picture form on screen. B-scan utilizes sound waves in a two-dimensional scanning procedure to display a two-dimensional image and real time scanning displays both two-dimensional structure images and movement with time. Use code 76700 to report ultrasound, B scan and/or real time, for the entire abdomen and 76705 for a single quadrant or organ of the abdomen.

76770–76775

Diagnostic ultrasound is an imaging technique bouncing sound waves far above the level of human perception through interior body structures. The sound waves pass through different densities of tissue and reflect back to a receiving unit at varying speeds. The unit then converts the waves to electrical pulses that are immediately displayed in picture form on screen. B-scan utilizes sound waves in a two-dimensional scanning procedure to display a two-dimensional image and real time scanning displays both two-dimensional structure images and movement with time. Use code 76770 to report ultrasound, B scan and/or real time, for a complete retroperitoneal exam and 76775 for a limited retroperitoneal exam.

76778

Diagnostic ultrasound is an imaging technique bouncing sound waves far above the level of human perception through interior body structures. The sound waves pass through different densities of tissue and reflect back to a receiving unit at varying speeds. The unit then converts the waves to electrical pulses that are immediately displayed in picture form on screen. B-scan utilizes sound waves in a two-dimensional scanning procedure to display a two-dimensional image and real time scanning displays both two-dimensional structure images and movement with time. Duplex studies combine real time with Doppler, which uses the frequency shifts of the emitted waves against their echoes to measure velocity, such as for blood flow. This code reports ultrasound of a transplanted kidney, with or without duplex Doppler studies.

76800

Diagnostic ultrasound is an imaging technique bouncing sound waves far above the level of human perception through interior body structures. The sound waves pass through different densities of tissue and reflect back to a receiving unit at varying speeds. The unit then converts the waves to electrical pulses that are immediately displayed in picture form on screen. Ultrasonography of the spinal canal and its contents includes imaging of the spinal cord, the vertebrae, and the intervertebral discs.

76805–76816

Diagnostic ultrasound is an imaging technique bouncing sound waves far above the level of human perception through interior body structures. The sound waves pass through different densities of tissue and reflect back to a receiving unit at varying speeds. The unit then converts the waves to electrical pulses that are immediately displayed in picture form on screen. B-scan utilizes sound waves in a two-dimensional scanning procedure to display a two-dimensional image and real time scanning displays both two-dimensional structure images and movement with time. Use code 76805 to report ultrasound, B scan and/or real time, on a pregnant uterus, complete, with both fetal and maternal evaluation. Use code 76810 for a complete exam, multiple gestation, after the first trimester; code 76815 for a limited evaluation, (fetal size, position, or

placental location); and code 76816 for a follow-up or repeat evaluation.

76818–76819

The health of a term or near-term fetus is assessed using ultrasound to monitor the fetus' movements, tone, and breathing, as well as to check amniotic fluid volume. The fetal heart rate is also monitored electronically in a biophysical profile. The physician conducts a non-stress test which monitors the baby's heart rate over a period of 20 minutes or more to look for accelerations with the baby's movement. Report 76819 if the fetal profile is done without non-stress testing.

76825–76826

Diagnostic ultrasound is an imaging technique bouncing sound waves far above the level of human perception through interior body structures. The sound waves pass through different densities of tissue and reflect back to a receiving unit at varying speeds. The unit then converts the waves to electrical pulses that are immediately displayed in picture form on screen. These codes report fetal echocardiography, real time, with or without M-mode recording. Real time scanning displays both two-dimensional structure images and movement with time. M-mode is a single dimension method of recording amplitude and velocity of a moving structure producing the echoes being studied. Report code 76825 for a complete evaluation of a fetal cardiovascular system and 76826 for a follow-up or repeat study.

76827–76828

Diagnostic ultrasound is an imaging technique bouncing sound waves far above the level of human perception through interior body structures. The sound waves pass through different densities of tissue and reflect back to a receiving unit at varying speeds. The unit then converts the waves to electrical pulses that are immediately displayed in picture form on screen. These codes report fetal doppler echocardiography by pulsed or continuous wave. Doppler echography uses the frequency shifts of the emitted waves against their echoes to measure velocity, such as for blood flow. Doppler may be pulsed or continuous wave. Pulsed wave transmits and records from a single source to determine a precise site of signal origin but not high velocity. Continuous wave uses two transducers, one to continually transmit and the other to record and can determine very high velocities. Report code 76827 for a complete evaluation of a fetal cardiovascular system and 76828 for a follow-up or repeat study.

76830

Diagnostic ultrasound is an imaging technique bouncing sound waves far above the level of human perception through interior body structures. The sound waves pass through different densities of tissue and reflect back to a receiving unit at varying speeds.

CPT® Lay Descriptions

The unit then converts the waves to electrical pulses that are immediately displayed in picture form on screen. This code reports transvaginal ultrasonography.

76831

Diagnostic ultrasound is an imaging technique bouncing sound waves far above the level of human perception through interior body structures. The sound waves pass through different densities of tissue and reflect back to a receiving unit at varying speeds. The unit then converts the waves to electrical pulses that are immediately displayed in picture form on screen. This code reports an ultrasound exam done on the uterus, with or without color flow Doppler. The addition of color flow Doppler monitors the behavior of a moving structure, such as flowing blood. The color image that is produced depicts the various levels of fluid concentration within a given area. In the case of hysterosonography, a small catheter is introduced into the cervical opening and a saline or liquid radiographic contrast material is injected into the endometrial cavity. This code reports only the radiological supervision and interpretation.

76856–76857

Diagnostic ultrasound is an imaging technique bouncing sound waves far above the level of human perception through interior body structures. The sound waves pass through different densities of tissue and reflect back to a receiving unit at varying speeds. The unit then converts the waves to electrical pulses that are immediately displayed in picture form on screen. B-scan utilizes sound waves in a two-dimensional scanning procedure to display a two-dimensional image and real time scanning displays both two-dimensional structure images and movement with time. Use code 76856 to report a complete pelvic evaluation (nonobstetric) and 76857 for a limited or follow-up pelvic evaluation.

76870

Diagnostic ultrasound is an imaging technique bouncing sound waves far above the level of human perception through interior body structures. The sound waves pass through different densities of tissue and reflect back to a receiving unit at varying speeds. The unit then converts the waves to electrical pulses that are immediately displayed in picture form on screen. This code reports ultrasonography of the scrotum and scrotal contents.

76872–76873

Diagnostic ultrasound is an imaging technique bouncing sound waves far above the level of human perception through interior body structures. The sound waves pass through different densities of tissue and reflect back to a receiving unit at varying speeds. The unit then converts the waves to electrical pulses that are immediately displayed in picture form on screen. Code 76872 reports transrectal

ultrasonography, or echography, and 76873 reports a prostate volume evaluation for planning brachytherapy treatment, which is applying radioelements to a treatment area.

76880

Diagnostic ultrasound is an imaging technique bouncing sound waves far above the level of human perception through interior body structures. The sound waves pass through different densities of tissue and reflect back to a receiving unit at varying speeds. The unit then converts the waves to electrical pulses that are immediately displayed in picture form on screen. B-scan utilizes sound waves in a two-dimensional scanning procedure to display a two-dimensional image and real time scanning displays both two-dimensional structure images and movement with time. The code reports ultrasonography of an extremity, nonvascular.

76885–76886

Diagnostic ultrasound is an imaging technique bouncing sound waves far above the level of human perception through interior body structures. The sound waves pass through different densities of tissue and reflect back to a receiving unit at varying speeds. The unit then converts the waves to electrical pulses that are immediately displayed in picture form on screen. Real time imaging displays both two-dimensional structure images and movement with time. 76885 reports dynamic ultrasonography of an infant's hips requiring physician manipulation involving compressing the leg at the knee and then prying the hip outwards as the sound wave transducer is applied to the hip area. 76886 reports static ultrasonography of an infant's hips requiring the legs to be still while the sound wave transducer is applied to the hip area.

76930

The physician drains fluid from the pericardial space around the heart guided by ultrasound. Ultrasound is an imaging technique bouncing sound waves far above the level of human perception through interior body structures. The sound waves pass through different densities of tissue and reflect back to a receiving unit which then converts the waves to electrical pulses that are immediately displayed in picture form on screen. The physician places a long needle below the sternum and directs it into the pericardial space. When fluid is aspirated, the physician may advance a guidewire through the needle into the pericardial space and exchange the needle over the guidewire for a drainage catheter. The physician removes as much pericardial fluid as is required. This code reports the imaging supervision and interpretation only for this procedure.

76932

The physician takes a biopsy of muscle tissue from within the heart guided by ultrasound. Ultrasound is an imaging technique bouncing sound waves far above the level of human perception through interior body structures. The sound waves pass through different densities of tissue and reflect back to a receiving unit which then converts the waves to electrical pulses that are immediately displayed in picture form on screen. The physician threads a special biopsy catheter up to the heart through a central intravenous line often inserted into the femoral vein and takes tissue samples of the heart's septum. This code reports the imaging supervision and interpretation only for this procedure.

76936

After sedation, the pseudoaneurysm or arteriovenous fistula is examined with a duplex scanner. The physician assesses the feasibility of compression repair by compressing the neck of the pseudoaneurysm. If the pseudoaneurysm can be completely ablated visually, therapeutic compression therapy is attempted. The physician applies directed pressure to ablate the pseudoaneurysm while blood flow is maintained. Continuous compression is maintained for 10-minute intervals (20-minute intervals if the patient is anticoagulated) until the pseudoaneurysm is thrombosed. If thrombosis has not occurred after four intervals, further attempts to noninvasively thrombose the aneurysm are usually abandoned. If successful ablation has occurred, the patient is kept flat in bed for 6-8 hours with a sandbag on the groin. At 24 hours, the patient is reexamined for evidence of pseudoaneurysm recurrence. At the completion of ablation, the arteries and veins are assessed for patency with the duplex scanner.

76941

The physician performs a blood transfusion to a fetus or inserts an amniocentesis needle through the abdominal wall into the umbilical vessels of the pregnant uterus and obtains fetal blood guided by ultrasound. Ultrasound is an imaging technique bouncing sound waves far above the level of human perception through interior body structures. The sound waves pass through different densities of tissue and reflect back to a receiving unit which then converts the waves to electrical pulses that are immediately displayed in picture form on screen. For fetal blood transfusion, the physician locates the umbilical vein. A needle is directed through the abdominal wall into the amniotic cavity. The umbilical vein is pierced and fetal blood is exchanged with transfused blood. This code reports the imaging supervision and interpretation only for this procedure.

76942

Ultrasonic guidance is used for guiding needle placement required for procedures such as breast biopsies, needle aspirations, injections, or placing localizing devices. Ultrasound is the process of bouncing sound waves far above the level of human perception through interior body structures. The

sound waves pass through different densities of tissue and reflect back to a receiving unit at varying speeds. The unit then converts the waves to electrical pulses that are immediately displayed in picture form on screen. Once the exact needle entry site is determined along with the depth of the lesion, the optimal route from the skin to the lesion is decided. The needle is inserted and advanced to the lesion under ultrasonic guidance. This code reports the imaging supervision and interpretation only for this procedure.

76945

The physician aspirates cells from the chorionic villus (early stage of the placenta) under ultrasonic guidance. Ultrasound is an imaging technique bouncing sound waves far above the level of human perception through interior body structures. The sound waves pass through different densities of tissue and reflect back to a receiving unit which then converts the waves to electrical pulses that are immediately displayed in picture form on screen. In the transcervical method, a sterile catheter is inserted through the cervix and into the uterine cavity toward the chorionic villus or early placenta. Aspirated cells are obtained for abnormal chromosome analysis. The procedure may also be done transvaginally or transabdominally. The transabdominal approach can be done throughout pregnancy while the other approaches are usually done between 9 and 12 weeks gestation. This code reports the imaging supervision and interpretation only for this procedure.

76946

The physician withdraws fluid from the amniotic sac under ultrasonic guidance. Ultrasound is an imaging technique bouncing sound waves far above the level of human perception through interior body structures. The sound waves pass through different densities of tissue and reflect back to a receiving unit which then converts the waves to electrical pulses that are immediately displayed in picture form on screen. Following preparation of the skin and administration of a local anesthetic, a small gauge needle is introduced into the amniotic sac and fluid aspirated. This code reports the imaging supervision and interpretation only for this procedure.

76948

The physician aspirates ova under ultrasonic guidance. Ultrasound is an imaging technique bouncing sound waves far above the level of human perception through interior body structures. The sound waves pass through different densities of tissue and reflect back to a receiving unit which then converts the waves to electrical pulses that are immediately displayed in picture form on screen. Following preparation of the skin and administration of a local anesthetic, a small gauge needle is introduced into the ovary and the ova are aspirated. This code reports the imaging supervision and interpretation only for this procedure.

CPT ® Lay Descriptions

76950

Ultrasound is used for placing radiation therapy fields. Ultrasound is an imaging technique bouncing sound waves far above the level of human perception through interior body structures. The sound waves pass through different densities of tissue and reflect back to a receiving unit which then converts the waves to electrical pulses that are immediately displayed in picture form on screen. Images of both normal and abnormal tissue structures are obtained and the treatment field area volume is determined. The normal tissues surrounding the treatment area are also defined. Acquiring this data is an important step in planning the patient's radiation treatment.

76965

Ultrasonic guidance is used for the accurate guiding and placement of an interstitial radioactive implant into a tumor during the course of brachytherapy for malignant neoplasms, such as in the prostate. Ultrasound is an imaging technique bouncing sound waves far above the level of human perception through interior body structures. The sound waves pass through different densities of tissue and reflect back to a receiving unit which then converts the waves to electrical pulses that are immediately displayed in picture form on screen. Radioactive implants may be enclosed in various apparatus modes such as tubes, needles, wires, or seeds. Common materials used are radium, cobalt-60, cesium-137, gold-198, and iridium-192.

76970

A follow-up study is performed after a previous ultrasonic study has been completed. The follow-up study may include a repeat A-scan, B-scan, or both. A-scan utilizes sound waves introduced in a straight line to display a single dimension image of vertical peaks and B-scan utilizes sound waves in a two-dimensional scanning procedure to display a two-dimensional image.

76975

The physician uses endoscopic ultrasound to examine the esophageal and gastric wall. Ultrasound is an imaging technique bouncing sound waves far above the level of human perception through interior body structures. The sound waves pass through different densities of tissue and reflect back to a receiving unit which then converts the waves to electrical pulses that are immediately displayed in picture form on screen. The physician passes an endoscope equipped with the ultrasound transducer through the patient's mouth into the esophagus. The entire esophagus, stomach, duodenum, and sometimes jejunum are viewed through ultrasonic images to help determine the extent of cancerous tissue. This code reports the imaging supervision and interpretation only for this process.

76977

Bone mineral density studies are used to evaluate diseases of bone and/or the responses of bone disease to treatment. Densities are measured at the wrist, hip, spine, or calcaneous. The studies assess bone mass or density associated with such diseases as osteoporosis, osteomalacia, and renal osteodystrophy. This code reports using low level ultrasound for measuring bone density instead of ionizing radiation.

76986

Intraoperative diagnostic ultrasonography is used to evaluate ocular abnormalities. Either A-mode, B-mode, or both types may be utilized. This procedure may be done to determine the location and depth of incisions to be made when keratorefractive surgery is performed. A-scan utilizes sound waves introduced in a straight line to display a single dimension image of vertical peaks and B-scan utilizes sound waves in a two-dimensional scanning procedure to display a two-dimensional image.

77261–77263

Treatment planning is conducted for radiation therapy. Treatment planning for oncology patients is the process of developing a complete plan for the course of radiation therapy. The best way to deliver the treatment to the malignancy while blocking the dose received by normal tissues must be determined. This requires localizing the tumor, determining its extent of malignancy and the volume to be treated, choosing the best method of treatment, the number and size of treatment ports, and calculating time and dosage among other procedures. A port is the site where the treatment beam will enter the skin and concentrate upon the malignant area(s). Simple planning, reported in 77261, consists of a single area of malignancy with a single port or opposing ports parallel to each other and basic or no blocking. Intermediate planning, reported in 77262, consists of two separate areas of malignancy with three or more ports that converge, multiple blocks, or special time or dosage considerations. Complex planning, reported in 77263, consists of three or more separate areas of malignancy with tangential ports, special wedges or compensators, complex blocking, a combination of two or more modes of treatment, or special rotating or other beam considerations.

77280–77290

Simulation-aided field setting is done prior to beginning the course of radiation treatment. This is done to determine the size and location of the ports to be used so that they surround the entire tumor. A port is the site where the treatment beam will enter the skin and concentrate upon the malignant area(s). Simulation can be done on a dedicated simulator, a radiation therapy treatment unit, an x-ray machine, or CT scanner. Simulation allows visualization and definition of the exact treatment area(s). Simple simulation, reported in 77280, is done for a single area of malignancy with a single port or opposing ports parallel to each other and basic or no blocking. Intermediate simulation, reported in 77280, is done for two separate areas of malignancy with three or more ports and multiple blocks. Complex simulation, reported in 77290, is done for three or more areas of malignancy with tangential ports and complex blocking that may require customized shielding blocks, rotation or arc therapy, brachytherapy source and hyperthermia probe verification, and use of contrast materials.

77295

Three dimensional simulation-aided field setting is done prior to beginning the course of radiation treatment. This is done to determine the size and location of the ports to be used so that they surround the entire tumor. A port is the site where the treatment beam will enter the skin and concentrate upon the malignant area(s). Simulation can be done on a dedicated simulator, a radiation therapy treatment unit, an x-ray machine, or CT scanner. Simulation allows visualization and definition of the exact treatment area(s). Three dimensional simulation involves using CT and/or MRI data to have computer-generated reconstructions of tumor volume and dose distribution of multiple or moving beams in three dimensional displays.

77300

Dosimetry is the calculation of the radiation dose to be delivered to the tumor. The physician chooses the energy level and modality of photon or electron beams to be used for each simulated port, even if only one treatment area is concerned. Once the tentative treatment fields have been determined, the dosimetry of the treatment portals can be calculated. A basic radiation dosimetry calculation is a photon calculation that includes central axis depth dose, time dose factor (TDF), nominal standard dose (NSD), gap calculation, off-axis and tissue inhomogeneity factors, as well as calculation of nonionizing radiation surface and depth dose. Dosimetry may be repeated during the course of treatment as required.

77301

Intensity modulated radiotherapy (IMRT) is capable of varying the intensity of radiation exposure in a portion of a field depending on whether tumor or critical normal structures are present in the beam pathway. The radiation therapy consists of multiple pencil thin beams or beamlets, calculated to hit tumors with high dose radiation beams and sensitive normal tissues with modulated lower intensity beams, leaving them mostly unaffected. Planning for IMRT involves the use of powerful computer programs that calculate the optimal arrangement of beam angle configurations and dosage intensities to deliver the best treatment. If the isodose distribution for target and critical structure partial tolerance specification and dose-volume histograms are not satisfactory, the optimization is repeated with modifications to clinical parameters, until an acceptable solution is reached.

77305–77315

For the initial setting of the treatment portals, an isodose distribution of the beams is required. Usually done by computer, a teletherapy isodose plan plots the lines of the same dosage levels to be delivered within the treatment field, usually from a combination of beams converging upon the treatment field. Only one plan may be reported per any therapy course to a specific treatment field. A simple teletherapy isodose plan, reported in 77305, consists of one or two parallel opposed ports directed to a single area of interest. An intermediate teletherapy isodose plan, reported in 77310, consists of three or more treatment ports directed to a single area of interest. A complex teletherapy isodose plan, reported in 77315, consists of tangential ports, the use of wedges, compensators, complex blocking, and rotating or special beam considerations.

77321

Special teletherapy port plans are usually done in connection with a complex level of treatment. These are electron calculations and cannot be submitted for the same field with a basic radiation dosimetry calculation, which is photon. Electron beams require extra special attention because of their characteristics in interacting with living tissue. A special teletherapy port plan calculates the dosage level of the treatment portal for the use of electrons or heavy particles when used in a portion of or as the main mode of treatment for the field of interest.

77326–77328

Brachytherapy is the application of radioactive isotopes for internal radiation. Some radioactive material is encapsulated in metal seeds, wires, tubes, or needles for intracavitary or interstitial implantation and some are prepared in solutions for instillation or oral administration. Sealed sources are inserted by the physician in or around the tumor. Sources are intracavitary or permanent interstitial placements and ribbons are temporary interstitial placements. Brachytherapy gives greater control over localized malignancy while preserving function and reducing damage to surrounding tissue. Brachytherapy isodose calculations are necessary to determine the amount of radiation that the tumor will absorb and the distribution of radiation around the sources. Report 77326 for simple calculation from a single plane, application of 1 to 4 sources/ribbons, remote afterloading, 1 to 8 sources. Report 77327 for intermediate calculation from multiplane doses, application of 5 to 10 sources/ribbons, remote afterloading, 9 to 12 sources. Report 77328 for complex calculation from multiplane doses, volume implant calculations, application of over 10 sources/ribbons, remote afterloading, over 12 sources, and special spatial reconstruction.

77331

Dosimetry is the calculation of the radiation dose to be delivered to the tumor. The physician chooses the energy level and modality of photon or electron beams to be used for each simulated port, even if only one treatment area is concerned. Once the tentative treatment fields have been determined, the dosimetry of the treatment portals can be calculated. Special dosimetry involves the use of special measuring and monitoring devices when the physician deems it necessary to calculate the total amount of radiation that a patient has received at any given point. The results help determine whether to uphold or alter the current treatment plan.

77332–77334

Treatment devices used in radiation oncology are customized blocks or shields to protect healthy tissue surrounding the treatment area and are made from a special energy-absorbing material such as cerrobend. Treatment device services contain a professional and technical component. The professional component is based upon the physician's participation in the actual design of the block. The technical component is based on each individual block requiring time and materials to be fabricated. 77332 reports a simple block; 77333 reports intermediate device services for multiple blocks; 77334 reports complex, irregular blocks, special shields, compensators, wedges, molds, or casts.

77336

This code reports ongoing medical physics consultation services to benefit patients undergoing radiation therapy. It includes quality assurance of dose delivery such as verification of dose calculation data, measuring for safe and effective use of software and equipment such as simulators, linear accelerators, and block devices. It also includes assessment of treatment parameters and review of treatment documentation, reported weekly during therapy.

77370

A special medical radiation physics consultation requires a thoroughly written analysis on the course of treatment and is done at direct request of the radiation oncologist when the complexity of the treatment plan is great. Problems analyzed may include photon and electron treatment plans and their consequences, complex dosage calculations because of interactions between multiple treatment fields, intensity modulating radiation, total body irradiation, special blocking procedures, or stereotactic or brachytherapy services.

77401

Radiation treatment delivery involves the delivery of a beam of radioactive electromagnetic energy from a treatment machine distanced from the treatment area. External radiation is very often delivered by linear accelerator which can deliver x-rays (photons) or electrons to a targeted area. Cobalt teletherapy units and cesium teletherapy units are also used to direct gamma rays from a distance to the targeted area. Photons can target deeper lying tumor tissue, while electrons are used for the maximum dose of radiation near the skin surface, making the method suitable to treat skin, superficial lesions, and shallow tumor volumes where underlying tissues need to be protected. Radiation treatment delivery codes are dependent upon the number and complexity of treatment areas as well as the energy level. Use this code to report superficial and/or orthovoltage energy levels, which are kilovoltage doses and usually treat superficial skin lesions.

77402–77406

Radiation treatment delivery involves the delivery of a beam of radioactive electromagnetic energy from a treatment machine distanced from the treatment area. External radiation is very often delivered by linear accelerator which can deliver x-rays (photons) or electrons to a targeted area. Cobalt teletherapy units and cesium teletherapy units are also used to direct gamma rays from a distance to the targeted area. Photons can target deeper lying tumor tissue, while electrons are used for the maximum dose of radiation near the skin surface, making the method suitable to treat skin, superficial lesions, and shallow tumor volumes where underlying tissues need to be protected. These codes are dependent upon the number and complexity of treatment areas as well as the energy level, measured in megavolts (MeV). Use 77402 to report a single treatment area, single port or parallel opposed ports, simple or no blocks; up to 5 MeV. Use 77403 for 6-10 MeV; use 77404 for 11-19 MeV; and use 77406 for 20 MeV or greater.

77407–77411

Radiation treatment delivery involves the delivery of a beam of radioactive electromagnetic energy from a treatment machine distanced from the treatment area. External radiation is very often delivered by linear accelerator which can deliver x-rays (photons) or electrons to a targeted area. Cobalt teletherapy units and cesium teletherapy units are also used to direct gamma rays from a distance to the targeted area. Photons can target deeper lying tumor tissue, while electrons are used for the maximum dose of radiation near the skin surface, making the method suitable to treat skin, superficial lesions, and shallow tumor volumes where underlying tissues need to be protected. These codes are dependent upon the number and complexity of treatment areas as well as the energy level, measured in megavolts (MeV). Use 77407 to report two separate treatment areas, three or more ports on a single treatment area, use of multiple blocks; up to 5 MeV. Use 77408 for 6-10 MeV; use 77409 for 11-19 MeV; and use 77411 for 20 MeV or greater.

77412–77416

Radiation treatment delivery involves the delivery of a beam of radioactive electromagnetic energy from a treatment machine distanced from the treatment area. External radiation is very often delivered by linear accelerator which can deliver x-rays (photons) or electrons to a targeted area. Cobalt teletherapy units and cesium teletherapy units are also used to direct gamma rays from a distance to the targeted area. Photons can target deeper lying tumor tissue, while electrons are used for the maximum dose of radiation near the skin surface, making the method suitable to treat skin, superficial lesions, and shallow tumor volumes where underlying tissues need to be protected. These codes are dependent upon the number and complexity of treatment areas as well as the energy level, measured in megavolts (MeV). Use 77412 to report three or more separate treatment areas, custom blocking, tangential ports, wedges, rotational beams, compensators, or special particle beams; up to 5 MeV. Use 77413 for 6-10 MeV; use 77414 for 11-19 MeV; and use 77416 for 20 MeV or greater.

77417

Therapeutic radiology port films are taken at regular intervals to verify correct positioning of all treatment portals on patients undergoing external beam radiation therapy, since discrepancies in the field placements can happen frequently and this negatively effects the treatment outcomes. The beam of the radiation treatment machine is used to make radiographic portal films. Portal images like a snapshot are taken for localization with a partial dose or recorded for the entire treatment for verification. Port film charges are a technical service only.

77418

Intensity modulated radiotherapy (IMRT) is capable of varying the intensity of radiation exposure in a portion of a field depending on whether tumor or critical normal structures are present in the beam pathway. The radiation therapy consists of multiple pencil thin beams or beamlets, calculated to hit tumors with high dose radiation beams and sensitive normal tissues with modulated lower intensity beams, leaving them mostly unaffected. By dividing the radiation beam into multiple slices, the beam-intensity in any slice can be varied by computer-controlled multileaf collimation (MLC) during the radiation exposure. MLC systems consist of multiple narrow leaves that are under computer control and allow custom-shaped beam apertures without fabricated blocks. During IMRT delivery, the leaves of the MLC are adjusted while the beam is on to modify the delivery of radiation across the portal.

77427

The physician reviews the port films. Then the dosimetry, dose delivery, and treatment parameters are reviewed. The treatment setup and positioning of the patient is evaluated including the assessment of immobilization devices, blocks, wedges, or other devices. The physician also provides care of infected skin, prescribes necessary medications, manages fluid and electrolytes as well as pain management. Nutritional counseling may be provided as necessary. This radiation treatment management code is accurately reported using units of five fractions or treatment sessions. All five sessions must be completed for use of this code.

77431

The physician reviews the port films. Then the dosimetry, dose delivery, and treatment parameters are reviewed. The treatment setup and positioning of the patient is evaluated including the assessment of immobilization devices, blocks, wedges, or other devices. The physician also provides care of infected skin, prescribes necessary medications, manages fluid and electrolytes as well as pain management. Nutritional counseling may be provided as necessary. This radiation treatment management code is used when the entire course of therapy consists of only one or two fractions (treatment sessions), excepting single application brachytherapy which does not require management.

77432

This service involves using multiple megavoltage treatment ports that are directed to a specific area within the brain. When a linear accelerator is used, the extremely narrow x-ray beam from the machine remains focused on the tumor volume of the cerebral lesion while the movement of the machine is carefully coordinated to distribute the beam entry points over a wider radius. Stereotactic treatment delivery requires the use of three-dimensional simulation for accuracy. This code is for a complete course of treatment consisting of one session and reports the radiation oncology services performed as part of the stereotactic radiosurgery procedure.

77470

This service covers the extra planning and monitoring effort involved in the use of special radiation therapy procedures such as total or hemibody irradiation or intraoperative cone irradiation.

77520–77525

Protons are positively charged particles that are particularly beneficial in treating malignancies and other neoplastic abnormalities near sensitive structures such as the optic nerve and spinal cord. Proton beam treatment delivers higher doses of radiation to tumors than photon beams and at the same time does not exceed radiation tolerance of normal, healthy tissue next to the targeted area. Because of the physical properties of the positively-charged protons, they stop short just at the target and do not deposit a dose beyond that boundary, making proton beam treatment advantageous for deep seated and solid tumors in any body site. Report 77520 for simple proton treatment delivery to a single treatment area utilizing a single non-tangential/oblique port and custom blocking without compensation and 77522 with compensation (custom-made devices attached to the treatment unit for manipulating the radiation dose). Report 77523 for intermediate proton delivery to one or more treatment areas utilizing two or more ports or one or more tangential/oblique ports, with custom blocks and compensators; and report 77525 for complex proton treatment delivery to one or more treatment areas utilizing two or more ports per treatment area with matching or patching fields and/or multiple isocenters, with custom blocks and compensators.

77600–77620

Hyperthermia involves the use of heat in an attempt to speed up cell metabolism. This is performed to increase potential cell destruction in the treatment of a malignancy by making tumors more susceptible to the therapy. The heat can be generated by a variety of sources, including microwave, ultrasound and radio frequency conduction. Report 77600 for hyperthermia, externally generated, superficial (i.e., heating to a depth of 4 cm or less) and 77605 for deep (i.e., heating to depths greater than 4 cm). For heat generated by interstitial probes acting like small antennae or microwave radiators placed directly into the tumor area, report 77610 for 5 or fewer interstitial applicators and 77615 for more than 5 interstitial applicators. For hyperthermia generated by intracavitary probes placed into a body cavity, report 77620.

77750

Brachytherapy is the application of radioactive isotopes for internal radiation. Radioactive material is either encapsulated for intracavitary or interstitial implantation or prepared in solutions for instillation or oral administration. For this brachytherapy procedure, the physician infuses or instills a radioactive solution to kill cancerous cells. The physician intravenously injects (e.g., Strontium -89) a radioactive substance in solution into a vein or the physician may instill a radioactive substance in solution into a body cavity. This type of brachytherapy may be referred to as unsealed internal radiation therapy.

77761–77763

Brachytherapy is the application of radioactive isotopes for internal radiation. Radioactive material is either encapsulated for intracavitary or interstitial implantation or prepared in solutions for instillation or oral administration. For intracavitary application, the physician inserts encapsulated radioactive elements (e.g., metal seeds, wires, tubes, or needles) into the affected body cavity using appropriate applicators, surgically inserted under ultrasound or fluoroscopic guidance. The physician may suture the

applicator into or near the tumor. A radioactive isotope, usually Cesium, Iridium, or Cobalt, is then placed in the applicator. The isotopes are left in place for two to three days, but may be left longer. This method provides radiation to a limited body area while minimizing exposure to normal tissue. Report 77761 for simple intracavitary application of 1-4 sources/ribbons; 77762 for intermediate intracavitary application of 5-10 sources/ribbons; and 77763 for complex intracavitary application of more than 10 sources/ribbons.

77776–77778

Brachytherapy is the application of radioactive isotopes for internal radiation. Radioactive material is either encapsulated for intracavitary or interstitial implantation or prepared in solutions for instillation or oral administration. For interstitial application, the physician inserts encapsulated radioactive elements (e.g., metal seeds, wires, tubes, or needles) directly into the affected tissue using appropriate applicators, surgically inserted under ultrasound or fluoroscopic guidance. The physician may suture the applicator into or near the tumor. A radioactive isotope, usually Cesium, Iridium, or Cobalt, is then placed in the applicator. The isotopes are left in place for two to three days, but may be left longer. Tiny seeds of radioactive material may be inserted directly into the tumor area and left there permanently. This method provides radiation to a limited body area while minimizing exposure to normal tissue. Report 77776 for simple interstitial application of 1-4 sources/ribbons; 77777 for intermediate interstitial application of 5-10 sources/ribbons; and 77778 for complex interstitial application of more than 10 sources/ribbons.

77781–77784

Brachytherapy is the application of radioactive isotopes for internal radiation. For remote afterloading high intensity brachytherapy, tiny catheters are used together with a single, high intensity radioactive material to produce the desired radiation distribution pattern around the tumor area. Extremely tiny catheters are fixed in place around the tumor and connected to the treatment machine. These catheters, or applicators, usually do not require surgical manipulation to set them in place. Once in position, the machine loads its radioactive source into each catheter, set at predetermined positions along each catheter for previously calculated dwelling times. The radioactive isotopes are left in place for a short period, usually only 3-5 minutes, due to the high radioactivity of the source that makes it thousands of times more powerful than normal brachytherapy sources. Report 77781 for 1-4 source positions or catheters; 77782 for 5-8 source positions or catheters; 77783 for 9-12 source positions or catheters; and 77784 for over 12 source positions or catheters.

77789

The physician performs a surface application of a radiation source. The physician places the radioactive source sealed in a small holder against a tumor. When surface application is used for treating pterygium, radioactive seeds are placed into a soft, plastic template, which is then inserted into an eye plaque that is implanted during surgery for a specified duration and then removed.

77790

The use of radiation sources for therapy requires special attention and preparations for proper and safe handling of the radioelement. This code reports the supervision, handling, and loading of the radiation source used for conventional brachytherapy, not depending on the number of sources or complexity of the source used. The care of instruments involved in radioelement usage is also included.

78000–78001

The uptake test is a measure of thyroid function to determine how much iodine the thyroid will take up and is expressed as the percentage of the administered radioiodine present in the thyroid gland at a given time after administration. A standard count must be taken of the Iodide-123 capsule before giving it to the patient by using an uptake probe, a sodium iodide counter within a lead shield. For a single, two-hour uptake exam, the neck is extended with the patient supine and the probe placed over the entire gland. A background count is also taken over the thigh by placing a probe over one leg. Net counts are obtained by subtracting background counts. Report 78001 if multiple determinations at 6 and 24-hour intervals are done.

78003

A suppression test involves administration of thyroid hormone to check if a nodule is acting autonomously or if it can be suppressed. A baseline radioiodide uptake and scan must first be obtained. The procedure requires giving the patient T3 hormone three times a day for eight days with radioiodide given orally on the seventh day. The determining uptake and scan are taken on the eighth day. Normal thyroid tissue that functions dependent on thyroid stimulating hormone will be suppressed by the T3. The stimulation test involves administering thyroid stimulating hormone (TSH) to check if a nonvisualized thyroid is present and active. A baseline radioiodide uptake and scan must first be obtained. The procedure requires giving the patient intramuscular injections of thyroid stimulating hormone (TSH) for three days along with a radioiodide tracer. A comparison uptake and scan are taken. Normal functioning thyroid tissue should show more than fifty percent increase in uptake following the simulation. This code does not include the initial uptake studies.

78006–78007

The thyroid imaging scan is performed for anatomical size and physiological evaluation. A radioactive tracer that will focus in the thyroid, such as an Iodide-123 capsule or a 99m-technetium injection is administered. With the patient supine, the neck is extended and the head immobilized. Images are scanned by a scintillation or gamma camera that detects the radiation from the tracer in the target tissue. The uptake test is a measure of thyroid function to determine how much iodine the thyroid will take up and is expressed as the percentage of the administered radioactivity present in the thyroid gland at a given time after administration. For a single, two-hour uptake exam, the neck is extended with the patient supine and the probe placed over the entire gland. A background count is also taken over the thigh by placing a probe over one leg. Net counts are obtained by subtracting background counts. Multiple determinations at 6 and 24-hour intervals may be done in addition to the 2-hour test. Report 78006 for imaging with single determination uptake and 78007 for imaging with multiple determination uptake.

78010–78011

The thyroid imaging scan is performed for anatomical size and physiological evaluation. A radioactive tracer that will focus in the thyroid, such as an Iodide-123 capsule or a 99m-technietium injection is administered. The physician palpates the patient's neck and outlines areas to be marked. With the patient supine, the neck is extended and the head immobilized. Images are scanned by a scintillation or gamma camera that detects the radiation from the tracer in the target tissue. Thyroid carcinoma functions much less than normal thyroid tissue and appears as a cold lesion with little or no accumulation of the radioiodide. Report 78011 for a vascular flow exam when a radioactive tracer is administered that will allow the blood flow and vascularity of the thyroid to be monitored by imaging at different intervals.

78015–78018

An imaging scan for thyroid cancer metastases is done only after ablation of normal thyroid tissue, 6-12 months after therapy treatment. Post-thyroidectomy patients with thyroid cancer are referred for whole body and area scanning to evaluate the thyroidectomy and demonstrate the presence and location of metastatic disease. Radioactive sodium iodide is given to the patient orally. The patient is placed supine with the neck extended and the head immobilized. Images are acquired of the neck, chest, or other clinically suspect areas with a scintillation or gamma camera that detects the radiation from the tracer in the target tissue. 78016 reports additional studies, such as a urinary recovery test in which urine is collected at intervals for radioactivity counts. Report 78018 for a whole body imaging scan.

78020

The uptake test is a measure of thyroid function to determine how much iodine the thyroid will take up and is expressed as the percentage of the administered radioactivity present in the thyroid gland at a given time after administration. An uptake for thyroid cancer metastases is done only after ablation of normal thyroid tissue. This is an add-on code. Radioactive iodine is given to the patient orally. The neck is extended with the patient supine and the probe placed over the entire gland. Since total thyroidectomy has been done to treat the cancer, and any remaining thyroid tissue would not be functioning, the radioactive iodine uptake noted to occur in the neck would be concentrated by metastatic lesions.

78070

Parathyroid imaging is a diagnostic tool for localizing parathyroid adenomas and hyperplastic glands by using dual radiotracer imaging and obtaining two sets of pictures. Thallium-210, which is taken up by the thyroid gland, is injected and the patient is placed supine with the neck extended and the camera centered over the neck. 60-second images are taken from 5 to 20 minutes following the injection. 99m-technetium is also injected and thyroid images taken from 5 to 10 minutes after injection. The images are normalized to each other and the technetium images are subtracted, distinguishing normal tissue from the parathyroid tissue. A thyroid image may be obtained 16 to 24 hours after oral administration of Iodine-123 and subtracted from thallium images to yield a more optimal subtraction image due to a better thyroid-to-background ratio.

78075

Nuclear adrenal imaging is used to evaluate biochemical evidence of adrenal cortical functioning. The adrenal cortex is responsible for steroid hormone production which is dependent on the availability and movement of cholesterol. Radiolabeled cholesterol is therefore the logical choice for adrenal cortex imaging. Depending on the underlying diagnosis, additional medications to aid in imaging are given at prescribed intervals and lengths of time in preparation for the study. After patients are injected with the radiocholesterol NP-59, they return for imaging a few days later. Optimal imaging intervals have also been empirically determined for different underlying diagnoses. All patients are given a solution to block thyroid uptake and a laxative to hasten excretion of the radiocholesterol metabolites. The patient is placed in the prone position for imaging and the gamma camera is centered to detect the radioactivity in the adrenal region.

78102–78104

Radiolabeled sulphur colloid is the most commonly used radiopharmaceutical for bone marrow imaging. The radiotracer is injected into the patient and images are obtained after a two or three-hour delay for optimal evaluation. A special camera, called a scintillation or gamma camera, takes planar images of the study area on computer screen or film by detecting the gamma radiation from the radionuclide that has traveled to the bone marrow as it "scintillates" or gives off energy in a flash of light when coming in contact with the camera's detector. The bone marrow scan provides information about the distribution of functioning bone marrow and any irregular pattern of marrow tissue expansion occurring in different clinical states such as malignancy or infection. Report 78102 for bone marrow imaging of a limited area; 78103 for multiple areas; and 78104 for whole body imaging.

78110–78111

The radiopharmaceutical volume-dilution technique is performed to determine the patient's plasma volume by using a radiolabeled protein tracer such as iodinated serum albumin. The tracer is injected intravenously into one arm and a blood sample is withdrawn from the opposite arm 15 minutes after the injection. A standard solution is prepared by diluting a known volume of the injected radiopharmaceutical with water to a known volume. The dilution factor is figured. The blood sample is centrifuged and divided into 5-ml aliquots for plasma calculation using a formula involving the dilution factor from the standard sample. Report 78110 for a single sampling and 78111 if multiple samplings are collected at 15, 25, and 35 minutes after the injection.

78120–78121

The red cell volume determination test is done by using radioactive chromium to label red blood cells (RBCs). One or two vials of blood are withdrawn from the patient, the RBCs are separated out of the sample, and mixed with the radioisotope. One sample is saved to prepare the standard sample by diluting the known volume of radiolabeled RBCs with water to a known volume. Another sample is injected back into the patient's arm and after a 15 minute delay, blood is withdrawn from the opposite arm. The red cell volume is calculated using a formula that applies the dilution factor from the standard. Report 78121 if multiple samplings are collected at 15, 25, and 35 minutes after the injection.

78122

The radiopharmaceutical volume-dilution technique is performed to determine the patient's plasma volume and red cell volume simultaneously by using a radiolabeled protein tracer such as iodinated serum albumin and autologous radiolabeled red blood cells. The procedure involves collecting blood and recording the blood counts to calculate the volumes using respective formulas that apply the dilution factor from a standard sample of each radiotracer. The radioactive protein tracer is injected intravenously into the arm as well as the radiolabeled autologous red blood cells and blood samples are withdrawn at 15, 25, and 35 minute intervals after the injection. Standard samples are prepared of each radiotracer by diluting a known volume with water until a known volume is reached. The blood samples are centrifuged and divided into 5-ml aliquots for separate red blood cell volume and plasma volume calculations which require different formulas.

78130–78135

A red cell survival study uses radioactive chromium to tag autologous red blood cells (RBCs) to evaluate the rate of red blood cell destruction, or lifespan, in patients with suspected hemolytic anemia. Prior to the procedure, the RBC volume is measured. Blood is withdrawn from the patient, the red blood cells are separated out, mixed with the radioisotope, and injected back into the patient. The initial blood sample is taken on the first day and then repeated at intervals for the next 2-3 weeks or until half of the initial radioactive chromium labeled RBCs are present. Whole blood samples are withdrawn and the hematocrit levels recorded. If a sequestration study is also performed (78135), an aliquot of initial labeled RBCs is saved and the patient's skin is marked over the liver and spleen for detector placement. Each day that the patient returns for the survival study, surface counting is performed over the desired locations with a probe, or scintillation counter, and the different ratios (organ-to-standard, liver-spleen) are compared.

78140

Red blood cell (RBC) sequestration if a test using Chromium-51 labeled autologous red blood cells to determine if the liver or spleen is the major site of sequestration. An aliquot of the patient's own radiolabeled RBCs is saved for a standard measurement and another is re-injected. The patient's skin is marked over the liver and spleen for detector placement. Over the following weeks, surface counting is performed at the desired locations with a probe, or scintillation counter, and the different ratios (organ-to-standard, liver-spleen) are compared. Since extravascular RBC destruction occurs mainly in the liver and spleen, the sequestration counts of radiolabeled RBC accumulation in the liver or spleen over time indicate the organs' related roles in RBC destruction.

78185

Radiolabeled sulphur colloid is the most commonly used radiopharmaceutical for spleen imaging. The radiotracer is injected into the patient and images are obtained after a 15-20 minute delay. A special camera, called a scintillation or gamma camera, takes planar images of the study area on computer screen or film by detecting the gamma radiation from the radionuclide that has traveled to the spleen as it "scintillates" or gives off energy in a flash of light when coming in contact with the camera's detector. The imaging is done first with a lead strip placed on

the left costal margin and then again after the strip is removed. If the imaging is done with a vascular flow study, radiolabeled damaged red blood cells are injected and their flow is followed in the spleen visualization. Splenic imaging is an indirect way of evaluation for liver disease since the disease will shunt the radiocolloid away from the liver.

78190

Once released from the bone marrow, platelets normally circulate in the blood for 8 to 10 days. In patients with certain types of chronic disease such as immune thrombocytopenic purpura (chronic ITP), an autoimmune disorder in which patients produce platelet autoantibodies that destroy blood platelets, the platelet survival time is shortened due to their destruction by the autoantibodies. The patient develops a low platelet count (thrombocytopenia). Platelet destruction occurs mainly in the spleen and to some extent in the liver and bone marrow. The tracer kinetic method involves using a radiolabeled biologically active compound to build a mathematical model for calculating the rate of platelet destruction. For this procedure, the tracer, radiolabeled plasma, is injected intravenously and a scintillation counter that detects the radiation from the plasma is used to follow the movement and destruction of platelets, and measure their concentration in specific organs or tissues.

78191

Once released from the bone marrow, platelets normally circulate in the blood for 8 to 10 days. In patients with certain types of chronic disease such as immune thrombocytopenic purpura (chronic ITP), an autoimmune disorder in which patients produce platelet autoantibodies that destroy blood platelets, the platelet survival time is shortened due to their destruction by the autoantibodies. The patient develops a low platelet count (thrombocytopenia). For the procedure, blood is withdrawn from the patient, the platelets are separated and labeled with Indium-111, and reinjected intravenously. Samples are withdrawn at intervals and the platelet levels recorded until a certain level of tagged platelets are left in circulation.

78195

Diagnostic nuclear lymphatic and lymph node imaging is a tool for studying diseases involving nodal tissue and evaluating lymphatic transport. The patient is placed in a supine position and radioactive antimony sulfide colloid is injected according to the lymph node to be visualized. For axillary and apical lymph nodes, for example, the injection is into the medial two interdigital webs of the hand and imaging is done two to four hours later. For the internal mammary lymph nodes, the injection is into the posterior rectus sheath below the rib cage and imaging is dependent upon the study. For the iliopelvic nodes, injection is into the perianal region with the patient in a knee to chest position. A special camera, called a scintillation or gamma camera, takes planar images of the study area on computer screen or film by detecting the gamma radiation from the radiopharmaceutical in the lymphatic tissue as it "scintillates" or gives off energy when coming in contact with the camera's detector.

78201

Diagnostic nuclear medicine involves the use of small amounts of gamma-emitting radioactive materials, or tracers, to determine the cause of the medical problem based on the function, or chemistry, of the organ or tissue. In a static test, the radionuclide travels to the intended organ. Radiolabeled sulphur colloid is the most commonly used radiopharmaceutical for liver imaging. The radioisotope is injected into a peripheral vein and then extracted by the liver. A special camera, called a scintillation or gamma camera, takes planar images of the study area on computer screen or film by detecting the gamma radiation from the radiopharmaceutical in the body tissue as it "scintillates" or gives off energy in a flash of light when coming in contact with the camera's detector, usually a sodium iodide crystal. Uniform distribution throughout the liver is normal; but an uneven distribution may indicate a tumor.

78202

Radiolabeled sulphur colloid is the most commonly used radiopharmaceutical for diagnostic nuclear imaging of the liver because it is taken up by the reticuloendothelial cells. The radioisotope is injected into a peripheral vein and then extracted by the liver. For imaging done with a vascular flow test, red blood cells are labeled to image the blood flow. A special camera, called a scintillation or gamma camera, takes images of the liver on computer screen or film by detecting the gamma radiation from the radiopharmaceutical in the tissue and the blood as it flows through the liver. This helps characterize lesions or tumors and determine vascular complications in the liver. Impaired blood flow and reticuloendothelial function can show up as patchy colloid uptake in the liver with preferential bone marrow and spleen uptake.

78205–78206

Tomographic SPECT (single photon emission computed tomography) imaging permits an in-depth evaluation of the complex anatomy and functional activity of the liver by introducing a radiolabeled sulphur colloid through an injection into a peripheral vein and then detecting the distribution of gamma radiation emitted from the radiopharmaceutical taken up by the reticuloendothelial cells of the liver. SPECT imaging differs from the usual planar scans of the gamma camera by rotating a single or multiple-head camera mounted on a gantry around the patient to give three-dimensional computer reconstructed views of cross-sectional slices of the liver. For imaging done

with a vascular flow test, red blood cells are labeled to enable imaging of the blood flow through the liver. Report 78205 for SPECT imaging of the liver without vascular flow and 78206 for SPECT imaging with vascular flow.

78215–78216

Radiolabeled sulphur colloid is the most commonly used radiopharmaceutical for diagnostic nuclear imaging of the liver. Radiolabeled heat-denatured red blood cells are used for detecting asplenia and polysplenia. The radioisotope is injected into a peripheral vein and then extracted by the liver and spleen. For imaging done with a vascular flow test, red blood cells are labeled to image the blood flow through the liver and spleen. A special camera, called a scintillation or gamma camera takes images of the liver and spleen on computer screen or film by detecting the gamma radiation from the radiopharmaceutical in the tissue and/or the blood as it flows through the study organs. This helps characterize lesions or tumors and determine vascular complications. Report 78215 for static liver and spleen imaging without vascular flow and 78216 for liver and spleen imaging with vascular flow.

78220

Special radiolabeled aminoacetic acids that are rapidly cleared by hepatocytes and excreted in the bile are used in a nuclear liver function study. The radiotracer is injected into a peripheral vein and then followed by serial imaging with a scintillation, or gamma camera, on computer screen or film by detecting the gamma radiation from the radiopharmaceutical in the liver and throughout the biliary tract as it is expelled. Biliary function scanning is used in diagnosing acute cholecystitis, cholestasis, obstructions, leaks, biliary-enteric fistulas, and cysts.

78223

For nuclear imaging of the hepatobiliary ductal system with gall bladder, special radiolabeled aminoacetic acids that are rapidly cleared by hepatocytes and excreted in the bile are injected into a peripheral vein. A special camera, called a scintillation or gamma camera, takes planar images of the ductal system on computer screen or film by detecting the gamma radiation from the radiopharmaceutical in the body tissue as it "scintillates" or gives off energy in a flash of light when coming in contact with the camera's detector. This imaging may be done with or without pharmacologic intervention to help aid in visualizing the gallbladder and/or measuring its function. An oral agent is administered that concentrates in the gallbladder after being absorbed in the intestine and excreted by the liver. The resulting opacification or even nonvisualization of the gallbladder can diagnose disease such as stones, polyps, and cholesterolosis. This code also includes calculations for a quantitative measurement of gallbladder function.

78230–78231

Diagnostic nuclear medicine involves the use of small amounts of gamma-emitting radioactive materials, or tracers, to determine the cause of the medical problem based on the function, or chemistry, of the organ or tissue. In a static test, the radionuclide travels to the intended organ. For salivary gland imaging, the patient is injected with a low-level radiotracer and immediately imaged with a special camera, called a scintillation or gamma camera, that takes planar images of the salivary, or parotid, gland by detecting the gamma radiation from the radiopharmaceutical in the body tissue. Report 78231 if the imaging is done by serial imaging and another set for comparison is taken after the patient has been given lemon candy to stimulate the salivary glands.

78232

In a nuclear imaging salivary gland function study, the patient is given a radiolabeled sulfur colloid mixture under the tongue that allows the visualization of the flow of saliva from the oral cavity through to the esophagus and the stomach. A gamma camera takes planar images by detecting the gamma radiation from the radiopharmaceutical in the saliva as it moves through the body. The test usually is conducted for an hour after the administration of the radiotracer to follow the saliva pathway.

78258

Diagnostic nuclear medicine involves the use of small amounts of gamma-emitting radioactive materials, or tracers, to determine the cause of the medical problem based on the function, or chemistry, of the organ or tissue. For esophageal motility imaging, a radioactive sulfur colloid in water is administered orally and followed by a scintillation, or gamma camera, that takes planar images by detecting the gamma radiation from the radiopharmaceutical as it gives off energy while being swallowed down the esophagus. This test is done to diagnose motility and neurodegenerative disorders, reverse peristalsis, and dysphagia.

78261

Radiolabeled pertechnetate is administered intravenously for a nuclear imaging study of gastric mucosa, especially in children. A scintillation, or gamma camera, scans a wide vision field from the xiphoid to the symphysis pubis and takes planar images by detecting the gamma radiation from the radiopharmaceutical. Gastric mucosa surfaces of the stomach will selectively collect and then secrete the pertechnetate. Gastric mucosa in an ectopic site, such as Meckel's diverticulum, will accumulate the radiotracer the same as in the stomach, and allow visualization of the ectopic area as long as there is sufficient mucosa to focally concentrate the tracer.

78262

Diagnostic nuclear medicine involves the use of small amounts of gamma-emitting radioactive materials, or tracers, to determine the cause of the medical problem based on the function, or chemistry, of the organ or tissue. For a gastroesophageal reflux study, a sulfur colloid radioisotope in liquid form such as milk is given to the patient to drink. A scintillation, or gamma camera, takes images on camera or film by detecting the gamma radiation from the radiotracer in the liquid in the stomach to visualize any gastroesophageal reflux. The test is usually done for an hour following ingestion of the material.

78264

Diagnostic nuclear medicine involves the use of small amounts of gamma-emitting radioactive materials, or tracers, to determine the cause of the medical problem based on the function, or chemistry, of the organ or tissue. For a gastric emptying study, a sulfur colloid radioisotope in liquid form such as milk is given to the patient to drink. A scintillation, or gamma camera, takes images on camera or film by detecting the gamma radiation from the radiopharmaceutical in the liquid as it moves through the stomach to measure the gastric emptying time. The test is usually done for an hour following ingestion of the material.

78267–78268

Diagnostic nuclear medicine involves the use of small amounts of gamma-emitting radioactive materials, or tracers, to determine the cause of the medical problem based on the function, or chemistry, of the organ or tissue. The urea breath test is a noninvasive method of diagnosing a Helicobacter pylori infection of the stomach. The patient swallows a pill containing a radiolabeled chemical, urea. The bacteria will produce an enzyme that breaks down the urea into ammonia and carbon dioxide gas if they are present. The gas is quickly absorbed into the bloodstream and expelled in the breath. Breath samples are taken 6, 12, and 20 minutes after swallowing the pill. The test may also be done with analysis of the radioactivity levels present in the breath which will rise by a predetermined amount if an H. pylori infection is present. Report 78268 for breath test analysis.

78270–78272

The Schilling test checks for vitamin B12 deficiency. The patient swallows a capsule that contains radioactive vitamin B12 and an hour later is given an injection of vitamin B12 that is not radioactively labeled. All urine excreted in the following 24 hours is collected and checked for radioactive B12 which will be present if it was absorbed. If the first test shows that it was not absorbed, then the same test is done again except that this time the patient also takes a capsule containing intrinsic factor. If there is now radioactive vitamin B12 in the urine, then an intrinsic factor deficiency is likely the cause of the vitamin B12 deficiency. Report 78270 for the Schilling test without intrinsic factor; 78271 for the Schilling test with intrinsic factor; and 78272 for combined vitamin B12 absorption studies both with and without intrinsic factor.

78278

Diagnostic nuclear medicine involves the use of small amounts of gamma-emitting radioactive materials, or tracers, to determine the cause of the medical problem based on the function, or chemistry, of the organ or tissue. For acute gastrointestinal blood loss imaging, a radioactive colloid is injected intravenously and images are scanned over a large field of vision including the abdomen and pelvis by a camera that detects the gamma radiation from the radioactive tracer introduced into the patient. Detection of a hemorrhage depends on the localization of radiotracer that has filtered out of the blood vessel and into the surrounding bowel lumen. Different angle images may be necessary to rule out bleeding that may be obstructed by other organs, such as the liver and spleen.

78290

Intestine imaging done with nuclear scintigraphy involves injecting the patient with radioactive sodium pertechnetate. With the patient supine, the scintillation, or gamma camera, scans a wide field of view covering the abdominal area and takes images on camera or film by detecting the gamma radiation from the radioactive tracer introduced into the patient. Structural abnormalities, such as ectopic gastric mucosa, diverticula, or twisting of the bowel causing obstruction may be detected and localized. Gastric mucosa surfaces in an ectopic site will selectively collect and then secrete the pertechnetate. Patients suspected of Meckel's diverticulum are given a medication to increase gastric uptake of the pertechnetate. When scanning for inflammatory disorders of the bowel, such as Crohn's disease and ulcerative colitis, autologous radiolabeled white blood cells, which focus at inflammation sites, are used as the radiotracer for imaging purposes.

78291

Diagnostic nuclear medicine imaging can test peritoneovenous shunt patency in patients with intractable ascites. The shunt is plastic tubing equipped with a pressure valve that is inserted to connect the peritoneal cavity to the internal jugular or subclavian vein and permit the return of ascites fluid and proteins to the venous system. Normal inspiration creates the necessary intra-abdominal versus intrathoracic pressure change that allows the pressure valve to open and drain the ascites fluid. The ascites fluid is radiolabeled and then followed by imaging with a camera that detects the gamma radiation from the radiotracer introduced into the patient. If the fluid is circulating into the systemic system correctly through a patent shunt, the radiotracer will appear in the cells of the liver.

78300–78315

Various radiopharmaceutical agents are used for diagnostic nuclear imaging of bones and/or joints. Gallium, a calcium analogue, is the radiopharmaceutical of choice when scanning for an inflammatory process because it accumulates in areas of bone mineral turnover, such as fractures, and localizes to infected or inflamed areas like inflammatory arthritis. Combining gallium with radiolabeled white blood cells, which also localize at infection sites, adds more diagnostic specificity when searching for acute osteomyelitis or osteoarthropathy. Radioactive diphosphonates are used for bony metastatic disease screening. A special camera scans the area of study and detects the gamma radiation from the radiotracer introduced into the patient to detect and localize the disease process. Report 78300 for bone and/or joint imaging of a limited area; 78305 for multiple areas; 78306 for a whole body scan; and 78315 for a three-phase scan.

78320

Tomographic SPECT (single photon emission computed tomography) imaging permits an in-depth evaluation of complex anatomy within body structures such as the bones and joints by introducing a special radionuclide and then detecting the distribution of gamma radiation emitted from the radiotracer with a single or multiple-head camera mounted on a gantry to rotate around the patient. SPECT images give three-dimensional computer reconstructed views of cross-sectional slices of the body. Gallium, a calcium analogue, is the radiopharmaceutical of choice when scanning for an inflammatory process in the bones or joints because it accumulates in areas of bone mineral turnover, such as fractures, and localizes to infected or inflamed areas like inflammatory arthritis. Combining gallium with radiolabeled white blood cells, which also localize at infection sites, adds more diagnostic specificity when searching for acute osteomyelitis or osteoarthropathy. Radioactive diphosphonates are used for bony metastatic disease screening.

78350–78351

Single and dual photon absorptiometry are both noninvasive techniques to measure the absorption of the mono or dichromatic photon beam by bone material. The painless study device is placed directly on the patient and uses a small amount of radionuclide to measure the bone mass absorption efficiency of the energy used. This provides a quantitative measurement of the bone mineral density of cortical bone in diseases like osteoporosis and can be used to assess an individual's response to treatment at different intervals. Report 78350 for single photon energy and 78351 for dual photon energy.

78428

For detecting right to left cardiac shunts, radiolabeled macroaggregated albumin is used, which is trapped by the lungs and will be identified in the systemic circulation if a right to left shunt is present. For left to right shunts, the first pass technique is used. A bolus of radionuclide is injected and rapid image frames are acquired as it moves in the venous system through the chambers of the heart. Early recirculation detected would identify a left to right shunt.

78445

Nuclear imaging for non-cardiac vascular flow studies may be performed to test for arterial or venous peripheral vascular diseases or injuries, graft patency, and even catheter malfunctions. In radionuclide angiography, for example, red blood cells from the patient are tagged with radioactivity and injected intravenously. A scintillation camera positioned over the arterial area of interest detects the radioactivity in the blood and takes a series of dynamic images every 2 to 3 seconds immediately after injection, followed by static images. These are recorded on computer and/or film to be studied at different frame rates, times, and intensities. Normal flow is demonstrated as swift and unimpeded. Luminal narrowing or widening, blood flow obstructions and occlusions, and extraluminal accumulation of the radioactive cells can be visualized for diagnostic purposes.

78455

Diagnostic nuclear imaging for a venous thrombosis study using radioactive fibrinogen is done to determine whether or not fibrinogen in the patient was localizing and forming a clot. After injection of the radiolabeled fibrinogen, different visits are required to monitor any clotting action and make a diagnosis. Images from a scintillation, or gamma camera, are taken by detecting the gamma radiation from the radiotracer in the fibrinogen as it localizes and forms clots.

78456

Diagnostic nuclear imaging for acute venous thrombosis imaging uses radiolabeled peptides. Peptides are short-string proteins that attach to platelets, which are essential in blood clotting, and then localize at sites where clots are present or beginning to form. Images from a scintillation, or gamma camera, are taken by detecting the gamma radiation from the radiotracer in the peptides attached to the blood component and these images can identify clots as soon as 10 minutes after the injection. Usually another set of images is done after 60 to 90 minutes following the injection as the image quality tends to improve with time after the injection. If a scan showed significantly increased uptake in any region of one leg compared to the other, or more intense uptake on delayed imaging, deep venous thrombosis is suspected.

78457–78458

A diagnostic nuclear venogram is done to identify the presence and location of thrombi (blood clots) within the venous system. An intravenous injection of a radiopharmaceutical into one or both extremities, most often the legs, is first performed. This is followed by rapid sequence imaging as the radiopharmaceutical passes through the venous system. Unilateral imaging for venous thrombosis is reported with 78457; bilateral imaging is reported with 78458. Bilateral studies may be performed even when only one leg is symptomatic for deep-vein thrombus as the normal extremity if used for comparison purposes.

78459

The cardiac muscle is imaged using data received from positron-emitting radionuclides administered to the patient. The collision of the positrons emitted by the radionuclide with the negatively-charged electrons normally present in tissue is then computer synthesized to produce an image, usually in color. This image will show the presence or absence of ischemic or fibrotic cardiac tissue and allow evaluation of metabolic functioning of cardiac tissue.

78460–78461

Stress is induced with the standard treadmill exercise test or pharmacologically with the infusion of a vasodilator. The patient then receives an intravenous injection of a radionuclide, usually thallium or technetium-99m, which will localize only in nonischemic tissue. Planar images of the heart are scanned immediately with a gamma camera that detects the radiation in the heart tissue to identify areas of infarction. In the nonstress version of the procedure, radionuclide is injected and images taken without stress induction. 78460 reports a single study, at rest or stress. In 78461, multiple procedures are done at rest and/or at stress with a second injection of radionuclide given again in the redistribution or resting phase just prior to resting images being taken.

78464–78465

Stress is induced with the standard treadmill exercise test or pharmacologically with the infusion of a vasodilator. The patient then receives an intravenous injection of a radionuclide, usually thallium or technetium-99m, which will localize only in nonischemic tissue. Tomographic SPECT (single photon emission computed tomographic) images of the heart are taken immediately to identify area of infarction. SPECT imaging differs from planar imaging by using a single or multiple-head camera that rotates around the patient to give three-dimensional tomographic imaging of the heart displayed in thin slices. In the nonstress version of the procedure, radionuclide is injected and images taken without stress induction. 78464 reports a single study at rest or stress. In 78465, multiple studies are done at rest and/or stress with a second injection of radionuclide given again in the redistribution or resting phase just prior to resting images being taken.

78466–78469

A radionuclide is injected intravenously that localizes in recently (under 72-hours) infarcted myocardial tissue. Multiple cardiac images are obtained between one and four hours after injection of the isotope. The location and extent of infarct can then be determined by the presence of the radionuclide in the heart tissue. In 78468, first-pass technique is utilized. In first-pass technique, a bolus of Technetium-99m or other radionuclide is injected and visualized as it moves through the venous system into the right atrium, right ventricle, pulmonary artery, lungs, left atrium, left ventricle, and aorta. Several cardia cycles are generally observed. Ejection fraction measurements from both the right and left ventricle are then calculated by determining the change in radioactivity over time. In 78469, SPECT images are obtained. SPECT images are tomographic reconstructions derived from either a single- or multiple-head gamma camera that rotates around the patient. Tomographic imaging displays the heart in thin slices allowing better separation of myocardial and nonmyocardial structures. SPECT imaging is particularly helpful in identifying small infarcts that are sometimes missed using planar imaging alone.

78472–78473

Radionuclide, which will adhere to the patient's red blood cells, is injected intravenously. Multiple images of the heart, synchronized with the electrocardiographic RR interval (ECG gated), are taken several minutes later, after the radionuclide has spread through the blood pool. These images are computer synthesized and data is generated to produce a video display of cardiac wall motion, calculation of left ventricular ejection fractions, and images based on computer manipulation of the data received. In 78472, the procedure is performed as a single study at either rest or stress, not both; in 78473, the procedure is performed at both rest and stress.

78478

This procedure is an additional service sometimes performed at the time of other myocardial perfusion studies. In this procedure, a radionuclide is injected intravenously and left ventricular muscle function and coronary artery blood distribution is evaluated with wall motion.

78480

This procedure is an additional service sometimes performed at the time of other myocardial perfusion studies. In this procedure, technetium pertechnetate or technetium-labeled albumin is used to evaluate the amount of the blood ejected from the ventricle during one cardiac cycle.

78481–78483

A bolus of radionuclide is injected intravenously for first pass technique. As the radioisotope passes through the cardiac chambers, rapid sequence imaging and computer generation of data and images is done to produce a video display of cardiac wall motion, calculation of ventricular ejection fractions, and images based on computer manipulation of the data received. This technique provides information about the functional status of the heart at rest or in response to stress. In 78481, the procedure is performed as a single study at either rest or stress, not both; in 78483, the procedure is performed at rest and stress.

78491–78492

The cardiac muscle is imaged using data received from positron-emitting radionuclides administered to the patient. The collision of the positrons emitted by the radionuclide with the negatively-charged electrons normally present in tissue is then computer synthesized to produce an image, usually in color, which will show the presence or absence of perfusion into normal or ischemic cardiac tissue. In 78491, the procedure is performed as a single study at either rest or stress, not both; in 78492, the procedure is performed at rest and stress.

78494

Radionuclide, which will adhere to the patient's red blood cells, is injected intravenously. Multiple SPECT (single photon emission computed tomography) images of the heart, synchronized with the electrocardiographic RR interval (ECG gated), are taken several minutes later, after the radionuclide has spread through the blood pool. These SPECT images are taken by a rotating single or multiple-head camera for three-dimensional views of cross-sectional slices and provide better contrast in imaging and greater accuracy than planar scans. The SPECT images are computer synthesized and data is generated to produce a video display of cardiac wall motion, calculation of ventricular ejection fractions, and images based on computer manipulation of the data received.

78496

A bolus of radionuclide is injected intravenously. As the radioisotope in the venous system passes through the cardiac chambers, rapid sequence imaging, synchronized with the electrocardiographic RR interval (ECG gated), is done. This first pass technique provides information for right ventricular ejection fraction calculation not possible with static gated images which do not show right ventricular count in isolation. This test for functional status of the heart is done as a single study at rest in addition to the primary procedure.

78580

Nuclear pulmonary perfusion imaging uses a venous injection of radioactive macroaggregated albumin particles which are too large to pass through the pulmonary capillary bed and accumulate there as they are strained out. A special camera, called a scintillation or gamma camera, takes planar images on computer screen or film by detecting the gamma radiation from the radiopharmaceutical in the lungs as it "scintillates" or gives off energy in a flash of light when coming in contact with the camera's detector. Localization of the radioactive particles is proportional to the blood flow and thereby maps lung perfusion. Standard perfusion imaging usually consists of 8 planar images from different projections with the posterior oblique views being most important since they image the lower lobes, the most common site for pulmonary embolism.

78584

Ventilation and perfusion imaging of the lungs is used to detect pulmonary embolism and the percentage of total perfusion and ventilation attributable to each lung. Perfusion imaging is done after a venous injection of radioactive macroaggregated albumin is given to the patient. The albumin particles are too large to pass through the pulmonary capillary bed and accumulate there as they are strained out. This localization of particles is proportional to the blood flow and thereby maps lung perfusion. A nuclear ventilation image is obtained to complement the perfusion image. For a single breath image, a posterior view of the thorax is taken as the patient inhales radiolabeled Xenon gas in a single breath and holds it as long as possible. This image obtained from the gamma camera that detects the radioactivity from the gas in the lungs will show well-ventilated areas having uniform activity and poorly ventilated areas with decreased or absent radioactivity.

78585

Ventilation and perfusion imaging of the lungs is used to detect pulmonary embolism and the percentage of total perfusion and ventilation attributable to each lung. For perfusion imaging, a venous injection of radioactive macroaggregated albumin is given to the patient. The albumin particles are too large to pass through the pulmonary capillary bed and accumulate there as they are strained out. This localization of particles is proportional to the blood flow and thereby maps lung perfusion. For complementary ventilation rebreathing and washout imaging, the patient breathes in a mixture of radioactive xenon gas and oxygen for a few minutes, allowing equilibration of the xenon in the airways. After rebreathing, single or multiple washin images are taken to reflect the total ventilated lung volume. Next, the patient breathes the room air and exhales the xenon gas while serial washout images are taken to visualize any focal retention of the radioactive particles that would demonstrate obstructive airway disease. This is done with or without single breath imaging upon initial inhalation of the radiolabeled gas.

78586–78587

Nuclear ventilation imaging of the lungs is designed to show the regional distribution of inspired air throughout the lung tissue and the uptake and clearance dynamics of the lungs. The patient is usually placed supine and breathes in a radioaerosol through a tube that is attached to a nebulizer. Once the aerosol is inhaled, the radioactivity stays in the area where it was deposited long enough to take images with a camera that detects the gamma radiation being given off from the aerosol in the air spaces. Increased central deposition occurs in severe obstructive airway disorders. Very rapid clearance from the lungs reflects interstitial lung disease, such as in smokers, where systemic absorption rises due to increased alveolar capillary permeability. Report 78586 for ventilation imaging from a single projection and 78587 for multiple projections such as anterior, posterior, and lateral views.

78588

Ventilation and perfusion imaging of the lungs is used to detect pulmonary embolism and the percentage of total perfusion and ventilation attributable to each lung. For perfusion imaging, an injection of radioactive macroaggregated albumin is given to the patient. The albumin particles are too large to pass through the pulmonary capillary bed and accumulate there as they are strained out. This localization of particles is proportional to the blood flow and thereby maps lung perfusion. For ventilation images, a series of single or multiple projection views, comparable to the perfusion views, are taken after the patient has inhaled a radiolabeled aerosol. The radioactivity stays in the area where it was deposited long enough to take images. If there is no obstruction, consistent appearance and disappearance of the radioactive gas in the air spaces of the lungs is shown.

78591

Nuclear ventilation imaging of the lungs is designed to show the regional distribution of inspired air throughout the lung tissue and the uptake and clearance dynamics of the lungs. For a single breath, single projection ventilation image, a posterior view of the thorax is taken as the patient inhales radiolabeled Xenon gas in a single breath and holds it as long as possible. This image obtained from the gamma camera that detects the radioactivity from the gas in the lungs will show well-ventilated areas having uniform activity and poorly ventilated areas with decreased or absent radioactivity.

78593–78594

Nuclear ventilation imaging of the lungs is designed to show the regional distribution of inspired air throughout the lung tissue and the uptake and clearance dynamics of the lungs. For rebreathing and washout imaging, the patient breathes in a mixture of radioactive xenon gas and oxygen for a few minutes, allowing equilibration of the xenon in the airways.

After rebreathing, single or multiple posterior washin images are taken to reflect the total ventilated lung volume. Next, the patient breathes the room air and exhales the xenon gas while serial washout images are taken to visualize any focal retention of the radioactive particles that would demonstrate obstructive airway disease. This is done with or without single breath imaging upon initial inhalation of the radiolabeled gas. Report 78593 if images are taken from a single projection only, usually posterior; and report 78594 if images include anterior, posterior, and/or lateral views.

78596

Ventilation and perfusion imaging of the lungs is used to detect pulmonary embolism and the percentage of total perfusion and ventilation attributable to each lung. Ventilation imaging of the lungs shows the regional distribution of inspired air throughout the lung tissue and the uptake and clearance dynamics of the lungs by having the patient inhale a radioaerosol or gas. Perfusion imaging uses an injection of radioactive albumin which are particles too big to pass through the pulmonary capillary bed and accumulate there, mapping blood perfusion as they are strained out. The two types of images complement each other for diagnosis purposes. When the data for these studies is acquired on a digital computer, lung ventilation and perfusion can be quantitated for gradient comparisons and function differential calculations.

78600, 78605

Diagnostic nuclear medicine involves the use of small amounts of gamma-emitting radioactive materials, or tracers, to determine the cause of the medical problem based on the function, or chemistry, of the organ or tissue. This is in contrast to diagnostic tests that determine disease presence based on structural appearance. In a static test, the radionuclide travels to the intended organ. The organ, tissue, or bone under study determines the type of radioactive material used and it is then introduced by injection, swallowing, or inhalation. A special camera, called a scintillation or gamma camera, takes planar images of the study area on computer screen or film by detecting the gamma radiation from the radiopharmaceutical in the body tissue as it "scintillates" or gives off energy in a flash of light when coming in contact with the camera's detector. Use 78600 for limited, static, imaging of the brain and 78605 for a static, complete imaging study of the brain.

78601, 78606

Diagnostic nuclear medicine involves the use of small amounts of gamma-emitting radioactive materials, or tracers, to determine the cause of the medical problem based on the function, or chemistry, of the organ or tissue. The organ, tissue, or bone under study determines the type of radioactive material used and how it is administered to the patient. In a static test,

the radionuclide travels to the intended organ and in a vascular flow test, the radionuclide labels red blood cells and therefore goes wherever the blood flows. A special camera, called a scintillation or gamma camera, takes images of the study area on computer screen or film by detecting the gamma radiation from the radiopharmaceutical in the tissue and blood as it flows through the study area. This helps characterize lesions or tumors and determine vascular complications in an organ. Use 78601 for limited imaging with vascular flow of the brain and 78606 for a complete imaging study with vascular flow of the brain.

78607

Tomographic SPECT (single photon emission computed tomography) imaging permits an in-depth evaluation of the complex anatomy and functional activity of the brain by introducing a radionuclide and then detecting the distribution of gamma radiation emitted from the radiopharmaceutical introduced into the brain tissue. SPECT images differ from the usual planar scans of the gamma camera by rotating a single or multiple-head camera mounted on a gantry around the patient to give three-dimensional computer reconstructed views of cross-sectional slices of the brain.

78608

Positron emission tomography (PET) produces thin slice images of the body that can be reassembled into three-dimensional representations by detecting positron-emitting radionuclides from a radiopharmaceutical introduced into the body. These radionuclides must be produced in a cyclotron or generator that can bombard chemicals with neutrons to produce unstable, short-lived radioisotopes, such as carbon-11, nitrogen-13, and oxygen-15. These can be readily incorporated into common and important, biological body compounds for administration. Data from the imaging yields metabolic or biochemical function information depending on the type of molecule tagged. In PET imaging of the brain with metabolic evaluation, the radionuclide in injected intravenously and carried to the brain where the scanner detects the radioactivity as the compound accumulates in different regions of the brain. By using specifically tagged compounds, information on glucose, oxygen, or drug metabolism in the brain is obtained.

78609

Positron emission tomography (PET) produces thin slice images of the body that can be reassembled into three-dimensional representations by detecting positron-emitting radionuclides from a radiopharmaceutical introduced into the body. These radionuclides must be produced in a cyclotron or generator that can bombard chemicals with neutrons to produce unstable, short-lived radioisotopes, such as carbon-11, nitrogen-13, and oxygen-15. These can be readily incorporated into common and important, biological body compounds for administration. Data from the imaging yields metabolic or biochemical function information depending on the type of molecule tagged. In PET imaging of the brain with perfusion evaluation, the radionuclide in injected intravenously and carried to the brain where the scanner detects the radioactivity as the tracer accumulates in different areas of the brain proportional to the rate of delivery of blood to that volume of brain tissue.

78610

Diagnostic nuclear medicine involves the use of small amounts of gamma-emitting radioactive materials, or tracers, to determine the cause of the medical problem based on the function, or chemistry, of the organ or tissue. In a vascular flow test, the radionuclide labels red blood cells and therefore goes wherever the blood flows. The radionuclide is administered to the patient and a special camera, called a scintillation or gamma camera, takes time-delayed, dynamic images of the study area on computer screen or film by detecting the gamma radiation from the radiopharmaceutical in the blood as it flows through the study area. This helps characterize lesions or tumors and determine vascular complications in an organ. Use this code for a vascular flow study only of the brain.

78615

For noninvasive cerebral vascular flow studies done in nuclear medicine, a radioactive tracer, Xenon-133, is mixed with air or saline solution and is administered either by inhalation or injection. After a few minutes of monitoring tracer concentration changes or clearance in the brain, local blood flow and flow-related values are calculated. Cerebral blood flow studies are applied to help evaluate vascular surgery, drug efficacy, mental functions, and the toxic effects of alcohol, solvents, and drugs.

78630

Diagnostic nuclear medicine involves the use of small amounts of gamma-emitting radioactive materials, or tracers, to determine the cause of the medical problem based on the function, or chemistry, of the organ or tissue. Cisternography is done to determine if there is any abnormal cerebral spinal fluid flow occurring in or around the brain. A lumbar puncture is necessary to inject the radiotracer into the lower spinal canal region. A special camera, called a scintillation or gamma camera, takes planar images of the study area on computer screen or film by detecting the gamma radiation from the radiopharmaceutical in the body tissue as it "scintillates" or gives off energy when coming in contact with the camera's detector. Cisternography is a multiple-day procedure requiring 6-hour, 24-hour, and 48-hour scan sessions.

78635

Diagnostic nuclear ventriculography is done to measure ventricular size in the brain, especially for patients with hydrocephalus who have shunts to drain abnormal accumulations of cerebrospinal fluid (CSF) in the brain due to ventricular obstruction of the normal cerebrospinal fluid pathways. A lumbar puncture may be necessary to inject the radiotracer into the lower spinal canal region or it may be injected into a reservoir or valve of the shunt. A special camera, called a scintillation or gamma camera, takes images of the study area on computer screen or film by detecting the gamma radiation from the injected radiopharmaceutical.

78645

A shunt is a tube placed in the interior ventricles of the brain that drains fluid by a pressure controlled valve away from the brain to another part of the body, usually the abdominal cavity, where it is reabsorbed. In order to detect any malfunction and asses the shunt's patency in a noninvasive manner, a radiotracer is injected into a reservoir or valve of the shunt. A special camera, called a scintillation or gamma camera, takes images of the head, chest, and abdomen by detecting the radiation from the injected radiopharmaceutical to determine the movement of the tracer from the shunt in the brain to the peritoneal cavity.

78647

Tomographic SPECT (single photon emission computed tomography) imaging permits an in-depth evaluation of complex anatomy or functional activity in the body by injecting a radionuclide and then detecting the distribution of gamma radiation emitted from the radiopharmaceutical introduced into the body tissues being studied. Cerebrospinal fluid (CSF) flow imaging will detect any abnormalities or injury occurring in the normal pathways of CSF. A lumbar puncture is necessary to inject the radiotracer into the lower spinal canal region. SPECT images differ from the usual planar scans of the gamma camera by rotating a single or multiple-head camera mounted on a gantry around the patient to give three-dimensional, computer-reconstructed views of cross-sectional slices of the body.

78650

Diagnostic nuclear medicine involves the use of small amounts of gamma-emitting radioactive materials, or tracers, to determine the cause of the medical problem based on the function, or chemistry, of the organ or tissue. Intracranial trauma, surgery, infection, malformation, or disease such as hydrocephalus or neoplasms can cause cerebrospinal fluid (CSF) to leak into and drain from nasal or oral cavities. A lumbar puncture may be necessary to inject the radiotracer into the lower spinal canal region. A special camera, called a scintillation or gamma camera, takes images of the study area on computer screen or film by

CPT ® Lay Descriptions

detecting the gamma radiation from the radiopharmaceutical to detect fluid levels in sinuses that suggest leakage and determine the leakage location.

78660

Dacryocystography is the radiographic evaluation of the lacrimal system to localize the site of an obstruction. In diagnostic nuclear medicine, a drop of a radiotracer is instilled in the eye and subsequent imaging by a special camera, called a scintillation or gamma camera, is performed to follow the passage of the radioactivity and the rate at which it disappears into the lacrimal system to assess if there is a stone or other blockage that interferes with normal tearing function.

78700

Diagnostic nuclear medicine involves the use of small amounts of gamma-emitting radioactive materials, or tracers, to determine the cause of the medical problem based on the function, or chemistry, of the organ or tissue. In a static test for kidney imaging, the radionuclide, 99mTc-DMSA, is commonly chosen because it will travel to the kidney and remain in the parenchymal tissue. It is injected into the patient and a special camera, called a scintillation or gamma camera, takes planar images of the kidney on computer screen or film by detecting the gamma radiation from the radiopharmaceutical in the renal tissue as it "scintillates" or gives off energy in a flash of light when coming in contact with the camera's detector.

78701

For diagnostic nuclear imaging of the kidney with a vascular flow test, the radionuclide, 99mTc-DTPA, is commonly chosen because it will follow the blood as it flows through the kidney and also identify any obstruction in the collecting system to determine the rate at which the kidney's are filtering. It is injected into the patient and a special camera, called a scintillation or gamma camera, takes planar images of the study area on computer screen or film by detecting the gamma radiation from the radiopharmaceutical as it flows through the kidney.

78704

Diagnostic nuclear medicine involves the use of small amounts of gamma-emitting radioactive materials, or tracers, to determine the cause of the medical problem based on the function, or chemistry, of the organ or tissue. This is in contrast to diagnostic tests that determine disease presence based on structural appearance. For an imaging renogram with function study, a special radiopharmaceutical, 99mTc-MAG3, is used to follow the normal pathway in urine production to study how well the tubules and ducts are functioning and how fast the tracer is excreted. A special camera, called a scintillation or gamma camera, takes images of the kidney on computer

screen or film by detecting the gamma radiation from the radiopharmaceutical as it flows through the kidney.

78707–78709

For a diagnostic nuclear imaging study of the kidney with vascular flow and function test, a special radiopharmaceutical is injected that follows the blood flow through the kidneys in the normal pathway for urine production. Obstructions in the collecting system are identified, along with the rate at which the kidney's are filtering the blood, and how well the tubules and ducts are functioning. A special camera, called a scintillation or gamma camera, scans the study area and takes images on computer screen or film by detecting the gamma radiation from the radiopharmaceutical as it flows through the kidney. If pharmacological intervention is used, a diuretic may also be injected that will increase urine flow during the exam. If the radiotracer accumulates and the kidney fails to clear it after diuretic administration, surgery may be necessary to correct the obstruction. Report 78707 for a single study without pharmacological intervention; 78708 for a single study with intervention; and 78709 for multiple studies, done with and without intervention.

78710

Tomographic SPECT (single photon emission computed tomography) imaging permits an in-depth evaluation of the complex anatomy and functional activity of the kidney by injecting a radionuclide and then detecting the distribution of gamma radiation emitted from the radiopharmaceutical introduced into the renal tissue. SPECT images differ from the usual planar scans of the gamma camera by rotating a single or multiple-head camera mounted on a gantry around the patient to give three-dimensional computer reconstructed views of cross-sectional slices of the kidney.

78715

Diagnostic nuclear medicine involves the use of small amounts of gamma-emitting radioactive materials, or tracers, to determine the cause of the medical problem based on the function, or chemistry, of the organ or tissue. This is in contrast to diagnostic tests that determine disease presence based on structural appearance. In a vascular flow test of the kidney, 99mTc-DTPA is injected. The radionuclide labels red blood cells for following blood flow through the kidneys. A special camera, called a scintillation or gamma camera, takes time-delayed, dynamic images of the study area on computer screen or film by detecting the gamma radiation from the radiopharmaceutical in the blood as it flows through the study area.

78725

A non-imaging radioisotopic study of kidney function requires the use of a radioisotope that is cleared from the body only by the glomerular filtration action of the kidneys. Measuring the glomerular filtration rate (GFR) is the best assessment of total renal function. The radioisotope is injected and blood samples are taken at 2, 3, and 4 hours for radioactive concentration counts. The filtration rate of the kidneys is proportional to the clearance rate of the radioisotope from the blood and is calculated using this information together with the distribution volume. The GFR can also be calculated by using urine collections but this method has more intrinsic complications than blood sampling.

78730

For a urinary bladder residual study, the patient is injected with 99mTc-DTPA to evaluate for obstructions or noncompliant bladder. Images are obtained with a gamma camera to record bladder activity for a set amount of time before voiding. The bladder is emptied and the volume that was discharged is measured. Bladder activity is then re-imaged for the same length of time after voiding. The residual urine volume is calculated using the amount of urine passed and the bladder counts both before and after voiding.

78740

A nuclear urethral reflex study is a voiding cystogram recorded with the use of a radiopharmaceutical that has been injected into the patient. Fluids are given into the bladder for half an hour through a Foley catheter and posterior images of activity are taken. According to the patient's need, the bladder is emptied while digital recordings are taken to the end of voiding and continued for another few minutes. Images are reconstructed from the digital data system to detect the presence and identify the grade of ureteric or intrarenal reflux which can lead to severe kidney damage. Time-activity curves may also by calculated to show increased renal activity during voiding due to the reflux.

78760–78761

For testicular diagnostic nuclear imaging, 99mTc-pertechnetate is injected into a vein in the arm and travels to the testicle where it accumulates. In a vascular flow test, the radionuclide labels red blood cells and therefore goes wherever the blood flows. A special camera, called a scintillation or gamma camera, takes images of the study area on computer screen or film by detecting the gamma radiation from the radiotracer concentrated in the testicle or the blood as it flows through the testicle. This test determines whether infection or twisting and infarction of the testis is occurring. Infection increases the blood supply and twisting, or torsion, cuts off the blood supply. One can be treated with antibiotics and the other requires surgical untwisting to keep the testicle viable. Report code 78760 for imaging only and 78761 for imaging with vascular flow study.

78800–78802

Diagnostic nuclear medicine involves the use of small amounts of gamma-emitting radioactive materials, or tracers, to determine the cause of the medical problem based on the function, or chemistry, of the organ or tissue. Monoclonal antibodies used for diagnosing certain cancers are developed from tumor-associated antigens and then radiolabeled for use as the radiopharmaceutical in tumor localization. After administration of the specialized radiotracer, a camera, called a scintillation or gamma camera, takes planar images of the study area on computer screen or film by detecting the gamma radiation from the radiopharmaceutical focused in the body tissue. Report 78800 for tumor localization within a limited area; 78801 for multiple areas; and 78802 for scanning over the whole body.

78803

Tomographic SPECT (single photon emission computed tomography) imaging permits an in-depth evaluation of complex anatomy and can localize tumors within organs and body structures by introducing a radionuclide and then detecting the distribution of gamma radiation emitted from the radiotracer introduced into the tissue being studied. Monoclonal antibodies used for diagnosing certain cancers are developed from tumor-associated antigens and then radiolabeled for use as the radiopharmaceutical in tumor localization. Tomographic SPECT images differ from the usual planar scans of the gamma camera by rotating a single or multiple-head camera mounted on a gantry around the patient to give three-dimensional computer reconstructed views of cross-sectional slices of the body.

78805–78806

Gallium, a calcium analogue, is the radiopharmaceutical of choice when scanning for an inflammatory process because it localizes to infected areas by attaching to plasma proteins found at infection sites and accumulating in areas of bone mineral turnover, such as fractures and inflammatory arthritis. Gallium is often combined with radiolabeled white blood cells, which also accumulate at infection sites but not at areas of increased bone replenishing, to augment accuracy in inflammatory localization. After administration of the specialized radiotracer, a camera, called a scintillation or gamma camera, takes planar images of the study area on computer screen or film by detecting the gamma radiation from the radiopharmaceutical in the body tissue as it "scintillates" or gives off energy when coming in contact with the camera's detector. Report 78805 for inflammatory process localization within a limited area and 78806 for scanning over the whole body.

78807

Tomographic SPECT (single photon emission computed tomography) imaging permits an in-depth evaluation of complex anatomy and can localize an inflammatory process within body structures by introducing a special radionuclide and then detecting the distribution of gamma radiation emitted from the radiotracer with a single or multiple-head camera mounted on a gantry to rotate around the patient and give three-dimensional computer reconstructed views of cross-sectional slices of the body. Gallium, a calcium analogue, is the radiopharmaceutical of choice when scanning for an inflammatory process because it localizes to infected areas by attaching to plasma proteins found at infection sites and accumulating in areas of bone mineral turnover, such as fractures and inflammatory arthritis. When combined with labeled white blood cells, which also accumulate at infection sites but not at areas of increased bone replenishing, accuracy in localizing an inflammatory process is increased.

78810

Positron emission tomography (PET) produces thin slice images of the body that can be reassembled into three-dimensional representations by detecting positron-emitting radionuclides from a radiopharmaceutical introduced into the body. The positron emitting radionuclides used in PET must be produced in a cyclotron or generator that can bombard chemicals with neutrons to produce unstable, short-lived radioisotopes, such as carbon-11 and oxygen-15. These can be readily incorporated into common and important, biological body compounds for administration. The data from the imaging yields metabolic or biochemical function information depending on the type of molecule tagged. In PET imaging of a tumor with metabolic evaluation, information on the tumor's glucose and oxygen utilization is obtained which gives information about the tumor's behavior compared to normal tissue or benign tumors.

78890–78891

The process reported in 78890 includes the nuclear physician's interpretation of data aided by computer generation with simple manipulations for less than 30 minutes. 78891 reports the nuclear physician's interpretation of data aided by computer generation with complex manipulations for more than 30 minutes.

78990

This code reports the provision of diagnostic radiopharmaceuticals which are reported separately from the nuclear medicine procedure.

79000–79001

The strategy for using radiopharmaceutical therapy is to combine high-energy, beta-particle emitters with relatively short half lives to specific tissue-seeking molecules that can be administered to the patient. Because iodine is taken into thyroid cells, radioactive iodine, I-131, is used to treat some types of thyroid

cancers and hormone overproduction (hyperthyroidism). The patient is given I-131 orally or intravenously. Once the iodine is in the patient, the urine is collected and treated as radioactive waste. Shielding lead barriers are used to protect staff and visitors. The patient may be kept in the hospital for several hours to days. After treatment, most patients require full thyroid hormone replacement therapy. Patients usually become hypothyroid within three months and begin receiving partial replacement doses about two months after receiving treatment. Use 79000 to report the initial therapy and patient evaluation and 79001 for subsequent therapy, each session.

79020

Changes in thyroid function can occur following major surgical procedures or in severe systemic illness. Patients have normal or decreased T4 levels, decreased T3 levels, and normal thyroid stimulating hormone (TSH). Thyroid suppression therapy is done to determine the autonomy of nodules or diffusely enlarged glands that might need surgical treatment. A pre-and post-intervention scan and uptake are performed which together show actual suppression. The patient is given T3, which will decrease the normal level of TSH production, resulting in decreased radiopharmaceutical uptake on the post-stimulation scan and uptake. If a nodule remains "hot" after suppression was attempted, this indicates it is not under normal hormonal control but is functioning autonomously and may need to be resected.

79030–79035

Because iodine is taken into thyroid cells, radioactive iodine, I-131, is the radiopharmaceutical used to treat some types of thyroid cancers. Large tumors usually require total or near-total thyroidectomy with postoperative radiopharmaceutical ablation of residual gland tissue. The patient is given the I-131 orally or intravenously. Once the iodine is in the patient, the urine is collected and treated as radioactive waste. Shielding lead barriers are used to protect staff and visitors. Repeat treatment may be required to achieve full ablation of any remaining thyroid tissue. After treatment, most patients will require full thyroid hormone replacement therapy. Report 79030 for the ablation of thyroid gland for carcinoma and 79035 when the therapy is done for metastases of thyroid carcinoma.

79100

Radiopharmaceutical therapy for polycythemia vera and chronic leukemia is done to slow down the rate at which bone marrow produces cells and have a state of remission occur. The strategy for using radiopharmaceutical therapy is to combine high-energy, beta-particle emitters with relatively short half lives to specific tissue-seeking molecules that can be administered to the patient. Radioactive phosphorous,

P-32, as sodium phosphate is administered intravenously. Phosphorus-32 has a high bone marrow toxicity and may have complications such as increased incidence of leukemia for those with polycythemia vera and damage to local tissues from infiltration of the skin at the injection site. If remission does not occur within a few months, the patient may be treated again with a dose 25 percent greater than the initial dose up to a certain limit. Report 79100 for each treatment.

79200

Colloids are a mixture in which one substance is divided into minute particles (called colloidal particles) and dispersed throughout a second substance. Colloidal solutions that contain natural or synthetic molecules are relatively impermeable to the vascular membrane and are useful in intracavity radioactive therapy. Intracavitary radiotherapy refers to the placement of radioactive sources into a body space or cavity, such as the esophagus, lung, vagina or uterus, to give high doses of radiation to the cancer, while giving only lower doses to the surrounding tissues.

79300

Colloids are a mixture in which one substance is divided into minute particles (called colloidal particles) and dispersed throughout a second substance. Colloidal solutions that contain natural or synthetic molecules are relatively impermeable to the vascular membrane and are good for interstitial radioactive therapy. Interstitial radiotherapy refers to the placement of radioactive sources into the affected body part or tissue, such as the prostate gland, to give high doses of radiation to the cancer, while giving only lower doses to the surrounding tissues. In rapid interstitial therapy, plastic tubes are inserted into the prostate, and rapid dose radioactive colloid solutions are placed in the tubes for several days. The sources and the tubes are removed after treatment.

79400

Nonthyroid and nonhematologic radiopharmaceutical therapy refers to the intravenous administration of Strontium, SR-89, for the palliative relief of bone pain in skeletal metastases from such diseases as breast and prostate cancer. Strontium Chloride, also known as Metastron, contains a small amount of radioactive Strontium that that goes directly to the diseased bone site, is absorbed at the metastasis, and begins irradiating it with minimal radiation spilling over to the normal surrounding bone and tissue. Administering this radiopharmaceutical also helps decrease the need for giving opioid narcotics as analgesics and can give relief for up to six months per injection.

79420

The goal of radiopharmaceutical therapy is to place a radionuclide for treatment in the body so as to enable it to deliver its energy close to, or even inside, the target cells. In balloon angioplasty, for instance, the inflated catheter used to open occluded arteries often tears the arterial wall as well. Some of the cells in the blood vessel respond to this injury by initiating repair, which often leads to reclosing of the artery; but radiation treatment of the lesion can inhibit the effect. For intravascular radiopharmaceutical therapy in the case of coronary angioplasty procedures, a catheter is inserted into the femoral artery and guided to the area of interest. Sealed sources of radionuclides are fed through the catheter and positioned in the artery at the lesion site to inhibit its growth.

79440

Each episode of joint bleeding causes inflammation and swelling of the synovial membrane. If bleeding occurs often or is not treated adequately, the inflammation may become chronic and can lead to the thickening of the synovial membrane and the release of substances that can destroy cartilage and bone. Radiopharmaceutical therapy destroys the membrane through radiation, rather than in a surgical procedure to remove the damaged membrane. A radioactive substance, such as phosphorus-32, is injected into the joint at a time when the patient has not been bleeding, and after a period of prophylactic therapy so that the swelling of the membrane is already reduced as much as possible.

79900

The provision of therapeutic radiopharmaceuticals refers to supplying patient-specific radioelements, such as Iridium-192, Iodine-125, or Gold-198, and not to the supply of such sources as Cobalt, Cesium, or Strontium, which are not patient-specific. The supply of patient-specific radioelements is a cost born by the facility or center that purchases such radiopharmaceuticals.

80048

A basic metabolic panel includes the following tests: calcium (82310); carbon dioxide (82374), chloride (83435), creatinine (82565), glucose (82947), potassium (84132), sodium (84295), urea nitrogen (BUN) (84520). Blood specimen is obtained by venipuncture. See the specific codes for additional information about the listed tests.

80050

A general health panel includes the following tests: albumin (82040), total bilirubin (82247), calcium (82310), carbon dioxide (bicarbonate) (82374), chloride (82435), creatinine (82565), glucose (82947), alkaline phosphatase (84075), potassium (84132), total protein (84155), sodium (84295), aspartate amino transferase (AST) (SGOT) (84450), urea nitrogen (BUN) (84520), thyroid stimulating hormone (84443). In addition, this panel includes a hemogram as described by either 85022 or 85025. Blood specimen is obtained by venipuncture. See specific codes for additional information about the listed tests.

80051

An electrolyte panel includes the following tests: carbon dioxide (82374), chloride (82435), potassium (84132), sodium (84295). Blood specimen is obtained by venipuncture. See specific codes for additional information about the listed tests.

80053

A comprehensive metabolic panel includes the following tests: albumin (82040), total bilirubin (82247), calcium (82310), carbon dioxide (bicarbonate) (82374), chloride (83435), creatinine (82565), glucose (82947), alkaline phosphatase (84075), potassium (84132), total protein (84155), sodium (84295), alanine amino transferase (ALT) (SGPT) (84460), aspartate amino transferase (AST) (SGOT) (84450), urea nitrogen (BUN) (84520). Blood specimen is obtained by venipuncture. See the specific codes for additional information about the listed tests.

80055

An obstetric panel includes the following tests: Hepatitis B surface antigen (HBsAg) (87340), rubella antibody (86762), syphilis test (VDRL, RPR, ART) (86592), RBC antibody screen (86850), ABO blood typing (86900), Rh (D) blood typing (86901). In addition, this panel includes a hemogram as described by either 85022 or 85025. Blood specimen is obtained by venipuncture. See specific codes for additional information about the listed tests.

80061

A lipid panel includes the following tests: total serum cholesterol (82465), high-density cholesterol (HDL cholesterol) by direct measurement (83718), triglycerides (84478). Blood specimen is obtained by venipuncture. See specific codes for additional information about the listed tests.

80069

A renal function panel includes the following tests: albumin (82040), calcium (82310), carbon dioxide (bicarbonate) (82374), chloride (83435), creatinine (82565), glucose (82947), inorganic phosphorus (phosphate) (84100), potassium (84132), sodium (84295), and urea nitrogen (BUN) (84520).

80074

An acute hepatitis panel includes the following tests: hepatitis A antibody (HAAb), IgM antibody (86709), hepatitis B core antibody (HbcAb), IgM antibody (86705), hepatitis B surface antigen (HbsAg) (87340), and hepatitis C antibody (86803).

80076

An hepatic function panel includes the following tests: albumin (82040), total bilirubin (82247), direct bilirubin (82248), alkaline phosphatase (84075),

protein, total (84155), alanine amino transferase (ALT) (SGPT) (84460), aspartate amino transferase (AST) (SGOT) (84450). Blood specimen is obtained by venipuncture. See the specific codes for additional information about the listed tests.

80090

The acronym TORCH stands for toxoplasmosis, other, rubella, cytomegalovirus, and herpes. These are infections known to have a detrimental effect on the fetus when contracted during pregnancy. A TORCH panel includes the following tests: cytomegalovirus antibody (CMV) (86644); herpes simplex antibody, nonspecific type test (86694); rubella antibody (86762); toxoplasma antibody (86777). Blood specimen is obtained by venipuncture. See specific codes for additional information about the listed tests.

80100

This test may be requested as a drug screen for multiple drug classes. Blood specimen is obtained by venipuncture. A random urine sample is obtained. The screening test must be performed by a chromatographic technique which has good sensitivity, although it may not be as specific as a confirmatory test. Thin-layer chromatography is a common chromatographic technique for drug screening tests. It is performed by applying a thin layer adsorbent to a rectangular plate in the stationary phase. The specimen is applied to the plate and the end of the plate is placed in a solvent. As the solvent rises along the adsorbent on the plate, the different components of the specimen are carried along at varying rates and deposited along the plate. The different components can then be separately visualized and analyzed. Positive tests are always confirmed with a second method.

80101

This test may be requested as a drug screen for a single drug class. The screening test should be performed by a technique which has good sensitivity, although it may not be as specific as a confirmatory test. Blood specimen is obtained by venipuncture. A random urine sample is obtained. A number of different methods are available to screen for single drugs or drug classes including very simple drug screening kits that rely on immunoassay for detection of a single specific drug or drug class. For example, Placidyl (aka ethchlorvynol), can be screened in urine with a very simple colorimetric test where equal parts of urine and a single reagent are mixed and observed for a visual color change. This would be reported with 80101. Positive tests are always confirmed with a second method.

80102

This test may be requested as drug screen confirmation. It is performed when the initial drug screen (80100-80101) is positive. Confirmatory tests must be both sensitive and specific and involve a different technique than the initial screen. For example, if the initial screen is performed by thin layer chromatography identifying a spot on the chromatogram which is the right color and in the right place to be consistent with a particular drug, it is confirmed with a more specific method, like high performance liquid chromatography (HPLC), gas chromatography-mass spectrometry (GC-MS), or immunoassay. If the drug suspected is a barbiturate, for example, a confirmatory HPLC method might be done to prove that the compound had the correct retention time, etc., and to identify it exactly as a particular barbiturate. This would be reported with 80102.

80103

Tissue is sometimes tested for the presence of drugs. This code reports the tissue preparation only.

80150

Amikacin is a type of antibiotic. Test specimens are frequently collected at peak and trough periods, which is shortly after administration of amikacin and again just before the next administration when serum concentration is at its lowest. This is an effective approach to determine a therapeutic level of drug. Method is radioimmunoassay (RIA) or high performance liquid chromatography (HPLC).

80152

Amitriptyline is a tricyclic antidepressant and the prototype brand name is Elavil. Test specimens are frequently collected at the trough period, which is about 12 hours after the last dose when serum concentration is at its lowest. This is an effective approach to determine a therapeutic level of drug. Drug overdose may be reason for the test as well. Method is typically high performance liquid chromatography (HPLC) or gas liquid chromatograph (GLC). This drug may be prescribed for disorders outside of depressive states, such as chronic pain.

80154

Benzodiazepines encompass a family of mild sedatives, including diazepam (Valium) and ativan. These drugs may be assayed to determine therapeutic levels, or sometimes to determine levels in the system following overdose. Test specimens are frequently collected at the trough period, which is about 12 hours after the last dose when serum concentration is at its lowest. Method is high performance liquid chromatography (HPLC), gas liquid chromatography (GLC), or radioimmunoassay (RIA). This family of drugs may be prescribed for numerous conditions and disorders. Alcohol withdrawal is a common use for diazepam, as are muscle spasms.

80156

This drug, also known as tegretol, is an enzyme inducer. Blood specimen collection is by venipuncture. CSF is obtained by spinal puncture which is reported separately. Test specimens for total levels are frequently collected at the trough period, which is about 12 hours after the last dose when serum concentration is at its lowest. This is an effective approach to determine a therapeutic level of drug. This drug is absorbed slowly and erratically by the GI tract and a total concentration may be required, depending on the treatment underway. Methods include high performance liquid chromatography (HPLC) or gas liquid chromatography (GLC). Tegretol may be administered for such conditions as trigeminal neuralgia, epilepsy, and manic disorders. It is known for its anticonvulsant and pain management properties.

80157

This drug, also known as tegretol, is an enzyme inducer. Specimen collection is by venipuncture. Test specimens for free drug concentrations may be collected near peak levels about 2 to 8 hours after ingestion. Methods include high performance liquid chromatography (HPLC) or gas liquid chromatography (GLC). This drug is absorbed slowly and erratically by the GI tract and a free plasma concentration may be assayed, depending on the type of treatment underway. Tegretol may be administered for such conditions as trigeminal neuralgia, epilepsy, and manic disorders. It is known for its anticonvulsant and pain management properties.

80158

This drug is also known as sandimmune. It is an immunosuppressant and is often carefully monitored to achieve desired results while avoiding nephrotoxicity. Test specimens are frequently collected at the trough period, which is typically about 12 hours after the last dose when serum concentration is at its lowest. Method is high performance liquid chromatography (HPLC) or fluorescence polarization immunoassay (FPIA).

80160

This drug is also known as norpramine and is among the tricyclic antidepressants. Steady state test specimens are frequently collected at the trough period, which is about 12 hours after the last dose when serum concentration is at its lowest. This is an effective approach to determine a therapeutic level of drug. Overdose is also a reason to run this test. Method is high performance liquid chromatography (HPLC) or gas liquid chromatography (GLC).

80162

This digitalis glycoside has numerous trade names: cystodigin, purodigin, lanoxin, etc. The drugs are used principally to treat conditions surrounding congestive heart failure, such as arrhythmias, atrial fibrillation, and tachycardia. Test specimens may be drawn during peak and trough periods, which is shortly after administration of digitalis and again just before the next administration when serum concentration is at its lowest. Method is high performance liquid chromatography (HPLC) or gas liquid chromatography (GLC).

80164

This drug is also known as depakene. This drug is often used to treat seizures. Test specimens are frequently collected at the trough period, which is about 12 hours after the last dose when serum concentration is at its lowest. This is an effective approach to determine a therapeutic level of drug. Method is gas liquid chromatography (GLC), gas chromatography-mass spectrometry (GC-MS), and enzyme immunoassay (EIA).

80166

This drug is also known as sinequam or adapin. This drug is classified as a tricyclic antidepressant (TCA). Steady state test specimens are frequently collected at the trough period, which is about 12 hours after the last dose when serum concentration is at its lowest. This is an effective approach to determine a therapeutic level of drug. Overdose may also prompt this test. Method is high performance liquid chromatography (HPLC), gas liquid chromatography (GLC), gas chromatography-mass spectrometry (GC-MS), and radioimmunoassay (RIA).

80168

This drug may also be known as zarontin. This is an anticonvulsant medication. Test specimens may be drawn during peak and trough periods, which is shortly after administration of zarontin and again just before the next administration when serum concentration is at its lowest. Methods include high performance liquid chromatography (HPLC), radioimmunoassay (RIA), and microbiology assay.

80170

This drug is classified as an aminoglycoside, an antibiotic. In its injectable form, the drug may be prescribed for gram-negative infections, septicemia and other serious infections, as well as unknown causative organisms. Common trade names include Garamycin and Gentacidin. A typical course will run seven to ten days. Monitoring may be initiated to measure drug clearance via the kidneys. Patients with impaired renal function may accumulate the drug. Peak serum concentrations can be expected about 30 to 60 minutes following an intramuscular injection. Trough concentrations occur just before the next dose. Dosage is highly dependent on the severity of infection. Methodology may include radioimmunoassay (RIA) and microbiological assay.

80172

This test may include the abbreviation for gold, Au, or the name myochrysine. Gold salts are sometimes used in the treatment of rheumatoid arthritis. Therapeutic levels may be difficult to determine. Method is atomic absorption spectrophotometry (AAS).

80173

This drug, also known as haldol, is a well established tranquilizer with antipsychotic and other properties. Blood concentrations of haloperidol do not correspond well with therapeutic dosages; therefore, assays may be performed to establish compliance or to measure the body's ability to metabolize the drug. Blood specimen is obtained by venipuncture. Methods may include high performance liquid chromatography (HPLC), gas liquid chromatography (GLC), and radioimmunoassay (RIA).

80174

This drug may also be known as Tofranil. The drug is classified as a tricyclic antidepressant (TCA). Steady state test specimens are frequently collected at the trough period, which is about 12 hours after the last dose when serum concentration is at its lowest. This is an effective approach to determine a therapeutic level of drug. Overdose may also prompt this test. Method is high performance liquid chromatography (HPLC), gas liquid chromatography (GLC), gas chromatography-mass spectrometry (GC-MS), and radioimmunoassay (RIA).

80176

This drug may also be known as Xylocaine, Dilocaine, L-caine, etc. Lidocaine is widely used in its various forms, including nonprescription ointments. However, lidocaine may be injected as an intravenous bolus as a treatment for ventricular arrhythmias and for cardiac manipulation. Any of a number of methods may be used, including high performance liquid chromatography (HPLC), gas liquid chromatography (GLC), gas chromatography-mass spectrometry (GC-MS), and fluorescence polarization immunoassay (FPIA).

80178

This drug may also be known as Eskalith. Lithium is a naturally occurring mineral and its salts may be used in the treatment of mental disorders, in particular bipolar depression. Steady state test specimens are frequently collected at the trough period, which is about 12 hours after the last dose when serum concentration is at its lowest. This is an effective approach to determine a therapeutic level of drug. Methods may include flame emission spectroscopy (FES), atomic absorption spectrophotometry (AAS), and ion-specific electrode (ISE).

80182

This drug may also be known as Aventyl or Pamelor. This drug is classified as a tricyclic antidepressant (TCA). Steady state test specimens are frequently collected at the trough period, which is about 12 hours after the last dose when serum concentration is at its lowest. This is an effective approach to determine a therapeutic level of drug. Overdose may also prompt this test. Any of a number of methods may be used, including high performance liquid chromatography (HPLC), gas liquid chromatography (GLC), and gas chromatography-mass spectrometry (GC-MS).

80184

This drug may also be known as Luminal. This drug may be administered to control seizures. Test specimens are frequently collected at the trough period, which is about 12 hours after the last dose when serum concentration is at its lowest. This is an effective approach to determine a therapeutic level of drug. Methodology may include gas liquid chromatography (GLC) and high performance liquid chromatography (HPLC).

80185–80186

This drug may also be known as Dilantin. This drug may be administered to control seizures. Steady state test specimens are frequently collected at the trough period, which is about 12 hours after the last dose when serum concentration is at its lowest. This is an effective approach to determine a therapeutic level of drug. Report 80185 for total serum levels and 80186 when free phenytoin is assayed. Methodology may include high performance liquid chromatography (HPLC), gas liquid chromatography (GLC), radioimmunoassay (RIA) fluorescence polarization immunoassay (FPIA). Free phenytoin is assayed by ultracentrifugation. Phenytoin is a known teratogen (cause of birth defects) and lowest therapeutic levels possible are often sought.

80188

This drug may also be known as Mysoline. This drug may be administered to control seizures. Test specimens are frequently collected at the trough period, which is about 12 hours after the last dose when serum concentration is at its lowest. This is an effective approach to determine a therapeutic level of drug. Methodology may include high performance liquid chromatography (HPLC), gas liquid chromatography (GLC), or enzyme immunoassay (EIA).

80190

This drug may also be known as Procan, Promine, or Pronestyl. This drug may be administered as an antiarrhythmic. Test specimens are frequently collected at the trough period, which is about 12 hours after the last dose when serum concentration is at its lowest. This is an effective approach to determine a therapeutic level of drug. Methodology may include high performance liquid chromatography (HPLC), gas liquid chromatography (GLC), and enzyme immunoassay (EIA).

80192

This procedure tests for Procan as well as metabolites, known as NAPA (n-acetyle procainamide).

80194

This drug may also be known as Duraquin, Quinate, Quinora, or Cardioquin. This drug is often administered as an antiarrhythmic. Test specimens are frequently collected at the trough period, which is about 12 hours after the last dose when serum concentration is at its lowest. This is an effective approach to determine a therapeutic level of drug. Methodology may include high performance liquid chromatography (HPLC) and gas liquid chromatography (GLC).

80196

This drug is known universally as aspirin and may also be referred to as a nonsteroidal antiinflammatory drug (NSAID). Specimen collection is at trough, which is the time just before the next dose of the drug when blood concentration is at its lowest. Overdose may also prompt this test. Methodology may include high performance liquid chromatography (HPLC) or gas liquid chromatography (GLC). Colorimetry and fluorometry may also be used.

80197

This drug is also known as Prograf. It is an immunosuppressant and may be prescribed for a number of conditions, including post-transplant therapies. Blood concentration monitoring may be ordered with this drug, particularly when delivered by IV. In this event, specimen collection may be random. Methodology may include high performance liquid chromatography (HPLC).

80198

This drug may also be known by numerous names, such as Aerolate, Bronkodyl, Sustaire, and Theophyl. This drug is available in several different forms, which may affect the type of assay run. Samples may be drawn about 30 minutes after oral administration. When delivered by IV, specimen collection may be random. The drug is widely used as a bronchodilator and to relieve bronchospasms. Methodology may include high performance liquid chromatography (HPLC) or gas liquid chromatography (GLC).

80200

This drug is also known as Nebcin. This drug has bactericidal properties and is usually injected. Specimen collection is at peak and trough. Peak will occur about one hour after an intramuscular injection and trough will occur about 12 hours after that. Method will often be by radioimmunoassay (RIA), microbiological assay, or high performance liquid chromatography (HPLC).

80201

This drug may also be known as Topimax. It is currently classified as an "orphan drug," a designation for certain drugs and biologicals used principally for very rare diseases. The product is kept in supply only in limited quantities for the limited number of patients requiring therapy. Distribution is not general. This particular drug is used primarily in the treatment of Lennox-Gastaut syndrome.

80202

This drug may also be known as Vancocin. Specimen collection may be drawn during the trough period. This occurs around 30 minutes prior to the next dose. It is sometimes also drawn at peak. Toxic and therapeutic dosages for vancomycin can be difficult to determine due to the way the drug is metabolized. Methods include radioimmunoassay (RIA), high performance liquid chromatography (HPLC), and microbiological assay.

80400

This test is sometimes ordered as corticotropin-releasing factor stimulation (or CRF) test, adrenocorticotropic hormone (ACTH) infusion test, rapid ACTH test, or cosyntropin test. Method is immunoassay. A chemistry test must be performed to determine baseline serum cortisol (serum ACTH may also be ordered). Shortly thereafter, cosyntropin, an ACTH-like drug, is administered to the patient, typically by IV bolus. Blood is again drawn and assayed for a change in serum cortisol. Variations are seen in administering a 24-hour test and a three-day test. This code reports the test for adrenal insufficiency (Addison's disease), which is an ordinary reason for the test. See code 82533 for serum cortisol testing specifics.

80402

This test may be ordered as an enzyme deficiency ACTH stimulation test. This code specifically cites 21-hydroxylase deficiency. The classic 21-hydroxylase deficiency is noted in ambiguous genitalia in neonates, but a later onset is also found. Cosyntropin, an ACTH-like drug, is administered to the patient, typically by IV bolus. Overproduction of the metabolite 17-hydroxyprogesterone is often associated with this condition and it is tested for as a baseline and following the ACTH stimulation injection. Cortisol levels are tested in a similar fashion in this panel.

80406

This test may be ordered as a 3B-HSD panel. The official description for the code is for 3 beta-hydroxydehydrogenase deficiency, or congenital adrenal hyperplasia. The panel may often be performed on infants and small children, but adult patients are also tested. The condition involves defects in steroid synthesis. A bolus infusion of ACTH is given to the patient after baseline cortisol and 17-hydroxypregnenolone have been drawn. Cortisol and 17-hydroxypregnenolone are drawn again and the results interpreted.

80408

This panel may be ordered as a saline infusion test. Specimen is drawn from the patient while in an upright position and the product saved for baseline aldosterone and renin testing. The patient is then administered saline, usually intravenously, while in a recumbent position. Specimen is again drawn for aldosterone and renin levels. In healthy individuals, aldosterone output is suppressed when the volume of blood is expanded. The test is useful in the evaluation of kidney function.

80410

This test may be ordered as human calcitonin test (HCT), or thyrocalcitonin panel. Calcitonin is a hormone secreted by the thyroid gland in response to elevated serum calcium levels. Calcitonin secretion causes the calcium to be excreted by the kidneys. A baseline calcitonin level is drawn. Stimulation of the thyroid for this panel is typically pentagastrin delivered by IV. Blood is again drawn at five and ten minutes from stimulation. The patient should be fasting.

80412

This test may be ordered as CRH "Stim" panel. This panel allows for multiple specimens to be drawn before administration of CRH. Orders may call for blood draws from both petrous sinus veins as well as from a peripheral source. Note the high number of cortisol and ACTH tests to be run. The timing of specimen draws for cortisol and ACTH may differ somewhat. The panel is useful to differentiate Cushing's disease and certain ACTH-secreting tumors, among other disorders.

80414

This test may be ordered as a HCG "Stim," or human chorionic gonadotropin panel. Blood specimens may be drawn on two separate mornings before HCG is administered, usually by intramuscular injection. Injections may be repeated on two following days. Blood collection times may vary following HCG administration. The test is useful in diagnosis of certain cases of hypogonadotrophism as well as certain steroid deficiencies.

80415

This test may be ordered as a HCG "Stim," or human chorionic gonadotropin panel. Blood specimens may be drawn on two separate mornings before HCG is administered, usually by intramuscular injection and sometimes in several sessions. Timing of blood draws may vary, but just prior to first administration of HCG and four hours after is common for women. Estradiol is among the more active endogenous estrogens. The panel is useful in the diagnosis of certain menstrual disorders, fertility problems, and estrogen-producing tumors.

80416–80417

This test may be ordered as renin "Stim" panel, renin activity panel, or plasma renin activity (PRA) panel. Baseline samples may be drawn from the renal vein (80416) or peripheral vein (80417) and tested for renin. Renin is an enzyme synthesized in the kidney. A renin-stimulating agent, such as the diuretics captopril and furosemide, is administered, usually orally and usually in several stages. The patient remains upright for several hours before again testing for renin, once again, usually in stages. The panel is a useful screen and diagnostic tool for various forms of hypertension, renal artery disorders, and other disorders of the renal/circulatory system.

80418

This series of tests may also be ordered as a pituitary panel, and many large facilities will have an internal code name for this panel. This is a complex panel with numerous tests. Facilities with proper capabilities can offer a rapid, combined series where stimulation agents (i.e., insulin, thyrotropin-releasing hormone, and luteinizing hormone-releasing hormone) are administered simultaneously on a single day. This panel may be used most often for suspected pituitary tumor. See individual code listings for specifics about portions of the panel.

80420

Baseline samples are usually drawn. Dexamethasone is the suppression agent and it is usually administered orally at night. The next morning a fasting blood sample is drawn and rendered to serum. The cortisol level is measured as described in code 82533. The free cortisol is a urine test as described in code 82530. This panel is a 48-hour work up to differentiate diagnoses; Cushing's syndrome from alcoholism, obesity, and depression.

80422

Arginine is a powerful stimulator of glucagon in healthy patients and may be administered as the stimulating agent for this panel. Baseline blood work is typically performed prior to stimulating glucagon. This glucagon tolerance panel tests for insulinoma, a type of benign tumor of cells in the islets of Langerhans portion of the pancreas. Insulinoma is a prime cause of the condition known as hypoglycemia. Glucagon is a hormone secreted in the pancreas in response to hypoglycemic conditions.

80424

Arginine is a powerful stimulator of glucagon in healthy patients and may be administered as the stimulating agent for this panel. Baseline blood work is typically performed prior to stimulating glucagon. Pheochromocytoma is a usually benign tumor of the adrenal gland. Glucagon is a hormone secreted in the pancreas in response to hypoglycemic conditions. Abnormally high levels of glucagon have been linked to pheochromocytomas. The panel includes a test for

fractionated catecholamines, as described by code 82384. This test helps to further differentiate a diagnosis of adrenal tumor from hypothymia and hypertension.

80426

This panel may be ordered as a GnRH "Stim." The panel tests for a variety of disorders, including pituitary disorders and premature sexual development in children. Baseline blood work is usually drawn. The gonadotropin-releasing hormone (GnRH) is typically administered by intravenous bolus. The peak response for follicle stimulating hormone (FSH) will be somewhat different than for luteinizing hormone (LH). Blood is often drawn at 30 minutes, 60 minutes, and 120 minutes.

80428

This panel may be ordered as a GH provocation test, insulin tolerance test (ITT), and as the Arginine test. Baseline blood work is typically drawn. Stimulation of growth hormone is often achieved through an intravenous infusion of arginine hydrochloride, L-dopa, or clonidine. This may be administered over about 30 minutes. Blood specimens are then collected at 15 minutes, 30 minutes, and 45 minutes. These samples will be tested for HCG as specified in code 83003.

80430

This panel may be ordered as a GH suppression test. Blood work is typically drawn before the test as a baseline. Glucose is the suppression agent for GH and administration may be orally. Blood is again drawn, often at 60 and 120 minutes for glucose, with one more specimen drawn for HCG.

80432

This panel may be ordered as connecting peptide insulin, insulin C-peptide, or proinsulin C-peptide. C-peptide is formed in the islets of Langerhans in the pancreas along with insulin. Both are released into the portal vein. C-peptide levels generally correlate to insulin levels and may reflect pancreatic function. Blood work is usually performed prior to the test to establish a baseline. Insulin is injected intravenously and blood is drawn at intervals for C-peptide and glucose; insulin is tested for only once.

80434

The insulin tolerance panel for ACTH insufficiency typically involves baseline blood work before testing. The insulin is administered following a fasting period, typically by an indwelling needle. The panel is specifically for adrenocorticosteroid hormone (ACTH). The cortisol test is an indirect but accurate measure of ACTH. The panel is useful to assess hypothalamic/pituitary/adrenal interaction.

CPT® Lay Descriptions

80435

The insulin tolerance panel for growth hormone insufficiency typically involves baseline blood work before testing. The insulin is administered following a fasting period, typically orally. The panel is specifically for growth hormone, or human growth hormone (GH or HGH). Glucose is administered, typically by IV bolus, and specimens are drawn at regular intervals following dosage. Note the number of times each component is drawn.

80436

The metyrapone panel typically involves baseline blood work before testing. The metyrapone is typically administered orally with the cortisol and 11 deoxycortisol tested for again the following morning. The test is sometimes administered outpatient and is useful in determining secondary adrenal insufficiencies, among other disorders.

80438–80439

This test is also known as TRH test or thyrotropin releasing factor (TRF) test. The thyrotropin-releasing hormone is typically administered by IV bolus shortly after collecting a sample to baseline for thyroid stimulating hormone. Report code 80438 for a one-hour version of the test, and 80439 for a two-hour version. Either test is useful in testing the anterior pituitary gland's ability to secrete TSH (normal response is for a rise in secretion following administration of TRH).

80440

This test may be called prolactin stimulation after TRH, or simply prolactin "Stim." Baseline blood work is performed before administration of thyrotropin releasing hormone. IV usually administers the TRH and blood is again drawn at 15 minutes and 30 minutes. The test is for hyperprolactinemia, or high levels of prolactin in the blood. This condition is sometimes linked to renal, thyroid, or liver problems.

80500–80502

A clinical pathology consultation is a service performed by a physician (pathologist) in response to a request from the attending physician regarding test results requiring additional medical interpretive judgment. Pharmacokinetic consultations regarding therapeutic drug levels may be reported with this code. Code 80500 reports a limited consultation not requiring review of the patient's history and medical records. Code 80502 reports a comprehensive consultation related to more complex diagnostic problems and requires review of the patient's history and medical records.

81000

This type of test may be ordered by the brand name product and the analytes tested. Although, screens are considered to show the presence of an analyte (qualitative), some newer products are semi-quantitative. Many are plastic strips that contain sites impregnated with chemicals that react with urine when the strip is dipped into a specimen. The result is a color change that is compared against a standardized chart. Most strips will test for numerous analytes, as well as for pH and specific gravity. Tablets work in a similar fashion. A drop of urine is placed on the tablet and a chemical reaction causes a color change that is compared to a standard chart. Usually only a single analyte is under consideration, per tablet. Code 81000 involves manual (nonautomated) test and includes a microscopic examination. Microscopy involves examination of the urine sediments or solids. The urine is first centrifuged in a graduated tube to concentrate the sediments. Samples (either wet or dry) are examined, usually under both high and low power, and abnormal constituents are noted. These may include a wide range of biological abnormalities, such as blood cells, casts, and bacteria, as well as chemical anomalies, such as crystals.

81001

This type of test may be ordered by the type of processor used and the analytes tested. The testing methodology is similar to the manual strips, except that the color change caused by the chemical reaction with urine is processed and read mechanically. The strip is exposed to the urine sample and is mechanically fed through a processor that reads the colors emitted by the reaction. The unit will be calibrated according to international standards and readings have a high degree of accuracy. The result may be displayed on a monitor, but is always printed or recorded in some form. Code 81001 also includes a microscopy. Microscopy involves examination of the urine sediments or solids. The urine is first centrifuged in a graduated tube to concentrate the sediments. Samples (either wet or dry) are examined, usually under both high and low power, and abnormal constituents are noted. These may include a wide range of biological abnormalities, such as blood cells, casts, and bacteria, as well as chemical anomalies, such as crystals.

81002

This type of test may be ordered by the brand name product and the analytes tested. Although usually considered screens to show the presence of an analyte (qualitative), some newer products are semi-quantitative. Many are plastic strips that contain sites impregnated with chemicals that react with urine when the strip is dipped into a specimen. The result is a color change that is compared against a standardized chart. Most strips will test for numerous analytes, as well as for pH and specific gravity. Tablets work in a similar fashion. A drop of urine is placed on the tablet and a chemical reaction causes a color change that is compared to a standard chart. Usually only a single analyte is under consideration per tablet, however. Code 81002 does not include a microscopic examination of the urine sample or its components.

81003

This type of test may be ordered by the type of processor used and the analytes tested. The testing methodology is similar to the manual strips, except that the color change caused by the chemical reaction with urine is processed and read mechanically. The strip is exposed to the urine sample and is mechanically fed through a processor that reads the colors emitted by the reaction. The unit will be calibrated according to international standards and readings have a high degree of accuracy. The result may be displayed on a monitor, but is always printed or recorded in some form. Code 81003 does not include a microscopic examination of the urine sample or its components.

81005

This test may be ordered by the type of processor used and the analytes under examination. The method will be any type of automated analyzer, usually colorimetry. The results of a semi-quantitative test indicate the presence or absence of an analyte and may be expressed as simply positive or negative. A qualitative result may be indicated as trace, 1+, 2+, etc.

81007

This type of test may be ordered by the brand name of the commercial kit used and the bacteria that the kit screens for. Human urine is normally almost entirely free of bacteria. However, bacteria can easily be introduced upon voiding. In addition, specimens containing any amount of pathological bacteria can have the organisms rapidly multiply after collection. For this reason, specimens are often examined shortly after collection. Method includes any method except culture or dipstick. The test is often performed by commercial kit. The type of kit used should be specified in the report.

81015

This test may be ordered as a microscopic analysis. Human urine is normally almost entirely free of bacteria. However, bacteria can easily be introduced upon voiding. In addition, specimens containing any amount of pathological bacteria can have the organisms rapidly multiply after collection. For this reason, specimens are often examined shortly after collection. The sample may first be centrifuged into a graduated tube to concentrate the sediments, or solid matter, held in suspension. Bacteria cells are comparatively small and a combination of stains and high power microscopy is usually employed. The concentration of bacteria will be noted.

81020

This test may be ordered as a two-glass or three-glass test, a MacConkey-blood agar test, an MC-blood agar test, or any of the previous with a gram-positive plate. This is a culture for bacteria and will typically involve a culture plate of 5 percent sheep's blood agar and a MacConkey plate (a medium containing differentiate for lactose and nonlactose fermenters). A third plate of gram-positive media may offer further discrimination of bacteria cultured. The test is useful in determining the types and prevalence of bacteria in the urine.

81025

This test may be ordered by any of the brand name kits available. The tests typically involve a dip stick impregnated with reagents that chemically react upon contact with urine. A change in color indicates positive or negative for the presence of hormones found in the urine of women in early pregnancy.

81050

This test may be ordered as simply a volume measurement, a flow study, uroflowmetry, or urodynamic study. Timed collections are typically collected over a given period (24 hours is common). This test may be performed as a preliminary study to determine the volume of urine voided per second. A flowmeter device may be used, or a simple timing of the flow into a graduated container may be employed. The test is sometimes also administered as a baseline or otherwise in conjunction with urinary tract procedures that might affect flow.

82000

This test is commonly ordered as acetaldehyde level. It is used to measure ethanol exposure/ingestion as ethanol is converted to acetaldehyde by alcohol dehydrogenase. Blood specimen is obtained by venipuncture, finger stick or heel stick. Methodology is gas-liquid chromatography (GLC).

82003

This test is commonly ordered as acetaminophen or Tylenol level. Specimen collection is obtained by venipuncture, finger stick and heel stick in infants. Method is immunoassay or UV spectrophotometry. Acetaminophen levels may be seen in overdose situations and measurement is useful to determine toxicity and potential liver damage. The expected half-life of acetaminophen is one to three hours.

82009–82010

This test is also referred to as blood ketone analysis or blood nitroprusside reaction. Specimen collection is obtained by venipuncture, finger stick, or heel stick in infants. Method is nitroprusside reaction (colorimetry). The test may be performed to assess suspected metabolic disorders or to determine absolute or relative starvation, especially in children. Qualitative analysis (82009) tests for the presence of acetone or other ketone bodies, while quantitative analysis (82010) measures the amount of acetone or other ketone bodies.

CPT® Lay Descriptions

82013

This test is also referred to as red blood cell (RBC) acetylcholinesterase, erythrocytic cholinesterase, or true cholinesterase. Specimen collection is by venipuncture, finger stick, or heel stick in infants. Method is colorimetric or spectrophotometric rate of hydrolysis determination. This test may be performed to help determine certain RBC disorders such as thalassemias, spherocytosis, and other anemias. It may also be used to determine toxicity or exposure to certain insecticides. For amniotic fluid specimen, a separately reportable amniocentesis is performed. The presence of acetylcholinesterase activity and increased alpha-fetoprotein in amniotic fluid are presumptive evidence of an open neural tube defect in the fetus.

82016–82017

These tests may be requested as qualitative acylcarnitine (carnitine esters) and quantitative acylcarnitine (carnitine esters). Acylcarnitine is a condensation product formed from carboxylic acid and carnitine. It has a variety of metabolic roles and may be an indicator of inborn errors of metabolism, chronic disease, or acute and critical illness. Blood specimen is obtained by venipuncture. A 24-hour urine specimen is required. The patient flushes the first urine of the day and discards it. All voided urine for the next 24 hours is collected and refrigerated. Methods include enzymatic, chromatography, and mass-spectrometry. Qualitative analysis (82016) tests for the presence of acylcarnitine while quantitative analysis (82017) measures the amount of acylcarnitine.

82024

This test is also referred to as adrenocorticotrophic hormone (ACTH) or corticotropin. Specimen collection is by venipuncture. Method is radioimmunoassay. This test may be performed to determine the presence of Cushing's disease, depression or pheochromocytoma, among other conditions.

82030

This test is also referred to as cyclic adenosine monophosphate (AMP) or cAMP. Specimen collection is by venipuncture for blood. Urine may be random, two-hour, or 24-hour. Methodology is radioimmunoassay (RIA). This test may be performed in the presence of hypercalcemia for determination of hyperparathyroidism.

82040

This test is often used to determine nutritional status, renal disease, and other chronic diseases. Specimen collection is by venipuncture, finger stick, or heel stick in infants. Method is colorimetry.

82042

This code reports quantitative analysis for albumin on urine, CSF, or amniotic fluid. Urine tests are usually performed on a 24-hour urine specimen to measure protein loss of patients with hypoalbuminemia. Patients typically perform specimen collection over a 24-hour period. Method is colorimetry. CSF analysis requires separately reportable spinal puncture and the test is performed using nephelometry. Amniotic fluid analysis requires separately reportable ultrasound guidance and amniocentesis and test is usually performed by autoanalyzer.

82043–82044

"Microalbuminuria" is defined as albuminuria of 30 to 300 mg/24 hours and is requested to determine early increase of proteinuria, usually in diabetes and in pre-eclampsia before protein becomes evident by conventional urinalysis. Patients commonly perform specimen collection over a 24-hour period. Methods include radioimmunoassay (RIA) or enzyme-linked immunosorbent assay (ELISA). Report code 82043 for quantitative microalbumin and 82044 for semi-quantitative or reagent strip microalbumin.

82055

This test may also be requested as ethanol, ethyl alcohol, or ETOH. If the specimen is blood (serum), collection is typically by venipuncture. Method is commonly enzymatic rate analysis (alcohol dehydrogenase). This test is typically performed to determine alcohol level for medical or legal purposes, to screen unconscious patients, to diagnose alcohol intoxication to determine appropriate therapy, and to monitor ethanol treatment for methanol intoxication.

82075

This test may be used primarily in screening for ethanol levels above the legal limit for driving. The legal limit varies from state to state with levels above 0.08-0.1 g/dL usually being defined as legally intoxicated.

82085

This test may also be requested as aldolase (ALD) or fructose biphosphate aldolase. Specimen collection is by venipuncture. Methods may include ultraviolet, kinetic, coupled enzymatic and colorimetric. This test can be useful in the identification of a variety of degenerative diseases, myopathies, and inflammations.

82088

For serum aldosterone, blood is obtained by post-fasting venipuncture. Extreme care must be taken in preparing the patient before specimen collection and handling the specimen in order to obtain an accurate measurement. Blood specimens are usually taken early in the morning and a notation is made as to whether the patient was sitting or supine. A second test may be performed approximately four hours later. A radioimmunoassay (RIA) is typically employed for analysis of the specimen. This test is most commonly used in the diagnosis of specific types of adrenal adenomas, or secondary aldosteronism caused by cirrhosis, congestive heart failure, nephrosis, potassium loading, toxemia of pregnancy, and other states of contraction of plasma volume. Urine aldosterone requires a 24-hour non-fasting urine specimen. The patient flushes the first urine of the day. All voided urine for the next 24 hours is collected. Method is radioimmunoassay.

82101

Alkaloids are nitrogenous substances found in plants, many of which are pharmacologically active. Common alkaloids include morphine, quinine, atropine, and strychnine. This test may be is used to measure (quantitate) the amount of a specific alkaloid present in a random urine specimen.

82103

This test may also be requested as A1 AT, AAT, Acute Phase Proteins, or -1-Antitrypsin. Specimen collection is by venipuncture. Method is by radial immunodiffusion (RID), or nephelometry. This test is used to detect hereditary decreases in the production of alpha1-antitrypsin, chronic obstructive lung disease, or liver disease.

82104

This test may also be requested as A1AT phenotype, AAT phenotype, and Pi phenotype. Specimen collection is by venipuncture. This test is used to detect hereditary decreases in the production of alpha1-antitrypsin by specific phenotype. There are more than 75 inherited variants of AAT. Two variants, Pi ZZ and Pi SZ phenotypes, represent severe deficiencies and are associated with chronic obstructive lung disease, liver disease, and hepatoma. Method is by radial immunodiffusion (RID).

82105

This test may be abbreviated as AFP. It may also be referred to as fetal alpha globulin. While this test is most often associated with pregnancy, it is also used to diagnose a variety of other conditions. During pregnancy, the test is normally performed between the 16th and 18th week of gestation. If levels are abnormal it may be repeated approximately one week after the first test. Blood is obtained by venipuncture. Analysis is normally performed by radioimmunoassay (RIA).

82106

The test may be abbreviated as AFP. The test is normally performed on pregnant women initially between the 16th and 18th week of gestation. An amniotic AFP may be performed when serum AFP (82105) results are abnormal to confirm a diagnosis. An ultrasound is performed to determine the exact location of the fetus. AFP levels are measured, generally by radioimmunoassay (RIA).

82108

This test may be abbreviated as Al. The test is used to monitor patients at risk for aluminum toxicity due to exposure or disease states, which cause aluminum accumulation (e.g., chronic renal failure). Blood specimen is obtained by venipuncture. A random urine sample is obtained. Method is atomic absorption spectrophotometry (AAS).

82120

This test is administered to determine the specific cause of vaginitis and may be performed following negative testing for yeasts or trichomonas. Disturbances in normal anaerobic flora are usually the etiological source. A saline wet slide is prepared and characteristic cells are identified microscopically, namely epithelial cells with bacilli clinging to the surfaces. A solution of potassium hydroxide (KOH) is added to the mount to activate amines. A characteristic odor is released when amines are present and become volatile.

82127–82128

This test may also be referred to as a metabolic screen for amino acids. Blood specimen is obtained by venipuncture. A random urine sample is obtained. Several methods may be used including thin layer chromatography (TLC), gas chromatography (GC), and ion-exchange chromatography. These tests determine whether an amino acid is or is not present (qualitative analysis). Code 82127 tests for the presence of single amino acids, while 82128 tests for the presence of multiple amino acids.

82131

This test may be requested as specific amino acid (e.g., cystine, tyrosine, methionine, proprionic acid). Blood specimen is obtained by venipuncture. A 24-hour urine specimen is used. The patient flushes the first urine of the day and discards it. All voided urine for the next 24 hours is collected and refrigerated. Method is ion-exchange chromatography. This test measures (quantifies) amounts of single specified amino acids.

82135

This test may be requested as aminolevulinic acid (ALA), delta ALA or DALA. Aminolevulinic acid is a precursor of heme, produced from glycine and succinyl-CoA. This test is used to diagnose genetic disorders that allow porphyrin products, specifically aminolevulinic acid, to accumulate in the liver or red blood cells. A 24-hour urine sample is required. The patient flushes the first urine of the day and discards it. All voided urine for the next 24 hours is collected and refrigerated. Methodology includes spectrophotometry or ion-exchange resin columns.

82136–82139

These tests may be requested as specific amino acids (e.g., cystine, tyrosine, methionine, proprionic acid).

CPT® Lay Descriptions

Blood specimen is obtained by venipuncture. A 24-hour urine specimen is required. The patient flushes the first urine of the day and discards it. All voided urine for the next 24 hours is collected and refrigerated. Method is ion-exchange chromatography. This test measures (quantifies) amounts of multiple specified amino acids. Report 82136 for two to five amino acids. Report 82139 for six or more.

82140

This test may be requested as NH3. Elevated levels may indicate that the liver is not able to detoxify ammonia from the blood due to severe liver disease. Blood is obtained by venipuncture or arterial puncture. A 24-hour urine specimen is required. The patient flushes the first urine of the day and discards it. All voided urine for the next 24 hours is collected and refrigerated. A number of methods are used including enzymatic, resin enzymatic, and ion-selective electrode (ISE).

82143

This procedure may be requested as an amniotic fluid analysis for hemolytic disease of a newborn, amniotic fluid spectral analysis, Liley test, and amniotic fluid OD 450 spectral analysis. An ultrasound is performed to determine the exact location of the fetus. Method is spectrophotometry. This test measures the amount of free bilirubin in the amniotic fluid.

82145

This test may be requested as a quantitative analysis of amphetamine/methamphetamine. Blood specimen is obtained by venipuncture. A random urine specimen is obtained. A number of methods are used. Methods used for blood include gas-liquid chromatography (GLC), gas chromatometry/mass spectometry (GC/MS), and radioimmunoassay (RIA). Methods used for urine include enzyme immunoassay (EIA), high performance liquid chromatography (HPLC), fluorescence polarization immunoassay (FPIA), and RIA. This test measures (quantifies) the amount of amphetamine or methamphetamine in the urine.

82150

This test may be requested as glucanohydrolase. Serum amylase is elevated in acute pancreatitis and is therefore a common test when abdominal pain, epigastric tenderness, nausea, and vomiting are present. Blood is obtained by venipuncture. A two-hour urine specimen is required. There are multiple methods of testing for amylase.

82154

This test may be requested as 3-Alpha-diol G. Androstanediol glucuronide is an androgen formed in the peripheral tissues. Elevated levels are frequently seen in females with hirsutism (excessive body hair). When androstanediol glucuronide is elevated, treatment of hirsutism is directed at the peripheral

tissue sites rather than at other sites that are sometimes responsible for overproduction of androgens (adrenal cortex, ovary). Blood is obtained by venipuncture. Method is radioimmunoassay (RIA).

82157

An androgenic steroid secreted by the testes, adrenal cortex, and ovaries. This test is used primarily to evaluate androgen production in females with hirsutism. Blood is obtained by venipuncture. Method is radioimmunoassay (RIA).

82160

Andosterone is a steroid hormone metabolite in the androgen series that is measured for evaluation of syndromes of androgen excess such as hirsutism and polycystic ovary syndrome. It has been measured typically by methods involving extraction and chromatography, followed by detection and quantification by colorimetric or immunometric techniques. Measurement of this compound has largely been replaced by determination of other specific plasma androgens (e.g. testosterone) by modern, sensitive assays.

82163

A hormone that acts as a powerful vasopressor, raising blood pressure and reducing fluid loss in the kidney by restricting blood flow. It also stimulates aldosterone secretion. Blood is obtained by venipuncture. The patient must remain in a recumbent position for 30 minutes prior to obtaining the specimen. Angiotensin II is difficult to measure accurately and great care must be taken in both collection and storage of the specimen. Method is radioimmunoassay (RIA). Degradation products and interfering peptides must be removed from the specimen prior to RIA.

82164

This test may be requested as ACE or peptidyl-dipeptidase A. ACE converts angiotensin I to angiotensin II. Blood is obtained by venipuncture. Method is spectrofluorometric combined with various synthetic substrates or radioimmunoassay (RIA).

82172

This test may be requested as Apolipoprotein A, Apolipoprotein A-1, Apolipoprotein B, Apolipoprotein E, Apo-A, Apo-A1, Apo-B, or Apo-E. Apolipoproteins are the components of lipoprotein complexes found in high density lipoprotein (HDL), low density lipoprotein (LDL), and very low density lipoprotein (VLDL). There are numerous variables that are designated as A, B, C, D, and E with some further subdivided (e.g., A1, A2, B48, B100, C1). Those of primary interest for laboratory testing are Apo-A1, Apo-B, and Apo-E. Multiple methods are used, including radioimmunoassay (RIA), radial immunodiffusion (RID), and enzyme-linked immunosorbent assay (ELISA).

82175

Arsenic is a toxic metallic element with exposure occurring either by inhalation or ingestion. Blood is obtained by venipuncture. Urine is the preferred specimen for acute exposure and when patient is symptomatic. A 24-hour urine specimen is required. The patient flushes the first urine of the day and discards it. All voided urine for the next 24 hours is collected. Method is colorimetry, atomic absorption spectrophotometry (AAS), or neutron activation analysis (NAA). This test measures (quantifies) the amount of arsenic present.

82180

This test is used to evaluate Vitamin C deficiency. It may be performed with or without Vitamin C saturation. When performed as a saturation test, megadoses of Vitamin C are given over a three-to-four day period. Blood is obtained by venipuncture. The amount of Vitamin C is measured (quantified).

82190

AAS is a method for detecting the absorption of specific wavelengths of light by analyte that have been vaporized in a flame. The analysis is performed using a specialized instrument known as an atomic absorption spectrometer. Analytes are typically pure elements, since each element has a specific absorption spectrum.

82205

This test may be requested as a quantitative analysis of barbiturates. Blood is obtained by venipuncture. A random urine specimen is obtained. A number of methods are used. Methods used for blood include gas-liquid chromatography (GLC), gas chromatometry/mass spectometry (GC/MS), and radioimmunoassay (RIA). Methods used for urine include enzyme immunoassay (EIA) and high performance liquid chromatography (HPLC). This test measures (quantifies) the amount of barbiturate.

82232

This test may be requested as Beta2M. Beta2M is a small (micro) nonpolymorphic protein. Blood is obtained by venipuncture. A 24-hour urine specimen is required with the patient being induced to produce alkaline urine prior to testing. The patient flushes the first urine of the day and discards it. All voided urine for the next 24 hours is collected and refrigerated. CSF is obtained by spinal puncture, which is reported separately. Method is by radioimmunoassay (RIA), enzyme immunoassay (EIA), or immunoradiometric assay (IRMA).

82239–82240

This is sometimes referred to as glycocholic acid. Bile acids are steroid acids derived from cholesterol. Cholylglycine is a bile salt formed by glycine and cholic acid. Blood is obtained by venipuncture. Method is enzymatic or gas-liquid chromatography

(GLC). Code 82239 reports total concentration of all bile acids. Code 82240 reports total concentration of cholylglycine only.

82247–82248

Bilirubin is a bile pigment formed by the breakdown of hemoglobin during both normal and abnormal erythrocyte destruction. Direct (conjugated) bilirubin is that portion of the bilirubin that has been taken up by the liver cells to form bilirubin diglucuronide. Indirect (unconjugated) bilirubin is that portion of the bilirubin that has not been taken up by the liver cells. Total bilirubin is the sum of direct and indirect bilirubin present in the specimen. Blood is obtained by venipuncture. Method is diazotization. Spectrophotometry may be used in neonates six weeks or younger. Report 82247 for total bilirubin. Report 82248 for direct bilirubin.

82252

Bilirubin is not normally present in feces, only in cases of rapid peristaltic movement of the gut or disturbances in normal intestinal flora. Detection may be useful in evaluation of some types of diarrhea. It can be detected with the dipstick or tablet tests commonly used for urine, by testing the supernatant fluid from watery feces, or adding water to solid feces.

82261

This test may be requested as an indirect test for biotin. Biotinidase is an enzyme required for the recycling of biotin. Biotinidase deficiency is a genetic condition. Newborn screening tests may include testing for deficiency of this enzyme. Blood specimen is obtained by venipuncture, finger stick, or heel stick. Method is colorimetry or enzymatic.

82270

This test may be requested as guaiac, stool, or by a variety of brand names. A random stool sample is obtained. Accuracy increases when three to six repeat tests are performed. Alternatively, a test kit may be sent home with the patient. When three samples have been obtained, the patient sends the kit to a prearranged lab for performance of the test. Method is peroxidase activity. This test reports the presence (qualitative analysis) of blood in the stool, but does not quantify the amount.

82273

This test may be requested as hemoglobin, urine. A random urine specimen is obtained. Method is dipstick, but microscopy may also be performed to identify red blood cells and red cell casts. This test reports the presence (qualitative analysis) of blood in the urine but does not quantify the amount.

82274

Fecal sample is dispersed in a diluent with antibodies for hemoglobin antigen to form a complex of antibody and antigen. A complex of antibody and

CPT® Lay Descriptions

antigen is separated from the specimen and exposed to a second antibody for the hemoglobin antigen, and a portion of the antibody. A sample from the first complex is bound to a solid carrier and a sample from the second antibody exposure is labeled with a detection agent to determine the presence of hemoglobin antigen in the original fecal specimen. This code requires three samples, which must be obtained from separate bowel movements, and each sample must be placed in a sterile leakproof container with a screw-cap lid for transport to the laboratory.

82286

Bradykinin is a biologically active peptide, found in plasma and many other tissues and fluids, important in the inflammatory response. A pathogenic role for Bradykinin has been suggested in diseases ranging from asthma to hereditary angioedema, as well as other kinds of swelling disorders and allergic-type diseases. It is measured in body fluids by techniques including immunoassay, capillary electrophoresis, chromatography and mass-spectrometry.

82300

Cadmium may be abbreviated as Cd. Cadmium is a bivalent metal. This test is used to evaluate toxic levels of cadmium after industrial exposure to cadmium fumes or ingestion of cadmium. A 24-hour urine specimen is recommended and must be collected in a plastic container. The patient flushes the first urine of the day and discards it. All voided urine for the next 24 hours is collected. Method is atomic absorption spectroscopy (AAS).

82306

This test may be requested as 25-OHD3, 25(OH) Calciferol, Vitamin D 25-Hydroxy, or Calciferol 25-Hydroxy. Blood specimen is obtained by venipuncture. Method is high performance liquid chromatography (HPLC), competitive protein binding (CPB), or radioimmunoassay (RIA).

82307

This test may be requested as cholecalciferol or Vitamin D3. Blood specimen is obtained by venipuncture. Method is high performance liquid chromatography (HPLC), competitive protein binding (CPB), or radioimmunoassay (RIA).

82308

This test may be requested as thyrocalcitonin. This test may be used to screen for specific malignant neoplasms. Blood specimen is obtained by venipuncture. A fasting specimen should be taken. The specimen is collected in a chilled tube and the test performed within 10 minutes of collection. Serum (plasma) is separated in a refrigerated centrifuge and frozen. The test is performed by assay or radioimmunoassay (RIA).

82310

May be abbreviated Ca. Blood is obtained by venipuncture or heel stick. Specimen is obtained in the morning and a fasting sample is preferable. Postural changes and venous stasis may provide misleading results. Accurate diagnosis may require obtaining additional specimens on subsequent days. Method is spectrophotometry or atomic absorption spectroscopy (AAS). The test may be used to assess thyroid and parathyroid function.

82330

This test may also be referred to as free calcium. It may be abbreviated Ca++ or Ca+2. Ionized or free calcium refers to calcium that is not bound to proteins in the blood. It is the metabolically active portion of the calcium in the blood. Blood is obtained by venipuncture and collected anaerobically. Method is by ion-selective electrode (ISE). The test may be used to assess thyroid and parathyroid function.

82331

The calcium infusion test is a provocative test for evaluation of medullary thyroid carcinoma (MTC). Calcitonin levels are measured following an IV infusion of calcium solution, and sometimes calcium levels are also measured to evaluate calcium incorporation or monitor hypercalcemia.

82340

This test may be abbreviated Ca++ or Ca+2. A 24-hour urine specimen is required. The patient flushes the first urine of the day and discards it. All voided urine for the next 24 hours is collected and refrigerated. Method is spectrophotometry or atomic absorption spectrometry (AAS).

82355–82360

This test may be requested as a calculus analysis or nephrolithiasis analysis. The specimen should be rinsed to remove any tissue or blood. Chemical analysis generally includes testing for the presence of calcium, carbonate, cystine, magnesium, oxalate, phosphates and urates. The analysis may be qualitative (82355), identifying only the chemicals that are present, or it may be quantitative (82360) measuring the amounts of each of the chemicals identified.

82365

This test may be requested as a calculus analysis or nephrolithiasis analysis. The specimen should be rinsed to remove any tissue or blood. The stone is analyzed for the presence of calcium, carbonate, cystine, magnesium, oxalate, phosphates, and urates. This code is specific for analysis by infrared spectroscopy, which is generally performed only by reference laboratories.

82370

This test may be requested as a calculus analysis or nephrolithiasis analysis. The specimen should be rinsed to remove any tissue or blood. The stone is analyzed for the presence of calcium, carbonate, cystine, magnesium, oxalate, phosphates, and urates. This code is specific for analysis by x-ray diffraction, which is generally performed only by reference laboratories. X-ray diffraction can separately analyze the nidus (center), which often differs chemically from the cortex (external layer).

82373

This test may be ordered as a CDT or CDT percentage. Blood specimen is obtained by venipuncture. The specimen is clotted and separated. Method is nephelometry or turbidometric immunnoassay. Carbohydrate deficient transferrin is a protein formed in the liver and abnormally high elevations are linked to a prolonged period of high alcohol use. The test may be ordered to confirm diagnosis of alcoholism or to measure compliance with an abstinence program.

82374

This test may be requested as HCO3 or bicarbonate. Bicarbonate (carbon dioxide) is an indicator of electrolyte and acid-base status (alkalosis, acidosis). It is elevated in metabolic alkalosis, compensated respiratory acidosis, and hypokalemia. It is decreased in metabolic acidosis, compensated respiratory alkalosis, and in diabetic ketoacidosis. Blood specimen is normally obtained by arterial puncture, but venipuncture may also be used. Bicarbonate is usually calculated using the Henderson-Hasselbalch equation (HCO3 = Total CO2 - H2CO3). However, it can also be determined by titration.

82375–82376

This test may be requested as carboxyhemoglobin, CO, or COHb. Carbon monoxide is a colorless, odorless, tasteless, poisonous gas formed by burning fuels, including natural gas, wood, and gasoline. These tests are used to identify the level of carbon monoxide poisoning in individuals with known or suspected exposure to the toxic gas. Blood specimen is obtained by venipuncture. Method is colorimetry, spectrophotometry, or gas-liquid chromatography (GLC). Report 82375 when testing for the amount (quantitative analysis) of carbon monoxide. Report 82376 when testing (qualifying) the presence of carbon monoxide.

82378

This test may be abbreviated as CEA. While CEA occurs normally in the gastrointestinal tract, it may be elevated for certain benign and malignant neoplasms and other diseases. CEA is used primarily to monitor patients with colorectal cancer and to a lesser extent advanced breast cancer. Blood specimen is obtained by venipuncture. Method is immunofluorescence,

enzyme immunoassay (EIA), and radioimmunoassay (RIA).

82379

Carnitine has a variety of metabolic roles and may be an indicator of inborn errors of metabolism, chronic disease, or acute and critical illness. Blood specimen is obtained by venipuncture. A 24-hour urine specimen is required. The patient flushes the first urine of the day and discards it. All voided urine for the next 24 hours is collected and refrigerated. Method is enzymatic. This test measures (quantifies) the amount of both total and free carnitine present.

82380

This test may also be requested as beta-carotene. Carotene is an isomeric pigment found in a number of vegetables and fruits. In the liver, carotene is converted to Vitamin A, which, in turn, is converted to retinal, the major molecule that enables vision. A fasting blood specimen is obtained by venipuncture. Method is high performance liquid chromatography (HPLC), colorimetry.

82382

Catecholamines are biogenic amines that include epinephrine, norepinephrine, and dopamine. This test is used to diagnose hypertension caused by increased levels of catecholamines secreted by specific types of tumors. A 24-hour urine specimen is preferred but shorter timed collections may also be used. The patient flushes the first urine of the day and discards it. All voided urine for the next 24 hours is collected and refrigerated. Method is fluorometry. Code 82382 reports total catecholamines and therefore does not differentiate between epinephrine, norepinephrine, and dopamine.

82383

Catecholamines are biogenic amines that include epinephrine, norepinephrine, and dopamine. This test is used to diagnose hypertension caused by increased levels of catecholamines secreted by specific types of tumors. Blood specimen is obtained by venipuncture. Preferred method is high performance liquid chromatography (HPLC), but radioimmunoassay (RIA) or radiochemical assay may also be used. Code 82383 tests for total catecholamines and does not differentiate between epinephrine, norepinephrine, and dopamine.

82384

Catecholamines are biogenic amines that include epinephrine, norepinephrine, and dopamine. This test is used to diagnose hypertension caused by increased levels of catecholamines secreted by specific types of tumors. Blood specimen is obtained by venipuncture. A 24-hour urine specimen is preferred but shorter timed collections may also be used. The patient flushes the first urine of the day and discards it. All voided urine for the next 24 hours is collected and refrigerated. Preferred method is high performance liquid chromatography (HPLC), but radioimmunoassay (RIA) or radiochemical assay may also be used. Code 82384 reports fractionated catecholamines and quantifies total epinephrine, norepinephrine, and dopamine separately. Most assays measure only free catecholamines, but some measure both free and conjugated types.

82387

Cathepsin D is an indicator of metastatic breast cancer. Neoplastic tissue must be dissected free of fat and normal breast tissue, sliced into small pieces, placed in a tube, and quick frozen in liquid nitrogen. The tissue is then analyzed by means of enzymatic immunoassay (EIA) or immunoradiometric assay (IRMA).

82390

This test may be requested as Cp, copper oxidase, or ferroxidase. Ceruloplasmin is a copper oxidase enzyme found in plasma. Decreased levels of ceruplasm are found in Wilson's disease, a disorder of copper metabolism. Blood specimen is obtained by venipuncture. A 24-hour urine specimen is preferred, but shorter timed collections may also be used. The patient flushes the first urine of the day and discards it. All voided urine for the next 24 hours is collected and refrigerated. Several methods may be used, including spectrophotometry, nephelometry, or radial immunodiffusion (RID) for blood specimens. RID is the method for urine.

82397

Chemiluminescent assay refers to a detection method, whereby a chemiluminogenic substrate is converted to a chemiluminescent (light emitting) product.

82415

This test may be requested as a chloramphenicol, chloromycetin, or Mychel-S level. Chloramphenicol is a broad spectrum antibiotic. This test is used to monitor therapeutic and toxic levels. Blood specimen is obtained by venipuncture. Several methods may be used, including high performance liquid chromatography (HPLC), gas-liquid chromatography (GLC), microbiological assay (MB), colorimetry, or enzymatic immunoassay (EIA).

82435

This test may be requested as Cl, blood. Chloride is a salt of hydrochloric acid and is important in maintaining electrolyte balance. Blood specimen is obtained by venipuncture. Methods include colorimetry, coulometry, and ion-selective electrode (ISE).

82436

This test may be requested as Cl, urine. Chloride is a salt of hydrochloric acid, the most common being sodium chloride (table salt). It is important in maintaining proper electrolyte balance. A 24-hour urine test is preferred, but shorter timed collections and random specimens may also be used. If a timed specimen is used, the patient flushes the first urine of the day and discards it. All voided urine for the next 24 hours (or shorter time increment) is collected and refrigerated. Methods include colorimetry, coulometry, and ion-selective electrode (ISE).

82438

This test may be requested as a cystic fibrosis sweat test or Cl, sweat. Saliva is sometimes used for cystic fibrosis evaluation, but is not as reliable as sweat. Chloride is a salt of hydrochloric acid, the most common being sodium chloride (table salt). Sweat is obtained from the forearm by pilocarpine iontophoresis, which is reported separately. Method is usually ion-selective electrode (ISE), but colorimetry, coulometry, Schales and Schales method, and Cotlove titration are also used.

82441

Chlorinated hydrocarbons are contained in solvents and are absorbed cutaneously and by inhalation. While they vary in toxicity, all are CNS depressants and can cause liver and kidney damage with prolonged exposure. This test is used to screen for toxic levels. Levels of one or more of the following substances are screened: carbon tetrachloride, chloroform, dichloromethane, trichloroethylene, and tetrachloroethylene. Testing methods include gas chromatography flame ionization detection (GC-FID) and gas chromatography electron capture detector (GC-ECD). Colorimetry measurement of metabolites may also be used but is nonspecific.

82465

Cholesterol level is a risk indicator for atherosclerosis and myocardial infarction. Blood specimen is obtained by venipuncture. Method is enzymatic. This test reports total cholesterol in serum or whole blood.

82480

This test may be requested as acylcholine acylhydralase, cholinesterase II, EC, PchE, psueodocholinesterase, SChE, or S-Pseudocholine Esterase. Cholinesterase is an enzyme of the hydrolase class with serum cholinesterase being specific to choline esters. Serum cholinesterase is requested primarily for diagnosis of an inherited hypersensitivity to the certain anesthetics or when organophosphate or carbamate insecticide poisoning is suspected. Blood specimen is obtained by venipuncture. Methods are colorimetry, kinetic enzyme with substrates, and fluorometry. This procedure is specific to serum cholinesterase.

82482

This test may be requested as acetylcholinesterase, cholinesterase I, erythrocytic cholinesterase, or true cholinesterase. Cholinesterase is an enzyme of the hydrolase class with RBC cholinesterase being specific to the substrate acetylcholine. RBC cholinesterase is requested when organophosphate or carbamate insecticide poisoning is suspected. Blood specimen is obtained by venipuncture. Methods include colorimetry, fluorometry, and spectrophotometry. This procedure is specific to RBC cholinesterase.

82485

Increased urine levels are found in certain mucopolysaccharidoses such as Hurler's syndrome. A 24-hour urine specimen is required. The patient flushes the first urine of the day and discards it. All voided urine for the next 24 hours is collected and refrigerated. Chondroitin B Sulfate has been measured using chromatographic techniques such as high performance liquid chromatography (HPLC).

82486

This code reports a specific chromatography technique for analyzing substances that are not specifically listed elsewhere in the chemistry section. Chromatography, itself, uses a number of different techniques to separate and analyze the specimen components. Code 82486 reports column chromatography, which uses a sorbent packed in a column. The specimen is dissolved in a solvent and poured into the column. Some of the specimen components bind to the sorbent and are retained in the column, while others escape. Subsequent washings with the same or different solvents cause more strongly bound components to escape. These components can then be individually analyzed. This code tests for the presence (qualitative analysis) of a single analyte.

82487–82488

These codes report specific chromatography techniques for analyzing substances that are not specifically listed elsewhere in the chemistry section. Chromatography uses a number of different techniques to separate and analyze the specimen components. Codes 82487 and 82488 report paper chromatography, which uses a special-grade filter paper in the stationary phase. The specimen is applied to the paper and the end of the paper is placed in a solvent. The solvent then rises along the paper, carrying and depositing the different components of the specimen along the filter paper. The different components can then be separately visualized and analyzed. These codes test for the presence (qualitative analysis) of a single analyte. Report 82487 for 1-dimensional and 82488 for 2-dimensional.

82489

This code reports a specific chromatography technique for analyzing substances that are not specifically listed elsewhere in the chemistry section. Chromatography uses a number of different techniques to separate and analyze the specimen components. Code 82489 reports thin-layer chromatography, which uses a thin layer adsorbent applied to a rectangular plate in the stationary phase. The specimen is applied to the plate and the end of the plate is placed in a solvent. As the solvent rises along the adsorbent on the plate, the different components of the specimen are carried along at varying rates and deposited along the plate. The different components can then be separately visualized and analyzed. This code tests for the presence (qualitative analysis) of a single analyte.

82491–82492

These codes report specific chromatography techniques for analyzing substances that are not specifically listed elsewhere in the chemistry section. Chromatography uses a number of different techniques to separate and analyze the specimen components. Codes 82491-82492 report column chromatography, which uses a sorbent packed in a column. The specimen is dissolved in a solvent and poured into the column. Some of the specimen components bind to the sorbent and are retained in the column, while others escape. Subsequent washings with the same or different solvents cause more strongly bound components to escape. These components can then be individually analyzed. Code 82491 measures (quantifies) the amount of a single analyte, while code 82492 measures (quantifies) the amount of multiple analytes.

82495

Blood specimen is obtained by venipuncture. A 24-hour urine specimen is required. The patient flushes the first urine of the day and discards it. All voided urine for the next 24 hours is collected and refrigerated. Hair samples must be cut close to the scalp. Methods used include atomic absorption spectrometry (AAS) and neutron activation analysis (NAA).

82507

Citrate determinations in urine are useful in evaluating nephrolithiasis. A 24-hour urine specimen is required. The patient flushes the first urine of the day and discards it. All voided urine for the next 24 hours is collected and refrigerated. Citrate may be measured using enzymatic/spectrophotometric methods or chromatography.

82520

Cocaine is a refined derivative of the coca plant and is a frequently abused drug. Blood specimen is obtained by venipuncture. A random urine specimen is collected. Multiple methods may be used including enzyme immunoassay (EIA), fluorescence polarization immunoassay (FPIA), radioimmunoassay (RIA), gas-liquid chromatography (GLC), high performance liquid chromatography (HPLC), and gas chromatography/mass spectrometry (GC-MS). The procedure measures (quantifies) the amount of cocaine or its metabolites in the sample.

82523

This test may be ordered as collagen crosslink N-telopeptide or pyridinium collagen crosslinks. Pyridinium includes pyrinoline and deoxypyridinoline. Collagen cross links are markers for bone resorption and are useful in evaluating and managing osteoporosis. A timed urine specimen is required. When testing for N-telopeptide, a two-hour specimen is usually obtained. Pyridinium, including pyrinoline and deoxypyridinoline, requires a 24-hour specimen. When a timed specimen is used, the patient flushes the first urine of the day and discards it. All voided urine for the next 24 hours (or shorter time increment) is collected and refrigerated. Method is enzyme-linked immunosorbent assay (ELISA) for N-telopeptide and high performance liquid chromatography (HPLC) for pyridinium.

82525

This test may be abbreviated as Cu. Copper is an essential trace mineral. Copper deficiency is rare, however, copper may accumulate to excessive levels in patients with Wilson's disease (a disorder of copper metabolism), primary biliary cirrhosis, and chronic extrahepatic biliary obstruction. Blood specimen is obtained by venipuncture. A 24-hour urine specimen is required. The patient flushes the first urine of the day and discards it. All voided urine for the next 24 hours is collected and refrigerated. Liver specimen is obtained by separately reportable liver biopsy. Methods include colorimetry and atomic absorption spectrometry (AAS).

82528

This test may be requested as Compound B. Corticosterone is a natural corticosteroid, similar to cortisol except that it does not possess anti-inflammatory qualities. Blood specimen is obtained by venipuncture. Method is radioimmunoassay.

82530

Cortisol is a naturally occurring glucocorticoid responsible for metabolism of glucose, protein, and fats and is important in immune system function. Urinary free cortisol is used in initial screening for Cushing's syndrome. A 24-hour urine specimen is required. The patient flushes the first urine of the day and discards it. All voided urine for the next 24 hours is collected and refrigerated. Amniotic fluid levels of free cortisol are useful in evaluating fetal lung maturation. To obtain an amniotic fluid specimen, an ultrasound is performed to determine the exact location of the fetus. Methods include high performance liquid chromatography (HPLC) for urine and radioimmunoassay (RIA) for amniotic fluid. This test measures free (unbound) cortisol only.

82533

Cortisol is a naturally occurring glucocorticoid responsible for metabolism of glucose, protein, and fats and is important in immune system function.

Blood specimen is obtained by venipuncture. To obtain an amniotic fluid specimen, an ultrasound is performed to determine the exact location of the fetus. The fluid is sent to the lab for analysis. Method is radioimmunoassay (RIA), competitive protein binding (CPB), or fluorescent assay. This test measures total cortisol (both free and bound).

82540

Creatine is measured in urine or serum to evaluate certain conditions involving increased muscle tissue breakdown. It has been measured in erythrocytes as an indicator of erythrocyte survival time in the evaluation of hemolytic disorders. Blood specimen is obtained by venipuncture. It can be measured by colorimetric or enzymatic/spectrophotometric methods.

82541–82542

These codes report specific chromatography techniques combined with mass spectrometry for analyzing substances that are not specifically listed elsewhere in the chemistry section. Chromatography uses different techniques to separate and analyze the specimen components. Codes 82541-82542 report column chromatography combined with mass spectrometry. Column chromatography uses a sorbent packed in a column. The specimen is dissolved in a solvent and poured into the column. Some of the specimen components bind to the sorbent and are retained in the column, while others escape. Subsequent washings with the same or different solvents cause more strongly bound components to escape. These components can then be individually analyzed. Mass spectrometry represents one of the most powerful new tools available for studying complex substances. Mass spectrometry isolates specific substances by sorting a stream of electrified particles (ions) based on their mass. Code 82541 screens for the presence (qualitative analysis) of an analyte using a single stationary and mobile phase, while code 82542 measures (quantifies) the amount of an analyte using a single stationary and mobile phase.

82543–82544

These codes report specific chromatography techniques combined with mass spectrometry for analyzing substances that are not specifically listed elsewhere in the chemistry section. Chromatography uses different techniques to separate and analyze the specimen components. Codes 82543-82544 report column chromatography combined with mass spectrometry. Column chromatography uses a sorbent packed in a column. The specimen is dissolved in a solvent and poured into the column. Some of the specimen components bind to the sorbent and are retained in the column, while others escape. Subsequent washings with the same or different solvents cause more strongly bound components to escape. These components can then be individually analyzed. Mass spectrometry represents one of the most powerful new tools available for studying complex substances. Mass spectrometry isolates specific substances by sorting a stream of electrified particles (ions) based on their mass. These two tests are also performed with a stable isotope dilution. Code 82543 measures (quantifies) a single analyte using a single stationary and mobile phase, while code 82544 measures (quantifies) the amount of multiple analytes using a single stationary and mobile phase.

82550

This test may be requested as creatine kinase (CK) or creatine phosphokinase (CPK). Blood specimen is obtained by venipuncture. Method is enzymatic, kinetic, or spectrophotometry. This code reports total CK. Creatine kinase is an enzyme found in striated muscle and it is released following injury. Elevated CK levels are primarily associated with myocardial infarction, trauma and surgery, but CK levels may be elevated with a number of other conditions as well.

82552

This test may be requested as creatine kinase (CK) isoenzymes or creatine phosphokinase (CPK) isoenzymes. Blood specimen is obtained by venipuncture. Method is electrophoresis (EP), column ion-exchange chromatography. Creatine kinase consists of three isoenzymes, each of which are composed of two units, muscle (MM), brain (BB), or muscle and brain (MB). CK1 (BB) is found primarily in the brain and smooth muscle, CK2 (MB) in cardiac muscle, and CK3 (MM) in skeletal muscle. Because elevated CK levels are indicative of injury to the cells, quantifying the levels of each isoenzyme may assist in pinpointing the injured site.

82553

This test may be requested as creatine kinase (CK) MB fraction, creatine phosphokinase (CPK) MB fraction, or CK2. Methods include immunochemical, fluorometric radial partition, microparticle enzyme immunoassay, immunoenzymetric, or chemiluminometric. Creatine kinase consists of three isoenzymes, which are each composed of two units, muscle (MM), brain (BB), or muscle and brain (MB). CK1 (BB) is found primarily in the brain and smooth muscle, CK2 (MB) in cardiac muscle, and CK3 (MM) in skeletal muscle. This code tests for the MB or CK2 fraction only. Blood specimen is obtained by venipuncture.

82554

This test may be requested as CK isoforms or CPK isoforms. Blood specimen is obtained by venipuncture. Methods include electrophoresis (EP), high performance liquid chromatography (HPLC), and isoelectric focusing (IEF). Creatine kinase consists of three isoenzymes, which are each composed of two units, muscle (MM), brain (BB), or muscle and brain (MB). CK1 (BB) is found primarily

in the brain and smooth muscle, CK2 (MB) in cardiac muscle, and CK3 (MM) in skeletal muscle. These isoenzymes can be further subdivided into isoforms which are designated by the isoenzyme (MM, MB, BB) followed by a number (e.g., 1, 2, 3) Examples include CK-MB1, CK-MB2.

82565

Serum creatinine is the most common laboratory test for evaluating renal function. Blood specimen is obtained by venipuncture (adults) or heel stick (pediatrics). Method is enzymatic or colorimetry.

82570

Urine creatinine levels are not normally used to evaluate disease processes except as part of a creatinine clearance test, but they are a good indicator of the adequacy of timed urine specimens. Amniotic fluid creatinine is used to evaluate fetal maturity. A 24-hour urine specimen is required. The patient flushes the first urine of the day. All voided urine for the next 24 hours is collected and refrigerated. For amniotic fluid specimen, a separately reportable amniocentesis is performed. Method is enzymatic, Jaffe reaction, or manual.

82575

This test may be requested as urea clearance or urea nitrogen clearance. Both blood and urine specimens are required. Blood specimen is obtained by venipuncture. A 24-hour urine specimen is preferred, but carefully timed shorter increments may also be acceptable. The patient flushes the first urine of the day. All voided urine for the next 24 hours (or other timed increment) is collected and refrigerated. Method is enzymatic or Jaffe reaction, or alkaline picrate. Creatinine clearance is a calculation of urine and serum creatinine content adjusted by urine volume and body size. The test is a general indicator of glomerular filtration function of the kidneys.

82585

Fibrinogen with an abnormal physical property causing it to precipitate in the cold (4° C) and dissolve again when warmed to 37° C is known as cryofibrinogen. This test is performed to evaluate cold intolerance. Blood specimen is obtained by venipuncture in a prewarmed tube and must be kept warmed. Method is cold precipitation.

82595

Cryoglobulin is a serum globulin with an abnormal physical property causing it to precipitate at cold temperatures (4° C) and dissolve again when warmed to 37° C. It is indicative of lymphoproliferative disorders, collagen vascular disease, and a variety of infections and other diseases. Blood specimen is obtained by venipuncture in a prewarmed tube and must be kept warmed. Method is cold precipitation.

82600

This test may be requested as CN, hydrocyanic acid, or potassium or sodium cyanide. Cyanide is poisonous, both as a gas (inhaled) and as a salt (ingested). It binds to cytochrome oxidase, preventing cellular respiration. Blood specimen is obtained by venipuncture. Multiple methods may be used, including colorimetry, spectrophotometry, microdiffusion, gas chromatography-mass spectrometry (GC-MS), and high performance liquid chromatography (HPLC).

82607

This test may be requested as antipernicious anemia factor, true cyanocobalamin, or Vitamin B12. It is essential for red blood cell maturation and for gastrointestinal and neurologic health. Decreased levels may be indicative of certain anemias. Blood specimen is obtained by venipuncture. Method is chemiluminescence, competitive protein binding (CPB) radioassay, or radioimmunoassay (RIA).

82608

This test may be requested as unsaturated Vitamin B12 binding capacity (UBBC) and Vitamin B12. It is essential for red blood cell maturation and for gastrointestinal and neurologic health. This test may be used to evaluate for certain anemias, myeloproliferative disorders, and the congenital absence of transcobalamin II or cobalophilin. Blood specimen is obtained by venipuncture. Method is radioimmunoassay (RIA).

82615

Cystine and homocystine are amino acids indicative of disease when found in the urine. A 24-hour urine specimen is preferred but random urine may also be used. If a timed urine specimen is requested, the patient flushes the first urine of the day and discards it. All voided urine for the next 24 hours is collected and refrigerated. Method is ion exchange chromatography or spectrophotometry.

82626

This test may be requested as unconjugated DHEA. Serum DHEA levels may be used to evaluate delayed puberty and hirsutism. Elevations may be indicative of ovarian disorders, neoplasm of the adrenal gland, Cushing's disease, or ectopic ACTH-producing neoplasm. Decreased levels in amniotic fluid may be indicative of congenital adrenal hypoplasia. Blood specimen is obtained by venipuncture. A 24-hour urine specimen is required. The patient flushes the first urine of the day and discards it. All voided urine for the next 24 hours is collected and refrigerated. For amniotic fluid specimen, a separately reportable amniocentesis is performed. Method is radioimmunoassay (RIA) or gas-liquid chromatography (GLC).

82627

This test may be requested as DHEA-S or DHEAS. Serum DHEA-S levels may be used to evaluate hirsutism. Elevations may be indicative of ovarian or adrenal disorders, neoplasm of the adrenal cortex, Cushing's disease, or ectopic ACTH-producing neoplasm. Decreased levels in amniotic fluid may be indicative of anencephaly. Blood specimen is obtained by venipuncture. For amniotic fluid speciment, an amniocentesis is performed. Method is typically radioimmunoassay (RIA).

82633

This test may be requested as DOC. Deoxycorticosterone is a hormone produced in small quantities by the adrenal cortex. A normal circadian rise and fall in levels is noted. Blood specimen is obtained by venipuncture. A 24-hour urine specimen is required. The patient flushes the first urine of the day and discards it. All voided urine for the next 24 hours is collected and refrigerated. Method is radioimmunoassay (RIA). The test may be ordered during pregnancy for a variety of reasons, including preeclampsia.

82634

This test may be requested as Compound S. This test may be ordered to evaluate adrenocortical function. Do not confuse with metyrapone stimulation panel (see comments). Blood specimen is obtained by venipuncture. Method is radioimmunoassay (RIA).

82638

This test may be requested as cholinesterase or pseudocholinesterase inhibition test. Dibucaine is used in this test as an inhibitor of cholinesterase to evaluate for unusual phenotypes with hypersensitivity to certain drugs. Individuals with these phenotypes experience apnea (cessation of breathing) when certain drugs are administered. Blood specimen is obtained by venipuncture. Method is enzymatic.

82646

This test may be requested as hydrocodone quantitative analysis. Dihydrocodeinone is an opioid having sedative and analgesic effects. Blood specimen is obtained by venipuncture. A random urine specimen is used. Methods include radioimmunoassay (RIA), gas-liquid chromatography (GLC), enzyme immunoassay (EIA), high-performance liquid chromatography (HPLC) for blood, and fluorescence polarization immunoassay (FPIA) for urine. This test measures (quantifies) the amount of dihydrocodeinone present.

82649

This test may be requested as hydromorphone or Dilaudid quantitative analysis. Dihydromorphinone is an opioid. Blood specimen is obtained by venipuncture. Methods include radioimmunoassay

(RIA), gas-liquid chromatography (GLC), and enzyme immunoassay (EIA).

82651

This test may be requested as DHT. Dihydroxytestosterone is a powerful androgenic hormone formed in the peripheral tissues. It is believed to be responsible for the development of most male secondary characteristics at puberty. Blood specimen is obtained by venipuncture. Method is radioimmunoassay (RIA).

82652

This test may be requested as 1,25 dihydroxy-calciferol, 1,25(OH)2 calciferol, and 1,25(OH)2D. This is the most active form of Vitamin D. It is formed by the renal cells and is essential for calcium absorption. Blood specimen is obtained by venipuncture. Method is radioimmunoassay (RIA) or competitive protein binding (CPB).

82654

This test may be requested as Methadone or Dolophine quantitative analysis. Dimethadione is an opioid. Blood specimen is obtained by venipuncture. Methods include radioimmunoassay (RIA), gas-liquid chromatography (GLC), enzyme immunoassay (EIA), and high-performance liquid chromatography (HPLC).

82657–82658

These codes report enzyme assays using a variety of different methods, some established and some relatively new. Code 82657 reports enzyme assay with nonradioactive substrate (substance upon which an enzyme acts), while 82658 reports enzyme assay with radioactive substrate.

82664

This code reports various electrophoretic techniques. Electrophoresis is a test method that uses an electrical field to move particles toward electrical poles. It separates ionic substances based on differences in their rates of migration toward the poles. Some types of electrophoresis include disc, gel, isoenzyme, and thin layer.

82666

Epiandosterone is a steroid hormone metabolite in the androgen series that is measured for evaluation of syndromes of androgen excess such as hirsutism and polycystic ovary syndrome. A 24-hour urine specimen is required. The patient flushes the first urine of the day and discards it. All voided urine for the next 24 hours is collected and refrigerated. It has been measured typically by methods involving extraction and chromatography, followed by detection and quantification by colorimetric or immunometric techniques. Measurement of this compound has largely been replaced by determination of other specific plasma androgens (e.g. testosterone) by modern, sensitive assays.

82668

This test may be requested as EPO or S-EPO. Eyrthropoietin is a hormone that regulates the production of erythrocytes (immature red blood cells). Blood specimen is obtained by venipuncture. Method is radioimmunoassay (RIA) or chemoluminescent immunoassay.

82670

This test may be requested as unconjugated estradiol (E2). Estradiol is derived from ovaries, testes, and the placenta and is the most active endogenous estrogen. Blood specimen is obtained by venipuncture. Method is radioimmunoassay (RIA).

82671

This test may be requested as fractionated estrogens. Estrogens are the female sex hormones and include estradiol, estrone, and estriol. Blood specimen is obtained by venipuncture. Method is radioimmunoassay. Fractionation involves separating total estrogen into its components.

82672

This test may be requested as total estrogen, serum or urine. Because the serum assay does not measure estriol levels, urine assay is perhaps more commonly ordered. Estrogens are the female sex hormones and include estradiol, estrone, and estriol. Blood specimen is obtained by venipuncture. A 24-hour urine specimen is required. The patient flushes the first urine of the day and discards it. All voided urine for the next 24 hours is collected and refrigerated. Method is spectroscopy or fluorometry.

82677

This test may be requested as estriol (E3). Estriol is a relatively weak estrogen, present in high concentrations during pregnancy. Low levels may be indicative of maternal complications (e.g., diabetes, preeclampsia), fetal growth retardation, or fetal anomaly (e.g., anencephaly). Blood specimen is obtained by venipuncture. A 24-hour urine specimen is required. The patient flushes the first urine of the day and discards it. All voided urine for the next 24 hours is collected and refrigerated. For amniotic fluid specimen, a separately reportable amniocentesis is performed. Method is radioimmunoassay (RIA) for serum or urine and gas-liquid chromatography (GLC) for amniotic fluid.

82679

This test may be requested as estrone (E1). Estrone is a moderately potent estrogen, derived primarily from oxidation of estradiol, but also secreted by the ovaries. Blood specimen is obtained by venipuncture. A 24-hour urine specimen is required. The patient flushes the first urine of the day and discards it. All voided urine for the next 24 hours is collected and refrigerated. For amniotic fluid specimen, a separately reportable amniocentesis is performed. Method is radioimmunoassay (RIA) for serum or urine and gas-liquid chromatography-mass spectrometry (GLC-MC) for amniotic fluid.

82690

This test may be requested as Placidyl quantitative analysis. Ethchlorvynol is a non-barbiturate sedative and hypnotic. Blood specimen is obtained by venipuncture. Method is gas-liquid chromatography (GLC) or colorimetry. This test measures (quantitates) the amount of the drug present.

82693

This test may be requested as 1,2-ethanediol. Ethylene glycol is toxic substance and a component of common automotive antifreeze. The substance has a natural sweet odor and exposure is by accidental or intentional ingestion. Blood specimen is obtained by venipuncture. A random urine specimen may be obtained. Methods include gas chromatography-flame ionization detection (GC-FID), liquid chromatography (LC), enzymatic assay, photometry, and fluorometry.

82696

Etiocholanolone is a steroid hormone metabolite in the androgen series that is measured for evaluation of syndromes of androgen excess such as hirsutism and polycystic ovary syndrome. A 24-hour urine specimen is required. The patient flushes the first urine of the day and discards it. All voided urine for the next 24 hours is collected and refrigerated. It has been measured typically by methods involving extraction and chromatography, followed by detection and quantification by colorimetric or immunometric techniques. Measurement of this compound has largely been replaced by determination of other specific plasma androgens (e.g. testosterone) by modern, sensitive assays.

82705

This test is used to evaluate steatorrhea, which is an abnormal amount of fat in the stool sometimes found with celiac disease and malabsorption syndromes. This is a qualitative test that assesses the presence of fat in the stool. A random stool specimen is obtained. Method is microscopic screen.

82710

This test is used to evaluate malabsorption and steatorrhea, which is an abnormal amount of fat in the stool. This test may be requested as 24-hour, 48-hour, or 72-hour stool collection for fat analysis. A 72-hour collection period is preferred. The patient is placed on a diet containing 50-150 grams of fat/day beginning at least two days prior to testing. All stool is then collected in a plastic container for the designated time period. Method is gravimetry or titrimetry.

82715

Quantitative fecal fat analysis is used in the evaluation of diarrhea and malabsorption. Differentiation of the types of fat excreted can be useful in identifying the cause of steatorrhea, such as differentiating pancreatic insufficiency from other causes of malabsorption. Generally, fecal fat is differentiated as neutral fat (triglycerides) and nonesterified fat (free fatty acids), but it may be more specifically differentiated as long or short chain fatty acids, and may include cholesterol analysis. Methods used for analysis include differential extraction with gravimetric quantification, enzymatic analysis of fecal extracts, or chromatography.

82725

This test may be requested as nonesterified fatty acids (NEFA) or free fatty acids (FFA). Blood specimen is obtained by venipuncture. Method is colorimetry, spectrophotometry, or enzymatic.

82726

Very long chain fatty acid levels are elevated in certain demyelinating diseases such as adrenoleukodystrophy and adrenomyeloneuropathy, and in several paroxysmal disorders including Zellweger syndrome and infantile Refsum's disease. Blood specimen is obtained by venipuncture. Skin fibroblasts may be obtained by scraping. Methods include new techniques such as capillary gas chromatography, mass spectrometry, and stable isotope dilution.

82728

Serum ferritin level measures available iron stores and is a reliable indicator of normal, as well as deficient, levels. Blood specimen is obtained by venipuncture. Method is radioimmunoassay (RIA), immunoradiometric assay (IRMA), enzyme immunoassay (EIA), or enzyme linked immunosorbent assay (ELISA).

82731

Fibronectin is an adhesive glycoprotein. The presence of fetal fibronectin in cervicovaginal secretions is an indicator that a pregnant woman will soon go into labor, and it is tested for the purpose of predicting premature labor. Rapid enzyme-linked immunosorbent assay (ELISA) tests are available to perform the assay on cervical swab specimens. The test is a semi-quantitative (positive or negative) test.

82735

Fluoride is available as hydrogen fluoride and its organic salts. These salts are used in industry and as components of insecticides. Fluoride is also given as a dietary supplement in areas where it is not available in drinking water. However, fluoride is toxic in excessive quantities. This test is performed to evaluate fluoride toxicity. Blood specimen is obtained by venipuncture. Method is fluoride specific electrode, ion-selective potentiometry, or gas-liquid chromatography (GLC).

82742

This test may be requested as Dalmane, quantitative analysis. Flurazepam is a benzodiazapine with sedative and hypnotic effects. Blood specimen is obtained by venipuncture. Method is gas chromatography (GC), gas chromatography-mass spectrometry (GC-MS), high performance liquid chromatography (HPLC), or thin layer chromatography (TLC). This test measures (quantitates) the amount of the drug present.

82746

This test may be requested as serum folate. This test is used to detect folic acid deficiency. Folic acid is a B vitamin necessary for normal red blood cell production. It is stored in the body as folates. Folic acid deficiency results in a form of megaloblastic anemia. Blood specimen is obtained by venipuncture. Method is competitive binding protein (CPB) radioimmunoassay, chemiluminescence, or microbiological assay.

82747

This test may be requested as RBC folate or red cell folate. It is used to detect folic acid deficiency. Folic acid is a B vitamin necessary for normal red blood cell production. It is stored in the body as folates. Folic acid deficiency results in a form of megaloblastic anemia. Blood specimen is obtained by venipuncture. Method is radioimmunoassay (RIA), competitive binding protein (CPB) radioimmunoassay, or chemiluminescence.

82757

This test may be requested as levulose analysis. Fructose is normally present in semen, but may be absent with some congenital anomalies of the male genital tract. A semen specimen is obtained. Method is colorimetry.

82759

Galactokinase is an enzyme necessary for galactose utilization. This test evaluates galactosemia resulting from galactokinase deficiency. Method is radioisotope.

82760

Galactose levels are normally measured shortly after a galactose-rich meal or a glass of milk. Blood specimen is obtained by venipuncture. Random urine or a specimen obtained two hours after ingestion of galactose-containing food is required. A five-hour urine specimen may be required for a galactose tolerance test. Method is enzymatic.

82775–82776

This test may be requested as UDP-G-1-P. Galactose-1-phosphate uridyl transferase is an enzyme necessary for utilization of galactose. This test is performed to

identify deficiency in this enzyme. Blood specimen is obtained by venipuncture. Method is radiometric or uridine diphosphoglucose (UDPG) consumption assay. Report 82775 when enzyme levels are measured (quantitated). Report 82776 when screening only for the presence (qualitative analysis) of the enzyme.

82784

This test may be requested as immunoglobulin, IgA, IgD, IgG, or IgM. Immunoglobulins are in the group of proteins classified as antibodies. Immunoglobulins are produced in response to foreign proteins referred to antigens. IgG is the most abundant immunoglobulin. It is produced in response to secondary exposure to viral and bacterial antigens. IgA is found primarily in the respiratory, gastrointestinal, and genitourinary tracts, as well as in tears and saliva. It is responsible for protecting the mucous membranes from viral and bacterial antigens. Congenital IgA deficiency is also associated with autoimmune disease. IgM is produced following primary exposure to an antigen and is active against rheumatoid factors, gram negative organisms, and the ABO blood group. IgD properties are not well understood but increases with chronic infection, connective tissue disorders, and some liver disease. Serum immunoglobulins may be tested for the four types (IgA, IgD, IgG, IgM) reported with this code. Blood specimen is obtained by venipuncture. Urine may be tested for IgA. A 24-hour urine specimen is required. The patient flushes the first urine of the day and discards it. All urine for the next 24-hours is collected and refrigerated. Saliva may be tested for IgA. CSF may be tested for IgA, IgD, IgG, and IgM. CSF is obtained by spinal puncture, which is reported separately. Method is dependent on specimen source and specific immunoglobulins being tested. Serum is usually analyzed using radial immunodiffusion (RID), enzyme linked immunosorbent assay (ELISA), nephelometry, or turbidimetry. Urine uses electroimmunodiffusion (EID). Saliva uses radial immunodiffusion (RID). CSF is analyzed with radioimmunoassay (RIA).

82785

This test may be requested as immunoglobulin, IgE. Immunoglobulins are in the group of proteins classified as antibodies. Immunoglobulins are produced in response to foreign proteins referred to as antigens. IgE is produced in response to allergic reactions and anaphylaxis. Blood specimen is obtained by venipuncture. CSF is obtained by spinal puncture, which is reported separately. Method is radioimmunoassay (RIA). Paper radioimmunosorbent test may also be used for serum specimen only.

82787

This test may be requested as immunoglobulin subclasses or IgG subclasses. There are four IgG subclasses, which are designated as IgG1, IgG2, IgG3, and IgG4. IgG is part of the body's defense system against infection. Deficiencies of single subclasses, particularly IgG1, can significantly impair this defense. Blood specimen is obtained by venipuncture. Method is radial immunodiffusion (RID), enzyme linked immunosorbent assay (ELISA), nephelometry, or turbidimetry.

82800

This test may be requested as blood pH. Blood pH is tested to identify acidemia or alkalemia. Arterial puncture is preferred, but venipuncture may also be performed. Method is glass pH electrode or potentiometry.

82803–82805

These tests may be requested as arterial blood gases (ABGs). Blood gases are usually requested to evaluate disturbances of acid-base balance, which may be caused by respiratory or metabolic disorders. Blood specimen is obtained by arterial puncture. Code 82803 reports any combination of pH, pCO_2, pO_2, CO_2, and HCO_3, including calculated O_2 saturation. Code 82805 reports any combination of the same gases, but O_2 saturation is performed by direct measurement. Method is selective electrode, potentiometry, or spectrophotometry (O_2 saturation).

82810

This test may be requested as O_2. Oxygen saturation is the percent of the oxygen in the blood that combines with hemoglobin. Blood specimen is obtained by arterial puncture. Method is spectrophotometry.

82820

This test may be requested as oxygen, P50 or as pO_2, P50. This test is performed to measure the affinity of hemoglobin for oxygen, which allows evaluation of oxygen delivery to body tissues. Blood specimen is obtained by arterial puncture. Method is spectrophotometry or potentiometry.

82926–82928

This test may be requested as hydrochloric acid (HCl) analysis. This code reports chemical analysis of gastric acid obtained by gastric intubation and aspiration. Chemical analysis evaluates free (unbound) HCl and total (bound and unbound) HCl. Report 82926 for analysis of free AND total gastric acid. Report 82928 for analysis of free OR total gastric acid.

82938

Gastrin stimulation test with secretin may be performed to evaluate patients with suspected gastrinoma and Zollinger-Ellison syndrome. Blood specimen is obtained by venipuncture. Blood specimen is obtained prior to secretin injection and at five-minute to 15-minute intervals over the next 30 to 60 minutes. Method is radioimmunoassay (RIA).

82941

Gastrin, produced by G cells in the antrum of the stomach, stimulates production of gastric acid. Gastrin may be measured to evaluate patients with suspected gastrinoma and Zollinger-Ellison syndrome. Blood specimen is obtained by venipuncture. Method is radioimmunoassay (RIA).

82943

Glucagon is a hormone secreted by the pancreas. It stimulates the conversion of glycogen stored in the liver to glucose. Glucagon levels may be requested to evaluate suspected diabetes mellitus or glucagonoma. Blood specimen is obtained by venipuncture. Method is radioimmunoassay (RIA).

82945

Glucose is the end product of carbohydrate metabolism, providing energy for living organisms. It is found in body fluids including joint fluid and CSF. Both elevated and decreased levels of glucose may be indicative of disease processes. Joint fluid specimen is obtained by separately reportable arthrocentisis. CSF specimen is obtained by separately reportable spinal puncture. Method is enzymatic.

82946

Glucagon is a hormone secreted by the pancreas. It stimulates the conversion of glycogen stored in the liver to glucose. Glucagon tolerance test may be requested to evaluate suspected diabetes mellitus or glucagonoma. Blood specimen is obtained by venipuncture. A fasting glucagon level is obtained. A high carbohydrate meal or an oral dose of glucose is given. Glucagon levels are then tested at 30, 60, and 120 minute intervals. Method is radioimmunoassay (RIA).

82947

This test may be requested as a fasting blood sugar (FBS). This quantative test is used to evaluate disorders of carbohydrate metabolism. The patient has ordinarily fasted for eight hours. Blood specimen is obtained by venipuncture. Method is enzymatic.

82948

This test is used to monitor disorders of carbohydrate metabolism. Blood specimen is obtained by finger stick. A drop of blood is placed on the reagent strip for a specified amount of time. When the prescribed amount of time has elapsed, the strip is blotted and the reagent strip is compared to a color chart. Method is reagent strip with visual comparison.

82950

This test may also be requested as glucose, postprandial (PP). This test is used to monitor disorders of carbohydrate metabolism. The patient consumes a high carbohydrate meal or an oral glucose solution. Blood specimen is obtained by venipuncture. Blood glucose levels are checked two hours after the meal or glucose solution. A one-hour postprandial screen may be used to evaluate pregnant women for gestational diabetes mellitus. Method is enzymatic.

82951–82952

This test may be requested as GTT, oral GTT, OGTT, intravenous GTT, or IVGTT. This test is used to monitor disorders of carbohydrate metabolism. This test is normally performed using an oral dose of glucose, but may also be performed using intravenous glucose. A blood specimen is obtained prior to glucose administration and at intervals following glucose administration. Code 82951 reports three specimens. Each additional specimen beyond three is reported with 82952. Method is enzymatic.

82953

This test may be requested as a tolbutamide tolerance test. It is used to evaluate pancreatic tumor and functional hypoglycemia. Baseline glucose and insulin levels are obtained. Tolbutamide is administered intravenously. Glucose and insulin levels are then obtained at 3, 30, 60, 90, 120, and 180 minutes following the tolbutamide administration.

82955–82960

These tests may be requested as G6PD quantitative or G6PD screen. This test is used to identify genetic G6PD deficiency, which causes hemolytic anemia after ingestion of certain drugs and foods and may also cause hemolytic disease of the newborn (HDN). Blood specimen is obtained by venipuncture. Method is methemoglobin reduction (Brewer's test), modified Bishop (ultraviolet), dye reduction, or ascorbic or fluorescent spot tests. Code 82955 is used to report measurement of amount (quantitation) of G6PD in erythrocytes, while 82960 reports screening (qualitative analysis) for the presence of G6PD only.

82962

This test is used to monitor disorders of carbohydrate metabolism. This test reports blood glucose monitoring by an FDA-approved device. While the code states that it is for home use, these devices may also be used in the physician office. Blood is obtained by finger stick. Method is enzymatic, electrochemical, or spectrophotometry by small portable device designed for home glucose testing.

82963

Deficiencies of this enzyme occur in metabolic disorders, particularly Gaucher disease. The enzyme is increased following liver ischemic injury, making it favorable to monitor serum levels for this condition. Blood specimen is obtained by venipuncture. Tissue is obtained by surgical excision or biopsy, reported separately. It can be measured by enzymatic methods using spectrophotometry.

82965

This test may be abbreviated as GLD or GLDH. GLD is an enzyme found primarily in the liver, but also in erythrocytes. GLD may be requested to evaluate liver and biliary disease as well as Reye's syndrome. Blood specimen is obtained by venipuncture. Method is spectrophotometry.

82975

This test may be abbreviated as Gln. Glutamine is an amino acid and is the most abundant amino acid found in CSF. This test may used to evaluate hepatic encephalopathy, Reye's syndrome, meningitis, rheumatoid arthritis, and other conditions. Blood specimen is obtained by venipuncture. A 24-hour urine specimen is required. The patient flushes the first urine of the day and discards it. All urine for the next 24-hours is collected and refrigerated. CSF is obtained by spinal puncture, which is reported separately. Method is ion-exchange chromatography or colorimetry.

82977

This test may be requested as GGT or glutamyl transpeptidase. GGT is an enzyme. This test may be used to evaluate liver disease in children or as a screening test for alcoholism. Blood specimen is obtained by venipuncture. Method is radioimmunoassay (RIA).

82978

Glutathione is a red blood cell tripeptide whose synthesis is generated by two enzymes. It is normally present in blood and serves an important role in protecting red blood cells against oxidant stress produced during infections and by certain drugs. A deficiency of glutathione is commonly associated with hemolytic anemia. Blood is obtained by venipuncture. Literature on methodology is somewhat unclear, but cyanide-ascorbate may be among the approaches.

82979

Glutathione reductase is an enzyme. This test may be performed to evaluate riboflavin deficiency or G6PD deficiency. Blood specimen is obtained by venipuncture. Method is enzymatic or spectrophotometry.

82980

This test may be requested as Doriden level. Glutethimide is a nonbarbituate similar to phenobarbitol and used as a sedative and hypnotic. Blood specimen is obtained by venipuncture. Method is gas-liquid chromatography (GLC), high performance liquid chromatography (HPLC), or gas chromatography-mass spectrometry (GC-MS). The test measures (quantifies) the amount of the drug.

82985

This test may be requested as serum fructosamine test. It is used to assess the level of blood glucose

CPT® Lay Descriptions

control in the recent past. It is useful in evaluating patient compliance and the accuracy of the patient's blood glucose self-monitoring. Blood specimen is obtained by venipuncture. Method is colorimetry, nitroblue tetrazolium (NBT).

83001

This test may be requested as FSH or follitropin. FSH is a gonadotropic hormone produced by the pituitary gland. It stimulates growth and maturation of the ovarian follicle in females and promotes spermatogenesis in males. This test may be requested in an infertility work-up. Blood specimen is obtained by venipuncture. A 24-hour urine specimen is required. The patient flushes the first urine of the day and discards it. All urine for the next 24-hours is collected and refrigerated. Method is immunoassay.

83002

This test may be requested as LH, lutropin, or interstitial cell-stimulating hormone (ICSH). LH is a gonadotropic hormone secreted by the pituitary gland. LH required for ovulation in females and stimulates testosterone production in males. LH may be ordered as part of an infertility work-up. Blood specimen is obtained by venipuncture. A 24-hour urine specimen is required. The patient flushes the first urine of the day and discards it. All urine for the next 24-hours is collected and refrigerated. Method is immunoassay.

83003

This test may be requested as GH, HGH, or somatotropin. This test may be used to evaluate pituitary gigantism or drawfism, acromegaly, hypopituitarism, adrenocortical hyperfunction, fetal anencephaly (amniotic fluid analysis), as well as other conditions. Blood specimen is obtained by venipuncture. Amniotic fluid sample is obtained by amniocentesis, which is reported separately. Method is radioimmunoassay.

83008

Cyclic guanosine monophosphate (cGMP) is a so-called "messenger" nucleotide, important in cell function. Levels have been measured in the evaluation of calcium metabolism disorders, including pseudohypoparathyroidism, and in certain other endocrine disorders. The most common method reported in the literature is radioimmunoassay.

83010

This test may be requested as Hp, HPT, hemoglobin-binding protein. Blood specimen is obtained by venipuncture. Method is turbidimetry or nephelometry. This procedure measures (quantifies) the amount of haptoglobin present in serum. Haptoglobin is a plasma glycoprotein. Haptoglobin prevents loss of free hemoglobin in the urine by binding with it and removing it to the liver. This test may be indicated to evaluate anemia or other

indicators of hemolysis, pregnancy induced hypertension, transfusion reactions, as well as other conditions.

83012

This test may be requested as Hp phenotype, HPT phenotype, or hemoglobin-binding protein phenotype. Haptoglobin is a plasma glycoprotein. Blood specimen is obtained by venipuncture. Method is turbidimetry or nephelometry. Haptoglobin prevents loss of free hemoglobin in the urine by binding with it and removing it to the liver. There are three common phenotypes, Hp 1-1, Hp 2-1, Hp 2-2. Hp 1-1 is a monomer, while Hp 2-1 and Hp 2-2 are polymers with much greater molecular weights. This is important in evaluating nephritic syndrome because Hp 1-1 is excreted resulting in a decreased haptoglobin level, while Hp 2-1 and Hp 2-2 are retained resulting in an increase. Blood specimen is obtained by venipuncture. Method is turbidimetry or nephelometry.

83013–83014

Helicobacter pylori (H. pylori), formerly referred to as Campylobacter pylori, is a gram-negative microaerophilic bacteria that causes gastritis and pyloric ulcers. Testing for H. pylori used to require a gastric or duodenal biopsy; however, this bacteria can now be identified using a simple breath test. An oral dose of of labeled urea is administered. The patient breathes into a collection device. The sample is then analyzed for isotopic CO_2 concentration. If urease (i.e. H. pylori) is present in the stomach, CO_2 is exhaled. Testing is by mass spectrometry. Report 83013 for breath test analysis only. Report 83014 for drug administration, sample collection, and breath test analysis.

83015

This test may be requested as a toxic metal or poisonous metal screen. Blood specimen is obtained by venipuncture. A 24-hour urine specimen is required. The patient flushes the first urine of the day and discards it. All urine for the next 24-hours is collected and refrigerated. Method is atomic absorption spectrometry (AAS), colorimetry, or neutron activation analysis (NAA). This test reports screening only (qualitative analysis) to detect and identify the presence of heavy metals.

83018

This test may be requested as a toxic metal or poisonous metal quantitation. Blood specimen is obtained by venipuncture. A 24-hour urine specimen is required. The patient flushes the first urine of the day and discards it. All urine for the next 24-hours is collected and refrigerated. Method is atomic absorption spectrometry (AAS), colorimetry,or neutron activation analysis (NAA). This test measures (quantifies) of the amount of each single metal present. Each metal quantified is reported separately.

83020

This test may be requested as Hb electrophoresis. Blood specimen is obtained by venipuncture. This test uses electrophoresis to test for several hemoglobin variants. It is used to identify the different types of hemoglobin present in the blood and measure (quantify) the amounts of each. The normal types of hemoglobin are Hb A1, Hb A2, and Hb F (fetal). When Hb F exceeds five percent of total hemoglobin after age 6 months, it may be an indicator of thalassemia. Increased amounts of Hb A2 may also indicate thalassemia. Abnormal variants which can be identified by electrophoresis include Hb S and Hb C. Hb S is the most common hemoglobin variant and is indicative of sickle cell anemia. Hb C is indicative of hemolytic anemia.

83021

This test may be requested as Hb chromatography. Blood specimen is obtained by venipuncture. This test uses chromatography to test for several hemoglobin variants. It is used to identify the different types of hemoglobin present in the blood and measure (quantify) the amounts of each. The normal types of hemoglobin are Hb A1, Hb A2, and Hb F (fetal). When Hb F exceeds five percent of total hemoglobin after age 6 months, it may be an indicator of thalassemia. Increased amounts of Hb A2 may also indicate thalassemia. Abnormal variants which can be identified by electrophoresis include Hb S and Hb C. Hb S is the most common hemoglobin variant and is indicative of sickle cell anemia. Hb C is indicative of hemolytic anemia.

83026

The copper sulfate method for measuring hemoglobin is performed by placing a drop of blood into each of a series of containers containing copper sulfate solutions of varying specific gravity. If the drop sinks, then the blood has greater specific gravity than the copper sulfate solution. The specific gravity of whole blood strongly correlates to the hemoglobin concentration, so the hemoglobin concentration may be accurately estimated. Specimen collection is by venipuncture.

83030

This is also known as Hb F. Specimen collection is by venipuncture. Hemoglobin F is the normal hemoglobin of the fetus. Most Hb F is replaced by hemoglobin A in the first days after birth. Hb F has an increased capacity to carry oxygen and is present in increased amounts in some pathologic conditions, including sickle cell anemia, aplastic anemia, and leukemia. Small amounts are produced throughout life.

83033

Hemoglobin F (Hb F) is the normal hemoglobin of the term fetus. Most Hb F is replaced by hemoglobin A in the first days after birth. Elevated levels after age 6 months may be indicative of blood disorder. Hb F has an increased capacity to carry oxygen and the test is also useful in determining whether bleeding disorders may have occurred preterm. Specimen collection is by venipuncture or neonate stool sample. Method for blood specimen is electrophoresis. Method for stool specimen may be by alkali denaturation visual screening. Hemoglobin F is alkali resistant. The procedure is used to examine fresh "red" blood taken from a fresh stool sample.

83036

This test may also be known as HbA1. Specimen collection is by venipuncture. Methods may include high performance liquid chromatography and ion exchange chromatography. Glycated hemoglobin is used to reflect the level of glucose in the blood stream over a relatively long period of time (four to eight weeks) to assess long-term glucose control in diabetes, especially in insulin-dependent diabetics whose blood and urine glucose measurements show significant daily variances.

83045

This test is performed after the onset of symptoms to detect the presence of the derivative methemoglobin in hemoglobin. Specimen collection is by venipuncture. This derivative occurs when the iron in hemoglobin is changed to different state due to certain compounds introduced into the blood stream (e.g., sulfonamides, chlorates, nitrates, nitrites, aniline). This is a qualitative test to determine the presence of methemoglobin. Method is typically co-oximetry (spectrophotometry).

83050

This test is performed after the onset of symptoms to detect and measure (quantitative) the percentage of total hemoglobin containing the derivative methemoglobin. Specimen collection is by venipuncture. This derivative occurs when the iron in hemoglobin is changed to a different state due to certain compounds introduced into the blood stream (e.g., sulfonamides, chlorates, nitrates, nitrites, aniline, and phenacetin). Methods may include co-oximetry (spectrophotometry).

83051

Specimen collection is by venipuncture. Method is spectrophotometry. Transferrin saturation plasma/blood tests measure the amount of stored irons in the blood. An excess of iron can result in hemochromatosis, or Iron Overload Disease (IOD). The extra iron can cause liver problems, arthritis, diabetes, and other diseases.

83055

This test is performed after the onset of symptoms to detects the presence of the derivative sulfhemoglobin in hemoglobin. Specimen collection is by venipuncture. Method is co-oximetry

CPT® Lay Descriptions

(spectrophotometry). The derivative occurs when certain compounds (e.g., phenacetin or sulfonamides) bind with hemoglobin. The hemoglobin is no longer able to transport oxygen. The condition is untreatable, except to wait until the affected red bloods are destroyed in their normal life cycle

83060

This test is performed after the onset of symptoms to measure (quantitative) the percentage of total hemoglobin containing the derivative sulfhemoglobin. Specimen collection is by venipuncture. Method is co-oximetry (spectrophotometry). The derivative occurs when certain compounds (e.g., phenacetin or sulfonamides) bind with hemoglobin.

83065

This is also known as the unstable hemoglobin heat denaturation test. Unstable hemoglobin is a chronic fall in the stable baseline of hemoglobin. Specimen collection is by venipuncture. Method is by heat denaturation. This test changes the physical properties of the globin (the protein constituent of hemoglobin) and the results in the subsequent loss of its biological activity

83068

This test screens for unstable hemoglobin (a fall in the stable baseline of hemoglobin). Specimen collection is by venipuncture. Method is to test the stability of the hemoglobin is checked against isopropanol hemoglobin prep solubility. Falling - or unstable hemoglobin - levels may indicate viral or bacterial infections or, in severe cases, there may be evidence of hepatic dysfunction and renal insufficiency due to anemia. Evaluation and treatment depends on changes in the hematologic levels from baseline and symptoms, rather than absolute values that are stable

83069

Specimen collection is by "clean-catch" ("midstream") urine. Method is spectrophotometry. It tests the presence of hemoglobin in the urine without the concurrent presence of red blood cells. Hemoglobin appears in urine only when levels in the blood are higher than the amount that can be reclaimed by the protein haptoglobin. Hemoglobin detected in the urine may indicate hemolytic anemia, or the hemolysis that can result from a transfusion reaction or other process.

83070

This test is performed to detect the presence (qualitative) of hemosiderin. Methods may include slide preparation and stain for microscopic examination. A sample from a morning collection of urine is preferable. Hemosiderin is an iron containing pigment derived from hemoglobin. The presence of hemosiderin may indicate immune hemolytic anemia

secondary to drugs (e.g., penicillins, cephalosporins, levodopa, methyldopa, quinidine, and sulfonamides).

83071

This test is performed to detect the presence of hemosiderin. Specimen collection is by random urine sample. A sample from a morning collection of urine is preferred. Hemosiderin is an iron containing pigment derived from hemoglobin. The presence of hemosiderin may indicate immune hemolytic anemia secondary to drugs (e.g., penicillins, cephalosporins, levodopa, methyldopa, quinidine, and sulfonamides).

83080

The test may be performed to detect hexosaminidase. Specimen collection is by venipuncture; if female, patient should not be pregnant. Methods may include chromatography, and automated heat inactivation/fluorometry. Levels of hexosaminidase can identify patients and carriers of Tay-Sachs disease. This genetic disorder results in degeneration of the central nervous system.

83088

This test detects the presence and measures the levels of histamine. Specimen collection is by venipuncture for blood or plasma; a random urine sample or 24-hour urine sample may also be collected. Method may be radioimmunoassay for blood or urine. Histamine is stored in mast cells and basophils and is released from cells in the tissues upon injury, causing local inflammation. Histamine also plays a part in controlling gastric secretions, smooth muscle control, cardiac stimulation, stimulation of sensory nerve endings and alertness. Certain medications may result in an excess of histamine in the blood stream, producing sedation, weight gain, and hypotension.

83090

This test may be requested as total homocystine (tHcy). The presence of homocystine in urine or blood may be indicative of metabolic disorders. More recently, plasma homocystine has been identified as a possible predictor for cardiovascular disease with risk increasing progressively with homocystine concentration. Blood specimen is obtained by venipuncture. Either a random urine sample or 24-hour urine specimen may be used. This code reports quantitative analysis of homocystine levels. Method is high performance liquid chromatography (HPLC), ion exchange chromatography, or spectrophotometry.

83150

This test is performed for the analysis of catecholamines or catecholamine metabolites homovanillic acid (HVA). Specimen collection is random or 24-hour urine. The patient flushes the first urine of the day. All voided urine for the next 24 hours is collected. Method may be high performance liquid chromatography. The test is performed to assist in diagnosing and monitoring pheochromocytoma or neuroblastoma. Catecholamines are produced by a part of the adrenal gland and metabolized to inactive substances excreted in the urine. They are also the main metabolites of neuroblastomas.

83491

This test is used to measure the cortisol metabolites (17-OCHS) for assessing adrenocortical function. Specimen collection is by 24-hour urine sample. A 24-hour test is necessary due to variations in cortisol metabolite excretion. The patient flushes the first urine of the day. All voided urine for the next 24 hours is collected. Method is commonly Porter-Silber. Low levels of 17-OCHS indicate hyposecretion of glucocorticoids that can result in Addison's disease (primary adrenal insufficiency). Elevated levels of 17-OCHS indicate hypersecretion of glucocorticoids, especially cortisol and cortisone, that can result in a condition called Cushing's syndrome.

83497

This test may be performed to measure the levels of 5-HIAA for detecting and following the clinical course of patients with carcinoid tumors. Specimen collection is urine, collected over a 24-hour period. The patient flushes the first urine of the day. All voided urine for the next 24 hours is collected. Method is high performance liquid chromatography. These tumors contain enteroendocrine cells that secrete stomach gastrin, a secretory hormone released upon nerve impulse. Neurohormones, such as gastrin, are metabolized by the liver and excreted in the urine. Rising levels of 5-HIAA may indicate a tumor is progressing; falling levels of 5-HIAA may indicate that a tumor is responding to antineoplastic therapy. This test measures (quantifies) the level of 5-HIAA present in the specimen.

83498

This test may also be known as 17-OHP. Specimen collection is by venipuncture for serum or separately reportable amniocentesis for amniotic fluid. Methodology may involve radioimmunoassay. This test is performed to diagnose and manage certain metabolic diseases. Insufficient amounts of hydroxyprogesterone can block the synthesis of cortisol, resulting in conditions such as adrenal hyperplasia, hirsutism (excessive body and facial hair, especially in women), and infertility.

83499

20-hydroxyprogesterone is a weakly active metabolite of progesterone with progestational activity. Levels have been measured in evaluation of ovulation, and gestagenic activity during the menstrual cycle and pregnancy. Typical methodology is column separation (chromatography) with radioimmunoassay detection.

83500

This test may also be known by the abbreviation Hyp. Specimen collection is by venipuncture for serum or

plasma; separately reportable lumbar puncture for CSF; or a 24-hour urine specimen. The patient flushes the first urine of the day. All voided urine for the next 24 hours is collected. Methods may include high performance liquid chromatography, ion-exchange chromatography, and colorimetry. This test detects the presence of free hydroxyproline, due to a defect in the enzyme hydroxyproline oxidase. A defect in the enzyme carried by both parent results in hyperhydroxyprolinemia. This condition has no effect on collagen metabolism.

83505

This test is performed to detect the percentage of total hydroxyproline. The patient collects a urine specimen over a 24-hour period. The patient flushes the first urine of the day. All voided urine for the next 24 hours is collected. Methods may include high performance liquid chromatography and colorimetry. This test may be useful in measuring response to therapy in Paget's disease.

83516–83518

Immunoassay uses highly specific antigen to antibody binding to identify specific chemical substances. This code reports a number of immunoassay techniques for identifying analytes (chemical substances) that are not specifically identified elsewhere, excluding infectious agent antibody or infectious agent antigen. More specific methods reported with these codes include enzyme immunoassay (EIA), and fluoroimmunoassay (FIA). This test identifies (qualitative analysis) the substance or roughly measures (semi-quantitative analysis) the amount of the substance. Code 83516 reports multiple step method, while 83518 reports single step method.

83519

Immunoassay uses highly specific antigen to antibody binding to identify specific chemical substances. This code reports measurement (quantitative analysis) using radiopharmaceutical immunoassay or radioimmunoassay (RIA) technique for identifying analytes (chemical substances) that are not specifically identified elsewhere, excluding infectious agent antibody or infectious agent antigen.

83520

Immunoassay uses highly specific antigen to antibody binding to identify specific chemical substances. This code reports measurement (quantitative analysis) using a technique other than radiopharmaceutical immunoassay or radioimmunoassay (RIA) for identifying analytes (chemical substances) that are not specifically identified elsewhere, excluding infectious agent antibody or infectious agent antigen.

83525

This test measures total insulin which includes both the protein bound and free hormone present in the blood. Blood specimen is obtained by venipuncture.

Method is radioimmunoassay (RIA). This test is used to evaluate hypoglycemia which may be caused by insulin producing neoplasm or islet cell hyperplasia.

83527

This test measures free insulin. Free insulin may also be referred to as active or unbound insulin. A fasting blood specimen is obtained by venipuncture. Method is radioimmunoassay. In rare instances, the level of total insulin (protein bound and unbound) may be normal or elevated when free insulin is actually low.

83528

Intrinsic factor (IF) is a glycoprotein secreted by the gastric glands and necessary for the absorption of vitamin B12. Blood specimen is obtained by venipuncture. Method is guinea pig intestinal mucosal homogenate (GPIMH) or radioassay. Indications are that this test is not frequently performed.

83540

This test may be requested as Fe. Iron is an essential constituent of hemoglobin which is present in foods and absorbed through the small bowel (duodenum and jejunum). Blood specimen is obtained by venipuncture. Method is colorimetry or atomic absorption spectrophotometry. This test is often used in combination with other tests to evaluate anemia, acute leukemia, lead poisoning, acute hepatitis, and vitamin B6 deficiency. It is also used to evaluate iron poisoning caused by accidental overdose (children) or excessive use of supplements.

83550

This test may be abbreviated as TIBC. Iron is an essential constituent of hemoglobin which is present in foods and absorbed through the small bowel (duodenum and jejunum). Blood specimen is obtained by venipuncture. Method is colorimetry or atomic absorption spectrophotometry. TIBC measures the total amount of iron capable of binding to the protein transferrin. This test is often used in combination with other tests to evaluate anemia, various neoplasms, acute hepatitis and other liver disease, hemochromatosis, thalassemia, and renal disease.

83570

This test may be abbreviated as ICD or IDH. Blood specimen is obtained by venipuncture. CSF is obtained by spinal puncture which is reported separately. Method is enzymatic or colorimetry. Isocitrate dehydrogenase is an enzyme. Elevated serum or plasma levels may indicate hepatitis, malignant neoplasm metastatic to liver, or other liver disease. Elevated CSF levels may indicate acute bacterial meningitis, vascular lesions of the brain, or malignant neoplasms of the cerebrospinal system.

83582

This test is may be referred to as a 17-KGS. Specimen collection is performed over a 24-hour period. The patient flushes the first urine of the day. All voided urine for the next 24 hours is collected and refrigerated. Method is Norymberski reaction, which is the Zimmerman color reaction after treatment with a strong oxidizing agent (e.g., periodate, bismuthate). This test is used to assess for increased adrenal function as in Cushing's Syndrome, stress, and some cases of adrenogenital syndrome, or decreased adrenal function as with Addison's disease and hypopituitarism. It measures 17-ketosteroids (KS) after cortols, cortolones, pregnanetriol, and 17-OHCS are oxidized to 17-KS. 17-KS are metabolites of the androgenic sex hormones (i.e., testosterone) that are secreted from the adrenal cortex and testes.

83586

This test is may be ordered as 17-KS. Specimen collection is performed over a 24-hour period. The patient flushes the first urine of the day. All voided urine for the next 24 hours is collected and refrigerated. Method is Zimmerman reaction, which is colorimetry after extractions. This test is used to assess for adrenal androgens. The 17-ketosteroids (KS) may be elevated in Cushing's Syndrome, some adrenal and gonadal tumors, pregnancy, and female pseudohermaphrodism. The 17-KS are metabolites of the androgenic sex hormones (i.e., testosterone) secreted from the adrenal cortex and testes. This test does not detect major androgens, testosterone, and dihydrotestosterone.

83593

This test may be ordered as 17-KS fractionation. Specimen collection is performed over a 24-hour period. The patient flushes the first urine of the day. All voided urine for the next 24 hours is collected and refrigerated. Method is column chromatography or gas-liquid chromatography (GLC). This test is for the quantitation of androsterone, etiocholanolone, and dehydroepiandrosterone (DHEA), the three major metabolites in the urine. It evaluates the presence of adrenal and gonadal abnormalities.

83605

This test is used to assess lactic blood levels to document the presence of tissue hypoxia, determine the degree of hypoxia, and monitor the effect of therapy in blood, plasma, or cerebrospinal fluid (CSF). Specimen collection is either CSF from a spinal puncture or arterial or venous blood. Hand clenching and the use of a tourniquet should be avoided to prevent the build-up of potassium and lactic acid. Method is enzymatic or gas chromatography (GS). This test may be used to determine lactic acidosis when unaccountable anion gap metabolic acidosis is detected.

83615

This test may also be ordered as LD or LDH. The test is a measure of LD or LDH, which is found in many body tissues, particularly the heart, liver, red blood cells, and kidneys. Specimen collection is by spinal puncture for cerebral spinal fluid (CSF), venous blood, or other body fluid, such as urine. Methods used are lactate to pyruvate or pyruvate to lactate. This test may be ordered for a wide variety of disorders, including renal diseases and congestive heart failure.

83625

This test may be ordered as LDH isoenzymes or LD isoenzymes. Specimen collection is collected in a series of three venipunctures: one initially and two more at six to eight-hour intervals. This differs from a total LDH (83615) in that several isoenzymes are individually identified (e.g., LDH1, LDH2). Method is by electrophoresis or immunochemical methods, including immunoprecipitation. This test may be ordered for a wide variety of reasons, and results may point to numerous diagnoses.

83632

This test may be called maternal serum hPL. Specimen collection is obtained by venipuncture. Method used is radioimmunoassay (RIA) or turbidimetric latex immunoassay. This test may be used to evaluate antepartum placental function and fetal health. It is also used as an indicator of intrauterine growth retardation in twin pregnancy, evaluation of placental function, and may be used to assess gestational age. Other uses are in detecting non-germ cell neoplasms.

83633

This is a diagnostic urine test to identify the presence of lactose in the small intestine. Specimen collection is by random urine sample. Method is gas chromatography. The absence of lactose implies a decrease in calcium absorption.

83634

This is a diagnostic urine test to extract and quantify (measure) the presence of lactose. Specimen collection is by random urine sample. Method may be by gas chromatography. The absence of lactose implies a decrease in calcium absorption.

83655

This test may be ordered using Pb, the chemical abbreviation for lead. A whole blood test may used to identify more recent lead exposures; the urine test is used to determine lead body burden, rather than to diagnose lead poisoning. In some instances, serum, hair samples, or bronchoalveolar lavage fluids may be tested. Specimen collection for urine is usually a 24-hour collection. Method used is source dependent, but commonly electrothermal atomic absorption spectrometry (AAS). Bronchoalveolar lavage

specimens may be tested by x-ray fluorescence spectrometry.

83661

Specimen collection is by amniocentesis, but amniotic fluid may be collected vaginally after rupture of the amniotic membrane. This test determines fetal pulmonary maturation and may be an indicator for the possibility of development of respiratory distress syndrome (RDS). Method used is thin-layer chromatography (TLC) and a 1D or 2D approach may be specified.

83662

This test may also be ordered as pulmonary surfactant or the "shake test." Specimen collection is by amniocentesis. Method involves diluting amniotic fluid with ethanol and then shaking the specimen. This test indicates fetal pulmonary maturation and newborn risk for respiratory distress syndrome. The test may also be useful in managing other conditions in both mother and fetus during late stages of pregnancy.

83663

Specimen collection is by amniocentesis. The amniotic fluid is then analyzed by fluorescent polarization (FPOL). A fluorescent phospholipid analogue is added to amniotic fluid and its fluorescence polarization is measured using a fluorescence polarimeter. The presence of increased amounts of surfactant indicating increased lung maturity result in lower polarization levels. Therefore, polarization values decrease during gestation in conjunction with maturation of the pulmonary surfactant system. This test indicates fetal pulmonary maturation and newborn risk for respiratory distress syndrome.

83664

Specimen collection is by amniocentesis. Lamellar body density is calculated by measuring the number of surfactant containing particles per microliter of amniotic fluid. Method is automated cell count. This test indicates fetal pulmonary maturation and newborn risk for respiratory distress syndrome.

83670

This test may also be ordered as LAP or leucyl aminopeptidase. Specimen collection is venipuncture. Urine samples are collected over a 24-hour period. The patient flushes the first urine of the day. All voided urine for the next 24 hours is collected. The ascitic fluid is obtained by paracentesis. Methods are commonly colorimetry, fluorometry, and enzyme assay. The test is commonly used to measure biliary excretory function for differential diagnoses of liver and pancreatic disorders.

CPT® Lay Descriptions

83690

This test may also be called triacylglycerol acylhydrolase. Specimen collection is by venipuncture for blood; thoracentesis for pleural fluid. Method is often by turbidimetric, a specialized processor. The test is used generally to indicate pancreatic, hepatic duct, and renal disorders.

83715

This test may also be known as lipoprotein phenotyping. Specimen collection is post-fasting venipuncture. The methodology is specified as electrophoresis, which reveals phenotypes as a classification of hyperlipoproteinemias. The testing assists in identifying various high-risk conditions, such as familial high cholesterol, hyperlipidemia, as well as premature vascular diseases. The test is sometimes performed on individuals at risk for developing heart disease.

83716

This test may be referred to as a Type III fractionation. Type III hyperlipoproteinemia is an inherited disorder whereby both cholesterol and triglycerides show high plasma concentrations. The condition can lead to premature congestive heart failure, claudication, and cerebral vascular accidents. This particular test, then, may be run subsequent to the previous test to further isolate abnormal beta-lipoprotein. Type III may be indicated when concentrations of very low-density lipoprotein cholesterol (VLDL-C) are high against triglycerides. Specimen collection is post-fasting venipuncture. Various methods may be employed, including ultracentrifugation, electrophoresis, and nuclear magnetic resonance. Often a combination of ultracentrifugation and electrophoresis is employed. A characteristic "band" may point toward a diagnosis.

83718

This test may be requested as HDL, HDLC, or HDL cholesterol. Lipoproteins are compounds composed of lipids bound to proteins, which are transported through the blood. High-density lipoprotein (HDL) is frequently referred to as "good cholesterol," or "friendly lipid," as it is responsible for decreasing plaque deposits in blood vessels. High levels of HDL decrease the risk of premature coronary artery disease. Blood specimen is post-fasting venipuncture. This code reports direct measurement only, normally performed using either an enzymatic or precipitation method.

83719

This test measures the amount of VLDLs, the lipoprotein that carries triglycerides in the blood. The test is useful to determine a patient's risk of arteriosclerotic occlusive disease, as well as other cholesterol-related disorders. Specimen collection is post-fasting venipuncture. The method used is electrophoresis and may first involve ultracentrifugation.

83721

This test may also be referred to as LDL-C. It measures the amount of low-density lipoproteins (LDLs), also known as "bad cholesterol." The test is useful to determine the patient's risk of coronary heart disease (CHD), among other disorders. Specimen collection is post-fasting venipuncture. Method may be by precipitation procedure with results derived by the Friedewald formula.

83727

This test may also be referred to as the LH-RH test. This test may be ordered to test for the presence of luteinizing releasing hormone (a congenital absence is known as Kallmann's syndrome; female patients cannot ovulate). Natural bursts of LH-RH govern the release of luteinizing hormone and follicular stimulating hormone, both essential to ovulation. The test, then, is useful in diagnosing problems in LH-RH transport or production, as well as associated fertility problems. Specimen collection is by venipuncture. Methodology may entail administration of a stimulation agent with a baseline blood sample drawn before the injection and several after. Samples may be tested by immunoassay.

83735

This test is used to determine magnesium levels and the chemical abbreviation Mg may be used. Specimen collection is post-fasting venipuncture or 24-urine collection. Cerebrospinal fluid (CSF) would be collected by a spinal puncture. Methods are atomic absorption spectrophotometry (blood and urine) and colorimetry (CSF). Other methods may also be employed. The test may be ordered for a wide variety of reasons.

83775

This test may also be known as MDH, or MD. This enzyme is widely distributed in the system's cellular makeup and levels follow lactate dehydrogenase activity. The test is probably considered of general usefulness and indications are that it is not frequently run. Specimen collection is by venipuncture for blood; surgical excision or biopsy for tissue. Methodology may be by electrophoresis.

83785

This test is usually performed to determine manganese toxicity, exposure, or poisoning. Specimen collection may be venipuncture, 24-hour urine collection, or random or spot urine samples. Hair is sometimes analyzed as is fluid from bronchoalveolar lavage. Methods are source dependent and include neutron activation and atomic absorption spectrophotometry (AAS) with Zeeman background correction for blood and urine. Hair may be processed with acetone and nitric acid before testing with AAS as well. Fluids are likely to be x-ray fluorescence spectrum.

83788

This test identifies the presence (qualitative) of specific analytes in protein. Specimen collection is finger stick and other collection methods for arterial blood samples. Method is mass spectrometry. The test is used for identifying the chemical makeup and structure of a substance. Tandem MS (MS/MS) is a method using sequential analysis to provide structural information by establishing relationships between substances. This test assists in analyzing viruses, sequencing and analyzing peptides and proteins, and providing information on such life-threatening diseases as AIDS and various types of skin cancers.

83789

This test is used for identifying the chemical makeup and structure of a substance. Specimen collection is by finger stick or other methods for arterial blood samples. Method is mass spectometry (MS). This test is used to analyze viruses, sequence and analyze peptides and proteins, and to provide information on such life-threatening diseases as AIDS and various types of skin cancers. This test quantifies (measures) the amount of analyte in the specimen.

83805

This test is performed to provide therapeutic monitoring and toxicity evaluation of this antianxiety agent (numerous trade names exist, including Equanil and Meprospan). Specimen collection is by venipuncture. Method used is gas-liquid chromatography or high performance liquid chromatography. Quantitative measurement may be taken for numerous reasons. The drug holds potential for abuse and dependence can occur.

83825

This test may also be ordered as Hg. Specimen collection for whole blood is typically venipuncture, urine sample is performed by patients over a 24-hour period, and hair specimens are cut close to the scalp. Methods are electrothermal atomic absorption, gold electrode deposition, or gas chromatography. Mercury toxicity may cause neurological defects, pneumonitis, and other problems depending on mode of entry into the body (e.g., vapor, ingestion) and which form it enters as: elemental, inorganic, and organic.

83835

The test is performed to determine metanephrine or normetanephrine concentrations. The patient performs specimen collection over a 24-hour period. The patient flushes the first urine of the day. All urine for the next 24-hours is collected. Method is high performance liquid chromatography (HPLC). Metanephrine or normetanephrine concentrations may be associated with neuroendocrine tumors. Other reasons for elevated concentrations include intense physical activity, life threatening illness and drug interferences.

83840

This test is used to measure toxicity and the determination of methadone in the system in cases of drug abuse. Specimen collection is by random urine sample. Methods for screening purposes are thin-layer chromatography and enzyme immunoassay; for confirmation, gas chromatography/mass spectrometry. This agent is widely used in the detoxification of opiate addicts.

83857

This test measures methemalbumin (hematin bound to serum albumin, which is formed in plasma when haptoglobin is depleted). It is representative of intravascular hemolysis. Specimen collection is by venipuncture for blood, or by amniocentesis for amniotic fluid. Methods may include Schumm test, ether, ammonium sulfide, EP for serum, and spectrophotometry for serum or plasma.

83858

This test is also known as methsuximide/normethsuximide. Specimen collection is by venipuncture. Methods may include gas-liquid chromatography and high-performance liquid chromatography. This test may be ordered to measure the amount of methsuximide, which is an anticonvulsant used in treating petit mal and psychomotor epilepsy.

83864–83866

This test may also be known as glycoaminoglycans, Keratosulfate, AMPS, and GAGS. The patient typically performs specimen collection over a 24-hour period. Methods may include turbidimetry, paper spot test, and colorimetry. This test may be used to detect the presence of mucopolysaccharides in solution. Mucopolysaccharides are important in the diagnosis of certain genetic metabolic disorders, such as Scheie's syndrome (also called a-L-iduronidase deficiency, Sheie type, and mucopolysaccharidosis IS).

83872

This test may also be referred to as a mucin coagulation test or joint fluid test, in addition to Rope's test. This test analyzes the hyaluronic acid in synovial fluid. Specimen collection is by arthrocentesis. Method involves adding a few drops of synovial fluid into a weak solution of acetic acid. The mixture is then evaluated for clumping and change of fluid opacity. Test results may be a general guide to numerous rheumatological disorders.

83873

This test may be ordered as an MBP assay. Specimen collection is by lumbar puncture. In rare instances, serum may be tested for myelin basic protein from patients with recent head injuries. Ordinarily, the CSF sample is taken when a patient is experiencing certain symptoms characteristic of disease activity, typically multiple sclerosis. Test methods include radial immunodiffusion (RIA), electroimmunodiffusion, immunofluorometry, immunoprecipitation, or immunonephelometry. This test is typically used as an evaluation of disease activity, rather than for diagnostic purposes.

83874

Myoglobin is a principle protein of skeletal and cardiac muscle tissue. Elevated serum levels may be found in severe muscle conditions, such as polymyositis and crushing traumas to muscle and bone. This test may be used in association with other disorders as well, such as acute myocardial infarct and infections. Specimen collection is by venipuncture for blood or random urine sample. Urine measurements may not prove as reliable as serum measurements. Methods include radioimmunoassay (RIA), fluorometric immunoassay, and immunoturbidimetry for blood. Urine specimens may be processed by antigen-antibody reaction nephelometry.

83883

Nephelometry is a method to measure the concentration of a suspension using an instrument (nephelometer) for assessing turbidity of a solution. For example, this code can be used to measure the concentration of albumin in body fluid. Albumins make up about 60 percent of plasma proteins, and exert considerable pressure in maintaining water balance between blood and tissues. Report this nephelometry test when the analyte is not specifically cited elsewhere in this section.

83885

This test may also be known as Nickel U or as Ni. Specimen collection is by venipuncture for blood. Urine specimens will typically be collected over 24-hours. A random stool sample is common for feces samples. Scalp-end hair may require treatment to remove contaminates. Methods may include atomic absorption spectrophotometry and x-ray fluorescence spectrometry. Measurement of nickel is useful to determine chronic environmental exposure of manufactured products containing nickel.

83887

Cotinine, a metabolite of nicotine, also may be detected by this test. Specimen collection is by venipuncture for blood. Random urine samples may be used, or specimens collected over a 24-hour period. The patient flushes the first urine of the day. All urine for the next 24-hours is collected. Methods may include gas chromatography, high performance liquid chromatography, colorimetry

83890

Molecular diagnostic assays can determine whether an individual carries a genetic mutation associated with specific diseases, without manifestation of the disease symptoms. They may also be used to interpret, diagnose and monitor disease states, and in screening and in preventive medicine to detect carriers or those predisposed to specific diseases. Molecular biology studies involve the isolation or extraction of the molecular sequence to be studied. Gene isolation may be used to study neurodegenerative diseases such as ataxia and Alzheimer's disease.

83891

Molecular diagnostic assays can determine whether an individual carries a genetic mutation associated with specific diseases, without manifestation of the disease symptoms. They may also be used to interpret, diagnose and monitor disease states, and in screening and in preventive medicine to detect carriers or those predisposed to specific diseases. The first step in most molecular biology studies involves the purification and isolation of nucleic acid. There are many techniques available, and the specific technique selected for a study depends on the type of research being conducted. The techniques may include extraction/precipitation, chromatography, centrifugation, and electrophoresis.

83892

Molecular diagnostic assays can determine whether an individual carries a genetic mutation associated with specific diseases, without manifestation of the disease symptoms. They may also be used to interpret, diagnose and monitor disease states, and in screening and in preventive medicine to detect carriers or those predisposed to specific diseases. Enzymatic digestion is a technique to degrade or modify DNA to hybridize a test strand of DNA against a reference.

83893

Molecular diagnostic assays can determine whether an individual carries a genetic mutation associated with specific diseases, without manifestation of the disease symptoms. They may also be used to interpret, diagnose and monitor disease states, and in screening and in preventive medicine to detect carriers or those predisposed to specific diseases. Dot/slot blot production involves detection methods in proteins.

83894

Molecular diagnostic assays can determine whether an individual carries a genetic mutation associated with specific diseases, without manifestation of the disease symptoms. They may also be used to interpret, diagnose and monitor disease states, and in screening and in preventive medicine to detect carriers or those predisposed to specific diseases. Electrophoresis separates nucleic acids by size. The process also is used to determine the size and purity of the nucleic acid. In some tests, DNA probes are anchored in polyacrylamide gel, which acts as a capture layer for complementary small nucleotides from the blood.

83896

Molecular diagnostic assays can determine whether an individual carries a genetic mutation associated with specific diseases, without manifestation of the disease symptoms. They may also be used to interpret, diagnose and monitor disease states, and in screening and in preventive medicine to detect carriers or those predisposed to specific diseases. Nucleic acid probes are used to locate, diagnose, and monitor inherited and infectious diseases.

83897

Molecular diagnostic assays can determine whether an individual carries a genetic mutation associated with specific diseases, without manifestation of the disease symptoms. They may also be used to interpret, diagnose and monitor disease states, and in screening and in preventive medicine to detect carriers or those predisposed to specific diseases. Fresh, frozen, or ethanol-fixed tissue may be used in Southern blot tests for possible diagnosis of immunoglobulin Heavy Chain and T-Cell Receptor Beta. A Southern blot test may be used to identify the presence of DNA sequences in totally isolated DNA (DNA isolated from tissue or cells).

83898

Molecular diagnostic assays can determine whether an individual carries a genetic mutation associated with specific diseases, without manifestation of the disease symptoms. They may also be used to interpret, diagnose and monitor disease states, and in screening and in preventive medicine to detect carriers or those predisposed to specific diseases. These methods of molecular diagnostic of nucleic acids amplifies specific nucleic acid sequences from extremely low levels to amounts which can be readily detected, such as through polymerase chain reaction (PCR). Fresh, frozen, ethanol-fixed or paraffin-embedded tissues are specimens required for PCR.

83901

Molecular diagnostic assays can determine whether an individual carries a genetic mutation associated with specific diseases, without manifestation of the disease symptoms. These methods of molecular diagnostic of nucleic acids amplify specific nucleic acid sequences from extremely low levels to amounts that can be readily detected.

83902

Molecular diagnostic assays can determine whether an individual carries a genetic mutation associated with specific diseases, without manifestation of the disease symptoms. They may also be used to interpret, diagnose and monitor disease states, and in screening and in preventive medicine to detect carriers or those predisposed to specific diseases. Transcription involves the transfer of information from a DNA molecule into an RNA molecule. It's a molecular process that occurs outside the nucleus. Reverse transcription is a method that reverses the normal flow of genetic information from the RNA molecule to

the DNA molecule and helps determine the sequence of nucleic acids in amino acids and protein.

83903

Molecular diagnostic assays can determine whether an individual carries a genetic mutation associated with specific diseases, without manifestation of the disease symptoms. They may also be used to interpret, diagnose and monitor disease states, and in screening and in preventive medicine to detect carriers or those predisposed to specific diseases. Various methods of mutation scanning are used to detect any mutation within a region of DNA. This code involves scanning of a single strand by physical properties.

83904

This method is a diagnostic test to detect alterations in DNA sequence that are known to be found in high frequency among individuals affected by the specific disorder. They may also be used to interpret, diagnose and monitor disease states, and in screening and in preventive medicine to detect carriers or those predisposed to specific diseases. Various methods of mutation scanning are used to detect any mutation within a region of DNA. This code is used for methods used in DNA sequence alterations, such as point mutations, deletions, insertions, and inversions.

83905

Molecular diagnostic assays can determine whether an individual carries a genetic mutation associated with specific diseases, without manifestation of the disease symptoms. They may also be used to interpret, diagnose and monitor disease states, and in screening and in preventive medicine to detect carriers or those predisposed to specific diseases. An allele is one of a pair of genes that control the same characteristic but have a different effect. This code identifies certain genetic mutations by allele transcription on a single segment of nucleic acid.

83906

Molecular diagnostic assays can determine whether an individual carries a genetic mutation associated with specific diseases, without manifestation of the disease symptoms. They may also be used to interpret, diagnose and monitor disease states, and in screening and in preventive medicine to detect carriers or those predisposed to specific diseases. An allele is one of a pair of genes that control the same characteristic but have a different effect. This code identifies certain genetic mutations by allele translation on a single segment of nucleic acid.

83912

Molecular diagnostic assays can determine whether an individual carries a genetic mutation associated with specific diseases, without manifestation of the disease symptoms. They may also be used to interpret, diagnose and monitor disease states, and in screening and in preventive medicine to detect carriers or those predisposed to specific diseases.

83915

This test is also known as 5'-N'TASE, and 5'-NT. Specimen collection is by venipuncture for blood or arthrocentesis for synovial fluid. Methods vary greatly, and may include molybdate color reaction, high performance liquid chromatography, and colorimetry. The activity is usually measured by hydrolysis of a particular nucleotide. The test may be ordered to assist in identifying the cause of increased 5'-nucleotidase, a liver-related enzyme.

83916

Specimen collection is by separately reportable lumbar puncture for the cerebrospinal fluid (CFS) and by venipuncture for the concurrent blood. Methods may include thin-gel agarose high-resolution electrophoresis and isoelectric focusing. This test may be used to identify diagnoses of inflammatory and autoimmune diseases of the CNS and other degenerative states.

83918

This test also may involve analyzing patterns of excretion for specific diagnosis. Specimen collection is by the patient over a 24-hour period. The patient flushes the first urine of the day. All urine for the next 24-hours is collected. Urine is the preferred specimen for organic acid screening due to concentration of the metabolites excreted by the kidney. Methods may include gas chromatography, followed by mass spectroscopy. There are many sources for organic acids, though most come from the metabolism of amino acids, fatty acids, carbohydrates, and cholesterol, and hormones such as steroids. Abnormal patterns of organic acids in excretion may be due to genetic metabolic disorders, vitamin deficiencies, and certain drugs.

83919

This test may involve analyzing patterns of excretion for specific diagnosis. Specimen collection is by the patient over a 24-hour period. The patient flushes the first urine of the day. All urine for the next 24-hours is collected. Urine is the preferred specimen for organic acid screening due to concentration of the metabolites excreted by the kidney, but blood testing may also be performed. There are many sources for organic acids, though most come from the metabolism of amino acids, fatty acids, carbohydrates, and cholesterol, and hormones such as steroids. Abnormal patterns of organic acids in excretion may be due to genetic metabolic disorders, vitamin deficiencies, and certain drugs. Organic acid analysis is useful for identification of inborn errors of metabolism. Qualitative screening tests are typically performed by thin layer chromatography, but may involve other chemical or chromatographic techniques.

83921

This test is a quantitative test for organic acids and the preferred specimen is urine, collected following a fast or at the height of symptoms. Urine is the preferred specimen for organic acid screening due to concentration of metabolites excreted by the kidney. Methods may include gas chromatography, followed by mass spectroscopy. The test may be performed on acutely ill neonates, suspected cases of Reye's syndrome, or failure-to-thrive syndrome. Any patient with metabolic acidosis, such as that associated with severe infections, may be tested.

83925

Specimen collection is by a random urine sample. Methods may include thin-layer chromatography, enzyme immunoassay, gas chromatography, and high performance liquid chromatography. This test measures the amount of a given opiate present. This test may be ordered to measure toxicity or possible drug abuse of opiates, such as morphine and meperidine (Demerol).

83930

This test is also known as osmolal gap and serum osmolality. Specimen collection is by venipuncture for adults; heel stick for children. Methodology may involve freezing point depression or vapor pressure techniques. The test measures the amount of molecules or ions (particles) in a solution of water or the presence of osmotically active molecules in serum. The results may be high or low serum osmolality, depending on the differential diagnosis.

83935

This test may also be known as osmolal gap. Specimen collection is by the patient over a 24-hour period or a random urine sample. The first-voided specimen may be used as the random sample. Method may be by freezing point depression. The test may be used to determine renal disease and disorders, electrolyte and water balance. The results may be high or low urine osmolality, depending on the differential diagnosis.

83937

Osteocalcin is a test developed to measure bone formation and for monitoring therapy of preexisting bone conditions. An imbalance between the two (formation and reabsorption) may account for many of the metabolic bone diseases, such as Paget's disease and osteomalacia. Specimen collection is by venipuncture. Methods may include enzyme-linked immunosorbent assay (ELISA).

83945

This test is also known as calcium oxalate. Specimen collection is over a 24-hour period, or first morning specimen collection may be taken as an estimate of daily output. The patient flushes the first urine of the day. All voided urine for the next 24 hours is collected. Methods may include colorimetry and high performance liquid chromatography. The test may be performed to determine patients at risk of forming oxalate calculi (stones), which are common in the urinary tract.

83970

This test may also be ordered as a PTH or parathyrin. Specimen collection is post-fasting venipuncture. Methods may include immunochemilunimomeric assay (ICMA), radioimmunoassay (RIA), and immunoradiometric assay (IRMA). Testing determines the PTH levels and may be used to differentiate between primary or secondary causes of parathyroid disorders.

83986

This test may also be called fecal pH, pleural fluid pH, or thoracentesis pH. Specimen collection for pleural fluid is by thoracentesis; for stool, fresh random sample; for urine, random sample; or ascitic fluid by paracentesis, etc. Methods may include a pH meter for pleural fluid; aqueous stool suspension with pH paper for stool; dipstick double indicator principal or pH meter for urine. The test may be ordered to differentiate among numerous diagnoses, depending on the sample taken and the method used.

83992

Specimen collection is by random urine sample. Methodology may include immunoassay, thin-layer chromatography (TLC), gas chromatography (GC), and gas chromatography/mass spectrometry (GC/TC), which quantifies the amount of drug. This test is performed to evaluate the presence of phencyclidine (also known as PCP, or angel dust), an illegal street drug.

84022

Derivatives of phenothiazine are numerous and most are classified as antipsychotics. A common one is Chlorpromazine, yet many more are seen. Specimen collection is by venipuncture for blood, or by random urine sample. Methods may include high performance liquid chromatography (HPLC), thin-layer chromatography (TLC), gas chromatography (GC) or fluorometry for blood; thin-layer chromatography (TLC), gas-liquid chromatography (GLC), or radioimmunoassay (RIA) for urine. The test is performed to evaluate the amount of phenothiazine present.

84030

This test may be ordered as a Guthrie, Phenylketonuria, or PKU test, or phenylalanine screen. Specimen collection is by venipuncture for adults and older children and heel stick for newborns and infants. Methods may include microbiologic inhibition assay, ion-exchange chromatography, and fluorometry. This test is performed to determine phenylalanine deficiency.

84035

This test detects the presence of phenylketone, a metabolite created in the breakdown of the amino acid phenylamine. Specimen collection is by venipuncture. Methods may include gas chromatography. The amino acid is essential to developing infants and normal protein metabolism throughout life. Reference ranges have been established for adults and newborns, and a test for phenylketonuria is part of the newborn screening. For newborns, a heel stick puncture is used to collect blood 12 hours after birth, or immediately prior to a blood transfusion. This is a qualitative screening test for the presence of phenylketones.

84060

This is also known as phosphoric monoester phosphohydrolase and PAP. Specimen collection is by post-fasting venipuncture. Methods may include radioimmunoassay (RIA), enzyme immunoassay (EIA), thymolphthalein monophosphate, and titrate inhibition. Phosphatase is an enzyme that is a catalyst in chemical reactions involving phosphate. This test may be used to identify phosphatase levels in individuals with diagnoses such as skeletal metastasis, and myelocytic leukemia. The test is useful in the staging of prostatic cancer rather than initial diagnosis of prostate cancer.

84061

Specimen collection is vaginal fluids. This test is performed to detect acid phosphatase, a constituent of semen, as part of evidence collection following a sex crime. Some specimens may be placed in glass tubes; others may be prepared as fixed smears. This test does not detect the presence of spermatozoa. Levels of phosphatase may be elevated due to vaginal infection, which may confuse test results.

84066

This test may also be known as ACP and prostatic phosphatase. Specimen collection is post-fasting venipuncture. Methods may include radioimmunoassay (RIA), enzyme monophosphate, alpha naphthylphosphate, and titrate inhibition. This test may be used to stage prostate cancer, assists in diagnosing metastatic prostate adenocarcinoma and to monitor treatment of patients already diagnosed with prostatic carcinoma

84075

This test may be requested as ALP or AP-EC. ALP is an enzyme. It is an indicator of liver cell damage. Amniotic fluid ALP may be screened for cystic fibrosis in mothers who have had a child affected with the disease. Blood specimen is obtained by venipuncture. For amniotic fluid specimen, a separately reportable amniocentesis is performed. Methods include a number of kinetic spectrophotometry and fluorescent techniques, as well as 4-nitrylphenophosphate (4-NPP) and diethanolamine (DEA).

84078

This may also be known as ALP and AP. Specimen collection is post-fasting venipuncture. Methodology may involve heat inhibition at 56°C. This test may be performed to identify general liver and bone diseases.

84080

This test may also be known as ALP isoenzymes and AP. Specimen collection is post-fasting venipuncture. Methods may include King-Armstrong phenyl phosphate, Bowers and McComb, and Kodak. This test may be ordered for patients with increased serum total alkaline phosphatase, or to compare total alkaline phosphatase to placental, liver, bone, and Regan isoenzymes.

84081

Specimen collection is by separately reportable amniocentesis. Methods may include thin-layer chromatography (TLC) and immunologic and enzymatic assays. These tests together are frequently ordered as LS/PG. Testing is performed in conjunction with an L/S (lecithin/sphingomyelin) ratio for assessment of fetal maturity based on pulmonary surfactant. This test may be performed to determine fetal lung maturity and to establish the possibility of the development of respiratory distress syndrome in the fetus.

84085

This test may also be known as 6-PGD. Specimen collection is by venipuncture. Methodology may involve spectrophotometry. The test may be performed to detect the presence and measure the levels of phosphogluconate, 6-, dehydrogenase, RBC, an enzyme present in the metabolic breakdown of sugars.

84087

This is also known as glucose-6-phosphate isomerase. Specimen collection is by venipuncture. Methods may include spectrophotometry and colorimetric. The test may be performed to detect the presence and measure the levels in serum of phosphohexose isomerase, an enzyme present in the breakdown of fructose.

84100

This test may be known as PG. This test may also be ordered as PO4. Specimen collection is post-fasting venipuncture. Methods may include phosphomolybdate - colorimetric and modified molybdate - enzymatic, and colorimetric. The testing may be performed to measure high or low levels of phosphorus to determine a variety of differential diagnoses. Potassium supplements increase phosphate levels. Also, phosphate levels may increase during the last trimester of pregnancy.

84105

Specimen collection is over a 24-hour period, or by random urine sample. Methods may include

enzymatic and colorimetric. This test is performed to identify the calcium/phosphorus balance. High values may be associated with primary hyperparathyroidism, vitamin D deficiency, and renal tubular acidosis; low values may be due to hypoparathyroidism, pseudohypoparathyroidism, and vitamin D toxicity. The test may also be used for nephrolithiasis assessment.

84106

This test may also be known as Watson-Schwartz and Hoesch tests. Specimen collection is by random urine sample. Methods are the Watson-Schwartz and Hoesch tests, and Ehrlich's reagent. The Hoesch test does not respond to urobilirubin. The test may be used to screen for acute intermittent porphyria. The test may also be ordered when acute attacks of abdominal and extremity pain is present.

84110

This test may also be known as Porphobilinogen (PBG), urine. Specimen collection is by the patient over a 24-hour period. The patient flushes the first urine of the day. All urine for the next 24-hours is collected. The urine sample may also be random. Urine colored amber-red or burgundy, which darkens in light, indicates the presence of abnormally high levels. This test may be used to detect levels of porphobilinogen associated in the diagnosis of genetic or drug-induced abnormal porphyrin metabolism. Methods may involve gas chromatography, colorimetry, and spectrophotometry. This test measures (quantifies) porphobilinogen present in the specimen.

84119

This test may be used to detect the presence (qualitative) of porphyria cutanea tarda (PCT). The patient typically performs specimen collection over a 24-hour period. The patient flushes the first urine of the day. All urine for the next 24-hours is collected. Methods may include high performance liquid chromatography. Urine porphyrins are useful for evaluating photosensitivity due to abnormal metabolism of the protein used in the synthesis of the iron (heme) in hemoglobin.

84120

Specimen collection is by the patient over a 24-hour period. Methods may include chromatography, fluorometry, and high performance liquid chromatography (HPLC). This test is performed for the quantitative evaluation (measurement) of porphyrias, which may include enzyme deficiencies that are necessary for heme synthesis and chemical porphyrias.

84126–84127

Specimen collection involves timed collections (24 to 72 hours) or liquid stools if examined for fecal porphyrins. Method is high performance liquid chromatography and fluorometry. Results may be used to measure the levels of coproporphyrin (a nitrogen-containing substance excreted in the feces from the breakdown of bilirubin from hemoglobin decomposition) and protoporphyrin (a form of porphyrin that combines with iron and protein to form organic molecules such as hemoglobin).

84132

This test may be requested as K or K+. Potassium is the major electrolyte found in intracellular fluids. Potassium influences skeletal and cardiac muscle activity. Extracellular potassium makes up about 2 percent of total potassium in the body and plays an important role in neuromuscular function. Very small fluctuations outside the normal range may cause significant problems, including muscle weakness and cardiac arrhythmias. Blood specimen is obtained by venipuncture. Methods include atomic absorption spectrometry (AAS), ion-selective electrode (ISE), and flame emission spectroscopy (FES).

84133

This test may be ordered as urine K+. Specimen collection is by the patient in a 24-hour period or by a random urine sample. The patient flushes the first urine of the day. All voided urine for the next 24 hours is collected. Methods may include flame emission photometry and ion-selective electrode (ISE). Potassium is the major electrolyte found within cells. The test may be ordered to determine elevated levels for the differential diagnoses of chronic renal failure, renal tubular acidosis, and for diuretic therapy.

84134

The test may also be known as PAB, thyroxine-binding prealbumin (TBPA), thyretin, and transthyretin. Specimen collection is by venipuncture for blood; a random urine sample or a 24-hour urine specimen may be required. The patient flushes the first urine of the day. All urine for the next 24-hours is collected. A separately reportable lumbar puncture is performed to obtain cerebrospinal fluid (CSF). Methods may include electrophoresis and nephelometry (serum). The plasma protein prealbumin plays a role in the transport and metabolism of vitamin A. Serum prealbumin can be used as an indicator of nutrition, liver injury, and chronic kidney disease. It may also be tested in the diagnosis of Hodgkin's disease.

84135

This test measures pregnanediol to evaluate progesterone production by the ovaries and placenta. Specimen collection is venipuncture for blood, random urine sample, or 24-hour urine specimen. For a 24-hour urine specimen, the patient flushes the first urine of the day. All urine for the next 24 hours is collected. A separately reportable amniocentesis is performed to obtain amniotic fluid. Methods may involve gas-liquid chromatography and

radioimmunoassay. Progesterone initiates the phase in ovulation that prepares the endometrium for implantation of a fertilized ovum. The serum and urine level of the progesterone metabolite pregnanediol increases rapidly during this phase, making it a useful measure in documenting and charting ovulation.

84138

The patient typically performs specimen collection over a 24-hour period; muscular exercise should be avoided before and during specimen collection due to the possible increase in urine pregnanetriol. The patient flushes the first urine of the day. All voided urine for the next 24 hours is collected. Methods may include extraction/gas-liquid chromatography (GLC) and spectrophotometry. This test may be performed to determine differential diagnoses of adrenogenital syndrome, tumors of ovary and adrenal cortices, Stein-Leventhal syndrome, and congenital adrenal hyperplasia, among others.

84140

This test is used for detecting and measuring the levels of pregnenolone, a steroid involved in the synthesis of numerous hormones. Specimen collection is by venipuncture, umbilical cord, and heel stick for blood; the patient collects urine sample over a 24-hour urine period. The patient flushes the first urine of the day. All urine for the next 24-hours is collected. Method is typically radioimmunoassay.

84143

Serum or urine may be examined using radioimmunoassay in this test for detecting and measuring the levels of 17-hydroxypregnenolone, a hormonal metabolite. Specimen collection is by venipuncture for blood; urine is collected over a 24-hour period. The patient flushes the first urine of the day. All urine for the next 24 hours is collected.

84144

Specimen collection is by venipuncture. Methods may include radioimmunoassay (RIA) and direct time-resolved fluorescence immunoassay. This test is performed to determine corpus luteum function, confirm ovulation, diagnose incompetent luteal phase, and insufficient progesterone production, which may be the cause of habitual abortions.

84146

Specimen collection is post-fasting venipuncture. Methods may include immunoassay and radioimmunoassay (RIA). Prolactin is a hormone secreted by the anterior pituitary gland. Prolactin level is helpful for monitoring the disease activity of pituitary adenomas. This test may be performed for the differential diagnoses of prolactinemia, galactorrhea (lactation disorder), pituitary prolactinoma and other pituitary tumors.

84150

This test may also be known as PG. Specimen collection is by venipuncture. Method is enzyme immunoassay. Prostaglandin (PG) is a potent unsaturated fatty acid that can act against organs in exceedingly low concentrations, and in their pharmaceutical form may be used for terminating pregnancy or treating asthma.

84152–84154

Specimen collection is by venipuncture. Methods may include radioimmunoassay (RIA) and monoclonal two-site immunoradiometric assay. These tests may be performed to determine the presence of cancer of the prostate, benign prostatic hypertrophy (BPH), prostatitis, post prostatectomy to detect residual cancer, and to monitor therapy. There are several forms of PSA present in serum. PSA may be complexed with the protease inhibitor alpha-1 antichymotrypsin (PSA- ACT). Complexed PSA is the most measurable form. PSA is also found in a free form. Free PSA is not complexed to a protease inhibitor. Higher levels of free PSA are more often associated with benign conditions of the prostate than with prostate cancer. Total PSA measures both complexed and free levels to provide a total amount present in the serum. A percentage of each form is sometimes calculated to help distinguish benign from malignant conditions. Code 84152 reports complexed PSA; code 84153 is for total serum PSA; code 84154 is for free (not complexed) PSA.

84155

This test may be performed to assess nutritional status. Serum protein is composed primarily of albumin and globulins. Blood specimen is obtained by venipuncture. A 24-hour urine specimen is required. The patient flushes the first urine of the day and discards it. All voided urine for the next 24 hours is collected and refrigerated. For amniotic fluid specimen, a separately reportable amniocentesis is performed. Aspiration of other body fluids (CSF, bronchial fluid, exudates) may also require separately reportable procedures. Method is biuret for blood (serum) and amniotic fluid. Method is turbidimetry or nephelometry for urine and CSF. For other body fluids, method is turbidimetry or biuret.

84160

Specimen collection is by venipuncture for adults and heel stick for specimen collection in children. Method is uses refractometry to determine the velocity of light through a refractive material (plasma). This test may also be used in combination with codes 84164, 86334, and 82784 in a test that may be ordered as protein electrophoresis, serum with reflex to immunofixation electrophoresis, serum. This combination test may be used to identify small M-proteins found in patients with amyloidosis, treated myeloma and macroglobulinemia, and solitary and extramedullary

plasmacytoma. Method is capillary electrophoresis/immunofixation electrophoresis.

84165

Specimen collection is by venipuncture for adults; heel stick for children. Methods may be cellulose acetate and agarose electrophoresis. The test is performed for the quantitation of albumin, alpha1, alpha2 beta, and gammaglobulins. CSF electropherosis may be useful in the diagnosis of tumors in the central nervous system or neurological illnesses.

84181–84182

Specimen collection is by venipuncture for blood; separately reportable lumbar puncture for cerebrospinal fluid (CSF). Methods may include enzyme immunoassay (EIA), enzyme-linked immunosorbent assay (ELISA), and indirect fluorescent (IFA) for sceening; Western blot for confirmation. For Western blot test, report 84181; for Western blot with immunological probe for band identification, report 84182. This test identifies serological response to the causative organism Borrelia burgdorferi and may be performed to assist in diagnosing Lyme disease

84202–84203

Specimen collection is by venipuncture for adults, heel stick for children. Methods may include hematofluorometry methods and high performance liquid chromatography. This test is performed to diagnose various anemias and lead toxicity. Code 84203 is a qualitative test used as a screen to determine if protoporphyrin is present in the specimen. Code 84202 measures (quantifies) the level of protoporphyrin present.

84206

Specimen collection is post-fasting venipuncture. Method is radioimmunoassay. This test may be performed for the differential diagnoses of insulinoma, renal failure, factitious hypoglycemia, and diabetes mellitus

84207

This test may also be known as PLP. Vitamin B6 is also known as pyridoxine and pyridoxal phosphate. Specimen collection is by venipuncture. Methods may include enzyme assay, high performance liquid chromatography (HPLC) with fluorometric detection, and immunoradiometric assay. This test may be performed to identify vitamin B6 deficiency, which may be an indicator of an underlying disease. Deficiency is often found in nutritional deficiencies as a result of other diseases including chronic alcoholism.

84210

This test is also known as pyruvic acid test. Specimen collection is by venipuncture or finger stick. Methods are usually enzymatic and colorimetry. This test measures the level of pyruvate in whole blood for possible diagnosis of an inherited disorder of metabolism. The abnormal breakdown of red blood cells and subsequent release of hemoglobin characterize a congenital deficiency of pyruvate.

84220

Specimen collection is by venipuncture; the erythrocytes are washed. Method is spectrophotometric kinetic assay. This test may be performed to identify pyruvate kinase deficiency and hemolytic anemia in newborns.

84228

Quinine is used in the treatment of malaria, atrial fibrillation, and other disorders of muscular tissues. Specimen collection is by the patient over a 24-hour period. The patient flushes the first urine of the day. All urine for the next 24-hours is collected. Method is thin-layer chromatography.

84233

Specimen collection is by separately reportable surgical removal. Methods may include biochemical measurement in cytosol fractions of tumor homogenate, dextranestradiol conjugate, immunoperoxidase using tissue sections, enzyme immunoassay (EIA), and in situ hybridization. This test may be ordered to assist in identifying a breast cancer patient's ability to respond to chemotherapy and endocrine therapy.

84234

Specimen collection is by separately reportable surgical removal. Methods may include sucrose density gradient, steroid binding assay, and enzyme immunoassay. This test assists in identifying a patient's ability to respond to treatment in breast and other cancers.

84235

The test may be used to predict or monitor patient response to hormonal therapy. Specimen collection is by venipuncture for whole blood and plasma; separately reportable biopsy or surgical excision for tumor tissue. Methods are radioimmunoassay (most commonly used technique), gas-liquid and liquid chromatography or electrophoresis.

84238

This test may also be known as AChR. This test may be used to predict or monitor patient response to therapy. Specimen collection is by venipuncture for whole blood; tumor tissue is by separately reportable biopsy or surgical excision. Methods include radioimmunoassay (most commonly used technique), gas-liquid and liquid chromatography or electrophoresis. The test is performed to determine the concentration of the target substance.

84244

This test may be ordered as plasma renin activity, or PRA. Specimen collection is by venipuncture. Certain medications such as beta-blockers, may affect testing outcome. Methodology may include radioimmunoassay.

84252

This test may be used primarily to determine nutritional deficiency of this vitamin. Blood specimen collection is by venipuncture; urine is a 24-hour specimen. The patient flushes the first urine of the day. All voided urine for the next 24 hours is collected. Methods may include high performance liquid chromatography (HPLC) or fluorometry.

84255

This test may also be known by the abbreviation Se. Specimen collection is by venipuncture for blood; urine specimens are collected over a 24-hour period. The patient flushes the first urine of the day and discards it. All voided urine for the next 24 hours is collected. Methods may include fluorometry and atomic absorption. The blood and the urine test may be performed simultaneously. This test may be ordered to monitor nutritional therapy and for possible toxic exposure.

84260

This test may also be called 5-HT or 5-Hydroxytryptamine. Specimen collection is by venipuncture for blood; a separately reportable lumbar puncture is performed to collect cerebrospinal fluid (CSF). Methods may include fluorometry, radioimmunoassay (RIA), and gas or liquid chromatography spinal puncture to obtain specimen is reported separately, see 62270. This test may be performed to diagnose carcinoid syndrome and severe depression.

84270

This test may also be ordered as SHBG. Specimen collection is by venipuncture for blood; separately reportable amniocentesis for amniotic fluid. Methods include radioimmunoassay. The test may be performed to determine the concentration of the hormone in serum. The test may be used to predict or monitor patient response to hormonal therapy and to assist in certain diagnoses, including hypothyroidism and hyperthyroidism.

84275

This test may also be known by Lipid Associated Sialic Acid or LASA. Specimen collection is by venipuncture. The term "sialic acids" comprises a group of natural neuraminic acid derivatives. The activity of the enzyme, neuraminidase, is also referred to as sialidase. Deficiency of the enzyme may result in the clinical disease sialidosis, a syndrome that may involve involuntary twitching of the muscular group affected and cherry-red spots on the skin. Methods include enzyme assay and spectrometry.

84285

Silica is a naturally occurring and common mineral found in sands, clays, and quartz deposits. Exposure is commonly by inhalation of dusts during rock mining and certain manufacturing. Deposition on the eyes and mucosal surfaces may also be a pathway of exposure. Most commonly, however, phagocytic cells may distribute the silica along lymph channels once the particles are inhaled and collect in lung alveoli. Long-term exposure is linked to numerous illnesses, including silicosis. But testing methods for silica in the system seem unclear in the literature.

84295

This test may be requested as Na. Sodium is an electrolyte found in extracellular fluid. Blood specimen is obtained by venipuncture. Methods include atomic absorption spectrometry (AAS), flame emission photometry, and ion-selective electrode (ISE).

84300

This test may also be ordered as urine Na. Specimen collection is often by the patient over a 24-hour period or by random urine sample. For a 24-hour urine specimen, the patient flushes the first urine of the day. All voided urine for the next 24 hours is collected. Methods may include flame emission photometry and ion selective electrode (ISE). Sodium is an electrolyte found in extracellular fluid. This test is used to identify increased (hypernatremia), and decreased (hyponatremia) levels of sodium due to various conditions or disease states.

84305

Somatomedin is a protein mainly produced in the liver. It is a peptide dependent on growth hormone for its actions. This test may be used to diagnose and evaluate response to therapy for a variety of growth disorders. The test may be performed to diagnose acromegaly, dwarfism, pituitary disease and disorders, nutritional deficiencies, and to monitor response to therapies. Specimen collection is by venipuncture. Methodology may use a process of dissociation from binding protein and chromatography, followed by radioimmunoassay (RIA).

84307

This test may be performed to measure somatostatin, a hormone found in the pancreas and in the gut. Specimen is by venipuncture. Method is usually radioimmunoassay. This hormone helps regulate the body's production of insulin, glucagon, gastrin, secretin, and renin. Somatostatin also may control how the body secretes insulin and glucagon.

84311

Specimen collection is by venipuncture for blood; or the patient collects urine over a 24-hour period; or a random urine sample is taken. Method is typically spectrophotometry, which provides a quantitative measure of the amount of a material in a solution absorbing applied light. Report this test for an analyte not elsewhere specified. Measuring the absorption of visible, ultraviolet or infrared light makes quantitative measurements of concentrations of reagents. For example, spectrophotometry can be used to measure the amount of sulfonamides in urine.

84315

Specimen collection is by the bodily fluid chosen as a sample (e.g., gastric secretions). Method is by specific gravity, which measures the concentration - or the weight of a substance - as compared to an equal volume of water. For laboratory testing, specific gravity shows the density of a specific material.

84375

This test is performed to separate chemical substances from particles and to measure the end products of carbohydrate (sugar) metabolism. Specimen collection is by the patient over a 24-hour period or a random urine sample. Methodology may include gas chromatography.

84376–84379

This test may be used for infants who are failing to thrive due to lactose, sucrose, or fructose imbalances. The patient performs specimen collection over a 24-hour period for urine. A separately reportable amniocentesis collects for amniotic fluid; a separately reportable lumbar puncture collects specimens for CSF; and paracentesis of posterior chamber of eye collects specimens for vitreous fluid. Methods include gas chromatography and mass spectrometry.

84392

Sulfates may be measured for the diagnosis of metachromatic leukodystrophy, an inherited lipid metabolism that results in the accumulation of metachromatic lipids in the tissues of the central nervous system, leading to paralysis and often death in early adolescence. The disease also is known as sulfatide lipidosis. The patient performs specimen collection over a 24-hour period. For a random sample; the first-voided specimen may be used. Method is spectrophotometry.

84402–84403

These tests may be used to evaluate testosterone levels. Testosterone is an androgenic hormone responsible for, among other biological activities, secondary male characteristics in women. Increased testosterone levels in women may be linked to a variety of conditions, including hirsutism. Code 84403 reports total testosterone, which includes both protein bound and free testosterone. Code 84402 reports testosterone as a free unbound protein. This test may be ordered to evaluate hirsute women; it may also be ordered to assist in diagnosis of hypogonadism, hypopituitarism, and Klinefelter's syndrome, among other disorders. Specimen collection is by venipuncture. Method may be by radioimmunoassay (RIA) and immunoassay (non-isotopic).

84425

This is also known as Vitamin B1. Specimen collection is by venipuncture for whole blood, serum, and erythrocytes; for urine, the sample is collected randomly or by the patient over a 24-hour period. The patient flushes the first urine of the day and discards it. All voided urine for the next 24 hours is collected and refrigerated. Methods are high performance liquid chromatography and thiochrome-fluorometry. This test determines the levels of thiamine, which decreased levels may identify alcoholism and beriberi.

84430

This drug may also be known as Nipride, Nitropusside, Thanite, Lethane, or KCN. Specimen collection is by venipuncture for blood or by random urine sample. Methods may include photometry or chromatography. The test may be ordered to evaluate thiocyanate toxicity, nitroprusside therapy and poisoning, or cigarette use.

84432

This test is also known as Tg. Specimen collection is by venipuncture. Method is immunoassay. This test is performed to determine thyroglobulin levels to identify thyroid disorders and tumors.

84436

This test may be ordered as a T4. Specimen collection is by venipuncture for adults, heel stick for newborns. Methods may include radioimmunoassay (RIA), enzyme-linked immunosorbent assay (ELISA), fluorescence polarization immunoassay (FPIA), and chemiluminescence assay (CIA). The test is performed to determine thyroid function screening test; total thyroxine makes up approximately 99% of the thyroid hormone.

84437

This test may be ordered as a neonatal T4. Specimen collection is by heel stick or taken from the umbilical cord. The specimen may be taken at the same time as a PKU (Phenylalanine) test. Method is typically radioimmunoassay (RIA). The test may be performed to determine hypothyroidism in newborns (performed in all 50 states) to prevent mental retardation and to monitor suppressive and replacement therapy.

84439

This test may be ordered as a FT4, free T4, FTI or FT4 index. Specimen collection is by venipuncture

and the serum is separated. Methods may include radioimmunoassay and equilibrium dialysis for reference method. Free thyroxine is a minimal amount of the total T4 level (approximately one percent). This test is not influenced by thyroid-binding abnormalities and perhaps correlates more closely with the true hormonal status. It may be effective in the diagnosis of hyperthyroidism and hypothyroidism.

84442

Specimen collection is by venipuncture for adults, heel stick for newborns. Methods may include chemiluminescent immunoassay. In addition, direct assays have been developed using equilibrium dialysis, ultrafiltration, and solid phase enzyme immunoassay (EIA) technology. Thyroxin binding globulin is a plasma protein that binds with thyroxine and transports it in the blood. TBG capacity has a regulatory and pronounced effect on the concentration of thyroid hormones. Elevated levels may be associated with pregnancy and newborn states, hepatitis, and other disorders. Decreased levels may be associated with liver diseases and acromegaly, among other disorders.

84443

TSH is produced in the pituitary gland and stimulates the secretion of thyrotropin (T3) and thyroxine (T4); these secretory products monitor TSH. Specimen collection is by venipuncture for adults; serum should be separated within four hours. Heel stick or umbilical cord sample is drawn from newborns and may be collected on a special paper. Methods may include radioimmunoassay (RIA), sandwich immunoradiometric assay (IRMA), fluorometric enzyme immunoassay with use of monoclonal antibodies, or microparticle enzyme immunoassay on IMx (MEIA). This test may be performed to determine thyroid function, to differentiate from various types of hypothyroidism (e.g., primary, and pituitary/hypothalamic), or to diagnose hyperthyroidism. The test may be ordered to evaluate therapy in patients receiving hypothyroid treatment, and in infants it may be used to detect congenital hypothyroidism.

84445

This test may also be ordered as TSI. This serum test measures the amount of thyroid stimulating antibody, which stimulates the thyroid to produce excessive amounts of thyroid hormone. Specimen collection is by venipuncture. Methods may include vitro bioassay and radioimmunoassay. The test may be useful in diagnosis of Grave's disease (hyperthyroidism).

84446

This test may also be known as a-tochopherol. Specimen collection is by venipuncture for adults; heel stick for newborns. Methods may include high performance liquid chromatography (HPLC), fluorometry after solvent extraction, and colorimetry. The test may be performed to determine vitamin E deficiency, to evaluate patients on long-term parenteral nutrition, and to evaluate numerous disorders.

84449

Cortisol-binding globulin (Transcortin) is a type of glycoprotein. This test is performed to measure transcortin, a chemical used to evaluate adrenal activity. It plays a role in fat and water metabolism. Specimen collection is by venipuncture for blood. The patient may perform urine collection over a 24-hour period. A random urine sample may be used. Method may include chemiluminescent. Levels of cortisol help in the diagnosis of Cushing's syndrome, and Addison's disease.

84450

This test is usually referred to as aspartate aminotransferase (AST), but may also be requested as serum glutamic oxaloacetic transaminase (SGOT). AST is an enzyme found primarily in heart muscle and the liver. Serum levels are low unless there is cellular damage, at which time large amounts are released into circulation. AST levels are increased following acute myocardial infarction (MI). Liver disease may also cause elevated levels of AST. Blood specimen is obtained by venipuncture. Method is spectrophotometry, kinetic assay, and enzymatic.

84460

This test is usually referred to as alanine aminotransferase (ALT), but may also be requested as serum glutamic pyruvic transaminase (SGPT). ALT is an enzyme found primarily in liver cells and elevations may be indicative of liver disease. Blood specimen is obtained by venipuncture. Method is spectrophotometry or enzymatic.

84466

This test may also be called a TRF, Tf, siderophilin, and pertains to a transferrin index or receptor. Specimen collection is by venipuncture. Urine is a 24-hour specimen. The patient flushes the first urine of the day. All urine for the next 24-hours is collected. Methods may include radial immunodiffusion (RID), and electro-immunodiffusion for urine, and rate nephelometry for serum. The test is performed to determine a patient's nutritional status. It may also be used to differentiate between iron deficiency anemia, acquired liver disorders and diseases, and kidney diseases.

84478

This test may be requested as TG. Triglycerides are blood lipids that are transported through the circulatory system by lipoproteins. Triglycerides contribute to atherosclerosis and other arterial diseases. Blood specimen is obtained by venipuncture. Method is enzymatic or colorimetry.

84479

This test may be requested as T3 uptake and T4 uptake or THBR. In the T3 or T4 uptake test, resin and radioactive T3 or T4 are added to the patient's serum and the proportion of the tracer (radioactive T3 or T4) bound by the solid matrix is measured. Method is chemiluminescent immunoassay. THBR is then calculated from the T3 or T4 uptake test as follows: THBR = % T uptake (patient serum) / % T uptake (control serum).

84480

This test may be ordered as a T3 (RIA) or total T3. A specimen collection is by venipuncture. Methods may include radioimmunoassay (RIA), immunochemiluminometric assay, and fluorometric immunoassay. This is a thyroid function test used to measure T3. Abnormal results may be diseases and disorders related to the thyroid.

84481

This test may also be known as FT3, or free T3. Specimen collection is by venipuncture, finger stick, heel stick, or umbilical cord. Method may involve equilibrium dialysis (tracer). This test may be used to identify thyroid dysfunction, such as hyperthyroidism and hypothyroidism.

84482

Reverse T3 (rT3) is an inactive form of the thyroid hormone T3, and is found in the blood of normal people. Measurement of rT3 has been suggested in differentiating euthyroid sick syndrome from true hypothyroidism, and in identifying factitious hyperthyroidism. RT3 is typically measured by radioimmunoassay.

84484

This test may also be known as troponin regulatory complex. Specimen collection is by venipuncture. Methods may include radioimmunoassay, enzyme-linked immunosorbent assay, and immunoenzymatic assay. This quantitative test measures the levels of troponin, found in muscle tissues. Elevated levels of troponin may be related to myocardial infarction and ischemic heart disease.

84485

This test may also be referred to as duodenal trypsinogen. Trypsin in duodenal aspirate has been measured by both radioimmunoassay and enzymatic methods. Measurement is useful in evaluation of pancreatic disease, such as primary biliary cirrhosis and cystic fibrosis, and malabsorption syndromes.

84488–84490

This test may be called fecal tryptic activity or immunoreactive trypsin. Specimen collection is fresh random stool sample. Methods may be kinetic and potentiometric, and x-ray film method. Trypsin is an enzyme that acts to degrade protein and it may be referred to as proteolytic enzyme, or proteinase. This test is performed to screen for pancreatic exocrine function and malabsorption syndromes in children under the age of four. Three specimens may be taken for an accurate assessment of pancreatic function. For qualitative screening, report 84488; for quantitative measurement, see 84490.

84510

This test may also be known by the abbreviation Tyr. Specimen collection is by venipuncture for serum or plasma; for urine, the specimen is typically collected by the patient over a 24-hour period. The patient flushes the first urine of the day. All voided urine for the next 24 hours is collected. For CSF, a separately reportable lumbar puncture is performed. Measurement of tyrosine is useful in the evaluation of certain amino-acidopathies or inborn errors of metabolism. Tyrosine has been measured by chromatographic techniques such as HPLC or gas chromatography combined with a variety of detection/evaluation technologies, including mass-spectrometry. This precursor of thyroid hormones, catecholamines, and melanin is measured to determine possible thyroid disorders and various other diseases.

84512

This may also be known as troponin regulatory complex. Specimen collection is by venipuncture. Cardiac tropinins are markers for myocardial muscle damage. Qualitative tests (positive/negative results) are primarily used to rule-in or rule-out myocardial infarction. Several bedside, point-of-care type assays are available. These tests are designed to be used at the point of care, such as in the emergency room or physician office. Methods are radioimmunoassay, enzyme-linked immunosorbent assay, and immunoenzymatic assay may also be seen.

84520

This test may be requested as blood urea nitrogen (BUN). Urea is an end product of protein metabolism. BUN may be requested to evaluate dehydration or renal function. Blood specimen is obtained by venipuncture. Method is colorimetry, enzymatic, or rate conductivity. This test measures (quantitates) the amount of urea in the blood.

84525

This test may also be ordered as a BUN. This test may provide useful information regarding carbohydrate metabolism (diabetes), kidney function, and acid-base balance. Specimen collection is by random urine sample. Method is reagent strip. The reagent strips react chemically with the urine sample taken that day to provide a standardized visible color reaction, which determines the level of urea nitrogen.

84540

This test may provide useful information regarding carbohydrate metabolism (diabetes), kidney function, and acid-base balance, in addition to dietary protein. Urea is a measure of protein breakdown in the body. Excretion of urea can be a reflection of kidney function. Urine urea excretion can be measured to obtain a ratio between the plasma (blood) urea and the urine urea; this ratio is an indicator of kidney function. The patient performs specimen collection over a 24-hour period. Methods may include enzymatic assay, colorimetry, and conductometric.

84545

This test is also known as BUN - blood urea nitrogen. Specimen collection is taken over a 24-hour period. Urea nitrogen is formed in the liver as an end product of protein metabolism. Increased or decreased levels of urea nitrogen can indicate renal disease, dehydration, congestive heart failure, and gastrointestinal bleeding, starvation, shock or urinary tract obstruction (by tumor or prostate gland).

84550

This test may be requested as urate. Uric acid may be ordered to evaluate gout, renal function and a number of other disorders. Blood specimen is obtained by venipuncture. Method is enzymatic or high performance liquid chromatography (HPLC).

84560

Uric acid is also known as urate. Specimen collection may be over a 24-hour period. Cerebrospinal fluid (CSF) is obtained by separately reportable lumbar puncture. Methods may include high performance liquid chromatography, uricase, and phosphotungstate. The test may be ordered to determine the possible occurrence of calculus formation, evaluate uric acid in gout, and to identify genetic defects and some malignancies.

84577

This also is known as the urobilinogen 48-hour feces test. Specimen collection is by random stool sample. Method is colorimetry. It is used to detect the presence of the yellow substance called urobilin that develops from the chemical breakdown of urobilinogen, which is excreted in the feces.

84578

This test is used to detect the presence of urobilinogen in urine. Specimen collection is by random urine sample. Urobilinogen determination in urine is a useful liver function test, and can be helpful in evaluating some hemolytic anemias. Urobilinogen can be detected qualitatively by a simple, visual colorimetric test or by urine dipstick. Methods may include Ehrlich's aldehyde reagent, para-dimethylaminobenzaldehyde reacts with urobilinogen with a color enhancer.

CPT® Lay Descriptions

84580–84583

These tests are used to report quantitative or semi-quantitative measurement of urobilinogen present in the urine. Specimen collection may be performed over a two-hour period. Urobilinogen is formed in the intestine by bacterial action and small amounts are eventually excreted in the urine. Elevated levels of urobilinogen can be early indicators of various types of liver disorders. Methods may include Ehrlich's aldehyde reagent, Watson's method, and Urobilistix. This test identifies some cases of liver diseases and hemolytic anemias, but not all. Report 84580 for a timed quantitative measurement urobilinogen; report 84583 for a semi-quantitative measurement of urobilinogen.

84585

This test is also called 3-methoxy-4-hydroxymandelic acid test, and also as VMA. Specimen collection is by the patient over a 24-hour period. The patient flushes the first urine of the day and discards it. All urine for the next 24-hours is collected. Methods may include colorimetry, spectrophotometry, gas chromatography, and high performance liquid chromatography (HPLC). The test may be performed to evaluate hypertensive states and to diagnose certain tumors and to monitor the efficacy of treatment modalities.

84586

VIP (vasoactive intestinal peptide) is found in and released from the central nervous system. It as found in the gut and affects the cells of the immune system. Specimen collection is post-fasting venipuncture. Method is radioimmunoassay. The test may be used to determine the concentration of vasoactive intestinal peptide (VIP) in serum.

84588

This test is also known as Arginine Vasopressin Hormone and Antidiuretic Hormone (ADH). Specimen collection is by venipuncture. Method is radioimmunoassay. The test is performed to determine the concentration of the hormone vasopressin, a substance that affects blood flow. Vasopressin increases blood pressure and the rate at which the kidneys absorb water. It is secreted by the hypothalamus and stored in and released by the posterior pituitary gland.

84590

This vitamin may is also known as retinol. Specimen collection is by venipuncture; patient should be fasting at least eight hours prior to collection. Methods are electrochemical, high performance liquid chromatography (HPLC), and fluorescence or UV/VIS spectroscopy. Serum levels of vitamin A can be increased in specific diseases and toxic states, and decreased levels are seen in other conditions, such as, nutritional deficiency.

84591

This test is used to analyze vitamin levels that are not specified elsewhere such as biotin and niacin. Blood specimen is obtained by venipuncture. A 24-hour urine specimen is required. Methods are dependent on the specific vitamin level being analyzed and on the type of specimen, but include microbiological assay (urine biotin levels), high performance liquid chromatography (HPLC) (urine niacine levels) solid phase (cellulose) binding assay (plasma biotin levels), chemoluminescence (serum biotin levels).

84597

This test is used to analyze vitamin K, a fat-soluble vitamin that plays an important role in blood clotting. Specimen collection is by venipuncture; patient should be fasting prior to specimen collection. Method is high-performance liquid chromatography A. A deficiency in vitamin K is characterized by the increased tendency to bleed, including internal bleeding. Such bleeding episodes may be severe in newborn infants.

84600

This is also known as volatile toxicology, which would include acetone, ethanol, isopropanol, and methanol. Specimen collection may be venipuncture for blood, random urine, and gastric juice samples. Gastric specimen may be collected by gastric lavage. Method may be gas-liquid chromatography (GLC). This test is performed to determine systemic alcohol levels and possibly as surveillance for drug abuse and to evaluate methanol and isopropanol toxicity.

84620

This test may also be known as a xylose tolerance test. Specimen collection is by venipuncture for blood or timed specimen for urine. Various timed tests for different categories of patients are required for this test. For adults, a five-hour urine and a one-hour serum sample may be common. Patients with intermediate renal insufficiency may call for a one-hour serum test only. Similarly, for children under the age of 12, only a serum test may be performed. Methods may be colorimetry, gas chromatography, and mass spectrometry. This test may be performed to evaluate the function of the jejunum.

84630

This test is also known as Serum Zn. Specimen collection is by venipuncture for blood or a 24-hour urine sample. The patient flushes the first urine of the day and discards it. All urine for the next 24-hours is collected. Methods may include atomic absorption spectrometry (AAS). Zinc is a trace mineral normally present in the body. It is linked to thyroid hormone function and to blood clotting. The test may be performed to determine nutrient levels for patients on total parenteral nutrition (TPN) and for burn victims and critically ill patients. The test may also be ordered to evaluate possible zinc toxicity.

84681

This test may also be known as a connecting peptide insulin test or a pro-insulin c-peptide. Specimen collection is by venipuncture for blood; urine is collected over a 24-hour period. The patient flushes the first urine of the day and all urine for the next 24-hours is collected. Methods may include radioimmunoassay (RIA). The test is primarily performed to determine hypoglycemia and to measure pancreatic beta cell secretory function. It may also be used to determine residual beta cell function in insulin-dependent diabetes, and to differentiate between insulin and non-insulin diabetics.

84702

This test may be ordered as hCG or as a serum pregnancy test. Specimen collection is by venipuncture. Method may be radioimmunoassay (RIA), two-site immunoradiometric assay (IRMA), two-site enzyme-linked immunosorbent assay (ELISA), and radioreceptor assay (RRA). This test is quantitative and measures the amount of hCG present, a determinate of pregnancy and certain tumors.

84703

This test is also known as a beta-subunit human chorionic gonadotropin. Specimen collection is by venipuncture for blood or random urine sample. Methods may include radioimmunoassay (RIA), immunoradiometric (IRMA), and enzyme immunoassay. The test may be ordered to determine pregnancy, ectopic pregnancy, and hCG tumors, and as a screening prior to select medical care (e.g., sterilization).

84830

This test is used for the qualitative detection of the luteinizing hormone (LH) in urine. Specimen collection is urine. Method is rapid chromatographic immunoassay. LH is always present in the blood and urine, though its levels are higher in urine during ovulation. The LH surge and actual release of the egg is considered as the most fertile time of the cycle, and the most likely time for becoming pregnant.

85002

This test may be ordered as a bleeding time or as an Ivy bleeding time. A small, superficial wound is nicked in the patient's forearm. Essentially, the amount of time it takes for the wound to stop bleeding is recorded at bedside. The Ivy bleeding time test is one standardized method. All methods are manual or point of care. A bleeding time is a rough measure of platelet (thrombocyte) function. The test is often performed on a pre-operative patient.

85007

This test may be ordered as a blood count with manual differential. Specimen collection is venipuncture, finger stick, or heel stick in infants.

Method is manual testing. A blood count typically includes measurement of white blood cells or leukocytes, hemoglobin, and hematocrit (volume of packed red cells or VPRC). In addition, this test includes a manual differential of white blood cells or "diff." The following leukocytes will be differentiated: neutrophils or granulocytes, lymphocytes, monocytes, eosinophils, and basophils. The platelet count will be estimated and red cell morphology will be commented on if abnormal.

85008

This test may be ordered as a manual blood smear examination without differential parameters, RBC smear, peripheral blood smear, or RBC morphology. Method is manual testing. A blood smear is prepared and examined for the presence of normal cell constituents, including white blood cells, red blood cells, and platelets. The white blood cell and platelet or thrombocyte counts are estimated and red cell morphology will be commented on if abnormal.

85009

This test may be ordered as a buffy coat differential or as a differential WBC count, buffy coat. Blood is obtained by venipuncture. Other collection types (e.g., finger stick or heel stick) do not yield the volume of blood required for this test. Method is manual testing. The whole blood is centrifuged to concentrate the white blood cells, which are then prepared as a blood smear and a manual WBC differential is performed. The following leukocytes will be differentiated: neutrophils or granulocytes, lymphocytes, monocytes, eosinophils, and basophils. The platelet count will be estimated and red cell morphology will be commented on if abnormal. This test does not include enumeration of the white blood cells or platelets. This test is usually performed when the number of WBCs or leukocytes is abnormally low and the presence of abnormal white cells (e.g., blasts or cancer cells) is suspected clinically.

85013

This test may be ordered as a microhematocrit, a spun microhematocrit, or a "spun crit." Specimen collection is finger stick or heel stick in infants. Method is manual testing. A spun microhematocrit only reports the volume of packed red cells or hematocrit. It is typically performed at sites where only limited testing is available, the patient is a very difficult blood draw, or on infants.

85014

This test may be ordered as a hematocrit, Hmt, or Hct. Specimen collection is venipuncture, finger stick, or heel stick in infants. Method is automated cell counter. The hematocrit or volume of packed red cells or VPRC is calculated by multiplying the red blood cell count or RBC times the mean corpuscular volume or MCV.

CPT ® Lay Descriptions

85018

This test may be ordered as hemoglobin, Hgb, or hemoglobin concentration. Specimen is commonly venipuncture, finger stick, or heel stick in infants. Method is usually automated cell counter but a manual method is seen in small labs with a limited test menu, blood bank drawing stations, and some limited testing physician office laboratories. Hemoglobin is an index of the oxygen-carrying capacity of the blood.

85021

Specimen collection is venipuncture, finger stick, or heel stick in infants. Method is automated cell counter. A hemogram typically includes measurement of erythrocytes (red blood cells or RBC), leukocytes (white blood cells or WBC), hemoglobin, hematocrit (volume of packed red blood cells or VPRC), and indices (mean corpuscular hemoglobin or MCH, mean corpuscular hemoglobin concentration or MCHC, mean corpuscular volume or MCV, and red cell distribution width or RDW). This code includes an automated hemogram with no WBC differential.

85022

This test may be ordered as a complete blood count (CBC) with manual differential. Specimen collection is venipuncture, finger stick, or heel stick in infants. Method is automated cell counter and manual differential. A hemogram typically includes measurement of leukocytes (white blood cells or WBC), erythrocytes (red blood cells or RBC), hemoglobin, hematocrit (volume of packed red blood cells or VPRC), and indices (mean corpuscular hemoglobin or MCH, mean corpuscular hemoglobin concentration or MCHC, mean corpuscular volume or MCV, and red cell distribution width or RDW). In addition, this test includes a manual differential of white blood cells or "diff." The following leukocytes will be differentiated: neutrophils or granulocytes, lymphocytes, monocytes, eosinophils, and basophils. The platelet count will be estimated and red cell morphology will be commented on if abnormal.

85023

This test may be ordered as a complete blood count (CBC) with platelets and manual differential. Specimen collection is venipuncture, finger stick, or heel stick in infants. Method is automated cell counter for the hemogram and platelet count with a manual WBC differential. The hemogram in this code includes measurement of leukocytes (white blood cells or WBC), erythrocytes (red blood cells or RBC), hemoglobin, hematocrit (volume of packed red blood cells or VPRC), platelet or thrombocyte count, and indices (mean corpuscular hemoglobin or MCH, mean corpuscular hemoglobin concentration or MCHC, mean corpuscular volume or MCV, and red cell distribution width or RDW). In addition, this test includes a manual differential of white blood cells or "diff." The following leukocytes will be differentiated:

neutrophils or granulocytes, lymphocytes, monocytes, eosinophils, and basophils. The platelet count will be estimated and red cell morphology will be commented on if abnormal.

85024

This test may be ordered as a complete blood count (CBC) with platelets and automated partial differential. Specimen collection is venipuncture, finger stick, or heel stick in infants. Method is automated cell counter. The hemogram in this code includes measurement of leukocytes (white blood cells or WBC), erythrocytes (red blood cells or RBC), hemoglobin, hematocrit (volume of packed red blood cells or VPRC), platelet or thrombocyte count, and indices (mean corpuscular hemoglobin or MCH, mean corpuscular hemoglobin concentration or MCHC, mean corpuscular volume or MCV, and red cell distribution width or RDW). In addition, this test includes an automated partial differential of white blood cells or "diff." The following leukocytes will be differentiated: neutrophils or granulocytes, lymphocytes, and monocytes.

85025

This test may be ordered as a complete blood count (CBC) with platelets and automated differential. Specimen collection is venipuncture, finger stick, or heel stick in infants. Method is automated cell counter. The hemogram in this code includes measurement of erythrocytes (red blood cells or RBC), leukocytes (white blood cells or WBC), hemoglobin, hematocrit (volume of packed red blood cells or VPRC), platelet or thrombocyte count, and indices (mean corpuscular hemoglobin or MCH, mean corpuscular hemoglobin concentration or MCHC, mean corpuscular volume or MCV, and red cell distribution width or RDW). In addition, this test includes an automated differential of white blood cells or "diff." The following leukocytes will be differentiated: neutrophils or granulocytes, lymphocytes, monocytes, eosinophils and basophils.

85027

Specimen collection is venipuncture, finger stick, or heel stick in infants. Method is automated cell counter. The hemogram in this code includes measurement of erythrocytes (red blood cells or RBC), leukocytes (white blood cells or WBC), hemoglobin, hematocrit (volume of packed red blood cells or VPRC), platelet or thrombocyte count, and indices (mean corpuscular hemoglobin or MCH, mean corpuscular hemoglobin concentration or MCHC, mean corpuscular volume or MCV, and red cell distribution width or RDW).

85031

This test may be ordered as a manual complete blood count, manual CBC, or manual hemogram. Specimen collection is venipuncture, finger stick, or heel stick in infants. Method is manual. The hemogram in this code includes measurement of erythrocytes (red blood cells or RBC), leukocytes (white blood cells or WBC), hemoglobin, hematocrit (volume of packed red blood cells or VPRC), platelet or thrombocyte count, and indices (mean corpuscular hemoglobin or MCH, mean corpuscular hemoglobin concentration or MCHC, and mean corpuscular volume or MCV). In addition, this test includes a manual differential of white blood cells or "diff." The following leukocytes will be differentiated: neutrophils or granulocytes, lymphocytes, monocytes, eosinophils, and basophils. The platelet count will be estimated and red cell morphology will be commented on if abnormal.

85041

This test may be ordered as red blood cell count or RBC. Specimen collection is venipuncture, finger stick, or heel stick in infants. Method is usually automated but, in some small laboratories with limited test menus, may be manual. Only the RBC is reported.

85044

This test may be ordered as a manual reticulocyte count or as a manual "retic." Specimen collection is venipuncture, finger stick, or heel stick in infants. Method is manual. A blood smear is prepared and stained with a dye that highlights the reticulum in these immature red blood cells, or reticulocytes. The reticulocytes are counted manually and reported as a percentage of total red blood cells.

85045

This test may be ordered as an automated reticulocyte count, an "auto retic," or a reticulocyte by flow cytometry. Specimen collection is venipuncture, finger stick, or heel stick in infants. Method is automated cell counter or flow cytometer. Reticulocytes are immature red blood cells that still contain mitochondria and ribosomes. When stained, the cells assume a peculiar structure enabling direct or automated identification. The reticulocytes are counted and reported as a percentage of total red blood cells.

85046

This test may be ordered as a reticulocyte count and hemoglobin concentration, "retics" and hgb, or as an "auto retic" and hemoglobin. Specimen collection is venipuncture, finger stick, or heel stick in infants. Method is automated cell counter. The hemoglobin concentration is determined and then the blood is stained with a dye that marks the reticulum in immature red blood cells or reticulocytes. The reticulocytes are counted and reported as a percentage of total red blood cells.

85048

This test may be ordered as a white blood cell or WBC count, white cell count, or leukocyte count. Specimen collection is venipuncture, finger stick, or

heel stick in infants. Method is usually automated cell count but this test may also be performed manually. The number of white blood cells or leukocytes are measured and reported.

85060

This test may be ordered as a peripheral blood smear with interpretation by a physician, with a written report. It would more usually be ordered following a hemogram with WBC differential where the technologist noted the presence of significant abnormalities and requested a pathology review. Although lacking specificity, peripheral smears also provide a quick and cost-effective screening for the presence of bacteremia. Specimen collection is venipuncture, finger stick, or heel stick in infants. The method is manual. A blood smear is prepared and reviewed by a physician/pathologist, who then submits a written interpretation of the findings.

85097

This test may be ordered as a bone marrow smear interpretation with or without differential cell count. Specimen collection is by aspiration with a syringe. The bone marrow aspirate may be collected from a variety of sites, including the posterior iliac crest (preferred) and the sternum. The method is manual. Slides or smears are prepared from the aspirate and stained. The slides are then reviewed by a physician/pathologist and a written interpretation of the findings is submitted. This report may include a differential count of the white blood cells present.

85130

This test may be ordered as a chromogenic substrate assay but would more likely be ordered as a specific clotting factor assay (e.g., factor V, fibrinogen, or antithrombin III) by chromogenic analysis. Specimen collection is venipuncture. The method is usually automated coagulation instrument but may be manual.

85170

This test may be ordered as a clot retraction or a clot retraction study. Specimen collection is by venipuncture. The method is manual. Clot retraction time is a measurement of blood platelet function. Specimen tubes are placed in a water bath and examined after about two hours. Normal blood begins to retract 30 to 60 minutes after collection. The test is an older method to measure platelet or thrombocyte function.

85175

This test may be ordered as a whole blood dilution clot lysis time. Specimen collection is by venipuncture. The method is manual. This is a non-specific test of fibrinolytic or clot-lysing activity. Blood specimens are allowed to clot in tubes. The tubes are examined at 24 and 48-hour intervals to assess degeneration of the clots. The test is rarely used today, as there are other specific assays that provide more useable information to the physician.

85210

This test may be ordered as a factor II, clotting factor II, or a prothrombin factor assay. Specimen collection is by venipuncture. The method is usually automated coagulation instrument but may be manual. This factor is one of several essential to clot formation. A decreased amount of this factor may be associated with clotting impairment.

85220

This test may be ordered as a factor V, clotting factor V, or labile factor assay. It may be ordered as a proaccelerin assay or an AcG factor assay. Specimen collection is by venipuncture. The method is usually automated coagulation instrument, but may be manual. This factor is one of several essential to clot formation. A decreased amount of this factor may be associated with blood clotting disorders.

85230

This test may be ordered as a factor VII assay, stable factor assay, or clotting factor VII assay. It may also be ordered as a proconvertin assay. Specimen collection is by venipuncture. The method is usually automated coagulation instrument, but may be manual. This factor is one of several essential to clot formation. A decreased amount of this factor may be associated with blood clotting disorders.

85240

This test may be ordered as a factor VIII assay, Factor VIII:C, or an anti-hemophilic globulin or AHG assay. Specimen collection is by venipuncture. The method is automated coagulation instrument, but may be manual. This factor is one of a number of factors essential for clot formation. A decreased amount, or absence, of this factor may be associated with blood clotting disorders. A factor VIII (AHG) deficiency is the most common clotting factor deficiency and is linked to hemophilia. This test is essentially an assay for the presence and quantity of the AHG.

85244

This test may be ordered as factor VIII related antigen or VIIIR:Ag. Specimen collection is by venipuncture. The method is automated coagulation instrument, but may be manual. The presence of Factor VIII related antigen is associated with carriers of the bleeding disorder hemophilia. The test may be useful for the detection of carriers of hemophilia A and in prenatal diagnoses.

85245

This test may be ordered as a ristocetin cofactor, VIIIR:Rco, or Von Willebrand factor ristocetin cofactor. Specimen collection is by venipuncture. The method is automated coagulation instrument, but may be manual. This test measures platelet aggregation in response to introduction of ristocetin into the tube. The resulting level of ristocetin cofactor may be interpreted to assess the function of the Von Willebrand Factor, which may be indicative of the presence of Von Willebrand's disease and the variant or type of the disorder.

85246

This test may be ordered as factor VIII related antigen, VIIIR:Ag, Von Willebrand factor or vWF, or Von Willebrand factor antigen vWF:Ag. Specimen collection is by venipuncture. The method is automated coagulation instrument, but may be manual. A deficiency or low level of Von Willebrand factor antigen is associated with a bleeding disorder called Von Willebrand's disease. A diminished VW factor antigen in combination with reduced function of VW factor can lead to a diagnosis of a variant of Von Willebrand's known as Type I. An absence of VW factor antigen, along with undetectable function of VW factor, can lead to a diagnosis of a variant of Von Willebrand's known as Type III.

85247

This test may be ordered as factor VIII assay with multimeric analysis of Von Willebrand factor, agarose gel electrophoresis of Von Willebrand factor, or vWF:Ag multimeric analysis. Specimen collection is by venipuncture. The method is agarose gel electrophoresis. This test is used to help provide a differential diagnosis for variants of Von Willebrand's disease. The absence of multimeric VW factor may be indicative of a variant of Von Willebrand's known as Type II.

85250

This test may be ordered as a factor IX assay, a PTC assay, or a Christmas disease assay. Specimen collection is by venipuncture. The method is automated coagulation instrument, but may be manual. This factor is one of a number of factors essential to clot formation. A decreased amount of this factor may be associated with a form of homeostasis disorder. A factor IX deficiency is the second most common clotting factor deficiency that results in a variant of hemophilia known by the suffix B or simply Christmas disease.

85260

This test may be ordered as a factor X assay or rarely as a Stuart-Prower assay. Specimen collection is by venipuncture. The method is automated coagulation instrument but may be manual. This factor is one of a number of factors essential for clot formation. A decreased amount of this factor may be associated with a systemic coagulation disorder known as Factor X deficiency.

85270

This test may be ordered as a factor XI assay or as a PTA assay or antihemophilic C assay. Specimen collection is by venipuncture. The method is automated coagulation instrument, but may be manual. This factor is one of a number of factors essential for clot formation. A decreased amount of this factor XI may be associated with systemic blood clotting disorder known as Hemophilia C.

85280

This test may be ordered as a factor XII assay or as a Hageman factor assay. Specimen collection is by venipuncture. The method is automated coagulation instrument, but may be manual. This factor is one of a number of factors involved in clot formation. A decreased amount of this factor may be associated with blood clotting problems.

85290

This test may be ordered as a factor XIII assay or as a fibrin stabilizing factor assay. Specimen collection is by venipuncture. The method is automated coagulation instrument but may be manual. This factor is one of a number of factors involved in clot formation. A decreased amount of this factor may be associated with clot dissolution and bleeding problems.

85291

This test may be ordered as a factor XIII solubility screen or a fibrin stabilizing factor solubility screen. Specimen collection is by venipuncture. The method is manual. This factor is one of a number of factors involved in clot formation. A decreased amount of this factor may be associated with clot dissolution and bleeding problems. This code does not measure the amount of factor XIII antigen but is a measure of factor XIII function.

85292

This test may be ordered as a prekallikrein assay or as a Fletcher factor assay. Specimen collection is by venipuncture. Finger stick or heel stick is not acceptable. The method is usually automated coagulation instrument but may be manual. A prekallikrein deficiency results in a prolonged clotting time but is not associated with abnormal bleeding.

85293

This test may be ordered as a high molecular weight kininogen or HMWK assay, a HMW kininogen assay, a Fitzgerald factor assay, or rarely as a Williams factor assay or a Flaujeac factor assay. Specimen collection is by venipuncture. The method is automated coagulation instrument, but may be manual. A Fitzgerald or HMWK factor deficiency results in a prolonged clotting time but is not associated with abnormal bleeding.

85300

This test may be ordered as an antithrombin III activity assay, an AT-III functional assay, or as a functional antithrombin III assay. Specimen collection

is by venipuncture. The method is automated coagulation instrument, but may be manual. A decrease in antithrombin III function or activity is associated with thrombosis or episodes of abnormal clot formation.

85301

This test may be ordered as an antithrombin III antigen assay, an immunological antithrombin III assay, or an AT-III antigen assay. Specimen collection is by venipuncture. The method is automated coagulation instrument but may be manual. Levels of antithrombin III antigen may be normal even though the antithrombin III activity is decreased, see 85300. Deficiencies of this antigen are associated with thrombosis or episodes of abnormal clot formation.

85302

This test may be ordered as a protein C antigen assay or an immunological protein C assay. Specimen collection is by venipuncture. The method is enzyme immunoassay. A decrease in protein C antigen levels is associated with thrombosis or episodes of abnormal clot formation.

85303

This test may be ordered as a protein C activity assay, or as a functional protein C assay. Specimen collection is by venipuncture. The method is enzyme immunoassay. A decrease in protein C activity or functional levels is associated with thrombosis or episodes of abnormal clot formation.

85305

This test may be ordered as a total protein S assay, protein S antigen assay, or immunological protein S antigen assay. Specimen collection is venipuncture. The method is enzyme immunoassay. A decrease in protein S antigen levels is associated with thrombosis or episodes of abnormal clot formation.

85306

This test may be ordered as a free protein S assay, a protein S functional assay, or a protein S activity assay. Specimen collection is by venipuncture. The method is enzyme immunoassay. A decrease in protein S activity or functional levels is associated with thrombosis or episodes of abnormal clot formation.

85307

This test may be requested as activated protein C (APC) resistance test. Blood specimen is obtained by venipuncture. Method is clotting assay. This test is used to evaluate patients with thrombosis. APC is an important natural anticoagulant present in the blood which functions by inactivating the coagulation factors FVa and FVIIIa. The APC resistance test consists of a standard activated partial thromboplastin time (APTT) test performed both in the absence and presence of commercially available activated protein C. In the normal response, the presence of APC will prolong the clotting time due to the anticoagulant action of this protein. Failure to prolong the clotting time in the presence of APC is an abnormality resulting from resistance to this protein. The results are reported as a ratio of the APC-APTT/APTT.

85335

This test may be ordered as a factor inhibitor test or a Bethesda qualitative test. The specific factor will be ordered (i.e., factor VIII). Specimen collection is by venipuncture. The method is automated coagulation instrument, but may be manual. This test is used to detect the presence of inhibitors or inactivators against a coagulation factor. It is rare but not impossible to exhibit inhibitors against more than one coagulation factor. This assay may be ordered several times before the inhibitor's target factor is identified.

85337

This test may be ordered as a thrombomodulin assay. Specimen collection is venipuncture. The method is usually automated coagulation instrument but may be manual. Thrombomodulin is a protein involved in activation of the clot dissolution or lysis process.

85345

This test may be ordered as a clotting time, a whole blood clotting time, or a Lee-White clotting time. Specimen collection is venipuncture. The method is manual. The Lee-White clotting time measures the ability of blood to clot and is performed at the patient's bedside to monitor anti-coagulant therapy such as heparin, warfarin, or coumadin.

85347

This test may be ordered as an activated clotting time, an activated whole blood clotting time, or an activated Lee-White clotting time. Specimen collection is by venipuncture. The method is manual. The activated clotting time measures the ability of blood to clot and is a precursor to the activated partial thromboplastin time (85730), or PTT.

85348

This test may be ordered as a clotting time. Specimen collection is by venipuncture finger stick or, in infants, heel stick. Methods vary, as the formal description implies. Point-of-care testing often involves a hand held instrument that gives some measurement of whole blood clotting time.

85360

This test may be ordered as a euglobulin lysis time, a euglobulin clot lysis time, or an EGT. Specimen collection is by venipuncture. The method is manual. This test is a measure of fibrinolytic or clot dissolving activity and is useful in the diagnostic workup for numerous disorders.

85362

This test may be ordered as fibrin (or fibrinogen) degradation products (FDP) or fibrin (or fibrinogen) split products (FSP). Specimen collection is venipuncture or urine sample. The test method is latex agglutination. The degradation products of fibrinogen have characteristic biological properties, including the inhibition of clotting. This test measures the products of fibrinolytic or clot dissolving activity. FDP tests on urine are performed primarily post kidney transplant and are helpful as a predictor of rejection.

85366

This test may be ordered as a protamine paracoagulation, fibrin monomer, ethanol gelation or ethanol gel, protamine sulfate, or protamine gelation test. Specimen collection is by venipuncture. The degradation products of fibrinogen have characteristic biological properties, including the inhibition of clotting. This test measures the products of fibrinolytic or clot dissolving activity. The test is not in common usage.

85370

This test may be ordered as quantitative fibrin (or fibrinogen) degradation products (FDP) or quantitative FDP, quantitative fibrin (or fibrinogen) split products (FSP). Specimen collection is by venipuncture. The method is radioimmunoassay (RIA). The degradation products of fibrinogen have characteristic biological properties, including the inhibition of clotting. This test measures the products of fibrinolytic or clot dissolving activity. The degradation products are quantitated.

85378–85379

These tests may be ordered as D-dimer, latex agglutination or slide D-dimer, semi-quantitative or qualitative. Specimen collection is by venipuncture. The degradation products of fibrinogen have characteristic biological properties, including the inhibition of clotting. Code 85378 is a semi-quantitative measure of two degradation fragments known as the D-dimer. The method typically includes latex agglutination, specific antisera. Code 85379 is a quantitative measure using enzyme-linked immunosorbent assay (ELISA).

85384

This test may be ordered as, Factor I, clotting Factor I, fibrinogen, or fibrinogen activity. Specimen collection is by venipuncture. The method is usually automated coagulation instrument but may be manual. This factor is one of a number essential to clot formation. A decreased amount of this factor may be associated bleeding disorders.

85385

This test may be ordered as Factor I, clotting Factor I, or fibrinogen antigen. Specimen collection is by venipuncture. The method is usually automated coagulation instrument but may be manual. This factor is one of a number essential to clot formation. A decreased amount of this factor may be associated with bleeding disorders.

85390

This test may be ordered as a fibrinolysin screen, as a coagulopathy screen, or as a disseminated intravascular coagulopathy (DIC) screen. Specimen collection is by venipuncture. The method combines automated coagulation instrument, latex agglutination, and automated cell counter. This test typically screens for intravascular coagulation disorders. A pathology interpretation and report is included with the screen.

85400

This test may be ordered as euglobulin lysis time, plasmin level, or plasmin activity. Specimen collection is by venipuncture. The method is chromogenic substrate. Plasmin is an important agent in the dissolution of clots. Increased plasmin levels are present during fibrinolytic or clot dissolving activity.

85410

This test may be ordered as alpha-2-antiplasmin. Specimen collection is by venipuncture The method is typically radial immunodiffusion. Increased alpha-2-antiplasmin levels are present during fibrinolytic or clot dissolving activity.

85415

This test may be ordered as plasminogen activator, plasminogen activator inhibitor (PAI), Specimen collection is by venipuncture. The method is chromogenic substrate or enzyme linked immunosorbent assay. These methods involve a two-stage process. First, a fixed amount of t-PA reacts with PAI in the test plasma. Other plasmin inhibitors are then destroyed by the introduction of an acidic compound. Next, the residual t-PA is measured. Increased plasminogen activator levels are present during fibrinolytic or clot dissolving activity.

85420

This test may be ordered as plasminogen level, functional plasminogen, or plasminogen activity. Specimen collection is by venipuncture. The method is chromogenic substrate. Increased plasminogen levels are present during fibrinolytic or clot dissolving activity, intrauterine death, and some metastatic cancers.

85421

This test may be ordered as plasminogen antigen level. Specimen collection is by venipuncture. The method is radial immunodiffusion. Increased plasminogen antigen levels may be present during fibrinolytic or clot dissolving activity, intrauterine death, and some metastatic cancers.

85441

This test may be ordered as a Heinz body stain, or a direct Heinz body stain. Heinz bodies are anomalous intracellular erythrocytic (red blood cell) inclusions that attach to the cell membrane. They are composed of denatured hemoglobin. Specimen collection is by venipuncture or finger stick in adults, or heel stick in infants. The method is phase contrast microscopy or supravital stain (e.g. methyl violet, crystal violet, and brilliant cresyl blue, new methylene blue). A blood smear is prepared and examined for the presence of Heinz bodies in the red blood cells. Elevated numbers of Heinz bodies are found following exposure to certain drugs and toxic chemicals, some enzyme deficiencies, and as a result of inherited disorders of blood hemoglobin.

85445

This test may be ordered as an induced Heinz body stain. Heinz bodies are anomalous intracellular erythrocytic (red blood cell) inclusions that attach to the cell membrane. They are composed of denatured hemoglobin. Specimen collection is by venipuncture or finger stick in adults, or heel stick in infants. The method is phase microscopy or supravital stain (e.g. methyl violet, crystal violet, and brilliant cresyl blue, new methylene blue). A blood sample is treated with a chemical (usually acetyl phenylhydrazine) and a blood smear is prepared and examined for the presence of Heinz bodies in the red blood cells. This test may be necessary to identify patients with certain types of unstable blood hemoglobin disorders.

85460

This test may be ordered as a Kleihauer-Betke stain or K-B stain, a Kleihauer-Betke stain for fetal hemoglobin, a Kleihauer-Betke stain for fetomaternal hemorrhage, acid-resistant fetal cells, or a differential lysis stain. Specimen collection is by venipuncture or finger stick. This test is not performed on infants. The method is semi-quantitative stain following acid elution. A blood smear is prepared and treated with an acid solution that elutes, or dissolves, the normal adult hemoglobin from normal adult red cells. The blood smear is stained and examined microscopically. The number of red cells containing fetal hemoglobin or acid-resistant hemoglobin red cells are counted and reported as a percentage of the normal adult hemoglobin-containing red cells. This test is usually performed on post-partum mothers to determine if the newborn bled during delivery. The number of acid-resistant, or fetal cells, present is useful in developing postpartum treatment plans, especially with Rh-negative mothers.

85461

This test may be ordered as a fetal hemoglobin screening test, a fetal red cell rosette, a FetalDex screen, or a fetal screen. Specimen collection is by venipuncture or finger stick. This test is not appropriate for infants. The blood is treated with a chemical (anti-D) which causes fetal cells to form a rosette, or circle, of cells. This test is a screen usually performed on Rh-negative post-partum mothers to determine if the newborn bled during delivery.

85475

This test may be ordered as an acid hemolysin test, positive acidified serum test, or as a Ham test. Specimen collection is by venipuncture or finger stick in adults, or heel stick in infants. The method is manual. The patient's red blood cells are incubated with a mildly acidic solution and observed for hemolysis. Patients with paroxysmal nocturnal hemoglobinuria (PNH) have a positive acid hemolysin test.

85520

This test may be ordered as a heparin assay, a quantitative heparin analysis, or as a heparin level. Specimen collection is by venipuncture. The method is chromogenic assay. This test measures the amount of heparin in a patient's blood and is usually ordered when the patient is on low-dose heparin therapy.

85525

This test may be ordered as a heparin neutralization test, a heparin-thrombin coagulation time test, or as protamine neutralization test. Specimen collection is by venipuncture. The method is manual. This test is used to determine the dose of protamine needed to neutralize heparin-induced bleeding.

85530

This test may be ordered as a heparin-protamine tolerance test. Protamine is given as an antidote to heparin overdose. However, some patients develop hypersensitivity to protamine and may go into anaphylactic shock if they receive a dosage. Method is point of care testing. This test is used to assess hypersensitivity to protamine and measures the amount of protamine that can be safely administered.

85536

This test may also be ordered as a Prussian blue stain, hemosiderin stain, or red cell iron stain. The test is performed to identify abnormal iron accumulations in peripheral red blood cells. The specimen is typically about 5 ml of blood drawn from a peripheral vein, stored unclotted. Method is slide preparation with Perl's Prussian blue stain and visual microscopy. The stain binds to iron in the blood cell and the test may be used to classify anemias as well as other disorders.

85540

This test may be ordered as a leukocyte alkaline phosphatase test (LAP), LAP score, or as a tartrate-inhibited acid phosphatase. Specimen collection is by venipuncture or finger stick in adults, or heel stick in infants. The method is enzyme reaction with leukocyte alkaline phosphatase liberating naphthol, which is then manually stained. Smears from freshly collected whole blood are prepared, stained, and examined microscopically. Cells are scored 0 to 4+ based on the amount of phosphatase activity identified. One hundred cells are counted and phosphatase activity scores totalled. The amount of leukocyte alkaline phosphatase present aids in the differential diagnosis of various leukemias.

85547

This test may be ordered as a red blood cell mechanical fragility test, or as a mechanical red cell fragility. Specimen collection by is venipuncture or finger stick in adults, or heel stick in infants. The method is manual. Some disorders of red blood cells cause variations in the cell membrane which may be demonstrated by stressing the red cells.

85549

This test may be ordered as a muramidase test, a myelomonocytic lysozyme test, or as a malignant lymphoma lysozyme test. Specimen collection is by venipuncture, bone marrow aspirate or 24-hour urine specimen. The method is flow cytometry, gel diffusion assay, radioimmunoassay, nephela (immunochemical). The presence of this protein aids in the differential diagnosis of certain leukemias and lymphomas.

85555

This test may be ordered as an osmotic fragility test, a red blood cell fragility, an uninucleated osmotic fragility, or as a red blood cell osmotic fragility. Specimen collection is by venipuncture. The method is manual. Certain diseases cause red cells to change from their normal shape, which may increase or decrease their ability to take up water without lysing. The red cells are diluted with increasing concentrations of sodium chloride. The concentration that demonstrates hemolysis, or bursting, of the red cells, is compared to a normal patient's red cells.

85557

This test may be ordered as an incubated osmotic fragility test, an incubated red blood cell fragility, or as an incubated red blood cell osmotic fragility. Specimen collection is by venipuncture. The method is manual. Certain diseases cause red cells that have been incubated at 37 degrees for 24 hours to change from their normal shape, which may increase or decrease their ability to take up water without lysing. The red cells are diluted with increasing concentrations of sodium chloride. The concentration that demonstrates hemolysis or bursting of the red cells is compared to a normal patient's red cells.

85576

This test may be ordered as a platelet aggregation study, or as an in vitro platelet aggregation study. Specimen is collected by venipuncture. The method may be platelet aggregometer. Platelet function is measured by observing the amount of platelet clumping that occurs when certain chemicals are added to a solution of platelets. Common agents include adenosine diphosphate (ADP), collagen, epinephrine, and ristocetin. These agents may be tested using different dilutions. The test is an in vitro enactment of the platelet aggregation that occurs naturally at the site of vascular injury. The test may be used to detect von Willebrand's disease or other inherited platelet disjunction diseases.

85585

This test may be ordered as platelet estimation, or as a smear estimation of platelets. Specimen collection is by venipuncture or finger stick in adults, or heel stick in infants. The method is manual stain. A blood smear is prepared and stained and then examined for the presence of platelets. This test is usually performed to verify an abnormal automated platelet count.

85590

This test may be ordered as a manual platelet count. Specimen collection is by venipuncture or finger stick in adults, or heel stick in infants. Method is manual. Whole blood is diluted in a fluid that bursts the red cells. The sample is then examined microscopically for platelets in a chamber that holds a specific volume. The number of platelets are counted and reported.

85595

This test may be ordered as an automated platelet count. Specimen collection is by venipuncture or finger stick in adults, or heel stick in infants. Method is automated cell counter. The number of platelets present is measured by an automated cell counter.

85597

This test may be ordered as a platelet neutralization test, or as a platelet neutralization test for lupus anticoagulant. Specimen collection is by venipuncture. Some patients with systemic lupus develop an anticoagulant that reacts with platelets. This test is very sensitive to this anticoagulant.

85610

This test may be ordered as a prothrombin time (PT), a prothrombin, or as simply PT. Specimen collection is by venipuncture. Method is one-stage using an automated device. The prothrombin time is prolonged when deficiencies of coagulation factors II, V, VII, or X are present. More commonly, this test monitors the effectiveness of the anticoagulant drug Coumadin or warfarin, prescribed to patients who have had blood clots or myocardial infarction.

85611

This test may be ordered as a diluted prothrombin time (PT), a prothrombin 1:1, or as plasma diluted PT. Specimen collection is by venipuncture. Addition or dilution with normal plasma helps differentiate between a clotting factor deficiency and a circulating anticoagulant. Prolonged prothrombin times due to a

clotting factor deficiency will shorten to normal with the addition of normal plasma while a prolonged prothrombin time due to a circulating anticoagulant may increase with the addition of normal plasma.

85612

This test may be ordered as a Stypven time, Russell viper venom time, or as an undiluted Russell viper venom time. Specimen collection is by venipuncture. Method is automated with a phospholipid being added to the test system to neutralize platelet activity. This test is used to confirm fibrinogen deficiency, deficiencies of Factors II and V, and some types of Factor X deficiency.

85613

This test may be ordered as a diluted Russell viper venom time. Specimen collection is by venipuncture. Method is automated. This test is used to confirm the presence of a lupus anticoagulant.

85635

This test may be ordered as a reptilase test or, more commonly, reptilase time (RT). Specimen collection is venipuncture. Method involves adding venom of pit viper to a sample of the patient's plasma and recording the clotting time. This test is most often used to monitor the effectiveness of thrombolytic or clot-lysing drugs such as streptokinase or urokinase. It may also be used to detect the presence of coagulation disorders such as dysfibrinogenemias (non-functional or abnormal fibrinogen) and clotting disorders such as disseminated intravascular coagulation (DIC).

85651

This test may be ordered as an erythrocyte sedimentation rate (ESR), a Westergren sedimentation rate, Wintrobe sedimentation rate, or simply as a "sed rate." Specimen collection is venipuncture. This test is a non-specific screening test for a number of diseases including anemia, disorders of protein production such as multiple myeloma, and other conditions that alter the size and/or shape of red cells or erythrocytes. This test may also be used to screen diseases that cause an increase or decrease in the amount of protein in the plasma or liquid portion of the blood. Further studies are often launched by ESR results. The method is manual. A variety of procedures have been used over time to study sedimentation rate. A common one performed manually is the Westergren tube. An amount of saline is placed in the tube by pipette. Mixed whole blood is added up to a second line level. The blood is allowed to sediment and is checked at 60 minutes. The distance between plasma meniscus and an indicator line is noted and compared against standardized values.

85652

This test may be ordered as a Zeta sedimentation rate or as a Zeta sed rate. Specimen collection is by venipuncture. Method is centrifugation; this is an automated test. This test is a non-specific screening test for a number of diseases including anemia, disorders of protein production such as multiple myeloma, and other conditions that alter the size and/or shape of red cells or erythrocytes. This test may also be used to screen diseases that cause an increase or decrease in the amount of protein in the plasma or liquid portion of the blood.

85660

This test may be ordered as a sickle cell metabisulfite test, a sickle cell reduction test, an erythrocyte (RBC) sickling test, or as an RBC reduction sickle cell test. Specimen collection is by venipuncture or finger stick in adults, or heel stick in infants. The method is manual. Whole blood is mixed with a reducing agent that causes erythrocytes that contain abnormal amounts of hemoglobin S to sickle or change their shape to an elongated 'sickle' cell. The solution is examined microscopically and the numbers of sickle cells are reported as a percentage of normal erythrocytes or RBCs.

85670

This test may be ordered as a thrombin time or as a TT. Specimen collection is by venipuncture. Finger stick or heel stick is unacceptable. The method is manual clotting. This test is used to measure the last stage of clotting which is the conversion of fibrinogen to fibrin following the addition of thrombin. This test is prolonged during heparin therapy, in the presence of fibrin split products, and other circulating anticoagulants, and in disorders of fibrinogen.

85675

This test may be ordered as a thrombin time titer or as a diluted thrombin time. Specimen collection is by venipuncture. Finger stick or heel stick is unacceptable. The method is manual clotting. This test is used to detect the presence of clotting inhibitors other than heparin. Dilutions of thrombin are used in 85670.

85705

This test may be ordered as a tissue thromboplastin inhibition test (TTI), or as a lupus anticoagulant (LA) test. Specimen collection is obtained by venipuncture. Extravascular tissue requires a biopsy, which is reported separately. The method is manual clotting. This test is used when the patient has prolonged prothrombin time (85610) and/or partial thromboplastin time (85730) not due to coagulation factor deficiencies or drug therapy, such as heparin or Coumadin. Some patients with suspected or diagnosed diseases such as lupus erythematosus and AIDS may be candidates for this test.

85730

This test may be ordered as a partial thromboplastin time or PTT, or as an activated partial thromboplastin

time or APTT. Specimen collection is by venipuncture. Finger stick or heel stick is unacceptable. The method is automated coagulation instrument. The partial thromboplastin time is prolonged when deficiencies of coagulation factors VIII, IX, XI, and XII are present. More commonly, this test is used to monitor the effectiveness of the anticoagulant drug heparin, which is prescribed for patients who have had blood clots or heart attacks.

85732

This test may be ordered as a diluted partial thromboplastin time, a PTT or APTT 1:1, or as a plasma diluted PTT or APTT. Specimen collection is by venipuncture. Finger stick or heel stick is not acceptable. The method is automated coagulation instrument. Addition of or dilution with normal plasma helps differentiate between a clotting factor deficiency and a circulating anticoagulant. Prolonged partial thromboplastin times due to a clotting factor deficiency will shorten to normal with the addition of normal plasma while a prolonged PTT due to a circulating anticoagulant may increase with the addition of normal plasma.

85810

This test may be ordered as a serum viscosity test or as a viscosity. Specimen collection is by venipuncture. Finger stick or heel stick is not acceptable. The method is viscometer. This test measures the viscosity or thickness of serum as compared to saline. Increased viscosity may be found in disorders such as Waldenström macroglobulinemia.

86000

This test may be ordered as febrile agglutinins or febrile agglute; or separately as Brucella antibody titers, Francisella Murine typhus antibody titers, Q fever antibody titers, Rocky Mountain spotted fever titers. . Specimen collection is by venipuncture and finger stick in adults, or heel stick in infants. Method is agglutination. If positive at a screening dilution, quantitation may be performed. Serologic agglutination may be used to identify and measure an antigen/antibody response to an infectious disease.

86001

This test may be requested as IgG RAST test. IgG is an immunoglobulin that may be a factor in some allergic reactions. Specimen collection is by venipuncture or finger stick in adults, or heel stick in infants. Allergen IgG testing may be performed by RAST (radioallergosorbent) methodology.

86003

This test may be ordered as a RAST (radioallergosorbent test). Specimen collection is by venipuncture or finger stick in adults, or heel stick in infants. Method may be by agar gel diffusion, ELISA, or Western blot. Immunoglobulin E (IgE) testing may be used when skin testing is unreliable due to generalized dermatitis or severe dermatographism, or when the patient is unable to discontinue use of antihistamines.

86005

This test may be ordered as a RAST (radioallergosorbent test) or by any of the several brand name products available. Blood specimen is obtained by venipuncture, finger stick or heel stick. The test is essentially a contact reagent method. A dipstick or a disk is exposed to the patient's blood. A change in color indicates the presence of antibodies, indicating an "allergic" status.

86021

This test may also be ordered as alloantibody identification, or alloagglutinin identification (the term "isoantibodies" is archaic). The term autoantibody may also be used. Leukocyte antibodies correlate closely to human leukocyte antigens, a complex genetic code for the immune system. The leukocyte antibody side of the equation may be referred to as alloagglutinins. This type of test is usually ordered to predict for one of several disorders: severe immune reactions from fetomaternal leukocyte incompatibility and/or neonatal incompatibilities, post-blood transfusion reactions, and poor blood component viability following transfusion. Alloantibodies arising from previous pregnancies and transfusions may be evident years after antigen exposure. Autoantibodies are usually identified with autoimmune disorders and infectious diseases. Methods may include agglutination and flow cytometry.

86022

This test may also be requested as serotonin release test. Platelets are small irregularly shaped cells, lacking a nucleus. Platelets serve a variety of functions, including providing a surface area for a variety of reactions. The presence of certain antibodies on the platelet surface can affect a variety of functions. Autoantibodies develop in response to the body's own platelets as a result of idiopathic thrombocytopenia. Alloantibodies develop following exposure to outside antigens, often from blood transfusions. Certain drugs may also induce platelet antibodies. Blood specimen is obtained by venipuncture. Methods include indirect immunofluorescence (IIF), flow cytometry, enzyme linked immunosorbent assay (ELISA).

86023

This test may be ordered as a platelet-associated IgG. Platelets are small irregularly shaped cells, lacking a nucleus. Platelets serve a variety of functions, including providing a surface area for a variety of reactions. The presence of certain antibodies on the platelet surface can affect a variety of functions. This test may be associated with idiopathic thrombocytopenia purpura (ITP), a serious disorder

involving low platelet counts. Method may commonly be by immunofluorescence (IF) or radial immunodiffusion (RID). IgG may also be detected by indirect assay involving interaction between patient blood product and normal platelets.

86038

This test may be ordered as antinuclear antibodies (ANA) test or, less commonly, nuclear binding antibody (NBA). Specimen collection is by venipuncture or finger stick in adults, or heel stick in infants. Methods include indirect immunofluorescent methodology and enzyme-linked immunoassay (ELISA). This test is used to measure autoantibodies to the nucleus of human cells and may be used as a screening test for autoimmune diseases such as systemic lupus erythematosus (SLE) and the family of diseases commonly known as scleroderma.

86039

This test may be ordered as antinuclear antibodies (ANA) titer or, less commonly, nuclear binding antibody (NBA) titer. Specimen collection is by venipuncture or finger stick in adults, or heel stick in infants. Methods include indirect immunofluorescent methodology and enzyme-linked immunoassay (ELISA). The test is used to measure autoantibodies in the nucleus of human cells and may be used as a screening test for autoimmune diseases such as systemic lupus erythematosus (SLE) and the family of diseases known as scleroderma.

86060

The test is ordered as antistreptolysin O (ASO) titer. Specimen collection is venipuncture or finger stick in adults, or heel stick in infants. Method is hemagglutination. The test is used for serological documentation of a group A streptococcal infection and may be used as a screening test for acute rheumatic fever, or glomerulonephritis.

86063

This test may be ordered as antistreptolysin O (ASO) screen. Specimen collection is by venipuncture or finger stick in adults, or heel stick in infants. Methods include hemagglutination and slide agglutination. The test is used for serological documentation of a group A streptococcal infection and may be used as a screening test for acute rheumatic fever or glomerulonephritis.

86077

This physician service is an assessment of crossmatch blood work and/or evaluation of irregular antibody(s) prior to transfusion. This type of physician review may be called for when anomalies arise in the antibody evaluation. An interpretation and written report are specifically required in the code description.

86078

This physician service is an assessment of transfusion reaction, including suspicion of transmissible disease. This type of assessment occurs following transfusion and an interpretation and written report are specifically required in the code description. Common reactions include fever and hives. Of greater concern are anaphylactic shock, graft-versus-host disease, and pulmonary edema.

86079

This physician service involves a written authorization to deviate from standard blood banking procedures. Many facilities maintain rare antigen variants well beyond recommended storage life simply to ensure availability. The code reports the authorization to transfuse this type of blood product, as well as product with incompatible Rh to the recipient. A written report is required.

86140

This test may be ordered as a C-reactive protein (CRP). Specimen collection is by venipuncture or finger stick in adults, or heel stick in infants. The test may be performed by one of several methods, including latex agglutination and enzyme-linked immunoassay (ELISA). Elevated levels of C-reactive protein may be used as a measure for nonspecific inflammatory response. High levels of CRP may be present in bacterial infection, some tumors and various types of tissue damage, but more commonly in acute rheumatic fever and rheumatoid arthritis.

86141

C-reactive protein is released into the bloodstream when the blood vessels leading to the heart are damaged, which qualifies it is a nonspecific marker of inflammation. Measurement of C-reactive protein by high sensitivity CRP (hsCRP) assays adds to the predictive value of other markers used to assess a variety of conditions which can lead to elevated serum concentration of CRP, including inflammation, infection, and malignancy. C-reactive protein, hsCRP is also used to assess cardiovascular and peripheral vascular disease. Either serum or plasma is used for the test; no matter the specimen, however, the serum or the plasma must be separated from cells within one hour after collection. CRP assay involves the coating of artificially produced particles (i.e., Latex) with an antibody specific to human CRP aggregate in the presence of CRP from the patient sample of formed immune complex. The immune complex causes an increase in light scattering that is proportional to the concentration of CRP in the sample. The light scattering is quantified optically by measuring turbidity.

86146

Beta 2 glycoprotein 1 antibody actually refers to a group of autoantibodies used as serological markers for antiphospholipid syndrome (APS). APS is characterized by recurrent arterial and venous thrombosis as well as recurrent fetal loss. These autoantibodies are natural regulators of the blood coagulation cascade. Blood specimen is obtained by venipuncture. Concentrations are measured in serum or citrated plasma. Method is enzye-linked immunoassay (ELISA). The test may be repeated at regular intervals.

86147

This test may also be ordered as antiphospholipid antibody or anticardiolipin antibodies (ACA). Specimen collection is by venipuncture or finger stick in adults, or heel stick in infants. Method is enzyme-linked immunoassay (ELISA). The test may be used to classify patients with recurrent venous or arterial thrombosis, thrombocytopenia (low platelet count), recurrent fetal loss, and acquired valvular heart disease, and systemic lupus erythematosus (SLE).

86148

Test may also be ordered as apoptotic cell assay or necrotic cell assay. Specimen collection is by venipuncture or finger stick in adults, or heel stick in infants. Various autoimmune diseases appear to be a consequence of a defective regulatory mechanism of apoptosis (cell death). Detection method may be by light scatter.

86155

This test may be ordered as phagocytic cell function evaluation, NBT slide assay, or DCF assay. Specimen collection is by venipuncture or finger stick in adults, or heel stick in infants. The method is gel agar diffusion. Whole blood is collected from the patient and concurrently from an individual unrelated to the patient (a control). Live neutrophils are required for a successful test. This test may be used for screening infections, perinatal abscesses, multiple episodes of pneumonia, or delayed wound healing may be tested. Patients under treatment for malignancy or those treated with immunosuppressive antiviral therapies may also be candidates.

86156

This test may be ordered as cold agglute or thermal amplitude assay. Specimen collection is by venipuncture or finger stick in adults, or heel stick in infants. Method is hemagglutination. The test may be used to provide an early detection of an immunoglobulin M (IgM) class antibody, which may be present in acute primary atypical pneumonia (Mycoplasma pneumoniae) and certain hemolytic anemias. Low levels of cold agglutinins have been demonstrated in malaria, peripheral vascular disease, and common respiratory diseases.

86157

This test may be ordered as cold agglute titer or thermal amplitude assay. Specimen collection is by venipuncture or finger stick in adults, or heel stick in infants. The method is hemagglutination. This test may be used to screen immunoglobulin M (IgM) class antibody, which may be present in acute primary atypical pneumonia (Mycoplasma pneumoniae) and certain hemolytic anemias. Low levels of cold agglutinins have been demonstrated in malaria, peripheral vascular disease, and common respiratory diseases.

86160

This test may be ordered as individual components 2-5 or Factor B. Specimen collection is venipuncture or finger stick in adults, or heel stick in infants. Methodology is radial immunodiffusion or nephelometry. Complement activation is a multi-component biological response function of the immune system present in inflammatory conditions; the degree of complement activation may be used to indicate the intensity of the inflammatory process. Syndromes associated with complement activation include rheumatoid arthritis, systemic lupus erythematosus (SLE), gram negative sepsis, and chronic hepatitis.

86161

This test may be ordered as individual component 1. Specimen collection is by venipuncture or finger stick in adults, or heel stick in infants. Methodology is radial immunodiffusion or nephelometry. Complement activation is a multi-component biological response function of the immune system present in inflammatory conditions; the degree of complement activation may be used to indicate the intensity of the inflammatory process. Syndromes associated with complement activation include rheumatoid arthritis, systemic lupus erythematosus (SLE), gram negative sepsis, and chronic hepatitis.

86162

This test may be ordered as complement CH50, total. Specimen collection is by venipuncture, or finger stick in adults, or heel stick in infants. Methodology involves an indicator system using predetermined amounts of sheep red blood cells coated with antibody. Specimen serum is introduced and the lysis of the coated cells is measured spectrophotometrically as the red color of hemoglobin is released into the solution. Complement activation is a multi-component biological response function of the immune system present in inflammatory conditions; the degree of complement activation may be used to indicate the intensity of the inflammatory process. Syndromes associated with complement activation include rheumatoid arthritis, systemic lupus erythematosus (SLE) gram negative sepsis and chronic hepatitis.

86171

This test may be ordered as a complement assay. The complementary system involves enzymes and regulatory proteins synthesized in the liver. Activation of the system triggers a cascading, or sequential, response that may lead to histamine release, inflammation, and other normal activities of the immune system. Blood specimen is obtained by venipuncture. Complement fixation is widely used test that relies on these principles. It usually involves two phases. The first phase involves antiserum reaction to test material in the presence of a known quantity of complement. The presence of an antigen will "fix" the complement. A second phase may involve the introduction of sheep blood coated with antibody cells. A lack of hemolysis during this stage further indicates fixation. The test may be used for a wide variety of suspected illnesses, including viral infections.

86185

This test may be ordered as a bacterial antigen test by CIE. It may also be referred to as countercurrent immunoelectrophoresis or counterelectrophoresis. A cerebrospinal fluid specimen is perhaps the most common, as it is used in cases of suspected bacterial meningitis, but other sources may also be used. Blood specimen is obtained by venipuncture. CSF specimen is obtained by separately reportable spinal puncture. A random urine specimen is obtained. Pleural fluid is obtained by separately reportable thoracentesis. The test methodology is similar to crossed immunoelectrophoresis (86327), since it involves a double electroimmunodiffusion. However, it differs from crossed immunoelectrophoresis because it is a one-dimensional as opposed to a two-dimensional technique. Antigen and antibody are placed in separate wells cut into the agar plate. Antigen is placed in wells cut toward the cathode (negative electrode), while antibody (antiserum) is placed in wells cut toward the anode (positive electrode). They are driven toward each other when an electrical field is applied and form precipitates when they meet in the area between the wells.

86215

This test may be ordered as DNA antibody. This test is probably a remnant of an earlier test to detect the DNA antibody and is not in common use.

86225

This test may be ordered as anti-DNA, anti-ds-DNA, ANDNA, dsDNA antibody, or anti-native DNA. Specimen collection is by venipuncture or finger stick in adults, or heel stick in infants. Methods include indirect immunofluorescent assay and enzyme-linked immunosorbent assay (ELISA). This test may be performed for patients previously diagnosed with systemic lupus erythematous (SLE). These patients may exhibit a high level of antibody against their own native double-stranded DNA, and results of the test may indicate renal involvement. This tests for the double-stranded DNA. Low levels of the antibody may be found in other autoimmune disorders such as

Sjogren's syndrome, mixed connective tissue disease, and progressive systemic sclerosis.

86226

This test may be ordered as ssDNA, antibody IgG, or anti-single stranded DNA. Specimen collection is by venipuncture or finger stick in adults, or heel stick in infants. Method is enzyme-linked immunosorbent assay (ELISA). Single stranded DNA antibodies are found in 20 to 30 percent of all cases of systemic lupus erythematosus (SLE), and less specific in the diagnosis of SLE compared to double-stranded DNA antibodies. Lower levels of double-stranded DNA antibodies are associated with chronic inflammatory processes, malignancy, drug-induced lupus, or cardiolipin antibodies (cross-reaction).

86235

Examples of antibodies covered by this code are listed in the CPT® description; however, other antibodies may also be reported with this code. The Sc170 or scleroderma antibody (now known as antitopoisomerase-1 or topo-1) is helpful in identifying diffuse scleroderma and CREST syndrome. CREST syndrome is an acronym to denote the presence of the following symptoms: subcutaneous calcinosis, Raynaud's phenomenon, esophageal dysmotility, sclerodactylia (a hardened, stiffened condition of the fingers), and telangiectasia. JO1 antibody is associated with myositis. RNP stands for ribonucleic protein. Identification of RNP antibody is useful in differentiating various autoimmune disorders including that known informally as lupus and scleroderma. Sjogren's syndrome (SS) is a complex autoimmune disorder that produces two distinct antibodies, SS-A and SS-B. These tests may be requested as Sjogren's antibodies. Methodology will vary according to the test. For example, methodology for JO1antibody is immunoblot assay or polyacrylamide gel electrophoresis, while Sc170 uses either a diffusion immunoprecipitin technique known as Ouchterlony or indirect fluorescent antibody (IFA) technique.

86243

Cell surfaces feature complex molecular structures to regulate activities with other cells. The Fc receptor is a site on certain cells (i.e., macrophages, eosinophils, etc.) to accommodate specific antigen/antibody activities. The Fc receptors may work in connection with specific immunoglobulins or classes. Three types are sometimes referred to: FcRI, FcRII, and FcRIII. A key function is to trigger phagocytes to feed and ingest antigens. Literature is unclear about testing methodology for Fc receptors.

86255–86256

These codes report detection of noninfectious agents using fluorescent agent antibody technique. A number of noninfectious agents are reported with codes 86255 and 86256. Some antibodies reported with these codes

include: acetylcholine receptor antibody (anti-AChR); adrenal cortex antibodies; anti D. S., DNA, IFA using C. Lucilae; mitochondrial antibody, liver; smooth muscle antibody; antineutrophil antibody; endomysial antibody; parietal cell antibody; and myositis-specific auto antibody. Code 86255 is a screen and reports the presence of the antibody only. Code 86256 is a titer and reports the level of antibody present.

86277

This test may also be ordered as somatotropin antibody, GH antibody test, or IGF (insulin-like growth factor) antibody. Portions of the pituitary gland secrete growth hormone. Serum levels normally rise and fall throughout the day. The literature is unclear about methodology for an antibody assay. However, radioimmunoassay is probably method of choice.

86280

This is a clinical lab test to detect the presence of certain hemagglutinating virus or other hemagglutinin antigen. Specimen collection is venipuncture. Method is typically hemagglutination. The test is based on the inability of red blood cells in the sample to clump together when the antibody to the virus or an antigen is added to the sample. If the virus or antigen is present, the antibody kills it and prevents the clumping of red blood cells to each other.

86294

This code is may be requested as single step qualitative or semi-quantitative immunoassay to identify the presence of a specific tumor antigen. Blood is obtained by venipuncture. Method is immunoassay.

86300

This test may also be requested as carbohydrate antigen 15-3. Blood specimen is obtained by venipuncture. Method is immunoassay. Quantitative analysis for CA 15-3 is used primarily to monitor patients for recurrence of breast cancer after diagnosis and initial treatment or to evaluate response to therapy. Elevated levels are often indicative of a recurrence or a failed treatment.

86301

This test may also be requested as carbohydrate antigen 19-9. Blood specimen is obtained by venipuncture. Method is immunoassay. Quantitative analysis for CA 19-9 is used primarily as a marker for pancreatic cancer. It is used both to help identify recurrence and monitor patients. It is also used to monitor gastrointestinal, head/neck, and gynecological cancer. It may be used to help in identifying recurrence of stomach, colorectal, liver, gallbladder, and urothelial malignancies.

86304

This test may also be requested as cancer antigen 125. Blood specimen is obtained by venipuncture. Method is immunoassay. CA 125 is found in ovarian cancers, and some endometrium and fallopian tube cancers. Testing for CA 125 is performed primarily to detect residual tumor in women who have been previously diagnosed with ovarian malignancy.

86308–86310

These tests may be requested as a heterophile antibody screen and/or titer. Common brand names include Monospot , Monosticon, Dri-Dot. Heterphile antibodies are commonly tested to diagnose infectious mononucleosis. Blood specimen is obtained by venipuncture. Method is agglutination. Code 86308 is a screen which identifies the presence of the antibody only; while 86309 is a titer which identifies the level of antibody present. Code 86310 reports a more specific methodology for testing heterophile titers using both beef cells and guinea pig kidneys. Heterophile antibodies can be absorbed by beef cells, but not by guinea pig kidneys.

86316

This test is an immunoassay for tumor antigen and may be requested by the specific antigen. Some of the more common tumor antigens include , carbohydrate antigen 549 (CA 549), carbohydrate antigen 72-4 (CA 72-4, TAG 72), and carbohydrate antigen 50 (CA 50). Each of these antigens is specific for certain types of cancer. CA 549 is found in Stage IV metastatic breast cancer and is used primarily to evaluate response to therapy. CA 72-4 is found in metastatic gastric carcinoma. Blood specimen is obtained by venipuncture. Method is immunoradiometric assay (IRMA).

86317

This code is may be requested to measure the amount of specific infectious disease antibodies in the blood that are not otherwise specified. It would normally be obtained subsequent to qualitative or semi-quantitative immunoassays (86318, 86602-86804) which identify the presence of specific antibodies but do not measure the amount of antibody present. Blood is obtained by venipuncture. Method is immunoassay.

86318

This code is may be requested as single step qualitative or semi-quantitative immunoassay to identify the presence of a specific infectious agent antibodies. Blood is obtained by venipuncture. Method is immunoassay. Single step methods frequently use a reagent strip for the specific antibody.

86320

This code may be abbreviated as serum IEP. Blood specimen is obtained by venipuncture. This code is used to report a technique most often used to identify monoclonal gammopathy or lymphoproliferative processes, specifically myelomas. It combines electrophoresis and immunodiffusion. Electrophoresis involves separating charged particles by moving them through a liquid medium in response to changes in an electric field. Charged particles move in a predictable fashion and are deposited in distinct bands. Immunodiffusion involves an antibody-antigen reaction which causes a visible precipitate to form. In this case, immunodiffusion is performed with monospecific antiserum to immunoglobulin and to specific heavy and light chains. This test is qualitative only.

86325

This code may be abbreviated as IEP. A random urine specimen is obtained. CSF is obtained by separately reportable spinal puncture. This code is used to report a technique most often used to identify monoclonal gammopathy or lymphoproliferative processes, specifically myelomas. It combines electrophoresis and immunodiffusion. Electrophoresis involves separating charged particles by moving them through a liquid medium in response to changes in an electric field. Charged particles move in a predictable fashion and are deposited in distinct bands. Immunodiffusion involves an antibody-antigen reaction which causes a visible precipitate to form. In this case, immunodiffusion is performed with monospecific antiserum to immunoglobulin and to specific heavy and light chains. This test is qualitative only.

86327

Two-dimensional or crossed immunoelectrophoresis (IEP) is similar to standard IEP as described in 86320 and 86325; however, following immunodiffusion, electrophoresis is performed a second time at right angles to the original separation.

86329–86331

This test may be abbreviated as ID. Immunodiffusion (86329) involves an antibody-antigen reaction which causes a visible precipitate to form. It is a technique used in identifying immunoglobulin. Ouchterlony gel diffusion (86331) involves evaluation of the precipitin reaction in a clear gel. An antigen is placed in a hole in the agar and allowed to diffuse into the medium. A visible ring forms where the antigen meets the antibody.

86332

Immune complex assays were once thought to be a promising diagnostic technique. However, they have generally been replaced with tests which are more specific, more standardized, and less expensive. Blood specimen is obtained by venipuncture. Method is a complement binding (CP) technique.

86334

Immunofixation electrophoresis (IFE) reports a method or technique as opposed to most laboratory codes which report testing for a specific analyte (substance) regardless of method or technique. It is the assay of choice in evaluating monoclonal gammopathies because it can more accurately identify biclonal gammopathies and small monoclonal gammopathies that cannot be detected by immunoelectrophoresis. Blood specimen is obtained by venipuncture. A 24-hour urine specimen is required. The patient flushes the first urine of the day and discards it. All voided urine for the next 24 hours is collected and refrigerated. IFE involves high resolution electrophoresis combined with immunoprecipitation. Electrophoresis involves separating charged particles by moving them through a liquid medium in response to changes in an electric field. Charged particles move in a predictable fashion and are deposited in distinct bands. Immunoprecipitation causes aggregation of an antigen in response to a specific antibody. In this case, antigen aggregation occurs when precipitin is added to the solution.

86337

This test may be requested as insulin antibody or anti-insulin Ab. It usually includes testing for antibodies to both beef and pork insulin. Insulin dependent diabetics sometimes develop IgG antibodies to insulin which can cause insulin resistance making larger doses of insulin necessary to achieve the same level of control. However, they may also develop IgA, IgM, IgD, and IgE antibodies. Most of these antibodies do not cause clinical problems. Blood specimen is obtained by venipuncture. Method is radioimmunoassay (RIA), radiobinding assay, or enzyme linked immunosorbent assay (ELISA).

86340

This test may be requested as intrinsic factor (IF) antibody. There are two types of IF antibody. Type I, blocking antibody, is the more common of the two. It prevents binding of B12 with intrinsic factor but will not react with complex intrinsic factor. Type II antibody, binding antibody, reacts with either free or complex IF. Blood specimen is obtained by venipuncture. Method is radioimmunoassay (RIA).

86341

This test detects the formation of antibodies to the pancreatic islet cell which causes destruction of those cells and, therefore, loss of an individuals ability to produce insulin. The presence of islet cell antibodies are helpful in establishing an initial diagnosis of Type I, insulin-dependent diabetes mellitus (IDDM) and in identifying those individuals at high risk of developing IDDM. It is also useful in identifying potential transplant donors for pancreatic islet cells. Blood specimen is obtained by venipuncture. Various methods are used.

86343

This test is performed to quantify the levels of histamine. Plasma specimen is obtained by venipuncture. Urine is collected by patient over a 24-hour period. Methods are fluirimetric, radioenzymatic, and immunoassay. Allergic and non-allergic intolerance to drugs, insect venom, paints or cosmetics, as well as heat or cold, or stress may induce histamine release. By using the histamine release test it is possible to identify a broad spectrum of a!lergies.

86344

Abnormalities in leukocyte phagocytosis may be used as a screen for a variety of disorders. Specimen collection is by venipuncture. Method is flow cytometry or fluorescence microscopy. Leukocytes protect against infection and immunological disease in a process called phagocytosis. It involves ingesting and killing invading microbes inside specialized biological compartments called phagolysosomes.

86353

This test may also be requested as lymphocyte mitogen response test or phytohemagglutinon (PHA) stimulation. Lymphocytes are normally produced early in an immune response. This test is used to determine the adequacy of early immune response using either nonspecific mitogens or specific antigens as transforming agents capable of inducing bastogenesis. Blastogenesis of lymphocytes involves transformation of small lymphocytes placed in tissue culture into large blast-like cells capable of undergoing mitosis by exposing the small lymphocytes to transforming agents, such as PHA or concanavalin. This process involves isolation of lymphocytes in peripheral blood and culture of the isolated lymphocytes in microtiter plates for three to seven days. Plates are set up with and without transforming agents (mitogen or antigens). Cell density and transforming agent concentration may also be varied to aid in establishing a dose-response curve. Prior to harvest of cultured cells, the lymphocytes are pulsed with triturated thymidine. Incorporated thymidine is then measured. Control values are then used to calculate a stimulation index.

86359

This test may also be referred to as T-cell assay, T-cell analysis, or T-cell study. It is used to quantitate total T-cell lymphocytes without providing absolute counts of the different types of lymphocytes. Examples of different types of lymphocytes included in the total count are CD3, CD4, CD8, CD20, CD38, etc. Specimen collection is by venipuncture. Whole blood is added to fluorochrome-labeled antibodies, also referred to as monoclonal antibodies, that bind specifically to cell surface antigens on lymphocytes. This is used in conjunction with flow cytometry to obtain the total T-cell count. This test is used to type and classify different types of lymphomas and lymphocytic luekemias as well as to monitor immunodeficiency states, including HIV infections.

86360

This test may also be requested as T4/T8 ratio, CD4/CD8 ratio, T-cell assay for CD4/CD8. It is used to quantitate CD4 and CD8 specifically, and from those counts to obtain a CD4 to CD8 ratio. Whole blood is added to fluorochrome-labeled antibodies, also referred to as monoclonal antibodies, that bind specifically to cell surface antigens on lymphocytes. This is used in conjunction with flow cytometry to obtain the CD4 and CD8 cell counts. This test is used primarily in staging HIV infection and monitoring the effects of treatment. It may also be useful in diagnosing and monitoring congenital immunodeficiciencies.

86361

This test may also be requested as T-cell assay for CD4. Specimen collection is by venipuncture. Whole blood is added to fluorochrome-labeled antibodies, also referred to as monoclonal antibodies, that bind specifically to cell surface antigens on lymphocytes. This is used in conjunction with flow cytometry to obtain the CD4 cell count. This test is used primarily in staging HIV infection and monitoring the effects of treatment. It may also be useful in diagnosing and monitoring congenital immunodeficiciencies.

86376

This test is performed to determine the presence of anti-thyroid microsomal antibodies. Specimen collection is by venipuncture. A hemagglutination test for thyroid antigens is used and, if that test is positive, it is followed by a fluorescent scan to show a decrease or absence of thyroid-stable iodine. Other methods include ELISA (enzyme linked immuno sorbent assay) or particle agglutination (PA). The anti-microsomal antibody or microsomal antibody test may be used to diagnose conditions such as Hashimoto's thyroiditis and other autoimmune disorders. Hashimoto's disease is an autoimmine thyroid disorder characterized by the production of antibodies in response to thyroid antigens. Normal thyroid structures are replaced by lymphocytes and lymphoid germinal centers.

86378

This test may be ordered as glycosylation-inhibiting factor (GLIF), macrophage migration inhibiting factor (MIF) test and the macrophage inhibition factor (MIF) test. Specimen collection is by venipuncture. Binding assay and immunocytochemical analysis have been used to detect the release and activation of MIF in inflammatory response. MIF is released by the pituitary and by macrophages during inflammatory response and has become an important immunotherapy target to treat a variety of inflammatory diseases and condition, such as rheumatoid polyarthritis and Crohn's disease.

86382

Blood specimen is collected by venipuncture. Tissue samples may be collected by biopsy. Fluorescent dye may be used to identify the target virus directly from clinical specimens or tissue. Neutralization tests are used in various serological tests to identify antibodies to the target virus in serum (i.e., Herpes simplex virus). The identification aids in the diagnosis of diseases caused by the virus.

86384

This code also may be ordered as Nitroblue Tetrazolium (NBT). Specimen collection is by venipuncture. A biochemical assay and simple laboratory equipment (microscope, incubator and centrifuge) are used to detect phagocytosis and intracelluar killing of microrganisms by normal polymorphonuclear neutrophils. The test has been found to have several applications, including the detection of certain immunodeficiency disorders (i.e., AIDS), Hodgkin's disease ,and chronic lymphocytic leukemia.

86403–86406

These tests may be ordered as PA. Specimen collection is by venipuncture. There are several methods used in tandem with PA tests, such as fluorescence enzyme assay and scattered light flow cytometry. Particle agglutination (PA) tests may be performed to evaluate immune status to and diagnosis certain viruses (i.e., measles virus infection). For example, antigen detection kits may contain antibody coated latex or gelatin particles and enzymes to detect the antigens of targeted viruses. Use 86403 to report each separate antibody screen, and 86406 to report each antibody tested according to titer.

86430

This test may be ordered as rheumatoid antibody (RA), arthritis screen, or rheumatoid factor (RF). Specimen collection is by venipuncture, finger stick, or heel stick in infants. The test is most significantly used as a qualitative measurement in evaluating patients with inflammatory polyarthritis. The presence of RF is not by itself usually considered sufficient to establish a diagnosis of rheumatoid arthritis. Rather, it usually serves as a contributing factor or a prognostic marker to a diagnosis. Testing methodology is by latex agglutination, ELISA, or nephelometry.

86431

This test may be ordered as rheumatoid antibody (RA) titer, arthritis screen, or rheumatoid factor (RF) titer. Specimen collection is by venipuncture, finger stick, or heel stick in infants. The test is most significantly used as a quantitative measurement in evaluating patients with inflammatory polyarthritis. The presence or quantity of RF is not by itself usually considered sufficient to establish a diagnosis of rheumatoid arthritis. Rather, it usually serves as a contributing factor or a prognostic marker to a diagnosis. Testing methodology is by latex agglutination, ELISA, or nephelometry.

86485

This test may be ordered as candida delayed hypersensitivity testing (DHT or DHR). The methods are: the intradermal test and the prick test. A nurse or technician typically performs the test. Candida albicans is a common environmental yeast, and this testing is usually a control for anergy or immunocompetence. A standardized concentration of the yeast is introduced into the skin of the arm, usually by needle or skin prick. The test site is examined within 30 minutes and again at 24, 48, and 72-hour intervals. Evidence of a reaction is carefully recorded.

86490

This test may be ordered as coccidioides delayed hypersensitivity testing (DHT or DHR). It may also be ordered as cocci skin test. Two testing methods are: the intradermal test and the prick test. A nurse or a technician typically performs the test. A standardized concentration of the antigen is introduced into the skin of the arm, usually by needle or skin prick. The test site is examined within 30 minutes and again at 24, 48, and 72-hour intervals. Evidence of a reaction is carefully recorded. This test has limited value diagnostically and usually provides supporting information only.

86510

This test may be ordered as histoplasma skin test. A nurse or technician typically performs the test. Two testing methods are: the intradermal test and the prick test. A standardized concentration of antigen is introduced into the skin of the arm, usually be needle or skin prick. The site is examined within 30 minutes and again at 24, 48, and 72- hour intervals. Evidence of a reaction is carefully recorded. This test has limited value diagnostically.

86580

This test may be ordered as TB skin test, TB delayed hypersensitivity testing (DHT or DHR), Tuberculin skin test, Mantoux test, or purified protein derivative test (PPD). A standardized concentration of tuberculin PPD is introduced into the skin of the arm. The method is intradermal. A nurse or a technician typically performs the test. The test may screen individuals in high-risk circumstances, or as routine surveillance among certain populations regularly exposed (i.e., health care workers). Patients showing certain signs or symptoms are also tested. Culture extracts of tuberculin proteins in a test dosage is injected intradermally (forearm). The test site is examined at 24, 48, and 72-hour intervals for evidence of induration. Evidence of a reaction is carefully recorded.

86585

This test may be ordered as TB tine test or prong test. The testing method is applied by a stainless steel disk with four prongs dipped in tuberculin. The disk is applied to the forearm of the patient. A nurse or a technician typically performs the test. The tine test requires almost no training for admission of the test. For this reason, the test is perhaps the more common TB test to screen large populations of asymptomatic individuals with low-risk of exposure. The test site is examined at 48 hours and 72-hours for evidence of induration and the results are recorded.

86586

This test may also be called skin testing, delayed hypersensitivity testing, or intradermal testing. The test is generic for skin testing to detect exposure to any antigens other than histoplasmosis, C. coccidioides, and tuberculosis. Typically, skin testing is performed for Blastyoycocis, Trichophyton, Mumps, Tetanus toxoid, and Streptokinase. The test may be used to assess prior exposure or also to assess immune status.

86590

This test is commonly ordered as anti-streptokinase. Specimen collection is by venipuncture, finger stick, or heel stick in infants. The test is useful for detection of antibody to an extracellular antigenic product of group A streptococci and commonly used to detect previous exposure to group A strep. The test may be performed by either latex agglutination or enzyme-linked immunosorbent assay (ELISA).

86592

This test is commonly ordered as RPR (rapid plasma reagin), STS (serologic test for syphilis), VDRL (venereal disease research laboratory), or ART (automated reagin test). It may also be ordered as standard test for syphilis. Specimen collection is by venipuncture, finger stick, or heel stick in infants. The test is commonly used to provide a diagnosis (screening test) for syphilis. The method is by nontreponemal rapid plasma reagin (RPR)-particle agglutination test. More recently, it is being performed by automated methodology, such as enzyme-linked immunosorbent assay (ELISA).

86593

This test is commonly ordered as quantitative RPR (rapid plasma reagin), STS (serologic test for syphilis), VDRL (venereal disease research laboratory), or ART (automated reagin test). May also be ordered as standard test for syphilis. Specimen collection is by venipuncture, finger stick, or heel stick in infants. It is most commonly used to provide a monitor for treatment, or to establish a diagnosis of re-infection with syphilis. The method is nontreponemal rapid plasma reagin-particle agglutination test or anticardiolipin antibodies. More recently, it is being performed by automated methodology, such as by enzyme-linked immunosorbent assay (ELISA).

86602

This test is commonly ordered as anti-actinomyces or actinomyces antibody titer. Specimen collection is by venipuncture, finger stick, or heel stick in infants. The test is used as a rapid serological method to diagnose for nocardial infections (infections caused by Nocardia, a genus of gram-positive bacteria). The methods are: complement fixation (CF), immunodiffusion, agglutination assay, and Western blot (immunoblot).

86603

This test is commonly ordered as anti-adenovirus titer or adenovirus antibody titer. Specimen collection is by venipuncture, finger stick, or heel stick in infants. The test is traditionally used as a rapid serological method to diagnose for adenovirus infections. The methods are: complement fixation (CF), immunofluorescent, and enzyme-linked immunosorbent assay (ELISA).

86606

This test is commonly ordered as anti-aspergillus titer or aspergillus antibody titer. Specimen collection is venipuncture, finger stick, or heel stick in infants. The test is used as a rapid serological method to diagnose for aspergillus infection. The methods are: complement fixation (CF), counterimmunoelectrophoresis, radioimmunoassay, immunofluorescence, enzyme-linked immunosorbent assay (ELISA), and immunodiffusion.

86609

This test is commonly ordered as a generic test for any bacterium that has not otherwise been specified. This test will usually utilize the words anti, titer, or antibody. Specimen collection is by venipuncture, finger stick, or heel stick in infants. The test is traditionally used as a rapid serological method to diagnose bacterial infections. The methods are: complement fixation (CF), immunofluorescence, and enzyme-linked immunosorbent assay (ELISA).

86611

This test may also be known as bacilliary angiomatosis (BA) or bacillary peliosis (BP) antibody. IgG testing may be used to identify current or past infection whereas IgM is more specific for current infection. Specimen is collected by venipuncture. Methods include enzyme immunoassay (EIA) and indirect fluorescence antibody test. The Bartonella genus of bacteria is implicated in a variety of life threatening infections. Exposure to the bacillus and presence of antibodies may remain asymptomatic. An opportunistic infection arising in some AIDS patients is linked to the Bartonella genus and is noted for vascular lesions.

86612

This test is commonly ordered as anti-Blastomyces or Blastomyces antibody titer. It may occasionally be ordered as "blasto" titer. Specimen collection is venipuncture, finger stick, or heel stick in infants. The test is used as a rapid serological method to diagnose for Blastomyces infections. The methods are: complement fixation (CF), immunodiffusion, agglutination assay, immunofluorescence, enzyme-linked immunosorbent assay (ELISA), and Western blot (immunoblot).

86615

This test is may be ordered as pertussis or whooping cough antibody. Bordetella pertussis is the causative agent of whooping cough. This test demonstrates antibodies, which is not a common approach to developing a clinical diagnosis due to the time required for seroconversion. However, it may be used to evaluate immunity following immunization. Blood specimen is obtained by venipuncture. Methods include enzyme-linked immunosorbent assay (ELISA), microhemagglutination, compliment fixation (CF), and toxin neutralization.

86617

This test may be ordered as a Lyme disease confirmation test. Borrelia burgdorferi is the causative agent of Lyme disease. A tick is the vector to humans. Antibodies usually build up in patients several weeks or longer into an infection. This test is confirmatory, meaning previous diagnostic work has been performed. Blood specimen is obtained by venipuncture. CSF specimen is obtained by spinal puncture that is reported separately. This test reports a second test for confirmation by immunoblot or Western blot. It may also be used to establish a diagnosis following indeterminate ELISA results.

86618

This test may be ordered simply as a Lyme disease antibody test. Borrelia burgdorferi is the causative agent of Lyme disease. A tick is the vector to humans. Antibodies usually build up in patients several weeks or longer into an infection. Blood specimen is obtained by venipuncture. CSF specimen is obtained by spinal puncture which is reported separately. Methods include enzyme-linked immunosorbent assay (ELISA), enzyme immunoassay (EIA), indirect fluorescent antibody (IFA), or specific IgG, IgM, and IgA by antibody capture.

86619

This test may be ordered as a relapsing fever antibody. Relapsing fever is caused by spirochetes of the genus Borrelia, and those infected suffer alternating fevers and chills. Ticks and body lice are the vectors to humans. Blood specimen is obtained by venipuncture.

CPT® Lay Descriptions

Literature is unclear about methods and reasons to order such testing. Indications are that this test is rarely performed.

86622

Brucellosis is a rare illness caused by bacteria from the genus Brucella. Humans contract the disease by ingesting meat or dairy products of infected cattle, sheep, or wild game animals. Direct infection from animals to humans may also occur and is found predominantly in workers in the livestock and meat processing industries. Blood specimen is obtained by venipuncture. Standard tube agglutination method is common. Other methods used include complement fixation (CF) and enzyme linked immunosorbent assay (ELISA). Because this disease is almost entirely eliminated from United States and Canadian cattle and sheep populations, this test is not commonly performed.

86625

Campylobacter is a genus of bacteria, some of which are responsible for a wide variety of illnesses in humans. Enteritis is among the more common illnesses. Campylobacter is also implicated in Guillain-Barre syndrome, a type of arthritis. Blood specimen is obtained by venipuncture. The literature is unclear about methods and reasons to order such testing. Most clinical cases of Campylobacter infection resolve themselves either spontaneously or following drug therapy.

86628

Candida is a ubiquitous genus of fungi, some species of which are pathogenic to humans. The range of illnesses is quite large. This test is performed primarily to evaluate suspected systemic invasions by Candida. If confirmed, tests may be obtained at biweekly intervals to assess effectiveness of drug therapy. Blood specimen is obtained by venipuncture. Methods include: latex agglutination (LA), immunodiffusion (ID), crossed (2-dimensional) immunoelectrophoresis, and enzyme-linked immunosorbent assay (ELISA).

86631

This test may be ordered as Chlamydia psittaci or LVG titer. Specimen collection is by venipuncture or finger stick in adults, or heel stick in infants. Methods are complement fixation (CF), enzyme-linked immunosorbent assay (ELISA), and immunofluorescent antibody (IFA). This test may be used to determine exposure to Chlamydia, though the test should not be used as a specific type. Chlamydomonas is a genus of algae that can cause nongonococcal urethritis, among other infections.

86632

This test may be ordered as Chlamydia IgM titer. Specimen collection is by venipuncture or finger stick in adults, or heel stick in infants. Complement

fixation (CF), enzyme-linked immunosorbent assay (ELISA) and immunofluorescent antibody (IFA) are methods commonly used to determine previous exposure to Chlamydia or a current infection. Chlamydomonas is a genus of algae that can cause nongonococcal urethritis, among other infections.

86635

This test may be ordered as Coccidioides titer, Coccidioides antibody titer, Cocci titer or Cocci precipitins. Specimen collection is by venipuncture or finger stick in adults, or heel stick in infants. Methods include complement fixation (CF), enzyme-linked immunosorbent assay (ELISA), immunofluorescent antibody (IFA), immunodiffusion, and precipitin test. The test may be performed to determine current infection or assess prognosis of Coccidioides immitis, a fungus that causes coccidioidomycosis.

86638

This test may be ordered as Q fever titer, Q fever antibody titer, or C. burnetti titer. Specimen collection is by venipuncture or finger stick in adults, or heel stick in infants. Methods are complement fixation (CF), enzyme-linked immunosorbent assay (ELISA), immunofluorescent antibody (IFA), immunodiffusion, or indirect hemagglutination (IHA). The test may be performed to determine Q fever due to Coxiella brunetii.

86641

This test may be ordered as cryptococcus antibody titer, cryptococcosis, and IFA. Specimen collection is by venipuncture or finger stick in adults, or heel stick in infants. Methods are complement fixation (CF), enzyme-linked immunosorbent assay (ELISA), and immunofluorescent antibody (IFA). This test may be performed to determine exposure and prognosis of cryptococcsis, an infectious disease caused by the fungus Cryptococcus neoformans characterized by nodular lesions or abscesses in the lungs, subcutaneous tissues, joints, and the brain and meninges.

86644

This test may be ordered as CMV-IFA, CMV titers, Cytomegalic inclusion titers, or CMV IgG. Specimen collection is by venipuncture or finger stick in adults, or heel stick in infants. Methods are complement fixation (CF), enzyme-linked immunosorbent assay (ELISA), immunofluorescent antibody (IFA), and latex agglutination. This test may be performed to determine current cytomegalovirus (CMV) infection. CMV is any of several viruses that can cause severe disease especially in newborns by infecting the salivary glands, brain, kidneys, liver, and lungs.

86645

This test is commonly ordered as CMV IgM antibody titer, CMV IgM titer, cytomegalovirus IGM antibody titer, or CMV IgM. Specimen collection is by venipuncture or finger stick in adults, or heel stick in infants. Methods are complement fixation (CF), enzyme-linked immunosorbent assay (ELISA), immunofluorescent antibody (IFA), and latex agglutination. This may be performed to determine previous exposure to cytomegalovirus (CMV) or an acute CMV infection. CMV is any of several viruses that can cause severe disease especially in newborns by infecting the salivary glands, brain, kidneys, liver, and lungs.

86648

This test may be ordered as Diphtheria antibody titer, or DPT titer. Specimen collection is by venipuncture or finger stick in adults, or heel stick in infants. Methods are complement fixation (CF), enzyme-linked immunosorbent assay (ELISA), immunofluorescent antibody (IFA), and latex agglutination. The test may be performed to determine exposure to Diphtheria, a bacterial disease that can cause inflammation to the heart and nervous system.

86651

This test may be ordered as La Crosse virus titer, California encephalitis titer, or bunyavirus titer. Specimen collection is by venipuncture or finger stick, or heel stick in infants. Methods are complement fixation (CF), or enzyme-linked immunosorbent assay (ELISA). This test may be performed to confirm the presence of the California encephalitis viral infection. There are several strains of the encephalitis virus that can cause inflammatory conditions, especially in the tissues of the brain.

86652

This test may be ordered as Eastern equine encephalitis titer. Specimen collection is by venipuncture or finger stick in adults, or heel stick in infants. Methods are complement fixation (CF), or enzyme-linked immunosorbent assay (ELISA). This test may be performed to confirm the presence of Eastern equine encephalitis. There are several strains of the encephalitis virus that can cause inflammatory conditions, especially in the tissues of the brain.

86653

This test may be ordered as St. Louis virus titer or St. Louis encephalitis titer. Specimen collection is by venipuncture or finger stick in adults, or heel stick in infants. Methods are complement fixation (CF), or enzyme-linked immunosorbent assay (ELISA). This test may be performed to confirm the presence of St. Louis encephalitis. There are several strains of the encephalitis virus that can cause inflammatory conditions, especially in the tissues of the brain.

86654

This test may be ordered as Western equine encephalitis titer. Specimen collection is by venipuncture or finger stick in adults, or heel stick in

infants. Methods are complement fixation (CF), or enzyme-linked immunosorbent assay (ELISA). This test may be performed to determine the presence of the Western equine encephalitis virus. There are several strains of the encephalitis virus that can cause inflammatory conditions, especially in the tissues of the brain.

86658

This test may be ordered as enterovirus antibody panel (IgG or IgM), coxsackie A titer, or poliovirus titer. The panel includes coxsackie, A and B, echovirus, and poliovirus. Specimen collection is by venipuncture or finger stick, or heel stick in infants. Methods are complement fixation (CF), viral neutralization, or enzyme-linked immunosorbent assay (ELISA). This test may be performed to determine presence of the coxsackie A virus, poliovirus, or other enteroviruses that typically occur in the gastrointestinal tract, but may also cause respiratory ailments, meningitis, and neurological disorders.

86663–86665

This test may be ordered as EBV-EA titer, EBNA (IgG or IgM) titer, or EBV - VCA (IgG or IgM), or EB-VCA (IgG or IgM) titer. Specimen collection is by venipuncture or finger stick in adults, or heel stick in infants. The test has been used as a serological method to detect previous exposure to EBV or acute EBV disease. Methods are complement fixation (CF) or enzyme-linked immunosorbent assay (ELISA), indirect fluorescent antibody, or immunofluorescent antibody (IFA). Code 86663 identifies an early antigen (short-lived); code 86664 is reported for nuclear antigen; code 86665 is used for viral capsid antigen (VCA). The VCA test may be the most effectual of the three tests for determining EB viral infection, which is the main cause of infectious mononucleosis.

86666

This test may also be ordered as Ehrlichia IgM or IgG. Specimen collection is by venipuncture. Methods include indirect fluorescent antibody (IFA) and immunofluorescent antibody (IFA). The Ehrlichia genus of rickettsia bacteria is implicated in a form of tick fever similar to Rocky Mountain Spotted Fever sometimes referred to as "spotless" fever. Testing may occur during acute or convalescent phases of illness.

86668

This test is also known as Tularemia antibody titer, rabbit fever antibodies, and Francisella tularensis antibodies. Specimen collection is by venipuncture or finger stick in adults, or heel stick in infants. Methods include complement fixation (CF), enzyme-linked immunosorbent assay (ELISA), or immunofluorescent antibody (IFA) agglutination, and hemagglutination. The test may be performed to determine the presence of the bacteria F. tularensis, a bacterium transmitted by insect bite that causes tularemia marked by toxemia.

86671

This code should be used to report antibody testing for fungi which do not have a more specific genus or species code listed in this section. For example, antibody testing for sporotrichosis would be reported with this code. Blood specimen is obtained by venipuncture. Methods are varied and may include: complement fixation (CF), immunodiffusion, latex agglutination (LA), immunofluorescence, Western blot (immunoblot), crossed (2-dimensional) immunoelectrophoresis, and enzyme-linked immunosorbent assay (ELISA).

86674

This test may be requested as Giardia antibody or Giardia titer. Giardia lamblia is the causative protozoal organism of the intestinal disorder known as Giardia. Blood specimen is obtained by venipuncture. Methods such as commercial kit, enzyme immunoassay (EIA), and indirect immunofluorescence may be employed.

86677

This test may be ordered as a H. Pylori antibody titer or Campylobacter pylori serology. Specimen collection is by venipuncture or finger stick in adults, or heel stick in infants. Method is enzyme-linked immunosorbent assay (ELISA). The test may be performed to determine the presence of Helicobacter Pylori, a common cause of intestinal disease and suspected as a cause of ulcerated stomach tissue.

86682

This code reports antibody testing for any of species of helminths not elsewhere classified in this section. Helminths are parasitic worms and many are further classified as nematodes. Helminthic infections may be intestinal or of tissues. Blood specimen is obtained by venipuncture. Test methodologies will vary according to the suspected parasite. Methods may include enzyme immunoassay (EIA) and bentonite flocculation. Tissue parasites are easier to assay for antibodies than are those affecting the GI tract.

86683

This test may also be ordered as a fecal occult blood antibody test. Sample may be collected from several consecutive stools. Each stool sample is then immediately applied to a specimen collection card. Methods include immunochromographic assay. This procedure tests for the presence of blood in the stool by detecting hemoglobin antibodies. This test may be performed to aid in the diagnosis of bleeding in the GI tract that might be caused by colon polyps, colorectal cancer. It may also be used to further investigate individuals with iron deficiency anemia.

86684

This test may be ordered as a H. Influenza (type A or B) antibody titer. Specimen collection is by venipuncture, finger stick, or heel stick in infants. Method is enzyme-linked immunosorbent assay (ELISA). This test is performed to determine the presence of H. Influenza, a common cause of chronic intestinal disease.

86687

This test is commonly ordered as HTLV-I antibody titer or Human T Cell Leukemia I Virus titer. Specimen collection is by venipuncture or in adults, or heel stick in infants. Methods are Western blot, radioimmunoprecipitation, and screen enzyme immunoassay. This test may be performed to determine the presence of HTLV-I virus and to screen blood and blood products used for transfusions.

86688

This test is commonly ordered as HTLV-II antibody titer or human T cell leukemia II virus titer. Specimen collection is by venipuncture or finger stick in adults, or heel stick in infants. Methods are Western blot, radioimmunoprecipitation, and screen enzyme immunoassay. This test may be performed to determine the presence of HTLV-II virus and to screen blood and blood products used for transfusions.

86689

This test is commonly ordered as HTLV or HIV by Western blot. Specimen collection is by venipuncture or finger stick, or heel stick in infants. This test may be performed as a confirmation of a positive test for human T cell leukemia II virus or human immunodeficiency virus (HIV), often by a previous enzyme-linked immunoassay (ELISA). Western blot is a protein-based test immunoblotting technique that involves separating antigens according to well-characterized molecular weights. The antibodies can then be detected as bands on the test results.

86692

This test may be ordered as hepatitis D antibody, hepatitis delta antibody, or superinfection antibody. Hepatitis D occurs concurrently with hepatitis B and may lead to more severe clinical symptoms than hepatitis B alone, a condition known as superinfection. Blood specimen is obtained by venipuncture. Methodology may involve enzyme immunoassay (EIA).

86694–86696

This test may be ordered as HSV antibody titer, HSV titer, herpes simplex antibody titer, or HSV IgG/IGM. Specimen collection is by venipuncture or finger stick in adults, or heel stick in infants. A number of methodologies have been employed, such as complement fixation (CF), enzyme-linked immunosorbent assay (ELISA), indirect fluorescent antibody (IFA), enzyme immunoassay, and latex agglutination. This test has been used as a serologic method to detect previous or recent exposure to herpes simplex. To report non-specific type testing, see 86694; testing for type 1, see 86695; testing for type 2, see 86696.

86698

This test may be requested as histoplasma antibody. Histoplasma capsulatum is a fungus that may be infectious in humans. Incidence seems tied to certain regions. Many infections are asymptomatic or feature mild symptoms. Blood specimen is obtained by venipuncture. Complement fixation (CF) is quantifiable and is considered one of the best methods. Immunodiffusion (ID), agar diffusion, latex agglutination (LA), radioimmunoassay (RIA), or enzyme immunoassay (EIA) may also be used.

86701

This test may be ordered as an HIV-1 serological test, an HIV-1 antibody, or by an internal code. HIV is a retrovirus and the causative agent of acquired immunodeficiency syndrome (AIDS). Blood specimen is obtained by venipuncture. Numerous kits are now available that use a variety of viral proteins and synthetic peptides as antigens. Methodology is enzyme immunoassay (EIA), enzyme-linked immunosorbent assay (ELISA), radioimmunoprecipitation assay (RIPA), or indirect fluorescent antibody (IFA). A negative test does not guarantee negative status and the test is often repeated several times.

86702

This test may be ordered as an HIV-2 serological antibody, or by an internal code. This is an antibody test for HIV-2. HIV-2 is a retrovirus closely related to simian AIDS and found initially in West African nations and Portugal, but with cases also being reported in the United States since 1987. Blood specimen is obtained by venipuncture. Specific kits are now available that use a variety of viral proteins and synthetic peptides as antigens to test for HIV-2. Methodology is enzyme immunoassay (EIA), enzyme-linked immunosorbent assay (ELISA), radioimmunoprecipitation assay (RIPA), or indirect fluorescent antibody (IFA). A negative test does not guarantee negative status and the test is often repeated several times.

86703

This test may be ordered as a combined HIV-1 and-2 serological, a combined HIV-1 and-2 antibody, or by an internal code. This is an antibody test that tests for both HIV-1 and HIV-2 in a single assay. Both are retroviruses. HIV-1 is the causative agent of acquired immunodeficiency syndrome (AIDS) while HIV-2 closely related to simian AIDS. Blood specimen is obtained by venipuncture. Specific kits are now available that use a variety of viral proteins and synthetic peptides as antigens to test for both HIV-1

and HIV-2. Methodology is enzyme immunoassay (EIA), enzyme-linked immunosorbent assay (ELISA), radioimmunoprecipitation assay (RIPA), or indirect fluorescent antibody (IFA). A negative test does not guarantee negative status and the test is often repeated several times.

86704

This test may be ordered as hepatitis Bc Ab (HBcAb), total. It may also be ordered as HBcAb, anti-HBc, HBVc Ab, anti-HBVc. This test identifies Hepatitis B core total antibodies (IgG and IgM) which are markers available to identify individuals with acute, chronic, or past infection of hepatitis B. The presence of high-titered IgM specific HBcAb is always indicative of an acute infection. The presence of IgG may indicate either acute or chronic infection. Blood specimen is obtained by venipuncture, finger stick, or heel stick in infants. Methods include radioimmunoassay (RIA) and enzyme-linked immunosorbent assay (ELISA).

86705

This test may be ordered as hepatitis Bc Ab (HBcAb), IgM. It may also be ordered as HBcAb, anti-HBc, HBVc Ab, anti-HBVc. This test identifies Hepatitis B core IgM antibodies, the presence of which always indicates an acute infection. Blood specimen is obtained by venipuncture, finger stick, or heel stick in infants. Methods include radioimmunoassay (RIA) and enzyme-linked immunosorbent assay (ELISA).

86706

This test may be requested as Hepatitis B surface antibody (HBsAb), Hepatitis Bs Ab, HBV surface antibody, or anti-HBs. The presence of HBsAb is indicative of a previous resolved infection or vaccination against hepatitis B. Blood specimen is obtained by venipuncture, finger stick, or heel stick in infants. Methods include radioimmunoassay (RIA), enzyme immunoassay (EIA), immunoradiometric assay (IRMA), and immunoenzymatic assay (IEMA).

86707

This test may be ordered as hepatitis Be antibody (HBeAb) as Hepatitis Be Ab, HBVe, or anti-HBe. The presence of HBeAb usually indicates a high likelihood of a lesser infectivity and usually points to a benign outcome, although some individuals with HBeAb have chronic hepatitis. Blood specimen is obtained by venipuncture, finger stick, or heel stick in infants. Methods include immunoradiometric assay (IRMA) and enzyme immunoassay (EIA).

86708

This test may be ordered as Hepatitis A Antibody (HAAb), HAV antibody, anti-Hep A or anti-HAV total (IgG and IgM). The presence of HAV IgG antibody may indicate acute infection or previous resolved infection, while IgM antibody always indicates acute infectious disease. Blood specimen is obtained by venipuncture, finger stick, or heel stick in infants. Methods include radioimmunoassay (RIA), enzyme immunoassay (EIA), immunoradiometric assay (IRMA), immunoenzymatic assay (IEMA), and microparticle enzyme immunoassay (MEIA).

86709

This test may be ordered as Hepatitis A Antibody (Haas), HAV IgM antibody, anti-Hep A IgM, or anti-HAV IgM. The presence of IgM antibody indicates acute infectious disease. Blood specimen is obtained by venipuncture, finger stick, or heel stick in infants. Methods include radioimmunoassay (RIA), enzyme immunoassay (EIA), immunoradiometric assay (IRMA), immunoenzymatic assay (IEMA), and microparticle enzyme immunoassay (MEIA).

86710

This test may be ordered as Flu A or Flu B, or Influenza A/B antibody titers. It may also be ordered as anti-Influenza A/B. The presence of IgG antibody usually indicates previous exposure, while IgM indicates a current acute infection. Blood specimen is obtained by venipuncture, finger stick, or heel stick in infants. Methods vary with hemagglutination inhibition (HI) (HAI) being preferred for influenza A and complement fixation (CF) for influenza B. Other methods currently in use are immunofluorescent assay (IFA), enzyme-linked immunosorbent assay (ELISA), radial immunodiffusion (RID), and enzyme immunoassay (EIA).

86713

This test may be ordered as Legionella antibody titers or as anti-Legionella. Both IgG and IgM antibodies should be tested. IgA testing may also be indicated. The presence of IgG antibody usually indicates previous exposure. The demonstration of IgM or IgA antibodies may establish the diagnosis of a current acute or recent Legionella infection. Blood specimen is obtained by venipuncture, finger stick, or heel stick in infants. Methods include: immunofluorescent assay (IFA) and enzyme-linked immunosorbent assay (ELISA).

86717

This test is ordered as Leishmania antibody titers or anti-Leishmania. This protozoan infection may also be referred to as kala-azar. The presence of IgG antibody usually indicates previous exposure. The demonstration of IgM or IgA antibodies may establish the diagnosis of a current acute or recent Leishmania infection. Blood specimen is obtained by venipuncture, finger stick, or heel stick in infants. Preferred methods are complement fixation (CF) and enzyme-linked immunosorbent assay (ELISA). However, a number of other methods are employed including indirect hemagglutination (IHA), immunofluorescent assay (IFA), immunoblot, and enzyme immunoassay (EIA).

86720

This test may be ordered as Leptospira antibody titers or anti-Leptospira. Blood specimen is obtained by venipuncture, finger stick, or heel stick in infants. The presence of IgG antibody usually indicates previous exposure. The demonstration of IgM or IgA antibodies may establish the diagnosis of a current acute or recent Leptospira infection. Methods include complement fixation (CF); hemagglutination, immunofluorescent assay (IFA) and enzyme-linked immunosorbent assay (ELISA).

86723

This test may be ordered as Listeria antibody titers or anti-Listeria. Blood specimen is obtained by venipuncture, finger stick, or heel stick in infants. The presence of IgG antibody usually indicates previous exposure. The demonstration of IgM or IgA antibodies may establish the diagnosis of an acute or recent Listeria infection. Methods include immunofluorescent assay (IFA) and enzyme-linked immunosorbent assay (ELISA).

86727

This test is ordered as LCM or LCMC antibody titers. It may also be ordered as anti-LCM. The presence of IgG antibody usually indicates previous exposure. The demonstration of IgM or IgA antibodies may establish the diagnosis of a current acute or recent LCM infection. Blood specimen is obtained by venipuncture, finger stick, or heel stick in infants. A separately reportable spinal puncture is used to collect CSF. Immunofluorescent assay (IFA), direct fluorescent antibody (DFA), and enzyme-linked immunosorbent assay (ELISA) methods are among those employed in identifying antibody response to the specific LCMC. A positive direct examination by electromicroscopy or direct fluorescent microscopy is indicative of active disease.

86729

This test is ordered as Chlamydia trachomatis antibody titers or LGV antibody titers. It may also be ordered as anti-LGV or anti-Chlamydia trachomatis. Lymphogranuloma Venereum is a sexually transmitted infection caused by C. trachomatis L1, L2, and L3 serovars. It is rarely reported in the United States. The presence of antibodies alone cannot positively differentiate LGV from other chlamydial infections. Testing must be correlated with clinical evidence of LGV. Blood specimen is obtained by venipuncture, finger stick, or heel stick in infants. Immunofluorescent assay (IFA) and complement fixation (CF) methods are employed in identifying an antibody response.

86732

This test may be ordered as Rhizopus antibody titer, Rhizomucor antibody titer, or Cunninghamella antibody titer. These are the common species of molds that cause mucormycosis, a rare opportunistic infection usually found in patients with pre-existing conditions. Blood specimen is obtained by venipuncture or finger stick. Literature is unclear, but immunofluorescent assay (IFA) is a common method to detect antibody responses.

86735

This test may be ordered as mumps antibody titers or anti-mumps titers. Testing may be performed to diagnose an acute infection or to evaluate immune status. The presence of IgG antibody alone usually indicates previous exposure and immunity. IgM antibodies in combination with IgG establish the diagnosis of a current acute or recent mumps infection. Blood specimen is obtained by venipuncture, finger stick, or heel stick in infants. Preferred methods include enzyme immunoassay (EIA) and virus neutralization test (NT). Other methods that may be employed include hemagglutination inhibition (HAI), complement fixation (CF), indirect fluorescent antibody (IFA), and hemolysis in gel.

86738

This test is ordered as Mycoplasma antibody titers. It may also be ordered as anti-walking pneumonia, primary atypical pneumonia (PAP), pleuropneumonia-like organism (PPLO), or anti-Mycoplasma titers. The presence of IgG antibody usually indicates previous exposure to Mycoplasma. The demonstration of IgM antibodies is required to establish the diagnosis of a current acute or recent Mycoplasma infection. Blood specimen is obtained by venipuncture, finger stick, or heel stick in infants. Methods include immunofluorescent assay (IFA), complement fixation (CF), and enzyme immunoassay (EIA), and IgM antibody agglutination.

86741

This test is ordered as N. meningitidis antibody titers. It may also be ordered as anti-Neisseria meningitidis. This is the causative agent of meningococcal meningitis. The presence of IgG antibody usually indicates previous exposure to N. meningitidis. The demonstration of IgM or IgA antibodies may establish the diagnosis of a current acute or recent N.meningitidis infection. Blood specimen is obtained by venipuncture, finger stick, or heel stick in infants. CSF is obtained by spinal puncture that is reported separately. Method is enzyme-linked immunosorbent assay (ELISA).

86744

This test is ordered as Nocardia antibody titers. It may also be ordered as anti-Nocardia titers. Pathogenic species of Nocardia include N. asteroides, N. brasiliensis, N. caviae, N. farcinica, N. transvalensis, and N. nova. These terms may be also used in ordering Nocardia antibody titers. Nocardiosis generally occurs only in immunosuppressed individuals and presents as suppurative or cavitary

pneumonia, cutaneous abscesses, or mycetoma formation on an extremity. The presence of IgG antibody usually indicates previous exposure to Nocardia. The demonstration of IgM or IgA antibodies may establish the diagnosis of a current acute or recent Nocardia infection. Blood specimen is obtained by venipuncture, finger stick, or heel stick in infants. Method is enzyme-linked immunosorbent assay (ELISA) or Western blot.

86747

This test may be ordered as Parvovirus antibody titers, anti-Parvovirus titers, or Parvo B19 antibody titers. The presence of IgG antibody usually indicates previous exposure to Parvovirus B19. The demonstration of IgM antibodies may establish the diagnosis of a current acute or recent Parvovirus B19 infection. Blood specimen is obtained by venipuncture, finger stick, or heel stick in infants. Enzyme-linked immunosorbent assay (ELISA), radioimmunoassay (RIA), and Western blot are among methods employed in identifying an antibody response to Parvovirus B19.

86750

This test is ordered as malaria antibody titers. This test is used primarily to screen blood donors. Blood specimen is obtained by venipuncture. Method is indirect immunofluorescence (IIF).

86753

This test is for antibodies to any of the clinically significant simple, single-celled organisms within the subkingdom of protozoa not specified by a more specific code in this section of CPT®. For example, detection of Entamoeba histolytica antibodies would be reported code 86753. Specimen collection is obtained by venipuncture, finger stick, or heel stick in infants. Enzyme-linked immunosorbent assay (ELISA), radioimmunoassay (RIA) complement fixation, Western Blot, indirect hemagglutination (IHA) are among the methods employed in identifying an antibody response to the specific protozoa.

86756

This test is ordered as RSV antibody titers. It may also be ordered as anti-respiratory syncytial viral titers, and anti-RSV titers. The presence of IgG antibody usually indicates previous exposure to respiratory syncytial virus. The demonstration of IgM antibodies may establish the diagnosis of a current acute or recent infection. Blood specimen is obtained by venipuncture, finger stick, or heel stick in infants. Enzyme-linked immunosorbent assay (ELISA), enzyme immunoassay (EIA), and complement fixation (CF) are among methodologies employed in identifying an antibody response.

86757

This test may also be ordered by the name of the suspected rickettsial pathogen (e.g., Rocky Mountain Spotted Fever, typhus). Blood is drawn by venipuncture. Methods include enzyme-linked immunoassay (ELISA) with indirect fluorescent antibody (IFA) confirmation.

86759

This test is ordered as rotavirus antibody titer. It may also be ordered as anti-rotavirus titer, Adenovirus 40-41 antibody titer, and anti-rotavirus titer. The presence of IgG antibody usually indicates previous exposure to rotavirus. The demonstration of IgM antibodies may establish the diagnosis of a recent or current rotavirus infection. Blood specimen is obtained by venipuncture, finger stick, or heel stick in infants. Enzyme-linked immunosorbent assay (ELISA) and radioimmunoassays (RIA) are among methods employed in identifying antibody response to the specific to rotavirus.

86762

This test is ordered as rubella antibody titers. It may also be ordered as German measles antibody titers, and anti-rubella titers. The test is used primarily to evaluate immune status. The presence of rubella IgG and IgM antibodies may indicate previous exposure, vaccination, or current acute infection. Blood specimen is obtained by venipuncture, finger stick, or heel stick in infants. Enzyme-linked immunosorbent assay (ELISA), enzyme immunoassay (EIA), and latex agglutination (LA) are among methods used in identifying antibody response, with ELISA being more common in larger, high volume laboratories.

86765

This test is ordered as rubeola antibody titers. It may also be ordered as measles antibody titers, anti-measles titers and anti-rubeola titers. This test is used primarily to evaluate immune status as clinical symptoms related to acute infection make laboratory testing unnecessary. CSF specimen is used for diagnosis of subacute sclerosing panencephalitis (SSPE). The presence of rubeola IgG antibody alone usually indicates previous exposure to rubeola. Both IgG and IgM antibodies are present with a current acute or recent rubeola infection. Blood specimen is obtained by venipuncture, finger stick, or heel stick in infants. CSF specimen is obtained by spinal puncture that is reported separately. Hemagglutination inhibition test (HAI) is the preferred method of testing for immune status. Enzyme-linked immunosorbent assay (ELISA), enzyme immunoassay (EIA), complement fixation (CF), and neutralization test (NT) are other methods commonly employed in identifying an antibody response.

86768

This test is ordered as Salmonella antibody titers. It may also be ordered as anti-Salmonella titers, S. typhi antibody titers or Salmonella typhi antibody titers. The presence of Salmonella IgG antibody usually indicates previous exposure to salmonella. The demonstration of Salmonella IgM antibodies may establish the diagnosis of a recent or current salmonella infection. Blood specimen is obtained by venipuncture, finger stick, or heel stick in infants. Enzyme-linked immunosorbent assay (ELISA) principles are most commonly employed in identifying an antibody response to the specific Salmonella. Agglutination principles may be utilized for the identification of S. typhi antibody.

86771

This test is ordered as Shigella antibody titers. It may also be ordered as anti-Salmonella titers. The presence of Shigella IgG antibody usually indicates previous exposure to Shigella. The demonstration of Shigella IgM antibodies may establish the diagnosis of a recent or current Shigella infection. Blood specimen is obtained by venipuncture, finger stick, or heel stick in infants. Enzyme-linked immunosorbent assay (ELISA) principles are most commonly employed in identifying an antibody response to the specific to Shigella. Agglutination principles may also be utilized for the identification of Shigella.

86774

This test is ordered as tetanus antibody titers. It may also be ordered as anti-tetanus titers, or Clostridium tetani antibody titers. This test is not commonly used as a diagnostic test for acute infection. It may be used to evaluate immune status. Blood specimen is obtained by venipuncture, finger stick, or heel stick in infants. Titration of tetanus antitoxin by mouse toxin neutralization principles is the most commonly employed method for identifying an antibody response. Agglutination, passive hemagglutination, or enzyme-linked immunosorbent assay (ELISA) principles may also be utilized for the identification of tetanus antibody.

86777

This test is ordered as Toxoplasma IgG antibody titers. It may also be ordered as anti-Toxoplasma IgG titers, or toxo IgG titers. The presence of Toxoplasma IgG antibody may indicate either current or past infection. Blood specimen is obtained by venipuncture, finger stick, or heel stick in infants. Amniotic fluid is collected by amniocentesis that is reported separately. Enzyme-linked immunosorbent assay (ELISA) or immunofluorescent assay (IFA) principles may be used for the identification of Toxoplasma antibody.

86778

This test is ordered as Toxoplasma IgM antibody titers. It may also be ordered as anti-Toxoplasma IgM titers, or toxo IgM titers. The demonstration of Toxoplasma IgM antibodies may establish the diagnosis of a recent or current infection. Blood specimen is obtained by venipuncture, finger stick, or heel stick in infants. Amniotic fluid is collected by amniocentesis that is reported separately. Enzyme-linked immunosorbent assay (ELISA) or immunofluorescent assay (IFA) principles may be used for the identification of toxoplasma IgM antibody.

86781

This test is commonly ordered as FTA (fluorescent Treponemal antibody). It may also be ordered as a confirmatory test for syphilis or as a confirmatory test for a positive venereal disease research lab test (VDRL), rapid plasma reagent (RPR) or serologic test (STS) for syphilis. Blood specimen is obtained by venipuncture, finger stick, or heel stick in infants. Fluorescent antibody (FA) or FTA principles are most commonly employed in identifying an antibody response to the specific syphilis. Agglutination or flocculation of cardiolipin principles may also be used for the identification of syphilis antibody.

86784

This test is ordered as trichinella antibody titers. It may also be ordered as trichinosis antibody titers. Trichinella antibody titers are to diagnosis infestation with the parasitic roundworm Trichinella spiralis that is transmitted by eating undercooked pork or bear meat. Blood specimen is obtained by venipuncture, finger stick, or heel stick in infants. Methods include bentonite flocculation test (BFT); indirect immunofluorescence (IIF), complement fixation (CF), latex agglutination (LA), enzyme immunoassay (EIA), and enzyme-linked immunosorbent assay (ELISA).

86787

This test may be requested as VZV antibody titers, chicken pox antibody titers, or herpes zoster antibody titers. This test is performed primarily to evaluate immune status. Blood specimen is obtained by venipuncture, finger stick, or heel stick in infants. Methods may include enzyme immunoassay (EIA), enzyme-linked immunosorbent assay (ELISA), complement fixation, and fluorescent antibody against membrane antigen (FAMA).

86790

This test is ordered as viral antibody titers not elsewhere specified. Specimen collection is obtained by venipuncture, finger stick, or heel stick in infants. The presence of viral IgG antibody usually indicates previous exposure, while viral IgM antibodies may establish the diagnosis of a recent or current infection. Methods include enzyme-linked immunosorbent assay (ELISA), indirect fluorescent antibody (IFA), and agglutination.

86793

This test is ordered as Yersinia antibody titers or by species name including Y. enterocolitica antibody and Y. pestis (bubonic plague) antibody. Blood specimen is obtained by venipuncture, finger stick, or heel stick in infants. A common method used is agglutination. However, newer techniques are also used that include a immunoblot, enzyme-linked immunosorbent assay (ELISA), indirect fluorescent antibody (IFA).

86800

This test is ordered as thyroglobulin antibody titers or anti-thyroglobulin. The presence of thyroglobulin antibody usually indicates presence of circulating autoantibodies in patients with endocrine disease (i.e., thyroiditis, Graves's disease). Specimen collection is obtained by venipuncture, finger stick, or heel stick in infants. Methods may include enzyme-linked immunosorbent assay (ELISA), tanned RBC agglutination test, radiobinding assay, and immunoradiometric assay (IRMA).

86803

This test may be ordered as Hepatitis C antibody titers. It may also be ordered as anti-hepatitis C titers, HCV Ab titers, and anti-HCV titers. This test is normally used initially to screen for Hepatitis C. Positive or unequivocal tests are repeated using different techniques that are reported separately. Blood specimen is obtained by venipuncture, finger stick, or heel stick in infants. Methods may include enzyme-linked immunosorbent assay (ELISA) or enzyme immunoassay (EIA).

86804

These tests may be ordered as hepatitis C antibody titers, anti-hepatitis C titers, HCV Ab titers, or anti-HCV titers. Specimen collection is by venipuncture or finger stick in adults, or heel stick in infants. Recombinant immunoblot assay (RIBA) principles may be employed in identifying an antibody response to the specific Hepatitis C virus. The presence of IgG antibody by RIBA is a confirmatory test (86805) for a previous ELISA hepatitis C antibody test (86804) and usually indicates previous exposure to hepatitis C virus.

86805–86806

These tests may also be referred to as compatibility tests or major histocompatibility complex (MHC) tests. These tests pertain primarily to matching potential donor tissues to transplant patients, but uses may also include bench research. Methodology involves mixing purified donor lymphocytes with recipient sera or known antibodies. Cytotoxic reaction (cell death) is visually monitored, usually by incubation method. Indicator dyes may be used to identify dead cells. Titration involves methodology to determine quantities. Report code 86805 for testing with titration; 86806 for testing without titration.

86807–86808

This test may be requested as PRA screen. This test is a preliminary screen to measure cytotoxicity, or cell death, when blood product is mixed. The standard method involves culturing and monitoring cytotoxicity, using marker dyes, and the corresponding buildup of antibodies, through replication and DNA. Code 86807 reports standard testing methods. Code 86808 reports a rapid method, where antibody growth and cytotoxicity are more immediately evident.

86812

This test may also be ordered as a histocompatibility antigen test, Class I (or Class III) antigen test, or according to a specific antigen (e.g., A10). This test pertains primarily to matching potential donor tissues to transplant patients. These human lymphocyte (or leukocyte) antigens (HLA) are genetically encoded, and are a barrier to allotransplantation (from sources other than the patient). This test helps to determine HLA compatibility of specific antigens. Method involves mixing purified donor lymphocytes with a known sera and complement. A culture is prepared and cytotoxic reaction (cell death) is monitored.

86813

This test may also be ordered as histocompatibility antigens test, Class I (or Class III) antigens test, or according to specific multiple antigens (e.g., A10-B-7). This test pertains primarily to matching potential donor tissues to transplant patients. These human lymphocyte (or leukocyte) antigens (HLA) are genetically encoded and are a barrier to allotransplantation (from sources other than the patient). This test determines HLA compatibility of multiple antigens. Method involves mixing purified donor lymphocytes with a known sera and complement. A culture is prepared and cytotoxic reaction (cell death) is monitored.

86816

This test may also be ordered as a Class II antigen test, or simply HLA-D antigen. This test pertains primarily to matching potential donor tissues to transplant patients. The D human lymphocyte antigens (HLA) are located separately from the Class I and Class III antigens on the chromosome. As with the Class I antigens, they are a barrier to allotransplantation (from sources other than the patient). Subregion names DR, DQ, and DP are described. This test determines HLA compatibility of a single Class II antigen. Method involves mixing purified donor lymphocytes with the sera and complement. A culture is prepared and cytotoxic reaction (cell death) is monitored.

86817

This test may also be ordered as a Class II antigens test, or simply HLA-D antigens. This test pertains primarily to matching potential donor tissues to transplant patients. The D human leukocyte antigens (HLA) are located separately from the Class I and Class III antigens on the chromosome. As with the Class I antigens, they are a barrier to allotransplantation (from sources other than the

patient). Subregion names DR, DQ, and DP are described. This test determines HLA compatibility for multiple Class II antigens. Method involves mixing purified donor lymphocytes with the sera and complement. A culture is prepared and cytotoxic reaction (cell death) is monitored.

86821

This test may also be ordered as a mixed lymphocyte culture (MLC) reaction, Class II antigen test, or simply HLA-D antigen. Donor and recipient blood samples are often collected at the same time. This test pertains primarily to matching potential donor tissues to transplant patients. The D human leukocyte antigens (HLA) are located separately from the Class I and Class III antigens on the chromosome and the MLC method is particularly good at identifying them. All of these antigens are a barrier to allotransplantation (from sources other than the patient). This test determines HLA compatibility of Class II antigens. The method is described in literature as mixing purified donor lymphocytes with the recipient's lymphocytes. A culture is prepared and the recipient's lymphocytic response is monitored. The greater the response, the greater the degree of antigen disparity.

86822

This test may also be ordered as a secondary mixed lymphocyte culture (MLC), a primed reaction Class II antigen test, or simply HLA-D primed. Donor and recipient blood samples are often collected at the same time. This test methodology is a rapid test and may take 24 to 36 hours to complete, rather than the seven to ten days for an MLC (86821). The test is specific to certain Class II antigens.

86850

This test may be ordered as an RBC antibody detection. The test is a screen for particular antibodies to red cell antigens that may present problems during a blood transfusion or childbirth. Blood specimen is obtained by venipuncture. The test may be performed using tubes, microtiter plates, or gel cards. Another method is agglutination.

86860

Elution is a technique for removing antibody from antibody/antigen complex on RBCs for identification purposes. Blood specimen is obtained by venipuncture. The process is usually part of a workup to aid in diagnosis of certain autoimmune disorders such as autoimmune hemolytic anemia, and for resolution of incompatible crossmatches due to unidentified antibodies, and to identify the antibody causing hemolytic disease of a newborn (HDN).

86870

This test is also known as an antibody panel. Blood specimen is obtained by venipuncture. The test identifies an antibody isolated by techniques reported by 86850 and/or 86860 above. The test may be performed using tubes, microtiter plates, or gel cards. This code can be reported up to four times during the same session for differences in technique necessary for identification (i.e., regular panel, cold-panel, pre-warmed panel, and enzyme treated panel). Techniques used are dependent on the isolated antibody.

86880

This test is also known as a direct Coombs or sometimes as a direct antiglobulin test (DAT). Blood specimen is collected by venipuncture or heel stick. Cord blood may also be used in neonates. The test is used to detect coating of the RBCs by antibody or complement. It is useful in diagnosis of hemolytic disease of the newborn (HDN), detection of autoimmune hemolytic anemia, investigation of transfusion reactions, and detection of red cell sensitization reactions caused by medication. Method may be by gel test, flow cytometry, or enzyme-linked immunosorbent assay (ELISA).

86885

This test is also known as an indirect Coombs, IAT, or sometimes as selectigen antibody screen. The indirect antiglobulin test indicates whether there is gamma globulin (antibody) in the serum, which will react to combine with a chemical structure on the red cell membrane (antigen). The test simply shows that an in vitro reaction has occurred. Uses for the IAT include: determining if there are IgG antibodies (coating antibodies) in the patient's serum; investigating the ability to sensitize red blood cells; crossmatching; detection of Du (weak D) antigen; and investigation of transfusion reactions. Blood specimen is obtained by venipuncture. Methodology includes agglutination, hemolysis of Type 0 test cells, flow cytometry, or enzyme-linked immunosorbent assay (ELISA).

86886

This test is also known as an antibody titer. The test determines the strength of antibody identified through test described in 86870. Blood specimen is obtained by venipuncture. Method is serial dilution with saline, enzyme, or low ionic strength saline followed by antiglobulin.

86890

This reports the donation of blood for one's own use. This procedure is used for patients requiring surgery who pre-deposit their own blood for use during the surgery. The procedure is most useful for patients with complex antibody production or extremely rare antibodies that make location of compatible blood nearly impossible.

86891

This procedure may also be known as a cell-saver. This is a device used in surgeries where large blood losses are inherent to the procedure (i.e., total hip, certain heart and lung procedures, liver and spleen

operations). The device aspirates spilled blood in the surgical cavity, washes it, and returns the RBCs to the patient. This reduces the need for stored blood. In postoperative patients, there may be major seepage and the patient is not physically up to additional surgery to correct the problem. The cell-saver washes the seepage and transfuses it back to the patient.

86900

This test may also be known as blood group. The test determines whether a patient is O, A, B, or AB. This typing of blood is the oldest and most widely recognized. It involves identifying the presence or absence of two antigens on red blood cells (A and B) and a reciprocal relationship to serum antibodies (anti-A and anti-B). The typing O indicates the state of having neither A nor B antigens. Blood specimen is obtained by venipuncture. The classic test method is by agglutination.

86901

This test is known as Rh type. The test determines whether a patient is "positive" or "negative" by identifying the presence (Rh positive) or absence (Rh negative) of Rh antigens on the RBC surface. Blood specimen is obtained by venipuncture. Method is enzyme-linked immunosorbent assay (ELISA), but may be performed by agglutination.

86903

This test is used to screen donated units of blood prior to a transfusion using reagent serum. The test confirms the absence of the antigen associated with the antibody(ies) identified by the test reported by 86870.

86904

This test is used to screen for compatible blood using patient serum when there is insufficient time to identify an antibody and then screen units for the associated antigen prior to transfusion. The test is also helpful when commercial antisera to the antigen is not available.

86905

This test is used to confirm the absence of antigens corresponding to antibodies identified by the antibody identification test (86870).

86906

Rh phenotyping may be required to assist in confirming the identity of an Rh antibody detected during screening, or when a family study is being undertaken for any number of reasons. Some donor centers maintain limited supplies of phenotyped blood to issue patients who have corresponding antibodies.

86910–86911

This test is a method to determine percentages of whether a particular male is the biological father of a

CPT® Lay Descriptions

particular child. These codes essentially group elements of 86900, 86901 and 86905 (MN refers to M antigen and N antigen, important in phenotyping). Code 86911 is reported when calculations using the antigen system in 86910 are indeterminate and additional systems must be analyzed. These codes also report all mathematical calculations of probability. These tests result in only a statistical probability of paternity. Today, tests for genetic markers can assist in resolving paternity issues.

86915

In certain cases of bone marrow transplant, acceptable donor bone marrow will not be ABO compatible. By washing the marrow with a starch solution, the donor's red blood cells can be removed from the marrow. The marrow is filtered through a nylon wool filter that also removes B-cell lymphocytes, T-cells, and metastatic carcinoma that are not desirable for transfusion.

86920

This test is one of the crossmatch components of tests ordered as "type and crossmatch." This step checks mainly for ABO compatibility of the unit being transfused. It may be the only step in the compatibility phase of the crossmatch when the patient has no demonstrated antibodies, or after a massive transfusion where very little of the patient's blood volume is his/her own.

86921

This test is one of the crossmatch components of tests ordered as "type and crossmatch." This test is an intermediate step using incubation technique, in a full major compatibility test (86920, 86921, and 86922). It is a crucial step in sensitization of IgG antigens.

86922

This test is the final step in a major crossmatch. A full, major crossmatch will always be performed when antibodies are present in the patient's serum, unless more than 10 units have been given in a 24-hour period.

86927

Fresh frozen plasma (FFP) is frozen within six hours of donation. It maintains clotting factors in the frozen state and for this reason is used to treat certain clotting disorders, such as over-medication with Coumadin, liver diseases (i.e., parenchymal liver disease), and disseminated intravascular coagulation (DIC). It may also be used for plasma exchanges to treat diseases like thrombotic thrombocytopenic purpura (TTP), Raynaud's disease, and glomerulonephritis. This code reports only the thawing process.

86930–86932

The preparation for freezing is also known as glycerolization. The process involves washing and mixing a unit of blood with a glycerol-based preservative prior to freezing. Freezing allows reasonably long-term storage of pre-deposited blood. The preparation of frozen blood with thawing is also known as deglycerolization. The product is thawed and washed to remove preservative. Certain cold-insoluble proteins, such as factor VIII and fibrinogen, may be removed when the blood is close to thawing. Report code 86930 for preparation for freezing only. Report code 86931 when preparations are made for both freezing and thawing the unit of blood product. And report 86932 when both preparation and freezing of the blood product are performed as well as the thawing.

86940–86941

These tests are used for screening (86940) or incubation (86941) of hemolysins and cold agglutinins. In transfusion medicine, cold agglutinins may mask antibodies that are not expected to be present in the blood. To determine if there are any significant antibodies present, the cold agglutinins are removed when the screening has indicated they may be interfering with examination for anomalous antibodies. Hemolysins are substances that lyse or dissolve red blood cells. In these tests hemolysins are subject to incubation with and without various additives, such as glucose to determine the degree that red blood cells will lyse. For other methods see individual tests listed in comments.

86945

Irradiation is used primarily to prevent graft versus host disease (GVHD) in certain immunosuppressed patients, newborns, and patients that share the same human lymphocyte antigen (HLA) haplotype as the donor. The process inactivates the lymphocytes. Irradiation is also required when the donor is a blood relation of the recipient (GVHD).

86950

Granulocyte transfusion is indicated in patients on chemotherapy for leukemia or those with severe infection whose absolute granulocyte count is less than 500/cu mm.

86965

Pooling in this sense means to blend blood product from a variety of sources. Platelets and cryoprecipitate require pooling of units in order to provide an adequate amount of product for the transfusion to be helpful. Platelets will be pooled from six or eight random units and cryoprecipitated from 10 random units. Cryoprecipitate is the harvesting of certain cold-insoluble proteins, such as factor VIII and fibrinogen. Cryoprecipitate is collected from frozen blood that is brought to thawing temperature.

86970

When a patient's direct Coombs (86880) test has demonstrated a drug induced autoimmune antibody, such as methyldopa, it is necessary to prove the existence of the drug. This is accomplished by taking reagent RBCs and incubating them with the suspected causative chemical. After the red blood cells have been coated another direct Coombs is performed on both the coated reagent cells and uncoated reagent cells from the same lot.

86971

The enzyme pretreatment of red blood cells is undertaken when there are multiple antibodies or one that is too weak to demonstrate without pre-treatment of the reagent RBCs. The enzyme used depends on the suspected antibody. Certain enzymes enhance particular antibodies while destroying others.

86972

In some red cell typing and antibody detection procedures it is desirable to exclude other cellular components of whole blood, such as white blood cells or platelets. Isolation of RBCs from whole blood may be accomplished by centrifugation in a density gradient.

86975

This method removes antibodies to certain drugs by using pre-treated red blood cells and the patient's serum. Serum is incubated with the treated RBCs (to attach the drug antibody) and centrifuged. The serum is removed and used in further testing.

86976

This is code is similar to 86975. There are times when the amount of antibody exceeds the amount of antigen attached to the RBCs. In these cases, the serum is diluted prior to adsorption or re-adsorption.

86977

In some instances, cell adsorption of the interfering substance will not work, and inhibitor is incubated with the patient's serum to "neutralize" the substance. The antibody to Sda is one of these substances.

86978

Incubation of the patient's cells and patient's serum together prior to testing can remove some autoimmune complexes. This can be done refrigerated for cold autoantibodies or warm for warm autoantibodies. In cases of multiple antibodies, each antibody may be absorbed out in turn by using reagent RBCs of known antigenicity.

86985

In transfusion cases where the patient is a child or where transfusion of a full unit of product will overload the circulatory system, a unit will be split into multiple smaller units.

87001

Animal inoculation with infected tissue, blood, or other specimen source is used in the diagnosis of several diseases, including rabies, Colorado tick fever, and infantile botulism. There are different specimen types for the different tests. Contact the reference lab that is performing the test for type of specimen and transport. Mice are inoculated with patient specimen to detect the presence of virus or toxin. If the test is positive, the mice die, there are however, more rapid tests to diagnose these diseases.

87003

Animal inoculation with infected tissue, blood, or other specimen source is used in the diagnosis of several diseases, including rabies, Colorado tick fever, and infantile botulism. There are different specimen types for the different tests. Contact the reference lab that is performing the test for type of specimen and transport. Mice are inoculated with patient specimen to detect the presence of virus or toxin. If the test is positive, the mice die. This test is used to observe signs of illness in mice for as long as three weeks and for the dissection of mice and preparation of tissue for microscopy to confirm diagnosis when mice become ill or die.

87015

Concentration may also be referred to as thick smear preparation. The source samples are treated to concentrate the presence of suspect organisms, usually through sedimentation or flotation. There are two common methods of concentration for ova and parasite exams: formalin concentration and zinc sulfate flotation. The two most common concentration methods for AFB stains or cultures are the N-acetyl-L cysteine method and the Zephiran-trisodium phosphate method.

87040

Blood cultures are drawn by venipuncture and usually consist of a set of bottles, an aerobic and an anaerobic bottle. The amount of blood drawn varies with the type and manufacturer of the bottles. Drawing at least two sets of cultures increases the effectiveness of the test. Manually, the blood culture test relies on gram staining and subculturing to solid media for detection of bacterial growth. Most labs employ one of the several automated systems that detect the presence of bacteria using colorimetric, radiometric, or spectrophotometric means. The purpose of blood culture tests is to detect the presence of aerobic and anaerobic bacteria in blood and to identify the bacteria.

87045

This test may be called a stool culture, culture for Salmonella and Shigella, or routine culture when stool is the specimen. The method is bacterial culture using specialized media for the recovery and detection of specific enteric pathogens. Stool specimens are collected in clean, leak-proof containers or a rectal swab in bacterial transport container. This test cultures specifically for the enteric pathogens Salmonella and Shigella.

87046

This test may be requested by the name of the suspected pathogenic organisms, including Campylobacter, Yersinia, Vibrio, E. coli 0157. The method is bacterial culture using specialized media for the recovery and detection of specific enteric pathogens. Stool specimens are collected in clean, leak-proof containers or a rectal swab in bacterial transport container.

87070

Common names for this test are numerous and may include routine culture, aerobic culture, or, using a body or source site, they may be referred to as vaginal culture, CSF culture, etc. The methodology is by bacterial culture and includes various identification procedures for the presumptive identification of any and multiple pathogens. The collection and transport of specimen is varied and specimen dependent.

87071

Common names for this test are numerous and may include routine culture, aerobic culture, or, using a body or source site, they may be referred to as vaginal culture, CSF culture, etc. The methodology is by bacterial culture and includes various identification procedures for the quantitation and presumptive identification of any and multiple pathogens. The collection and transport of specimen is varied and specimen dependent.

87073

The most common name for this procedure is anaerobic culture. It is a procedure for the isolation quantitation and presumptive identification of anaerobic bacteria. Tissues, fluids, and aspirations are collected in anaerobic vials or with anaerobic transport swabs and transported immediately. Anaerobic bacteria are very sensitive to oxygen and cold.

87075

The most common name for this procedure is anaerobic culture. The procedure is for isolation and presumptive identification of anaerobic bacteria. Tissues, fluids, and aspirations are collected in anaerobic vials or with anaerobic transport swabs and transported immediately. Anaerobic bacteria are very sensitive to oxygen and cold.

87076

Anaerobic organism identification is for definitive identification of an already-isolated anaerobic bacterium. It involves the use of traditional special media and biochemicals for the identification of anaerobic bacteria.

87077

Aerobic organism identification is for definitive identification of an already-isolated aerobic bacterium. It involves the use of traditional special media and biochemicals for the identification of aerobic bacteria.

87081

This is a presumptive screening culture for one or more pathogenic organisms. The methodology is by culture and the culture should be identified by type (e.g., anaerobic, aerobic) and specimen source (e.g., pleural, peritoneal, bronchial aspirates). If a specific organism is suspected, the client will typically use common names, such as strep screen, staph screen, etc., to specify the organism for screening.

87084

This is a presumptive screening culture for one or more pathogenic organisms, which includes an estimation of the number of organisms based on a density chart. The methodology is by culture and the culture should be identified by type (e.g., anaerobic, aerobic) and specimen source (e.g., pleural, peritoneal, bronchial aspirates). If a specific organism is suspected, the client will typically use common names, such as strep screen, staph screen, etc., to specify the organism for screening.

87086

The common name is urine culture. Urine from clean catch, catheter, or suprapubic collection transported in a sterile, leak-proof container provides acceptable specimens. Specimen is generally refrigerated. The methodology is presumptive identification by bacterial culture with colony count.

87088

The common name is urine culture. This test includes isolation and presumptive identification of a urine pathogen. The methodology may be traditional biochemical tests or by commercial kit.

87101

Dermatophyte culture and fungal culture are common names for this test. Fungi are divided into two broad categories, yeasts and molds. Yeast pathogens are single-celled, rounded fungi that produce by budding. Molds are filamentous fungi that can cause severe, life-threatening infections in immunocompromised individuals. Skin, hair or nail scrapings from infected site are transported in a sterile, dry container at room temperature. The scrapings are transferred to appropriate agar. Growth and confirmation by microscopic methods identify, or confirm, a presumptive identification of fungus isolated. Alternately, the scrapings are dropped onto dermatophyte test media (DMT) at the time of collection. The media changes color to indicate dermatophyte growth.

87102

Fungal culture, yeast culture, and mold culture are common names for this procedure. Fungi are divided into two broad categories: yeasts and molds. Yeast pathogens are single-celled, rounded fungi that reproduce by budding. Molds are filamentous fungi that can cause severe, life-threatening infections in immunocompromised individuals. Collection is as varied as the sources and the same specimen may be used for other tests. This test is to culture and isolate fungi (yeast or mold) with presumptive identification. Presumptive identification may include fungi (yeast or mold) present or a genus name with no species (e.g. Aspergillus sp.).

87103

Fungal blood culture or blood culture for yeast are common names for this procedure. Fungi are divided into two broad categories: yeasts and molds. Yeast pathogens are single-celled, rounded fungi that reproduce by budding. Molds are filamentous fungi that can cause severe, life-threatening infections in immunocompromised individuals. Blood is subcultured to fungal media. This test procedure is a culture to isolate fungi (yeast or mold) with presumptive identification. Presumptive identification may include fungi (yeast or mold) present or a genus name with no species (e.g. Aspergillus sp.).

87106

This test is commonly known as a fungal yeast identification. Fungal yeast pathogens are single-celled, rounded fungi that produce by budding. Yeast isolates from fungal cultures are further tested for definitive identification. This code reports testing only for yeast pathogens. Various identification procedures, including growth patterns, and macroscopic and microscopic characteristics, are employed. Examples of fungal yeast pathogens that might require definitive identification include: Histoplasma, Coccidioides and Blastomyces

87107

This test is commonly known as a mold Identification. Molds are filamentous fungi that can cause severe, life-threatening infections in immunocompromised individuals. Mold isolates from fungal cultures are further tested for definitive identification. Various identification procedures, including growth patterns, and macroscopic and microscopic characteristics, are employed. Examples of conidium- forming filamentous fungi species that might require definitive identification include: Aspergillus sp., Fusarium sp., Rhizopus arrhizus, Scedosporium apiospermum and Sporothrix schenckii.

87109

A common name for this test is Mycoplasma culture. Specimens are typically transported in viral transport media (VTM). Mycoplasma culture methods are

employed. This procedure is for the isolation and identification of Mycoplasma.

87110

This test is commonly known as a Chlamydia culture. A swab of the infected site is placed in a vial of sucrose transport media containing antibiotics and glass beads. The specimen is generally kept refrigerated. The test method is by cell culture, fluorescent stain. The cell culture technique is to isolate for Chlamydia.

87116

Common names include AFB culture, TB culture, mycobacterium culture, and acid-fast culture. Collection methods are source dependent. The methodology is by culture for the isolation and presumptive identification of mycobacterium. An acid-fast smear should be done at the time the specimen is cultured. Media for isolation should include both solid and liquid types.

87118

This procedure is a definitive identification of mycobacterial organisms isolated by procedure 87116. This procedure may be performed by a reference laboratory after isolation by a primary lab. Methodology is traditional biochemical tests for identification of mycobacterium.

87140

Specific antisera are combined with a fluorescent dye and used to stain slides of organisms. Stained slides are scanned with a fluorescent microscope to look for fluorescing organisms. Typing of organisms by immunofluorescent technique is usually to determine whether an organism is of a more pathogenic strain, to determine a treatment, or for epidemiological purposes.

87143

This procedure is performed to provide more specific typing of cultured pathogenic organisms. The methodology is gas liquid chromatography (GLC) or high pressure liquid chromatography (HPLC) to analyze byproducts of rapidly growing organisms. GLC is an automated technique in which the culture specimen is dissolved in a solvent, vaporized, and transported by an inert gas through an adsorbent gas-liquid column containing detectors that analyze and graph the components of the specimen. HPLC is similiar to GLC except that the liquid is forced under high pressure through a column packed with sorbent and separated by various methods including adsorption, gel filtration, ion-exchange, or partition. This procedure is performed on an isolated organism as in the definitive identification of mycobacterium.

87147

This test is used for more specifically dentifying cultured specimens using an immunologic method other than immunofluorescence. For example, agglutination technique may be used to more specifically identify Salmonella usually to a group level since there are more than 2,000 serovar of Salmonella. The different species have been grouped by common antigens and are tested with polyvalent antisera and reported by group (e.g., Salmonella Group D).

87149

Nucleic acid probes may be used to diagnose and monitor infectious diseases. These probes can be used to detect fungi and other organisms after they have been grown in culture. Culturing is required for many organisms because direct staining does not produce accurate results. The organism may be cultured for as little as 2-3 hours or may require as long as 16-24 hours after which the nucleic acid probe is introduced. Specificity using this culture technique is nearly 100% for many organisms.

87152

This test may also be known by the acronym PFGE (pulsed field gel electrophoresis), or CHEF (contour-clamped homogeneous electronic), or a combination of the two. A bacterial culture and nucleic acid isolation precedes the test and cells are harvested by centrifugation and washing. The PGFE method resolves and separates very large DNA molecules for cloning and direct visualization of small chromosomes (among other genetic analysis). Unlike conventional electrophoresis, PGFE produces a pulsing electric field through an agarose matrix of gel that separates larger from smaller DNA molecules for physical mapping. This emerging method provides information about macromolecular structure and function and has been used to detect in vivo chromosome breakage and degradation, the number and size of chromosomes, and to identify invasive infection in humans.

87158

Any methodology that would identify a microbial organism to the species level or a type level that does not involve the use of biochemical substrates (traditional bacteriology), antigen specific fluorescent stain, gas chromatography, phage testing, or agglutination or precipitation from antigen-antibody reactions. Lectin assays and bacteriocin typing are two tests that fit in this procedure description.

87164–87166

Names commonly used include dark field for syphilis and dark field exam. Dark field microscopic exams have generally been limited to the bacteria called spirochetes. Treponema pallidum, the agent of syphilis, Borrelia burgdorferi, the agent of Lyme disease; and Leptospira are among the better known spirochetes. Specimens for dark field exam are

typically examined within 30 minutes of collection. Certain immunological tests have rendered this method to be somewhat outdated. The term "dark field" refers to the staining method. If the lab is responsible for specimen collection, report 87164. If the lab is not responsible for collection of the specimen, report 87166.

87168

This test is performed to identify arthropods that might be vectors of disease causing organisms in man. Arthropods are small animals having a hard, jointed exoskeleton and paired legs. This group of animals includes lice and ticks. Method is visual examination (macroscopic) of the source specimen.

87169

This test is performed to identify parasites other than arthropods that might be vectors of disease causing organisms in man. Method is visual examination (macroscopic) of the source specimen.

87172

This test may be requested as pinworm examination. Clear tape is applied to the perianal area. The tape is removed and submitted to the laboratory on a clean slide. Method is microscopic examination.

87176

This test may be called grinding or homogenization of tissue. The methodology is mechanical disruption of the tissue to enhance extraction of endotoxin. It may involve the use of sterile equipment, such as scissors, mortar and pestle, or disposable grinders.

87177

Common names for this procedure are ova and parasite exam, or O & P. Stool is collected in a clean, leak-proof container (when processed within 1 hour) or the specimen is added to formalin or fixative (both available in commercial kits). The methodology of an ova and parasite exam for stools includes a direct smear, and smear of concentrated material, such as formalin concentration technique or zinc flotation method. Identification is by observing parasites with the aid of a microscope.

87181

A susceptibility study is performed to determine the susceptibility of a bacterium to an antibiotic. The methodology is agar diffusion (the E test is a method of agar diffusion). The specific antibiotics could be chosen and limited. The test is reported per antibiotic tested. The agar dilution is reported as minimum inhibitory concentration (MIC), which is a method of measuring the exact amount of antibiotic needed to inhibit an organism.

87184

This is commonly called a Kirby-Bauer or Bauer-Kirby sensitivity test. It is a sensitivity test to determine the susceptibility of a bacterium to an antibiotic. The methodology is disk diffusion and results are reported as sensitive, intermediate, or resistant. As many as 12 antibiotic disks may be used per plate and the procedure is billed per plate not per antibiotic disk.

87185

Bacteria produce enzymes that can inactivate some types of antibiotics. This susceptibility test identifies those bacteria that will be resistent to certain types of antibiotics by detecting the presence of these enzymes. For example, almost all gram negative bacteria produce enzymes that catalyze the beta-lactam rings found in penicillins and cephalosporins rendering these antibiotics inactive against the pathogenic bacteria.

87186

This procedure may be called an MIC, or a sensitivity test. It is a sensitivity test to determine the susceptibility of a bacterium to an antibiotic. The methodology is microtiter dilution (several commercial panels use this method). Results are given as a minimum inhibitory concentration (MIC) with an interpretation of sensitive, intermediate, or resistant. The antibiotics on commercial plates are numerous, but predetermined. The procedure is charged by plate not by antibiotic.

87187

This test may be called an MBC (minimum bactericidal concentration). The MIC (minimum inhibitory concentration) measures the dilution of antibiotic needed to inhibit an organism while the MBC is the dilution of antibiotic needed to kill the bacteria. MICs are tube dilutions read visually. Tubes that may visually appear to have no growth are cultured to solid media to detect a concentration of antibiotic where no organisms grow. This is the MBC.

87188

This test may be referred to as an MIC (minimum inhibitory concentration). It is a susceptiblity test to determine the sensitivity of a bacterium to an antibiotic. The methodology is macrobroth dilution. Results are given as a minimum inhibitory concentration (MIC) with an interpretation of sensitive, intermediate, or resistant. The procedure is charged per antibiotic tested.

87190

Mycobacterium susceptibility test is a procedure done only on mycobacterium (e.g., M. tuberculosis, M. marinum, etc.). Proportion method is used and involves testing of a panel of antibiotics used only for the treatment of mycobacterium. Results are given as sensitive or resistant.

87197

This procedure is called a serum cidal level, a serum bactericidal titer, or a Schlichter test. This test cannot

be performed without a bacterial organism that has been previously isolated from the same patient. The killing power of the patient's serum against the isolated pathogen is measured. Blood is usually drawn and tested at peak and trough level of the antibiotic. This is similar to a tube dilution test, but uses serum, which may be a combination of more than one antibiotic and host defenses, instead of an antibiotic.

87198

Cytomegalovirus is a herpesvirus that infects directly through mucous membrane contact, tissue transplant, or blood transfusion. In a direct fluorescent antibody test, cytomegalovirus (CMV) antibodies that have been stained by a fluorescent dye are added to a sample of the patient's serum. The flagged antibodies form a complex with specific antigens, which is indirectly identified by the presence of a reaction against the known, flagged antibody.

87199

Diagnosis is by viral culture, generally done on sputum from a nasal aspiration, respiratory secretion, throat washing, stool sample may be obtained for the laboratory test. A sputum sample is obtained by coughing into a specimen container. In the laboratory, enterovirus antibodies that have been stained by a fluorescent dye are added to the sample. The flagged antibodies will form a complex with the enterovirus antigen. The enterovirus antigen is indirectly identified by the presence of a reaction against a known, flagged antibody.

87205

Any smear done on a primary source (e.g., sputum, CSF, etc.) to identify bacteria, fungi, and cell types. An interpretation of findings is provided. Bacteria, fungi, WBCs, and epithelial cells may be estimated in quantity with an interpretation as to the possibility of contamination by normal flora. A gram stain may be the most commonly performed smear of this type.

87206

A fluorescent or acid-fast stain for bacteria, fungi, parasites, viruses or cell types. These are special stains usually for specific groups of organisms (e.g., mycobacterium and Nocardia). Identification of Cryptosporidium and related parasites are examples of parasites that can be identified by fluorescent or acid fast stain. An interpretation is included.

87207

This is a special stain to look for inclusion bodies or parasites inside body cells (e.g., blood to look for Malaria inside red cells). Its use to detect herpes has been outdated by amplification and immunological methods. An interpretation is included.

87210

This test may be requested as a KOH prep. A wet mount is prepared from a primary source to detect bacteria, fungi, or ova and parasites. Motility of organisms is visible on wet mounts and the addition of a simple stain, such as iodine, India ink, or simple dyes, may aid detection of bacteria, fungi, and parasites. An interpretation of findings is included.

87220

Potassium hydroxide (KOH) prep and calcofluor stains are the most common methods of looking for hyphal elements and or yeast in tissue. The KOH causes a clearing of the specimen to make fungus more visible. A wet mount is prepared by adding KOH to small pieces of specimen on a microscope slide and allowing the slide to sit for several minutes to several hours before viewing. A calcofluor is prepared the same way except that the preparation is enhanced for microscopic observation by adding a drop of calcofluor, a type of fluorescent dye, to the slide and reading the preparation with a fluorescent microscope.

87230

This procedure is a toxin assay for diagnosis of toxin producing organisms, such as Clostridium difficile, E. coli 0157, enterotoxigenic E. coli, and Vibrio cholerae. Stool is collected for testing. Filtrates of the stool are inoculated into cell cultures and observed for CPE (cytopathic effect) microscopically. Confirmation of toxin production may be done by toxin neutralization. Different cell cultures are used to test for different toxins, so organism must be specified.

87250

Embryonated egg or small animal inoculation with specimen source is used in the diagnosis of some viruses. There are different specimen types for the different viruses. Contact the reference lab that is performing the test for type of specimen and transport. Mice are inoculated with patient specimen to detect the presence of virus, and if the test is positive the mice become ill or die. There are, however, more rapid tests to diagnosis for most viral infections. This code includes observation for signs of illness in mice for as long as three weeks and dissection of mice and preparation of tissue for microscopy to confirm diagnosis when mice become ill or die.

87252

Cell culture is a procedure used particularly for viral detection. There is a general viral culture which can detect most viruses, but when a specific agent is suspected such as CMV, HSV, Influenzae A or B, mumps, or varicella zoster, more specific and rapid culture techniques can be used. This procedure provides presumptive identification by cytopathic effect only. Specimens may be collected by swab, washings and fluids, and blood draw.

87253

This code reports additional tissue culture studies required for specific virus identification and is reported for each isolate.

87254

This test may also be ordered as a an SV culture, a rapid shell assay, or an immediate early antigen test. Specimen collection is by separately reportable appropriate procedure. Shell vial isolation cultures offer more immediate results (often 48-hours) than conventional cultures. The technique is particularly useful in identification of respiratory organisms. Flat-bottomed shell vial tubes containing t-Mk and human diploid cells and medium are inoculated. The medium is centrifuged following a culture period. Antibody is added to detect viruses, usually one to three days post-infection. Immunofluorescence is a technique in which antibody reacts with an antigen on a fixed slide. The antibody in turn reacts with antihuman globulins for the diagnosis of infectious diseases. The fluorescence is best viewed with a laser-scanning confocal microscope.

87260

This test may be requested as adenovirus by DFA or by immunofluorescence. It is most commonly used to diagnose serotypes that cause infantile gastroenteritis. A random stool sample is obtained. Infectious agent antigen detection by immunofluorescence includes direct and indirect fluorescent antibody technique and involves nonculture (primary source) detection of infected cells using monoclonal antibodies and immunofluorescence microscopy. Cellular material must be obtained from the site for immunofluoresence to be an effective diagnostic technique.

87265

This test may be requested as Bordetella pertussis or parapertussis by DFA or by immunfluorescence. Bordetella pertussis is the causative agent of whooping cough. Infectious agent antigen detection by immunofluorescence includes direct and indirect fluorescent antibody technique and involves nonculture (primary source) detection of infected cells using monoclonal antibodies and immunofluorescence microscopy. Cellular material must be obtained from the site for immunofluoresence to be an effective diagnostic technique.

87270

This test may be requested as Chlamydia trachomatis or C. trachomatis by DFA or by immunofluorescence. C. trachomatis is a frequently occurring sexually transmitted disease. It may cause nonspecific urethritis or pelvic inflammatory disease (PID), although it is frequently asymptomatic in women.

Another serotype also causes conjunctivitis. Infectious agent antigen detection by immunofluorescence includes direct and indirect fluorescent antibody technique and involves nonculture (primary source) detection of infected cells using monoclonal antibodies and immunofluorescence microscopy. Cellular material must be obtained from the site for immunofluoresence to be an effective diagnostic technique.

87272

This procedure may be referred to as a direct fluorescent antibody (DFA) or immunofluorescent stain for Cryptosporidium and Giardia. These parasites infect the gastrointestinal tract causing symptoms such as diarrhea, weight loss, fever, and abdominal pain. Infectious agent antigen detection by immunofluorescence includes direct and indirect fluorescent antibody technique and involves nonculture (primary source) detection of infected cells using monoclonal antibodies and immunofluorescence microscopy. Some commercial kits have combined monoclonal antibodies for detection of both parasites in one test.

87273

This test may be requested as HSV 2 by DFA or HSV 2 by immunofluorescence. Herpes simplex is classified by HSV type. HSV 2 is a sexually transmitted disease with lesions occurring primarily in the genitourinary tract. Infectious agent antigen detection by immunofluorescence includes direct and indirect fluorescent antibody technique and involves nonculture (primary source) detection of infected cells using monoclonal antibodies and immunofluorescence microscopy. Cellular material must be obtained from the site for immunofluorescence to be an effective diagnostic technique.

87274

This test may be requested as HSV 1 by DFA or HSV 1 by immunofluorescence. Herpes simplex is classified by HSV type. HSV 1 is primarily responsible for oral lesions frequently referred to as fever blisters or cold sores. Infectious agent antigen detection by immunofluorescence includes direct and indirect fluorescent antibody technique and involves nonculture (primary source) detection of infected cells using monoclonal antibodies and immunofluorescence microscopy. Cellular material must be obtained from the site for immunofluoresence to be an effective diagnostic technique.

87275

This test may be requested as influenza B by DFA or by immunofluorescence. Influenza B is less common than other types of influenza although the symptoms of type A and type B influenza are indistinguishable. Infectious agent antigen detection by

immunofluorescence includes direct and indirect fluorescent antibody technique and involves nonculture (primary source) detection of infected cells using monoclonal antibodies and immunofluoresence microscopy. Cellular material must be obtained from the site for immunofluoresence to be an effective diagnostic technique.

87276

This test may be requested as influenza A by DFA or by immunofluorescence. Type A influenza is the most common strain. The causative agent is subject to wide variation in antigenic type. This is referred to as antigen shift and causes new variations of the Type A virus to appear at two to three year intervals. Infectious agent antigen detection by immunofluorescence includes direct and indirect fluorescent antibody technique and involves nonculture (primary source) detection of infected cells using monoclonal antibodies and immunofluorescence microscopy. Cellular material must be obtained from the site for immunofluoresence to be an effective diagnostic technique.

87277

This procedure may be requested as Legionella micdadei by direct fluorescent antibody (DFA) stain or by immunofluorescence. L. micdadei is the second most commonly isolated member of Legionella. This bacterium can cause the same flu-like symptoms and pneumonia which characterize an L. pneumophila infection. Infectious agent antigen detection by immunofluorescence includes direct and indirect fluorescent antibody technique and involves nonculture (primary source) detection of infected cells using monoclonal antibodies and immunofluorescence microscopy. Cellular material must be obtained from the site for immunofluoresence to be an effective diagnostic technique. For DFA procedure it is acceptable to prepare and send two air-dried smears. This method may be a rapid diagnosis, but is not as accurate as cultured tests.

87278

This procedure may be requested as Legionella pneumophila by direct fluorescent antibody (DFA) stain or by immunofluorescence. L. pneumophila is the bacterium associated with Legionnaires' disease and Pontiac fever. Legionnaires' disease is characterized by a gradual onset of flu-like symptoms with severe pneumonia and involvement of other body systems developing in some cases. The flu-like symptoms are also seen in Pontiac fever but pneumonia does not develop and infection does not spread beyond the lungs. Infectious agent antigen detection by immunofluorescence includes direct and indirect fluorescent antibody technique and involves noncunure (primary source) detection of infected cells using monoclonal antibodies and immunofluorescence microscopy. Cellular material must be obtained from the site for immunofluoresence to be an effective diagnostic technique. For DFA procedure it is acceptable to prepare and send two air-dried smears. This method may be a rapid diagnosis, but is not as accurate as cultured tests.

87279

This test may be requested as parainfluenza virus by DFA or by immunofluorescence. Parainfluenza is a group of viruses that cause upper respiratory infections that are often the causative agents in croup, bronchitis and bronchiolitis. Infectious agent antigen detection by immunofluorescence includes direct and indirect fluorescent antibody technique and involves nonculture (primary source) detection of infected cells using monoclonal antibodies and immunofluorescence microscopy. Cellular material must be obtained from the site for immunofluoresence to be an effective diagnostic technique.

87280

This test may be requested as DFA or immunofluorescent stain for respiratory syncytial virus (RSV). RSV causes respiratory disease that can be particularly severe in infants. Infectious agent antigen detection by immunofluorescence includes direct and indirect fluorescent antibody technique and involves nonculture (primary source) detection of infected cells using monoclonal antibodies and immunofluorescence microscopy. Cellular material must be obtained from the site for immunofluoresence to be an effective diagnostic technique.

87281

This test may be requested as pneumocystis carinii or PCP by DFA or by immunofluorescence. The microorganism Pneumocystis carinii causes lung infection or pneumonia in premature infants, cancer patients, patients being treated with immunosuppressive medications for the management of organ transplantation or cancer, and AIDS patients. Infectious agent antigen detection by immunofluorescence includes direct and indirect fluorescent antibody technique and involves nonculture (primary source) detection of infected cells using monoclonal antibodies and immunofluorescence microscopy. Cellular material must be obtained from the site for immunofluoresence to be an effective diagnostic technique.

87283

This test may be requested as rubeola stain or rubeola IFA. Rubeola, more commonly referred to as measles,

is characterized by fever, coryza, cough, and conjunctivitis after which Koplik's spots appear appear in the mouth with pharyngitis and inflammation of the laryngeal and tracheobronchial musoca. Infectious agent antigen detection by immunofluorescence includes direct and indirect fluorescent antibody technique and involves nonculture (primary source) detection of infected cells using monoclonal antibodies and immunofluorescence microscopy. Cellular material must be obtained from the site for immunofluoresence to be an effective diagnostic technique.

87285

The spirochete Treponema pallidum is the causative agent of syphilis. Infectious agent antigen detection by immunofluorescence includes direct and indirect fluorescent antibody technique and involves nonculture (primary source) detection of infected cells using monoclonal antibodies and immunofluorescence microscopy. Cellular material must be obtained from the site for immunofluorescence to be an effective diagnostic technique.

87290

This test may be requested as direct fluorescent stain for varicella zoster virus. This is the causative agent of chickenpox. Infectious agent antigen detection by immunofluorescence includes direct and indirect fluorescent antibody technique and involves nonculture (primary source) detection of infected cells using monoclonal antibodies and immunofluorescence microscopy. Cellular material must be obtained from the site for immunofluoresence to be an effective diagnostic technique. This test has a high specificity, but sensitivity is dependent on adequacy of the sample collected. A negative sample should be cultured.

87299

This code reports immunofluorescent technique of specific infectious agents not identified by more specific codes. Infectious agent antigen detection by immunofluorescence includes direct and indirect fluorescent antibody technique and involves nonculture (primary source) detection of infected cells using monoclonal antibodies and immunofluorescence microscopy. Cellular material must be obtained from the site for immunofluorescence to be an effective diagnostic technique.

87300

This code reports immunofluorescent technique to identify multiple strains of bacteria or other infectious organisms in a single test. Infectious agent antigen detection by immunofluorescence includes direct and indirect fluorescent antibody technique and involves nonculture (primary source) detection of infected cells using monoclonal antibodies and immunofluorescence microscopy. Cellular material must be obtained from the site for immunofluorescence to be an effective diagnostic technique.

87301

This test may be requested as adenovirus enteric types 40/41 by EIA. These serotypes cause infantile gastroenteritis. A random stool sample is obtained. Enzyme immunoassay (EIA) refers to a technique which utilizes a chemical bond between an enzyme and an antigen or antibody as a label to identify specific chemical or infectious agents.

87320

This test may be requested as Chlamydia trachomatis or C. trachomatis by enzyme immunoassay (EIA). C. trachomatis is a frequently occurring sexually transmitted disease. It may cause nonspecific urethritis or pelvic inflammatory disease (PID), although it is frequently asymptomatic in women. Another serotype also causes conjunctivitis. Enzyme immunoassay refers to a technique which utilizes a chemical bond between an enzyme and an antigen or antibody as a label to identify specific chemical or infectious agents. Special reagents and equipment are required for C. trachomatis EIA. Sensitivity of EIA is approximately 75-85%.

87324

This test may be requested as enzyme immunoassay (EIA) for the detection of Clostridium difficile toxin(s) or more simply referred to as a C. difficile toxin test. Enzyme immunoassay refers to a technique which utilizes a chemical bond between an enzyme and an antigen or antibody as a label to identify specific chemical or infectious agents. A random stool sample is obtained. Fresh stool should be kept refrigerated and transported in clean leak proof container.

87327

This test may be requested as enzyme immunoassay (EIA) for the detection of Cryptococcus neoformans. Blood is obtained by venipuncture. CSF is obtained by separately reportable lumbar puncture. Enzyme immunoassay refers to a technique which utilizes a chemical bond between an enzyme and an antigen or antibody as a label to identify specific chemical or infectious agents. Cryptococcosis is a life threatening infection of the meninges in patients with compromised immune systems du to diseases such as acquired immune deficiency syndrome (AIDS). This test is most effective when performed on CSF of patients with symptoms of cryptococcal meningitis; however, serum may also contain detectable levels of antigen.

87328

This procedure is for the detection of Cryptosporidium or Giardia by EIA (Enzyme Immunoassay). These parasites infect the gastrointestinal tract causing symptoms such as diarrhea, weight loss, fever, and abdominal pain. Enzyme immunoassay refers to a technique which utilizes a chemical bond between an enzyme and an antigen or antibody as a label to identify specific chemical or infectious agents. A random stool sample is obtained. Transport fresh or preserved stool in clean leak proof container.

87332

This test may be requested as cytomegalovirus (CMV) by enzyme immunoassay (EIA). CMV is part of the viral family that includes herpes zoster, Epstein-Barr, and Varicella zoster infections. CMV usually causes only mild symptoms except in fetal infection or immunosuppressed patients, including AIDS and transplant patients. Blood specimen is obtained by venipuncture. Enzyme immunoassay refers to a technique which utilizes a chemical bond between an enzyme and an antigen or antibody as a label to identify specific chemical or infectious agents. EIA is often used in conjunction with culture.

87335

This test may be requested enzyme immunoassay (EIA) for the detection of Escherichia Coli (E. Coli) 0157. E. Coli 0157 is the causative agent of hemorrhagic colitis in food borne epidemics. Enzyme immunoassay refers to a technique which utilizes a chemical bond between an enzyme and an antigen or antibody as a label to identify specific chemical or infectious agents. A random stool sample is obtained. Stool or rectal swabs may be transported in Carey-Blair transport media. Fresh stool can be sent in clean leak proof container, but if transport time exceeds 2 hours the specimen should be frozen at -70 C.

87336

This test may be requested as enzyme immunoassay (EIA) for the detection of Entamoeba histolytica dispar group. E histolytica is an enteric protozoan that exists in either trophozoite or cyst form. Three to six stool examinations are recommended, each permanently stained using a trichrome stain. Biopsies may be obtained by separately reportable open or endoscopic procedure. Enzyme immunoassay refers to a technique which utilizes a chemical bond between an enzyme and an antigen or antibody as a label to identify specific chemical or infectious agents.

87337

This test may be requested as enzyme immunoassay (EIA) for the detection of Entamoeba histolytica group. E histolytica is an enteric protozoan that exists in either trophozoite or cyst form. Three to six stool examinations are recommended, each permanently stained using a trichrome stain. Biopsies may be

CPT® Lay Descriptions

obtained by separately reportable open or endoscopic procedure. Enzyme immunoassay refers to a technique which utilizes a chemical bond between an enzyme and an antigen or antibody as a label to identify specific chemical or infectious agents.

87338

This test may be ordered as an H. pylori antibody titer, stool. Specimen collection is from a stool sample, particularly drawn from mucous in the specimen. Method is multiple step, qualitative or semiquantitative, enzyme immunoassay (EIA) or enzyme-linked immunosorbent assay (ELISA). H. pylori may be found along the gastric mucosa and on the mucosal cells of the GI tract and its presence is linked to several serious disorders of the stomach.

87339

This test may be ordered as an H. pylori antibody titer. Method is multiple step, qualitative or semiquantitative, enzyme immunoassay (EIA) or enzyme-linked immunosorbent assay (ELISA). H. pylori may be found along the gastric mucosa and on the mucosal cells of the GI tract and its presence is linked to several serious disorders of the stomach.

87340

This test may be requested as HBsAg by enzyme immunoassay (EIA). Hepatitis B is a retrovirus which can cause persistent infection leading to cirrhosis and hepatocellular carcinoma. HBsAg is a lipoprotein that coats the surface of the hepatitis B virus. Blood specimen is obtained by venipuncture. Enzyme immunoassay refers to a technique which utilizes a chemical bond between an enzyme and an antigen or antibody as a label to identify specific chemical or infectious agents.

87341

This test may be requested as HBsAg by enzyme immunoassay (EIA) confirmation. This assay is performed only when a specimen is repeatedly reactive for Hepatitis B surface antigen. Elevated HBsAg levels beyond 6 months may indicate a chronic carrier (i.e., chronic hepatitis). The HBsAg neutralization test is performed to identify false positives. False positives on a standard HBsAg test will not neutralize with anti-HBs in the confirmatory assay. Hepatitis B is a retrovirus which can cause persistent infection leading to cirrhosis and hepatocellular carcinoma. HBsAg is a lipoprotein that coats the surface of the hepatitis B virus. Blood specimen is obtained by venipuncture. Enzyme immunoassay refers to a technique which utilizes a chemical bond between an enzyme and an antigen or antibody as a label to identify specific chemical or infectious agents.

87350

This test may be requested as HBeAg by enzyme immunoassay (EIA). Hepatitis B is a retrovirus which

can cause persistent infection leading to cirrhosis and hepatocellular carcinoma. HBeAg is normally tested only on individuals who are chronically HBsAg positive. Blood specimen is obtained by venipuncture. Enzyme immunoassay refers to a technique which utilizes a chemical bond between an enzyme and an antigen or antibody as a label to identify specific chemical or infectious agents.

87380

This test may be requested as hepatitis delta agent (HDAg) by enzyme immunoassay (EIA). Hepatitis delta agent is normally tested only on individuals who are chronically HBsAg positive or have an exacerbation of their hepatitis as HDAg requires the presence of HBsAg to become an infectious virus. Blood specimen is obtained by venipuncture. Enzyme immunoassay refers to a technique which utilizes a chemical bond between an enzyme and an antigen or antibody as a label to identify specific chemical or infectious agents.

87385

This test may be requested as Histoplasma capsulatum by enzyme immunoassay (EIA). Histoplasma capsulatum infection results from inhalation or ingestion of spores and is common in the Midwestern United States. It is usually asymptomatic, but on occasion causes acute pneumonia, disseminated reticuloendothelial hyperplasia with hepatosplenomegaly and anemia, or influenza-like symptoms with joint effusion and erythema nodosum. Reactivated infection is common is immunocompromised individuals affecting lungs, meninges, heart, peritoneum and adrenal glands. Blood specimen is obtained by venipuncture. Enzyme immunoassay refers to a technique which utilizes a chemical bond between an enzyme and an antigen or antibody as a label to identify specific chemical or infectious agents.

87390

This test may be requested as human immunodeficiency virus Type 1 (HIV-1) by EIA. HIV-1 is the causative agent of acquired immunodeficiency syndrome (AIDS). Blood specimen is obtained by venipuncture. Enzyme immunoassay refers to a technique which utilizes a chemical bond between an enzyme and an antigen or antibody as a label to identify specific chemical or infectious agents. If EIA is positive, it is repeated. Two out of three tests must be positive before the test is reported as positive. All positive EIA tests are confirmed with a additional test using a different technique, usually Western blot, which is reported separately.

87391

This test may be requested as human immunodeficiency virus Type 2 (HIV-2) by EIA. HIV-2 is a retrovirus closely related to simian AIDS and found initially in West African nations and Portugal, but with cases also being reported in the United States since 1987. Blood specimen is obtained by venipuncture. Enzyme immunoassay refers to a technique which utilizes a chemical bond between an enzyme and an antigen or antibody as a label to identify specific chemical or infectious agents. If EIA is positive, it is repeated. Two out of three tests must be positive before the test is reported as positive. All positive EIA tests are confirmed with a additional test using a different technique, usually Western blot, which is reported separately.

87400

This test may be requested as Influenza A EIA or Influenza B EIA. Serum specimen is collected by venipuncture. Other specimens may be collected by separately reportable procedures. In a classic enzyme immunoassay, plastic plates, paddles, or beads are coated with the antigen (in this case, Influenza A or B). Specific antibody present in the serum reacts to form an antigen-antibody complex. The plate or bead is incubated with an enzyme-labeled antibody conjugate. If antibody is present, the conjugate reacts with the antigen-antibody complex. Enzyme activity is measured spectrophotometrically or visually by a change in color. Influenza A and B are a genus of the virus that causes the acute respiratory illness known as influenza. The designation is based on antigenic testing. Testing may occur during the acute phase of illness and again 10 to 14 days after onset of symptoms.

87420

This test may be requested as respiratory syncytial virus (RSV) by enzyme immunoassay (EIA). RSV causes respiratory disease which can be particularly severe in infants. Blood specimen is obtained by venipuncture. Enzyme immunoassay refers to a technique which utilizes a chemical bond between an enzyme and an antigen or antibody as a label to identify specific chemical or infectious agents.

87425

This test may be requested as rotavirus by enzyme immunoassay (EIA). Rotavirus causes sometimes severe infectious gastroenteritis in infants and young children. Adults may contract a milder infection. Blood specimen is obtained by venipuncture. Enzyme immunoassay refers to a technique which utilizes a chemical bond between an enzyme and an antigen or antibody as a label to identify specific chemical or infectious agents.

87427

This test may be ordered as a Shigella Type 1 by EIA or S. dysenteriae test by EIA. Serum is collected by venipuncture. In a classic enzyme immunoassay, plastic plates, paddles, or beads are coated with the antigen (in this case, Influenza A or B). Specific antibody present in the serum reacts to form an antigen-antibody complex. The plate or bead is incubated with an enzyme-labeled antibody conjugate. If antibody is present, the conjugate reacts with the antigen-antibody complex. Enzyme activity is measured spectrophotometrically or visually by a change in color. Shigella is an enteric pathogen known for its ability to produce protein toxins that cause acute gut inflammation and dysentery. Serology tests are usually conducted during the acute phase of illness.

87430

This test may be requested as Streptococcus A by enzyme immunoassay (EIA). Streptococcus A is a form of beta hemolytic streptococcus which causes pharyngitis. Untreated infection may lead to rheumatic fever or glomerulonephritis. Enzyme immunoassay refers to a technique which utilizes a chemical bond between an enzyme and an antigen or antibody as a label to identify specific chemical or infectious agents.

87449–87451

These codes report enzyme immunoassay (EIA) of infectious agents which are not specifically identified elsewhere. Enzyme immunoassay refers to a technique which utilizes a chemical bond between an enzyme and an antigen or antibody as a label to identify specific chemical or infectious agents. Code 87449 reports testing for a single organism using a multiple step method; 87450 reports testing for a single organism using a single step method; and 87451 reports testing for mutiple organisms using a multiple step method and a polyvalent antiserum. The term polyvalent when used in reference to microbiology denotes an antibody molecule with multiple antigen binding sites.

87470

This test may be requested as B. henselae or B. quintana. These organisms are gram-negative bacilli that infect the red blood cells and epithelial cells of the lymph nodes, liver, and spleen. Blood specimen is obtained by venipuncture. Tissue specimen requires a separately reportable biopsy. The specimen is treated to isolate the nucleic acid. Nucleic acid is analyzed using direct probe technique.

87471

This test may be requested as B. henselae or B. quintana. These organisms are gram-negative bacilli that infect the red blood cells and epithelial cells of the lymph nodes, liver, and spleen. Blood specimen is obtained by venipuncture. Tissue specimen requires a separately reportable biopsy. The specimen is treated to isolate the nucleic acid (DNA, RNA) and eliminate substances which inhibit amplification. The nucleic acid is then amplified using specific primers for B. henselae and B. quintana sequences.

87472

This test may be requested as B. henselae or B. quintana. These organisms are gram-negative bacilli that infect the red blood cells and epithelial cells of the lymph nodes, liver, and spleen. Blood specimen is obtained by venipuncture. Tissue specimen requires a separately reportable biopsy. The specimen is treated to isolate the nucleic acid (DNA, RNA). This code reports quantification only and is used primarily to assess extent of disease or disease progression.

87475

This test may be requested as DNA direct probe for Lyme disease. Borrelia burgdorferi is a bacteria transmitted by tick bite and the causative agent of Lyme disease, acrodermatitis chronica atrophicans, and erythema chronicum migrans. Blood specimen is obtained by venipuncture. CSF requires a spinal puncture which is reported separately. Synovial fluid is obtained by arthrocentesis and is reported separately. A random urine specimen is obtained. DNA from spirochete Borrelia burgdorferi is analyzed using direct probe technique.

87476

This test may be requested as DNA amplified probe for Lyme disease. Borrelia burgdorferi is a bacteria transmitted by tick bite and the causative agent of Lyme disease, acrodermatitis chronica atrophicans, and erythema chronicum migrans. Blood specimen is obtained by venipuncture. CSF requires a spinal puncture which is reported separately. Synovial fluid is obtained by arthrocentesis and is reported separately. A random urine specimen is obtained. DNA from spirochete Borrelia burgdorferi is analyzed using amplified probe technique. The specimen is treated to isolate the DNA and eliminate substances which inhibit amplification. The DNA is then amplified using specific primers for Borrelia burgdorferi sequences.

87477

This test may be requested as Lyme disease quantification using DNA. Borrelia burgdorferi is a bacteria transmitted by tick bite and the causative agent of Lyme disease, acrodermatitis chronica atrophicans, and erythema chronicum migrans. Blood specimen is obtained by venipuncture. CSF requires a spinal puncture which is reported separately. Synovial fluid is obtained by arthrocentesis and is reported separately. A random urine specimen is obtained.

87480

This test is used to diagnosis an infection by any species of Candida, but usually C. albicans. This test would normally be performed to diagnosis systemic (invasive) candidiasis. Blood is obtained by venipuncture. The specimen is treated to isolate nucleic acid (DNA, RNA). Nucleic acid is analyzed using direct probe technique.

87481

This test is used to diagnosis an infection by any species of Candida, but usually C. albicans. This test would normally be performed to diagnosis systemic (invasive) candidiasis. Blood is obtained by venipuncture. The specimen is treated to isolate the nucleic acid (DNA, RNA) and eliminate substances which inhibit amplification. The nucleic acid is then amplified using specific primers for Candida sequences.

87482

This test is used to diagnosis an infection by any species of Candida, but usually C. albicans. This test would normally be performed to diagnosis systemic (invasive) candidiasis. Blood is obtained by venipuncture. The specimen is treated to isolate the nucleic acid (DNA, RNA). This code reports quantification only and is used primarily to assess extent of disease or disease progression.

87485

Chlamydia pneumoniae causes both upper and lower respiratory tract infections and is a causative agent in many community acquired pneumonia. Blood is obtained by venipuncture. Sputum may be obtained by deep coughing or aerosol induced technique. The specimen is treated to isolate nucleic acid (DNA, RNA). Nucleic acid is analyzed using direct probe technique.

87486

Chlamydia pneumoniae causes both upper and lower respiratory tract infections and is a causative agent in many community acquired pneumonia. Blood is obtained by venipuncture. Sputum may be obtained by deep coughing or aerosol induced technique. The specimen is treated to isolate the DNA and eliminate substances which inhibit amplification. The DNA is then amplified using a technique such as polymerase chain reaction (PCR).

87487

Chlamydia pneumoniae causes both upper and lower respiratory tract infections and is a causative agent in many community acquired pneumonia. Blood is obtained by venipuncture. Sputum may be obtained by deep coughing or aerosol induced technique. The specimen is treated to isolate the nucleic acid (DNA, RNA). This code reports quantification only and is used primarily to assess extent of disease or disease progression.

87490

This test may be requested as Chlamydia trachomatis or C. trachomatis by direct DNA probe. C. trachomatis is a frequently occurring sexually transmitted disease. It may cause nonspecific urethritis or pelvic inflammatory disease (PID), although it is frequently asymptomatic in women. Another serotype also causes conjunctivitis. The specimen is treated to isolate the DNA using direct probe.

87491

This test may be requested as Chlamydia trachomatis or C. trachomatis by polymerase chain reaction. C. trachomatis is a frequently occurring sexually transmitted disease. It may cause nonspecific urethritis or pelvic inflammatory disease (PID), although it is frequently asymptomatic in women. Another serotype also causes conjunctivitis. The specimen is treated to isolate the DNA and eliminate substances which inhibit amplification. The DNA is then amplified using a technique such as polymerase chain reaction (PCR).

87492

This test may be requested as Chlamydia trachomatis or C. trachomatis DNA quantification. C. trachomatis is a frequently occurring sexually transmitted disease. It may cause nonspecific urethritis or pelvic inflammatory disease (PID), although it is frequently asymptomatic in women. Another serotype also causes conjunctivitis. This code reports quantification only.

87495

This test may be requested as cytomegalovirus (CMV) direct DNA probe technique. CMV is part of the viral family that includes herpes zoster, Epstein-Barr, and varicella zoster infections. CMV usually causes only mild symptoms except in fetal infection or immunosuppressed patients, including AIDS and transplant patients. Blood specimen is obtained by venipuncture. A random urine specimen is obtained. A separately reportable tissue biopsy is obtained. The specimen is treated to isolate the DNA using direct probe.

87496

This test may be requested as cytomegalovirus (CMV) by polymerase chain reaction. CMV is part of the viral family that includes herpes zoster, Epstein-Barr, and varicella zoster infections. CMV usually causes only mild symptoms except in fetal infection or immunosuppressed patients, including AIDS and transplant patients. Blood specimen is obtained by venipuncture. A random urine specimen is obtained. A separately reportable tissue biopsy is obtained. The specimen is treated to isolate the DNA and eliminate substances which inhibit amplification. The DNA is then amplified using a technique such as polymerase chain reaction (PCR).

87497

This test may be requested as cytomegalovirus (CMV) quantification. CMV is part of the viral family that includes herpes zoster, Epstein-Barr, and varicella zoster infections. CMV usually causes only mild symptoms except in fetal infection or immunosuppressed patients, including AIDS and

transplant patients. Blood specimen is obtained by venipuncture. A random urine specimen is obtained. A separately reportable tissue biopsy is obtained. This code reports quantification only and is usually performed following amplification which is reported separately.

87510

This test may also be requested as haemophilus vaginalis by direct nucleic acid probe. Gardnerella vaginalis is a gram-negative bacteria which causes an infection of the female genital tract producing a gray or yellow discharge. The specimen is treated to isolate nucleic acid (DNA, RNA). Nucleic acid is analyzed using direct probe technique.

87511

This test may also be requested as haemophilus vaginalis by amplified nucleic acid probe. Gardnerella vaginalis is a gram-negative bacteria which causes an infection of the female genital tract producing a gray or yellow discharge. The specimen is treated to isolate the nucleic acid (DNA, RNA) and eliminate substances which inhibit amplification. The nucleic acid is then amplified using specific primers for Gardnerella vaginalis sequences.

87512

This test may also be requested as haemophilus vaginalis. Gardnerella vaginalis is a gram-negative bacteria which causes an infection of the female genital tract producing a gray or yellow discharge. The specimen is treated to isolate the nucleic acid (DNA, RNA). This code reports quantification only and is used primarily to assess extent of disease or disease progression.

87515

This test may be requested as HBV DNA direct probe. Hepatitis B is a retrovirus which can cause persistent infection leading to cirrhosis and hepatocellular carcinoma. Molecular (DNA) tests are useful in identifying potentially infectious individuals as well as chronic progression of the disease. Blood specimen is obtained by venipuncture. A liver biopsy is required for analysis of liver tissue and is reported separately. The specimen is treated to isolate the DNA using direct probe.

87516

This test may be requested as HBV DNA by polymerase chain reaction. Hepatitis B is a retrovirus which can cause persistent infection leading to cirrhosis and hepatocellular carcinoma. Molecular (DNA) tests are useful in identifying potentially infectious individuals as well as chronic progression of the disease. Blood specimen is obtained by venipuncture. A liver biopsy is required for analysis of liver tissue and is reported separately. The specimen is treated to isolate the DNA and eliminate substances which inhibit amplification. The DNA is then amplified using a technique such as polymerase chain reaction (PCR).

87517

This test may be requested as HBV DNA quantification. Hepatitis B is a retrovirus which can cause persistent infection leading to cirrhosis and hepatocellular carcinoma. Blood specimen is obtained by venipuncture. A liver biopsy is required for analysis of liver tissue and is reported separately. Quantification is used primarily to monitor response to therapy in chronic hepatitis B. This code reports quantification only.

87520

This test may be requested as HCV RNA direct probe. Hepatitis C is also referred to as non-A non-B (NANB) hepatitis. Blood specimen is obtained by venipuncture. A liver biopsy is required for analysis of liver tissue and is reported separately. The specimen is treated to isolate the RNA using direct probe.This test is relatively difficult and expensive to perform and is used primarily by research facilities.

87521

This test may be requested as HCV RNA amplified probe or as HCV RNA RT-PCR. Hepatitis C is also referred to as non-A non-B (NANB) hepatitis. Blood specimen is obtained by venipuncture. A liver biopsy is required for analysis of liver tissue and is reported separately. Testing for HCV by amplified probe requires a molecular method referred to as reverse transcription polymerase chain reaction (RT-PCR). This test is relatively difficult and expensive to perform and is used primarily by research facilities.

87522

This test may be requested as HCV RNA quantification using molecular technique. Hepatitis C is also referred to as non-A non-B (NANB) hepatitis. Blood specimen is obtained by venipuncture. A liver biopsy is required for analysis of liver tissue and is reported separately. This code reports quantification only.

87525

This test may be requested as HGV-RNA direct probe. Blood specimen is obtained by venipuncture. A liver biopsy is required for analysis of liver tissue and is reported separately. The specimen is treated to isolate the RNA using direct probe. This test is relatively difficult and expensive to perform and is used primarily by research facilities. The precise role of HGV/GB-C in human disease is currently under investigation; however, HGV is associated with acute and chronic hepatitis and active infection has been observed to persist for up to nine years. HGV is transmissible via blood transfusion and also can be acquired by exposure to blood and blood products.

87526

This test may be requested as HGV RNA amplified probe or as HCGV RNA RT-PCR. Blood specimen is obtained by venipuncture. A liver biopsy is required for analysis of liver tissue and is reported separately. Testing for HGV by amplified probe requires a molecular method referred to as reverse transcription polymerase chain reaction (RT-PCR). This test is relatively difficult and expensive to perform and is used primarily by research facilities. The precise role of HGV/GB-C in human disease is currently under investigation; however, HGV is associated with acute and chronic hepatitis and active infection has been observed to persist for up to nine years. HGV is transmissible via blood transfusion and also can be acquired by exposure to blood and blood products.

87527

This test may be requested as HGV RNA quantification using molecular technique. Blood specimen is obtained by venipuncture. A liver biopsy is required for analysis of liver tissue and is reported separately. This code reports quantification only. The precise role of HGV/GB-C in human disease is currently under investigation; however, HGV is associated with acute and chronic hepatitis and active infection has been observed to persist for up to nine years. HGV is transmissible via blood transfusion and also can be acquired by exposure to blood and blood products.

87528

This test may be requested as HSV by direct DNA probe. Herpes simplex may be classified as HSV type 1 (HSV 1) or HSV type 2 (HSV 2). HSV 1 is primarily responsible for oral lesions frequently referred to as fever blisters or cold sores. HSV 2 is a sexually transmitted disease with lesions occurring primarily in the genitourinary tract. Lesion swab/scrapings are obtained. CSF is obtained by spinal puncture. Blood specimen is obtained by venipuncture. The specimen is treated to isolate the DNA using direct probe. Detection and typing (HSV1, HSV2) by direct DNA probe is superior to culture methods.

87529

This test may be requested as HSV by amplified DNA probe. Herpes simplex may be classified is HSV type 1 (HSV 1) or HSV type 2 (HSV 2). HSV 1 is primarily responsible for oral lesions frequently referred to as fever blisters or cold sores. HSV 2 is a sexually transmitted disease with lesions occurring primarily in the genitourinary tract. Lesion swab/scrapings are obtained. CSF is obtained by spinal puncture. Blood specimen is obtained by venipuncture. The specimen is treated to isolate the DNA and eliminate substances which inhibit amplification. The DNA is then amplified using a technique such as polymerase chain reaction (PCR). Detection and typing (HSV 1, HSV 2) by amplified DNA probe is superior to culture methods.

87530

This test may be requested as HSV quantification by molecular technique. Herpes simplex may be classified is HSV type 1 (HSV 1) or HSV type 2 (HSV 2). HSV 1 is primarily responsible for oral lesions frequently referred to as fever blisters or cold sores. HSV 2 is a sexually transmitted disease with lesions occurring primarily in the genitourinary tract. Lesion swab/scrapings are obtained. CSF is obtained by spinal puncture. Blood specimen is obtained by venipuncture. This code reports quantification only.

87531

This test may be requested as HHV-6 direct DNA probe. Human herpes virus-6 is most commonly associated with roseola in children, but also causes pnuemonitis, encephalitis, and hepatitis in immunosuppressed individuals. Sputum is obtained by deep coughing or by separately reportable aerosol induced technique. Respiratory fluids may also be obtained endoscopically using bronchial alveolar lavage which is reported separately. CSF is obtained by spinal puncture which is reported separately. Blood specimen is obtained by venipuncture. Liver tissue is obtained by biopsy which is also reported separately. The cells are lysed and DNA is extracted. HHV-6 DNA is identified by direct probe.

87532

This test may be requested as HHV-6 amplified DNA probe. Human herpes virus-6 is most commonly associated with roseola in children, but also causes pnuemonitis, encephalitis, and hepatitis in immunosuppressed individuals. Sputum is obtained by deep coughing or by separately reportable aerosol induced technique. Respiratory fluids may also be obtained endoscopically using bronchial alveolar lavage which is reported separately. CSF is obtained by spinal puncture which is reported separately. Blood specimen is obtained by venipuncture. Liver tissue is obtained by biopsy which is also reported separately. The cells are lysed and DNA is extracted. HHV-6 DNA is then amplified using specific primers.

87533

This test may be requested as HHV-6 quantification using nucleic acid technique. Human herpes virus-6 is most commonly associated with roseola in children, but also causes pnuemonitis, encephalitis, and hepatitis in immunosuppressed individuals. Sputum is obtained by deep coughing or by separately reportable aerosol induced technique. Respiratory fluids may also be obtained endoscopically using bronchial alveolar lavage which is reported separately. CSF is obtained by spinal puncture which is reported separately. Blood specimen is obtained by venipuncture. Liver tissue is obtained by biopsy which is also reported separately. The cells are lysed and DNA is extracted. This code reports quantification only.

87534

This test may be requested as human immunodeficiency virus Type 1 (HIV-1) by direct nucleic acid (DNA, RNA) probe. HIV is the causative agent of acquired immunodeficiency syndrome (AIDS). Blood specimen is obtained by venipuncture. A random urine sample is obtained. Tissue is obtained by separately reportable biopsy procedure. The specimen is treated to isolate the DNA using direct probe.

87535

This test may be requested as human immunodeficiency virus Type 1 (HIV-1) by amplified nucleic acid (DNA, RNA) probe or HIV-1 by PCR. HIV is the causative agent of acquired immunodeficiency syndrome (AIDS). Blood specimen is obtained by venipuncture. A random urine sample is obtained. Tissue is obtained by separately reportable biopsy procedure. The specimen is treated to isolate the DNA and eliminate substances which inhibit amplification. The DNA is amplified using a technique such as polymerase chain reaction (PCR).

87536

This test may be requested as human immunodeficiency virus Type 1 (HIV-1) nucleic acid (DNA, RNA) quantification. HIV is the causative agent of acquired immunodeficiency syndrome (AIDS). Blood specimen is obtained by venipuncture. A random urine sample is obtained. Tissue is obtained by separately reportable biopsy procedure. This code reports quantification only.

87537

This test may be requested as human immunodeficiency virus Type 2 (HIV-2) by EIA. HIV-2 is a retrovirus closely related to simian AIDS and found initially in West African nations and Portugal, but with cases also being reported in the United States since 1987. Blood specimen is obtained by venipuncture. The specimen is treated to isolate the DNA using direct probe.

87538

This test may be requested as human immunodeficiency virus Type 2 (HIV-2) by EIA. HIV-2 is a retrovirus closely related to simian AIDS and found initially in West African nations and Portugal, but with cases also being reported in the United States since 1987. Blood specimen is obtained by venipuncture. Infectious agent antigen detection by amplified DNA probe technique involves nonculture detection of infected cells. The specimen is treated to isolate the DNA and eliminate substances which inhibit amplification. The DNA is then amplified using a technique such as polymerase chain reaction (PCR).

CPT® Lay Descriptions

87539

This test may be requested as human immunodeficiency virus Type 2 (HIV-2) by EIA. HIV-2 is a retrovirus closely related to simian AIDS and found initially in West African nations and Portugal, but with cases also being reported in the United States since 1987. Blood specimen is obtained by venipuncture. This code reports quantification only.

87540

This test may also be requested as nucleic acid probe for Legionnaire's disease. The bacteria responsible for the disease, Legionella pneumophila, causes a fulminating pneumonia. It can also cause an influenza-like illness known as Pontiac fever. Sputum is obtained by deep coughing or by separately reportable aerosol induced technique. The specimen is treated to isolate nucleic acid using direct probe.

87541

This test may also be requested as nucleic acid probe for Legionnaire's disease. The bacteria responsible for the disease, Legionella pneumophila, causes a fulminating pneumonia. It can also cause an influenza-like illness known as Pontiac fever. Sputum is obtained by deep coughing or by separately reportable aerosol induced technique. The specimen is treated to isolate nucleic acids, in this case either the macrophage infectivity potentiator (mip) gene or the 5S rRNA gene, and eliminate substances which inhibit amplification. The nucleic acid is amplified using a technique such as polymerase chain reaction (PCR).

87542

This test may also be requested as nucleic acid quantification for Legionnaire's disease. The bacteria responsible for the disease, Legionella pneumophila, causes a fulminating pneumonia. It can also cause an influenza-like illness known as Pontiac fever. Sputum is obtained by deep coughing or by separately reportable aerosol induced technique. This code reports quantification only.

87550

This test may be requested as Mycobacterial direct DNA probe. Blood specimen is obtained by venipuncture. A random urine sample is obtained. Sputum is obtained by deep coughing or by separately reportable aerosol induced technique. Tissue is obtained in a separately reportable biopsy procedure. DNA is isolated directly from the specimen or following culture. The specimen is then treated to isolate the Mycobacterial species. The DNA probe is hybridized and the excess probe removed. The bound probe is then analyzed using chemiluminescence, color detection, or autoradiography.

87551

This test may be requested as Mycobacterial amplified DNA probe or Mycobacterial polymerase chain reaction (PCR). Blood specimen is obtained by

venipuncture. A random urine sample is obtained. Sputum is obtained by deep coughing or by separately reportable aerosol induced technique. Tissue is obtained in a separately reportable biopsy procedure. DNA is isolated directly from the specimen or following culture. The specimen is then treated to isolate the Mycobacterial species. DNA amplification is performed using PCR or transcription-based techniques. DNA amplification assay provides increased accuracy in diagnosis.

87552

This test may be requested as Mycobacterial nucleic acid quantification. Blood specimen is obtained by venipuncture. A random urine sample is obtained. Sputum is obtained by deep coughing or by separately reportable aerosol induced technique. Tissue is obtained in a separately reportable biopsy procedure. DNA is isolated directly from the specimen or following culture. The specimen is then treated to isolate the Mycobacterial species. This code reports quantification only.

87555

This test may be requested as tuberculosis (TB) test by direct nucleic acid probe. Tuberculosis was once diagnosed only by conventional culture techniques which required four to six weeks for identification of mycobacteria tuberculosis. Nucleic acid probes allow for accurate identification in as little as 36-48 hours. Sputum is obtained by deep coughing or by separately reportable aerosol induced technique. The specimen is treated to isolate nucleic acid using direct probe.

87556

This test may be requested as tuberculosis (TB) test by amplified nucleic acid probe. Tuberculosis was once diagnosed only by conventional culture techniques which required four to six weeks for identification of mycobacteria tuberculosis. Nucleic acid probes allow for accurate identification in as little as 36-48 hours. Sputum is obtained by deep coughing or by separately reportable aerosol induced technique. The specimen is treated to isolate nucleic acid using an amplified probe technique such as polymerase chain reaction (PCR). To enhance sensitivity PCR may be followed by oligonucleotide hybridization or nested PCR studies.

87557

This test may be requested as tuberculosis (TB) quantification by nucleic acid technique. Tuberculosis was once diagnosed only by conventional culture techniques which required four to six weeks for identification of mycobacteria tuberculosis. Nucleic acid probes allow for accurate identification in as little as 36-48 hours. Sputum is obtained by deep coughing or by separately reportable aerosol induced technique. This code reports quantification only.

87560

This test may be requested as Mycobacterial avium-intracellulare direct DNA probe. Blood specimen is obtained by venipuncture. A random urine sample is obtained. Sputum is obtained by deep coughing or by separately reportable aerosol induced technique. Tissue is obtained in a separately reportable biopsy procedure. DNA is isolated directly from the specimen or following culture. The specimen is treated to isolate Mycobacterial avium-intracellulare DNA. The DNA probe is hybridized and the excess probe removed. The bound probe is then analyzed using chemiluminescence, color detection, or autoradiography.

87561

This test may be requested as Mycobacterial avium-intracellulare amplified DNA probe or Mycobacterial avium-intracellulare polymerase chain reaction (PCR). Blood specimen is obtained by venipuncture. A random urine sample is obtained. Sputum is obtained by deep coughing or by separately reportable aerosol induced technique. Tissue is obtained in a separately reportable biopsy procedure. DNA is isolated directly from the specimen or following culture. The specimen is treated to isolate the Mycobacterial avium-intracellulare DNA. DNA amplification is performed using PCR or transcription-based techniques. DNA amplification assay provides increased accuracy in diagnosis.

87562

This test may be requested as Mycobacterial avium-intracellulare nucleic acid quantification. Blood specimen is obtained by venipuncture. A random urine sample is obtained. Sputum is obtained by deep coughing or by separately reportable aerosol induced technique. Tissue is obtained in a separately reportable biopsy procedure. DNA is isolated directly from the specimen or following culture. The specimen is then treated to isolate the Mycobacterial avium-intracellulare. This code reports quantification only.

87580

This test may be requested as Mycoplasma pneumoniae direct DNA probe. Mycoplasma pneumoniae is responsible for anywhere from one to eight percent of all community acquired pneumonias diagnosed each year. Infection may be mild to severe, but is rarely fatal. Sputum is obtained by deep coughing or by separately reportable aerosol induced technique. Specimen may also be obtained endoscopically using bronchial alveolar lavage which is reported separately. Direct nucleic acid probe is a rapid and sensitive test for Mycoplasma pneumoniae nucleic acids, specifically rRNA, in respiratory fluids. Cells must be lysed to release the Mycoplasma pneumoniae specific rRNA.

87581

This test may be requested as Mycoplasma pneumoniae amplified DNA probe. Mycoplasma pneumoniae is responsible for anywhere from one to eight percent of all community acquired pneumonias diagnosed each year. Infection may be mild to severe, but is rarely fatal. Sputum is obtained by deep coughing or by separately reportable aerosol induced technique. Specimen may also be obtained endoscopically using bronchial alveolar lavage which is reported separately. Nucleic acid probe is a rapid and sensitive test for Mycoplasma pneumoniae nucleic acids, specifically rRNA, in respiratory fluids. Cells must be lysed to release the Mycoplasma pneumoniae specific rRNA. They are then amplified using polymerase chain reaction (PCR).

87582

This test may be requested as Mycoplasma pneumoniae nucleic acid quantification. Mycoplasma pneumoniae is responsible for anywhere from 1-8% of all community acquired pneumonias diagnosed each year. Infection may be mild to severe, but is rarely fatal. Sputum is obtained by deep coughing or by separately reportable aerosol induced technique. Specimen may also be obtained endoscopically using bronchial alveolar lavage which is reported separately. Nucleic acid probe is a rapid and sensitive test for Mycoplasma pneumoniae nucleic acids, specifically rRNA, in respiratory fluids. Cells must be lysed to release the Mycoplasma pneumoniae specific rRNA. This code reports quantification only.

87590

This test may be requested as gonorrhea direct DNA probe, gonorrhea molecular probe assay, or DNA detection of gonorrhea. Neisseria gonorrhea is one of the most common sexually transmitted infections. In the past it was commonly diagnosed using conventional culture techniques. However, molecular (nucleic acid probe) techniques offer rapid, accurate identification of Neisseria gonorrhea. While an a cervical or urethral swab is preferred, molecular techniques are sensitive enough to detect the organism in urine also. Neisseria gonorrhea can be detected by DNA, RNA, or rRNA probes.

87591

This test may be requested as gonorrhea amplified DNA probe, gonorrhea molecular probe assay, or DNA detection of gonorrhea. Neisseria gonorrhea is one of the most common sexually transmitted infections. In the past it was commonly diagnosed using conventional culture techniques. However, molecular (nucleic acid probe) techniques offer rapid, accurate identification of Neisseria gonorrhea. While an a cervical or urethral swab is preferred, molecular techniques are sensitive enough to detect the organism in urine also. Neisseria gonorrhea can be detected by DNA or rRNA probes. Amplification can be performed using a number of techniques.

CPT ® Lay Descriptions

Polymerase chain reaction (PCR) and ligase chain reaction (LCR) detect gonorrhea DNA. An assay is also available which detects gonorrhea ribosomal RNA (rRNA)

87592

This test may be requested as gonorrhea nucleic acid quantification. Neisseria gonorrhea is one of the most common sexually transmitted infections. In the past it was commonly diagnosed using conventional culture techniques. However, molecular (nucleic acid probe) techniques offer rapid, accurate identification of Neisseria gonorrhea. While an a cervical or urethral swab is preferred, molecular techniques are sensitive enough to detect the organism in urine also. Neisseria gonorrhea can be detected by DNA or rRNA probes. This code reports quantification only.

87620

This test may be requested as human papillomavirus (HPV) direct DNA probe. Human papillomaviruses are a genus of viruses that causes warts (benign neoplasms of skin and mucous membranes). There are at least 58 known types which are identified as HPV-1 to HPV-58. HPV is commonly associated with both plantar and genital warts. HPV infection of the cervix is of particular concern as it may be associated with cervical cancer. The specimen is treated to encourage attachment of HPV DNA to filters. It is then probed with commercially available DNA probes for specific HPV types. DNA probes are specific for HPV types 6, 11, 16, 18, 31, 33, and 35.

87621

This test may be requested as human papillomavirus (HPV) amplified DNA probe. Human papillomaviruses are a genus of viruses that causes warts (benign neoplasms of skin and mucous membranes). There are at least 58 known types which are identified as HPV-1 to HPV-58. HPV is commonly associated with both plantar and genital warts. HPV infection of the cervix is of particular concern as it may be associated with cervical cancer. The specimen is treated to encourage attachment of HPV DNA to filters. DNA is then amplified by polymerase chain reaction (PCR) and probed for specific HPV types. DNA probes are only able to detect a limited number of HPV types, including types 6, 11, 16, 18, 31, 33, and 35.

87622

This test may be requested as human papillomavirus (HPV) amplified DNA probe. Human papillomaviruses are a genus of viruses that causes warts (benign neoplasms of skin and mucous membranes). There are at least 58 known types which are identified as HPV-1 to HPV-58. HPV is commonly associated with both plantar and genital warts. HPV infection of the cervix is of particular concern as it may be associated with cervical cancer. The specimen

is treated to encourage attachment of HPV DNA to filters. This code reports quantification only.

87650

This test may be requested as Streptococcus A by direct nucleic acid probe. Streptococcus A is a form of beta hemolytic streptococcus which causes pharyngitis. Untreated infection can cause rheumatic fever or glomerulonephritis. The specimen is treated to isolate the DNA using a direct probe.

87651

This test may be requested as Streptococcus A by amplified nucleic acid probe. Streptococcus A is a form of beta hemolytic streptococcus which causes pharyngitis. Untreated infection can cause rheumatic fever or glomerulonephritis. The specimen is treated to isolate the DNA and eliminate substances which inhibit amplification. The Streptococcus A DNA is amplified using specific primers.

87652

This test may be requested as Streptococcus A nucleic acid quantification. Streptococcus A is a form of beta hemolytic streptococcus which causes pharyngitis. Untreated infection can cause rheumatic fever or glomerulonephritis. This code reports quantification only.

87797

This code reports infectious agent detection by nucleic acid (DNA, RNA) direct probe for microorganisms that are not identified with a more specific code in range 87470-87652. Nucleic acid detection, also referred to as molecular pathology, is a rapidly developing diagnostic technique that is especially useful in identifying microorganisms which require tedious isolation and incubation and/or those which cannot be cultured. Another advantage of molecular methods is that they are able to detect infectious agents at much lower levels than required using other techniques. Direct probe involves isolating and identifying the infectious agent DNA or RNA. This involves cell lysis and extraction of the DNA using phenol or chloroform.

87798

This code reports infectious agent detection by nucleic acid (DNA, RNA) amplified probe for microorganisms that are not identified with a more specific code in range 87470-87652. Nucleic acid detection, also referred to as molecular pathology, is a rapidly developing diagnostic technique that is especially useful in identifying microorganisms which require tedious isolation and incubation and/or those which cannot be cultured. Another advantage of molecular methods is that they are able to detect infectious agents at much lower levels than required using other techniques. Amplified probe involves isolating and identifying the infectious agent DNA or RNA. This involves cell lysis and extraction of the

DNA using phenol or chloroform. The nucleic acids are then amplified using one of several techniques. Polymerase chain reaction (PCR) is the most frequently used amplification technique. Other techniques include ligase chain reaction (LCR) and the signal detection method (bDNA).

87799

This code reports infectious agent quantification using nucleic acid (DNA, RNA) technique for microorganisms that are not identified with a more specific code in range 87470-87652. Nucleic acid detection, also referred to as molecular pathology, is a rapidly developing diagnostic technique that is especially useful in identifying microorganisms which require tedious isolation and incubation and/or those which cannot be cultured. Another advantage of molecular methods is that they are able to detect infectious agents at much lower levels than required using other techniques. Quantification may be performed following direct or amplified probe. It measures the amount of the microorganism DNA/RNA present.

87800–87801

Code 87800 reports multiple infectious agent detection by nucleic acid (DNA or RNA) using direct probe technique. Nucleic acid detection, also referred to as molecular pathology, is a rapidly developing diagnostic technique that is especially useful in identifying microorganisms that require tedious isolation and incubation and/or those that cannot be cultured. Another advantage of molecular methods is that they are able to detect infectious agents at much lower levels than required using other techniques. A nucleic acid probe is a short strand of the unique DNA or RNA that is complementary for the base sequence of the test target. Cell lysis using phenol or chloroform is employed to extract the pathogenic DNA. The test is useful in that absolute specifity of hard-to-identify organisms can be attained. Report 87801 when the multiple DNA target sequences are amplified using any of several techniques, such as polymerase chain reaction (PCR), or ligase chain reaction (LCR), or signal detection (bDNA).

87802

Enzyme immunoassays (EIA) are methods for identifying organisms, extracellular toxins, and viral agents using protein and polysaccharide antigens. The test may my performed directly on clinical samples or after growth on agar plates or in viral cell cultures. The basis of detection is antigen-antibody binding. Cultures and impression smears for both aerobic and anaerobic infectious agents are commonly taken from involved lymph nodes, sputum, pleural fluid, cerebrospinal fluid (CSF), and spleen. EIA systems involve antibodies coupled to an enzyme in which antigen is detected by the development of a color when colorless substrate is converted to a colored product after an antigen-antibody reaction has

occurred. Direct optical microscopic observation allows for continuous direct observation of low-light or low-contrast samples in the presence of fluorescence.

87803

Clostridium difficile is the major cause of antibiotic-associated diarrhea and colitis and is the cause for virtually all cases of pseudo-membranous colitis (PMC). The organism is found in stools of most patients with these diseases. One gram of stool is collected and sent to the laboratory unpreserved. The fecal sample is dispersed in a diluent with antibodies for *Clostridium difficile* antigen to form a complex of antibody and antigen. A complex of antibody and antigen is separated from the specimen and exposed to a second antibody for the antigen, and a portion of the antibody. A sample from the first complex is bound to a solid carrier and a sample from the second antibody exposure is labeled with a detection agent to determine the presence of *Clostridium difficile* antigen in the original fecal specimen.

87804

Influenza, a highly contagious, acute viral infection of the respiratory tract, is caused by a single-strand RNA virus known as an influenza virus. An infection may be identified by direct detection of the virus in respiratory secretions (usually, collected within one week of onset of symptoms) using enzyme immunoassay with monoclonal antibodies to detect viral antigen in the sample.

87810

This test may be requested as an optical immunoassay for Chlamydia trachomatis. C. trachomatis is a frequently occurring sexually transmitted disease. It may cause nonspecific urethritis or pelvic inflammatory disease (PID), although it is frequently asymptomatic in women. Another serotype also causes conjunctivitis. This test reports detection using a competitive protein binding assay, where an antigen binds to an antibody which is fixed to a reflecting surface. This change in reflection can be observed directly as a color change.

87850

This test may be requested as an optical immunoassay for Neisseria gonorrhea. N. gonorrhea is one of the most common sexually transmitted infections. This test reports detection using a competitive protein binding assay where an antigen binds to an antibody which is fixed to a reflecting surface. This change in reflection can be observed directly as a color change.

87880

This test may be requested as an optical immunoassay for Streptococcus A. Streptococcus A is a form of beta hemolytic streptococcus which causes pharyngitis. Untreated infection can cause rheumatic fever or glomerulonephritis.This test reports detection using a competitive protein binding assay where an antigen binds to an antibody which is fixed to a reflecting surface. This change in reflection can be observed directly as a color change.

87899

This test may be requested as an optical immunoassay. This test reports detection using a competitive protein binding assay where an antigen binds to an antibody which is fixed to a reflecting surface. This change in reflection can be observed directly as a color change. This code should be reported when the infectious agent being tested does not have a more specific code.

87901–87904

Treatment of HIV requires the use of multiple antiviral drugs administered in combination to suppress viral replication. However, over time, the HIV virus can become resistent to one or more of the drugs used in the treatment regimen. This can be identified by increases in viral load and declines in CD4 counts. These codes are used to report assays that help identify HIV antiviral drug resistance. Code 87901 reports a genotype assay that can predict expected HIV drug resistance for most individuals. In code 87902, HCV DNA is isolated from patient specimens and amplified by polymerase chain reaction; one distinct gene segment shows amplification if HCV DNA is present. Anti-HBc IgM can be detected at about the same time clinical symptoms appear. Code 87903 reports a phenotype assay that may be required when newer drugs are being considered for treatment of HIV as newer drugs sometimes do not have sufficient data to predict expected outcomes based on genotype studies alone. Phenotype analysis reported by code 87903 includes drug resistance tissue culture analysis of up to 10 drugs. Report 87904 for each additional drug tested for a maximum of 5 additional drugs.

88000

This code reports the examination of a body after death. The body is dissected. The organs and tissues (excluding the brain and central nervous system) are systematically examined and described. This is usually done to determine the cause of death, to improve diagnosis and treatment of diseases, or to benefit family members in cases of heritable illnesses.

88005

This code reports the examination of a body after death. The body is dissected. The organs and tissues are systematically examined and described, including the brain. This is usually done to determine the cause of death, to improve diagnosis and treatment of diseases, or to benefit family members in cases of heritable illnesses.

88007

This code reports the examination of a body after death. The body is dissected. The organs and tissues

are systematically examined and described, including the brain and spinal cord. This is usually done to determine the cause of death, to improve diagnosis and treatment of diseases, or to benefit family members in cases of heritable illnesses.

88012

This code reports the examination of an infant's body after death (birth through 12th month). The body is dissected. The organs and tissues are systematically examined and described, including the brain. This is usually done to determine the cause of death, to improve diagnosis and treatment of diseases, or to benefit family members in cases of heritable illnesses.

88014

This code reports the examination of a newborn's body after death (birth through 28th day), or the examination of a stillborn fetus. The body is dissected. The organs and tissues are systematically examined and described, including the brain. This is usually done to determine the cause of death, to improve diagnosis and treatment of diseases, or to benefit family members in cases of heritable illnesses.

88016

This code reports the examination of a stillborn fetus whose body tissues have become softened, as happens when there is a delay from the time of death in utero to the delivery. The body is dissected. The organs and tissues are systematically examined and described, including the brain. This is usually done to determine the cause of death, to improve diagnosis and treatment of diseases, or to benefit family members in cases of heritable illnesses.

88020

This code reports the examination of a body after death. The body is dissected. The organs and tissues are systematically examined (gross and microscopic) and described (except the brain and central nervous system). Representative samples from the organs are taken and microscopically examined and described. Laboratory tests may also be performed on tissue samples. This is usually done to determine the cause of death, to improve diagnosis and treatment of diseases, or to benefit family members in cases of heritable illnesses.

88025

This code reports the examination of a body after death. The body is dissected. The organs and tissues are systematically examined (gross and microscopic) and described (including the brain). Representative samples from the organs are taken and microscopically examined and described. Laboratory tests may also be performed on tissue samples. This is usually done to determine the cause of death, to improve diagnosis and treatment of diseases, or to benefit family members in cases of heritable illnesses.

88027

This code reports the examination of a body after death. The body is dissected. The organs and tissues are systematically examined (gross and microscopic) and described (including the brain and spinal cord). Representative samples from the organs are taken and microscopically examined and described. Laboratory tests may also be performed on tissue samples. This is usually done to determine the cause of death, to improve diagnosis and treatment of diseases, or to benefit family members in cases of heritable illnesses.

88028

This code reports the examination of an infant's body after death (birth through 12th month). The body is dissected. The organs and tissues are systematically examined (gross and microscopic) and described (including the brain). Representative samples from the organs are taken and microscopically examined and described. Laboratory tests may also be performed on tissue samples. This is usually done to determine the cause of death, to improve diagnosis and treatment of diseases, or to benefit family members in cases of heritable illnesses.

88029

This code reports the examination of a newborn's body after death (birth through 28th day), or the examination of a stillborn fetus. The body is dissected. The organs and tissues are systematically examined (gross and microscopic) and described (including the brain). Representative samples from the organs are taken and microscopically examined and described. Laboratory tests may also be performed on tissue samples. This is usually done to determine the cause of death, to improve diagnosis and treatment of diseases, or to benefit family members in cases of heritable illnesses.

88036

This code reports the examination of a body after death. The body is dissected. Certain organs and tissues within a system or region of the body are systematically examined (gross and microscopic) and described. Representative samples from the organs are taken and microscopically examined and described. Laboratory tests may also be performed on tissue samples. This is usually done to determine the cause of death, to improve diagnosis and treatment of diseases, or to benefit family members in cases of heritable illnesses.

88037

This code reports the examination of a body after death. The body is dissected. A single organ and its related tissues are systematically examined (gross and microscopic) and described. Representative samples from the organ are taken and microscopically examined and described. Laboratory tests may also be performed on organ tissue samples. This is usually done to determine the cause of death, to improve

diagnosis and treatment of diseases, or to benefit family members in cases of heritable illnesses.

88040

This code reports the examination of a body after death. The body is dissected. The organs and tissues are systematically examined (gross and microscopic) and described. Representative samples from the organs are taken and microscopically examined and described. Laboratory tests may also be performed on tissue samples. This is usually done for the purpose of gathering and preserving evidence for presentation in a court of law.

88045

A coroner is a public official, either elected or appointed, who investigates the causes and circumstances of deaths that occur within a specific legal jurisdiction (i.e., county). Coroners may be called only to deaths that may have resulted from unnatural causes. However, in many jurisdictions coroners must present themselves and sign death certificates of all persons who die while not under the care of a physician. In some instances, a preliminary gross exam is performed on-site and procedural arrangements are made for a more thorough examination under laboratory conditions. As with all codes in the postmortem examination range, 88045 reports physician services. Only four states require coroners to be physicians. A medical examiner is a physician.

88099

This code reports the examination of a body after death that in some aspect fails to fit any of the above categories.

88104–88107

This test has many different names, depending on the type of specimen obtained for analysis (e.g. bronchial cytology, esophageal cytology, etc). Specimen is obtained by separately reportable washing or brushing procedure. Code 88104 reports cytopathology evaluation of smear specimens, including alcohol fixed, Papanicolaou, direct smear with 95 percent ethanol, or liquid fixative; 88106 is for filter method only and 88107 reports cytopathology evaluation of specimen(s) using both smear and filtration techniques.

88108

This test may also be identified as bronchial aspirate cytology and bronchial wash cytology. Specimen collection is by bronchoscopy. Post-bronchoscopy specimen is recommended. An expectorant cough sample may be taken. Method is concentration technique, such as Saccomanno; specimen is collected in a cytologic fixative and an antibiotic. Sputum is collected into a solution of 50 percent ethanol and two percent polyethelene glycol.

CPT® Lay Descriptions

88125

Biological samples are studied using techniques common to DNA testing, such as fluorescent staining techniques. Forensic pathology is the pathology application to legal purposes. Forensic scientists study biological evidence at crime scenes, such as hair samples, blood, and sperm for DNA testing to assist in the inclusion or the exclusion of an individual in the crime.

88130

This screening test will identify the presence or lack of sex chromatin. Specimen collection is by buccal mucosa scraping, though the first scraping should be discarded. Specimen should be fixated with 95 percent ethanol. Method is by smear and microscopy. Examination of cells obtained by amniocentesis for the presence or absence of sex chromatin is a technique used to determine the infant's sex prior to birth.

88140

Fluorescent staining techniques are used to identify a Barr body in a polymorphonuclear leukocyte. In females one of the two X chromosome remains tightly coiled. In some nuclei the coiled chromosome is visible as a small dense mass known as a Barr body. The Barr body in the inner aspect of the nuclear membrane, but in the lobulated nucleus of the polymorphonuclear leukocyte it can be seen as a protrusion, often in the shape of a "drumstick."

88141

This test is for the interpretation by a physician of a Papanicolaou (Pap) smear.

88142–88145

This test may be identified by the name "thin prep." Specimen collection is by cervical or endocervical scraping or aspiration of vaginal fluid. This method saves physician time by eliminating the need for the physician to prepare a smear. The physician obtaining the specimen places the specimen in a preservative suspension. Then at the laboratory, special instruments take the cells in the preservative suspension and "plate-out" a monolayer for screening. Screening, defined as the careful review of the specimen for abnormal cells, may then be accomplished by any of four different methods, including the relatively new method of computer imaging. Code selection is based on the screening process used, with manual screening under physician supervision being reported with code 88142, manual screening and rescreening under physician supervision with code 88143, manual screening and computer-assisted rescreening under physician supervision with code 88144, manual screening and computer-assisted rescreening using cell selection and review under physician supervision with code 88145.

88147–88148

These tests may be identified as a cervical smear, Pap smear, or vaginal cytology. Specimen collection is by cervical or endocervical scraping or aspiration of vaginal fluid. Method is microscopy examination of a spray or liquid fixated smear. Screening, defined as the careful review of the specimen for abnormal cells, may then be accomplished by any of two different methods both of which involve the use automated systems. Code 88147 should be used to report smears screened by automated system under physician supervision, while code 88148 reports automated screening with manual rescreening under physician supervision.

88150–88154

This test may also be identified as a cervical smear, Pap smear, or vaginal cytology. Specimen collection is by scraping or brushing the cervix or endocervix, or aspiration of vaginal fluid. Method is microscopy examination of a spray or liquid fixated smear. Screening, defined as the careful review of the specimen for abnormal cells, may then be accomplished by any of four different methods, including the relatively new method of computer imaging. These codes should be reported when the any system other than the Bethesda System of evaluating and describing cervical/vaginal cytopathology slides is used. One such reporting system involves designating the level cervical intraepithelial neoplasia (CIN) with designations defined as follows: CIN 1 (mild and mild-to-moderate dysplasia), CIN 2 (moderate and moderate-to-severe dysplasia), CIN 3 (severe dysplasia and carcinoma in situ). Code selection is based on the screening process used, with manual screening under physician supervision being reported with code 88150, manual screening and computer-assisted rescreening under physician supervision with code 88152, manual screening and rescreening under physician supervision with code 88153, manual screening and computer-assisted rescreening using cell selection and review under physician supervision with code 88154.

88155

This test may also be identified as the maturation index and cytologic estrogen effect. Specimen collection is by tongue depressor or wooden spatula of the lateral vaginal wall. Method is microscopy examination of a spray or liquid fixated smear. The test may be used to determine the balance of estrogen and progesterone of the vaginal squamous epithelium.

88160–88162

Specimen collection is by separately reportable percutaneous needle biopsy. Methods include microscopy examination of smears or a centrifuge specimen. These codes report the pathology examination portion of the procedure only. Code 88160 reports screening and interpretation only. Code 88161 reports preparation, screening and interpretation. Code 88162 reports an extended study involving over 5 slides and/or multiple stains.

88164–88167
This test may be identified as a cervical smear, Pap smear, or vaginal cytology. Specimen collection is by scraping or brushing the cervix or endocervix, or aspiration of vaginal fluid. Method is microscopy examination of a spray or liquid coated smear. Screening, defined as the careful review of the specimen for abnormal cells, may then be accomplished by any of four different methods, including the relatively new method of computer imaging. These codes should be reported when the Bethesda System of evaluating and describing cervical/vaginal cytopathology slides is used. The Bethesda System includes evaluation of the following: adequacy of specimen, general categorization (optional), descriptive diagnosis, and description of any epithelial cell abnormalities (squamous and glandular cells). Code selection is based on the screening process used, with manual screening under physician supervision being reported with code 88164, manual screening and rescreening under physician supervision with code 88165, manual screening and computer-assisted rescreening under physician supervision with code 88166, manual screening and computer-assisted rescreening using cell selection and review under physician supervision with code 88167.

88172–88173
These codes are used to report the pathology examination portion of the fine needle aspirate procedure only. Code 88172 reports the immediate cytohistologic evaluation to determine the adequacy of the specimen(s). Code 88173 reports the final interpretation and report.

88180–88182
This test may also be identified as lymphocyte immunophenotyping or fluorescence activated cell sorting. Specimen collection is by biopsy or needle biopsy for tissue and bone marrow; blood is drawn by venipuncture. Methodology may involve flow cytometry investigation of a fluorochrome-stained single cell. For each cell surface, cytoplasmic or nuclear marker, report 88180; for cell cycle or DNA analysis, report 88182.

88230
This code is used to report lymphocyte culture for nonneoplastic disorders, which would include chromosome analysis as well as other cytogenetic studies. Cytogenetics is the branch of genetics that studies cellular (cyto) structure and function as it relates to heredity (genetics). White blood cells, specifically T-lymphocytes, are the most commonly used specimen for chromosome analysis. A peripheral blood specimen is obtained by venipuncture. The blood is then separated into its cellular constituents

and the white blood cells are extracted. The white blood cells are then placed in a tissue culture medium. White blood cells, specifically T-lymphocytes, are then stimulated with phytohemaglutinnin (PHA) and grown in the tissue culture.

88233
This code is used to report culturing of skin cells or other solid tissue cells for evaluation of nonneoplastic disorders, which would include chromosome analysis as well as other cytogenetic studies. Cytogenetics is the branch of genetics that studies cellular (cyto) structure and function as it relates to heredity (genetics). Skin cells may be obtained by buccal smear or separately reportable biopsy. Solid tissue specimen requires separately reportable biopsy. Skin or other solid tissue cells are then placed in a tissue culture medium. The cells are stimulated and grown in the tissue culture.

88235
This code is used to report culturing of fetal cells for evaluation of nonneoplastic disorders, which would include chromosome analysis as well as other cytogenetic studies. Cytogenetics is the branch of genetics that studies cellular (cyto) structure and function as it relates to heredity (genetics). Fetal cells are normally cultured to detect chromosome abnormalities and sex-linked disorders. A separately reportable amniocentesis or chorionic villus sampling is performed. Fetal cells are then placed in a tissue culture medium. The cells are stimulated and grown in the tissue culture. Culture and growth of an adequate number of fetal cells for analysis may require two to three weeks.

88237
This code is used to report tissue culture only of bone marrow or blood cells for the purpose of evaluating neoplastic, usually malignant, disorders. Many neoplastic disorders have a genetic origin and therefore cytogenetic studies aid in diagnosis and are prognostic indicators. In addition, they may help identify individuals at high risk for developing certain cancers. Bone marrow is obtained by separately reportable biopsy. Blood specimen is obtained by venipuncture. The marrow and blood cells may be separated by cell type. The cells are then placed in a tissue culture medium, which stimulates cell growth.

88239
This code is used to report tissue culture only of solid tumor cells for the purpose of evaluating neoplastic, usually malignant, disorders. Many neoplastic disorders have a genetic origin and therefore cytogenetic studies aid in diagnosis and are prognostic indicators. Translocations and deletions of nuclear DNA are especially common in the chromosomes of tumor cells, which makeup is different from that of normal somatic cells. This code reports cell culture

prepared from a biopsied or resected solid tumor. The cells are placed in a tissue culture medium, which stimulates cell growth.

88240

Cryopreservation is a technique of freezing and maintaining cells at extremely low temperatures to preserve the genetic and metabolic properties of the cell. Cryopreservation is performed to allow storage of cells for subsequent culture and analysis at a reference laboratory. Report this code for each cell line. A cell line is considered one that holds the potential for indefinite subculture in a lab setting.

88241

Cells frozen by cryopreservation are thawed and expanded (amplified) for study. Report each aliquot separately. An aliquot refers to the equal division of a sample of a substance, with each part related quantitatively to each other and to the sample as a whole.

88245

This cytogenetic study may be requested as a chromosome breakage analysis, sister chromatid exchange (SCE) study, or a chromosome instability test. This test involves evaluation for increased sister chromatid exchange (SCE) of 20 to 25 cells. This exchange refers to the crossing over of genetic information between the sister chromatids. Chromatids are the identical threadlike filaments of a chromosome joined by a common centromere, which are present during cell division. This analysis is specifically for chromosome breakage syndromes, which are characterized by an increased rate of SCE during cell division where exact duplication of the genetic information in each chromatid fails to occur. Instead, genetic information is rearranged between the sister chromatids during cell division. This test would normally use more traditional techniques, such as direct microscopic analysis of cells arrested in metaphase.

88248

This test may be requested by the name of the specific breakage syndrome being evaluated. Examples include Ataxia-telangiectasia (A-T) breakage study, Fanconi anemia (FA) breakage study, Fragile X breakage study, and Xeroderma pigmentosum (XP) chromosome breakage study. It may also be requested simply as a chromosome breakage study or chromosome instability study. Chromosome breakage syndromes are characterized by fragile sites along the chromosome that may appear as bent or partially detached fragments. The specific location of the fragile site determines the characteristics of the specific syndrome. For example, Fragile X is a breakage syndrome found in males carrying an X chromosome that has a fragile site at the bands of chromosome q27 and q28. The syndrome is associated with a moderate degree of intellectual

delay. The procedure includes collecting 50 to 100 cells, counting 20, and performing two karyotypes. Karyotype is the full chromosome set that genetically defines an individual. The term is also used for the standardized visual maps of chromosomal makeup, a technique used in identifying and organizing abnormalities. This test would normally use more traditional techniques, such as direct microscopic analysis of cells arrested in metaphase.

88249

This code reports a specific technique for analysis of breakage syndromes involving clastogen stress. Clastogen is a substance (e.g., chemical or radiation) that causes chromosome breakage when applied to the cell. Some substances that can be used as clastogens include diepoxybutane, mitomycin C, ionizing radiation, and UV radiation. When applied to the cells, these clastogens will identify fragile sites on the chromosome. The location of the fragile site is used to diagnose the specific breakage syndrome. The code includes the scoring of 100 cells.

88261–88262

These codes are reported for chromosome analysis to detect certain inherited disorders or syndromes, excluding breakage syndromes. The chromosomes of individuals with suspected genetic anomalies and neoplastic disorders are analyzed to provide definitive diagnosis. In addition, suspected carriers may be analyzed for recessive traits that may affect, or have affected, their offspring. Code 88261 should be reported for a five-cell count and one karyotype, with banding. Code 88262 should be reported for a 15 to 20 cell count and two karyotypes, with banding. Karyotype is the full chromosome set that genetically define an individual. The term is also used for the standardized visual maps of chromosomal makeup, a technique used in identifying and organizing abnormalities. Banding refers to the appearance of stripes on stained paired bundles of chromosomes. DNA bands are arranged in a vertical column and are typically composed of one DNA band representing the maternal chromosome and one representing the paternal chromosome. This test would normally use more traditional techniques, such as direct microscopic analysis of cells arrested in metaphase.

88263

This code is reported for chromosome analysis of 45 cells for the presence of mosaicism. It includes two karyotypes with banding. Mosaicism refers to alterations in chromosomes that do not affect every somatic (non-sex cell) chromosome, but are manifested during embryonic development. The individual is said to have two or more cell lines of different genetic or chromosomal make-up. Karyotype is the full chromosome set that genetically define an individual. The term is also used for the standardized visual maps of chromosomal makeup, a technique used in identifying and organizing abnormalities.

Banding refers to the appearance of stripes on stained paired bundles of chromosomes. DNA bands are arranged in a vertical column and are typically composed of one DNA band representing the maternal chromosome and one representing the paternal chromosome. This test would normally use more traditional techniques, such as direct microscopic analysis of cells arrested in metaphase.

88264

This test reports chromosome analysis related to malignant neoplasms (cancer). Cancer cytogenetics requires complete analysis (not just counting) of 20-25 cells. Chromosome analysis is performed to identify specific chromosomal anomalies, which can aid in diagnosis and provide prognostic indicators for certain cancers. In addition, identification of aberrant chromosomal bands provides information on the specific genes affected in certain malignancies. Individuals with family histories indicating a high risk for certain types of cancer can be tested to determine whether they carry the aberrant bands.

88267

This is a prenatal technique used to analyze chromosomes from cells of extracted amniotic fluid or chorionic villus for possible genetic abnormalities that can be detected during embryonic development. The code includes a 15-cell count, one karyotype, with banding. Karyotype is the full chromosome set that genetically define an individual. The term is also used for the standardized visual maps of chromosomal makeup, a technique used in identifying and organizing abnormalities. Banding refers to the appearance of stripes on stained paired bundles of chromosomes. DNA bands are arranged in a vertical column and are typically composed of one DNA band representing the maternal chromosome and one representing the paternal chromosome. This test would normally use more traditional techniques, such as direct microscopic analysis of cells arrested in metaphase with Giemsa or quinacrine banding techniques.

88269

This is a prenatal technique used to analyze intact chromosomes within the cells of amniotic fluid for possible genetic abnormalities that can be detected during embryonic development. The code includes a cell count from six to 12 colonies, one karyotype, with banding. Karyotype is the full chromosome set that genetically define an individual. The term is also used for the standardized visual maps of chromosomal makeup, a technique used in identifying and organizing abnormalities. Banding refers to the appearance of stripes on stained paired bundles of chromosomes. DNA bands are arranged in a vertical column and are typically composed of one DNA band representing the maternal chromosome and one representing the paternal chromosome. By studying the occurrence of different DNA bands in the

population, one can calculate the probability of two DNA samples matching one another. Any number of methods may be used, including polymerase chain reaction (PCR), restriction fragment length polymorphism (RFLP), and Northern or Southern blot.

88271

Molecular cytogenetics represent relatively new techniques capable of detecting changes in chromosomes that cannot be detected by traditional microscopic techniques. This code reports the use of a DNA probe to identify chromosomal abnormalities. Fluorescent in situ hybridization (FISH), is one type of DNA probe. It allows chromosomes and genes to be analyzed simultaneously. It utilizes fluorescent molecules to dye chromosomes or portions of chromosomes. The fluorescent dye is the genetic or DNA probe. When applied to the specimen, the very specific fluorescent genetic probe will attach itself only to its exact copy. For example, a probe containing a specific colon-cancer gene will attach to and light up only an identical colon-cancer gene. In situ hybridization involves treating native double-stranded DNA to render it single-stranded. The strand is then incubated to allow the strand to recognize complementary bases and to reform as a double-strand (hybridization). When a strand is radioactively marked, it is the "probe." The specificity to which the hybridization takes place is carefully analyzed.

88272–88273

Molecular cytogenetics represent relatively new techniques capable of detecting changes in chromosomes that cannot be detected by traditional microscopic techniques. In situ hybridization is the base pairing of a sequence of DNA to chromosomes on a microscope slide. The technique involves printing thousands of protein-coded DNA (cDNA) clones on a single microscope slide. Fluorescent cDNA probes prepared from any cell or tissue source of interest are paired to provide a large scale view of gene expression. In situ hybridization is used to determine the consequences of a given genetic alteration on gene expression. Report 88272 when three to five cells are analyzed usually to identify derivatives and markers. A genetic marker is a segment of DNA with an identifiable physical location on a chromosome. Markers are often used as an indirect way of tracking the hereditary pattern of genes, since DNA segments that lie near each other on a chromosome tend to be inherited together. Report 88273 when 10 to 30 cells are analyzed usually for the purpose of identifying microdeletions. A microdeletion involves the removal or acquired absence of one or more nucleotides from a gene or chromosome.

88274–88275

Molecular cytogenetics represent relatively new techniques capable of detecting changes in chromosomes that cannot be detected by traditional microscopic techniques. In situ hybridization is the base pairing of a sequence of DNA to chromosomes on a microscope slide. The technique involves printing thousands of protein-coded (cDNA) clones on a single microscope slide. Fluorescent cDNA probes prepared from any cell or tissue source of interest are paired to provide a large scale view of gene expression. In situ hybridization is used to determine the consequences of a given genetic alteration on gene expression. Report 88274 for in situ hybridization techniques used during interphase (resting phase) of cell division, for analyzing 25 to 99 cells. When 100 to 300 cells are analyzed report 88275.

88280

This code is reported for chromosome analysis to detect certain disorders or syndromes that may be inherited. The chromosomes of individuals with suspected genetic anomalies and neoplastic disorders are analyzed to provide definitive diagnosis. In addition, suspected carriers may be analyzed for recessive traits that may affect, or have affected, their offspring. This code is used for each additional karyotype beyond the number stipulated in other chromosome analysis codes in this same section of CPT® 1999. Karyotype is the full chromosome set that genetically define an individual. The term is also used for the standardized visual maps of chromosomal makeup, a technique used in identifying and organizing abnormalities. This test would usually involve more traditional microscopic techniques.

88283–88285

These codes are used for chromosome analysis to detect certain disorders or syndromes that may be inherited. The chromosomes of individuals with suspected genetic anomalies and neoplastic disorders are analyzed to provide definitive diagnosis. In addition, suspected carriers may be analyzed for recessive traits that may affect, or have affected, their offspring. Code 88283 is used for each additional karyotype specialized banding technique, such as NOR and C-banding. Banding refers to the appearance of stripes on stained paired bundles of chromosomes. DNA bands are arranged in a vertical column and are typically composed of one DNA band representing the maternal chromosome and one representing the paternal chromosome. C-banding is a method of identifying banding patterns based on nucleic acid content and staining. Report 88285 for additional cells counted, each study. This test would usually involve more traditional microscopic techniques.

88289

This code is used for chromosome analysis to detect certain disorders or syndromes that may be inherited. The chromosomes of individuals with suspected genetic anomalies and neoplastic disorders are analyzed to provide definitive diagnosis. In addition,

suspected carriers may be analyzed for recessive traits that may affect, or have affected, their offspring. This code is used for each additional high resolution study.

88291

This code is used to report physician interpretation and report of complex cytogenetic and molecular cytogenetic tests or when abnormal cytogenetic tests require complex interpretations.

88300

This procedure may be called a gross pathology exam or gross exam of tissue. The exam may not be specifically ordered ahead of time; rather, the tissue is harvested in the course of a surgery and sent for routine lab evaluation. Tissue is submitted in a container labeled with the source, preoperative diagnosis, and patient identification information. Specimens from separate sites must be submitted in separate containers, each labeled with the tissue source.

88302

This examination may be ordered as a gross and microscopic pathology exam or a gross and microscopic tissue exam. The exam may not be specifically ordered ahead of time; rather, the tissue is harvested in the course of a surgery and sent for routine lab evaluation. Tissue is submitted in a container labeled with the tissue source, preoperative diagnosis, and patient identification information. Specimens from separate sites must be submitted in separate containers, each labeled with the tissue source. This procedure is used to describe examination of tissues presumed normal. It includes both a gross and microscopic examination with the microscopic exam mainly to confirm the tissue is free of disease. Examples of its use might include tissues from a fallopian tube or vas deferens performed in the course of sterilization procedures, newborn foreskin following circumcision, hernia sac, hydrocele sac, etc.

88304–88309

This examination would be ordered as a gross and microscopic pathology exam or a gross and microscopic tissue exam. Tissue is submitted in a container labeled with the tissue source, preoperative diagnosis, and patient identification information. Specimens from separate sites must be submitted in separate containers, each labeled with the tissue source. Codes 88304-88309 describe levels of service for specimens requiring additional levels of work due to a presumed presence of disease. Code 88304 describes the lowest level of complexity for diseased or abnormal tissue with each subsequent code (88305, 88307, and 88309) describing in ascending order higher levels of complexity and physician work. Specific types of disease and tissue sites are listed for each code in the CPT® description.

88311

This procedure is performed in addition to the basic surgical pathology examination (88302-88309) on specimens requiring decalcification for accurate evaluation. When calcium is present in the tissue, the specimen is too hard to be properly sectioned for microscopic evaluation. Using an acid solution, calcareous matter is removed from bone and other tissue (decalcification). The specimen is then bathed in a solution to remove calcium ions via an ion exchange. This process may take hours or days depending on the specimen. Decalcification is commonly performed in bone marrow biopsy.

88312–88314

These codes report special stains used in the evaluation of some tissue specimens. Depending on the type of specimen and the reason for the pathology examination, different stains may be required to highlight or outline cells for identification. Code 88312 reports Group I stains for microorganisms; 88313 reports Group II stains for all other conditions excluding immunocytochemistry and immunoperoxidase. Examples of Group II stains include Ziehl-Neelsen, acid phosphatase stain with and without tartrate, alpha-naphthyl esterase stain with and without fluoride, amyloid, ASD chloroacetate esterase stain, nonspecific esterase, PAS stain, and sudan black stain. Code 88314 reports histochemical staining with frozen sections.

88318–88319

These codes report additional histochemistry services performed with basic pathology services. Code 88318 reports determinative tests for chemical components (e.g., copper, zinc), while 88319 reports determinative tests for enzyme constituents, each constituent. An example of a specimen that might require histochemistry for enzyme constituents (88319) is a muscle biopsy.

88321–88325

A pathology consultation involves an opinion or advice on the presence or absence of diseased or abnormal tissue provided at the request of another physician. These three codes report consultations and written interpretations on slide(s) or material(s) referred from another facility or source. Code 88321 reports a consultation and written report on slide(s) prepared by another source; 88323 reports a consultation and written report on material referred from another source requiring routine preparation of slides by the consultant; and 88325 reports a comprehensive consultation with review of records, evaluation of specimens requiring more complex slide preparation, and a written report.

88329

The procedure may also be referred to as an intraoperative pathology exam. A pathology consultation involves an opinion or advice on the presence or absence of diseased or abnormal tissue provided at the request of another physician. This code describes a pathology consultation during the course of a surgery, and includes only a gross examination of tissue without concurrent microscopic examination. Intraoperative consultations are performed to assist the surgeon in determining immediate surgical course.

88331–88332

These procedures may also be referred to as an intraoperative pathology exam with frozen section (FS). A pathology consultation involves an opinion or advice on the presence or absence of diseased or abnormal tissue provided at the request of another physician. These codes describe such a pathology consultation during the course of a surgery. The codes include a gross examination of tissue and frozen sections, including a written interpretation of findings. The specimen is immediately frozen in a cold liquid or cold environment (-20 to -70 C) to facilitate sectioning with a microtome. The specimen is sectioned using a cryostat which is a refrigerated box containing a microtome. Once sectioned, the tissues are placed on a slide, stained and examined microscopically. Code 88331 reports examination of a single block of tissue; 88332 reports each additional block of tissue from the same specimen. Intraoperative consultations are performed to assist the surgeon in determining immediate surgical course.

88342

This procedure is also referred to as immunostain or peroxidase-antiperoxidase (PAP). It is a technique used to identify specific antigens found in tumor cells. It is used primarily for the diagnosis of poorly differentiated neoplasms. There are several methods of performing immunocytochemistry tests; however, all involve treating the specimen with a tumor specific antibody, incubation, and subsequent washing of the specimen to remove unbound antibody. The specimen is then examined for positive and negative responses. Multiple immunostains are normally performed on each specimen to more specifically identify the suspect neoplasm by providing known positive and negative responses specific to that neoplasm.

88346–88347

Immunofluorescent studies may be performed using either a direct or indirect technique. The direct method, also referred to as a direct fluorescent antibody (DFA), involves the use of biopsied tissues. The indirect method, also referred to as indirect fluorescent antibody (IFA), involves the use of serum. Both involve introduction of fluorescein-tagged antibodies. Antibodies used are dependent upon tissue being examined and the suspected diagnosis, but may include IgG, IgM, IgA, C3, C4, C1q, properdin, fibrin, fibrinogen, and albumin. The specimen is then examined under fluorescent microscopy for intensity, pattern, and distribution of immunoglobulins.

88348–88349

These procedures are also referred to as electron microscopy (EM), transmission electron microscopy, or ultrastructural study. They are used primarily for the diagnosis of neoplasms when other techniques have failed to provide a definitive diagnosis. Tissues are prepared and fixed in a plastic polymer. Initially, thick sections (1 micron) are cut and stained to identify best specimen sites for further study. Subsequently, thin sections are cut and prepared with electron dense stain. The specimens are then examined using electron microscopy. Code 88348 reports diagnostic EM. Code 88349 reports scanning EM.

88355–88358

These procedures may also be referred to as histomorphometry. Methodology is by flow cytometry or quantitative image analysis system. Cells are stained and the histologic organization, including structure, composition, and function, is evaluated.

88362

Teased fiber evaluation is a technique used in specialty neuropathology labs. Peripheral nerves are often encased in a myelin sheath. This lipid-like substance is important to nerve function and can be an element in diagnostic evaluation. The technique involves biopsy collection, usually under local anesthetic. Light and electron microscopy are usually employed. Individual nerve fibers are "teased" from surrounding tissues to analyze myelinated nerve fiber size, distribution, and density.

88365

Also known as DNA-to-DNA homology, or simply ISH. In situ hybridization involves comparing double-stranded DNA from a test strain with that of a control strain. Both samples are treated to render them single-stranded. The test strand is marked, often with a radioisotope marker. The control DNA may be treated with a separately reportable nylon-type support process before mixing of the two strains. Pairing (or hybridization) of the single strands then occurs. The amount of pairing is measured and is indicative of the genomic relationship between the two. Techniques will include light microscopy and neutral buffered formalin-fixed paraffin-embedded tissues.

88371–88372

Western blot is an immunoassay technique that detects and confirms certain viral antibodies. Protein analysis of tissue involves separation of protein and glycoprotein components by electrophoresis. For certain diagnoses, polyacrylamid gel electrophresis is used to create substrate bands that are transferred by electrophoretic blotting to a membrane. Patient serum is placed on the substrate strips and any of the targeted antibodies present will bind to the viral antigens. Report 88372 when the protein analysis of tissue by Western blot includes an immunological probe for band identification. The band patterns are visualized by immunohistochemical methods. Either service requires interpretation and written report.

88380

Laser capture microdissection (LCM) is a method for procuring pure cells from specific microscopic regions of tissue sections to study developing disease lesions in actual tissue. A transfer film is applied to the surface of the tissue section. Under the microscope, the diagnostic pathologist or researcher views the thin tissue section and chooses microscopic clusters of cells to study. When the cells of choice are in the center of the field of view, a pulsed laser beam activates a spot on the transfer film immediately above the cells of interest. At this location the film melts and fuses with the underlying cells. When the film is removed, the chosen cells are held, while the rest of the tissue is left behind. This allows multiple homogeneous samples within the tissue section to be targeted for analysis. Under the microscope, tissues are heterogeneous structures with hundreds of different cell types locked in units that adhere to adjacent cells, connective stroma, blood vessels, glandular and muscle components, adipose cells, and inflammatory or immune cells. In normal or developing organs, specific cells express different genes and undergo molecular changes in response to internal control signals, signals from adjacent cells, and humoral stimuli. In disease pathologies, the diseased cells, such as precancerous cells, are surrounded by heterogeneous tissue elements.

88400

Bilirubin is a bile pigment produced through the breakdown of blood components. High concentrations in the blood is found in some newborns and others and is known as jaundice. Transcutaneous bilirubinometry uses subcutaneous tissue photometry to measure bilirubin concentration, particularly in newborns. The optic head of the photometric analyzer is pressed against the infant's skin (often the forehead or upper part of the sternum) for a measurement that takes several seconds. Additional measurements may be taken nearby and averaged. Calibration is in units of Transcutaneous Bilirubin Index (TcBI), according to international practice. Measurements of infants with jaundice may be taken at least four times a day to monitor the condition and check efficiency of therapy.

89050–89051

CSF cell count may also be referred to as a CSF analysis or spinal fluid analysis; joint fluid cell count may also be refered to as synovial fluid analysis. In 89050, a manual nucleated blood cell count using a hemacytometer is performed on fluids obtained during a separately reportable spinal puncture or arthrocentesis. In 89051, a differential cell study using manually prepared smears or a cytocentrifuge is performed in addition to the cell count. Depending on the suspected condition, a number of separately reportable additional tests may be performed.

89060

A fluid sample is obtained. A variety of different methods may be used to process the specimen depending on the source. The fluid is analyzed for the presence of crystals using either direct light or polarized light microscopy. A newer technique using atomic force microscopy (AFM) may be available in some laboratories.

89100–89105

A tube is inserted orally or nasally and positioned in the duodenum. When a single specimen is obtained (89100), the duodenal contents are simply aspirated. When multiple specimens are obtained (89105), either pancreatic or gallbladder stimulation is required and the following procedure is used. Intravenous administration of either synthetic C-terminal octapeptide of cholecystokinin or cholecystokinin pancreozymin is performed. Duodenal fluid is then collected over a period of 20-30 minutes. Specimens are usually collected in multiple containers with the bile from each source being identified as common duct origin (yellow in color), gallbladder origin (viscous, green or green brown color), and hepatic duct origin (lighter in color than the other two sources). Alternately, the bile may be pooled into a single specimen.

89125

Prior to obtaining the stool specimen the patient is placed on a diet containing at least 60 gm of fat/day. A random stool specimen is obtained. A small amount of stool is prepared with Sudan III stain and examined microscopically. A random urine sample is obtained. Urine sediment is stained with Sudan III or IV and analyzed using light and polarized microscopy. Respiratory secretions may be obtained by separately reportable bronchoscopy and are stained and analyzed using techniques similar to those for other types of specimens.

89130–89132

The patient is not allowed to take anything by mouth except water after the evening meal on the day prior to the study. A tube is inserted orally or nasally and positioned in the stomach. Correct placement is verified using separately reportable fluoroscopy or x-ray. Gentle suction is applied and gastric contents aspirated. The contents are sent to the lab where chemical and/or cytopathology analysis is performed. When the procedure is performed without stimulation report 89130, with stimulation report 89132.

89135–89141

The patient is not allowed to take anything by mouth except water after the evening meal on the day prior to the study. A tube is inserted orally or nasally and positioned in the stomach. Correct placement is verified using separately reportable fluoroscopy or x-ray. Gentle, constant suction is applied and gastric contents aspirated. Secretions acquired during the first 15-30 minutes of suction are discarded. A Toomey syringe is used to aspirate all contents for the next 60-120 minutes. The specimens are obtained over 15-minute increments and placed into four to eight separate containers. These constitute the basal acid output (BAO). When only a BAO is obtained report 89135 for a one-hour study or 89136 for a two-hour study. Codes 89140 and 89141 include all services in a BAO. However, in addition to BAO, gastric stimulation is accomplished using pentagastrin or Histalog. Post-stimulation contents are then aspirated for a minimum of 60 minutes. These specimens are also collected in 15-minute increments and stored in separate specimen containers. For gastric secretory study including stimulation, report 89140 if total duration of study is two hours and 89141 if total duration is three hours.

89160

An adequate intake of red meat is required for 24-72 hours prior to testing. A stool specimen is obtained. The specimen is mixed with 10 percent solution of eosin in ethanol and stained on a slide for three minutes and cover-slipped. It is then analyzed microscopically for rectangular striated muscle fibers.

89190

Two slides are normally obtained. Wright's stain is applied and the specimens are examined microscopically for the presence of eosinophils.

89250–89251

Eggs (oocytes) are aspirated transvaginally using ultrasound guidance in a separately reportable procedure. These eggs are fertilized in the laboratory, using the partner's sperm, approximately four hours after aspiration. The eggs are kept in an incubator in a petri dish culture for two to six days after fertilization. Code 89251 is reserved for those instances when co-culture techniques over and above those normally required are performed.

89252

This test involves injection of a single sperm into the egg (oocyte) to enable fertilization when sperm counts are very low or when sperm are non-motile. It requires micromanipulation of the sperm, which is also referred to as microtechnique. The usual method involves intracytoplasmic sperm injection (ICSI). Using ICSI technique, the mature egg is held in place with a holding pipette. A very delicate, sharp, hollow needle is used to immobilize and pick up a single sperm. This needle is inserted through the egg's outer shell (zona pellucida) into the cytoplasm of the egg. The sperm is injected into the cytoplasm and the needle removed. The eggs are checked the next day for evidence of fertilization.

89253

Assisted embryo hatching is performed in selected cases on the day of embryo transfer. A pipette is placed on one side of the embryo to keep it from moving. A very delicate, hollow needle called a hatching needle is placed on the other side of the embryo. An acidic solution is expelled from the needle against the outer shell (zona pellucida) of the embryo. The acidic solution digests a small area of the outer shell. The embryo is then washed and replaced in the culture solution in the incubator.

89254

Because the egg (oocyte) is microscopic, only the follicle (fluid filled structure surrounding the egg) can be seen during the ultrasound guided retrieval. Upon aspiration of the follicle, specially trained personnel use a microscope to search for the oocyte-cumulus complex, which includes the egg and surrounding cumulus cells from the ovary. This is accomplished by pouring the collected fluid into flat dishes and using a microscope to search for eggs.

89255

After the embryos have been cultured for two to six days, three to four healthy embryos are selected for transfer. Selected embryos are loaded into a transfer catheter. In a separately reportable procedure, the catheter is placed in the cervical canal and the embryos are transferred into the uterine cavity.

89256

Previously frozen embryos are thawed. Since only two-thirds of embryos generally survive the freeze-thaw process, they must be first be examined to determine viability. The healthiest embryos are then selected and prepared for transfer.

89257

A separately reportable testicular biopsy with aspiration is performed to obtain sperm. This may be required in cases where azoospermia is due to suspected obstruction to the spermatic ducts or in instances where the patient has had a failed reversal of a vasectomy. This procedure reports microscopic examination of aspirated fluid for the presence of sperm. If sperm are identified, further evaluation services may be performed and would be reported separately.

89258

After ovarian stimulation, more healthy eggs (oocytes) may be produced than required for current transfer. Storing of embryos may also be done for women of childbearing age who face cancer therapies that may diminish fertility. Because eggs cannot be frozen, all healthy eggs are generally fertilized and any embryos not required for the current transfer are frozen using a process referred to as cryopreservation. Pre-implantation embryo storage is a relatively new procedure as compared to sperm storage, but more than two-thirds of the embryos survive the cryopreservation process and can be preserved for an indefinite period of time.

89259

A cryoprotectant, usually glycerol or Dimethyl Sulfoxide (DMSO), is mixed with the semen to help prevent damage to sperm during the freezing process. The semen specimen is then placed in a vial and frozen in liquid nitrogen at -196 C. This halts all biologic and metabolic processes allowing the sperm to be preserved for many years.

89260

Prior to insemination or further diagnostic studies, the sperm go through a spinning and washing process in a series of solutions. The purpose of this is to separate sperm from seminal fluids, allowing the sperm to go through a process referred to as capacitation. Capacitation is an invisible change mature spermatozoa must undergo to acquire accelerated movement, allowing them to navigate through the uterus and fallopian tube. In addition, this procedure checks the ability of the sperm to swim in a forward progressive fashion. This procedure includes a semen analysis (count, motility, volume and differential).

89261

Prior to insemination or further diagnostic studies, the sperm go through a spinning and washing process in a series of solutions. The purpose of this is to separate sperm from seminal fluids, allowing the sperm to go through a process referred to as capacitation. Capacitation is an invisible change mature spermatozoa must undergo to acquire accelerated movement, allowing them to navigate through the uterus and fallopian tube. This complex prep includes a Percoll gradient and albumin gradient. This procedure includes a semen analysis (count, motility, volume and differential).

89264

A separately reportable testicular biopsy is performed to obtain sperm. A small amount of testicular tissue is taken for microscopic evaluation for the presence of sperm. This test is used only when no other means is available of obtaining a sperm sample because of the possibility of causing further testicular damage.

89300–89321

Semen analysis must be performed in specialized infertility/andrology laboratories. Sexual activity culminating in ejaculation should be avoided for a minimum of 48 hours prior to testing. In 89300, a post coital specimen is obtained using a cervical swab.

The test is timed to coincide with ovulation. Semen is tested for the presence (quantity) and/or motility of sperm. In 89310-89321, semen is collected postcoitus using a condom-like seminal fluid collection device or by masturbation into a sterile container. In 89310, only sperm movement (motility) and number (count) are performed. Code 89320 reports a complete semen analysis which includes: volume, number (count, concentration) and structure (shape) of sperm, sperm movement (motility), direction of movement (forward motility). In addition, fluid thickness, acidity, and sugar content are evaluated. Code 89321 tests only for the presence (quantity) and/or motility of sperm. Tests reported with 89300-89321 may be accomplished using a variety of methods including semen function tests and computer-assisted sperm morphology/motility studies.

89325

This procedure tests for antisperm antibodies in both the male and female. Semen and cervical mucus are placed together in a special medium. Antisperm antibodies bind with the sperm inhibiting movement and their ability to fertilize. The sperm will appear clumped together on microscopic examination.

89329

This test is also called sperm penetration assay (SPA) or hamster zona free ovum (HZFO) and tests the ability of the sperm to penetrate a hamster egg which has been stripped of the zona pellucida (outer membrane). The patient should abstain from sexual activity culminating in ejaculation for a minimum of 48 hours. Semen is collected postcoitus using a condom-like seminal fluid collection device or by masturbation into a sterile container. Upon receiving the specimen in the laboratory, the sperm is washed and placed in a special culture medium along with a single hamster egg. It is then examined periodically using phase contrast microscopy. The test measures the ability of sperm to capacitate (invisible change which allows sperm to navigate rapidly forward), acrosome react (structural change fusing the outer membrane of the acrosome with the plasma membrane of the sperm head freeing enzymes in the acrosome which facilitate entry into the ovum) , and fuse with the ovum.

89330

Sperm mucus interaction is assessed in vitro. Either human or bovine ovulatory mucus is placed in a capillary tube. Sperm penetration is measured over a period of 90 minutes. Sperm progression defined as those sperm which have progressed the farthest down the tube is then measured. Patient sperm penetration can be compared with fertile sperm specimens using in vitro methods.

89350

Aerosol induced sputum collection involves use of an aerosol mist which is inhaled into the lungs to loosen secretions making them easier to expectorate.

89355

A random stool sample is collected. It is examined microscopically for the presence of starch granules.

89360

Iontophoresis involves the introduction of ions of soluble salts into the tissue by direct current. It is also referred to as pilocarpine iontophoresis. It is employed to stimulate the production of sweat, usually on the forearm. The sweat is then collected in a previously weighed gauze pad.

89365

This procedure is also referred to as the antidiuretic hormone (ADH) suppression test or vasopressin suppression test. The patient is given a water load. Output is then measured to determine whether the water load is being excreted. Urine osmolity is also measured.

90281

This code identifies the Immune globulin (IG), human, for intramuscular use. An immune globulin is a passive immunization agent obtained from pooled human plasma. Report with the appropriate administration code, 90780–90784.

90283

This code identifies the Immune globulin (IGIV), human, for intravenous use. An immune globulin is a passive immunization agent obtained from pooled human plasma. Report with the appropriate administration code, 90780–90784.

90287

This code identifies the Botulinum antitoxin, equine, administered by any route. The vaccine stimulates antitoxin antibodies that neutralize tissue, destroying bacterial exotoxins. Report with the appropriate administration code, 90780–90784.

90288

This code identifies the Botulism immune globulin, human, for intravenous use. An immune globulin is a passive immunization agent obtained from pooled human plasma. Report with the appropriate administration code, 90780–90784.

90291

This code identifies the Cytomegalovirus immune globulin (CMV-IGIV), human, for intravenous use. An immune globulin is a passive immunization agent obtained from pooled human plasma. Report with the appropriate administration code, 90780–90784.

90296

This code identifies the Diphtheria antitoxin, equine, administered by any route. The vaccine stimulates antitoxin antibodies that neutralize tissue, destroying bacterial exotoxins. Report with the appropriate administration code, 90780–90784.

90371

This code identifies the Hepatitis B immune globulin (HBIG), human, for intramuscular use. An immune globulin is a passive immunization agent obtained from pooled human plasma. Report with the appropriate administration code, 90780–90784.

90375

This code identifies the Rabies immune globulin (RIG), human, for intramuscular and/or subcutaneous use. An immune globulin is a passive immunization agent obtained from pooled human plasma. Report with the appropriate administration code, 90780–90784.

90376

This code identifies the Rabies immune globulin, heat-treated (RIG-HT), human, for intramuscular and/or subcutaneous use. An immune globulin is a passive immunization agent obtained from pooled human plasma. Report with the appropriate administration code, 90782.

90378

This code identifies the respiratory syncytial virus immune globulin (RSV-IgIM), for intramuscular use, 50 mg. each. An immune globulin is a passive immunization agent obtained from pooled human plasma. Report with the appropriate administration code, 90782.

90379

This code identifies the respiratory syncytial virus immune globulin (RSV-IGIV), human, for intravenous use. An immune globulin is a passive immunization agent obtained from pooled human plasma. Report with the appropriate administration code, 90784.

90384

This code identifies the Rho(D) immune globulin (RhIG), human, full-dose, for intramuscular use. An immune globulin is a passive immunization agent obtained from pooled human plasma. Report with the appropriate administration code, 90782.

90385

This code identifies the Rho(D) immune globulin (RhIG), human, mini-dose, for intramuscular use. An immune globulin is a passive immunization agent obtained from pooled human plasma. Report with the appropriate administration code, 90782.

90386

This code identifies the Rho(D) immune globulin (RhIGIV), human, for intravenous use. An immune globulin is a passive immunization agent obtained from pooled human plasma. Report with the appropriate administration code, 90784.

90389

This code identifies a tetanus immune globulin (TIG), human, for intramuscular use. An immune globulin is a passive immunization agent obtained from pooled human plasma. Report with the appropriate administration code, 90782.

90393

This code identifies the vaccinia immune globulin, human, for intramuscular use. An immune globulin is a passive immunization agent obtained from pooled human plasma. Report with the appropriate administration code, 90782.

90396

This code identifies varicella-zoster immune globulin, human, for intramuscular use. An immune globulin is a passive immunization agent obtained from pooled human plasma. Report with the appropriate administration code, 90782.

90399

This code identifies an immune globulin not listed. An immune globulin is a passive immunization agent obtained from pooled human plasma. Report with the appropriate administration code, 90799.

90471

A physician, nurse, or medical assistant administers an injectable (includes percutaneous, intradermal, subcutaneous, intramuscular) or jet injection immunization to the patient. It may be one or more vaccines or toxoids in a single immunization (e.g., diphtheria, pertussis, and tetanus toxoids are in a single DPT immunization). Report 90471 for the administration of one immunization. Report 90472 to identify each additional vaccine or toxoid administration after the first. Use 90472 in conjunction with 90471.

90471–90472

A physician, nurse, or medical assistant administers an injectable (includes percutaneous, intradermal, subcutaneous, intramuscular) and/or jet injection immunization to the patient. It may be one or more vaccines or toxoids in a single immunization (e.g., diphtheria, pertussis, and tetanus toxoids are in a single DPT immunization). Report 90471 for one vaccine. Report 90472 for each additional vaccine (single or combination vaccine/toxoid).

90472

A physician, nurse, or medical assistant administers an immunization to a patient. This can be an injection or an oral dose. It may be a single or multiple vaccine or toxoid. This code may be reported multiple times to identify each additional vaccine or toxoid administration after the first which is reported with 90471.

90473–90474

A physician, nurse, or medical assistant administers an immunization to a patient via intranasal route (e.g., a nasal spray) or via an oral route (e.g., a liquid that is swallowed). It may be a single or multiple vaccine or toxoid (e.g., adenovirus, Rotavirus, typhoid, poliovirus). Report 90473 for one vaccine. Report 90474 for each additional vaccine (single or combination vaccine/toxoid).

90476

A vaccine induces the immune system to produce immunity against specific microorganisms/viruses. This vaccine is an oral preparation to immunize a patient against a type 4 adenovirus. This vaccination — live — contains the actual virus. An adenovirus causes diseases of the upper respiratory tract and conjunctivae, and is also present in latent infections in normal persons. Types 3, 4, 7, 14, and 21 have been isolated from patients with acute respiratory disease. Report with the appropriate administration code, 90471, 90472.

90477

A vaccine induces the immune system to produce immunity against specific microorganisms/viruses. This vaccine is an oral preparation to immunize a patient against a type 7 adenovirus. This vaccination — live — contains the actual virus. An adenovirus causes diseases of the upper respiratory tract and conjunctivae, and is also present in latent infections in normal persons. Types 3, 4, 7, 14, and 21 have been isolated from patients with acute respiratory disease. Report with the appropriate administration code, 90471, 90472.

90581

A vaccine induces the immune system to produce immunity against specific microorganisms/viruses. This vaccine is prepared for subcutaneous use to immunize a patient against anthrax. Cutaneous anthrax is the most common among humans, and is usually acquired by injection of the bacterial Bacillus anthracis or its spores from contact with infected animals or their waste material. The most fatal form is inhalational anthrax that can cause pneumonia. Report with the appropriate administration code, 90471, 90472.

90585

A vaccine induces the immune system to produce immunity against specific microorganisms/viruses. This vaccine is prepared for percutaneous use to immunize a patient against bladder cancer using Bacillus Calmette-Guerin (BCG). This vaccination —

live — contains the actual pathogen. Calmatte-Guerin is an organism of the strain Mycobacterium boviss is used for immunization of humans against tuberculosis and in cancer chemotherapy. Report with the appropriate administration code, 90471, 90472.

90586

A vaccine induces the immune system to produce immunity against specific microorganisms/viruses. This vaccine is prepared for intravenous use and contains the actual pathogen. Calmatte-Guerin is an organism of the strain Mycobacterium bovis. This vaccination is for treating bladder cancer. Report with proper administration code, 90471, 90472.

90632

A vaccine prepared from the blood plasma of asymptomatic human carriers of the viral hepatitis caused by the hepatitis A virus or through recombinant DNA technology is prepared for intramuscular use, adult dose, to achieve immunity. Report with the appropriate administration code, 90471, 90472.

90633

A vaccine prepared from the blood plasma of asymptomatic human carriers of the viral hepatitis caused by the hepatitis A virus or through recombinant DNA technology is prepared for intramuscular use, pediatrics/adolescent 2-dose schedule, to achieve immunity. Report with the appropriate administration code, 90471, 90472.

90634

A vaccine prepared from the blood plasma of asymptomatic human carriers of the viral hepatitis caused by the hepatitis A virus or through recombinant DNA technology is prepared for intramuscular use, pediatrics/adolescent 3-dose schedule, to achieve immunity. Report with the appropriate administration code, 90471, 90472.

90636

A vaccine prepared from the blood plasma of asymptomatic human carriers of the viral hepatitis caused by the hepatitis A and the hepatitis B virus (HepA-HepB) or through recombinant DNA technology is prepared for intramuscular use, adult dose, to achieve immunity. Report with the appropriate administration code, 90471, 90472.

90645

A vaccine induces the immune system to produce immunity against specific microorganisms/viruses. The Hemophilus influenza b vaccine (Hib) HbOC conjugate vaccine is prepared for intramuscular use, in a 4-dose schedule, to immunize a patient against hemophilus influenza. Hemophilus influenza is caused by the bacteria Haemophilus and the strain used for this vaccine is of the species once thought to be the cause of the great flu epidemic among humans.

Report with the appropriate administration code, 90471, 90472.

90646

A vaccine induces the immune system to produce immunity against specific microorganisms/viruses. The Hemophilus influenza b vaccine (Hib) PRP-D conjugate vaccine is prepared for intramuscular use, booster only, to immunize a patient against hemophilus. Hemophilus influenza is caused by the bacteria Haemophilus and the strain used for this vaccine is of the species once thought to be the cause of the great flu epidemic among humans. Report with the appropriate administration code, 90471, 90472.

90647

A vaccine induces the immune system to produce immunity against specific microorganisms/viruses. A Hemophilus influenza b vaccine (Hib) PRP-OMP conjugate vaccine is prepared for intramuscular use, in a 3-dose schedule, to immunize a patient against hemophilus. Hemophilus influenza is caused by the bacteria Haemophilus and the strain used for this vaccine is of the species once thought to be the cause of the great flu epidemic among humans. Report with the appropriate administration code, 90471, 90472.

90648

A vaccine induces the immune system to produce immunity against specific microorganisms/viruses. A Hemophilus influenza b vaccine (Hib) PRP-Tconjugate vaccine is prepared for intramuscular use, in a 4-dose schedule, to immunize a patient against hemophilus. Hemophilus influenza is caused by the bacteria Haemophilus and the strain used for this vaccine is of the species once thought to be the cause of the great flu epidemic among humans. Report with the appropriate administration code, 90471, 90472.

90657

A vaccine induces the immune system to produce immunity against specific microorganisms/viruses. A split suspension of the prevalent strains of influenza virus is prepared for intramuscular use or by jet injection in a dosage for an infant/toddler from six months to 35 months of age. The vaccine induces active immunity to the highly contagious infection of the respiratory tract caused by a myxovirus and transmitted by airborne droplet infection. Report with the appropriate administration code, 90471, 90472.

90658

A vaccine induces the immune system to produce immunity against specific microorganisms/viruses. A split suspension of the prevalent strains of influenza virus is prepared for intramuscular use or by jet injection in a dosage for age 3 years and older. The vaccine induces active immunity to the highly contagious infection of the respiratory tract caused by a myxovirus and transmitted by airborne droplet

infection. Report with the appropriate administration code, 90471, 90472.

90659

A vaccine induces the immune system to produce immunity against specific microorganisms/viruses. A suspension of the prevalent strain of influenza virus is prepared for intramuscular use or by jet injection to induce active immunity to the highly contagious infection of the respiratory tract caused by a myxovirus and transmitted by airborne droplet infection. Report with the appropriate administration code, 90471, 90472.

90660

A vaccine induces the immune system to produce immunity against specific microorganisms/viruses. A suspension of the prevalent strain of influenza virus is prepared for intranasal use to induce active immunity to the highly contagious infection of the respiratory tract caused by a myxovirus and transmitted by airborne droplet infection. This vaccination — live — contain the actual pathogen. Report with the appropriate administration code, 90471, 90472.

90665

A vaccine induces the immune system to produce immunity against specific microorganisms/viruses. A vaccine to protect the adult patient from Lyme disease is prepared for intramuscular use. Lyme disease is an acute inflammatory infection transmitted by a tickborne bacteria Borrelia burgdorferi. Report with the appropriate administration code, 90471, 90472.

90669

A vaccine induces the immune system to produce immunity against specific microorganisms/viruses. An active suspension containing antigens of the 14 types of Pneumococcus associated with 80 percent of the cases of pneumococcal pneumonia is prepared for intramuscular use, in children under five years.

90675

A vaccine induces the immune system to produce immunity against specific microorganisms/viruses. A vaccine for immunization against and postexposure spread of rabies is prepared for intramuscular use. The vaccine is prepared from a sterile suspension of killed rabies virus prepared from duck embryo. Report with the appropriate administration code, 90471, 90472.

90676

A vaccine induces the immune system to produce immunity against specific microorganisms/viruses. A vaccine for immunization against and postexposure spread of rabies is prepared for interdermal use. The vaccine is prepared from a sterile suspension of killed rabies virus prepared from duck embryo. Report with the appropriate administration code, 90471, 90472.

90680

A vaccine induces the immune system to produce immunity against specific microorganisms/viruses. A vaccine for immunization against a rotavirus is prepared for oral use. This vaccination — live — contains the actual virus. A rotavirus replicates in the cells of the intestine and causes acute diarrhea, particularly in infants. Report with the appropriate administration code, 90471, 90472.

90690

A vaccine induces the immune system to produce immunity against specific microorganisms/viruses. A Typhoid vaccine for immunization against a bacterial infection usually caused by Salmonella typhi is prepared for oral use. This vaccination — live — contains the actual pathogen. The bacterial infection is transmitted by contaminated milk, water, and food and causes high fever, diarrhea, and rash. Report with the appropriate administration code, 90471, 90472.

90691

A vaccine induces the immune system to produce immunity against specific microorganisms/viruses. A Typhoid vaccine Vi capsular polysaccharide (ViCPs) for immunization against a bacterial infection usually caused by Salmonella typhi is prepared for intramuscular use. The bacterial infection is transmitted by contaminated milk, water, and food and causes high fever, diarrhea, and rash. Report with the appropriate administration code, 90471, 90472.

90692

A vaccine induces the immune system to produce immunity against specific microorganisms/viruses. A Typhoid vaccine, heat- and phenol-inactivated (H-P) for immunization against a bacterial infection usually caused by Salmonella typhi is prepared for subcutaneous or intradermal use. The bacterial infection is transmitted by contaminated milk, water, and food and causes high fever, diarrhea, and rash. Report with the appropriate administration code, 90471, 90472.

90693

A vaccine induces the immune system to produce immunity against specific microorganisms/viruses. A Typhoid vaccine acetone-killed, dried (AKD) for immunization against a bacterial infection usually caused by Salmonella typhi is prepared for subcutaneous use or by jet injection (U.S. military). The bacterial infection is transmitted by contaminated milk, water, and food and causes high fever, diarrhea, and rash. Report with the appropriate administration code, 90471, 90472.

90700

A toxoid stimulates specific antitoxin antibodies that destroy toxins secreted by bacteria, and provides immunity that is effective and long-lasting. A vaccine induces the immune system to produce immunity

against specific microorganisms/viruses. This code describes an immunization against diphtheria, tetanus, and pertussis (in acellular form — synthetic). A combined DTaP is a routine immunization for infants at two, four, six, and 18 months, and again between the ages of four to six years, by intramuscular use. Report with the appropriate administration code, 90471, 90472.

90701

A toxoid stimulates specific antitoxin antibodies that destroy toxins secreted by bacteria, and provides immunity that is effective and long-lasting. A vaccine induces the immune system to produce immunity against specific microorganisms/viruses. This code describes an immunization against diphtheria, tetanus, and pertussis (in whole cell form). A combined DTaP is a routine immunization for infants at two, four, six, and 18 months, and again between the ages of four to six years, by intramuscular use. Report with the appropriate administration code, 90471, 90472.

90702

A toxoid stimulates specific antitoxin antibodies that destroy toxins secreted by bacteria, and provides immunity that is effective and long lasting. This code describes an immunization against diphtheria and tetanus, absorbed for intramuscular use, in individuals younger than seven years.

90703

A toxoid stimulates specific antitoxin antibodies that destroy toxins secreted by bacteria, and provides immunity that is effective and long-lasting. This code describes an immunization against tetanus for intramuscular or jet injection use. Report with the appropriate administration code, 90471, 90472.

90704

A vaccine induces the immune system to produce immunity against specific microorganisms/viruses. A mumps vaccine is a routine immunization given to infants at 12 months or younger. This code is for subcutaneous or jet injection use. Report with the appropriate administration code, 90471, 90472.

90705

A vaccine induces the immune system to produce immunity against specific microorganisms/viruses. A measles vaccine is a routine immunization administered to infants at 12 months or younger. This code is for subcutaneous or jet injection. Report with the appropriate administration code, 90471, 90472.

90706

A vaccine induces the immune system to produce immunity against specific microorganisms/viruses. A rubella vaccine is a routine immunization administered to infants at 12 months or younger. This code is for subcutaneous or jet injection. Report with the appropriate administration code, 90471, 90472.

90707

A vaccine induces the immune system to produce immunity against specific microorganisms/viruses. This code combines the measles, mumps, and rubella (MMR), live, for subcutaneous or jet injection use. Report with the appropriate administration code, 90471, 90472.

90708

A vaccine induces the immune system to produce immunity against specific microorganisms/viruses. This code combines the measles and rubella, live, for subcutaneous or jet injection use. Report with the appropriate administration code, 90471, 90472.

90709

A vaccine induces the immune system to produce immunity against specific microorganisms/viruses. This code combines the rubella and mumps, live, for subcutaneous use. Report with the appropriate administration code, 90471, 90472.

90710

A vaccine induces the immune system to produce immunity against specific microorganisms/viruses. This code combines the measles, mumps, rubella and varicella (MMRV), live, for subcutaneous use. Report with the appropriate administration code, 90471, 90472.

90712

A vaccine induces the immune system to produce immunity against specific microorganisms/viruses. This code describes the polio virus vaccine, inactivated, (OPV), for oral use. An oral polio vaccine is routinely administered to infants at two, four, six and 18 months and again between the ages of four to six years. Report with the appropriate administration code, 90471, 90472.

90713

A vaccine induces the immune system to produce immunity against specific microorganisms/viruses. This code describes the polio virus vaccine, inactivated, (IPV), for subcutaneous use. A polio vaccine is routinely administered to infants at two, four, six and 18 months and again between the ages of four to six years. Report with the appropriate administration code, 90471, 90472.

90716

A vaccine induces the immune system to produce immunity against specific microorganisms/viruses. This code describes the varicella vaccine for subcutaneous use. The vaccine is routinely administered once between the ages of one to 12 years. Report with the appropriate administration code, 90471, 90472.

90717

A vaccine induces the immune system to produce immunity against specific microorganisms/viruses. This code describes the immunization against yellow fever, live, for subcutaenous use. Report with the appropriate administration code, 90471, 90472.

90718

A toxoid stimulates specific antitoxin antibodies that destroy toxins secreted by bacteria, and provides immunity that is effective and long lasting. This code describes an immunization against tetanus and diphtheria, absorbed, for intramuscular or jet injection, in individuals seven years or older.

90719

A toxoid stimulates specific antitoxin antibodies that destroy toxins secreted by bacteria, and provides immunity that is effective and long-lasting. This code describes an immunization against diphtheria for intramuscular use. Report with the appropriate administration code, 90471, 90472.

90720

A toxoid stimulates specific antitoxin antibodies that destroy toxins secreted by bacteria, and provides immunity that is effective and long-lasting. A vaccine induces the immune system to produce immunity against specific microorganisms/viruses. This code describes an immunization combining diphtheria and tetanus toxoids, and whole blood pertussis vaccine, and Hemophilus influenza B vaccine (DTP-Hib), for intramuscular use. Report with the appropriate administration code, 90471, 90472.

90721

A toxoid stimulates specific antitoxin antibodies that destroy toxins secreted by bacteria, and provides immunity that is effective and long-lasting. A vaccine induces the immune system to produce immunity against specific microorganisms/viruses. This code describes an immunization combining diphtheria and tetanus toxoids, and acellur pertussis vaccine, and Hemophilus influenza B vaccine (DTaP-Hib), for intramuscular use. Report with the appropriate administration code, 90471, 90472.

90723

A toxoid stimulates specific antitoxin antibodies that destroy toxins secreted by bacteria, and provides immunity that is effective and long lasting. A vaccine induces the immune system to produce immunity against specific microorganisms/viruses. This code describes an immunization combining diphtheria and tetanus toxoids, and acellular pertussis vaccine, and Hepatitis B, and poliovirus vaccine, inactivated (DTaP-HepB-IPV), for intramuscular use.

90725

A vaccine induces the immune system to produce immunity against specific microorganisms/viruses.

This code describes a cholera vaccine prepared for injectable use. Report with the appropriate administration code, 90471, 90472.

90727

A vaccine induces the immune system to produce immunity against specific microorganisms/viruses. The code describes a plaque vaccine for intramuscular or jet injection. Report with the appropriate administration code, 90471, 90472.

90732

A vaccine induces the immune system to produce immunity against specific microorganisms/viruses. This code describes a pneumococcal polysaccharide vaccine, 23-valent, adult or immunosuppressed patient dosage, 2 years or older, for subcutaneous or intramuscular use.

90733

A vaccine induces the immune system to produce immunity against specific microorganisms/viruses. The code describes a meningococcal polysaccharide vaccine (any group(s)), for subcutaneous or jet injection use. Report with the appropriate administration code, 90471, 90472

90735

A vaccine induces the immune system to produce immunity against specific microorganisms/viruses. The code describes a Japanese encephalitis virus vaccine for subcutaneous use. Report with the appropriate administration code, 90471, 90472.

90740–90744

A vaccine induces the immune system to produce immunity against specific microorganisms/viruses. These codes describe a Hepatitis B vaccine prepared for dialysis or immunosuppressed patient dosage (three-dose schedule), adolescent (two-dose schedule), and pediatric/adolescent dosage (three-dose schedule) for intramuscular use.

90746

A vaccine induces the immune system to produce immunity against specific microorganisms/viruses. The code describes a hepatitis B vaccine, prepared in an adult dosage, for intramuscular use. Report with the appropriate administration code, 90471, 90472.

90747

A vaccine induces the immune system to produce immunity against specific microorganisms/viruses. This code describes a hepatitis B vaccine, prepared in a dialysis or immunosuppressed patient dosage (four-dose schedule), for intramuscular use.

90748

A vaccine induces the immune system to produce immunity against specific microorganisms/viruses. The code describes a combined hepatitis B and hemophilus influenza B (HepB-Hib)) vaccine for intramuscular use. Report with the appropriate administration code, 90471, 90472.

90749

This code reports a vaccine or toxoid preparation that is not listed. Report with the appropriate administration code, 90471, 90472.

90780

A physician or an assistant infuses a therapeutic or diagnostic medication for up to one hour through an intravenous catheter inserted by needle into a patient's vein. The code applies to the physician administering the drug or supervising an assistant infusing the drug.

90781

A physician or an assistant infuses a therapeutic or diagnostic medication through an intravenous catheter inserted by needle into a patient's vein. The code requires a physician administering the drug or supervising an assistant infusing the drug. The code applies to an infusion for each additional hour up to eight hours beyond the first hour.

90782–90784

The physician injects a therapeutic, prophylactic or diagnostic substance into the patient. Report 90782 if subcutaneous or intramuscular; report 90783 if intra-arterial; report 90784 if intravenous. These codes report the injection service only. The drug or other substance is reported separately.

90788

The physician performs an intramuscular injection to instill an antibiotic.

90801

The physician examines the patient. This examination may include an interview including history, mental status, or disposition. The examination may include discussion of the patient's state with the family and interpretation of medical tests.

90802

The physician examines the patient. This examination may include an interview including history, mental status, or disposition. The examination may include discussion of the patient's state with the family and interpretation of medical tests. It may also include play equipment, physical devices, a language interpreter, and other mechanisms of communication.

90804–90805

The physician provides psychotherapy in an office or outpatient facility using support, suggestion, persuasion, reeducation, reassurance, and the occasional aid of medication. Several treatment modalities exist, including behavioral, brief, existential, insight oriented, and supportive. Use this code to report face-to-face sessions of 20 to 30 minutes. Use 90805 to report psychotherapy with medical evaluation and management services furnished on the same day.

90806–90807

The physician provides psychotherapy in an office or outpatient facility using support, suggestion, persuasion, reeducation, reassurance, and the occasional aid of medication. Several treatment modalities exist, including behavioral, brief, existential, insight oriented, and supportive. Use this code to report face-to-face sessions of 45 to 50 minutes. Use 90807 to report psychotherapy with medical evaluation and management services furnished on the same day.

90808–90809

The physician provides psychotherapy in an office or outpatient facility using support, suggestion, persuasion, reeducation, reassurance, and the occasional aid of medication. Several treatment modalities exist, including behavioral, brief, existential, insight oriented, and supportive. Use this code to report face-to-face sessions of 75 to 80 minutes. Use 90809 to report psychotherapy with medical evaluation and management services furnished on the same day.

90810–90811

The physician provides individual, interactive, psychotherapy using play equipment, physical devices, a language interpreter, and other mechanisms of communication. Several treatment modalities exist, including behavioral, brief, existential, insight oriented, and supportive. Use this code to report sessions of 20 to 30 minutes performed in an office or outpatient facility. Use 90811 to report psychotherapy with medical evaluation and management services furnished on the same day.

90812–90813

The physician provides individual, interactive, psychotherapy using play equipment, physical devices, a language interpreter, and other mechanisms of communication. Several treatment modalities exist, including behavioral, brief, existential, insight oriented, and supportive. Use this code to report sessions of 45 to 50 minutes performed in an office or outpatient facility. Use 90813 to report psychotherapy with medical evaluation and management services furnished on the same day.

90814–90815

The physician provides individual, interactive, psychotherapy using play equipment, physical devices, a language interpreter, and other mechanisms of communication. Several treatment modalities exist, including behavioral, brief, existential, insight oriented, and supportive. Use this code to report sessions of 75 to 80 minutes performed in an office or outpatient facility. Use 90815 to report sychotherapy

with medical evaluation and management services furnished on the same day.

90816–90817

The physician provides individual, insight oriented, psychotherapy using behavioral and supportive modalities. Use this code to report sessions of 20 to 30 minutes performed in an office or outpatient facility. Use 90817 to report psychotherapy with medical evaluation and management services furnished on the same day.

90818–90819

The physician provides individual, insight oriented, psychotherapy using behavioral and supportive modalities. Use this code to report sessions of 45 to 50 minutes performed in an office or outpatient facility. Use 90819 to report psychotherapy with medical evaluation and management services furnished on the same day.

90821–90822

The physician provides individual, insight oriented, psychotherapy using behavioral and supportive modalities. Use this code to report sessions of 75 to 80 minutes performed in an inpatient hospital, partial hospital, or residential care setting. Use 90822 to report psychotherapy with medical evaluation and management services furnished on the same day.

90823–90824

The physician provides individual, interactive psychotherapy using play equipment, physical devices, language interpreter, or other mechanisms of non-verbal communication. Use this code to report sessions of 25 to 30 minutes performed in an inpatient hospital, partial hospital, or residential care setting. Use 90824 to report psychotherapy with medical evaluation and management services furnished on the same day.

90826–90827

The physician provides individual, interactive psychotherapy using play equipment, physical devices, language interpreter, or other mechanisms of non-verbal communication. Use this code to report sessions of 45 to 50 minutes performed in an inpatient hospital, partial hospital, or residential care setting. Use 90827 to report psychotherapy with medical evaluation and management services furnished on the same day.

90828–90829

The physician provides individual, interactive psychotherapy using play equipment, physical devices, language interpreter, or other mechanisms of non-verbal communication. Use this code to report sessions of 75 to 80 minutes performed in an inpatient hospital, partial hospital, or residential care setting. Use 90829 to report psychotherapy with medical evaluation and management services furnished on the same day.

90845

The physician utilizes methods of eliciting a patient's past experiences to discover how these experiences pilot the patient's current behavior. The physician will perform continuing diagnostic evaluation and possible drug therapy.

90846

The physician meets with the patient's family without the patient present to help evaluate and treat the patient's condition. Attention is also given to the impact the patient's condition has on the family, with therapy aimed at improving the interaction between the patient and family members.

90847

The physician meets with the patient and the patient's family to evaluate and treat the patient's condition. Attention is also given to the impact the patient's condition has on the family, with therapy aimed at improving the interaction between the patient and family members. Continuing evaluation and drug management may be indicated.

90849

The physician meets with several patients' families to evaluate and treat patients' conditions. Attention is also given to the impact the patients' condition has on the family, with therapy aimed at improving the interaction between the patients and family members. Continuing evaluation and drug management may be indicated.

90853

The physician(s) or psychologist(s) facilitate emotional and rational cognitive interactions in a group setting in an effort to change the individual behavior of each person in the group through interpersonal exchanges. The group may be made up of patients with separate and distinct maladaptive disorders or share some facet of a disorder with other people in the group (e.g., drug abuse, victims of violence). This code should be used for group psychotherapy involving patients other than the patients' family.

90857

The physician treats mental disorders in groups using support, suggestion, persuasion, reeducation, reassurance, and the occasional aid of medication. Several modalities exist, including behavioral, brief, existential, insight oriented, and supportive.

90862

The physician manages the patient's medications — including prescription, use, and review.

90865

A hypnotic drug known as sodium Amytal or amobarbital is injected into the patient for psychotherapeutic treatment to help in managing some mental disorders and alcohol aversion therapy. It can also be used partly as a diagnostic aid. Injection of this drug allows recall of past traumatic events that can be discussed in another setting.

90870–90871

The physician initiates a seizure using electroconvulsive therapy (ECT), most often to combat chronic or profound depression. The physician anesthetizes the patient with a barbiturate and a muscle relaxant. Electrodes are placed on the patient's skull, and a measured electrical dose is applied to commence the seizure. Report 90870 if a single seizure is initiated. Report 90871 if multiple seizures are initiated. Report by day.

90875–90876

The physician utilizes biofeedback with psychotherapy to modify physiological behavior. The physician prepares the patient with a sensor that reads and displays blood pressure, muscle tension, or brain wave activity, and the physician teaches the patient to control these physiological functions through relaxation techniques. Management of the physiological functions is indicated by the sensors; patients learn to recognize and manipulate the functions displayed. Biofeedback is used for treatment of conditions including high blood pressure, incontinence, Raynaud's syndrome, and anticipatory nausea due to chemotherapy. Report 90875 for sessions of 20–30 minutes; report 90876 for sessions of approximately 45–50 minutes.

90880

The physician uses hypnosis as a modality for psychotherapy. The physician induces an altered state of conscious in the patient, evaluating the patient and altering behavior patterns while the patient is under a state of heightened awareness and lowered critical judgement.

90882

The physician uses this code to charge time spent initiating medical management activities with agencies, employers, or institutions on the patient's behalf.

90885

The physician evaluates the patient's hospital records, other psychiatric reports such as psychometric and projective tests, and other pertinent data for a possible medical diagnosis associated with or provides insight into the patient's condition.

CPT® Lay Descriptions

90887

The physician uses this code to charge time spent explaining the patient's condition to family members, either in an explanatory or advisory fashion.

90889

The physician uses this code to report time spent preparing reports on a patient's mental condition for legal, insurance, medical, and other entities.

90901

Biofeedback trains patients to control their autonomic or involuntary nervous systems to help regulate vital signs such as heart rate, blood pressure, temperature, and muscle tension. Monitors of various types are used to indicate body responses, which the patient learns to control in serial sessions. The code applies to any of several modalities of biofeedback training.

90911

Biofeedback trains patients to control their autonomic or involuntary nervous systems to help regulate vital signs like heart rate, blood pressure, temperature and muscle tension. The code applies to biofeedback training that uses the monitoring of the anus and/or rectum — including electromyography (measures muscle contractions) and manometry (measures pressure).

90918

Dialysis is a process to remove toxins from the blood and to maintain fluid and electrolyte balance when the kidneys no longer function. The patient's blood is removed through a previously placed catheter, pumped through a dialysis machine and returned to the patient through a second catheter. The code applies to dialysis services each month for end stage renal disease and includes the physician's evaluation and management such as assessing nutrition and growth and parental counseling for patients younger than two years of age.

90919

Dialysis is a process to remove toxins from the blood and to maintain fluid and electrolyte balance when the kidneys no longer function. The patient's blood is removed through a previously placed catheter, pumped through a dialysis machine, and returned to the patient through a second catheter. The code applies to dialysis services each month for end stage renal disease, and includes the physician's evaluation and management such as assessing nutrition and growth and parental counseling for patients between two and 11 years of age.

90920

Dialysis is a process to remove toxins from the blood and to maintain fluid and electrolyte balance when the kidneys no longer function. The patient's blood is removed through a previously placed catheter, pumped through a dialysis machine and returned to the patient through a second catheter. The code applies to dialysis services each month for end stage renal disease, and includes the physician's evaluation and management such as assessing nutrition, growth, and parental counseling for patients between 12 and 19 years of age.

90921

Dialysis is a process to remove toxins from the blood and to maintain fluid and electrolyte balance when the kidneys no longer function. The patient's blood is removed through a previously placed catheter, pumped through a dialysis machine and returned to the patient through a second catheter. The code applies to dialysis services each month for end stage renal disease and includes the physician's evaluation and management such as assessing nutrition and growth and parental counseling for patients 20 years of age and older.

90922

Dialysis is a process to remove toxins from the blood and to maintain fluid and electrolyte balance when the kidneys no longer function. The patient's blood is removed through a previously placed catheter, pumped through a dialysis machine and returned to the patient through a second catheter. The code applies to dialysis services each day for end stage renal disease and includes the physician's evaluation and management such as assessing nutrition and growth and parental counseling for patients under two years old.

90923

Dialysis is a process to remove toxins from the blood and to maintain fluid and electrolyte balance when the kidneys no longer function. The patient's blood is removed through a previously placed catheter, pumped through a dialysis machine and returned to the patient through a second catheter. The code applies to dialysis services each day for end stage renal disease and includes the physician's evaluation and management such as assessing nutrition and growth and parental counseling for patients between two and 11 years old.

90924

Dialysis is a process to remove toxins from the blood and to maintain fluid and electrolyte balance when the kidneys no longer function. The patient's blood is removed through a previously placed catheter, pumped through a dialysis machine and returned to the patient through a second catheter. The code applies to dialysis services each day for end stage renal disease and includes the physician's evaluation and management such as assessing nutrition and growth and parental counseling for patients between 12 and 19 years old.

90925

Dialysis is a process to remove toxins from the blood and to maintain fluid and electrolyte balance when the kidneys no longer function. The patient's blood is removed through a previously placed catheter, pumped through a dialysis machine and returned to the patient through a second catheter. The code applies to dialysis services each day for end stage renal disease and includes the physician's evaluation and management such as assessing nutrition and growth and parental counseling for patients 20 years of age and older.

90935

Hemodialysis is a process to remove toxins from the blood and to maintain fluid and electrolyte balance when the kidneys no longer function. The procedure involves placing a previously placed catheter in either an artery or vein, withdrawing the patient's blood, circulating the blood through a dialysis machine and transfusing the blood back to the patient. The code applies to one hemodialysis treatment for a diagnosis other than end stage renal disease (see 90918–90925) and includes the physician's evaluation.

90937

Hemodialysis is a process to remove toxins from the blood and to maintain fluid and electrolyte balance when the kidneys no longer function. The procedure involves placing a previously placed catheter in either an artery or vein, withdrawing the patient's blood, circulating the blood through a dialysis machine and transfusing the blood back to the patient. The code applies to repeated hemodialysis treatments for a diagnosis other than end stage renal disease (see 90918–90925) and includes the physician's evaluation.

90939

A hemodialysis access flow study is performed to determine blood flow in a graft or arteriovenous fistula. The health care provider performs the test after approximately 30 minutes of treatment and after turning off ultrafiltration. In the direct dilution method (also known as the urea-based measurement of recirculation method), arterial and venous line samples are drawn and the blood rate is reduced to 120 mL/minute. The blood pumped is turned off 10 seconds after reducing the blood flow rate and an arterial line is clamped above the sampling port. Systemic arterial samples are drawn, the line is disconnected, and dialysis is resumed. Measurements of BUN in the arterial, venous, and arterial sample are taken and the percent recirculation is calculated.

90940

A specially trained hemodialysis nurse or other staff member monitors the blood flow in a graft or arteriovenous fistula during hemodialysis using an ultrasound indicator dilution method. A dialysis staff member uses clips to attach one ultrasound sensor to the arterial line and one ultrasound sensor to the venous line of a graft or arteriovenous fistula. A bolus of normal saline, as an indictor is infused into the graft or fistula. Transducers in the sensors allow ultrasonic signals to pass back and forth; intersecting the flow of the diluted blood as it passes through the arterial and venous portions of the graft or fistula. Information from the sensors is relayed, captured, measured, and displayed, in real-time on a computer monitor. This code includes the hook-up, measurement (during the study), and disconnection.

90945

Dialysis is a process to remove toxins from the blood and to maintain fluid and electrolytes balance when the kidneys no longer function. This code applies to one dialysis procedure with a single physician evaluation using a technique other than hemodialysis. In peritoneal dialysis, a fluid is introduced into the peritoneal cavity that removes toxins and electrolytes that passively leach into the fluid. Hemofiltration, similar to hemodialysis, incorporates a special filtration process to remove excess fluid. Other continuous renal replacement therapies may be employed.

90947

Dialysis is a process to remove toxins from the blood and to maintain fluid and electrolytes balance when the kidneys no longer function. This code applies to one dialysis procedure that requires repeated physician evaluations, with or without substantial revision of a dialysis prescription, using a technique other than hemodialysis. In peritoneal dialysis, a fluid is introduced into the peritoneal cavity that removes toxins and electrolytes that passively leach into the fluid. Hemofiltration, similar to hemodialysis, incorporates a special filtration process to remove excess fluid. Other continuous renal replacement therapies may be employed.

90989

The physician or healthcare provider trains the patient or patient's caregiver to help with dialysis. The code applies to completing the entire course.

90993

The physician or healthcare provider trains the patient or patient's caregiver to help with dialysis. The code applies to one session of the complete course.

90997

Hemoperfusion is a technique to remove toxins from the blood and to maintain fluid and electrolyte balance when the kidneys no longer function. The physician draws the patient's blood, perfuses the blood through activated charcoal or resin and transfuses the blood back into the patient using needle and catheter.

91000

The physician inserts a tube into the patient's esophagus to collect fluid and cell samples, occasionally adding a fluid such as saline to increase the sample yield. The sample is preserved and mounted on a slide for microscopic viewing.

91010

The physician inserts a tube with sensors into the patient's esophagus to measure the fluid and gas pressure and motility waves associated with swallowing. The physician removes the tube. Pressure measurements are expressed as millimeters of mercury, millimeters of water, or torr.

91011

The physician inserts a tube with sensors into the patient's esophagus to measure the fluid and gas pressure and motility waves associated with swallowing. Pressure measurements are expressed as millimeters of mercury, millimeters of water, or torr. The physician removes the tube. The code applies to use of a stimulant.

91012

The physician inserts a tube with sensors into the patient's esophagus to measure the fluid and gas pressure and motility waves associated with swallowing. Pressure measurements are expressed as millimeters of mercury, millimeters of water, or torr. The physician removes the tube. The code applies to the test in conjunction with acid perfusion studies.

91020

The physician inserts a tube with sensors into the patient's esophagus to measure the fluid and gas pressure and motility waves associated with swallowing. Pressure measurements are expressed as millimeters of mercury, millimeters of water, or torr. The physician removes the tube. The code applies to testing that includes the lower esophageal sphincter.

91030

The physician inserts a tube and hydrochloric acid into the patient's esophagus to recreate the patient's complaints of pain. A positive result (pain) confirms gastroesophageal reflux.

91032

The physician inserts a tube into the patient's esophagus to evaluate for gastroesophageal reflux. The code applies to the pH level — acidity of the esophagus — measured by a sensor on the tip of the probe. The physician removes the tube.

91033

The physician inserts a tube into the patient's esophagus to evaluate for gastroesophageal reflux. The code applies to a prolonged recording of the pH level — acidity of the esophagus — measured by a sensor

on the tip of the probe. The physician removes the tube.

91052

The physician draws fluid from a patient's stomach through a tube to determine the acidity of stomach secretions. The physician inserts the tube to the stomach and adds a substance — histamine, insulin, pentagastrin, calcium, and secretin — to stimulate acidic secretion for measuring both baseline and stimulated states.

91055

The physician inserts a tube into the patient's stomach to collect fluid and cells to determine the acidity of stomach secretions. A fluid such as saline may be added to increase the sample yield. The sample is preserved and mounted on a microscope for evaluation. The physician removes the tube in a separately reported procedure.

91060

The physician inserts a tube and a fluid such as saline into the patient's stomach to check for an obstruction at the stomach outlet. The residual fluid is withdrawn 30 minutes later to determine the extent of the obstruction. The physician removes the tube.

91065

The physician measures the amount of hydrogen in a patient's breath after the patient ingests a lactase solution. The code applies to determining lactase deficiency.

91100

The patient lies on the left side and the physician passes a small flexible or semi-rigid gastrointestinal tube through the mouth and guides it to the duodenum (upper intestine) to monitor and suppress bleeding of the upper intestine. The device includes a hemostatic bag, irrigation and aspiration catheter, rectal catheter, and gastrointestinal string and tubes to locate internal bleeding.

91105

A nasogastric or orogastric tube is inserted into the patient's stomach for use in suctioning out the stomach's contents. A fluid such as saline may be used to increase the effectiveness. The physician removes the tube. The code applies to evacuating stomach contents often after a patient ingests poisons.

91122

The physician inserts a tube into the patient's anus and/or rectum to measure the pressure of liquid or gas. The physician removes the tube. Millimeters of mercury or millimeters of water or torr are the standard measurements.

91123

Abnormalities in the rectal emptying can lead to disorders of defecation. In severe cases of impaction, hospital admission is necessary for pulsed rectal irrigation. Pulsed Irrigation Evacuation (PIE) is an automated enema that has been used for bowel management of chronic constipation patients without voluntary bowel control (e.g., quadriplegics, paraplegics, spina bifida). The PIE system consists of a speculum, tubing, a disposable collection container, and an electrical unit that delivers positive and negative air pressure through the tubing. During the procedure, small pulses of warm tap water are delivered into the rectum, serving to rehydrate feces and promote peristalsis.

91132–91133

In electrogastrography (EGG) electrodes are placed on the skin over the stomach at a specific distance from each other, and the other end of the electrodes are attached to a computer. The electrical activity of the initiated by the distal two-thirds of the stomach (gastric electrical activity - GEA) is recorded and analyzed by the computer. Report 91132 when diagnostic electrogastrography is performed alone. Report 91133 when diagnostic EGG is performed in conjunction with the administration of a drug in an attempt to manipulate conditions and provoke a measurable abnormality.

92002

The physician reviews the new patient's medical history, general medical observation, external ocular and adnexal examination and other diagnostic procedures like ophthalmoscopy, biomicroscopy or tonometry. The visit may include mydriasis (the dilation of the patient's pupils). Generally, the patient has a complicated problem or two diagnostic problems.

92004

The physician makes a complete visual system examination including history, general medical observation, external and ophthalmoscopic examination, gross visual fields and basic sensorimotor examination of the new patient. The physician may also include biomicroscopy, examination with cycloplegia (temporary immobilization of the ciliary body) or mydriasis (the dilation of pupils), and tonometry. Near visual acuity testing, keratometry, tear testing, corneal staining, corneal sensitivity, fundus examination, and exophthalmometry may also be employed. A comprehensive exam always includes initiation of diagnostic and treatment programs. It may take more than one patient encounter to complete the service.

92012

The physician reviews the established patient's history, general medical observation, external ocular and adnexal examination, and other diagnostic procedures like ophthalmoscopy, biomicroscopy, or tonometry. The visit may include the use of mydriasis (dilation of the patient's pupils). Generally, the patient has a complicated problem or two diagnostic problems.

92014

The physician makes a complete visual system examination including history, general medical observation, external and ophthalmoscopic examination, gross visual fields, and basic sensorimotor examination of the established patient. The physician may also include biomicroscopy, examination with cycloplegia (immobilization of the ciliary body) or mydriasis (dilation of the patient's pupils), and tonometry. Near visual acuity testing, keratometry, tear testing, corneal staining, corneal sensitivity, fundus examination, and exophthalmometry may also be employed. A comprehensive exam always includes initiation of diagnostic and treatment programs. It may take more than one patient encounter to complete the service.

92015

The examiner determines the prescription required for the patient's eyeglasses or contact lenses by evaluating the effectiveness of a series of lenses through which the patient is asked to view an eye chart. This is usually accomplished with a phoropter, a device that contains a range of lens powers which can be quickly changed, allowing the patient to compare various combinations when viewing the eye chart. A prescription is issued; no fitting for eyeglasses or contact lenses occurs at this time.

92018–92019

The physician examines the eyes of a patient under general anethesia who has significant injury or who cannot otherwise tolerate the examination while conscious. This examination may include manipulation of the globe and gonioscopy in a complete examination (e.g., 92018), or a limited examination without manipulation of the globe (e.g., 92019).

92020

The gonioscope examines the trabecular meshwork, located at the "angle" of the eye where the iris and cornea meet. The examiner observes the angle of the anterior chamber of the eye with the goniolens, a contact lens with a reflecting mirror or prism. The procedure is noninvasive.

92060

The examiner utilizes a series of vertical and horizontal prism bars or individual handheld prisms to measure ocular deviation. The patient is asked to focus on either a distant or near object. An occluder is alternately used to cover one eye until enough prism power in front of the opposite eye neutralizes movement.

92065

The physician prescribes exercises to correct ocular problems, most frequently ocular muscle imbalances. Then the physician or a technician trains the patient to perform these therapeutic exercises. These exercises frequently include repetitive tasks with prisms, color cards, or rods. A near object is moved progressively closer to improve convergence.

92070

The physician measures the patient's cornea for the fitting of a soft contact lens that has no refractive properties, or in the case of keratoconus, with refractive properties. This soft contact lens, often called a collagen shield, is placed over the cornea as a bandage, to protect a damaged eye, to cushion a painful cornea, or to reshape the cornea in keratoconus.

92081

This test measures the extent of the field of vision during daylight conditions, documenting any peripheral loss or blind spots in a patient's vision. The blind spots are plotted on visual field charts.

92082

This test measures the extent of the field of vision during daylight conditions, documenting any peripheral loss or blind spots in a patient's vision. This describes an intermediate procedure and may involve the use of specialized methods. The Goldmann perimeter may be used with at least two isopters. An isopter is defined as a boundary which is mapped out and is specific for that target. A hollow white spherical bowl is positioned a set distance from the patient. A variable size and intensity light is used by the examiner in either static or kinetic fashion. This method can test the full limit of peripheral vision.

92083

This test measures the extent of the field of vision during daylight conditions, documenting any peripheral loss or blind spots in a patient's vision. This describes an extended procedure and may involve the use of specialized methods. The Goldmann, perimeter may be used with at least three isopters. An isopter is defined as a boundary which is mapped out and is specific for that target. A hollow, white, spherical bowl is positioned a set distance from the patient. A variable size and intensity light is used by the examiner in either static or kinetic fashion. This method can test the full limit of peripheral vision.

92100

Though constantly flushed and renewed, the overall pressure of aqueous is constant in a healthy eye's anterior chamber. Too little or too much fluid can cause permanent damage. In tonography, the physician measures the outflow of aqueous from the eye. A constant pressure is applied to the globe while the progressive decrease in ocular tension is measured. This determines if fluids in the eye are at proper levels and circulating properly. Serial tonometry involves multiple pressure checks over the course of a day, usually in cases of diurnal curve or acute angle closure. Among the tonography testing equipment are Goldmans applanation, MacKay-Marg, and Schoitz's tonometers.

92120

Though constantly flushed and renewed, the overall pressure of aqueous is constant in a healthy eye's anterior chamber. Too little or too much fluid can cause permanent damage. In tonography, the patient is hooked up to a tonometric device that records the intraocular pressure over the course of a day. This determines if fluids in the eye are at proper levels and circulating properly.

92130

Though constantly flushed and renewed, the overall pressure of aqueous is constant in a healthy eye's anterior chamber. Too little or too much fluid can cause permanent damage. In water provocation tests, the patient drinks one quart of water after fasting and is hooked up to a tonometric device that records the intraocular pressure changes. This determines if fluids in the eye are at proper levels and circulating properly.

92135

This procedure involves scanning computerized ophthalmic diagnostic imaging. One type of scanning laser currently in use for early detection of glaucoma is known as a scanning laser glaucoma test (SLGT). The SLGT analyzes the nerve fiber layer in the posterior portion of the eye using a confocal scanning laser ophthalmoscope and/or polarimetry. During the examination the patient fixates on a light. A technician aligns and focuses the scanning instrument. The retinal nerve fiber layer (RNFL) that is the only part of the retina that can alter the state of polarized light is scanned with a low power laser beam that double-passes the RNFL. The instrument measures the change in polarization (retardation) that is directly related to the thickness of the tissue. A computer analyzes the measurements compared to standardized norms. Results are displayed and the data is stored in the computer for use as a comparison for future testing of the patient.

92136

In A-scan biometry, one thin, parallel sound beam is emitted from the ultrasound probe tip at a frequency of 10 MHz, with an echo bouncing back into the probe tip as the sound beam strikes each part of the eye (e.g., the solid cornea, the liquid aqueous, the solid lens, the liquid vitreous, the solid retina, choroid, sclera, and the orbital tissue). The probe transmits echoes that are picked up by a receiver, and a biometer attached to the receiver converts the echoes into spikes. Spike height along the baseline is affected by the difference in density as it travels through the eye (the greater the density of the structure it is passing through, the greater the amount of absorption). Partial coherence interferometry (PCI) measures the depth of the anterior chamber of pseudophakic patients, whose visual acuity is decreased due to a postrefractive error, such as the inability of the IOL to change shape, as shown by an IOL power calculation.

92140

Though constantly flushed and renewed, the overall pressure of aqueous is constant in a healthy eye's anterior chamber. Too little or too much fluid can cause permanent damage. In a test for glaucoma, the patient drinks one quart of water after fasting. The physician then measures intraocular pressure with a tonometer. The patient may also be placed in a dark room, where the physician rechecks the eyes once they have sufficiently dilated. This determines if fluids in the eye are at proper levels. Among the tonography testing equipment are Goldmann's applanation, MacKay-Marg, and Schoitz's tonometers.

92225–92226

Opthalmoscopy allows a complete view of the back of the eye. After the pupils have been dilated, views of the retina are seen with the direct ophthalmoscope, the indirect ophthalmoscope, or both. The exam is extended. The direct ophthalmoscope allows the highly magnified view of the posterior portion of the retina; indirect gives a broader view that includes posterior and anterior retina and vitreous. An extended ophthalmoscopy can also be performed with a contact lens, ruby lens, or 90 diopter lens. Both eyes are viewed, and the physician sketches views of the patient's retinas and their defects. The initial exam (92225) may be insufficient for diagnosis. The follow-up is reported with 92226.

92230

Opthalmoscopy allows a complete view of the back of the eye. This procedure is for detection of abnormalities of retinal blood vessels. The patient's eyes are dilated. The angioscopy begins when a small amount of fluorescein dye is injected into the arm. The dye is transported to the eye through the blood vessels. As the dye traverses the retinal vessels, the retina is viewed through the ophthalmoscope using filters that enhance the fluorescence of the eye.

92235

Opthalmoscopy allows a complete view of the back of the eye. This procedure is for detection of abnormalities of retinal blood vessels. The patient's eyes are dilated. The angioscopy begins when a small amount of fluorescein dye is injected into the arm. The dye is transported to the eye through the blood vessels. As the dye traverses the retinal vessels, a motorized camera attached to an opthalmoscope

photographs a sequence, documenting the dye's progress through the vessels of the retina. Both eyes are photographed. The photographs are black and white. The circulation takes seconds, but photography continues in 10- to 30-minute intervals to check for late leakage of recirculating dye. The physician reviews the film and makes a diagnostic evaluation of the patient's retina.

92240

Ophthalmoscopy allows viewing of the eyeball's interior through the pupil. Indocyanine-green (ICG) dye flouresces through blood and pigment, and is used for detecting abnormalities in the vascular choroid which lies between the retina and sclera. The patient's eyes are dilated. The angioscopy begins when a small amount of ICG is injected into the arm, and transported to the eye through the blood vessels. Rapid injection is essential. As the dye transverses the choroid, a motorized camera attached to an opthalmoscope photographs a sequence, documenting the dye's progress through the choroidal vessels. The photography is generally performed bilaterally, but may be performed unilaterally. Photographs are in black and white. Timing for photography is determined by arm to retinal time. This is estimated at about 10 seconds in young patients, and 12 to 18 seconds in older patients.

92250

Opthalmoscopy allows a complete view of the back of the eye. The physician or technician aligns the fundus camera, which is attached to an ophthalmoscope, along the patient's optical axis after the patient's pupil has been dilated. The 35 mm camera is, in effect, a large ophthalmoscope that allows viewing of the retina and a light flash system for producing color photographs of the retina. Both eyes are photographed. The results are interpreted by the physician.

92260

The physician exerts pressure on the sclera with a spring plunger while observing with an ophthalmoscope the vessels of the optic disk. Ophthalmodynamometry gives a measurement of the relative pressures in the central retinal arteries. It is also an indirect means of assessing carotid artery flow on either side.

92265

The physician or technician applies concentri needle electrodes to the patient's extraocular muscles to record muscle actions. This procedure is mostly applied for research into eye movement.

92270

A normal retina has a predictable electrical response to light. The EOG records metabolic changes in the retinal pigment epithelium by evaluating the retina's response to light. The physician or technician places electrodes on the skin around the eye so that eye movements of both eyes can be recorded separately or together. The EOG is often used in cases where the electroretinography isn't sensitive enough to pick up macular degeneration. The physician interprets the results of the test.

92275

A normal retina has a predictable electrical response to light. To determine if the retina is damaged, the physician places an ocular fitted contact lens electrode on the patient's eye and another electrode on the forehead so that the retina's electrical responses to external stimuli can be recorded under light-adapted conditions. This procedure, often abbreviated ERG, is repeated in dark-adapted conditions. The ERG waves are then analyzed by the physician.

92283

This test describes an extended color vision examination involving an anomaloscope, which is an instrument used to diagnose abnormalities of color perception in which one-half of a field of color is matched by mixing two other colors.

92284

This exam tests the function of the two photoreceptors: the rods and the cones. Rods are most sensitive in dim illumination and are responsible for night vision. The cones are more sensitive in bright luminations and are responsible for day vision. The eye to be tested is exposed to a bright light and then the room is darkened. At 30-second intervals, the light is increased and the effect of the stimulus on the retina is measured by a Goldmann-Weekers machine.

92285

These photos are often referred to as anterior segment photography, and are used to document abnormalities of the anterior segment that do not require magnification to be seen in the lids, cornea, anterior chamber, lens, and iris. The physician photographs the eye using a free-standing camera, a camera affixed to a slit lamp, or a stereo-photography.

92286

The physician performs this microscopy, often called endothelial cell count, to check the integrity and density of the endothelial cells that comprise the innermost layer of the cornea.

92287

The physician performs this microscopy to examine the iris. This procedure includes fluorescein angiography which is for detection of abnormalities of retinal blood vessels. The angioscopy begins when a small amount of fluorescein dye is injected into the arm. The dye is transported to the eye through the blood vessels. As the dye traverses the vessels in the iris, the iris is viewed through the scope using filters that enhance the fluorescence of the eye. This test most often is used to deliniate fine neovascularization of tumors in the anterior segment.

92310

Using a keratometer, the technician determines the patient's corneal curvatures. The lenses are fitted for power, size, curvature, flexibility and lens type. The fitting includes instruction and training of the wearer and incidental revision of the lens during the training period, which ranges from six to 12 weeks.

92311–92312

Using a keratometer, the technician determines the patient's corneal curvature. The lens is fitted for power, size, curvature, flexibility and lens type. The fitting includes instruction and training of the wearer and incidental revision of the lens during the training period, which ranges from six to 12 weeks.

92313

Using a keratometer, the technician determines the patient's corneal curvature. The corneoscleral lens is fitted for power, size, curvature, flexibility and lens type. The fitting includes instruction and training of the wearer and incidental revision of the lens during the training period, which ranges from six to 12 weeks.

92314

The lens is fitted for power, size, curvature, flexibility and lens type. The fitting includes instruction and training of the wearer and incidental revision of the lens during the training period, which ranges from six to 12 weeks.

92315–92316

The lens is fitted for power, size, curvature, flexibility and lens type. The fitting includes instruction and training of the wearer and incidental revision of the lens during the training period, which ranges from six to 12 weeks. Report 92315 if one eye is fitted or 92316 for both eyes.

92317

The lens is fitted for power, size, curvature, flexibility and lens type. The fitting includes instruction and training of the wearer and incidental revision of the lens during the training period, which ranges from six to 12 weeks.

92325

The physician or technician uses a grinder to flatten or polish the contact lens or lens edge to provide a more comfortable fit.

92326

The ophthalmologist meets with the patient to discuss replacement of contact lenses, which may be due to wear and tear of the existing pair, loss, or discomfort. A new prescription is a separately reported service.

92330

The physician measures dimensions, selects colors and any modifications, and provides an ocular prosthesis of glass or plastic shaped and colored to specifications to resemble the anterior portion of the patient's normal eye. The physician inserts the artificial eye into the patient's eviscerated or enucleated eye or eye socket.

92335

An independent technician prescribes and directs the fitting of a ready-made or custom-made prosthesis of glass or plastic shaped and colored to specifications to resemble the anterior portion of the patient's normal eye, for insertion for cosmetic reasons into the socket or of an enucleated or eviscerated eye. The physician supervises the patient's adaptation to the prosthesis.

92340–92342

The physician or technician measures the patient's anatomical facial characteristics, records the laboratory specifications, and performs the final adjustment of the monofocal (e.g., for 92340), bifocal (e.g., for 92341), or multifocal (e.g., for 92342) spectacles to the visual axes and anatomical topography.

92352–92353

The physician or technician measures the aphakic patient's anatomical facial characteristics, records the laboratory specifications, and performs the final adjustment of the monofocal (e.g., for 92352) or multifocal (e.g., for 92353) spectacles to the visual axes and anatomical topography.

92354

Some low vision aids are simply a convex lens mounted to spectacles. The physician or technician measures the patient's anatomical facial characteristics, records the laboratory specifications, and performs the final adjustment of the monofocal spectacles to the visual axes and anatomical topography.

92355

A focusable Galilean or Keplarian (internal prism) system in a spectacle frame is a popular choice. The fitting the the spectacles is separate from the prescription of the spectacles, which is considered part of the eye exam. The fitting includes measurement of anatomical facial characteristics, the writing of laboratory specifications, and the final adjustment of the spectacles to the visual axes and anatomical topography. The supply of materials is a separate component, as is the prescription.

92358

The physician or technician procures or provides a temporary, ready-made contact lens to a patient, whose natural intraocular lens had been previously removed surgically.

92370–92371

The physician or technician repairs or refits a pair of spectacles. Adjustments may be made to the ear or nose pieces, or plastic frames may be heated and bent to better fit the patient, who has natural or artificial intraocular lenses. Report 92370 if the patient is not aphakic, and 92371 if the patient is aphakic.

92390

The physician or technician assembles or procures a pair of spectacles using established measurements for physical and optical characteristics for the patient who has natural or artificial intraocular lenses.

92391

The physician or technician creates or procures contact lenses using established measurements for physical and optical characteristics for the patient who has natural or artificial intraocular lenses.

92392

The physician or technician assembles or procures a pair of low vision aids using established measurements for physical and optical characteristics for the patient who has severe refractive error.

92393

The physician or technician creates or procures a prosthesis of glass or plastic. The prosthesis is shaped and colored to resemble a normal eye. In the case of an eviscerated eye, the prosthesis may simply be a small disc simulating a pupil and iris.

92395

The physician or technician assembles or procures a pair of spectacles for the aphakic patient using established measurements for physical and optical characteristics.

92396

The physician or technician creates or procures a contact lens for the aphakic patient using established measurements for physical and optical characteristics.

92502

Occasionally, a child or an adult is uncooperative and a otolaryngologic examination cannot be performed until the patient is placed under general anesthesia. At other times, as in the case of a trauma victim, the patient is already anesthetized. At this time, a thorough examination of the ear, nose, and pharynx is completed.

92504

The physician uses an operating binocular microscope to examine the ear and occasionally the nose for direct, detailed visualization.

92506

The physician takes a history of the patient, including speech and language development, hearing loss, and physical and mental development. A physical examination is performed. Hearing tests and speech/language evaluations are performed. Assessment of deficits and a plan for the patient are made. These plans may involve speech therapy, hearing aids, etc.

92507–92508

Under direction of a physician, the patient undergoes developmental programs such as speech therapy, sign language, or lip reading instruction or hearing rehabilitation following placement of a cochlear implant. The program is for the individual in 92507 or in a group setting in 92508.

92510

Aural rehabilitation is auditory training or therapy conducted by a physician, speech and language therapist, or teacher of the hearing impaired. This post-surgical training program should be initiated after the speech processor component has been programmed by the audiologist of the cochlear implant team. After programming, the patient is assessed through a series of listening inventories and phonetic discrimination testing to determine the patient's level of meaningful sound perception. The patient is taught a logical progression of auditory skills to maximize communication abilities and increase the use of residual hearing. The auditory training goals range from awareness of environmental sound to progressively higher levels of speech discrimination.

92511

The examination is performed with the patient lying on his back and under local anesthetic with topical Lidocaine that is sprayed onto the back of the throat and into the nasal passages. The physician introduces the flexible fiberoptic endoscope through the nose and advances it into the pharynx to determine whether there are any fixed blockages such as a deviated septum, nasal polyps, or enlarged adenoids and tonsils. The physician may position the tip of the endoscope at the level of the hard palate and instruct the patient to perform simple manoeuvres that demonstrate airway activity under conditions that promote or help prevent collapse. The test may be performed to identify anatomic factors contributing to sleep disorder, stability of the upper airway, and determining treatments.

92512

Nasal function studies are performed for analyzing nasal resistance during breathing. In rhinomanometry, the physician uses a tubular probe to generate and transmit an audible sound signal into the patient's nasal cavity through an anatomically fitted nose piece. A microphone picks up the sound from the nasal cavity and the data is analyzed by computer to determine area distance in the nasal cavity.

92516

Facial nerve functions studies, such as electroneuronography (EnoG) are used to diagnose facial paralysis disorders, such as Bell's palsy (a unilateral or bilateral facial paralysis due to a viral attack on the facial nerve). These tests include an ENoG or an electromyogram that measure nerve conduction to diagnose degenerative disorders. In an electromyogram, the physician attaches small disc electrodes to the skin surface over the muscle or nerve by inserting small metal needles into the areas. The needle or electrode may be changed as needed for a complete study. An oscilloscope displays and records the data.

92520

The physician inserts a laryngoscope through the mouth or nose to examine the larynx. An indirect laryngoscope uses mirrors to view the larynx, while a direct laryngoscope is done with a fiberoptic scope. The function studies are used to diagnose the reason for laryngeal dysfunction such as swallowing disorders, chronic hoarseness, or an obstruction.

92525

The physician may prescribe any of a variety of tests to access swallowing disorders, which may be caused by neuromuscular disorders such as Parkinson's disease or tumors. Simple bedside evaluation of swallowing can serve as an initial screen for swallowing disorders. A more detailed examination may require the assistance of a speech pathologist testing swallowing substances of various textures. Further evaluation focuses on the function of structures in the throat and mouth. Finally, the physician may choose a video recording of barium being swallowed may define abnormalities from the mouth to the stomach.

92526

The treatment of swallowing disorders is aimed at finding the specific cause of the dysfunction to treat the problem, such as, anti-reflux medications to decrease stomach acidity or improve esophageal motility. Patients who have had strokes and cannot be treated surgically or by drugs for swallowing dysfunctions may require assistance from a rehabilitation specialist. In severe cases, the physician may elect to insert a feeding tube through the nose or in the stomach through the abdomen.

92531

Nystagmus is uncontrolled rapid movement of the eyeball in a horizontal, vertical, or rotary motion. It can be a symptom of a disturbance in the patient's vestibular system, and can be induced to measure the difference between the patient's right and left vestibular functions. The patient's eyes are observed for spontaneous nystagmus as the patient is asked to look straight ahead, 30 degrees to 45 degrees to the right, and 30 degrees to 45 degrees to the left. No electrodes are used and no recording made.

92532

A positional nystagmus test measures whether the eyes can maintain a static position when the head is in different position, which helps in documenting and quantifying patient complaints of dizziness in certain positions. The test also may be performed as a diagnostic tool to determine if an abnormality is associated with the central nervous system or the peripheral nervous system. The patient is placed in a variety of positions including supine with head extended dorsally, left and right, and sitting in an attempt to induce nystagmus. This is done with the patient's eye open so that eye movements can be observed directly. No recording electrodes are used to record the nystagmus.

92533

Nystagmus is uncontrolled rapid movement of the eyeball in a horizontal, vertical, or rotary motion. It can be a symptom of a disturbance in the patient's vestibular system, and can be induced to measure the difference between the patient's right and left vestibular functions. In this test, each ear is separately irrigated with cold water and then warm water to create nystagmus in the patient. The physician or audiologist observes the patient to detect any difference between the reaction of the right side and the left side. Four irrigations occur: a warm and cold irrigation for both the right and the left ear.

92534

A rotating drum made of alternating light and dark vertical stripes is placed in front of the patient and the patient is instructed to stare at the drum without focusing on any one stripe. The eyes are observed for nystagmus while the drum is rotated in one direction. The direction of the drum is then reversed. No electrodes are used.

92541

Nystagmus is uncontrolled rapid movement of the eyeball in a horizontal, vertical, or rotary motion. It can be a symptom of a disturbance in the patient's vestibular system, and can be induced to measure the difference between the patient's right and left vestibular functions. ENG (electronystagmography) electrodes are placed and the patient is asked to look straight ahead, 30 degrees to 45 degrees to the right, and 30 degrees to 45 degrees to the left. Recordings are made to detect spontaneous nystagmus.

92542

Nystagmus is uncontrolled rapid movement of the eyeball in a horizontal, vertical, or rotary motion. It can be a symptom of a disturbance in the patient's vestibular system, and can be induced to measure the

difference between the patient's right and left vestibular functions. The patient is placed in a variety of positions including supine with head extended dorsally, left and right; and sitting in an attempt to induce nystagmus. With the patient's eyes closed, an ENG recording is made to detect nystagmus.

92543

Nystagmus is uncontrolled rapid movement of the eyeball in a horizontal, vertical, or rotary motion. It can be a symptom of a disturbance in the patient's vestibular system, and can be induced to measure the difference between the patient's right and left vestibular functions. In this test, each ear is separately irrigated with cold water and then warm water to create nystagmus in the patient. ENG recordings are evaluated to detect any difference between the nystagmus of the right side and the left side. Four irrigations occur: a warm and cold irrigation for both the right and the left ear.

92544

Nystagmus is uncontrolled rapid movement of the eyeball in a horizontal, vertical, or rotary motion. It can be a symptom of a disturbance in the patient's vestibular system, and can be induced to measure the difference between the patient's right and left vestibular functions. This test is usually done with a rotating drum of alternating light and dark vertical stripes. The drum is placed in front of the patient and the patient is instructed to stare at the drum without focusing on any one stripe. The drum is then rotated in one direction and then reversed and rotated in the opposite direction. ENG electrodes are used to record nystagmus.

92545

Nystagmus is uncontrolled rapid movement of the eyeball in a horizontal, vertical, or rotary motion. It can be a symptom of a disturbance in the patient's vestibular system, and can be induced to measure the difference between the patient's right and left vestibular functions. With ENG electrodes in place, the patient is asked to follow a swinging object such as a ball on a string. A recording is made of the eye tracking the motion. The recording is then analyzed for smoothness.

92546

Nystagmus is uncontrolled rapid movement of the eyeball in a horizontal, vertical, or rotary motion. It can be a symptom of a disturbance in the patient's vestibular system, and can be induced to measure the difference between the patient's right and left vestibular functions. The patient is seated in a rotary chair with the head bent forward 30 degrees. ENG electrodes are placed to measure nystagmus while the chair is rotated with the patient's eyes closed. A recording is made and studied to determine an abnormal labyrinthine response on one side or the other.

92547

ENG electrodes are placed to measure vertical and rotary nystagmus. List 92547 separately in addition to the code for the primary procedure, and use 92547 in conjunction with 92541–92546.

92548

Computerized dynamic posturography tests a patient's sensory organization, motor control, evoked postural responses (EMG), and sway patterns to assess balance and postural instability by systematic manipulation of somatosensory and visual information. The patient is placed in the posturography system. The system is made up of a force plate which controls foot support and a visual surround reference that can be controlled. Force transducers measure the vertical and horizontal force output of the patient's feet. The patient's center-of-force is used as an estimate of body sway during testing. A sway bar and potentiometer at the pelvis and shoulder measure anterior-posterior position and displacement of the visual surround is changed or as the ankle angle is changed. In the posture portion of posturography, the support surface rotates faster than the body can move, producing a sway and ankle rotation that is opposite of what normally occurs in a standing position on a fixed surface. This exaggerated sway produces a stretching of the ankle joint which is recorded as three surface EMG signals from the gastrocnemius and tibialis anterior muscles of the legs to a computer which records the data. Patients with normal function will maintain balance while patients with a disturbance of balance will elicit abnormal results. The EMG portion of posturography along with the sensory organization and motor control tests help differentiate between the possible diagnoses causing the patient's imbalance and postural instability.

92551

Earphones are placed and the patient is asked to respond to tones of different pitches and intensities. This is a limited study using a few different pitches and intensities. If a patient fails to respond appropriately, additional testing is indicated.

92552–92553

Often, physicians or technicians can diagnose a cause of hearing loss through tests using an audiometer. Many causes of hearing loss have characteristic threshold curves. In pure tone audiometry, earphones are placed and the patient is asked to respond to tones of different pitches (frequencies) and intensities. The threshold, which is the lowest intensity of the tone that the patient can hear 50 percent of the time, is recorded for a number of frequencies on each ear. Bone thresholds (e.g., for 92553) are obtained in a similar manner except a bone oscillator is used on the mastoid or forehead to conduct the sound instead of tones through earphones. The air and bone thresholds are compared to differentiate between conductive, sensorineural, or mixed hearing losses.

92555–92556

Often, physicians or technicians can diagnose a cause of hearing loss through tests using an audiometer. Many causes of hearing loss have characteristic threshold curves unique to that specific diagnosis. In speech audiometry, earphones are placed and the patient is asked to repeat bisyllabic (spondee) words. The softest level at which the patient can correctly repeat 50 percent of the spondee words is called the speech reception threshold. The threshold is recorded for each ear in 92555. This process occurs in 92556, in addition to a discrimination test. There, the word discrimination score is the percentage of spondee words that a patient can repeat correctly at a given intensity level above his or her speech reception threshold. This is also measured for each ear.

92557

Often, physicians or technicians can diagnose a cause of hearing loss through tests using an audiometer. Many causes of hearing loss have characteristic threshold curves. In comprehensive audiometry, earphones are placed and the patient is asked to respond to tones of different pitches (frequencies) and intensities. The threshold, which is the lowest intensity of the tone that the patient can hear 50 percent of the time, is recorded for a number of frequencies on each ear. Bone thresholds are obtained in a similar manner except a bone oscillator is used on the mastoid or forehead to conduct the sound instead of tones through earphones. The air and bone thresholds are compared to differentiate between conductive, sensorineural, or mixed hearing losses. With the earphones in place, the patient is also asked to repeat bisyllabic (spondee) words. The softest level at which the patient can correctly repeat 50 percent of the spondee words is called the speech reception threshold. The threshold is recorded for each ear. The word discrimination score is the percentage of spondee words that a patient can repeat correctly at a given intensity level above his or her speech reception threshold. This is also measured for each ear.

92559

Often, physicians or technicians can diagnose a cause of hearing loss through tests using an audiometer. Many causes of hearing loss have characteristic threshold curves. In audiometric testing of groups, many people are tested concurrently usually by pure tone screening. Earphones are placed and the patient is asked to respond to tones of different pitches and intensities. This is a limited study using a few different pitches and intensities.

92560–92561

Often, physicians or technicians can diagnose a cause of hearing loss through tests using an audiometer. Bekesy audiometry is a complex and rarely used diagnostic test. A special audiometer is used to deliver pulsing and continuous tones to the patient through earphones. The patient makes an audiogram by pushing and relaxing a button to indicate whether or not the tone was heard at changing intensity levels. In 92560, the audiograms are used as a screening tool to determine hearing thresholds. In 92561, the tracings are then analyzed and categorized into several different hearing patterns.

92562

Earphones are placed and tones of the same pitch but different intensities are presented to each ear (binaural). Or tones of different intensities and pitches are presented to the same ear (monaural). The patient is asked to compare the loudness of the tones. Differences in intensities that are perceived by the patient as the same are measured.

92563

Earphones are placed and a tone is presented to the patient at a volume above the patient's lowest hearing level for that tone. Measurements are made of the time the tone is audible or the increase in volume needed to maintain an audible tone over time. These measurements are compared to established norms and can be reported at different tone frequencies.

92564

Earphones are placed and tones are presented to the patient. The loudness of the tones is increased in small increments. The patient is tested on the ability to detect slight changes in loudness. A percentage of the correctly identified loudness changes is recorded.

92565

This test is for unilateral pseudohypacusis (malingering). It is based on the principle that if two sounds of the same frequency but different intensities are presented simultaneously to both ears, only the louder tone will be heard. Tones are presented to the "good ear" at a level above that ear's threshold to obtain a response. Tones are presented to the "poor ear" simultaneously. The intensity of the sound in the "poor ear" is then increased while the intensity presented to the "good ear" remains the same. The patient will respond until the intensity of the tones in the "poor ear" exceeds that of the "good ear." At that point, the patient will not respond because the patient is not supposed to hear out of the "poor ear." However, the patient should still respond as the intensity of presentation to the "good ear" has not changed.

92567

Using an ear probe, the eardrum's resistance to sound transmission is measured in response to pressure changes. Tympanometry varies the pressure in the external ear canal and identifies the pressure at which maximum sound transmission occurs. This corresponds to current middle ear pressure status. The pressures are recorded and compared to normal values.

92568

The audiologist places a probe in one ear (ipsilateral ear) to measure the impedance of the middle ear and places an earphone on the patient's opposite ear (contralateral ear). A loud sound is presented in either the contralateral or ipsilateral ear, and the change in impedance caused by the contraction of the stapedinus is measured.

92569

The audiologist places a probe to measure impedance in one ear (ipsilateral ear) and places an earphone on the other ear (contralateral ear). A loud tone is presented to one of the ears and maintained for 10 seconds. The impedance change (acoustic reflex) is measured by the probe. In a normal ear, the reflex persists for 10 seconds. In an abnormal ear, the reflex diminishes at least 50 percent in the first five seconds.

92571

The patient is presented monosyllabic words which are low pass filtered allowing only the parts of each word below a certain frequency (pitch) to be presented. A score is given on the number of correct responses. This test is most commonly used to identify central auditory dysfunction.

92572

With the patient wearing earphones, the audiologist presents bisyllabic (spondee) words in groups of two words. The first syllable of the first word is given to one ear (first word ear) then the last syllable of the first word is given to the same ear at the same time the first syllable of the second word is given to the opposite ear (second word ear). The second syllable of the second word is then presented alone to the second word ear. The patient is asked to identify the words presented to each ear and a score is given for each ear.

92573

This is principally a test for pseudohypacusis (malingering). The patient reads a passage into a microphone while the audiologist makes noise (masking) in earphones the patient is wearing. The patient's voice volume while reading is measured as the masking level is increased. If the patient increases his or her voice volume with the increase in masking as is normal, it is assumed that the noise (masking) was heard by the patient. This level may prove to be lower than the patient had previously volunteered.

92575

The audiologist places earphones on the patient and presents tones to the patient at different volumes and different frequencies (pitches). The volume at each frequency where the patient responds correctly 50 percent of the time is the threshold at that frequency. The sounds presented through the earphones are air-conduction. The air-conduction thresholds are then measured in the presence of noise (masking) through a bone vibrator on the side of the head (bone-conducted masking). The masked and unmasked air-conduction thresholds are then compared.

92576

Using earphones, seven-word sentences that do not follow normal rules of grammar are presented to one ear while a taped story is presented to the other ear simultaneously (competition). The patient is scored on the ability to correctly identify the seven-word sentences. This test is principally used for central hearing disorders.

92577

This is a test for unilateral pseudohyphensis (malingering). It is based on the principle that if two sounds of the same frequency and different intensities are presented simultaneously to both ears, only the louder will be heard. Bisyllabic (spondee) words are presented to the "good ear" at a level above that ear's threshold to respond. Then words are presented simultaneously to the "poor ear." The intensity of the sound in the "poor ear" is then increased while the intensity presented to the "good ear" remains the same. The patient will respond until the intensity of the words in the "poor ear" exceeds that of the "good ear." At that point, the patient will not respond because the patient is not supposed to hear out of the "poor ear." However, the patient should still respond as the intensity of presentation to the "good ear" has not changed.

92579

Visual reinforcement audiometry (VRA) is used to test hearing in infants and in both difficult-to-test children and adults. The process includes case history and otologic examination, typically conducted in a sound booth. Lighted toys are used as reinforcement for response to auditory stimuli. Stimuli may include frequency-specific signals, calibrated noises, or live voice. The results are usually recorded on an audiogram. The interpretation of the testing addresses the type and the severity of hearing loss and any recommendations.

92582

Often, physicians or technicians can diagnose a cause of hearing loss through tests using an audiometer. Many causes of hearing loss have characteristic threshold curves. Conditioning play audiometry tests pure tone air and bone conduction and speech thresholds in children. Test sounds can be presented with earphones or sound field testing (pure tone air conduction only). The child is conditioned to perform a simple task (i.e., drop a block in a bucket) when the test sound is heard.

92583

Often, physicians or technicians can diagnose a cause of hearing loss through tests using an audiometer. Many causes of hearing loss have characteristic

threshold curves. In select picture audiometry, the patient is placed in a booth with or without earphones. The patient is asked to identify different pictures with the instructions given at different intensity levels. A threshold level for speech, which is the intensity level at which the patient responds correctly 50 percent of the time, is obtained.

92584

An electrode is placed through the tympanic membrane into the promontory of the inner ear. The ear is stimulated and recordings are made of the electrical response of the cochlear nerve. This can be done under local, topical, or general anesthesia.

92585–92586

Electrodes are placed in various locations on the scalp and electrical recordings are made in response to auditory stimulations. The origin of the electrical response is believed to be from the auditor nerve and brain stem. The physician interprets the results of the tests. Report 92585 if the procedure is limited. Report 92586 if the test is comprehensive.

92587–92588

A probe tip is placed in the ear canal. The probe tip emits a repeated clicking sound. The clicking sound passes through the tympanic membrane, middle ear, and then to the inner ear. In the inner ear, the sound is picked up by the hair cells in the cochlea. Computerized equipment is then able to record an echo off the hair cell in the cochlea. Report 92587 if the test is limited to a single stimulus level. Report 92588 if the test is comprehensive or a diagnostic evaluation.

92589

There are numerous methods to test central auditory function including techniques using pure tones, monosyllabic words, bisyllabic (spondee) words, and sentences. These tests are used to help differentiate central from peripheral hearing loss and occasionally to identify the site of a lesion in the central nervous system.

92590–92591

The physician takes a history of hearing loss. The patient's ears are examined. Medical or surgical treatment is offered if possible. The appropriate type of hearing aid is selected to fit the patient's pattern of hearing loss. Report 92590 if one ear is fitted with a hearing aid and 92591 if both ears receive aids.

92592–92593

The audiologist inspects the hearing aid and checks the battery. The aid is cleaned and the power and clarity are checked using a special stethoscope, which attaches to the hearing aid. Report 92592 if a monaural hearing aid is check and 92593 if both hearing aids are checked.

92594–92595

A printout from a hearing aid analyzer is used to compare the electroacoustical characteristics of a monaural hearing aid with the specifications for that aid in 92594 or a binaural hearing aid with specifications for that aid in 92595.

92596

This test can be performed in one of several ways. One method is to check the speech or pure tone threshold, which is the intensity at which the patient responds correctly 50 percent of the time, with and without ear protection (ear plugs or earphones) while the patient is in a soundproof booth.

92597

A communication device such as an amplifier is used to augment speech for a patient with complete or partial speech loss. The code applies to evaluating and/or fitting the device often by a speech therapist or physician.

92598

A communication device such as an amplifier is used to augment speech for a patient with complete or partial speech loss. This code applies to the modification of an existing device often by a speech therapist or physician.

92950

Cardiopulmonary arrest occurs when the patient's heart and lungs suddenly stop. In a clinical setting, cardiopulmonary resuscitation, the attempt at restarting the heart and lungs, is usually directed by a physician or another healthcare provider who is certified in Advanced Cardiac Life Support (ACLS). The patient's lungs are ventilated by mouth-to-mouth breathing or by a bag and mask. The patient's circulation is assisted using external chest compression. An electronic defibrillator may be used to shock the heart into restarting. Medications used to restart the heart include epinephrine and lidocaine.

92953

A temporary pacemaker is placed on the patient's heart to regulate heartbeats considered dangerously irregular. The physician applies electrodes to the chest wall. The electrodes give small electronic shocks through the chest to pace the heart as controlled by the physician.

92960–92961

The physician may administer an electronic shock to the patient's chest to regulate heartbeats considered dangerously irregular. The physician uses a defibrillator machine and places two paddles on the patient's chest and/or back. A measured electric shock is delivered through the chest to the heart to convert the heartbeat to a regular rhythm. Report 92960 for external cardioversion, and 92961 when the procedure is performed internally.

92970

In internal circulatory assist the femoral artery is cannulated and a catheter with balloon or other device is inserted into the aorta. Various devices may be used to assist circulation. This code should be reported for the internal insertion of such a device, but should not be used to report inta-aortic balloon pump (IABP), or implantation of ventricular assist devices which are reported elsewhere.

92971

Devices are placed at the outside of the body to assist circulation. One example of external circulatory assist is Military Anti-Shock Trousers (MAST) which apply counterpressure around the legs and abdomen. The artificial peripheral resistance helps coronary perfusion. In a related procedure pressure cuffs are used to assist circulation. The patient is placed on a treatment table where their lower extremities are wrapped in a series of three compressive air cuffs, which inflate and deflate in synchronization with the patient's cardiac cycle. During diastole the three sets of air cuffs are inflated sequentially (distal to proximal) compressing the vascular beds within the muscles of the calves, lower thighs and upper thighs. This action results in an increase in diastolic pressure, generation of retrograde arterial blood flow and an increase in venous return. The cuffs are deflated simultaneously just prior to systole, which produces a rapid drop in vascular impedance, a decrease in ventricular workload and an increase in cardiac output. The augmented diastolic pressure and retrograde aortic flow appear to improve myocardial perfusion, while systolic unloading appears to reduce cardiac workload and oxygen requirements. The increased venous return coupled with enhanced systolic flow appears to increase cardiac output.

92973

The physician percutaneously removes a blood clot from a native or grafted coronary artery. A double lumen catheter is passed to the area of the clot. A high-pressure saline stream (via a pump) is introduced through a lumen that has multiple jet orifices located at the distal tip. The low-pressure zone created by the jets causes the clot to break-up into small pieces and be pushed through the catheter with a force that drives debris from the thrombus through the other lumen (exhaust) and out of the body. The procedure is useful to clear fatty and degenerated arteries and to modify plaques in preparation for more definitive treatment with adjunctive balloon angioplasty or stenting.

92975–92977

The physician places a hollow catheter in the aorta from the arm or leg. A small incision is made. Using fluoroscopic guidance, the physician advances the catheter tip to the coronary artery to be treated, and confirms the presence of thrombus (blood clot) in the artery by injecting contrast material through the catheter into the artery. The physician infuses a thrombolytic agent (urokinase, for example), into the affected artery in order to dissolve the thrombus. The physician may perform contrast injections to assess the size and extent of the thrombus after infusion of the thrombolytic agent. The catheter is removed from the patient's body. Pressure is placed over the incision for 20 to 30 minutes to stem bleeding. The patient is observed for a period afterward. Report 92977 if intravenous infusion is used.

92978–92979
Intravascular ultrasound may be used during diagnostic evaluation of coronary vessel or graft. It may also be used both before and after a therapeutic intervention upon a coronary vessel or graft to assess patency and integrity of the vessel or graft. A needle is inserted through the skin and into a blood vessel. A guide wire is threaded through the needle into a coronary blood vessel or graft. The needle is removed. An intravascular ultrasound catheter is placed over the guide wire. The ultrasound probe is used to obtain images from inside the vessel to assess area and extent of disease prior to interventional therapy as well as adequacy of therapy after interventional therapy. The ultrasound probe provides a two-dimensional cross-sectional view of the vessel or graft as the probe is advanced and withdrawn along the area of interest. When the ultrasound examination is complete, the catheter is removed. Code 92978 is reported for the initial vessel or graft. In 92979, the physician advances the ultrasound catheter into additional vessels or grafts to assess patency and structure. The catheter and guide wire are removed, and pressure is applied over the puncture site to stop bleeding.

92980–92981
A stent is used to hold open a blocked or collapsed blood vessel in the heart. The physician makes a small incision in the arm or leg. Two catheters are placed. A central venous catheter is inserted through the femoral or brachial artery and a second catheter is threaded up to the heart. Any obstruction is first treated by inflating a balloon at the tip of the second catheter (PTCA) and/or by using a rotary cutter (atherectomy) to flatten or remove the obstruction.. A stent is introduced through a special catheter and placed under radiographic guidance. Pressure is placed over the incision for 20 to 30 minutes to stem bleeding. The patient is observed for a period afterward. Report 92980 for one coronary vessel. Report 92981 for each additional vessel.

92982–92984
The physician makes a small incision in the arm or leg. Two catheters are placed. A central venous catheter is inserted through the femoral or brachial artery and a second catheter with a balloon tip is threaded up to the heart. The physician inflates the balloon at the tip of the second catheter to flatten plaque obstructing the artery against the walls of the

artery. If sufficient results are not obtained after the first inflation, the physician may reinflate the balloon for a longer period of time or at greater pressure. The catheter is removed. Pressure is placed over the incision for 20 to 30 minutes to stem bleeding. The patient is observed for a period afterward. Report 92982 for the balloon catheterization of one blocked vessel. Report 92984 for each additional vessel treated.

92986–92990
Valvuloplasty is a procedure for opening a blocked valve. The physician makes a small incision in the arm or leg. Two catheters are placed — a central venous catheter and a second catheter threaded up to the heart. The physician inflates a balloon at the tip of the second catheter to open the blocked valve. The catheter is removed. Pressure is placed over the incision for 20 to 30 minutes to stem bleeding. The patient is observed for a period afterward. The code applies to the procedure performed on the aortic valve. Report 92987 if the procedure is performed on the mitral valve. Report 92990 if the procedure is performed on the pulmonary valve.

92992
Certain congenital heart defects, particularly those involving transposition of the great vessels, require surgical creation or enlargement of an opening in the interatrial septum (wall) that separates the upper right and left chambers of the heart. The physician makes a small incision in the arm or leg. Two catheters are placed — a central venous catheter and a second catheter threaded up to the heart. When the foramen ovale has not closed, a deflated balloon (Rashkind-type) is passed through the foramen ovale, inflated, and pulled through the atrial septum, enlarging the opening and improving oxygenation of the blood. When the septum is intact, the deflated balloon (Rashkind-type) is passed from the right atrium through the septum to the left atrium, inflated and then withdrawn, creating an interatrial septal defect and improving oxygenation of the blood. The catheters are removed. Pressure is placed over the incision for 20 to 30 minutes to stem bleeding. A cardiac catheterization may be included. The patient is observed for a period afterward.

92993
The purpose of this procedure is to increase blood flow across the atrial septum in children with certain forms of cyanotic congenital heart disease. This procedure is used as an alternative to the Rashkind procedure (balloon method of atrial septostomy), typically in infants older than one month of age. The physician makes a small incision in the femoral vein. The physician places a transseptal sheath in the right femoral vein using standard methods, advancing the sheath to the superior vena cava under fluoroscopic or echocardiographic guidance. The physician uses a transseptal needle to cross the atrial septum, entering

the left atrium. The physician introduces a guidewire into the left atrium, removes the transseptal catheter while leaving the wire in place. The physician advances a special septostomy catheter over the wire into the left atrium. This catheter has a retracted blade, which the physician extends. The physician pulls the blade slowly across the atrial septum from the left into the right atrium, under fluoroscopic or echocardiographic guidance. The physician may make several passes with the blade catheter in this fashion. The physician removes the septostomy catheter and venous sheath. Pressure is placed over the incision for 20 to 30 minutes to stem bleeding. The patient is observed for a period afterward.

92995–92996

The physician removes the atherosclerotic plaque blocking the coronary artery. The physician makes a small incision in the arm or leg. Two catheters are placed. A central venous catheter is inserted through the femoral or brachial artery and a second catheter threaded up to the heart blockage. The blockage is removed using a rotary cutter introduced through a special catheter under radiographic guidance. The blockage may also require subsequent inflation of the balloon on the tip of the second catheter to flatten any remaining plaque. The catheters are removed. Pressure is placed over the incision for 20 to 30 minutes to stem bleeding. The patient is observed for a period afterward. Report 92995 for the first vessel. Report 92996 for each additional vessel.

92997

The purpose of this procedure is to use a balloon to expand a narrowed pulmonary artery. The physician places an introducer sheath in the femoral vein, using percutaneous puncture. The physician places a special angioplasty catheter through the introducer sheath into the femoral vein and advances it under fluoroscopic guidance to the right ventricle and out into the main pulmonary artery. The physician advances the angioplasty balloon into the narrowed pulmonary artery, using injections of x-ray contrast material to guide the way. The physician inflates the balloon to expand the pulmonary artery, sometimes using several balloon inflations. The physician removes the catheter and sheath from the femoral vein. Vessel hemostasis is achieved using manual pressure. Pressure is placed on the wound for 20 to 30 minutes to stem bleeding.

92998

Following single vessel percutaneous transluminal pulmonary artery balloon angioplasty (code 92997), the physician redirects the balloon angioplasty catheter to an additional pulmonary artery. The physician may change to a different sized balloon catheter if the additional pulmonary artery is of different size. The physician inflates the balloon to expand the pulmonary artery, sometimes using several balloon inflations. The physician removes the catheter

and sheath from the femoral vein. Pressure is placed on the wound for 20 to 30 minutes to stem bleeding.

93000

Twelve electrodes are placed on a patient's chest to record the electrical activity of the heart. A physician interprets the findings. This code is used to report the combined technical and professional components of an ECG.

93005

Twelve electrodes are placed on a patient's chest in a standard patter to record the electrical activity of the heart. This code is used to report the technical component only.

93010

A physician interprets a previously acquired recording of the heart's electrical activity acquired by placing 12 electrodes on the patient's chest. This code is used to report only the professional component.

93012

A patient uses a portable unit to record the electrical activity of the heart. Following a symptomatic episode, the recording is transmitted by telephone to the physician for printing. This code is reported one time per every 30 days. This code is used to report the technical component only.

93014

A patient uses a portable unit to record the electrical activity of the heart. The recording is transmitted by telephone to the physician for printing. This code applies to the physician's interpretation of the printed report.

93015

A continuous recording of electrical activity of the heart is acquired by an assistant supervised by a physician while the patient is exercising on a treadmill or bicycle and/or given medicines. The stress on the heart during the test is monitored. This code includes the test, physician supervision, and physician interpretation of the report.

93016

An assistant supervised by a physician makes a continuous recording of the electrical activity of a patient's heart while the patient is exercising on a treadmill or stationary bicycle with or without medication. The code applies only to the physician's supervision of the test.

93017

An assistant supervised by a physician makes a continuous recording of the electrical activity of a patient's heart while the patient is exercising on a treadmill or stationary bicycle with or without medication. The code applies only to acquiring the test.

CPT® Lay Descriptions

93018

An assistant supervised by a physician records the electrical activity of a patient's heart while the patient is exercising on a treadmill or stationary bicycle with or without medication. The code applies to the physician's interpretation of a previously acquired report.

93024

The purpose of the study is to evaluate for coronary artery spasm. If ergonovine is not available, certain other ergot medications may be infused for the same purpose. Following baseline coronary angiography (coded elsewhere), the physician infuses gradually escalating doses of ergonovine into a peripheral vein, while monitoring for chest discomfort and electrocardiographic changes. Repeat angiography is performed during ergonovine infusion to assess the size of the coronary lumen. If the patient develops symptomatic coronary spasm, the physician may directly infuse vasodilating medications through the intracoronary catheter to relieve the problem.

93025

T-Wave Alternans testing is an electrocardiographic method of measuring the alternating electrical amplitude from beat to beat on an electrocardiogram and is used as a method of evaluating ventricular arrhythmia risk. Microvolt T-wave alternans can be measured during exercise or pharmacologic stress, or during cardiac pacing, using a spectral analytic method with equipment that is able to detect as little as one microvolt of T-wave alternans. In electrode placement for a 12-lead ECG, the health care provider positions the leads either on the wrists and ankles or shoulders and groins. Left leg electrodes are placed below the heart (but not on the chest), preferably below the umbilicus. The sensing electrodes look at the inferior surface of the heart, the left or lateral side of the heart, and at the right side of the heart.

93040

One to three electrodes placed on a patient's chest are used to record electrical activity of the heart. The physician interprets the report.

93041

An assistant records the electrical activity of the heart by placing one to three electrodes on a patient's chest in a predetermined pattern. This code describes the tracing only.

93042

A physician interprets a recording of electrical activities of a patient's heart acquired by placing one to three electrodes on the patient's chest.

93224

The purpose of this study is to evaluate the patient's ambient heart rhythm during a full daily cycle. The physician instructs the patient in the use of the electrocardiographic (ECG) recorder (also known as a Holter monitor). A technician places ECG leads on the patient's chest and the patient wears the recorder for 24 hours. The patient returns the device, and the recorded heart rhythm is played back into digital format by a technician. The technician uses visual superimposition scanning to classify different ECG waveforms and to generate a report. The generated report describes the overall rhythm and significant arrhythmias. Rhythm strips are also generated. The physician reviews these data and provides the final interpretation in a report.

93225

The purpose of this study is to evaluate the patient's ambient heart rhythm during a full daily cycle (24 hours). The physician instructs the patient in the use of the electrocardiographic (ECG) recorder (also known as a Holter monitor). A technician places ECG leads on the patient's chest and the patient wears the recorder for 24 hours. The patient returns the device, and the recorded heart rhythm is played back into digital format by a technician. The technician uses visual superimposition scanning to classify different ECG waveforms and to generate a report. The generated report describes the overall rhythm and significant arrhythmias. Rhythm strips are also generated.

93226

The purpose of this study is to evaluate the patient's ambient heart rhythm during a full daily cycle. The physician instructs the patient in the use of the electrocardiographic (ECG) recorder (also known as a Holter monitor). A technician places ECG leads on the patient's chest and the patient wears the recorder for 24 hours. The patient returns the device, and the recorded heart rhythm is played back into digital format by a technician. The technician uses visual superimposition scanning to classify different ECG waveforms and generate a report. The generated report describes the overall rhythm and significant arrhythmias. Rhythm strips are also generated. This code does not include physician review and interpretation.

93227

The purpose of this study is to evaluate the patient's ambient heart rhythm during a full daily cycle. The physician instructs the patient in the use of the electrocardiographic (ECG) recorder (also known as a Holter monitor). A technician places ECG leads on the patient's chest and the patient wears the recorder for 24 hours. The patient returns the device, and the recorded heart rhythm is played back into digital format by a technician. The technician uses visual superimposition scanning to classify different ECG waveforms and generate a report (coded separately, 93226; or together with physician interpretation, 93224). The generated report describes the overall rhythm and significant arrhythmias. Rhythm strips are also generated. The physician reviews these data and provides the final interpretation in a report. This code does not include scanning analysis with report (see codes 93224 and 93226).

93230–93233

The purpose of this study is to evaluate the patient's ambient heart rhythm during a full daily cycle. The physician instructs the patient in the use of the electrocardiographic (ECG) recorder (also known as a Holter monitor). A technician places ECG leads on the patient's chest and the patient wears the recorder for 24 hours. The patient returns with the device, which is disconnected. This code includes hook-up, recording, and disconnection. Analysis/report is coded separately (93232); as is physician review and interpretation (93233). If all of these services are to be billed together, use code 93230

93235–93237

The purpose of this study is to evaluate the patient's ambient heart rhythm, usually during hospitalization. A technician places ECG leads on the patient's chest and the electrocardiographic signals are monitored for 24 hours. A computer classifies different ECG waveforms in real time. Intermittent full-sized waveform tracings are generated when the computer flags an abnormal rhythm, or possibly when the patient activates the device. A report is generated by the computer, often with the help of a technician. If this is done without physician review and interpretation, use code 93236. If physician review and interpretation is billed separately, use code 93237. If monitoring and data analysis with report is to be billed together with physician review and interpretation, use code 93235.

93268

The purpose of this study is to evaluate the patient's ambient heart rhythm during symptoms. The physician instructs the patient in the use of a portable rhythm monitor. A technician places ECG leads on the patient's chest and the monitor uses a continuous loop mechanism to constantly record the patient's rhythm. During symptoms, the patient activates the monitor by pressing a button. The resulting recording includes ECG activity prior to and during symptoms. The patient uses the device to transmit the recording over the telephone line, allowing a rhythm printout to be generated. The physician reviews and interprets this rhythm strip. Report this code one time per every 30 days.

93270

The purpose of this study is to evaluate the patient's ambient heart rhythm during symptoms. The physician instructs the patient in the use of a portable rhythm monitor. A technician places ECG leads on the patient's chest and the monitor uses a continuous loop mechanism to constantly record the patient's rhythm. During symptoms, the patient activates the

monitor by pressing a button. The resulting recording includes ECG activity prior to and during symptoms. The patient returns the device, which is disconnected. The recording is played back, allowing a rhythm printout to be generated.

93271–93272

The purpose of this study is to evaluate the patient's ambient heart rhythm during symptoms. The physician instructs the patient in the use of a portable rhythm monitor. A technician places ECG leads on the patient's chest and the monitor uses a continuous loop mechanism to constantly record the patient's rhythm. During symptoms, the patient activates the monitor by pressing a button. The resulting recording includes ECG activity prior to and during symptoms. The patient uses the device to transmit the recording over the telephone line, allowing a rhythm printout to be generated and analyzed. Hook-up, recording, and disconnection are coded separately as 93270; physician review and interpretation is coded separately as 93272.

93278

Electrodes placed on a patient's chest record the heart's electrical activity. This technique uses signal-averaged electrocardiography (SAECG) and may include a standard electrocardiogram.

93303

Transducers are placed on the patient's chest to record an echocardiograph, which uses ultrasound to visualize the heart's function, blood flow, valves, and chambers. The code applies to an evaluation for congenital defects.

93304

Transducers are placed on a patient's chest to record an echocardiograph, which uses ultrasound to visualize the heart's function, blood flow, valves, and chambers. The code applies to a follow-up or a limited evaluation for congenital defects.

93307–93308

A noninvasive study that uses ultrasound to visualize the heart's function, blood flow, valves, and chambers. Two dimensional echocardiography also referred to as "real-time" imaging is performed using multiple transducers or a rotating transducer and these images are recorded on videotape. Computer reconstruction provides the two-dimensional image of specific planes of the heart. M-mode provides additional detail of specific portions of the heart. A stationary ultrasound beam is directed at the area of the heart requiring additional study. 93307 applies to a complete evaluation. 93308 should be used for a follow-up or limited study.

93312–93314

Transesophageal echocardiograpy (TEE) is an invasive technique whereby the transducer is placed at the tip

CPT® Lay Descriptions

of an endoscope and introduced into the patient's esophagus to record a two-dimensional echocardiograph. This set of codes should be used for TEE used to diagnose cardiac sources of emboli, prosthetic heart valve malfunction, endocarditis, aortic dissection, cardiac tumors, and valvular heart disease excluding congenital heart disease. Code 93312 applies to a complete evaluation including probe placement, image acquisition, and the physician's interpretation. Report 93313 for probe placement only. Report 93314 for image acquisition, physician interpretation and report only.

93315–93317

Transesophageal echocardiograpy (TEE) is an invasive technique whereby the transducer is placed at the tip of an endoscope and introduced into the patient's esophagus to record a two-dimensional echocardiograph. This set of codes should be used for TEE used to diagnose cardiac sources of emboli, prosthetic heart valve malfunction, endocarditis, aortic dissection, cardiac tumors, and valvular heart disease excluding congenital heart disease. The set of codes is specific to evaluations for congenital defects. 93315 applies to a complete evaluation for congenital defects including probe placement, image acquisition, and the physician's interpretation. Report 93316 for probe placement only. Report 93317 for image acquisition, physician interpretation and report only.

93318

Transesophageal echocardiography (TEE) is an invasive technique whereby the transducer is placed at the tip of an endoscope and introduced into the patient's esophagus to record a two-dimensional echocardiograph. TEE provides high-quality, real-time images of the beating heart and mediastinal structures. This code reports ongoing hemodynamic monitoring using TEE. TEE may be used to monitor critically ill patients in the intensive care unit as well as patients in certain operative settings. In both the intensive care unit and the operating room, it is used to monitor cardiac function including cardiac preload, contractility and valve function in patients with acute hemodynamic decompensation. In addition, TEE may also be used to assess and monitor mediastinal, heart, lung, and aortic injury resulting from blunt chest trauma even in patients undergoing other life-saving procedures.

93320–93321

Transducers are placed on a patient's chest to record a Doppler echocardiograph, which uses ultrasound to visualize blood flow velocity, direction, and type of flow in different locations in the heart. Doppler studies can be displayed on either a strip chart of videorecorder. Report 93320 for a complete evaluation. Report 93321 for limited or follow-up studies. List separately in addition to codes for 93303, 93304, 93307, 93308, 93312, 93314, 93315, 93317, and 93350.

93325

The technique for Doppler color flow velocity mapping is similar to that of other echocardiographs with transducers being placed on the patients chest to record cardiac activity. Color Doppler is two-dimensional Doppler in which the signal is encoded with color to more clearly identify flow direction. List separately in addition to code for echocardiography 76825, 76826, 76827, 76828, 93303, 93304, 93307, 93308, 93312, 93314, 93315, 93317, 93320, 93321, and 93350.)

93350

Transducers are placed on a patient's chest to record a two-dimensional echocardiograph, which uses ultrasound to visualize the heart's function, blood flow, valves, and chambers. The code applies to the echocardiography completed while the patient is at rest and exercising on a treadmill or stationary bicycle with or without medication.

93501

The physician threads a catheter to the heart most frequently through an introducing sheath placed percutaneously into the femoral vein. However, the physician may elect to use the subclavian, internal jugular, or antecubital vein instead. The catheter is then threaded into the right atrium, through the tricuspid valve into the right ventricle and across the pulmonary valve into the pulmonary arteries. ECG monitoring for the entirety of the procedure is included. Blood samples, pressure and electrical recordings, and/or other tests are performed through the catheter. The code applies to catheterizing the heart's right side only. The appropriate stress testing code from the 93015–93018 series should be reported in addition to this code.

93503

The physician threads a catheter to the right heart through a central intravenous line often inserted up the femoral vein to take blood samples, pressure and electrical recordings, and/or other tests. The code applies to the insertion or a flow directed catheter such as the Swan-Ganz device used for measuring pressure and related parameters.

93505

The physician threads a catheter to the heart through a central intravenous line often inserted up the femoral vein to take tissue samples of the heart's septum.

93508

The physicians performs a catheter placement in coronary arteries, arterial coronary conduits, and/or venous coronary bypass grafts for coronary angiography without concomitant left heart catheterization. The physician places an introducer sheath in an artery, typically the femoral artery, using percutaneous puncture. The physician advances an angiography catheter through the introducer sheath into ascending aorta and advances it under fluoroscopic guidance to the opening (os) of the coronary artery, arterial coronary conduit, or venous coronary bypass graft. The physician injects radiopaque contrast material through the catheter into the vessel while recording a cineangiogram. The physician removes the catheter and sheath from the femoral artery. Pressure is placed on the wound for 20 to 30 minutes to stem bleeding. This code does not include measurement of left heart pressures or left ventriculography.

93510–93511

The physician threads a catheter to the heart most frequently through an introducing sheath placed percutaneously into the femoral, brachial, or axillary artery using retrograde technique. Using this technique, the catheter passes through the aortic valve into the left ventricle. Blood samples, pressure and electrical recordings, and/or other tests are performed. ECG monitoring for the entirety of the procedure is included. 93510 should be used for percutaneous catheter placement. 93511 should be used when surgical dissection or a cutdown is required to locate the artery.

93514

This physician uses this approach to the left heart when standard approaches cannot be performed, usually due to abnormal anatomy or the presence of prosthetic heart valves. The physician locates the left ventricular apex using palpation, fluoroscopy, and possibly echocardiography. The physician anesthetizes the skin overlying the ventricle, using local anesthetic. The physician punctures the skin and chest wall with a large bore needle, aimed into the left ventricular cavity. The physician introduces a guide wire through the needle into the left ventricle and removes the needle backwards over the guide wire. The physician advances a dilator, a catheter, over the needle and into the left ventricular cavity. The physician manipulates the catheter to record left heart pressures and may inject radiographic contrast through the catheter to obtain a left ventriculogram.

93524

The physician threads a catheter to the heart using combined retrograde and transeptal techniques to evaluate left heart function. The retrograde portion is performed through an introducing sheath placed percutaneously into the femoral, brachial, or axillary artery. The catheter is then passed through the aortic valve into the left ventricle. Transeptal catheterization involves passing a catheter from the right femoral vein to the right atrium. The interatrial wall or septum is punctured and the catheter is passed into the left atrium through the mitral valve and into the left ventricle. Blood samples, pressure, electrical recordings, and/or other measurements are made.

93526

This procedure is performed to evaluate both right and left heart function. To accomplish right heart catheterization, the physician threads a catheter through an introducing sheath placed percutaneously into the femoral, subclavian, internal jugular, or antecubital vein. The catheter is then threaded into the right atrium, through the tricuspid valve into the right ventricle and across the pulmonary valve into the pulmonary arteries. Left heart catheterization is also performed in this case using retrograde technique. The catheter is inserted through an introducing sheath placed percutaneously into the femoral, brachial, or axillary artery. The catheter is passed through the aortic valve into the left ventricle. ECG monitoring for the entirety of the procedure is included. Blood samples, pressure and electrical recordings, and/or other tests are performed through the catheter.

93527

This procedure is performed to evaluate both right and left heart function. To accomplish right heart catheterization, the physician threads a catheter through an introducing sheath placed percutaneously into the femoral, subclavian, internal jugular, or antecubital vein. The catheter is then threaded into the right atrium, through the tricuspid valve into the right ventricle and across the pulmonary valve into the pulmonary arteries. Left heart catheterization is also performed using transeptal technique. A catheter is threaded into the right atrium where the interatrial septum (wall) is punctured and the catheter is inserted into the left atrium, passed through the mitral valve and into the left ventricle. Retrograde left heart catheterization may also be performed. When retrograde technique is used, a catheter is inserted through an introducing sheath placed percutaneously into the femoral, brachial or axillary artery. The catheter is passed through the aortic valve into the left ventricle. ECG monitoring for the entirety of the procedure is included. Blood samples, pressure and electrical recordings, and/or other tests are performed through the catheter.

93528

This procedure is performed to evaluate both right and left heart function. To accomplish right heart catheterization, the physician threads a catheter through an introducing sheath placed percutaneously into the femoral, subclavian, internal jugular, or antecubital vein. The catheter is then threaded into the right atrium, through the tricuspid valve into the right ventricle and across the pulmonary valve into the pulmonary arteries. To evaluate left heart function a direct percutaneous puncture into the left ventricle is performed. Retrograde left heart catheterization may also be performed. When retrograde technique is used, a catheter is inserted through an introducing sheath placed percutaneously into the femoral, brachial or axillary artery. The catheter is passed through the aortic valve into the left ventricle. ECG monitoring for the entirety of the procedure is included. Blood samples, pressure, electrical recordings, and/or other measurements are made.

93529

This procedure is performed to evaluate both right and left heart function. To accomplish right heart catheterization, the physician threads a catheter through an introducing sheath placed percutaneously into the femoral, subclavian, internal jugular, or antecubital vein. The catheter is then threaded into the right atrium, through the tricuspid valve into the right ventricle and across the pulmonary valve into the pulmonary arteries. Left heart catheterization is also performed using transeptal technique. In this case a catheter is threaded into the right atrium and passed through an existing septal opening into the left atrium. It is then passed through the mitral valve and into the left ventricle. Retrograde left heart catheterization may also be performed. When retrograde technique is used, a catheter is inserted through an introducing sheath placed percutaneously into the femoral, brachial or axillary artery. The catheter is passed through the aortic valve into the left ventricle. ECG monitoring for the entirety of the procedure is included. Blood samples, pressure and electrical recordings, and/or other tests are performed through the catheter.

93530

The physician performs a right heart catheterization for congenital cardiac anomalies. The physician investigates congenital cardiac anomalies by measuring pressures, taking blood samples for oximetry, and/or injecting contrast to assess chamber size and function. The physician places an introducer sheath in a vein (typically the femoral vein), using percutaneous puncture. The physician places a lumen catheter through the introducer sheath into the femoral vein and advances it under fluoroscopic guidance to the heart chamber(s) receiving venous circulation. The physician may use the fluid filled catheter to record intracardiac pressures, withdraw blood samples, or inject radiopaque contrast material. The physician removes the catheter and sheath from the femoral vein. Pressure is placed on the wound for 20 to 30 minutes to stem bleeding.

93531

The purpose of this procedure is to investigate congenital cardiac anomalies by measuring pressures, taking blood samples for oximetry, and/or injecting contrast to assess chamber size and function. The physician places an introducer sheath in a vein (typically the femoral), using percutaneous puncture. The physician places a lumen catheter through the introducer sheath into the femoral vein and advances it under fluoroscopic guidance to the heart chamber(s) receiving venous circulation. The physician places an introducer sheath in an artery

(typically the femoral), using percutaneous puncture. The physician places a lumen catheter through the introducer sheath into the femoral artery and advances it under fluoroscopic guidance through the aorta to the heart chamber(s) providing arterial circulation. The physician may use the fluid filled catheters to record intracardiac pressures, withdraw blood samples, or inject radiopaque contrast material. The physician removes the catheters and sheaths from the femoral vessels. Pressure is placed on the wound for 20 to 30 minutes to stem bleeding.

93532

The purpose of this procedure is to investigate congenital cardiac anomalies by measuring pressures, taking blood samples for oximetry, and/or injecting contrast to assess chamber size and function. The physician places an introducer sheath in a vein (typically the femoral), using percutaneous puncture. The physician places a lumen catheter through the introducer sheath into the femoral vein and advances it under fluoroscopic guidance to the heart chamber(s) receiving venous circulation. The physician exchanges this catheter over a wire for a transseptal puncture needle, dilator, and sheath. The physician advances the transseptal puncture apparatus to the right atrium and punctures the intraatrial septum with the needle. The physician advances the needle, dilator, and transseptal sheath into the left atrium. The physician may also perform retrograde left heart catheterization as follows: The physician places an introducer sheath and lumen catheter in an artery (typically the femoral), using percutaneous puncture. The physician advances the lumen catheter under fluoroscopic guidance through the aorta to the heart chamber(s) providing arterial circulation. The physician may use the fluid filled catheters to record intracardiac pressures, withdraw blood samples, or inject radiopaque contrast material. The physician removes the catheters and sheaths from the femoral vessels. Pressure is placed on the wound for 20 to 30 minutes to stem bleeding.

93533

The purpose of this procedure is to investigate congenital cardiac anomalies by measuring pressures, taking blood samples for oximetry, and/or injecting contrast to assess chamber size and function. The physician places an introducer sheath in a vein (typically the femoral), using percutaneous puncture. The physician places a lumen catheter through the introducer sheath into the femoral vein and advances it under fluoroscopic guidance to the heart chamber(s) receiving venous circulation. The physician directs this catheter through an existing septal opening into the left atrium. The physician may also perform retrograde left heart catheterization as follows: The physician places an introducer sheath and lumen catheter in an artery (typically the femoral), using percutaneous puncture. The physician advances the lumen catheter under fluoroscopic guidance through the aorta to the heart chamber(s) providing arterial circulation. The physician may use the fluid filled catheters to record intracardiac pressures, withdraw blood samples, or inject radiopaque contrast material. The physician removes the catheters and sheaths from the femoral vessels. Pressure is placed on the wound for 20 to 30 minutes to stem bleeding.

93539

The physician injects dye through a previously placed and separately reportable catheter threaded through a central line. The code applies to injecting dye into arterial conduits to check patency with fluoroscopy. Any required repositioning of catheters or use of automatic power injectors are included in this procedure.

93540

The physician injects dye through a previously placed and separately reportable catheter threaded through a central line. The code applies to injecting dye into bypass grafts of coronary arteries to check patency with fluoroscopy. The catheter is removed and pressure applied to the wound. Any required repositioning of catheters or use of automatic power injectors are included in this procedure.

93541

The physician injects dye through a previously placed and separately reportable catheter threaded through a central line. The code applies to injecting dye into the pulmonary artery to evaluate function with fluoroscopy. The catheter is removed and pressure applied to the wound. Any required repositioning of catheters or use of automatic power injectors are included in this procedure.

93542

The physician injects dye through a previously placed and separately reportable catheter threaded through a central line. The code applies to injecting dye into the right ventricle or atrium to evaluate function with fluoroscopy. The catheter is removed and pressure applied to the wound. Any required repositioning of catheters or use of automatic power injectors are included in this procedure.

93543

The physician injects dye through a previously placed and separately reportable catheter threaded through a central line. The code applies to injecting dye into the left ventricle or atrium to evaluate function with fluoroscopy. Any required repositioning of catheters or use of automatic power injectors are included in this procedure.

93544

The physician injects dye through a previously placed and separately reportable catheter threaded through a central line. The code applies to injecting dye into the aorta to evaluate function with fluoroscopy. Any

required repositioning of catheters or use of automatic power injectors are included in this procedure.

93545

The physician injects dye through a previously placed and separately reportable catheter threaded through a central line. The code applies to injecting dye into the coronary arteries to evaluate function with fluoroscopy. Any required repositioning of catheters or use of automatic power injectors are included in this procedure.

93555

During separately reportable cardiac catheterization and injection procedures, the physician supervises imaging and interprets the findings in a written report. The code applies to imaging supervision for injection procedures of atrial and ventricular spaces.

93556

During separately reportable cardiac catheterization and injection procedures, the physician supervises imaging and interprets the findings in a written report. The code applies to imaging supervision for injection procedures of the pulmonary vessels, aorta, and heart blood vessels including venous bypass grafts and arterial conduits.

93561

The physician threads a catheter through a central line leading to the heart to take blood samples, pressure and electrical recordings, and other measurements. The code applies to dye or thermal dilution studies of coronary arteries and veins to evaluate heart functions, including cardiac output.

93562

The physician threads a catheter through a central line leading to the heart to take blood samples, pressure and electrical recordings, and other measurements. The code applies to dye or thermal dilution studies of coronary arteries and veins to take a subsequent measurement of cardiac output.

93571–93572

A diagnostic angiography is the x-ray visualization of the heart and blood vessels after the introduction of a radiopaque contrast medium. Testing for patient hypersensitivity to the iodine content of the medium is advised before the radiopaque substance is used. The physician injects the contrast medium into a catheter inserted into a peripheral artery and threaded through the vessel to the visceral site. A Doppler ultrasound records blood velocity and pressure by measuring the frequency of ultrasonic waves reflected from moving surface. This code reports the Doppler measurements of the initial vessel; a second code reports the primary coronary angiography procedure. Report 93572 for each additional vessel beyond the initial vessel.

93600

The physician places a venous sheath, usually in a femoral vein, using standard techniques. The physician advances an electrical catheter through the venous sheath and into the right heart under fluoroscopic guidance. The physician attaches the catheter to an electrical recording device to allow depiction of the intracardiac electrograms obtained from electrodes on the catheter tip. The physician moves the catheter tip to the bundle of His, on the anteroseptal tricuspid annulus, and obtains recordings. Alternatively, the physician may obtain similar recordings by placing a catheter into the left ventricular outflow tract via the aorta.

93602

The physician places a venous sheath, usually in a femoral vein, using standard techniques. The physician advances an electrical catheter through the venous sheath and into the right heart under fluoroscopic guidance. The physician attaches the catheter to an electrical recording device to allow depiction of the intracardiac electrograms obtained from electrodes on the catheter tip. The physician moves the catheter tip to the right atrium, and obtains recordings. The physician may obtain left atrial recordings by crossing the interatrial septum. Alternatively, the physician may obtain left atrial recordings by placing an arterial catheter into the aorta and crossing both the aortic and mitral valves in a retrograde fashion.

93603

The physician places a venous sheath, usually in a femoral vein, using standard techniques. The physician advances an electrical catheter through the venous sheath and into the right heart under fluoroscopic guidance. The physician attaches the catheter to an electrical recording device to allow depiction of the intracardiac electrograms obtained from electrodes on the catheter tip. The physician moves the catheter tip to the right ventricle, and obtains recordings.

93609

The physician places an appropriate arterial or venous sheath, usually femoral, to allow access to the chamber to be mapped. The physician advances an electrical catheter through the sheath and into the appropriate chamber under fluoroscopic guidance. The physician attaches the catheter to an electrical recording device to allow depiction of the intracardiac electrograms obtained from electrodes on the catheter tip. The physician moves the catheter tip throughout the chamber to be mapped, and obtains recordings. The physician compares activation times from different sites in order to identify the origin of the tachycardia.

93610

The physician places a venous sheath, usually in a femoral vein, using standard techniques. The physician advances an electrical catheter through the venous sheath and into the right heart under fluoroscopic guidance. The physician attaches the catheter to an electrical pacing device to allow transmission of pacing impulses through the catheter to the right atrium. The physician may pace the left atrium by placing the catheter in the coronary sinus or by crossing the interatrial septum. Alternatively, the physician may pace the left atrium by placing an arterial catheter into the aorta and crossing both the aortic and mitral valves in a retrograde fashion.

93612

The physician places a venous sheath, using standard techniques. The physician advances an electrical catheter through the venous sheath and into the right ventricle under fluoroscopic guidance. The physician attaches the catheter to an electrical pacing device to allow transmission of pacing impulses through the catheter to the right ventricle. Alternatively the physician may pace the left ventricle by placing the catheter in the right atrium, crossing the intraatrial septum and mitral valve. Finally, the physician may pace the left ventricle by advancing a catheter through an arterial sheath, via the aorta, across the aortic valve into the left ventricle.

93613

Electrophysiologic studies use electric stimulation and monitoring in the diagnosis of conduction abnormalities that predispose patients to bradyarrhythmias and to determine a patient's chance of developing ventricular and supraventricular tachyarrhythmias. The physician inserts an electrode catheter percutaneously into the right subclavian vein and, under fluoroscopic guidance, positions the electrode catheter at the right ventricular apex, both for recording and stimulating the right atrium and the right ventricle. A second is inserted percutaneously into the right femoral vein and positioned across the tricuspid valve for recording the His bundle electrogram. For mapping, a third electrode catheter is inserted percutaneously from the right femoral artery and advanced into the left ventricle. Ventricular tachycardia is induced by programmed ventricular stimulation from both the right and left ventricular apexes. The earliest activation site is determined and the diastolic pressure is recorded on the endocardial activation mapping during the ventricular tachycardia. Intracardiac electrograms with surface electrocardiograms are simultaneously displayed and recorded on a multichannel oscilloscopic photographic recorder.

93615

The physician places electrodes into the esophagus via either the oropharyngeal or nasopharyngeal route. The physician attaches the catheter to an electrical recording device to allow depiction of the esophageal electrograms obtained from electrodes on the catheter tip. The physician moves the catheter tip to the esophageal site that provides the optimal signal, and obtains recordings. The physician compares the esophageal and surface electrograms to help identify the mechanism of the arrhythmia.

93616

The physician measures the heart's electrical function using a catheter placed into the patient's esophagus. The recording electrode at the end of the probe measures electrical activity of the atrium by pacing with or without recording activity of the ventricle.

93618

The physician places an appropriate arterial or venous sheath, usually femoral, to allow access to the chamber to be studied. The physician advances an electrical catheter through the sheath and into the appropriate chamber under fluoroscopic guidance. The physician attaches the catheter to an electrical pacing device to allow transmission of pacing impulses through the catheter to the heart chamber of interest. The physician stimulates the heart with rapid pacing or programmed electrical stimulation until the arrhythmia is induced.

93619

The physician places three venous sheaths, usually in one or both femoral veins, using standard techniques. The physician advances three electrical catheters through the venous sheaths and into the right heart under fluoroscopic guidance. The physician attaches the three catheters to an electrical recording device to allow depiction of the intracardiac electrograms obtained from electrodes on the catheter tips. The physician moves the tips of the three catheters to the right atrium, the bundles of His, and the right ventricle, and obtains recordings.

93620

The physician places three venous sheaths, usually in one or both femoral veins, using standard techniques. The physician advances three electrical catheters through the venous sheaths and into the right heart under fluoroscopic guidance. The physician attaches the three catheters to an electrical recording device to allow depiction of the intracardiac electrograms on the catheter tips. The physician moves the tips of the three catheters to the right atrium, the bundles of His, and the right ventricle, and obtains recordings. The physician attaches the catheters to an electrical pacing device to allow transmission of pacing impulses through the catheters to the different heart chambers. The physician stimulates the heart with rapid pacing or programmed electrical stimulation in an attempt to induce an arrhythmia.

93621

The physician places four central venous sheaths, using standard techniques. The physician advances four electrical catheters through the venous sheaths and into the right heart under fluoroscopic guidance. The physician attaches the four catheters to an electrical recording device to allow depiction of the intracardiac electrograms obtained from electrodes on the catheter tips. The physician moves the tips of the four catheters to the right atrium, the bundle of His, the coronary sinus, and the right ventricle, and obtains recordings. The physician may attach the catheters to an electrical pacing device to allow transmission of pacing impulses through the catheters to the different heart chambers. The physician may stimulate the heart with rapid pacing or programmed electrical stimulation in an attempt to induce an arrhythmia.

93622

The physician places three central venous sheaths and an arterial sheath, using standard techniques. The physician advances four electrical catheters through these sheaths and into the heart under fluoroscopic guidance. The physician attaches the four catheters to an electrical recording device to allow depiction of the intracardiac electrograms obtained from electrodes on the catheter tips. The physician moves the tips of the four catheters to the right atrium, the bundle of His, the right ventricle, and the left ventricle, and obtains recordings. The physician may attach the catheters to an electrical pacing device to allow transmission of pacing impulses through the catheters to the different heart chambers. The physician may stimulate the heart with rapid pacing or programmed electrical stimulation in an attempt to induce an arrhythmia.

93623

Programmed stimulation and pacing after intravenous drug infusion (Use this code with 93620, 93621, 93622). The physician places an appropriate arterial or venous sheath, usually femoral, to allow access to the chamber to be studied. The physician advances an electrical catheter through the sheath and into the appropriate chamber under fluoroscopic guidance. An intravenous drug, such as isoproterenol, is infused. The physician attaches the catheter to an electrical pacing device to allow transmission of pacing impulses through the catheter to the heart chamber of interest. The physician stimulates the heart with rapid pacing or programmed electrical stimulation in an attempt to induce an arrhythmia.

93624

Following administration of therapy (antiarrhythmic drugs, surgery, ablation, etc.), the physician places an appropriate arterial or venous sheath, usually femoral, to allow access to the chamber to be studied. The physician advances an electrical catheter through the sheath and into the appropriate chamber under fluoroscopic guidance. An intravenous drug, such as isoproterenol, is infused. The physician attaches the catheter to an electrical pacing device to allow transmission of pacing impulses through the catheter to the heart chamber of interest. The physician stimulates the heart with rapid pacing or programmed electrical stimulation in an attempt to induce an arrhythmia.

93631

The purpose of this procedure is to localize the site of tachycardia during open-heart surgery, to allow surgical correction of the tachycardia. The physician may place pacing or mapping catheters inside the heart prior to or during surgery using a standard transvenous approach. Additionally, the surgeon will place electrical probes on the outside (epicardium) of the heart in order to allow additional mapping. The physician attaches the catheters and probes to an electrical recording device to allow depiction of the electrograms obtained from electrodes on the catheter and probe tips. The surgeon's electrical probe can be moved around the outside of the heart to allow comparison of electrical activation times from different regions. The physician may attach the catheters to an electrical pacing device to allow transmission of pacing impulses through the catheters to the different heart chambers. The physician may stimulate the heart with rapid pacing or programmed electrical stimulation in an attempt to induce an arrhythmia.

93640

The purpose of this study is to ensure that the cardioverter-defibrillator (ICD) leads are positioned well and working properly, to ensure proper function of this device in the future. Leads are typically placed in the heart via the subclavian vein, but occasionally defibrillation patches are placed on the epicardium or under the skin. To test the leads, the physician records cardiac electrical signals from the leads and paces the heart through the leads. The physician may test the leads using the actual ICD or by hooking the lead to an external device. The physician uses the lead to pace the heart into an arrhythmia such as ventricular tachycardia or fibrillation. The ICD or external device detects the arrhythmia and shocks the heart through the ICD lead. The physician may perform this test with several different levels of shock to ensure that the ICD can reliably terminate the arrhythmia.

93641

The purpose of this study is to ensure that the cardioverter-defibrillator (ICD) and ICD leads are positioned well and working properly, to ensure proper function of this device in the future. Leads are typically placed in the heart via the subclavian vein, but occasionally defibrillation patches are placed on the epicardium or under the skin. To test the leads, the physician records cardiac electrical signals from the leads and paces the heart through the leads. The

physician attaches the leads to the ICD generator. The physician uses the ICD pulse generator to pace the heart into an arrhythmia such as ventricular tachycardia or fibrillation. The ICD detects the arrhythmia and shocks the heart through the ICD lead. The physician may perform this test with several different levels of shock to ensure that the ICD can reliably terminate the arrhythmia.

93642

The purpose of this study is to ensure that the cardioverter-defibrillator (ICD) and ICD leads are positioned well and working properly, to ensure proper function of this device in the future. The physician records cardiac electrical signals from the leads and paces the heart through the leads to determine pacing threshold. The physician uses the ICD pulse generator to pace the heart into an arrhythmia such as ventricular tachycardia or fibrillation. The ICD detects and terminates the arrhythmia, using pacing or shocking the heart through the ICD lead. The physician may reprogram the ICD's treatment parameters to optimize the device function to best treat the patient's arrhythmia.

93650

The purpose of this procedure is to create complete heart block, usually for control of the ventricular rate during atrial arrhythmias. The physician places a venous sheath, usually in a femoral vein, using standard techniques. The physician advances an electrical catheter through the venous sheath and into the right heart under fluoroscopic guidance. The physician attaches the catheter to an electrical recording device to allow depiction of the intracardiac electrograms obtained from electrodes on the catheter tip. The physician moves the catheter tip to the bundle of His, on the anteroseptal tricuspid annulus, and obtains recordings. Alternatively, the physician may obtain similar recordings by placing a catheter into the left ventricular outflow tract via the aorta. The physician maps the His bundle area and ablates the His bundle by sending cautery (radiofrequency) current through the catheter. The physician may also place a temporary pacing catheter in the right ventricle for this procedure.

93651

The purpose of this procedure is to ablate an arrhythmogenic focus or pathway to cure supraventricular arrhythmias. The ablation is typically done following a more complex electrophysiologic study, coded elsewhere. The physician places an introducer sheath, typically in a femoral vein, using standard techniques. The physician advances an electrical catheter through the sheath and into the heart under fluoroscopic guidance. The physician attaches the catheter to an electrical recording device to allow depiction of the intracardiac electrograms obtained from electrodes on the catheter tip. The physician moves the catheter tip to the arrhythmogenic focus or pathway while guided by electrical recordings and fluoroscopic views. The physician ablates the focus or pathway by sending cautery (radiofrequency) current through the catheter.

93652

The purpose of this procedure is to ablate an arrhythmogenic focus or pathway in the right or left ventricle, to cure ventricular tachycardia. The ablation is typically done following a more complex electrophysiologic study, coded elsewhere. The physician places an introducer sheath, typically in a femoral artery or vein, using standard techniques. The physician advances an electrical catheter through the sheath and into the right or left ventricle under fluoroscopic guidance. The physician attaches the catheter to an electrical recording device to allow depiction of the intracardiac electrograms obtained from electrodes on the catheter tip. The physician moves the catheter tip to the arrhythmogenic focus or pathway while guided by electrical recordings and fluoroscopic views. The physician ablates the focus or pathway by sending cautery (radiofrequency) current through the catheter.

93660

The purpose of this procedure is to evaluate the patient's susceptibility to neurocardiogenic syncope. The physician secures the patient to the tilt table and attaches ECG leads to the chest. The physician also attaches an intermittent blood pressure monitor. The physician tilts the table, with the patient on it, and monitors the patient's symptoms, heart rhythm, and blood pressure. The physician may infuse medication, such as isoproterenol, through a standard intravenous catheter, and repeat the tilt test.

93662

During separately reportable electrophysiologic evaluation or intracardiac catheter ablation of arrhythmogenic focus, intracardiac echocardiography (ICE) is performed. ICE uses intravascular ultrasound imaging systems in the cardiac chambers providing direct endocardial visualization. A single rotating transducer that provides a 360-degree field of view in a plane transverse to the long axis of the catheter is introduced through a long vascular sheath. Access is typically via the femoral vein. The transducer is then directed to various sites within the heart. During electrophysiologic evaluation, ICE is used to guide placement of mapping and stimulating catheters. During intracardiac ablation procedures, ICE allows for precise anatomic localization of the ablation catheter tip in relation to endocardial structures. Since the focus of some arrhythmias can be anatomically determined it also allows the ablative procedure to be performed using anatomic landmarks.

93668

An exercise physiologist or nurse supervises rehabilitation exercises in a patient diagnosed with peripheral arterial disease (PAD). Rehabilitation for PAD is provided using either a motorized treadmill or a track. The patient is supervised during physical exercise sessions lasting between 45 minutes to 60 minutes in order to achieve symptom-limited claudication. The supervising provider monitors the patient's claudication threshold and other cardiovascular limitations and adjusts the level of activity in order to reduce claudication symptoms and increase exercise tolerance.

93701

Bioimpedance is a noninvasive, continuous measurement of blood flow, respiration, and other cardiopulmonary dynamics, using a patient's thorax as an impedance transducer. The health care provider attaches the patient to the bioimpedance system with solid-gel electrodes placed along the widest dimension of the thorax. The electrical bioimpedance measurement current is passed through the thorax in a direction parallel with the spine between a pair of electrodes placed on upper neck and a pair of electrodes placed on upper abdomen. On its way through the thorax, the measurement current seeks the shortest and the most conductive pathway. As a result, the majority of the thoracic electrical bioimpedance (TEB) measurement current flows through the thoracic aorta and superior and inferior vena. The measurement current produces a high-frequency voltage across the impedance of the thorax, sensed by two other pairs of electrodes placed at the beginning of the thorax and the end of the thorax. The sensing electrodes also detect the ECG signal. The heart rate is derived from the R-R intervals of the ECG signal.

93720–93722

Plethysmography measures and records changes in the volume of a body part in response to variations in the amount of blood passing through or contained in that body part. Total body plethysmography involves the use of a chamber enclosing the entire body and is used primarily to assess respiratory function. 93720 should be used to report the complete procedure, including physician interpretation and report. 93721 is used to report the tracing or technical component only, and 93722 is for the physician interpretation and report only.

93724

Patients with previously implanted pacemakers require periodic analysis of pacemaker function. The code applies to routine electronic analysis of pacemakers used to control irregularly fast heartbeats (antitachycardial) and includes electrocardiogram, programming, tests, and physician interpretation of the tests.

93727

In a previously reported procedure (33282) a patient-activated cardiac recorder has been implanted. This code is reported when the physician uses a special "programmer" to retrieve the information (events) that have been recorded by the patient. This code includes information retrieval, review, interpretation of ECG data, and reprogramming.

93731

Patients with previously implanted pacemakers require periodic analysis of pacemaker function. The code applies to routine electronic analysis of a dual-chambered pacemaker and includes an electrocardiogram, tests, and physician's interpretation of the tests. The code excludes reprogramming.

93732

Patients with previously implanted pacemakers require periodic analysis of pacemaker function. The code applies to routine electronic analysis of a dual-chambered pacemaker and includes an electrocardiogram, reprogramming, tests, and physician's interpretation of the tests.

93733

Patients with previously implanted pacemakers require periodic analysis of pacemaker function. The code applies to routine electronic analysis of a dual-chambered pacemaker and includes an electrocardiogram, tests, physician's interpretation of the tests, and telephone analysis.

93734

Patients with previously implanted pacemakers require periodic analysis of pacemaker function. The code applies to routine electronic analysis of a single-chambered pacemaker and includes an electrocardiogram, tests, and physician's interpretation of the tests. The code excludes reprogramming.

93735

Patients with previously implanted pacemakers require periodic analysis of pacemaker function. A pacemaker may be implanted to control a patient's irregular heartbeat. The code applies to routine electronic analysis of a single-chambered pacemaker and includes an electrocardiogram, reprogramming, tests, and physician's interpretation of the tests.

93736

Patients with previously implanted pacemakers require periodic analysis of pacemaker function. A pacemaker may be implanted to control a patient's irregular heartbeat. The code applies to routine electronic analysis of a single-chambered pacemaker and includes an electrocardiogram, tests, and physician's interpretation of the tests and telephone analysis.

93740

Temperature gradient studies assess heart or circulatory functions by contrasting temperatures of certain vessels via an intravenous catheter.

93741

Patients with previously implanted cardio-defibrillators require periodic analysis of their function. This code applies to routine electronic analysis of a single chamber pacing cardioverter-defibrillator. The code includes interrogation, evaluation of pulse generator status, evaluation of programmable parameters at rest and during activity, using electrocardiographic recording and interpretation of recordings at rest and during exercise, and the analysis of event markers and device response. The code does not include reprogramming.

93742

Patients with previously implanted cardio-defibrillators require periodic analysis of their function. This code applies to routine electronic analysis of a single chamber pacing cardioverter-defibrillator. The code includes interrogation, evaluation of pulse generator status, evaluation of programmable parameters at rest and during activity, using electrocardiographic recording and interpretation of recordings at rest and during exercise, and the analysis of event markers and device response, including reprogramming.

93743

Patients with previously implanted cardio-defibrillators require periodic analysis of their function. This code applies to routine electronic analysis of a dual chamber pacing cardioverter-defibrillator. The code includes interrogation, evaluation of pulse generator status, evaluation of programmable parameters at rest and during activity, using electrocardiographic recording and interpretation of recordings at rest and during exercise, and the analysis of event markers and device response. The code does not include reprogramming.

93744

Patients with previously implanted cardio-defibrillators require periodic analysis of their function. This code applies to routine electronic analysis of a single chamber pacing cardioverter-defibrillator. The code includes interrogation, evaluation of pulse generator status, evaluation of programmable parameters at rest and during activity, using electrocardiographic recording and interpretation of recordings at rest and during exercise, and the analysis of event markers and device response, including reprogramming.

93760

A thermogram is a method of recording the body's heat differentials, often in relation to blood flow. In most cases, this technique is performed with a camera called a thermograph, which identifies hot and cold by color-coding the image. This code applies to the head region.

93762

A thermogram is a method of recording the body's heat differentials, often in relation to blood flow. In most cases, this technique is performed with a camera called a thermograph, which identifies hot and cold by color-coding the image. This code applies to the extremities.

93770

Venous blood pressure is measured to assess heart and circulatory system functions. This code applies to the peripheral measurement.

93784

Blood pressure is monitored and recorded over a 24-hour period on an outpatient basis for the physician's analysis and interpretation. 93784 should be used for the complete procedure including physician interpretation and report.

93786

The purpose of this study is to evaluate the patient's ambient blood pressure during a 24 hour period. A technician attaches the blood pressure monitor to the patient, who wears the monitor for 24 hours. During this period, the device obtains blood pressure measurements and records them on magnetic tape or computer disk. This code does not include scanning analysis with report (coded 93788) or physician review with interpretation and report (coded 93790).

93788

The purpose of this study is to evaluate the patient's ambient blood pressure during a 24 hour period. A technician attaches the blood pressure monitor to the patient, who wears the monitor for 24 hours. During this period, the device obtains blood pressure measurements and records them on magnetic tape or computer disk. A technician scans the data and generates a data summary. This code does not include recording(coded 93786).

93790

The purpose of this study is to evaluate the patient's ambient blood pressure during a 24 hour period. A technician attaches the blood pressure monitor to the patient, who wears the monitor for 24 hours. During this period, the device obtains blood pressure measurements and records them on magnetic tape or computer disk. A technician scans the data and generates a data summary. The physician reviews and interprets the data and generates a report. This code does not include recording (coded 93786) or scanning analysis with report (coded 93788).

93797

Patients with severe cardiac disease, particularly those who have had myocardial infarctions, surgery on the coronary vessels, and other occlusive coronary artery diseases, often require outpatient rehabilitation. A physician supervises outpatient cardiac rehabilitation

in areas of exercise, diet, and related modalities. Report 93797 if this code excludes continuous electrocardiogram monitoring. Report 93798 if this code includes continuouse ECg monitoring.

93798

Patients with severe cardiac disease, particularly those who have had myocardial infarctions, surgery on the coronary vessels, and other occlusive coronary artery diseases, often require outpatient rehabilitation. A physician supervises outpatient cardiac rehabilitation in areas of exercise, diet, and related modalities. This code includes continuous electrocardiogram monitoring.

93875

The physician or an assistant performs an ultrasound scan of the extracranial arteries in the head and neck to evaluate vascular blood flow in relation to blockage. Ultrasound uses high frequency sound waves to provide an image. This code applies to a bilateral evaluation using multiple noninvasive modalities to include blood flow, pneumoplethysmography, and ultrasound.

93880

The physician or an assistant performs a Duplex ultrasound scan, which is a combination of real-time and Doppler studies, of the extracranial arteries in the head and neck to evaluate vascular blood flow in relation to blockage. Ultrasound uses high frequency sound waves to provide an image. This code applies to both sides of the head and neck.

93882

The physician or an assistant performs a Duplex ultrasound scan, which is a combination of real-time and Doppler studies, of the extracranial arteries in the head and neck to evaluate vascular blood flow in relation to blockage. Ultrasound uses high frequency sound waves to provide an image. This code applies to a unilateral (one side of the head or neck) or limited study.

93886

The physician or an assistant performs a Doppler ultrasound scan of the extracranial arteries in the head and neck to evaluate vascular blood flow in relation to blockage. This code applies to a complete study of the intracranial arteries.

93888

The physician or an assistant performs a Doppler ultrasound scan of the extracranial arteries in the head and neck to evaluate vascular blood flow in relation to blockage. This code applies to a limited study of the intracranial arteries.

93922–93923

The physician or assistant evaluates the arteries of the arms or legs to check blood flow in relation to blockage. In one example, the physician places a transducer on each leg at a prescribed level and measures the change in blood-handling characteristics during constriction by pneumatic cuffs. Technique is similar — the constriction and measuring of tension in the vascular system — but the medium may change. 93922 applies to ultrasound, plethysmography, and oxygen tension measurements in a bilateral evaluation limited to one level. 93923 includes multiple levels and provocative functional maneuvers.

93924

The physician or assistant evaluates the arteries of the arms or legs to check blood flow in relation to blockage. This code applies to ultrasound and oxygen tension measurements in a bilateral evaluation that occurs before and after a treadmill stress test.

93925–93926

The physician or assistant evaluates the arteries of the legs bilaterally to check blood flow in relation to blockage,by use of Duplex ultrasonography, which is a combination of real-time and Doppler studies. 93925 refers to a complete bilateral study. 93926 applies to studies of one leg or limited areas of both legs.

93930

A diagnostic study is performed on the upper extremity arteries or arterial bypass grafts. A duplex scan involves a two-dimensional ultrasonic scan, which provides a two-dimensional display of the structure. This procedure is a complete bilateral study and is not intended to report unilateral procedures.

93931

A diagnostic study is performed on a specific site or area of the upper extremity arteries. A duplex scan involves a two-dimensional ultrasonic scan, which provides a two-dimensional display of the structure. This reports limited or follow-up ultrasounds.

93965

The physician or assistant evaluates the veins in the arms and legs. This code applies to a complete bilateral evaluation including blood flow, plethysmography, and ultrasound.

93970

The physician or assistant performs a Duplex ultrasound scan, which is a combination of real-time and Doppler studies, of the veins in the arms or legs to evaluate vascular blood flow in relation to blockage. This code applies to complete responses to compression and other tests and includes both sides.

93971

The physician or assistant performs a Duplex ultrasound scan, which is a combination of real-time and Doppler studies, of the veins in the arms or legs to evaluate vascular blood flow in relation to blockage. This code applies to complete responses to compression and other tests and includes one side or limited areas of both sides.

93975

The physician or assistant performs a Duplex ultrasound scan, which is a combination of real-time and Doppler studies, of the arteries and veins in the abdominal, pelvic, or genitorectal areas to evaluate vascular blood flow in relation to blockage. This code applies to a complete bilateral evaluation.

93976

The physician or assistant performs an Duplex ultrasound scan, which is a combination of real-time and Doppler studies, of the arteries and veins in the abdominal, pelvic, or genitorectal areas to evaluate vascular blood flow in relation to blockage. This code applies to a limited evaluation.

93978

The physician or assistant performs a Duplex ultrasound scan, which is a combination of real-time and Doppler studies, of the arteries and veins in the aorta, inferior vena cava, or iliac areas to evaluate vascular blood flow in relation to blockage. This code applies to a complete bilateral evaluation.

93979

The physician or assistant performs a Duplex ultrasound scan, which is a combination of real-time and Doppler studies,of the arteries and veins in the aorta, inferior vena cava, or iliac areas to evaluate vascular blood flow in relation to blockage. This code applies to one side or limited areas of the sides.

93980

The physician or assistant performs a Duplex ultrasound scan, which is a combination of real-time and Doppler studies, of the arteries and veins in the penis to evaluate vascular blood flow in relation to blockages. This code applies to a complete evaluation.

93981

The physician or assistant performs a Duplex ultrasound scan, which is a combination of real-time and Doppler studies, of the arteries and veins in the penis to evaluate vascular blood flow in relation to blockages. This code applies to a follow-up or limited evaluation.

93990

The physician or assistant performs a Duplex ultrasound scan, which is a combination of real-time and Doppler studies, of an arterial-venous dialysis catheter to evaluate vascular blood flow in relation to blockage.

94010

A spirometer in a pulmonary lab is used to measure functions of the lungs including amount of air in the lungs, rate of expiration, and the amount of air a patient respires. The physician interprets the results of the spirometry and a graphic record is obtained.

94014–94016

A spirometer is an instrument that measures and records the volume of inhaled and exhaled air and used to assess pulmonary function. This range of codes is used to report a patient initiated spirometric recording up to a 30-day period. Report 94014 when the procedure includes teaching the patient how to use a spirometer, recording the volume of air exhaled and inhaled, analyzing the data, recalibrating the unit, and the physician's analysis of the pulmonary function. Report 94015 when the procedure involves recording the data (hook-up, continued education, data transmission and capture, trend analysis and periodic recalibration) without the physician's analysis of the pulmonary function. Report 94016 when the physician reviews and interprets the information only.

94060

A spirometer in a pulmonary lab is used to measure functions of the lungs including amount of air in the lungs, rate of expiration, and the amount of air a patient respires. The physician interprets the results of the spirometry. This code applies to a spirometry completed both before and after administering a bronchodilating medicine to evaluate bronchospasm.

94070

A spirometer in a pulmonary lab is used to measure functions of the lungs including amount of air in the lungs, rate of expiration, and the amount of air a patient respires.This code applies to spirometry conducted multiple times to evaluate bronchospasms after exposing the patient to a bronchodilating antigen, exercise, cold air, methacholine or other agents. This test usually follows performance of 94010 where reduced airflow is indicated.

94150

This procedure measures the largest volume of air a patient can expire from his lungs. The patient amount of air inhaled and exhaled is measured and calculated with body size to determine the capacity of the lungs. This test is important for determining the threshold of capacity needed for vitality in patients with compromised respiration. For men, this is typically four to five liters; for women this is normally three to four liters. It is normally performed as a part of a larger procedure and should only be billed separately when performed alone.

94200

This code applies to measuring maximum breathing capacity or maximal voluntary ventilation (the largest volume of air that a patient can inhale and exhale in 60 seconds). The patient inhales to the maximum vital capacity then exhales into a spirometer. The physician measures the maximal expiratory flow at 50% of expired vital capacity and at 75% of expired vital capacity.

94240

Pulmonary function testing is performed in a pulmonary lab using helium, nitrogen open circuit, or another method to check lung functions to include residual capacity or residual volume, the volume of air remaining in the lung after a patient exhales. The physician interprets the report.

94250

Pulmonary function testing is performed in a pulmonary lab using helium, nitrogen open circuit, or another method to check lung functions to include residual capacity or residual volume, the volume of air remaining in the lung after a patient exhales. The physician interprets results. This code applies to collecting and, in a separately reportable procedure, evaluating expired air.

94260

Pulmonary function testing is performed in a pulmonary lab using helium, nitrogen open circuit, or another method to check lung functions to include residual capacity or residual volume, the volume of air remaining in the lung after a patient exhales. The physician interprets results. This code applies to the total volume of thoracic gas.

94350

Pulmonary function testing is performed in a pulmonary lab using helium, nitrogen open circuit, or another method to check lung functions to include residual capacity or residual volume, the volume of air remaining in the lung after a patient exhales.The physician interprets results. The code applies to the distribution of inspired gas using multiple breath nitrogen washout curves and including alveolar nitrogen or helium equilibration time.

94360

Pulmonary function testing is performed in a pulmonary lab using helium, nitrogen open circuit, or another method to check lung functions to include residual capacity or residual volume, the volume of air remaining in the lung after a patient exhales. The physician interprets results. The code applies to measuring the resistance to airflow using oscillatory or plethysmographic methods.

94370

Pulmonary function testing is performed in a pulmonary lab using helium, nitrogen open circuit, or another method to check lung functions to include residual capacity or residual volume, the volume of air remaining in the lung after a patient exhales. The physician interprets results. The code applies to measuring the total airway closing volume in a single breath.

CPT® Lay Descriptions

94375

Pulmonary function testing is performed in a pulmonary lab using helium, nitrogen open circuit, or another method to check lung functions to include residual capacity or residual volume, the volume of air remaining in the lung after a patient exhales. The physician interprets results. The code applies to measuring the respiratory flow volume loop.

94400

Pulmonary function testing is performed in a pulmonary lab using helium, nitrogen open circuit, or another method to check lung functions to include residual capacity or residual volume, the volume of air remaining in the lung after a patient exhales. The physician interprets results. The code applies to the patient breathing in carbon dioxide and measuring the resultant lung response.

94450

Pulmonary function testing is performed in a pulmonary lab using helium, nitrogen open circuit, or another method to check lung functions to include residual capacity or residual volume, the volume of air remaining in the lung after a patient exhales. The physician interprets results. The code applies to a patient's response to low amounts of oxygen.

94620

Pulmonary function testing is performed in a pulmonary lab using helium, nitrogen open circuit, or another method to check lung functions to include residual capacity or residual volume, the volume of air remaining in the lung after a patient exhales. Basic ventilation studies are performed with a spirometer and recording device as the patient breathes through a mouthpiece and connecting tube, a nose clip prevents nasal breathing. The physician interprets results. Report 94620 for a patient's breathing during stress and prolonged exercise. Report 94621 for detailed measuring of carbon dioxide output, oxygen consumption and an electrocardiogram.

94640

A nonpressurized inhalation treatment is applied for an acute obstruction of the airway preventing the patient from taking in sufficient air on his or her own.

94642

An antimicrobial medication called pentamidine is given in cases of pneumocystis carinii pneumonia treatment or prophylaxis in high risk groups. The patient breathes the aerosolized medication into his lungs.

94650

A mechanical ventilator is applied with a mask over the nose and mouth or through a tube placed into the trachea for patients requiring help breathing due to a lung disorder. Intermittent positive pressure breathing uses positive pressure during the inspiration phase of breathing. The code applies to the initial evaluation.

94651

A mechanical ventilator is applied with a mask over the nose and mouth or through a tube placed into the trachea for patients requiring help breathing due to a lung disorder. Intermittent positive pressure breathing uses positive pressure during the inspiration phase of breathing. The code applies to the physician's evaluation beyond the first treatment.

94652

A mechanical ventilator is applied with a mask over the nose and mouth or through a tube placed into the trachea for patients requiring help breathing due to a lung disorder. Intermittent positive pressure breathing uses positive pressure during the inspiration phase of breathing. The code applies to newborns.

94656

A mechanical ventilator is applied with a mask over the nose and mouth or through a tube placed into the trachea for patients requiring help breathing due to a lung disorder. Intermittent positive pressure breathing uses positive pressure during the inspiration phase of breathing. The code applies to ventilation assistance using adjustments in volume and pressure in the initial day of treatment.

94657

A mechanical ventilator is applied with a mask over the nose and mouth or through a tube placed into the trachea for patients requiring help breathing due to a lung disorder. Intermittent positive pressure breathing uses positive pressure during the inspiration phase of breathing. The code applies to ventilation assistance using adjustments in volume and pressure in days subsequent to the initial treatment.

94660

A mechanical ventilator is applied with a mask over the nose and mouth or through a tube placed into the trachea for patients requiring help breathing due to a lung disorder. Intermittent positive pressure breathing uses positive pressure during the inspiration phase of breathing. The code applies to initial evaluation or application of continuous positive airway pressure for ventilation assistance with positive pressure during inspiration and exhalation.

94662

A mechanical ventilator is applied with a mask over the nose and mouth or through a tube placed into the trachea for patients requiring help breathing due to a lung disorder. Intermittent negative pressure breathing uses negative pressure during the inspiration phase of breathing. The code applies to subsequent evaluation or application of continuous negative airway pressure for ventilation assistance with negative pressure during inspiration and exhalation.

94664

Inhaling aerosols or vapors can help mobilize sputum, dilate the bronchi and improve sputum production when sputum is collected for evaluation. The code applies to the initial evaluation and treatment.

94665

Inhaling aerosols or vapors can help mobilize sputum, dilate the bronchi and improve sputum production when sputum is collected for evaluation. The code applies to subsequent evaluation and treatment.

94667

A respiratory therapist supervised by a physician manipulates the chest wall — cupping, vibration, and percussion — to help mobilize secretions and improve breathing for some lung disorders. The code applies to initial evaluation and treatment.

94668

A respiratory therapist supervised by a physician manipulates the chest wall — cupping, vibration, and percussion — to help mobilize secretions and improve breathing for some lung disorders. The code applies to subsequent evaluation and treatment.

94680

Pulmonary testing supervised by a physician in a lab measures functions of the lungs. The code applies to collecting expired air and evaluating oxygen uptake using direct methods during rest and exercise.

94681

Pulmonary testing supervised by a physician in a lab measures functions of the lungs. The code applies to collecting expired air and evaluating oxygen uptake, carbon dioxide output, and percentage oxygen extracted.

94690

Pulmonary testing supervised by a physician in a lab measures functions of the lungs. The code applies to collecting expired air and evaluating oxygen uptake using indirect methods during rest.

94720

Pulmonary testing supervised by a physician in a lab measures functions of the lungs. The code applies to measuring carbon monoxide diffusing capacity when the patient inhales carbon dioxide and the physician compares the inhaled and exhaled amounts.

94725

Pulmonary testing supervised by a physician in a lab measures functions of the lungs. The code applies to measuring membrane diffusing capacity when the patient inhales a gas such as carbon monoxide and the physician compares the inhaled and exhaled amounts.

94750

Pulmonary testing supervised by a physician in a lab measures functions of the lungs. The code applies to measuring compliance of the lungs using various methods.

94760

A sensor is placed on either the ear lobe or finger to measure oxygen levels in the blood for a pulse oximetry. A light shines through the capillary bed for the measurement. The code applies to a single measurement.

94761

A sensor is placed on either the ear lobe or finger to measure oxygen levels in the blood for a pulse oximetry. A light shines through the capillary bed for the measurement. The code applies to multiple measurements.

94762

A sensor is placed on either the ear lobe or finger to measure oxygen levels in the blood for a pulse oximetry. A light shines through the capillary bed for the measurement. The code applies to continuous overnight measurement.

94770

A pulmonary lab assistant performs pulmonary function testing to measure various aspects of the lungs. A physician interprets the report. The code applies to using an infrared light device to measure the carbon dioxide amounts in expired air.

94772

A pulmonary lab assistant performs pulmonary function testing to measure various aspects of the lungs. A physician interprets the report. The code applies to measuring the circadian respiratory pattern of an infant over a 12 to 24 hour period (pediatric pneumogram).

95004

A physician scratches, punctures, or pricks the skin to introduce specific allergy extracts to determine a patient's allergies. The immediate skin reaction is documented.

95010

A physician scratches, punctures, or pricks the skin to introduce drugs, venoms or other biological agents to determine a patient's allergies. The immediate skin reaction is documented.

CPT® Lay Descriptions

95015

A physician injects drugs, venoms, or other biological substances into the skin to determine the patient's allergies. The immediate reaction is documented.

95024

A physician injects suspected allergenic substances into the skin to determine the patient's specific allergies. The immediate skin reaction is documented.

95027

A physician uses skin end point titration to determine specific allergies. The code applies to the special technique used in allergy testing to measure skin response.

95028

A physician injects suspected allergenic substances into a patient to determine the patient's specific allergies. The delayed skin reaction is documented.

95044

A physician applies a patch containing specific allergenic substances to a patient's arm to determine the patient's specific allergies. The reaction is documented.

95052

A physician applies a patch containing specific allergenic substances to a patient's arm and exposes the area to ultraviolet light to determine a patient's specific allergies. The reaction is documented.

95056

A physician exposes an area of the patient's skin to ultraviolet light to determine the patient's allergic reactions. The reaction is documented.

95060

A physician introduces specific allergy extracts to the patient's eye mucus membranes to determine the patient's specific allergic reactions. The reaction is documented.

95065

A physician introduces specific allergy extracts to the patient's mucus membrane in the nose to determine the patient's specific allergic reactions. The reaction is documented.

95070

A physician has the patient inhale histamines, methacholamines or other medications to determine the patient's specific allergies. The reaction is documented.

95071

A physician has the patient inhale specific allergenic substances to determine the patient's specific allergies. The reaction is documented.

95075

A physician has the patient ingest specific substances such as food or drugs to determine the patient's specific allergies. The reaction is documented.

95078

A physician applies directly to the patient's skin a certain number of suspected allergenic substances to determine the patient's specific allergies. The reaction is documented. The procedure often used to confirm a diagnosis.

95115

A physician injects small but increasing dosages of a substance to which the patient is allergic for desensitization. This code applies to a single injection of the allergen and does not include the provision of the substance.

95117

A physician injects small but increasing dosages of a substance to which the patient is allergic for desensitization. This code applies to two or more injections of the allergen and does not include the provision of the substance.

95120

A physician injects small but increasing dosages of a substance to which the patient is allergic for desensitization. This code applies to a single injection of the allergen and includes the provision of the substance.

95125

A physician injects small but increasing dosages of a substance to which the patient is allergic for desensitization. This code applies to two or more injections of the allergen and does include the provision of the substance.

95130

A physician injects small but increasing dosages of insect venom to which the patient is allergic for desensitization. The code applies to the injection of one venom and includes the provision of the venom.

95131

A physician injects small but increasing dosages of insect venom to which the patient is allergic for desensitization. The code applies to the injection of two venoms and includes the provision of the venoms.

95132

A physician injects small but increasing dosages of insect venom to which the patient is allergic for desensitization. The code applies to the injection of three venoms and includes the provision of the venoms.

95133

A physician injects small but increasing dosages of insect venom to which the patient is allergic for desensitization. The code applies to the injection of four venoms and includes the provision of the venoms.

95134

A physician injects small but increasing dosages of insect venom to which the patient is allergic for desensitization. The code applies to the injection of five venoms and includes the provision of the venoms.

95144

The physician supervises the preparation and provision of antigen for allergen immunotherapy. This code applies to a single dose vial. The number of vials must be specified.

95145

The physician supervises the preparation and provision of single stinging insect venom. The number of vials must be specified.

95146

The physician supervises the preparation and provision of two stinging insect venoms. The number of doses must be specified.

95147

The physician supervises the preparation and provision of three stinging insect venoms. The number of doses must be specified.

95148

The physician supervises the preparation and provision of four stinging insect venoms. The number of doses must be specified.

95149

The physician supervises the preparation and provision of five stinging insect venoms. The number of doses must be specified.

95165

The physician supervises the preparation and provision of antigens for allergen immunotherapy. This code applies to single or multiple antigens. The number of doses must be specified.

95170

The physician supervises the preparation and provision of antigens for allergen immunotherapy. This code applies to whole body extract of biting insect or other arthropod. The number of doses must be specified.

95180

A physician administers small but increasing dosages of a substance that causes a patient's allergic reaction to desensitize the patient and to develop the patient's tolerance to the substance. This code applies to a certain number of hours of rapid desensitization to a medication such as insulin, penicillin, or equine serum. This code should be reported for each hour of desensitization.

95250

The physician monitors glucose levels by continuous recording and storage of glucose values. The physician inserts a glucose sensor in the subcutaneous tissue in the lower abdomen or other area. The sensor measures the change in intracellular fluid (ICF) and sends the information from the sensor to a small monitor that stores the information for 72 hours. Each day the patient calibrates the monitor by entering three separate blood glucose levels obtained from a glucose monitor. Other information, such as insulin dosage and meals, is also entered into the monitor. After 72 hours, the sensor is removed and the information from the monitor is downloaded into a computer. Special computer software interprets the information and the interpretation is printed.

95805

Physiological parameters of a patient asleep in a lab setting are monitored for at least six hours. A physician interprets the results. The code applies to multiple sleep latency testing during periods of napping to assess sleepiness.

95806

Physiological parameters of a patient asleep in a lab setting or home are monitored for at least six hours. Cardiorespiratory and oxygen saturation measurements are made during the test. A physician interprets the results.

95807

Physiological parameters of a patient asleep in a lab setting are monitored for at least six hours. A physician interprets the results. The code applies to testing of several parameters including ventilation, respiratory effort, ECG or heart rate, oxygen saturation by a technologist.

95808

Physiological parameters of a patient asleep in a lab setting are monitored for at least six hours for polysomnography studies. In contrast to sleep studies, polysomnography details measurements such as sleep staging with electroencephalogram (EEG), electro-oculogram and submental electromyogram. The code applies to sleep staging with one to three additional measurements such as respiration, air flow, oximetry, muscle activity, vital signs, and snoring.

95810–95811

Physiological parameters of a patient asleep in a lab setting are monitored for at least six hours for polysomonography studies. In contrast to sleep studies, polysomnography details measurements such as sleep staging with electroencephalogram (EEG), electro-oculogram and submental electromyogram. The code applies to sleep staging with four or more additional measurements such as respiration, air flow, oximetry, muscle activity, vital signs, and snoring. Report 95811 if with the initiation of continuous positive airway pressure therapy or bi-level ventilation, attended by a technologist.

95812

Sensors are placed on a patient's head in an electroencephalogram (EEG) to measure and record the brain's electrical activity. Brain waves are captured on paper or electronic medium for study. The code applies to an EEG acquired in one hour or less.

95813

Sensors are placed on a patient's head in an electroencephalogram (EEG) to measure and record the brain's electrical activity. Brain waves are captured on paper or electronic medium for study. The code applies to an EEG acquired in more than one hour.

95816

Sensors are placed on a patient's head in an electroencephalogram (EEG) to measure and record the brain's electrical activity. Brain waves are captured on paper or electronic medium for study. The code applies to a patient awake and drowsy during the EEG and hyperventilating and/or light stimulated.

95819

Sensors are placed on a patient's head in an electroencephalogram (EEG) to measure and record the brain's electrical activity. Brain waves are captured on paper or electronic medium for study. The code applies to a patient intermittently awake then asleep during the EEG and hyperventilating and/or light stimulated.

95822

Sensors are placed on a patient's head in an electroencephalogram (EEG) to measure and record the brain's electrical activity. Brain waves are captured on paper or electronic medium for study. The code applies to a patient sleeping during the EEG.

95824

Sensors are placed on a patient's head in an electroencephalogram (EEG) to measure and record the brain's electrical activity. Brain waves are captured on paper or electronic medium for study. The code applies to checking a patient for brain activity and determining whether the patient is "brain dead." This involves evaluation by isoelectric encephalogram for a minimum of 30 minutes with no EEG change in response to sound or pain.

95827

Sensors are placed on a patient's head in an electroencephalogram (EEG) to measure and record the brain's electrical activity. Brain waves are captured on paper or electronic medium for study. The code applies to a patient sleeping through the night during the EEG testing.

95829

Sensors are placed directly on the brain's surface during surgery in an electrocorticogram to measure and record the brain's electrical activity. Brain waves are captured on paper or electronic medium for study in a separately reported procedure.

95830

The physician places sensors in or near the sphenoid process. Any electroencephalographic (EEG) recording is separately reportable.

95831

Muscles or muscle groups are tested for strength. The code applies to manually testing the arm, leg, or trunk by the physician.

95832

Muscles or muscle groups are tested for strength. The code applies to manually testing the hands by the physician.

95833

Muscles or muscle groups are tested for strength. The code applies to manually testing the body exclusive of the hands by the physician.

95834

Muscles or muscle groups are tested for strength. The code applies to manually testing the body inclusive of the hands by the physician.

95851

Testing determines active and passive range of motion for extremities and joints. The code applies to manually testing each arm or leg or sections of the spinal muscles in a separately reported procedure.

95852

Testing determines active and passive range of motion for extremities and joints. The code applies to manually testing the hands.

95857

This test for myasthenia gravis involves injecting Tensilon (edrophonium chloride) intravascularly. After administration by a physician, eye muscle abnormalities will markedly decrease within two minutes after injection in individuals with myasthenia gravis.

95858

This test for myasthenia gravis involves injecting Tensilon (edrophonium chloride) intravascularly. After administration by a physician, eye muscle abnormalities will markedly decrease within two minutes after injection in individuals with myasthenia gravis. An electromyogram (a measurement of the muscle's electrical activity) is performed with the Tensilon injection.

95860–95864

Needle electromyography (EMG) records the electrical properties of muscle using an oscilloscope. Recordings, which may be amplified and heard through a loudspeaker, are made during needle insertion, with the muscle at rest, and during contraction. Code 95860 should be used when one extremity (arm or leg) is tested, 95861 for tests of two extremities, 95863 for tests of three extremities and 95864 for tests of four extremities.

95867–95868

Needle electromyography (EMG) records the electrical properties of muscle using an oscilloscope. Recordings, which may be amplified and heard through a loudspeaker, are made during needle insertion, with the muscle at rest, and during contraction. These codes are specific to the twelve nerves which emerge from or enter the cranium. 95867 should be used for unilateral studies and 95868 for bilateral studies.

95869–95870

Needle electromyography (EMG) records the electrical properties of thoracic paraspinal muscles (95869) using an oscilloscope. Recordings, which may be amplified and heard through a loudspeaker, are made during needle insertion, with the muscle at rest, and during contraction. Report 95870 for a limited study of muscles in one extremity or non-limb (axial) muscles other than thoracic paraspinal or cranial supplied muscles or sphincters.

95872

Needle electromyography (EMG) records the electrical properties of muscle using an oscilloscope. Recordings, which may be amplified and heard through a loudspeaker, are made during needle insertion, with the muscle at rest, and during contraction. This procedure uses a single fiber electrode to obtain additional information on specific muscles, including quantitative measurement of jitter, blocking, and/or fiber density.

95875

Needle electromyography (EMG) records the electrical properties of muscle using an oscilloscope. Recordings, which may be amplified and heard

through a loudspeaker, are made during needle insertion, with the muscle at rest, and during contraction. This procedure tests electrical properties of ischemic limb during exercise and includes lactic acid determination.

95900–95904

Nerve testing uses sensors to measure and record nerve functions including: conduction, amplitude, and latency/velocity. Nerves are stimulated with electric shocks along the course of the muscle. The time required to initiation of contraction is measured and recorded. Measurements of distal latency, the time required to traverse the segment nearest the muscle, and conduction velocity, the time required for an impulse to travel a measured length of nerve, are also recorded. 95900 applies to motor testing without F-wave studies. 95903 applies to motor testing with F-wave studies. 95904 if the test is of sensory response. Each nerve tested can be billed separately.

95920

This code is used when an evoked potential study is required during surgery. This is often necessary to determine what effect a surgery is having on specific nerve functions. In some cases, continuous monitoring is necessary. Report this code per hour.

95921

The physician uses an indwelling catheter, usually inserted in the right radial artery, to test the parasympathetic system's ability to monitor the cardiovascular system and to analyze the arterial blood gas. The patient is semi-reclined and horizontal to ECG, pulse oximetry and NIBP monitoring. The cannula is connected to the pressure monitoring. The test measures deep breathing with recorded R-R intervals and the Valsalva ration (the amount of air expelled against a closed glottis).

95922

To test the sympathetic nervous system's ability to regulate blood pressure, the physician places an electronic blood pressure monitor on the patient. The patient is placed supine and asked to perform the Valsalva maneuver (expelling air against a closed glottis) while blood pressure is checked between heartbeats. The patient is asked to cease the maneuver and is tilted using the table for at least five minutes. Beat by beat blood pressure measurements are taken and evaluated to determine the nervous system's ability to respond to the test.

95923

These tests are performed to gauge the damage to the autonomic nerves serving the skin. In the silastic sweat imprint (method of Minor), the patient lies on the stomach or back. An iodine/castor oil mixture is painted on the area to be tested and left to dry. The area is dusted with powdered starch. The physician injects pilocarpine to stimulate sweating, and remains

CPT® Lay Descriptions

for 20 to 30 minutes to evaluate the sweating, its amount, and distribution. As the patient sweats, the starch dissolves and reacts with the iodine to produce a dark purple color. Areas not stained indicate impaired sympathetic reactions. The patient is cleaned after the test.

95925–95927

The physician uses somatosensory-evoked potential to provide information about the integrity of the peripheral nerves, spinal cord, brain stem, and the cortex. Evoked potentials require low voltages and the placement of electrodes on the scalp near the parts of the nervous system where the signals are generated. The physician may place electrical stimulation at the median nerve of the wrist or the posterior tibial nerve at the ankle, or the physician may stimulate points between these and the central nervous system. Many applications may be necessary to screen background "noise" to measure the interval between stimulation and generated response. Report 95925 if the upper limbs are being tested; report 92926 for tests of the lower limbs; report 95927 for tests of the trunk or head.

95930

The physician uses sensors to measure and record nerve functions such as conduction and amplitude and, in this code, for using visual evoked potentials (VEP) to test the central nervous system. The code applies to the checkerboard or flash technique.

95933

The physician uses sensors to measure and record nerve functions such as conduction and amplitude. The code applies to testing the blink reflex.

95934

The physician uses sensors to measure and record nerve functions such as conduction and amplitude. The code applies to testing the amplitude and latency (H-reflex) of the lower leg muscles.

95936

The physician uses sensors to measure and record nerve functions such as conduction and amplitude. The code applies to testing the amplitude and latency (H-reflex) of muscles other than the lower leg muscles.

95937

The physician uses sensors to measure and record nerve functions such as conduction and amplitude. The code applies to measure the junction between nerves and muscles for one nerve.

95950

The physician places sensors on a patient's head in an electroencephalogram (EEG) to measure and record the brain's electrical activity. The code applies to an 8-channel EEG to evaluate a cerebral seizure for each 24-hour period of monitoring.

95951

The physician places sensors on a patient's head in an electroencephalogram (EEG) to measure and record the brain's electrical activity. The code applies to a 16-channel telemetry EEG to evaluate presurgical localization of the specific area where the cerebral seizure emanates, and applies to each 24 hour period of monitoring.

95953

The physician places sensors on a patient's head in an electroencephalogram (EEG) to measure and record the brain's electrical activity. The code applies to a 16-channel telemetry EEG using video recordings to evaluate a cerebral seizure for each 24-hour period of monitoring.

95954

The physician places sensors on a patient's head in an electroencephalogram (EEG) to measure and record the brain's electrical activity. The code applies to a patient stimulated by medications or physical activity.

95955

The physician places sensors on a patient's head in an electroencephalogram (EEG) to measure and record the brain's electrical activity. The code applies to an EEG during surgery exclusive of surgery to the brain.

95956

The physician places sensors on a patient's head in an electroencephalogram (EEG) to measure and record the brain's electrical activity. The code applies to a 16-channel telemetry EEG to evaluate a cerebral seizure over each 24 hour period of monitoring.

95957

The physician places sensors on a patient's head in an electroencephalogram (EEG) to measure and record the brain's electrical activity. The code applies to computer digital analysis of an EEG as in cases of epilepsy.

95958

The physician places sensors on a patient's head in an electroencephalogram (EEG) to measure and record the brain's electrical activity. The code applies to a Wada activation test to evaluate function of the brain hemispheres.

95961

Sensors record the response of electrodes placed on the brain and stimulated during surgery. The procedure maps the brain's surface to determine the focus of a seizure or other abnormality. The code applies to the first hour of physician attendance.

95962

Sensors record the response of electrodes placed on the brain and stimulated during surgery. The procedure maps the brain's surface to determine the focus of a seizure or other abnormality. The code applies to every hour of physician attendance after the first.

95965–95967

Magnetoencephalography (MEG) provides functional mapping information about how the brain processes sensory stimulation by measuring the associated magnetic fields emanating from the outer surface of the brain. MEG can be used both as a tool for fundamental study of the brain and for assessing patients with specific neurological disorders. The biomagnetometer is commonly housed in a shielded room; the recording device contains magnetic detection coils continuously bathed in liquid helium to superconducting temperatures of -269 degrees Celsius. The spontaneous (95965) or evoked (95967) magnetic fields emanating from the brain induce a current in these coils, which in turn produce a magnetic field in a device called a superconducting quantum interference device (SQUID), which makes images every 1/1000 of a second. MEG helps to identify where in the brain the electrical current is flowing in response to the stimulus. For example, MEG can be used to determine the millimeters of the brain responsible for fingertip sensation and movement, which can be crucial in surgeries involving neuroresection.

95970

A previously placed neurostimulator pulse generator is tested to verify that is it functioning properly. The neurostimulator may be either a simple or complex brain, spinal cord, or peripheral device. Functions which may be tested include: rate, pulse amplitude and duration, configuration of wave form, battery status, electrode selectability, output modulation, cycling, impedance, and patient compliance. This code reports testing without reprogramming of the device.

95971

A previously placed neurostimulator pulse generator is tested to verify that is it functioning properly. In this case, a simple brain, spinal cord, or peripheral device is tested. A simple device affects only three or fewer of the following: pulse amplitude, pulse duration, pulse frequency, eight or more electrode contacts, cycling, stimulation train duration, train spacing, number of programs, number of channels, phase angle, alternating electrode polarities, configuration of wave form, more than one clinical feature. All of the functions that apply may be tested intraoperatively or on subsequent occasions. This code reports testing with reprogramming of the device.

95972–95973

A previously placed neurostimulator pulse generator is tested to verify that is it functioning properly. In this case, a complex brain, spinal cord or peripheral device is tested. A complex device affects more than three of the following: pulse amplitude, pulse duration, pulse frequency, eight or more electrode contacts, cycling, stimulation train duration, train spacing, number of programs, number of channels, phase angle, alternating electrode polarities, configuration of wave form, more than one clinical feature. All of the functions that apply may be tested intraoperatively or on subsequent occasions. Report code 95972 for the first hour of testing and reprogramming of the device. Report 95973 for each additional 30 minutes of testing and reprogramming.

95974–95975

This range of codes involves a complex neurostimulator, a device that provides chronic electrical stimulation to the nerves of the central or peripheral nervous system and, for these two codes, implanted in the cranial nerve. The stimulation affects the pulse (amplitude, duration, frequency) to treat, for example, the tremors characteristic of Parkinson's disease. Report 95974 for electronic analysis of a complex cranial nerve neurostimulator pulse generator/transmitter with intraoperative or subsequent programming. The procedure may include nerve interface testing and the code is used for the first hour, while 95975 is reported for each additional 30 minutes beyond the first hour.

96000–96001

Human motion analysis has several applications including biomedical and athletic performance. To conduct a biomedical analysis, patient movements are recorded, digitized, copied on computer, and processed. For example, when calculating net joint moments, the joint center is calculated using a local coordinate system created from body markers. When tracking markers in 3D using video, two or more cameras are used to identify the markers. After all parameters are found (e.g., linear acceleration, angular acceleration, ground reaction forces) and gathered using stereo X-rays or MRI techniques, the resultant net joint forces and moments can be calculated. In 3-D kinematics, joint centers are digitized for the first few frames of the sequence recorded. Linear parameters of movement can be measured to assess horizontal and vertical motion. Also, angular parameters can measure the degrees of movement of the joints to analyze specific joint motion. In 96001, while taking dynamic plantar pressure measurements, data is collected using a pressure sensor platform positioned on a walkway. The patient walks along the walkway so pressure data can be analyzed in areas of the foot: (i.e., the heel, metatarsal heads, and the hallus). The peak pressure is determined in all areas and the highest pressure of all sites (i.e., peak pressure foot) is measured. Report

96004 in addition to each of these codes for physician review and interpretation of results, which includes the physician's written report.

96002

Electrodes placed on the muscle belly, parallel to the grain of the muscle fiber, detects an electrical signal that comes from active muscles (the patient is in motion during the test). The strength and pattern of the signal is seen on a computer screen and the data is collected in a software program that is able to run various analyses of the data to create useful reports regarding muscle function. For example, gait analysis allows the clinician to analyze time normal activation patterns separately for stance and swing phases between conditions or against data base values. Report 96002 for a study of 1 to 12 muscles. Report 96004 in addition to this code for physician review and interpretation of results, which includes the physician's written report.

96003

Electrodes placed on the muscle belly, parallel to the grain of the muscle fiber, detects an electrical signal that comes from active muscles (the patient is in motion during the test). The strength and pattern of the signal is seen on a computer screen and the data is collected in a software program that is able to run various analyses of the data to create useful reports regarding muscle function. For example, gait analysis allows the clinician to analyze time normal activation patterns separately for stance and swing phases between conditions or against data base values. Use 96003 to report one minute of activity for analysis. Report 96004 in addition to this code for physician review and interpretation of results, which includes the physician's written report.

96004

The physician reviews and interprets computer-based motion analysis, dynamic plantar pressure measurements, dynamic surface electromyography during walking or other functional activities, and dynamic fine wire electromyography performed using codes 96000, 96001, 96002, and 96003 to report the service.

96100

The physician or other healthcare professional administers and interprets the results of psychological testing. The testing in written, oral, or combined formats measures personality, emotions, intellectual functioning, and psychopathology. The code applies to each hour of testing.

96105

The physician or other healthcare professional administers tests to measure communication problems such as speech and writing in an aphasic patient. The code applies to each hour of testing.

96110

The physician or other healthcare professional measures cognitive, psychomotor and other abilities characteristic to development through written, oral, or combined format testing. The code applies to limited testing.

96111

The physician or other healthcare professional measures cognitive, motor, social, language, and other abilities characteristic to development through written, oral, or combined format testing. The code applies to extended testing per hour.

96115

The physician or other healthcare professional evaluates aspects of thinking, reasoning, and judgment to evaluate a patient's behavioral abilities. The code applies to each hour of examination.

96117

The physician or other healthcare professional administers a series of tests in thinking, reasoning and judgment to evaluate the patient's behavioral abilities. The code applies to each hour of examination.

96150–96151

These report assessment of psychological, behavioral, emotional, cognitive, and relevant social factors that can help to prevent, treat, or manage physical health problems. The assessment must be associated with an acute or chronic illness, the prevention of a physical illness or disability, and the maintenance of health. The initial assessment (96150) and re-assessment (96151) apply to each 15-minute direct, face-to-face session with the patient. Report 96150 for the initial assessment; while the reassessment (96151) is reported to obtain objective measures of goals formulated in the initial assessment and to modify plans as is indicated to support the goals.

96152–96155

These are interventional services prescribed to modify the psychological, behavioral, emotional, cognitive, and social factors relevant to affecting the patient's physical health problems. Each code applies to a 15-minute session of direct face-to-face intervention. Report 96152 for the initial assessment with the individual/patient only. Report 96153 for intervention attended by a group (two or more patients). Report 96154 for intervention that includes the family with the patient present. Report 96155 for intervention with the family without the patient's presence.

96400

The physician or supervised assistant prepares and administers medication to combat diseases such as malignant neoplasms or microorganisms. This code applies to medication injected under the skin (subcutaneous) or into a muscle (intramuscular) often in the arm or leg.

96405

The physician or supervised assistant prepares and administers medication to combat diseases such as malignant neoplasms or microorganisms. The code applies to medication injected directly into the lesion or up to seven lesions.

96406

The physician or supervised assistant prepares and administers medication to combat diseases such as malignant neoplasms or microorganisms. The code applies to medication injected directly into more than seven lesions.

96408

The physician or supervised assistant prepares and administers medication to combat diseases such as malignant neoplasms or microorganisms. The code applies to medication injected through a catheter placed in a vein.

96410–96412

The physician or supervised assistant prepares and administers medication to combat diseases such as malignant neoplasms or microorganisms. The code applies to medication injected slowly through a catheter placed in a vein. 96410 should be used for the first hour and 96412 for each additional hour up to eight hours.

96414

The physician or supervised assistant prepares and administers medication to combat diseases such as malignant neoplasms or microorganisms. The code applies to use of a implantable or portable pump to infuse medication slowly for more than eight hours through a catheter placed in a vein.

96420

The physician or supervised assistant prepares and administers medication to combat diseases such as malignant neoplasms or microorganisms. The code applies to medication injected through a catheter placed in an artery. Placement of the intra-arterial catheter should be reported separately.

96422–96423

The physician or supervised assistant prepares and administers medication to combat diseases such as malignant neoplasms or microorganisms. The code applies to medication injected slowly through a catheter placed in an artery. Placement of the intra-arterial catheter should be reported separately. Report 96422 for the first hour and 96423 for each additional hour up to eight hours.

96425

The physician or supervised assistant prepares and administers medication to combat diseases such as malignant neoplasms or microorganisms.The code applies to use of a implantable or portable pump to infuse medication slowly through a catheter placed in an artery for more than eight hours. Placement of the intra-arterial catheter should be reported separately.

96440

The physician or supervised assistant prepares and administers medication to combat diseases such as malignant neoplasms or microorganisms. The code applies to medication injected into the lung cavity through a catheter placed into the pleura.

96445

The physician or supervised assistant prepares and administers medication to combat diseases such as malignant neoplasms or microorganisms. The code applies to medication injected into the abdominal cavity through a catheter placed in the peritoneum.

96450

The physician or supervised assistant prepares and administers medication to combat diseases such as malignant neoplasms or microorganisms. The code applies to medication injected into the spinal cord through a catheter placed through the space between the lower back bones (lumbar puncture).

96520

The physician or supervised assistant prepares and administers medication to combat diseases such as malignant neoplasms or microorganisms. The code applies to maintaining or refilling portable pumps used for prolonged infusions.

96530

The physician or supervised assistant prepares and administers medication to combat diseases such as malignant neoplasms or microorganisms. The code applies to maintaining or refilling an implantable pump or reservoir used for prolonged infusions.

96542

The physician or supervised assistant prepares and administers medication to combat diseases such as malignant neoplasms or microorganisms. The code applies to medication infused into the central nervous system through a catheter leading from a subcutaneous reservoir of medication in the brain's subarachnoid or intraventricular space.

96545

The physician or supervised assistant prepares medication to combat diseases such as malignant neoplasms or microorganisms. The code applies to chemotherapeutic medication.

96570–96571

In Photodynamic Therapy (PDT), the physician injects the photosensitizing agent into the patient's bloodstream where it is absorbed by cells all over the body. The agent remains in cancer cells for a longer time than it does in normal cells. When the treated cancer cells are exposed to laser light, the photosensitizing agent absorbs the light and produces an active form of oxygen that destroys the treated cancer cells. Light exposure must be timed carefully so that it occurs when most of the photosensitizing agent has left healthy cells but is still present in the cancer cells. The fiber-optic used in the procedure can be directed through a bronchoscope into the lungs for the treatment of lung cancer or through an endoscope into the esophagus for the treatment of esophageal cancer. Report 96570 for the first 30 minutes, and 96571 for each additional 15 minutes. The endoscopy or bronchoscopy procedures for the lung and esophagus are reported separately.

96900

The physician uses ultraviolet light to treat skin ailments.

96902

The physician examines by microscope hairs plucked or clipped from a patient's scalp to determine telogen and anagen counts. The physician also looks for structural hair shaft deformities. Results of the test help determine if hair loss is result of short-term biological changes, malnutrition, medication, or hereditary.

96910

The physician uses photosensitive chemicals and light rays to treat skin ailments. This code applies to either tar and ultraviolet B rays (Goeckerman treatment) or petrolatum and ultraviolet B rays.

96912

The physician uses photosensitive chemicals and light rays to treat skin ailments. This code applies to psoralens and ultraviolet A rays (PUVA).

96913

The physician uses photosensitive chemicals and light rays to treat skin ailments. This code applies to tar and ultraviolet B rays (Goeckerman treatment) and/or psoralens and ultraviolet A rays (PUVA) used for severe skin problems requiring between four to eight hours of care under a physician's direct supervision.

97001

The PT examines the patient/client. This includes taking a comprehensive history, systems review and tests and measures. Tests and measures may include but are not limited to tests of range of motion, motor function, muscle performance, joint integrity, neuromuscular status and review of orthotic or prosthetic devices. The PT formulates an assessment, prognosis and note anticipated intervention.

97002

The PT re-examines the patient/client to obtain objective measures of progress towards stated goals. Tests and measures include but are not limited to

those noted in 97001. The PT modifies the treatment plan as is indicated to support medical necessity of skilled intervention.

97003

The occupational therapist evaluates the patient. Various movements required for activities of daily living are examined. Dexterity, range of movement, and other elements may also be studied.

97004

The occupational therapist re-evaluates the patient to gauge progress of therapy. Various movements required for activities of daily living are examined. Dexterity, range of movement, and other elements may also be studied.

97005

The health care provider examines the patient, which includes taking a comprehensive history, systems review, and obtaining tests of range of motion, motor function, muscle performance, joint integrity, and neuromuscular status. The physical therapist formulates an assessment, prognosis, and notes the anticipated intervention.

97006

The health care provider re-examines the patient to obtain objective measures of progress toward stated goals. Tests include, but are not limited to, range of motion, motor function, muscle performance, joint integrity, and neuromuscular status. The physical therapist modifies the treatment plan as is indicated to support medical necessity of skilled intervention.

97010

The clinician applies heat (dry or moist) or cold to one or more body parts with appropriate padding to prevent skin irritation. The patient is given necessary safety instructions. The treatment requires supervision only and one unit may be billed per day.

97012

The clinician applies sustained or intermittent mechanical traction to the cervical and/or lumbar spine. The mechanical force produces distraction between the vertebrae thereby relieving pain and increasing tissue flexibility. Once applied, the treatment requires supervision and one unit may be billed per day.

97014

The clinician applies electrical stimulation to one or more areas in order to stimulate muscle function, enhance healing, and alleviate pain and/or edema. The clinician chooses which type of electrical stimulation is appropriate. The treatment is supervised after the electrodes are applied and only one unit may be billed per day.

97016

The clinician applies a vasopneumatic device to treat extremity edema (usually lymphedema). A pressurized sleeve is applied. Girth measurements are taken pre- and post- treatment. This code can only be billed one unit per day.

97018

A clinician uses a paraffin bath to apply superficial heat to a hand or foot. The part is repeatedly dipped into the paraffin forming a "glove." Use of paraffin facilitates treatment of arthritis and other conditions that cause limitations in joint flexibility. Once the paraffin is applied and the patient instruction provided, the procedure requires supervision. This code can only be billed one unit per day.

97020

The clinician applies microwave as a form of superficial heat to one or more body parts to help alleviate pain and increase circulation. Once applied and safety instructions provided, the treatment requires supervision. This code can only be billed one unit per day.

97022

The clinician uses a whirlpool to provide superficial heat in an environment that facilitates tissue debridement, wound cleaning and/or exercise. The clinician decides the appropriate water temperature, provides safety instruction and supervises the treatment. This code can only be billed one unit per day.

97024

The clinician uses diathermy as a form of superficial heat for one or more body areas. After application and safety instructions have been provided, the clinician supervises the treatment. This code can only be billed one unit per day.

97026

The clinician uses infrared light as a form of superficial heat that will increase circulation to one or more localized areas. Once applied and safety instructions have been provided, the treatment is supervised. This code can only be billed one unit per day.

97028

The clinician applies ultraviolet light to treat dermatological problems. Once applied and safety instructions have been provided, the treatment is supervised. This code can only be billed one unit per day.

97032

The clinician applies electrical stimulation to one or more areas to promote muscle function, wound healing edema and/or pain control. This treatment requires direct contact by the provider and can be billed in multiple 15 minute units.

97033

The clinician uses electrical current to administer medication to one or more areas. Iontophoresis is usually prescribed for soft tissue inflammatory conditions and pain control. This code requires constant attendance by the clinician and can be billed in 15-minute units.

97034

The clinician uses hot and cold baths in a repeated, alternating fashion to stimulate the vasomotor response of a localized body part. This code requires constant attendance and can be billed in 15-minute units.

97035

The clinician applies ultrasound to increase circulation to one or more areas. A water bath or some form of ultrasound lotion must be used as a coupling agent to facilitate the procedure. The delivery of corticosteroid medication via ultrasound is called phonophoresis. Ultrasound or phonophoresis requires constant attendance and can be billed in 15-minute units.

97036

Hubbard tank is used when it is necessary to immerse the full body into water. Care of wounds and burns my require use of the Hubbard tank to facilitate tissue cleansing and debridement. This code requires constant attendance and can be billed in 15-minute units.

97110

The clinician and/or patient perform(s) therapeutic exercises to one or more body areas to develop strength, endurance, and flexibility. This code requires direct contact and may be billed in 15-minute units.

97112

The clinician and/or patient perform(s) activities to one or more body areas that facilitate reeducation of movement, balance, coordination, kinesthetic sense, posture, and proprioception. This code requires direct contact and may be billed in 15-minute units.

97113

The clinician directs and/or performs therapeutic exercises with the patient/client in the aquatic environment. The code requires skilled intervention by the clinician and documentation must support medical necessity of the aquatic environment. This code can be billed in 15-minute units.

97116

The clinician instructs the patient in specific activities that will facilitate ambulation and stair climbing with or without an assistive device. Proper sequencing and safety instructions are included when appropriate. This code requires direct contact and may be billed in 15-minute units.

97124

The clinician uses massage to provide muscle relaxation, increase localized circulation, soften scar tissue or mobilize mucous secretions in the lung via tapotement and/or percussion. This code requires direct contact and can be billed in 15-minute units, regardless of number of body parts treated.

97139

This code may be used if the clinician performs a therapeutic procedure to one or more body areas that is not listed under the current codes. A narrative descriptor should be noted on the claim. This code can be billed in 15-minute units.

97140

The clinician performs manual therapy techniques including soft tissue and joint mobilization, manipulation, manual traction and/or manual lymphatic drainage to one or more areas. This code requires direct contact with the patient and can be billed in 15-minute units.

97150

The clinician supervises group activities (two or more patients/clients) of therapeutic procedures on land or the aquatic environment. The patients/clients do not have to be performing the same activity simultaneously, however, the need for skilled intervention must be documented. This code can be billed in 15-minute units.

97504

The clinician fits and/or trains the patient in use of an orthotic device for one or more body parts. This does not include fabrication time, if appropriate, or cost of materials. This code can be billed in 15-minute increments.

97520

The clinician fits and/or trains the patient in use of a prosthetic device for one or more body parts. This does not include fabrication time, if appropriate, or cost of materials. This code is billed in 15-minutes units.

97530

The clinician uses dynamic therapeutic activities designed to achieve improved functional performance (e.g., lifting, pulling, bending). This code requires direct contact and can be billed in 15-minute units.

97532

An occupational therapist or rehabilitation specialist works one-on-one with an individual to assist in the development of cognitive skills in individuals with inherited learning disabilities or in individuals who have lost these skills as a result of illness or brain injury. The individual often needs to develop compensatory methods of processing and retrieving information when disability, illness or injury has affected these cognitive processes. Cognitive skill development includes mental exercises that assist the patient in areas such as attention, memory, perception, language, reasoning, planning, problem-solving, and related skills.

97533

Sensory experiences include touch, movement, body awareness, sight, sound, and the pull of gravity. The process of the brain organizing and interpreting this information is called sensory integration. Sensory integration provides a crucial foundation for later, more complex learning and behavior. An occupational therapist or rehabilitation specialist works one-on-one with individuals with sensory integration disorders to provide techniques for enhancing sensory processing and adapting to environmental demands. Sensory integration disorders may be the result of a learning disability, illness, or brain injury.

97535

The clinician instructs and trains the patients in self-care and home management activities (e.g., ADL and use of adaptive equipment in the kitchen, bath and/or car). Direct contact is required. This code can be billed in 15-minute units.

97537

The clinician instructs and trains the patient/client in community re-integration activities (e.g., work task analysis and modification, safe accessing of transportation). This requires direct supervision and can be billed in 15-minute units.

97542

The clinician instructs and trains the patient in proper wheelchair skills (e.g., propulsion, safety techniques). This requires direct contact and is billed in 15-minute units.

97545–97546

This code is used for a procedure where the injured worker is put through a series of conditioning exercises and job simulation tasks in preparation for return to work. Endurance, strength, and proper body mechanics are emphasized. The patient is also educated in problem solving skills related to job task performance and employing correct lifting and positioning techniques. Report 97546 for each additional hour after the initial two hours.

97601–97602

The physician performs wound care management to promote healing using either selective or non-selective debridement techniques to remove devitalized tissue. Selective techniques are those in which the physician has complete control over which tissue is removed and which is left behind. Selective techniques include high-pressure waterjet and sharp debridement techniques using scissors, scalpel, or tweezers. Another newer method of selective debridement is autolysis, which uses the body's own enzymes and moisture to re-hydrate, soften, and finally liquefy hard eschar and slough. Autolytic debridement is accomplished using occlusive or semi-occlusive dressings that keep wound fluid in contact with the necrotic tissue. Types of dressings used in autolytic debridement include hydrocolloids, hydrogels, and transparent films. Non-selective debridement techniques are those in which both necrotic and healthy tissue is removed. Non-selective techniques sometimes, referred to as mechanical debridement, include wet-to-moist dressings, enzymatic chemicals, and abrasion. Wet-to-moist debridement involves allowing a dressing to proceed from moist to wet, then manually removing the dressing, which removes both the necrotic and healthy tissue. Chemical enzymes are fast acting products that produce slough of necrotic tissue. Selective debridement is reported with 97601 and non-selective with 97602.

97703

The clinician evaluates the effectiveness of an existing orthosis or prosthetic device and makes necessary recommendations for changes, as appropriate. This code can be billed in 15 minute units.

97750

The clinician performs a test of physical performance evaluating function of one or more body areas and evaluates functional capacity. A written report is included. This is in addition to a routine evaluation or re-evaluation (97001–97004). This code can be billed in 15-minute increments.

97780–97781

The physician applies acupuncture using one or more needles. The physician inserts a fine needle as dictated by acupuncture meridians to relieve pain. More than one needle may be used as needed. The needles may be twirled or manipulated (97780), or electrical stimulation may be employed by energizing the needles (97781) with micro-current.

97802–97804

A dietetic professional provides medical nutrition therapy assessment or re-assessment and intervention in a face-to-face or group patient setting. After nutritional screening identifies patients at risk preventive or therapeutic dietary therapy is initiated to induce a positive result in the role nutrition plays in improving health outcomes. Report 97802 for the initial assessment and intervention face-to-face with an individual patient for each 15 minutes of medical nutrition therapy. Report 97803 for re-assessment and intervention with an individual patient for each 15 minutes of medical nutrition therapy. Report 97804

for group medical nutrition therapy provided for two or more individuals, each 30 minutes.

98925–98929

The physician uses these codes to report osteopathic manipulation, unique manual treatments that are used to treat somatic dysfunction and related disorders. Several techniques exist. Body regions included are head, cervical thoracic, lumbar, sacral, pelvic, extremities, rib cage, abdomen and viscera. Report 98925 if one to two body regions are involved; report 98926 if three to four body regions are involved; report 98927 if five to six body regions are involved; report 98928 if seven to eight body regions are involved; report 98929 if nine body regions are involved.

98940–98943

The chiropractor uses these codes to report the unique manual treatments used to influence joint and neurophysiological function. Several modalities exist. Report 98940 if treatment is spinal, one to two regions; report 98941 if treatment is spinal, three to four regions; report 98942 if treatment is spinal, five regions; and report 98943 if treatment is extraspinal (head, extremities, rib cage, and abdomen), one or more regions.

99000

This code is adjunct to basic services rendered. The physician reports this for the handling and/or conveyance of a specimen from the physician's office to a laboratory.

99001

This code is adjunct to basic services rendered. The physician reports this code for the handling and/or conveyance of a specimen from the patient in other than the physician's office to the laboratory.

99002

This code is adjunct to basic services rendered. The physician reports this code regarding handling, conveyance, and/or any other service in connection with implementation of devices such as orthotic, protective, and prosthetic fabricated by an outside laboratory and fitted by the attending physician.

99024

The physician reports this code to indicate a postoperative follow-up visit, included in global service.

99025

This code is adjunct to basic services rendered. The physician reports this code to indicate an initial visit when a starred surgical procedure constitutes a major service at that visit.

CPT® Lay Descriptions

99050

This code is adjunct to basic services rendered. The physician reports this code to indicate services after office hours in addition to basic service.

99052

This code is adjunct to basic services rendered. The physician reports this code to indicate services requested between 10:00 p.m. and 8:00 a.m. in addition to basic service.

99054

This code is adjunct to basic services rendered. The physician reports this code to indicate services requested on Sundays and holidays in addition to basic service.

99056

This code is adjunct to basic services rendered. The physician reports this code to indicate typical office services provided at the request of a patient in a location other than the physician's office.

99058

This code is adjunct to basic services rendered. The physician reports this code to indicate services provided on an emergency basis.

99070

This code is adjunct to basic services rendered. The physician reports this code to indicate supplies and materials provided by the physician over and above those usually included with the office visit or other services rendered. This code does not include eyeglasses; report 92390–92395 if eyeglasses are provided. List drugs, trays, supplies, and other materials provided when using this code.

99071

This code is adjunct to basic services rendered. The physician reports this code to indicate educational supplies provided by the physician for the patient's education.

99075

This code is adjunct to basic services rendered. The physician reports this code to indicate medical testimony.

99078

The physician provides educational services to patients in a group setting. The topics vary according to the group but can include prenatal care, diet, diabetic instruction, and smoke cessation.

99080

This code is adjunct to basic services rendered. The physician reports this code to indicate special reports such as insurance forms, more than the information in standard communications methods or forms.

99082

This code is adjunct to basic services rendered. The physician reports this code to indicate unusual travel for the purpose of transportation or accompanying the patient.

99090

This code is adjunct to basic services rendered. The physician reports this code to indicate analysis of clinical data stored in computers.

99091

This is the collection and interpretation of physiologic data by the physician or other qualified health care professional. The data (e.g., blood pressure) is stored digitally and may be transmitted by the patient and/or their caregiver to the physician. The report should contain the time it took the provider to acquire the physiologic data, review and interpret the data, and modify any care plan due to the additional data acquisition. A minimum of 30 minutes of time must be spent in the collection and interpretation of data to report this service.

99100

This code is adjunct to basic services rendered. The physician reports this code to indicate qualifying circumstances regarding anesthesia for a patient under one year or over seventy.

99116

This code is adjunct to basic services rendered. The physician reports this code to indicate qualifying circumstances regarding anesthesia complicated by utilization of total body hypothermia.

99135

This code is adjunct to basic services rendered. The physician reports this code to indicate qualifying circumstances regarding anesthesia complicated by utilization of controlled hypotension.

99140

This code is adjunct to basic services rendered. The physician reports this code to indicate qualifying circumstances regarding anesthesia complicated by emergency conditions. Specify emergency conditions encountered when submitting claim.

99141–99142

A physician or trained healthcare professional administers medication that allows a decreased level of consciousness but does not put the patient completely asleep into a state called conscious sedation. This allows the patient to breathe without assistance and respond to commands. This is used for less invasive procedures and/or a second medication for pain. 99141 is used when the sedative is administered via intravenous, intramuscular, or inhalation routes. 99142 is used when the sedative is administered orally, nasally, or rectally.

99170

The physician inserts the colposcope into or around the anogenital area to magnify and directly observe the condition of living tissues in cases of suspected child sexual abuse. This examination allows a better view of any problem area, such as very small tears in and around the anus since the colposcope magnifies from 6 to 40 times.

99172

There are several parts to this screening exam. For visual acuity, the physician asks the patient to stand at a specified distance (20 feet for Snellen eye chart) away from the chart. The patient is instructed to cover the left eye with the left hand, or hold a card in front of the lens for those patients wearing eyeglasses. The patient reads the letters on the chart to test the visual acuity of the right eye. If the patient can read the smallest line of letters, visual acuity of the right eye is measured at 20/20. To measure the visual acuity of the left eye, the patient is asked to repeat the steps beginning with covering the right eye in the same manner as the left. Ocular alignment is checked by determining whether the eyes work together in the same direction. The patient is positioned in front of a screen, looking ahead, and the non-tested eye is covered in a field of vision screening. The provider flashes objects in various areas in the field of vision and the patient is asked to respond to where the see the object. The patient's response creates a map of the visual field. To test color vision the patient looks at cards with many different colored dots that make specific shapes. The patient with normal color vision will be able to discern the shapes within the colors. This exam helps identify possible vision problems. It does not replace the examination by an ophthalmologist or optometrist and is used as a screening test only.

99173

The physician asks the patient to stand at a specified distance (20 feet for Snellen eye chart) away from the chart. The patient is instructed to cover the left with the left hand, or hold a card in front of the lens for those patients wearing eyeglasses. The patient reads the letters on the screen to test the visual acuity of the right eye. If the patient can read the smallest line of letters, visual acuity of the right eye is measured at 20/20. To measure the visual acuity of the left eye, the patient is asked to repeat the steps beginning with covering the right eye in the same manner as the left. This exam helps identify possible vision problems; it does not replace the examination by an ophthalmologist or optometrist and is used as a screening test only.

99175

The physician administers ipecac or a similar substance to induce vomiting and observes the patient until the stomach is adequately emptied of poison.

99183

The physician attends and supervises hyperbaric oxygen therapy. Report per session. Report procedures provided in conjunction with hyperbaric oxygen therapy separately.

99185–99186

The physician lowers the temperature of part (99185) or all (99186) of a patient's body to help facilitate surgery requiring the suppression of the patient's metabolism.

99190–99192

The physician assembles and operates a pump with an oxygenator or heat exchanger. Report 99190 to identify each hour; report 99191 to report 3/4 hour; report 99192 to report 1/2 hour.

99195

The physician draws blood from the patient to help right dramatically imbalanced blood levels (i.e., hemoglobin, potassium salts). The procedure is similar to drawing blood from a donor, but a number of pints may be taken to reduce the imbalance. Actual blood removal may be performed by a clinician under a physician's direction.

99274

Using an X-ray machine in a cardiac catheterization laboratory, the physician places the delivery catheter in the coronary artery at the site of the in-stent restenosis (re-blockage in the artery). The transfer delivery device is connected to the delivery catheter; the transfer delivery device is used to deliver the radioactive seeds to the location. There are various methods for transcatheter placement, but commonly the methods involve the use of a guiding catheter. The radioactive seeds are positioned at the location for an appropriate length of time to administer radiation to the artery. At the completion of the radiation treatment, the radioactive seeds are returned to the transfer device.

99500

The home health provider may visit patients with prenatal complications once a week during the first month, and every other week until the birth of the baby. The home nurse may obtain vaginal-anorectal/cervical cultures, perform a non-stress test, draw blood for serology (including offering of AFP/HIV testing), and other tests (e.g., glucose screening at 24 to 28 weeks gestation). A fetoscope may be used at 18 to 20 weeks to check the fetal heart rate.

99501

The home visit for postnatal assessment may include a review of plans for future health maintenance and care, including routine infant immunizations, identification of illness and periodic health evaluations, and to link the family with other sources of support (e.g., social services, parenting classes, lactation consultants) as necessary.

99502

Postpartum early discharge is defined as six hours to 36 hours after uncomplicated vaginal delivery or 72 hours after uncomplicated cesarean delivery. Specialized nursing helps the family make the transition from hospital to home. The home health visit is not intended to replace a complete evaluation by a physician, but focuses on aspects that require early intervention (e.g., feeding problems, jaundice, signs of infection, etc.).

99503

A trained respiratory therapist or other health care professional provides care for patients with temporary or chronic respiratory conditions. The health care professional may provide pulmonary evaluations, patient and family education and counseling, and instruction in self-care. The visit is designed to assist the physician in caring for the patient by avoiding complications, infections, disease progression, and to ultimately reduce hospitalizations. The visit may also include evaluation and monitoring of the equipment used, including diagnostics and calibration of the equipment; changes in medications (e.g., bronchodilator); and/or advice and education about dosage and the use of a particular medication.

99504

A respiratory therapist or other home health care professional visits a patient's home when the patient is receiving mechanical ventilation. The health care professional instructs the patient and family members on the ventilator equipment, including checking the machine and the settings. During the home health visit, related equipment or issues, such as oxygen and tracheostomy care (when present), is discussed.

99505

The home health care provider measures vital signs, inspects incisions, assesses mobility and appetite, and determines if there are problems or situations that could require a surgeon's intervention. The provider checks the stoma site and the stoma's function. The home health provider teaches and answers questions the patient may have about the care and maintenance of the colostomy and/or cystostomy. The home health provider also administers medications or draws blood so that the surgeon can continue to monitor the patient's condition. Most patients who have had a colostomy or cystostomy will be seen by a home health provider one or more times after discharge.

99506

The home health provider visits a patient's home to perform an intermuscular injection of medication per a physician's or another valid order. The home health provider brings supplies and medications that are necessary to accomplish the injection to the patient's home, including a syringe, needle, liquid disinfectant, cotton ball, and adhesive tape. The procedure involves inserting the needle, aspiration and slow injection, and at the end of the procedure a cotton ball is placed over the injection site. Adhesive tape is applied over the cotton ball.

99507

The home health provider may visit the patient daily or up to twice daily, with frequency determined by physician orders and assessment of patient condition and needs. Skilled procedures required for the home visit include venipuncture for lab, therapeutic drug levels; Foley catheter, suprapubic catheter, and nasogastric tube insertion/management; gastrostomy tube changes/management; dressing changes and assessment of wounds; ureterostomy care; management of open or draining wounds, ulcers, or fistulae; suture/staple removal; drainage tube pouching/management; and administering IM, IV, and subcutaneous medications, including chemotherapy; management of implanted ports/pumps, external pumps for pain management or chemotherapy administration, and urinary incontinence management.

99508

A polysomnogram is a sleep study that involves using electroencephalography (EEG) to monitor the brain and muscle activity, heart rhythm, and breathing of a sleeping patient. A portable recorder used in the home measures nasal/oral airflow, chest wall movement, cardiac rhythm, and blood oxygen saturation. During the home health visit, the technician assists in setting up the portable equipment for home monitoring.

99509

In order to qualify for home assistance with activities of daily living and personal care, the patient must be unable to perform two or more "activities of daily living," such as eating, toileting, transferring, bathing, dressing, and continence. When a referral is made, a health care provider visits the home to conduct a comprehensive assessment of the patient's needs. The plan of care is developed in conjunction with the client, their physician, and family. Acting as a liaison with the client's physician, and other community programs, the case manager responds to all client requests, questions, and concerns and reports frequently on the client's status and progress.

99510

A home health professional makes an initial visit to the home to evaluate specific needs. If home health care would be of benefit, a plan of care is developed based on medical orders from the patient's provider. For example, a plan might specify one or more visits from a therapist. The provider regularly reviews progress reports.

99511

A home health visit includes assistance with dietary management and bowel management/retraining (i.e., use of prescribed medication as well as establishing a habit regimen to treat constipation). The home health caregiver may manually remove the impaction or administer an enema. The length of time it takes to administer an enema depends on the amount of fluid to be infused. The amount of fluid administered depends on the age and size of the person receiving the enema. If necessary, a specimen is collected for diagnostic evaluation.

99512

A home health nurse commonly visits the patient three times a week to provide hemodialysis. Each treatment lasts from two hours to four hours. Before treatment, access is made to the bloodstream to provide a way for blood to be carried from the patient to the dialysis machine that filters outs wastes and extra fluids and to return the newly cleaned blood back again. The access may be under the skin or outside the body. During treatment, the patient can read, write, sleep, talk, or watch TV.